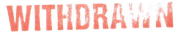

Introduction to Management and Leadership for Nurse Managers
Third Edition

Russell C. Swansburg, RN, PhD
Consultant in Nursing and Hospital Administration
San Antonio, Texas

Richard J. Swansburg, RN, BSN, MSCIS
Systems Software Specialist II
University of South Alabama
Mobile, Alabama

JONES AND BARTLETT PUBLISHERS
Sudbury, Massachusetts
BOSTON   TORONTO   LONDON   SINGAPORE

World Headquarters
Jones and Bartlett Publishers
40 Tall Pine Drive
Sudbury, MA 01776
978-443-5000
info@jbpub.com
www.jbpub.com

Jones and Bartlett Publishers Canada
2406 Nikanna Road
Mississauga, ON L5C 2W6
CANADA

Jones and Bartlett Publishers International
Barb House, Barb Mews
London W6 7PA
UK

Copyright © 2002 by Jones and Bartlett Publishers, Inc.

ISBN 0-7637-1644-8

Production Credits
Chief Executive Officer: Clayton Jones
Chief Operating Officer: Don W. Jones, Jr.
Sponsoring Editor: Penny Glynn
Associate Editor: Thomas Prindle
Marketing Manager: Alisha Barry
Production Manager: Amy Rose
Associate Production Editor: Tara McCormick
Manufacturing Buyer: Amy Duddridge
Design, Editorial Production Service, Typesetting: Nova Graphic Services, Inc.
Cover Design: Philip Regan
Printing and Binding: D.B. Hess Company
Cover Printing: D.B. Hess Company

Library of Congress Cataloging-in-Publication Data
CIP data unavailable at time of printing

Printed in the United States of America
05 04 03   10 9 8 7 6 5 4 3 2

To Laurel Clark Swansburg, RN

Contents

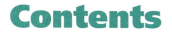

5   The Planning Process

6   Mission, Philosophy, Objectives, and Management Plans

7   Staffing and Scheduling

11   Managing a Clinical Practice Discipline

12   Decision-Making and Problem-Solving

13   Implementing Planned Change

25   Total Quality Management

26   Quality Management

27   Legal Principles of Nursing

28   Performance Appraisal

29   Pay for Performance

Preface

> Management exists for the sake of the institution's results. It has to start with the intended results and has to organize the resources of the institution to attain these results. It is the organ to make the institution, whether business, church, university, hospital, or a battered women's shelter, capable of producing results outside of itself.
>
> P. F. Drucker[1]

This book is organized around the four major management functions: planning, organizing, directing or leading, and controlling or evaluating. It is designed for management development of professional nurses in the twenty-first century. *Introduction to Management and Leadership for Nurse Managers, Third Edition*, is suitable for an introductory course in nursing administration in graduate programs. This book also can be used in upper-level baccalaureate programs in which students complete a basic course in essentials of management before their senior year. This text is also designed for staff development of nurse managers in the service setting. The theory and principles of *Introduction to Management and Leadership for Nurse Managers, Third Edition*, apply to the entire spectrum of health care institutions and settings.

Introduction to Management and Leadership for Nurse Managers, Third Edition, provides theoretical and practical knowledge that will aid professional nurses in meeting the demands of constantly changing patient care services. Because the demand for nurses in some specialties and geographic areas is currently exceeding supply, it is essential that management processes provide the environment for high morale, motivation, and productivity. Financial considerations have increasingly dominated the health care industry, making the job of managing costly human and material resources ever more important.

All chapters have been updated. Chapters have been added on managed care and the legal principles of nursing. Because of its importance and relevance in the total management spectrum, critical thinking has been separated from other areas and placed in the front of the book as a separate chapter.

Health care institutions have been restructured, demassed, and decentralized along with other business and industrial institutions. This book has been revised to provide the best management concepts and theory of management available from the fields of generic management as well as nursing management sources. The current shortages of students in generic nursing programs and graduate nurses in practice require application of sound management principles to recruit and retain nurses in these areas.

NOTE

1. *Management Challenges for the 21st Century* (New York: HarperCollins, 1999).

Contributors

Chapter 3   Theory of Nursing Management
Linda Roussel, DSN, RN, CNA
Associate Professor
LSU Health Sciences Center School of Nursing
New Orleans, Louisiana

Chapter 9   Collective Bargaining
C. Phillip Kendrick, PhD, CRNA
CRNA Supervisor
University of South Alabama Hospitals
Mobile, Alabama

Chapter 18   Leadership
Sharon Farley, PhD, RN
Professor and Executive Associate Dean for Academic Affairs
School of Nursing
Indiana University
Indianapolis, Indiana

Chapter 21   eNursing
Richard J. Swansburg, RN, BSN, MSCIS,
Systems Software Specialist II
University of South Alabama
Mobile, Albama

Chapter 22   The Nurse Manager of Staff Development
Nancy C. McDonald, EdD, RN
Distinguished Teaching Professor
School of Nursing
Auburn University Montgomery
Montgomery, Albama

Chapter 23   Conflict Management
Enrica Kinchen Singleton, DrPH, MBA, RN
Professor of Nursing
Southern University and A & M College
Baton Rouge, Louisiana

Chapter 26   Quality Management
Beverly Blain Wright, RNC, CNA, CPHQ
Quality Management Project Coordinator
University of South Alabama Medical Center
Mobile, Alabama

CHAPTER 1

Critical Thinking

Russell C. Swansburg, PhD, RN

> The ideal critical thinker is habitually inquisitive, well informed, trustful of reason, open minded, flexible, fair minded in evaluation, honest in facing personal biases, prudent in making judgments, willing to reconsider, clear about issues, orderly in complex matters, diligent in seeking relevant information, reasonable in the selection of criteria, focused in inquiry, and persistent in seeking results which are as precise as the subject and circumstances of inquiry permit.
>
> P. A. Facione[1]

LEARNING OBJECTIVES AND ACTIVITIES

- Compose an illustration of a definition of critical thinking.
- Use a decision-making process to make a personal decision confronting you.
- Evaluate a situation in which public officials are involved in debate and argumentation (critical thinking). Relate it to health care policy in the public domain.
- Do a concept analysis of critical thinking.

CONCEPTS: Critical thinking, concept analysis, debate.

MANAGER BEHAVIOR: Promote critical thinking within the parameters of organizational policies and procedures.

LEADER BEHAVIOR: Coach staff to become critical thinkers and to use critical thinking to promote positive patient outcomes and effective interpersonal relationships. Reward personnel for fixing system failures.

Introduction

Nurses use critical thinking for several reasons including applying professional and technical knowledge and skills in caring for clients. In these applications, critical thinking is the best guarantee that nurses will have successful outcomes. In the tenth edition of their book entitled *Argumentation and Debate*, Freeley and Steinberg indicate that competency in critical thinking is necessary for developing one's ability to participate effectively in human affairs, pursue higher education, and succeed in the highly competitive world of business and the professions. These authors also indicate that the ability to reach successful decisions is based on accurate evidence and valid reasoning.[2] Behaviors based on critical thinking are essential to a nurse's role as clinician, manager, researcher, or teacher.

Freeley identifies seven methods of critical thinking:

1. **Debate.** Debate involves inquiry, advocacy, and reasoned judgment on a proposition. A person or group may debate or argue the pros and cons of a proposition in coming to a reasoned judgment. A debate usually entails opposing positions and specific rules.
2. **Individual decisions.** An individual may debate a proposition in his or her mind using problem-solving or decision-making processes. When consent or cooperation of others is needed, the individual may use group discussion, persuasion, propaganda, coercion, or a combination of these methods.
3. **Group discussion.** Five conditions for reaching decisions through group discussion are that "the group members (1) agree that a problem exists, (2) have comparable standards of value, (3) have compatible purposes, (4) are willing to accept the consensus of the group, and (5) are relatively few in number."[3]
4. **Persuasion.** Persuasion is communication to influence the acts, beliefs, attitudes, and values of others by reasoning, urging, or inducement. Debate and advertising are two forms of communication whose intent is to persuade.
5. **Propaganda.** Propaganda can be good or bad. It is multiple media communication designed to persuade or influence a mass audience. Propagandists may debate and argue. Their tactics need to be subjected to critical analysis.

6. **Coercion.** Threat or use of force is the communication of coercion. An extreme example is brainwashing, in which subjects are completely controlled physically for an indefinite period of time.

7. **Combination of methods.** Some situations require a combination of the forgoing communication techniques to reach a decision.[4]

A general consensus is emerging that critical thinking should underlie the nursing process within nursing education programs. Critical thinking generally is regarded by academicians as essential to the educated mind and superordinate to problem-solving in the nursing process.[5] The nursing process should involve critical thinking in problem-solving and decision-making. Exhibit 1-1 lists several definitions and characteristics of critical thinking from which one can see the relationship of the concept of critical thinking to decision-making, problem-solving, and standards.

Research

A number of research studies have been done relative to critical thinking and nursing education. Using the Health Care Professional Attitude Inventory to measure professionalism and the Watson–Glaser Critical Thinking Appraisal (CTA) to measure general critical thinking abilities, Brooks and Shepherd sampled 200 associate degree, diploma, generic, and upper-division baccalaureate nursing students and found the following:

- Seniors in upper-division and generic programs exhibited significantly higher critical thinking abilities than did seniors in associate degree and diploma programs.
- A positive correlation between critical thinking abilities and professionalism was almost as strong in seniors with generic and associate degrees compared with seniors in upper division programs.
- Seniors in diploma programs exhibited the lowest levels of professionalism and critical thinking.
- Seniors in upper-division programs achieved higher professionalism scores than did seniors in the 4-year generic programs; these two groups showed almost identical levels of critical thinking abilities.[6]

Saarmann and co-authors used the Watson–Glaser CTA scale on a sample of 32 subjects in each of the following groups: nurses in a nursing faculty, registered nurses with a bachelor of science degree, ADN-prepared registered nurses, and nursing students entering their sophomore year in Southern California. The authors found that "the critical thinking ability of faculty was not significantly higher than that of sophomore nursing students when the influence of age was controlled statistically. The values of all three groups of nurses were strikingly similar, although faculty valued achievement most highly (P = .0001), while sophomore students valued goal orientation most highly (P = .001). All subjects valued support highly, but only sophomore students valued benevolence highly."[7]

Hickman analyzed 18 studies of critical thinking in nursing education and reached the conclusion that "there is not a strong research base supporting a relationship between nursing curricula and critical thinking."[8] However, nursing schools strive to meet mandates that require program outcomes of critical thinking, communication, and therapeutic nursing interventions.

> **Nurse administrators and managers need to do their own teaching of critical thinking skills and research of the effects of experience on the level of critical thinking.**

Other research studies reached the following conclusions:

1. Critical thinking skills increased among sophomore and senior collegiate nursing students as measured by the California Critical Thinking Skills Test. Significant increases also were seen in the overall scores of these same student, and in subtest scores in truth-seeking, analyticity, self-confidence, and inquisitiveness, as measured by the California Critical Thinking Disposition Inventory.[9]

2. In a study to examine the relationship between critical thinking and clinical competence, May and colleagues used an exploratory nonexperimental design with a heterogeneous sample consisting of two graduating nursing classes ($N = 143$). "While the group of participants was able to think critically and practice competently according to set standards, there were no statistically significant correlations between critical thinking and clinical competence total scores. One conclusion for these findings is that critical thinking may not emerge as an associated factor with clinical competence until some time after nursing students become practicing nurses."[10]

3. In another study involving 15 qualified nurses, Bell and Procter came to the following conclusion: "Engaging in research activities does not always result in the development of practice; however, there appears to be a link between practice development and critical thinking."[11]

More descriptive research studies are needed in nursing management. Fulfilling this need will require

EXHIBIT 1-1
Critical Thinking

DEFINITIONS

The word *critical* is derived from the Greek and means to question, to discuss, to choose, to evaluate, to make judgment.

Greek *kritein*—to choose, to decide

Greek *krites*—judge

English *criterion*—a standard, rule, or method

- Critical thinking is reflecting on a situation, a plan, an event under the rule of standards and antecedent to making a decision. (McKenzie)
- "Critical thinking is both a philosophical orientation toward thinking and a cognitive process characterized by reasoned judgment and reflective thinking." (Jones and Brown)
- "[Critical thinking] is an investigation whose purpose is to explore a situation, phenomenon, question, or problem to arrive at a hypothesis or conclusion about it that integrates all available information and that can be convincingly justified." (Kurfiss)
- "Critical thinking is (1) an attitude of being disposed to consider in a thoughtful way, the problems and subjects that come within the range of one's experiences, (2) knowledge of the methods of logical inquiry and reasoning, and (3) some skill in applying those methods." (Glaser)
- "Critical thinking abilities include defining a problem, selecting pertinent information for the solution, recognizing stated and unstated assumptions, formulating and selecting relevant and promising hypotheses, drawing conclusions, and judging the validity of the inferences." (Hickman; Watson and Glaser)
- "Critical thinking is the intellectually disciplined process of actively and skillfully conceptualizing, applying, analyzing, synthesizing, and evaluating information gathered from or generated by observation, experience, reflection, reasoning, and communication, as a guide to belief and action." (National Council for Excellence in Critical Thinking Instruction)

CHARACTERISTICS

- Critical thinking is a multidimensional cognitive process. It requires a skillful application of knowledge and experience for the sophisticated judgment and evaluation needed in complex situations. It is interactive—individual with interpretations made of the world.
- It is process-oriented.
- It uses structure as a means rather than an end.
- It is a framework within which to interpret knowledge, challenge assumptions of theory and practice, generate contradictory hypotheses, and develop modifications. (Jones and Brown; Boychuk Duchscher)

- It is affective learning, including moral reasoning and development of values guiding decisions and activities.
- It is awareness of self as the basis for building relationships with a client; conscious awareness of feelings, beliefs, values, and attitudes.
- It is empathy and empowerment. (Woods; Reilly and Oermann)
- It includes social learning theory.
- It is an important outcome of professional socialization.
- It involves cognitive skills of comprehension, application, analysis, synthesis, and evaluation. (Saarmann and co-authors)
- It is an attitude of critical inquiry that enhances professionalism. (Brooks and Shepherd; Boychuk Duchscher)
- It is fallible.
- It may lead to bad decisions and errors in judgment.
- It will consistently lead to superior decisions but is sometimes imperfect.
- It includes feelings, images, and intuitional prompts.
- It employs psychological as well as logical or linear patterns. (McKenzie)
- It teaches how to think as a means of dealing with relentless information development and change. (Daly)

Sources: L. McKenzie. "Critical Thinking in Health Care Supervision." *Health Care Supervisor* (June 1992), 1–11; S. A. Jones and L. N. Brown. "Alternative Views on Defining Critical Thinking Through the Nursing Process." *Holistic Nurse Practitioner* (April 1993), 71–76; J. G. Kurfiss. *Critical Thinking: Theory and Practice* (Washington, DC: Association for the Study of Higher Education, 1988), 2; E. M. Glaser. *An Experiment in the Development of Critical Thinking* (New York, NY: Teacher's College, 1941), 5–6; J. S. Hickman. "A Critical Assessment of Critical Thinking in Nursing Education." *Holistic Nurse Practitioner* (April 1993), 36–47; G. Watson and E. M. Glaser. *Watson–Glaser Critical Thinking Appraisal Manual* (New York, NY: Harcourt, Brace & World, 1964); National Council for Excellence in Critical Thinking Instruction. *Critical Thinking: Shaping the Mind of the 21st Century* (Rohnen Park, CA: Sonoma State University Center for Critical Thinking and Moral Critique, 1992), 7; J. E. Boychuk Duchscher. "Catching the Wave: Understanding the Concept of Critical Thinking." *Journal of Advanced Nursing* (March 1999), 572–583; J. H. Woods. "Affective Learning: One Door to Critical Thinking." *Holistic Nurse Practitioner* (April 1993), 64–70; D. E. Reilly and M. H. Oermann. "Affective Learning in the Clinical Setting." In D. E. Reilly and M. H. Oermann, eds., *Clinical Teaching in Nursing Education* (New York, NY: National League for Nursing, 1992), Publication 15-2471; L. Saarmann, L. Freitas, J. Rapps, and B. Riegel. "The Relationship of Education to Critical Thinking Ability and Values Among Nurses: Socialization into Professional Nursing." *Journal of Professional Nursing* (January–February 1992), 26–34; K. L. Brooks and J. M. Shepherd. "Professionalism versus General Critical Thinking Abilities of Senior Nursing Students in Four Types of Nursing Curricula." *Journal of Professional Nursing* (March–April 1992), 87–95; W. M. Daly. "Critical Thinking as an Outcome of Nursing Education. What Is It? Why Is It Important to Nursing Practice?" *Journal of Advanced Nursing* (August 1998), 323–331.

that more nurse managers be trained in nursing research and suggests that the members of the nursing community should unify to implement a theory of nursing management encompassing critical theory. Nurse managers employing a critical thinking approach would determine how their subordinates interpret organizational phenomenon. They would discuss possible falsities of interpretations with their associates, bringing out illusions and delusions.[12]

Applications of Critical Thinking

Concept analysis is advocated as a strategy for promoting critical thinking.[13] Concept analysis uses critical thinking to advance the knowledge base of nursing management and nursing practice.

The rudiments of critical thinking are recalling facts, principles, theories, and abstractions to make deductions, interpretations, and evaluations in solving problems, making decisions, and implementing changes.

A class of nursing students developed a method of concept analysis using critical thinking. The students did literature searches before each class in preparation for concept analysis. In their first session, they developed the following format for concept analysis:

1. Identify and clarify the concept, including the philosophy and content analysis.
2. List the characteristics and attributes of the concept, for example, concrete or abstract, the quality, and quantity.
3. Obtain perceptions, that is, what people think or their interpretations about selling, marketing, and customers (determine whom the concept affects and what is perceived as needed).
4. Identify the use or application and the policies, procedures, practices (skills), and knowledge required.
5. Perform a researchable and synergistic evaluation to promote change, create energy, and validate theory.

This format was used to study and analyze concepts such as organizational climate, legal and ethical nursing practices, nursing care delivery systems, theory of nursing management, standards of nursing practice, evaluation of patient care, and research in nursing administration.[14]

Application of critical thinking theory to nursing management requires that the nurse manager have knowledge of the theory. Nursing staff development faculty also must have knowledge of the theory and the teaching skills that will stimulate critical thinking and test it at the highest cognitive, affective, and psychomotor domains, not only in process but also in outcomes. Lectures are the least effective method for teaching critical thinking. Teaching methods to develop and test the higher level of the cognitive domain and competencies of the affective and psychomotor domains should be a part of the staff development process.[15] Critical thinking skills can be developed through the study of logic, problem-solving observation, analytic reading of books and articles about nursing and management, and group discussion.[16] (See Exhibit 1-2.)

Futurist John Naisbitt describes *high tech* as technology that embodies both good and bad consequences. "High touch is embracing the primeval forces of life and death. High touch is embracing that which acknowledges all that is greater than we."[19] Professional nurses are high-tech–high-touch people whose work requires the cognitive abilities of synthesis and analysis. Professional nurses are critical thinkers.

Summary

Critical thinking has been advocated in education for many decades; however, lately it has been receiving attention in defining nursing curricula. Critical thinking is consistent with the nursing process and should be evident in higher level learning objectives in the cognitive, affective, and psychomotor domains.

EXHIBIT 1-2

Activities and strategies for promoting critical thinking include problem-solving, decision-making, clinical judgment, reflective thinking, questioning, dialogue, dialectical thinking, concept mapping, concept analysis, inquiry-based learning, script theory, two-way talks, case studies, clinical pathways, research findings, clinical rounds, peer review, shift reports, information processing, skills acquisition theory, conferences, context-dependent test items, and cognitive apprenticeship.

Models for studying critical thinking include

- Loving's competence validation model.[17]
- The cognitive apprenticeship model.[18]

APPLICATION EXERCISES

EXERCISE 1-1

In your own words, write a definition of *critical thinking*. Relate it to your use of the nursing process in caring for clients.

EXERCISE 1-2

We all make personal decisions daily that relate to work, home, family, community, or other aspects of our lives. State a personal problem facing you. Identify the outcome that you want. Determine the means available to achieve this outcome. List the pros and cons of each means, and decide which you will use. Do it!

EXERCISE 1-3

Refer to your daily newspaper. Identify an issue being discussed related to local (city or county) government.

- What are the arguments involved?
- Which do you support?
- What can you do about them?

Debate the issue. Form a group of your peers and do the following:

1. Determine the pros and cons of the issue.
2. Elect a team captain for each side of the issue.
3. Identify the members of each team.
4. Set rules for the debate: decide on a monitor, determine the speaking sequence and length of time each team member may speak, decide whether the team captains will give summaries, determine who will judge the debate, and decide when and where the debate will take place.
5. Do an evaluation.

Note: If you wish to do a more formal debate, refer to the Freely and Steinberg book of note 1, particularly pages 310–311.

NOTES

1. P. A. Facione, *The Delphi Report. Critical Thinking: A Statement of Expert Consensus for Purposes of Educational Assessment and Instruction*, Executive Summary (Milbrae, CA: The California Academic Press, 1990), 2.
2. A. J. Freeley and D. L. Steinberg, *Argumentation and Debate*, 10th ed. (Belmont, CA: Wadsworth, 1999), 1–3.
3. Ibid., 8.
4. Ibid., 9–12.
5. S. A. Jones and L. N. Brown, "Alternative Views on Defining Critical Thinking Through the Nursing Process," *Holistic Nurse Practitioner* (April 1993), 71–76.
6. K. L. Brooks and J. M. Shepherd, "Professionalism Versus Critical Thinking Abilities of Senior Nursing Students in Four Types of Nursing Curricula," *Journal of Professional Nursing* (March–April 1992), 87–95.
7. L. Saarmann, L. Freitas, J. Rapps, and B. Riegel, "The Relationship of Education to Critical Thinking Ability and Values Among Nurses: Socialization Into Professional Nursing," *Journal of Professional Nursing* (January–February 1992), 26–34.
8. J. S. Hickman, "A Critical Assessment of Critical Thinking in Nursing Education," *Holistic Nurse Practitioner* (April 1993), 36–47.

9. P. McCarthy, P. Schuster, P. Zehr, and D. McDougal, "Evaluation of Critical Thinking in a Baccalaureate Nursing Program," *Journal of Nursing Education* (March 1999), 142–144.
10. B. A. May, V. Edell, S. Butell, J. Doughty, and C. Langford, "Critical Thinking and Clinical Competence: A Study of Their Relationship in BSN Seniors," *Journal of Nursing Education* (March 1999), 100–110.
11. M. Bell and S. Procter, "Developing Nurse Practitioners to Develop Practice: The Experience of Nurses Working on a Nursing Development Unit," *Journal of Nursing Management* (March 1998), 61–69.
12. B. D. Steffy and A. J. Grimes, "A Critical Theory of Organizational Science," *Academy of Management Review* (April 1986), 332–336.
13. V. H. Kemp, "Concept Analysis as a Strategy for Promoting Critical Thinking," *Journal of Nursing Education* (November 1985), 382–384.
14. Graduate students in the master's program in nursing management at Louisiana State University School of Nursing, New Orleans, LA, Fall 1993.
15. J. H. Woods, "Affective Learning: One Door to Critical Thinking," *Holistic Nurse Practitioner* (April 1993), 64–70.

16. L. McKenzie, "Critical Thinking in Health Care Supervision," *Health Care Supervisor* (June 1992), 2.
17. S. Bos, "Perceived Benefits of Peer Leadership as Described by Junior Baccalaureate Nursing Students," *Journal of Nursing Education* (April 1998), 189–191.
18. K. L. Taylor and W. D. Care, "Nursing Education as Cognitive Apprenticeship: A Framework for Clinical Education," *Nurse Educator* (July–August 1999), 31–36.
19. J. Naisbitt, *High Tech High Touch* (New York: Broadway Books, 1999), 24–26.

REFERENCES

Adams, M. H., L. M. Stover, and J. F. Whitlow. "A Longitudinal Evaluation of Baccalaureate Nursing Students' Critical Thinking Abilities." *Journal of Nursing Education* (March 1999), 139–141.

Beitz, J. M. "Concept Mapping. Navigating the Learning Process." *Nurse Educator* (September–October 1998), 35–41.

Bradshaw, M. J. "Clinical Pathways: A Tool to Evaluate Clinical Learning." *Journal of the Society of Pediatric Nurses* (January–March 1999), 37–40.

Bittner, M. P., and E. Tobin. "Critical Thinking: Strategies for Clinical Practice." *Journal of Nursing Staff Development* (November–December 1998), 267–272.

Brock, A., and J. B. Butts. "On Target: A Model to Teach Baccalaureate Nursing Students to Apply Critical Thinking." *Nursing Forum* (July–September 1998), 5–10

Brown, H. N., and J. M. Sorrell. "Connecting Across the Miles: Interdisciplinary Collaboration in the Evaluation of Critical Thinking." *Nursing Connections* (summer 1999), 43–48.

Colucciello, M. L. "Relationships Between Critical Thinking Dispositions and Learning Styles." *Journal of Professional Nursing* (September–October 1999), 294–301.

Fowler, L. P. "Improving Critical Thinking in Nursing Practice." *Journal of Nursing Staff Development* (July–August 1998), 183–187.

Greenwood, J. "Critical Thinking and Nursing Scripts: The Case for the Development of Both." *Journal of Advanced Nursing* (February 2000), 428–436.

Hanson, E. J., J. Tetley, and A. Clarke. "Respite Care for Frail Older People and Their Family Caregivers: Concept Analysis and User Group Findings of a Pan-European Nursing Research Project." *Journal of Advanced Nursing* (December 1999), 1396–1407.

Jones, D. C., and M. E. Sheridan. "A Case Study Approach: Developing Critical Thinking Skills in Novice Pediatric Nurses." *Journal of Continuing Education in Nursing* (March–April 1999), 75–78.

Keenan, J. "A Concept Analysis of Autonomy." *Journal of Advanced Nursing* (March 1999), 556–562.

Leppa, C. J. "Standardized Measures of Critical Thinking. Experiences with the California Critical Thinking Tests." *Nurse Educator* (September–October 1997), 29–33.

Massarweh, L. J. "Promoting a Positive Clinical Experience." *Nurse Educator* (May–June 1999), 44–47.

Oermann, M. H. "How to Assess Critical Thinking in Clinical Practice." *Dimensions of Critical Care Nursing* (November–December 1998), 322–327.

Oermann, M. H. "Two-Way Talks." *Nursing Management* (June 1999), 56–58.

Platzer, H., D. Blake, and D. Ashford. "An Evaluation of Process and Outcomes from Learning Through Reflective Practice Groups on a Post-Registration Nursing Course." *Journal of Advanced Nursing* (March 2000), 689–695.

Schell, K. "Promoting Student Questioning." *Nurse Educator* (September–October 1998), 8–12.

Sedlak, C. A., and M. O. Doheny. "Peer Review Through Clinical Rounds. A Collaborative Critical Thinking Strategy." *Nurse Educator* (September–October 1998), 42–45.

Smith, L. S. "Concept Analysis: Cultural Competence." *Journal of Cultural Diversity* (spring 1998), 4–10.

Wade, G. H. "Professional Nurse Autonomy: Concept Analysis and Application to Nursing Education." *Journal of Advanced Nursing* (August 1999), 310.

Whitley, G. G. "Processes and Methodologies for Research Validation of Nursing Diagnosis." *Nursing Diagnosis* (January–March 1999), 5–14.

Yurkovich, E., and T. Smyer. "Shift Report: A Time for Learning." *Journal of Nursing Education* (December 1998), 401–403.

CHAPTER 2

Introduction to Managed Care

Russell C. Swansburg, PhD, RN

> The HMO revolution has already forced some 53 million people from Marcus Welby–style medicine into the Wal-Mart model of health care.
>
> E. Spragins[1]

LEARNING OBJECTIVES AND ACTIVITIES

- Discuss the comparative costs of various health care services based on information from a variety of sources.
- Demonstrate the development of health insurance influences on health care delivery in today's world.
- Describe the changes occurring in the U.S. health care system.
- Describe the elements of managed care and their impact on patients.
- Explain the effects of managed care relative to managers, nurses, physicians, health care organizations, and other providers.

CONCEPTS: Managed care, fee-for-service reimbursement, indemnity insurance plans, health maintenance organization (HMO), capitation, preferred provider organization (PPO), contracting.

MANAGER BEHAVIOR: Solve problems resulting from managed care and promote interests of patients and personnel.

LEADER BEHAVIOR: Assist personnel in maximum understanding of their health care benefits, including wellness benefits. Empower professional nurses to produce quality outcomes for patients, personnel, and insurers within an environment influenced by managed care.

Introduction

Headlines and topics related to the high cost of health care have emerged as a major impetus for evolution of the health care system into one of managed care. A nurse manager need only examine a few days' mail to note the importance of this occupational phenomenon. New publications abound, having titles such as *Inside Medicaid Managed Care* and *Managed Care Quarterly*.

All major health care publications carry articles on managed care that posit questions such as "Will the Cost Cutting in Health Care Kill You?"[2] Major newspapers and news weeklies include articles entitled "HMOs Tell Courts They Aren't Liable," and "Does Your HMO Stack Up?"[3] Writers have reported that the cost of quality health care is wreaking havoc on the budgets of consumers, companies, and the federal government. As a result, managed care has become the dominant health care delivery system in the United States.

> Investor-owned HMOs typically use 15% to 25% of premiums for corporate costs and profits, inevitably limiting services. Business people and investors do not take the Hippocratic oath and cannot be expected to put the interests of the patient or community before profits.[4]

Health Care Costs

National health expenditures have risen from $12.7 billion, or 4.4%, of the gross domestic product (GDP) in 1950 to $1,092.4 billion, or 12.8%, of the GDP in 1997. (See Exhibit 2-1.) In 1999, more than 90.5% of federal spending went to national defense, payments to individuals, Social Security, Medicare, Medicaid, and interest on the national debt. Medicare is financed almost exclusively by payroll taxes, with expenditures growing at a faster rate than is the wage-based tax. The primary contribution to this disparity, once again, is rising medical costs. Solutions to the problem include reduced health care cost increases, higher cost-sharing by beneficiaries, reduced provider reimbursement, and increased payroll taxes.

Expenditures of Health Care Dollars

During the years 1950 to 1997, the amount of private health expenditures went from $8.9 billion to $585.3 billion, an increase of 6,576%. Public expenditures rose from $2.8 billion to $507.1 billion, an increase of 18,111%. The ratio of public to private expenditures actually decreased from approximately 1:3.2 to 1:1.2. (See Exhibit 2-1.)

Although direct patient (out-of-pocket) payments rose from $7.1 billion in 1950 to $187.6 billion in 1997, they actually decreased from 79.8% to 32.1% of the total private health expenditures. Insurance premiums rose from $1.3 billion to $348.0 billion during the same period. (See Exhibit 2-1.)

In the public domain, the health care dollar is spent on Medicare, Medicaid, the Veterans Administration, public health services, and other public assistance programs. Medicare increased from $7.7 billion in 1970 to approximately $214.6 billion in 1997. Public assistance, mostly Medicaid, rose from $6.3 billion to an estimated $165.2 billion between 1970 and 1997. Exhibit 2-2 shows hospital care and physician service expenditures from 1980 to 1997. Exhibit 2-3 shows consumer price indexes for medical services and commodities from 1990 to 1998.

> The ultimate solution to control costs has become managed care.

The U.S. Health Care System

One could argue that the health care system of the United States is a non-system. Rising health care costs have spawned health care policy issues to control them and to encourage wellness or fitness care as a viable alternative to illness care. Ambulatory care also continues to expand as an alternative to inpatient care.

During the twentieth century, heart disease and cancer (which account for nearly 60% of all deaths) have surpassed infectious and parasitic diseases (which once accounted for over 40% of deaths) as the major causes of death. Antibiotics are widely used to treat and prevent infections and parasites, urban water supplies are filtered and chlorinated, milk is pasteurized, and persons with infectious diseases are effectively treated using isolation procedures. Many safe, efficient, and cost-effective vaccines are available, such as the vaccine for rubella for children between the ages of 17 and 35 months, that are not being used to their full potential.[5]

Life expectancy at birth increased from 54.1 years in 1920 to 76.5 years in 1997. Life expectancy is predicted to increase to 77.4 years in 2010 (74.1 for males and 80.6 for females).[6] Increased life expectancy changes the nature of health care as older persons develop more degenerative diseases.

EXHIBIT 2-1
National Health Expenditures from 1950 to 1997

				PRIVATE			PUBLIC			
YEAR	TOTAL ($, BILLIONS)	PER CAPITA ($, DOLLARS)	GDP %	TOTAL ($, BILLIONS)	OUT-OF-POCKET PAYMENTS TOTAL ($, BILLIONS)	INSURANCE PREMIUMS ($, BILLIONS)	TOTAL ($, BILLIONS)	MEDICARE ($, BILLIONS)	PUBLIC ASSISTANCE ($, BILLIONS)	MEDICAID ($, BILLIONS)
50	12.7	0	4.4	8.9	7.1	1.3	2.8	—	0.1	—
55	17.7	0	4.4	12.9	9.1	3.2	4.0	—	0.2	—
60	26.9	141	5.1	19.5	13.1	5.9	5.7	—	0.5	—
65	41.1	202	5.7	29.4	18.5	10.0	8.3	—	1.7	—
70	73.2	341	7.1	43.0	24.9	16.3	24.9	7.7	6.3	5.1
75	130.7	582	8.0	72.3	38.1	31.3	50.1	16.4	14.5	12.3
80	247.2	1,002	8.9	142.5	60.3	69.7	104.8	37.5	28.0	23.3
85	428.2	1,666	10.2	253.9	100.6	132.3	174.3	72.2	44.4	37.5
90	697.5	2,588	12.1	413.1	148.4	232.4	284.3	112.1	80.4	64.8
95	988.5	3,509	13.7	532.1	182.6	310.6	456.4	187.0	146.4	120.1
97	1,092.4	3,800	12.8	585.3	187.6	348.0	507.1	214.6	165.2	123.6

The Medicaid column is part of the public assistance column total.

Source: U.S. Bureau of the Census. *Statistical Abstract of the United States* 1999, 119th ed. Washington, D.C., 1999.

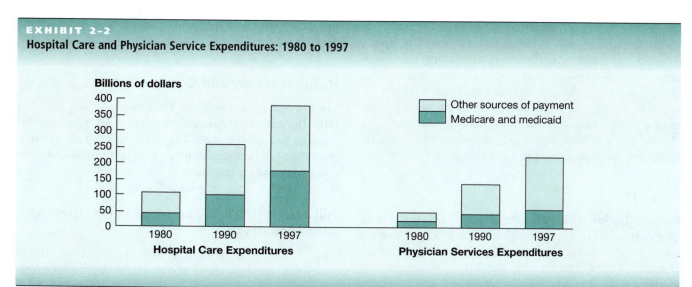

EXHIBIT 2-2
Hospital Care and Physician Service Expenditures: 1980 to 1997

Billions of dollars

Other sources of payment
Medicare and medicaid

Hospital Care Expenditures   Physician Services Expenditures

Source: Chart prepared by U.S. Census Bureau.

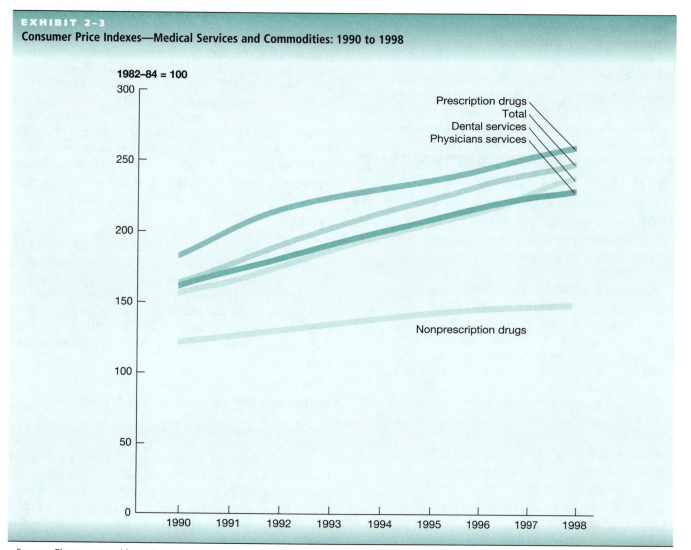

EXHIBIT 2-3
Consumer Price Indexes—Medical Services and Commodities: 1990 to 1998

1982–84 = 100

Prescription drugs
Total
Dental services
Physicians services

Nonprescription drugs

Source: Chart prepared by U.S. Census Bureau.

Maintenance of community health is affected by social, economic, and political factors. Suicides, homicides, and accidents are among the leading causes of death among persons aged 1 to 39 years. Suicide and homicide rates doubled among those aged 10 to 24 years from 1961 to 1994.[7] Solutions to these problems must take the behavioral component into account.

Exhibit 2-4 outlines the sequential development of health care insurance in the United States.

Blue Cross

Prepaid health care plans began in 1929 with Blue Cross. By the 1940s, one-fifth of the U.S. population was covered, and by 1966, one-third. By 1984, approximately 57% of the U.S. population was covered by employer- or employer-union–provided group plans. By 1997, government or private insurance covered 269.1 million persons, or 83.9% of the population, and 43.4 million or 16.1% were not insured.[8]

For updates on these and previous data go to the Internet site (http://census.gov/)

Social Security

The Social Security Act of 1935 provided funds for maternal and child health services, education and training of public health workers, research in nutri-

---

EXHIBIT 2-4
Historical Development of Health Care Insurance

1929 Blue Cross

1935 Social Security Act

1946 Hospital Survey and Construction Act (Hill–Burton)

1964 Hill–Harris Hospital and Medical Facilities Amendments

1965 Public Law 89-97, Medicare and Medicaid

1982 Public Law 97-248, Tax Equity and Fiscal Responsibility Act (TEFRA)

1983 Public Law, 98-21, Social Security Amendments Prospective Payment System

1985 Consolidated Omnibus Budget Reconciliation Act (COBRA)

1986 Gramm–Rudman Deficit Reduction Amendment and Omnibus Budget Reconciliation Act

1987,

1988 Omnibus Budget Reconciliation Act (OBRA)

1989 Physician Payment Review Commission

1994 Medicare Choice Act

1996 Health Insurance and Accountability Act

1997 Balanced Budget Act

---

tion and industrial hygiene, and aid to children with disabilities.[9]

Hospital Survey and Construction Act

The Hospital Survey and Construction Act of 1946 (Hill–Burton) stimulated construction of hospitals in areas of severe shortage. This act equalized the relative availability of hospital facilities between urban and rural areas and among the states.[10]

Hill–Harris Hospital and Medical Facilities Amendments

The Hill–Harris Hospital and Medical Facilities Amendments, enacted in 1964, dealt with modernization grants, area-wide planning, and long-term care facilities.[11]

Social Security Amendments of 1965

In 1965, Public Law 89-97 created Medicare and Medicaid. With this law, the federal government assumed a major role in health care financing. As a result, approximately one-tenth of the U.S. population was aided in 1965. This number represented about one-third of hospital patient days, bringing the proportion covered by third-party payers to two-thirds at the time the law went into effect. By 1997, approximately 35.6 million persons were covered by Medicare and 29.0 million by Medicaid. These figures represented over 24% of the U.S. population.[12]

TEFRA

The Tax Equity and Fiscal Responsibility Act (TEFRA), was passed by Congress in 1982 and went into effect in 1983. It ushered into effect the Prospective Payment System (PPS), because it made reimbursement for patients on Medicare prospective, creating a system of cost-per-case limits. This system was the prelude to the diagnosis-related groups (DRGs) reimbursement system.

Social Security Amendments of 1983

President Reagan signed Public Law 98-21, the Social Security Amendments of 1983, in April 1983. It was enacted to head off potential deficits in the Hospital Insurance Trust Fund of the Social Security program. This law established a prospective payment system (PPS) for hospital care based on DRGs. Prospective payment means the expected payment for a particular DRG.

COBRA

The Omnibus Budget Reconciliation Acts of 1986, 1987, and 1988 followed the Consolidated Omnibus Budget Reconciliation Act (COBRA) of 1985. These acts modify the reimbursement provisions of the prospective payment system.

Physician Payment Review Commission

The Physician Payment Review Commission was created in 1989. This system introduced a new payment system for Medicare by limiting amounts physicians could charge above a resource-based fee schedule within a neutral budgetary environment.

Medicare Choice Act

The Medicare Choice Act of 1994 allows seniors to opt out of Medicare and into integrated health plans. It allows for choice of Medicare fee-for-service, employer-sponsored, or other managed care health plans during open enrollment periods.

Health Insurance and Accountability Act

Signed into law on August 21, 1996, the Health Insurance and Accountability Act established favorable federal tax treatment for the benefits and premiums of qualified long-term care services. Benefits received from a qualified long-term care insurance policy are not taxable. Premiums for qualified long-term care insurance policies (up to a specified limit based on age) and expenses not reimbursed for qualified long-term care services are tax-deductible, similar to medical expenses. This act also protects the portability of health insurance for employees changing jobs and establishes law for medical savings accounts.

Balanced Budget Act

President Clinton signed into law the Balanced Budget Act on August 5, 1997. This act offers a new level of health care options called Medicare plus Choice. Among these choices are preferred provider organizations (PPOs) and provider-sponsored organizations (PSOs). Other changes include redistributed payments between rural and urban areas and restricted movement among plans.[13]

The Balanced Budget Act covers multiple years, and hospital administrators complain of budget deficits requiring personnel cutbacks because of reduced federal payments. An ambulatory payment classification system was implemented in 2000 by the Health Care Financing Administration for all ambulatory care procedures. This system replaced the current fee schedule.

The result of these third-party payer programs has been a mixed blessing. Many people enjoy good health and good health care because such programs insure them. Out-of-pocket costs to these persons have been dramatically reduced, but third-party payer programs have been weak incentives to consumers, who have seldom questioned the need for many services or sought out less costly providers or styles of care.

Components of the U.S. Health Care System

The U.S. health-care system has many components: patients, insurers, and employers; providers such as hospitals, ambulatory care services, home health services, long-term care facilities, physicians, nurses, allied health personnel, pharmacists and pharmacies, providers of durable medical equipment; and federal, state, and local public health services. As costs have increased, physicians who have been reimbursed based on fees for services are increasingly being reimbursed by capitation through contracts with managed care insurers or have become employees of the managed care insurers. Employees have switched from indemnity insurance plans to managed care plans.

Indemnity insurance plans cover bills from most providers and pay most health care bills by charges or costs, with some deductibles or copayments. Indemnity plans are fast disappearing as employers and governments switch to managed care plans. As health care costs have soared, employers have increased employees' share of indemnity insurance premiums. Indemnity insurance plans do not keep costs down. Indemnity insurers are changing to become organizers and administrators of managed care networks and subsequently deliverers of health care. This transformation is reducing the number of insurers.[14]

> **The heart of the managed care revolution is money, not medicine.**
>
> *George Anders*[15]

In the new managed care environment, many providers are integrated into insurance plan services through individual contracts and subcontracts. Clients accept the providers of these contract services, thus limiting their choices regarding most health care provider services. Clients receive a total package of health care dictated by the contracts between employers and insurers.

Managed Care

Managed care is a patient care system that includes insurance companies, employers, providers, and clients. Most enrollees of managed care plans are employees of businesses that contract for health insurance as a benefit. Many plans accept individual enrollees, particularly plans that enroll Medicare beneficiaries. Managed care is also the process by which health care benefits are monitored for purposes of cost management, resulting in limitation of benefit coverage and access to health care benefits. Managed care organizations manage the distribution of health care dollars, use of services, and access to benefits.

Organizations and Alternative Delivery Systems

Patients now accept health care plans that limit their freedom of choice. The following sections discuss some of these plans.

Health Maintenance Organizations

Financing of health maintenance organizations (HMOs) is done by *capitation*, in which there is a predetermined payment per patient or per service. Managed care is designed to cut costs.

The HMO is defined as "a prepaid health plan delivering comprehensive care to members through designated providers, having a fixed periodic payment for health care services, and requiring members to be in a plan for a specified period of time (usually 1 year). A group HMO delivers health services through a physician group that is controlled by the HMO unit or contracts with one or more independent group practices to provide health services. An individual practice association (IPA) HMO contracts directly with physicians in independent practice, and/or contracts with one or more associations of physicians in independent practice, and/or contracts with one or more multispecialty group practices. Data are based on a consensus of HMOs."[16]

HMOs have the following characteristics:

- Utilization risks are shifted from payer to provider.
- Competition draws consumers to less costly services when they have a choice of plans.
- Use of preventive care and ambulatory facilities decreases hospital admission rates, lowering insurance costs by 10% to 40%.
- Use of primary care physicians and nurse practitioners at fixed salaries decreases the use of expensive surgeons and specialists.
- HMOs eliminate unneeded facilities such as hospitals, operating rooms, and radiation therapy units.

- Paperwork and overhead are reduced.
- HMOs provide organized, cooperative care for individuals and families.
- Enrollees make appointments with gatekeeper physicians or nurses, mostly family practice physicians, internists, and pediatricians.
- Gatekeepers control all referrals to specialists.
- Enrollees pay a small fee per visit and for medications.
- Gatekeepers control unneeded procedures, both diagnostic and therapeutic.
- HMO plans contract for discounted prices with various providers, such as hospitals, laboratories, radiologists, physician specialists and pharmacists.
- HMO plans emphasize complete patient care, management of chronic illnesses, education, disease prevention, and wellness. (See Exhibit 2-5.) Oxford Health Plans hired 20 nurse practitioners because they are trained to provide services for disease prevention and health promotion. These registered nurse practitioners perform more preventive care and are reimbursed at the same rate as physicians.
- HMOs make physicians business-oriented practitioners.
- HMO plans do mass customization to give each of a mass of customers what the customer desires.

EXHIBIT 2-5
Wellness Example

A 91-year-old patient in a nursing home existed in a terrified state, requiring oxygen and medication to sustain her breathing. She refused to leave her room. Then, the Eden Alternative was introduced to change the environment of nursing homes. This alternative brings pets—cats, birds, and fish—into the resident's environment. In this new environment, the patient–resident cares for a cat and a parakeet. She lunches with friends and participates in activities with other residents. She no longer needs an oxygen tank, and her medications have been reduced. Other modifications of this environment include interior decoration, large and luxurious indoor plants, raised flower beds and bird feeders outside, and validation therapy. All these modifications are designed to include the residents. Autonomous, self-directed teams of nurses, housekeepers, aides, and therapists manage the nursing home. Families participate. Employee turnover is reduced. There is a playground where residents can watch children of employees and relatives of residents play. Schoolchildren visit with residents. The environment is one in which wellness prevails over illness. Spirits are nurtured and soar over apathy. This is holistic care that raises the quality of residents' lives.

Source: A. McDonald. "Nursing Homes Teach Elders to Live Again." *San Antonio Express-News* (14 April 1997), 1D, 10D.

- HMOs offer capitated payments, one price per enrollee.
- HMOs reduce the risks of unneeded procedures, such as caesarian sections and hysterectomies.
- Half of HMO physicians are paid flat fees that are incentives to reduce care.

Pilot programs of Medicare HMOs indicate that hospitalization of clients on Medicare could be decreased by 30%. HMO membership increased from 9.1 million in 1980 to 64.8 million in 1998.

Hospitals that do not succeed in the growing competitive atmosphere will be faced with empty beds, unused ancillary services, decreasing reimbursement revenues, closings, and layoffs. Hospital administrators will learn not to respond to physicians at all costs. Many will employ physicians, give up beds and services, seek out special markets and relationships, and adopt aggressive marketing strategies and techniques. Hospitals will save management fees by managing their own HMOs.

Wolfe indicates that HMOs do not decrease costs, because they increase profits. In 1994, eight insurance companies owned 45% of HMOs. Their average profit from first quarter 1992 to first quarter 1993 was 40%.[17]

As HMOs expand, health costs increase. In California, with 80% of employees covered under managed care plans, costs are 19% above the national average and increasing more rapidly than elsewhere in the country.[18]

Although HMOs are the most common type of managed care organization, many more millions of people belong to other types, which are discussed in the following paragraphs.

Preferred Provider Organizations

In a PPO, a group of providers acts as health care brokers providing services to a group of patients at reduced fees. PPOs have the following characteristics:

- PPOs contract with consumers through employers and insurers and with providers, including physicians, hospitals, and allied services.
- PPO services are discounted, and patients have no out-of-pocket expenses.
- In PPOs, patients are limited to using the listed providers or paying larger fees for out-of-network providers.
- PPOs are intermediaries between payer and subscriber groups, furnishing marketing and administrative services.
- PPOs set their own size, number of staff specialists, geographic availability, time limits for claims and payments, and other features.
- PPOs place hospitals but not physicians at risk. Physicians are paid discounted rates for a steady flow of patients.

Arguments that the traditional physician–patient relationship will be destroyed are relatively inconsequential because these relationships will soon disappear. Working people want efficiency; they do not want to sit in a physician's office waiting for hours past their appointed time. Given adequate information, they will make choices about their care, and they should. The old concept of withholding information is outmoded and dangerous and in some cases illegal (e.g., re informed consent). The objective of all competitive health care plans is to provide good quality care less expensively. There are approximately 1036 PPOs in the United States and more than 50.2 million enrollees.[19]

Health Care Cost Coalitions

Health care cost coalitions (HCCCs) are organizations of employers, and sometimes unions, that effectively bargain for better rates and parity with Medicare, Medicaid, and other insurers. They work to develop PPOs and utilization review programs.

Prudent Buyer Systems

Prudent buyer systems are characterized by joint purchasing arrangements, purchasing consortia composed of multiple providers, and competitive bidding for exclusive contracts.

Health Promotion and Wellness Programs

Increased education and awareness enable these programs to emphasize illness prevention.

Hospital Physician Organizations

The hospital physician organization (HPO) is a relatively new entity. Its objective is to combine and reduce overhead, which can be done by sharing services such as billing.

Provider-Sponsored Organizations (PSOs)

Provider-sponsored organizations (PSOs) are networks of physicians and hospitals that are their owners. Approximately 84 PSOs exist in the United States. Supporters of PSOs say they are health providers engaged in treating patients, while HMOs are insurance companies that invest in stocks, bonds, and other liquid assets. PSOs offer less risk to providers than do HMOs because providers receive only part of their income from the PSO.[20]

Managed care is a fact of life. It will not go away. Most Americans eventually will belong to a managed care plan.

Enrollment

More than 64 million people were enrolled in HMOs in 1998, with more than 140 million estimated today. This number includes 7.8 million of the 38 million plus beneficiaries of Medicare. The average Medicare HMO patient is 12% healthier than is the average patient on Medicare. More than three-fourths of active employees are enrolled in managed care plans. Average annual premiums went from $3,741 in 1994 to $3,915 in 1996.[21] HMO enrollments are shown in Exhibit 2-6.

Advantages

Managed care has a number of advantages, including the following:

- Managed care has reined in skyrocketing medical costs. Medical care inflation, the lowest since 1973, has increased since 1997 to pay for 2 years of rollbacks and decreasing profits.
- Managed care puts patients first by making clinical decisions before economic ones.
- Managed care limits patients' time to get appointments.
- Managed care offers fast-track treatment for life-threatening conditions.
- The U.S. Department of Health and Human Services is responsible for ensuring due process for Medicare HMO enrollees. It can require written notice describing the reason for denial of a service, provide clear information on how to appeal an HMO decision, and require expedited consideration in time-sensitive medical situations.
- Managed care holds the interests of third parties at bay.
- Medicare rules limit financial penalties against physicians in managed care plans for referrals or expensive procedures.

EXHIBIT 2-6
HMO Enrollments for 1980 to 1998

YEAR	NUMBER OF PLANS	ENROLLMENTS (IN THOUSANDS)
1980	236	9,100
1985	393	18,894
1989	590	32,493
1990	556	33,622
1991	559	35,052
1992	559	27,199
1993	540	39,783
1994	547	43,443
1995	550	46,182
1998	651	64,800

- By law, new mothers in managed care plans cannot be forced out of hospitals in less than 48 hours.
- Law can limit gag rules.
- Most HMO enrollees receive the care they need. Sixty percent are highly satisfied (this number ranged from 45% to 77% depending on the HMO). Of enrollees, 10% would not recommend HMOs.[22]
- Some plans pay for prescription drugs.
- Changes in federal law would allow HMOs to be sued for malpractice and held accountable for mistakes.
- Profit motives may be checked.
- Managed care plans receive better quality report cards than indemnity insurance plans.
- Managed care plans can keep out physicians who have malpractice judgments.

Strengths

If improvements are made, managed care will lead to better-informed consumers. Treatment guidelines for managed care plans will be developed that people can trust. Conservative treatment may cost less and have better outcomes. For example, $1,000 worth of physical therapy may be better for a herniated disk than would a $15,000 operation. In a study of Californians under 65 years of age who had appendicitis, 25.8% of HMO members had ruptured appendices versus 29.3% of patients in fee-for-service plans. Patients in managed care plans have a place to voice complaints. Of women HMO members at Scripps Clinic, La Jolla, California, 95% receive mammograms, whereas the national average is about 75%. Mammograms can detect breast cancer and result in earlier treatment.[23]

Problems

The following are among the problems associated with managed care:

- Medicare enrollees in HMOs may not regain Medigap insurance if they choose to return to fee-for-service plans.
- Gag clauses in contracts between the plan and physician forbid disclosures that advise patients medically necessary but expensive treatment options. Gag clauses limit care, undermine trust, and are negative to clinical independence. Presidential orders prohibit gag rules for Medicare patients (5.7 million or 8.8% of beneficiaries) and 7.8 million recipients of Medicaid. The managed care industry has promised not to restrict patient–doctor communications.
- Managed care limits choices by denial of referral to specialists.

- Managed care performs less research.
- Managed care plans have conflicting formularies and incompatible information systems.
- Physicians must pursue approvals and correct inappropriate denials.
- Physicians are rewarded for providing less care.
- Money goes to corporate salaries and profits (20%).
- High-risk patients are screened out. Services to sick and disabled persons are limited. Patients are dumped into public facilities. The poor, the sick, and the elderly have limited access, low satisfaction, and poor outcomes.
- Medical service accounts are opposed by managed care insurers because unused money in the savings account goes to the employee, and not the insurance company.
- Women have a harder time getting needed medical care from HMOs.
- Because more people are now in the managed care system, they have a harder time accessing needed care and therefore visit doctors more frequently because they become sicker.
- Members with rare medical conditions sometimes encounter problems in obtaining appropriate treatment. This problem can be solved with a point-of-service option that permits clients to go to any physician by paying an additional fee.
- Patients are being moved through the system by decisions of clerks rather than nurses. For example: A patient was observed in the recovery room for 45 minutes and then was moved to the floor against the nurse's better judgment. The patient had complications and then had to be moved to the intensive care unit.
- Plans have a tendency to look only at statistical averages and fail to understand the individuality of patients. As a result, plans fail to recognize that complex medical problems cannot always be standardized into predetermined treatment paths.
- HMO enrollees with mental health problems often receive poorer detection and treatment.

Solutions

Some of these managed care problems have solutions. In 1996, 400 bills representing backlash legislation against managed care were introduced in state legislatures. Among the goals of such bills are the following:

- Managed care programs would be forced to pay the physician or the hospital used by the client.
- Clients would see specialists without preapproval.
- Emergency room care would be paid for even when the visit is not deemed an emergency.

- HMOs would be banned from paying physicians for withholding treatments.
- Gag clauses would be outlawed.
- HMOs would not be able to fire physicians who speak out against policies they believe endanger patients.[24]

In 1997, the Texas state legislature passed, and the governor signed into law, a bill making managed care plans responsible when they withhold medical treatment. Texas is the first state to pass legislation allowing managed care groups to be sued for withholding treatment with resultant harm to the client. About 4.3 million Texans are enrolled in managed care plans.[25]

To be financially viable, the provider must negotiate a contract that will balance a budget, which requires sound financial acumen.

Contracts

Under managed care, contracts are a way of life for insurers, employers, health care providers, and consumers. Consumers usually obtain their contracts through employers and should carefully study the provisions of their contract coverage. Insurers have contracts with both employers and health care providers. To avoid legal pitfalls and maximize profits, health care providers must have a thorough knowledge of the terms of their contracts with insurers. Contract terms include coverage limits, criteria for authorization of services, identification of all the provider parties to the contract, automatic renewal, criteria for termination of contracts, credentialing processes, criteria for accepting or rejecting patients, liability insurance requirements, grievance procedures, provision for contract changes, utilization review requirements, provision for timely payment of claims, provision for continuity of care and payment when contracts are terminated, avoidance of unnecessary record-keeping, and provision for assignments when insurers are bought and sold. Providers of health care need to know all state laws regulating managed care insurers.[26]

Nurses are frequently providers of services, and particularly home care services, under managed care contracts. Other nurses are case managers for insurers and employers. Nurses involved in negotiating managed care contracts need access to good cost data, including fixed and variable costs. Other needed data include the benefits package, and patient and physician demographics, including practice patterns. Legal counsel is a necessity in contract negotiations under managed care. All nurse managers need knowledge of managed care contracts affecting their patients.

In an HMO, the client may have the option of choosing a primary care provider who is a nurse. This nurse may receive a monthly fee (capitation) to provide appropriate primary care services, including prior approval for specialty care, hospitalization, surgery, and simple emergencies. The nurse provider has a contract negotiated with the HMO. When nurse providers reduce the costs of health care, they benefit from bonuses paid by the HMO for reducing costs, provided the nurse providers have such clauses in their contracts. Nurse providers may consider negotiating contracts that provide an exclusive relationship with the HMO whereby they contract only with that HMO. Other contract negotiations include sign-on bonuses and additive fee-for-service payments for particular services such as transportation, intensive outreach, and health education.[27] See Exhibit 2-7 for a managed care contract checklist.

Economic Implications

Managed care, whether by for-profit or not-for-profit organizations, has a number of economic implications. Profits of mental health managed care plans are enormous. Administrative and profit-loading costs are seldom below 40%.[28] Unnecessary mastectomies, heart bypass procedures, and prostate surgeries are reduced under managed care plans. Health care premiums rose only 2% in 1995. Some companies encourage workers to choose the best HMOs by discounting monthly premiums.[29] Overuse of medical services and administrative inefficiencies result in $200 million in unnecessary costs each year.[30]

Whether the organization is designated as not for profit or for profit, profit is the ultimate goal of managed care. The not-for-profit organization needs to make a profit to stay in business. By law, any profits must be reinvested in the business or used to reduce premiums. For-profit organizations want to make profits for their shareholders. Business is about providing employment, providing value for customers, developing skills of employees, developing capabilities of suppliers, and earning money for shareholders.

Having reached maximum savings through managed care health care costs are expected to rise. This increase will be partly a result of higher costs for technology and drugs, which have risen three times faster than other components of health care. Also, legislators and employers tell the insurers they must cover a certain minimum level of service and a minimum number of persons who have preexisting or serious conditions. Physicians are demanding higher compensation.[31]

Managed care organizations are making tremendous profits. Oxford Health Plans, an HMO, has more than $2 billion in annual sales. The company is growing by 125% annually, and its earnings are compounded

---

EXHIBIT 2-7
Questions to Ask When Choosing a Managed Care Plan

1. Are your physicians on salary or captiation?
2. Do your physicians get bonuses for keeping costs down?
3. How does your plan address the need for basic medical research?
4. How does your plan address the need for education of health professionals?
5. How does your plan measure quality?
6. What have been the results of measuring quality?
7. How does your plan credential physicians? Are all specialists board certified?
8. What other health professionals does your plan credential?
9. What is the average time for a person to get an appointment with a physician?
10. What is covered by the plan? Prescription drugs? Preventive care? Hearing and eye care? Dental care? Podiatry? Mental health care? Chiropractic care? Medical supplies and equipment? Home health care? Nursing home care? Rehabilitation?
11. What is not covered by the plan? What are the specific exclusions?
12. What copayments are required by the plan? Deductions? Specify.
13. What are the costs of the plan? How much is my employer paying?
14. Is there a point-of-service option allowing care by certain providers outside the plan? How does it work?
15. Are there maximum amounts the plan will pay for particular services?
16. Who are the physicians in the plan? Is there access to specific specialists and hospitals, or is such access restricted?
17. Are physicians' offices conveniently located?
18. Do the hospitals affiliated with the plan meet my needs?
19. Do enrollees like the plan? Check with consumer groups, the media, and other employees.
20. How many members disenrolled during the past 3 years? Why?
21. How many primary care physicians left the plan during the past 3 years? Why?
22. How does the plan handle emergency or urgent care?
23. How does the plan handle emergency or urgent care outside the service area?
24. Is the plan accredited? (http://www.ncqa.org.)
25. How does the plan handle complaints?

---

at over 75%. In 4 years, the price of company stock went from $4 a share to over $47 a share. Other big earners are medical device companies and national health care providers. Healthsouth Treasure Coast Rehabilitation Hospital, Vero Beach, Florida, does $6 billion worth of rehabilitation and outpatient surgery a year at 1,000 locations. Its specialty is sports medicine. Heart valves cost less than $1,000 to manufacture but sell for $3,000. St. Jude Medical, St. Paul, Minnesota, designs, manufactures, and distributes medical devices. The company holds the patents on and has FDA approval for many of its products; it also has few competitors. PhyCor, which buys and runs physician practices, imposes management practices that cut costs.[32]

Managed care is creating an economic upheaval.

Ethical Implications

Successful managed care organizations will recognize all players as stakeholders in a community. These organizations will conduct business in an ethical manner. They will make long-term commitments to employees, customers, suppliers, and other stakeholders. Doing so will give these organizations a competitive advantage.

Whether myth or fear, the following are some of the ethical questions raised by managed care:

- Will pressure of legalization for physician-assisted suicide and cost management by managed care organizations affect patient outcomes?
- Will the poor, the elderly, and the uninsured continue to be forced to accept fewer costly procedures and face early death?
- Will patients' rights force physicians to inform patients of the right to physician-assisted suicide?
- Should people, including those in need, receive uncompensated care?

Implications for Consumers

Most consumers are not in managed care plans voluntarily but because of choices made by their employers. Consumers need to be informed and vigilant so they use the services effectively and efficiently. Many physicians belong to several plans, and several plans have many physicians from whom to choose. Thus, physician choice for consumers is broadened.

The following are some examples of managed care problems for the consumer:

- A 61-year-old woman waited 4 hours in an HMO hospital emergency room while a blood clot starved her body of oxygen. She had no call button and was not monitored. Her daughter blamed her death on the HMO-owned hospital.[33]
- A woman claimed that an HMO stopped an orthopedist from mending her broken, infected leg because it would cost too much. Approval for treatment took much persuasion by the doctor. The HMO recommended amputation; the orthopedist saved the leg.[34]

- Patients become sicker waiting 6 to 10 weeks to see a cancer specialist or get a computed tomography (CT) scan.[35]
- The parents of a 6-month-old baby who is feverish, moaning, and panting call a hotline nurse. The nurse refers them to an HMO contract hospital 42 miles away. They drive through torrential rain and past a nearby non-HMO hospital on their way to the designated hospital. Because of the delay, a potential fatal infection results in amputation of the child's hands and feet.[36]
- "In Massachusetts, 22% of HMO patients are afraid that their doctors would not provide needed care, and only two-thirds have confidence in their physicians."[37]
- "Twenty percent of Medicare HMO enrollees dropped out within 12 months of joining."[38]
- "Your policy may say you'll get quality treatments and hospitalization, but in the brave new world of managed care your actual treatments will probably be determined by someone who never saw you."[39]

Practice Implications

Nurse-midwife numbers are increasing. Physicians and hospitals are hiring nurse-midwives. Because nurse midwives are less expensive than are physicians and they score high in patient satisfaction, managed care organizations are interested in hiring them. Nurse-midwives provide quality time and personal attention and apply their expert state-of-the-art skills to patient care.

In other areas, less skilled employees are replacing registered nurses. Shifts are understaffed. Inferior supplies include surgical gloves that break more easily, smaller alcohol sponges, and chest suction with valves that do not indicate whether they are on or off.

HMOs also are determining practitioners' credentials and setting practice guidelines that result in less well-qualified providers and less stringent rules.

Education Implications

Education is unprofitable in the managed care environment. Future generations of caregivers may push distance-learning technology, which has inconveniences such as compressed videos, logistical or mechanical problems, lack of spontaneous reactions, and distracted students. Research indicates, however, that students learn as well as or better than they do on-site, and there is a wider audience with distance education, but distance education still has a long way to go.[40]

Research Implications

Research is unprofitable in the managed care environment. Because research expands the frontiers of medical knowledge, less funding for research has serious implications for health care.

Quality Implications

A system for rating HMO quality allows "consumers to differentiate between an HMO that's great at answering the phone from one that's doing a great job of detecting breast cancer."[41]

Criteria for rating HMOs may include the following:

- Meets industry standards of accreditation by the National Committee for Quality Assurance (NCQA). The Health Plan Employer Data and Information Set (HEDIS) measures aspects of plans such as checking on physicians' credentials, affiliation with the Joint Commission on Accreditation of Healthcare Organizations accredited hospitals, and board certification.
- Measures satisfaction of physicians and members.
- Tracks members' health, measuring and addressing risk-taking behavior.
- Uses hard-nosed outcomes measures, including morbidity and mortality.
- Develops prevention and screening tools to keep people healthy through early detection.
- Encourages perinatal care during first trimester of pregnancy, resulting in low caesarian section rates and high rates of normal delivery.
- Allows employers to perform independent surveys of contract plans using outcomes measures.[42]

Quality isn't examined very closely when most employers choose group health insurance plans. In a recent study of the chronically ill, the elderly and the sickest poor fared much worse in three urban HMOs than their counterparts did in traditional plans.

Jane Bryant Quinn[43]

The three major contenders in the movement for health care quality are[44]:

1. The National Committee for Quality Assurance which judges 50 different characteristics.
2. John Ward's Medical Outcomes Survey. The survey evaluates the general health of persons. It may be effective over time.
3. The Foundation for Accountability (FACCT). FACCT develops standards for judging how well HMOs handle specific illnesses.

It is difficult for different persons to agree on and thus to standardize quality measurements. Insurers and providers often select treatment based on the least expensive outcome rather than on morbidity and mortality rates. If they are to access quality care, consumers need knowledge of ways in which providers deliver care without increasing costs; of how consumers can be assertive about obtaining needed services; about data linked to expected care and treatment outcomes; about best practices that are benchmarks, including critical paths for specific diagnoses and procedures; and about data on morbidity and mortality related to all health care providers.[45]

Health maintenance organizations with thick rosters of physicians may be laggards in providing quality care. These contracted physicians practice medicine in the way in which the HMO dictates. The best HMOs may have fewer physicians and a central office. Aetna U.S. Healthcare has large numbers of physicians and offers financial incentives to keep costs down. In 1996, the average physician worked for 13 HMOs, with 13 sets of criteria. Physicians who are on salary use treatments that work best and thus maintain quality. This fact can be proven; for example, Kaiser Permanente HMO scores higher on quality measures than does Aetna U.S. Healthcare.[46]

How the consumer can find quality care:
1. **Learn the best medical technique for the procedure or treatment you are facing.**
2. **Check public information about the providers who will be caring for you.**
3. **Check member satisfaction surveys before choosing an HMO.**
4. **Assert yourself in dealing with your HMO, and file a grievance when dissatisfied.**
5. **Switch health plans if dissatisfied. If unable to switch, nag your boss.**

Hospitals are beginning to use a program developed by General Motors for measuring quality, called Purchased Input Concept Optimization with Suppliers (PICOS). PICOS purports to eliminate waste, streamline operations, and improve customer satisfaction. A hospital using PICOS guides a small team of 8 to 10 key employees to examine a process, identify waste, and redesign the process to reduce or eliminate the waste. Health care providers look at waiting times, billing procedures, and duplication of work.[47]

Patients may be satisfied with physicians and access to them, although physicians may not know the latest treatment for a patient's condition. It is easy to find satisfied customers who are healthy.

Self-surveys may inflate customer satisfaction. Independent surveys are best, although the results may comply with the wishes of those who pay for them.

Among good independent surveyors are the Sachs Group, Evanston, Illinois; Care Data; *Center for the Study of Services Annual Guide*, which rates 400 HMOs; and the NCQA HEDIS 3.0 Report.

Management Implications

As managed care plans and enrollments increase, managers of all health care provider organizations face the need to maintain financial stability. To do this, they become experts in negotiating contracts, planning new ventures, and reorganizing their organizations to make maximum use of human resources. Successful managers provide leadership that empowers employees to provide maximum quality outcomes for their patients. As managers pursue these functions, they oversee evaluation techniques that are simple to administer and lead to quality improvement.

Summary

Managed care is fast replacing fee-for-service and indemnity insurance plans. The objectives of this transformation are reduced costs and increased profits. Although many problems exist in managed care, they are gradually being solved—some with federal and state legislation. The most prominent form of managed care is the HMO. Managed care has important implications for practice, research, education, and management.

APPLICATION EXERCISES

EXERCISE 2-1   Choose several managed care products. Identify the costs to the patient enrolled in a managed care plan and compare them with the costs to a patient in an indemnity health insurance plan.

EXERCISE 2-2   Attend a marketing session given by a managed care company. Analyze the presentation. What are the advantages and disadvantages for the patient?

EXERCISE 2-3   From information in this chapter, prepare a short questionnaire (10 to 15 questions) pertaining to the services provided for managed care enrollees. Identify and interview two persons, one who is a managed care plan enrollee and one an indemnity insurance plan enrollee. Compare the problems and advantages of the two plans.

EXERCISE 2-4   John Kay, director designate of Oxford University's new School of Management Studies, asks the question: "What is a company's purpose if it is not to maximize shareholder value?"[48] With a group of your peers, discuss how the values evident in a world of managed care can be integrated to meet the goals of this statement with the goals of quality health care for clients.

EXERCISE 2-5   Locate and read five recent articles on managed care published in nursing journals. Summarize the implications for the nursing profession.

NOTES

1. E. Spragins, "Does Your HMO Stack Up?" *Newsweek* (24 June 1996), 56–61, 63.
2. E. Faltermayer, "Will the Cost Cutting in Health Care Kill You?" *Fortune* (31 October 1994), 221–222, 224, 226, 228, 230, 232.
3. "HMOs Tell Courts They Aren't Liable," *San Antonio Express-News* (17 November 1996), 28A.
4. A. S. Relman, Editor-in-Chief Emeritus, *New England Journal of Medicine* © American Media Passage, 1995. Reprinted from *Physician's Weekly*.
5. U.S. Bureau of the Census, *Statistical Abstract of the United States 1999*, 118th ed. Washington, D.C., 1999, 149.
6. Ibid., 93.
7. Ibid.
8. Ibid., 127; T. C. Tillock, "Cost Containment in the Health Care Industry," *Aging & Leisure Service* (February 1981), 5–15.
9. Tillock, op. cit.
10. Ibid.
11. Ibid.
12. U.S. Bureau of the Census, op. cit., 127.
13. J. Rother, "Managed Care and Medicare Part 1," *Modern Maturity* (November–December 1997), 34–43, 75–76, 80.
14. C. J. Loomis, "The Real Action in Health Care," *Fortune* (11 July 1994), 149–153, 155–157.
15. Book Review: "How HMOs Are Destroying Medical Trust," G. Anders, *Health Against Wealth: HMOs and the Breakdown of Medical Trust* (Boston, MA: Houghton Mifflin, 1996), in *Public Citizen Health Research Group Health Letter* (January 1997), 1–4.
16. U.S. Bureau of the Census, op. cit., 130.
17. S. M. Wolfe, ed. "$1.06 Trillion for Health in 1994, $1.2 Trillion by 1995, $2 Trillion by 2000," *Public Citizen Health Research Group Health Letter* (February 1994), 1–2.
18. J. Canham-Clyne, S. Woolhandler, and D. Himmelstein, *The Rational Option for a National Health Care Program* (Stony Creek, CT: Pamphleteer's Press, 1995), 400.
19. www.thirteen.org/archive/mhc.
20. "Health Care Battle Pits Doctors Against Insurance Firms," *San Antonio Express-News* (30 March 1997), 13A.
21. "Health Premiums Will Go Up This Year and Next, Study Says," *Healthweek* (10 February 1997), 24; B. B. Gray, "Managed Care Enrollment: Big and Getting Bigger," *Healthweek* (16 December 1996), 1; www.aahp.org.
22. "Study Says Health Care Costs, Access Troubling to Many," *San Antonio Express-News* (23 October 1996), 6A.
23. E. Faltermayer, op. cit.
24. "HMO Backlash Spurs Wave of Restrictive Legislation," *San Antonio Express-News* (15 March 1996), 10B.
25. L. Tolley, "Bush Clears Bill to OK HMO Suits," *San Antonio Express-News* (23 May 1997), 1E, 3E.
26. E. E. Hogue, "Contracting with Managed Care Providers," *Journal of Home Health Care Practice*, 6(2), 1994, 17–23.
27. M. Jenkins and D. L. Torrisi, "Nurse Practitioners, Community Nursing Centers, and Contracting for Managed Care," *Journal of the American Academy of Nurse Practitioners* (March 1995), 119–123.
28. C. Olian, "HMO: Managed or Mangled?" *Public Citizen Health Research Group Health Letter* (March 1997), 3–5.
29. "HMO Backlash," op. cit.
30. C. J. Loomis, op. cit.
31. P. Lamiell, "With Savings Peaked, Health-Care Costs May Rise," *Austin American-Statesman* (12 April 1997), D2.
32. A. E. Serwer, "Health Care Stocks: The Hidden Growth Stars," *Fortune* (14 October 1996), 74, 79–80, 82.
33. "HMO Backlash," op. cit.
34. Ibid.
35. Ibid.
36. "Book Review," op. cit.
37. S. Woolhandler and D. H. Himmelstein, "Annotation: Patients on the Auction Block," *Public Citizen Health Research Group Health Letter* (March 1997), 1–2.
38. Ibid.
39. C. Olian, op. cit.
40. S. Gandy, "Distance Learning May Take You Where You Want to Go, but It's Still a Bumpy Ride," *Healthweek Houston–San Antonio* (21 April 1997), 1, 10.
41. E. E. Spragins, "Does Your HMO," op. cit.
42. Ibid.
43. J. B. Quinn, "Is Your HMO OK—or Not?" *Newsweek* (10 February 1997), 52.
44. Ibid.
45. G. Anders, op. cit.
46. E. E. Spragins, "Take My Freedom, Please!" *Newsweek* (7 April 1997), 81.
47. K. Driscoll, "Hospitals Take Lesson in Quality Improvements from GM," *San Antonio Express-News* (13 April 1997), 3H.
48. J. Kay, "Shareholders aren't Everything," *Fortune* (17 Februry 1997), 133–134.

REFERENCES

Allen, E. "Baptist Health Systems Lays Off about 100 Staffers." *San Antonio Express-News* (12 January 2000), 2E.

Bauerhaus, P. I. "Creating a New Place in the Competitive Market." *Nursing Policy Forum* (March–April 1996), 18–20.

Bunch, D. "The Next Frontier in Managed Care." *AARC Times* (December 1995), 48–49.

Butler, K. "Managed Care: Emerging Issues in Clinical Ethics." *ASHA* (summer 1996), 7.

Cericola, S. A. "Facing Challenges of Managed Care." *Plastic Surgical Nursing* (winter 1995), 219.

Coile, R. C. Jr. "Integration, Capitation, and Managed Care: Transformation of Nursing for 21st Century Health Care." *Advanced Practice Nursing Quarterly* (fall 1995), 77–84.

Conway-Welch, C. "Trends in Health Care Impact on Nursing Education." *NSNA Imprint* (April–May 1996), 37–38.

Corder, K. T., J. Phoon, and M. Barter. "Managed Care: Employers' Influence on the Health Care System." *Nursing Economics* (July–August 1996), 213–217.

D'Andrea, G. "Introduction to Managed Care." *Journal of AHIMA* (January 1996), 42–46.

Davidson, J. R., and T. Davidson. "Confidentiality and Managed Care: Ethical and Legal Concerns." *Health and Social Work* (August 1996), 208–215.

Davis, G. S. "Learning the Ropes of Contracting." *Provider* (July 1996), 32–34.

Day, B. "BHS Lays Off 290 Workers." *San Antonio Express-News* (14 April 2000), 1D, 8D.

Emery, D. W. "Global Theory and the Nature of Risk, Part 2. Towards a Choice-Based Model of Managed Care." *Physician Executive* (July–August 1999), 62–66.

Flaherty, M. "Fight Over Rights." *HealthWeek* (17 August 1998), 1, 30.

Goodroe, J. H., and Murphy, D. A. "The Algebra of Managed Care." *Hospital Topics* (fall 1994), 14–18.

Gray, B. "Managed Health Care Plans Pose Employment Risk for NPs." *NP News*, 3(3), 1995, 1, 8.

Grimaldi, P. L. "HMOs and Medicare." *Nursing Management* (April 1985), 16, 18, 20.

"HMOs Win Physician Support but Quality Questions Remain." *Medical Staff News* (July 1985), 3.

Hutchins, B. "Managing Cost and Quality." *REHAB Management* (April–May 1996), 25–26.

Kin, C. S. "Managed Care: Is It Moral?" *Advanced Practice Nursing Quarterly* (winter 1995), 7–11.

Mackelprang, R., and P. B. Johnson. "Managed Care: Balancing Costs, Quality and Access." *SCI Psychosocial Process* (November 1995), 175–178.

Maturen, V., and L. Van Dyke. "Using Outcome-Based Critical Pathways to Improve Documentation." *Home Health Care Management Practice* (February 1996), 48–58.

Mendlen, J., S. Goss, and K. Heist. "Managing Data for Managed Care." *Provider* (July 1996), 66–68.

Moore, K. F. "Cost or Quality When Selecting a Health Plan?" *Nursing Policy Forum* (March–April 1996), 24.

Netzel, L. "A Primer On Capitation: Another Step in Managed Care." *The Surgical Technologist* (November 1995), 16–18.

"Negotiating Managed Care Contracts." *Laboratory Medicine* (September 1996), 587–596.

Osley, M. "Legislative Update." *Journal of Legal Nurse Consulting* (October 1995), 12–13.

Petersen, B. A. "Nurse-Midwifery in a Managed Care Environment." *Journal of Nurse Midwifery* (July–August 1996), 267–268.

Phoon, J., K. Corder, and M. Barter. "Managed Care and Total Quality Management: A Necessary Integration." *Journal of Nursing Care Quality* (January 1996), 25–32.

Potter, L. "The Managed Care Contract: Survival or Closure." *Nursing Administration Quarterly* (summer 1999), 58–62.

Roybal, H., S. J. Baxendale, and M. Gupta. "Using Activity-Based Costing and Theory of Constraints To Guide Continuous Improvement in Managed Care." *Managed Care Quarterly* (winter 1999), 1–10.

Rulon, V. "Measurement Systems Beyond HEDIS: The Evolution of Healthcare Data Analysis in Managed Care." *Journal of AHIMA* (February 1996), 48, 50–52.

Sandler, R. H. "Managed Costs, Mismanaged Care." *Health Letter* (February 2000), 1–2.

Sparer, M. S. "Medicaid Managed Care and the Health Reform Debate: Lessons from New York and California." *Journal of Health Politics, Policy and Law* (fall 1996), 433–460.

Spitzer-Lehman, R. "Managed Care: What's Ahead." *Surgical Services Management* (January 1995), 18–21.

Talone, P. "Ethics and Managed Care: Beyond Helplessness," *MEDSURG Nursing* (June 1996), 212–214.

Towers, J. "What Do You Know About NCQA?" *Nursing Policy Forum* (May–June, 1996), 30.

CHAPTER 3
Theory of Nursing Management

Linda Roussel, DSN, RN, CNA

LEARNING OBJECTIVES AND ACTIVITIES

- Define the terms *manager, managing, management,* and *nursing management.*
- Differentiate among concepts, principles and theory.
- Describe critical theory.
- Discuss general systems theory.
- Illustrate selected principles of nursing management.
- Describe roles for nurse managers differentiating among levels.
- Distinguish between two cognitive styles: intuitive thinking and rational thinking. Give examples of each.

CONCEPTS: Management theory, nursing management theory, critical theory, general systems theory, nursing management, management principles, management development, nursing management roles, role development, cognitive styles, intuitive thinking, rational thinking, management levels.

MANAGER BEHAVIOR: Applies traditional management theory to organizational operations.

LEADER BEHAVIOR: Examines the possibility of developing application of a nursing management theory by creating a business plan that incorporates a pilot study. Works with representatives of the professional nursing staff to develop and test the pilot study.

What Is Management?

Modern management theory evolved from the work of Henri Fayol, who identified the activities or functions of the administrator as planning, organizing, coordinating, and controlling.[1] Fayol defined management in these words[2]:

To manage is to forecast and plan, to organize, to command, to coordinate, and to control. To foresee and provide means [of] examining the future and drawing up the plan of action. To organize means building up the dual structure, material and human, of the undertaking. To command means binding together, unifying and harmonizing all activity and effort. To control means seeing that everything occurs in conformity with established rule and expressed demand.

Although some persons believed these were technical functions that could be learned only on the job, Fayol believed that they could be taught in an educational setting if a theory of administration could be formulated.[3] He also stated that the need for managerial ability increases in relative importance as an individual advances in the chain of command.[4]

Fayol listed the principles of management as follows[5]:

1. Division of work
2. Authority
3. Discipline
4. Unity of command
5. Unity of direction
6. Subordination of individual interests to the general interests
7. Remuneration
8. Centralization
9. Scalar chain (line of authority)
10. Order
11. Equity
12. Stability or tenure of personnel
13. Initiative
14. Esprit de corps.

Another theorist in the development of the science and art of management was L. Urwick, who believed that administrative skill was a practical art that improved with practice and required hard study and thinking. According to Urwick, the administrator must master intellectual principles, with the process being reinforced by general reflection about actual problems. From his work, Urwick concluded that there are three principles of administration. He described the first principle as investigation and stated that all scientific procedure is based on investigation of the facts. Investigation leads to planning. The second principle is appropriateness, which underlines forecasting, enters into the process with organization, and takes effect in coordination. Exercising the third principle, the administrator looks ahead and organizes resources to meet future needs. Planning enters into the process with command and is effected in control.[6]

Throughout management literature, the original functions of planning, organizing, directing (command and coordination), and controlling as defined by Fayol, Urwick, and others have been accepted as the principal functions of managers. Managing means accomplishing the goals of the group through effective and efficient use of resources. The manager creates and maintains an internal environment in an enterprise in which individuals work together as a group. Managing is the art of doing, and management is the body of organized knowledge underlying the art. In modern management, staffing is frequently separated from the planning function, directing has been labeled leading, and *controlling* is used interchangeably with *evaluating*. The American Nurses Association (ANA) standards for nursing administration are based on these principles, which support the science of nursing administration.

Theory, Concepts, and Principles

The knowledge base of management science includes theory, which in turn includes concepts, methods, and principles. The principles are related and can be observed and verified to some degree when they are translated into the art or practice of management. *Concepts* are thoughts, ideas, and general notions about a class of objects that form a basis for action or discussion. Concepts tend to be true but are not always true. *Principles* are fundamental truths, laws, or doctrines on which other notions are based. *Principles* provide guidance to concepts and to thought or action in a situation.[7] In nursing management, research—Urwick's "investigation of facts"—becomes part of the theory of the field.

If nursing is going to base its theory on laws, nurses will need to validate principles through research, a difficult task, as theorists in the social sciences have discovered. It is difficult to reduce human behavior to laws. Nurses deal with human behavior in all roles but particularly so in nursing management.

White explores a viewpoint on nursing theories in which she addresses "prescriptive theories." She notes that their use as practice guidelines "must be broad enough to encourage a wide range of practice situations but not so broad as to be meaningless." A theory of decision-making might be more beneficial than a theory of nursing in the practice arena. Nurses believe that for nursing to be a real profession, it should have a scientific and theoretical base. Nursing is thus a practice profession based on the physical and social sciences.[8]

Nurse managers learn to merge the disciplines of human relations, labor relations, personnel management, and industrial engineering into a unifying force for effective management. Many nurse managers would add the theory of nursing to this list. A successful synthesis of these disciplines can promote employee commitment, increased productivity, enhanced competency, good labor relations, and competitiveness in health care. The work force is poorly managed when these goals are not achieved.

> **Management is the specific and distinguishing organ of any and all organizaztions.[9]**

Contradictions exist in management theory because of a lack of agreement about sets of ideas and concepts among and within disciplines.[10] Two common approaches are described in the following sections.

Critical Theory Versus Critical Thinking

Steffy and Grimes note that a strict natural science approach to social science is naïve, because subjective or qualitative analysis is important to quantitative research. This holds true for management and, consequently, nursing management. Health care organizational models are not objective and value-free. Steffy and Grimes suggest using a critical theory approach to organizational science, rather than a phenomenological or hermeneutic approach.

A phenomenological approach uses second-order constructs or "interpretations of interpretations." This approach requires researchers to become participants in the organization and to suspend all judgments and preconceived ideas about possible meanings. The nurse manager would interpret the meaning of nursing management experiences or observations and arrive at a nursing management theory from the aggregate of meanings.

Hermeneutics is the art of textual interpretation. The nurse manager as researcher would view herself or himself as a historically produced entity and would recognize personal biases in doing research. She or he would consider the specific context and historic dimensions of data collected and would reflect on the relationship between theory and history.[11]

Critical theory is an empirical philosophy of social institutions. Decision-makers, in this case nurse managers, translate theories into practice. Theories in use are behavioral technologies that include organizational development, management by objectives or results, strategic planning, planned change, performance appraisal, and other practice-oriented activities performed by managers. Critical theory aims

1. to critique the ideology of scientism, "the institutionalized form of reasoning which accepts the idea that the meaning of knowledge is defined by what the sciences do and thus can be adequately explicated through analysis of scientific procedures," and

2. "to develop an organizational science capable of changing organizational processes."

These aims are compatible with a theory of nursing management. Nurses are using science to legitimize the practice of clinical nursing and nursing management.[12]

Critical theory is a contemporary school of thought that strenuously criticizes oppressive established values and instructions. "In a more moderate form, critical theory maintains the necessity of examining the hidden assumptions that undergird thinking."[13]

General Systems Theory

General systems theory is an organismic approach to the study of the general relationships of the empirical universe of an organization and human thought. It grew out of biology as an analogy between an organism and a social organization. Boulding describes nine levels of a general systems theory,[14] which are given here with nursing management applications:

1. A static structure—the framework. Nursing is a discipline with an aggregate population of registered nurses educated at several levels (including those with hospital diplomas and those with degrees from associate through doctoral levels), licensed practical nurses, and unlicensed assistive personnel (e.g., aides, orderlies, attendants, nursing assistants, and clerks). They function within a dynamic and flattening structure that may change frequently. Superior–subordinate relationships are giving way to decentralized, participatory, and transformational management at the practice level. Flat organizations usually have a top administrator, first-line man-

agers, and practitioners. These nursing persons usually function in an environment in which the focus of attention is the client. One approach to a framework in nursing is that nursing persons apply the nursing process in giving care to patients. Many similarities exist between the nursing process and nursing management. (See Exhibit 3-1.)

2. A moving level of necessary predetermined motions—the clockwork. Nurse managers process the knowledge and skills of management—planning, organizing, leading, and evaluating—to produce nursing care through nursing management. The function of nursing management is the use of personnel, supplies, equipment, clinical knowledge, and skills to give nursing care to clients within varying environments. The nurse manager may also have other ancillary personnel to manage, such as therapists, housekeepers, and social workers, adding to the complexity of the system in providing overall quality services for client care. One of these environments is the hospital physical plant. Nursing planning (NP) + nursing organizing (NO) + nursing leading (NL) + nursing evaluating (NE) = nursing management (NM): NP + NO + NL + NE = NM. To this we may add that nursing management (NM) + nursing practice (NP) = nursing care of clients (NCC), or NM + NP = NCC. The move is toward equilibrium.

3. A control mechanism level—the thermostat. In nursing administration, this thermostat could be the top administrator or any first-line manager. This person maintains a management information system that transmits and interprets information and communication to and from employees. Production of nursing care of satisfactory quality and quantity depends on the manager maintaining an environment satisfactory to employees.

4. An open system or self-maintaining structure—the cell. Nursing management will survive and maintain the nursing organization by being open to new ideas, new management techniques, and the input of human and material resources to produce the nursing care needed by clients. An open system will reproduce itself by keeping up to date and by developing replacements. Keep up to date by adding nursing education (NE): NM + NP + NE = NCC.

5. The genetic-societal level. There is a division of labor even within nursing management, but especially among nursing personnel who produce the nursing care of patients. Further integrating multiskill level personnel into the mix offers more comprehensive complimentary care in meeting clients' health care needs. The raw materials, that is, the human and material resources, are *input*. These

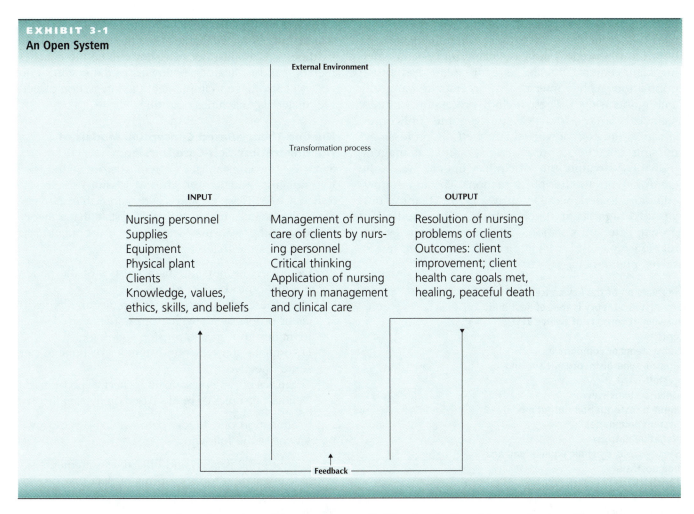

EXHIBIT 3-1
An Open System

External Environment

Transformation process

INPUT

Nursing personnel
Supplies
Equipment
Physical plant
Clients
Knowledge, values,
ethics, skills, and beliefs

Management of nursing
care of clients by nurs-
ing personnel
Critical thinking
Application of nursing
theory in management
and clinical care

OUTPUT

Resolution of nursing
problems of clients
Outcomes: client
improvement; client
health care goals met,
healing, peaceful death

Feedback

resources are processed as *throughput* by a group of nursing personnel with varying knowledge and skills using a theory-based nursing care delivery system. The *output* is resolution of the nursing needs and problems of clients, with their improvement, their health care goals having been met, then healing, or their having succumbed to a peaceful death.

6. The "animal" level. This level has increased mobility, teleological (designing or purposeful) behavior, and self-awareness. Some evidence is emerging that nursing management is reaching this level. As nurse managers learn the knowledge and skills of the business and industrial world, they are adapting them to the management of health care services. This puts nursing management and nursing practice on a much more scientific basis, the end result of which may be that nurses will be able to demonstrate empirically and theoretically that what they do affects client outcomes.

7. The "human" level. The nurse manager develops an increased awareness, a self-consciousness and knows that he or she can process the knowledge and skills of management to produce specific results.

8. The level of social organization. Nurse managers at this level distinguish themselves from other groups of managers. Nurse managers operate within complex roles; their functions are made effective by communication, relationships, and other interpersonal processes.

9. Transcendental systems. At this level nurse managers ask questions for which there are as yet no answers. Theoretical models of nursing management extend to level 4 (the cell), the level of application of most other models. Empirical knowledge is deficient at nearly all levels. Descriptive models are needed to catalogue events in nursing. The movement toward decentralization and participatory and service line management, while still a very simple system, is growing each year as nurse scientists develop and apply new nursing administration models and theories of nursing. General systems theory is the skeleton of a science. Adding nursing research (NR) gives: NM + NP + NE + NR = NCC.

Disciplines and sciences have bodies of knowledge that grow with meaningful information. The empirical universe provides general phenomena relevant to many different disciplines; these phenomena can be built into theoretical models, including one for nursing management. Nursing as a discipline has varied populations (phenomena) that interact dynamically among themselves. These include professional nurses, technical nurses, practical nurses, and unlicensed assistive nursing personnel, as well as professional nursing teachers, researchers, and managers. Individuals within the discipline interact with the environment (another phenomenon). Through knowledge and experience they grow, growth being a universally significant phenomenon. The media for growth are information, interpersonal processing, relationships, and communication, which are themselves phenomena.[15]

Another version of the key concepts of general systems theory is that of Kast and Rosenzweig. It consists of twelve key concepts[16]:
1. **Subsystems or components**
2. **Holism, synergism, organicism, and gestalt**
3. **Open-systems view**
4. **Input-transformation-output model**
5. **System boundaries**
6. **Negative entropy**
7. **Steady state, dynamic equilibrium, and homeostasis**
8. **Feedback**
9. **Hierarchy**
10. **Internal elaboration**
11. **Multiple goal-seeking**
12. **Equifinality of open system**

With the emerging changes in health care systems, nurse leaders will need to accelerate changes in nursing organizations. The goal may be nursing modules centered on closely related operations, such as differentiated practice delivery models matched with intensity of care or specialized services. Standardization and flexibility can be melded together to develop systems based on a requirement for a theory of nursing practice as a foundation for all modules, but with different theories being used in different modules chosen by professional clinical nurses.[17]

The test of nursing for the next decade will be its ability to make alliances outside the profession rather than to become circumscribed.

Full realization of systems theory is as far in the future for nursing as it is for manufacturing. Nursing is a "head, heart, and hands" discipline. Nursing management and practice are what tie the parts of the health care system together. Transformational nurse leaders will be fully knowledgeable about the work being done by their constituents, because they will be the coaches, mentors, and facilitators. Followers of the systems concept will also have to implement the integration of people, materials, machines, and time.[18]

Nursing-Theory-Based Conceptual Models of Administration: Self-Care Nursing.

Sarah E. Allison established Orem's theory as the basis for nursing practice at the Mississippi Methodist Rehabilitation Hospital and Center more than 30 years ago. Allison, McLaughlin, and Walker state that a theory-based nursing systems design for a population of patients does the following:

- Describes the nursing characteristics of the patient population to be served
- Uses these characteristics to predict the types of client problems for which nursing is needed
- Identifies appropriate nursing technologies
- Determines the types and number of nursing personnel needed
- Organizes nursing personnel for effective performance
- Defines outcomes or results based on nursing theory.[19]

Examination of a theory-based nursing system will be evident in the following:

- Mission, philosophy, and objectives statements
- Documentation tools or forms of data that provide a nursing database
- Standards of care and practice
- Staff education and development
- Quality assurance outcomes audits
- Patient acuity systems
- Position descriptions and performance evaluation
- Policies and procedures
- Career development programs that attract and retain the best nurses by motivating and clarifying the role of the nurse
- Support given by nursing administration commitment.[20]

A conceptual model for nursing administrative practice will assist in solving problems associated with change. The model will serve as a visual image to guide planning, decision-making, and communicating. The Iowa Model of Nursing Administration "provides for the critical interdependence of both clinical activities and management activities or outcomes." The Iowa model may be used to guide decision-making and evaluating change.[21] It is depicted in Exhibit 3-2 and the terms are defined in Exhibit 3-3.

A third systems-perspective model of nursing is that of Scalzi and Anderson. It comprises three elements: the nursing domain, the management domain, and the

EXHIBIT 3-2

The Iowa Model of Nursing Administration

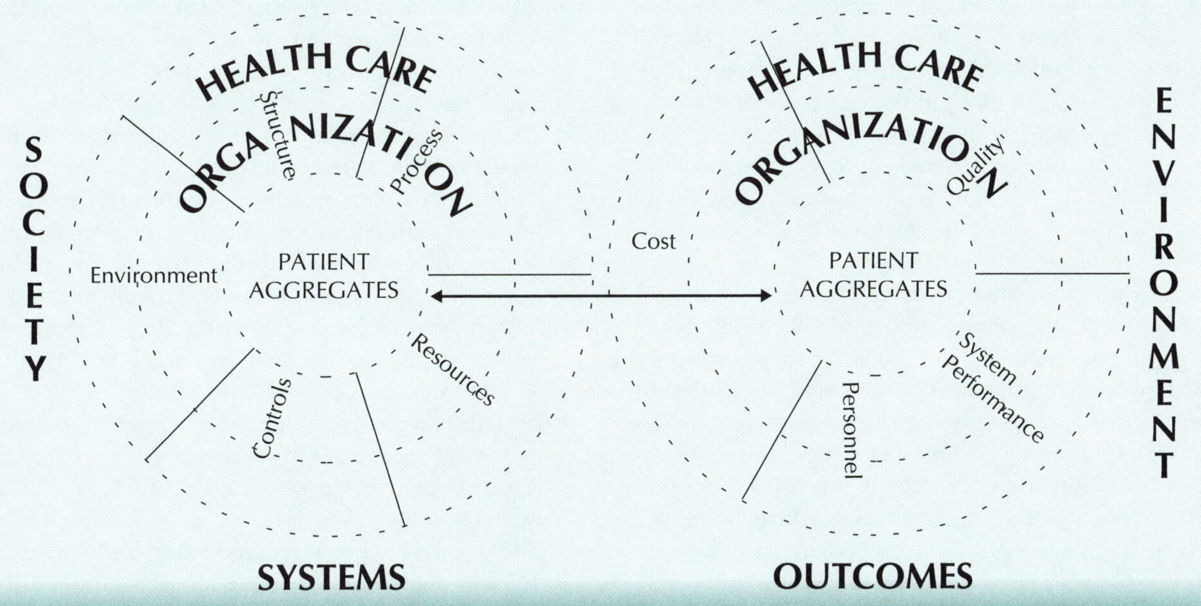

Source: Copyright 1990 by the NSA Program, The University of Iowa College of Nursing. Reprinted with permission.

EXHIBIT 3-3

Definitions Applied to the Iowa Model of Nursing Administration

Patient aggregates	A grouping of patients who have similar basic care characteristics (e.g., medical diagnosis) within a nursing unit
Organization	A group of employees acting together to achieve the goals of the employing institution (e.g., quality patient care)
Health care system	All financial, political, legal, and professional groups in the United States involved in the delivery of health-care services to the public
Systems	A set of interrelated and interdependent parts that form a complex whole or work together to deliver health care to the public
Outcomes	Desired results; the degree to which goals and objectives are met in the delivery of health care to the public

Source: D. L. Gardner, K. Kelly, M. Johnson, J. C. McCloskey, and M. Maas. "Nursing Administration Model for Administrative Practice." *Journal of Nursing Administration* (March 1991), 38. Reprinted with permission of J. B. Lippincott, Williams and Wilkins.

interval where the two domains interact, that is, systems concerns.[22]

Nursing Management

In nursing, management relates to performing the functions of planning, organizing, staffing, leading (directing), and controlling (evaluating) the activities of a nursing enterprise and departmental subunits. A nurse manager performs these management functions to deliver health care to patients. Nurse managers or administrators work at all levels to put into practice the concepts, principles, and theories of nursing management. They manage the organizational environment to provide a climate optimal to the provision of nursing care by clinical nurses and ancillary staff.

Management knowledge is universal; so is nursing management knowledge. It uses a systematic body of knowledge that includes concepts, principles, and theories applicable to all nursing management situations. A nurse manager who has applied this knowledge successfully in one situation can be expected to do so in new situations. Nursing management occurs at unit and executive levels. At the executive level, it is frequently termed *administration*.

However, the theories, principles, and concepts remain the same.

With decentralization and participatory management, the supervisor or middle management level has been largely eliminated. Nurse managers of clinical units are being educated in management theory and skills at the master's level. Clinical nurses are being educated in management skills that empower them to take action in managing groups of employees as well as clients and families. Clinical nurse managers are doing more of the coordinating duties among units, departments, and services.

Nursing administration is the application of the art and science of management applied to the discipline of nursing. Nursing management consists of a group of nurse managers who manage the nursing organization or enterprise. Finally, nursing management is the process by which nurse managers practice their profession. Although many nursing management jobs do not require specialty certification, such certification is available. The ANA awards two levels of management certification: Certified Nurse Administration and Certified Nurse Administration, Advanced. The American Organization of Nurse Executives has in the past certified nurse managers at the nominee, candidate, and fellow levels. Both programs require education, experience, and examinations.

Who Needs Nursing Management?

All types of health care organizations need nursing management, including nursing homes, hospitals, assisted living facilities, residential care programs, home health care agencies, ambulatory care centers, student infirmaries, and many others. Even the nurse working with one client and family needs management knowledge and skills to help people work together to accomplish a common goal. A primary nurse working with several clients must prioritize care, with the goal of assisting them to improved health, healing, or sometimes, having a peaceful death.[23]

"The new assumption on which management, both as a discipline and as a practice, will increasingly have to base itself is that the scope of management is not legal. It has to be operational. It has to embrace the entire process. It has to be focused on results and performance across the entire economic chain."[24]

General Principles

The following are some major principles of nursing management, which are discussed in more detail in subsequent chapters.

- Planning is a major function of nursing management and is primary to all other management activities or functions.
- Effective utilization of time is essential to effective nursing management, which performs in the present while planning for future performance, growth, and change.
- Decision-making is a primary element of nursing management at every level.
- Nurse managers manage a clinical practice discipline in which professional nurses are primarily knowledge workers, applying their knowledge to gathering data, making nursing diagnoses and nursing prescriptions, supervising the implementation of the nursing care plan by skilled workers, and evaluating and adjusting the plan.
- Social goals are formulated by nurse managers and achieved by clinical nurses.
- Organizing is a second major function of nursing management.
- Change is a major element in nursing management; exponentially increasing change is the only constant in today's world.
- Organizational cultures should be managed to reflect values and beliefs, with managers in nursing having a common purpose of making productive the values, aspirations, and traditions of employees who are individuals as well as members of communities and of society.
- Directing or leading is a third major function of nursing management, empowering employees, improving quality, and leading to excellence of production.
- Motivation is a basic element of the directing function of nursing management. Satisfactory performance results from job satisfaction, quality of work life, and organizational commitment, conditions that require nurse managers to stimulate motivation of nurse employees.
- Effective communication and management are primary elements of nursing management that result in fewer misunderstandings and give employees a common vision, common understanding, and unity of direction and effort.
- Staff development is an important element of the directing function of nursing management that serves to maintain the competency of all practicing nurses.
- Controlling or evaluating is the fourth major function of nursing management and includes the processes of evaluating the given directives and how well the adopted plan was carried out, establishing principles and standards, comparing performance with standards, evaluating patterns, and correcting deficiencies.

All of the major functions of nursing management operate independently and interdependently.

Management Development

Management development is big business: in the 1980s, 500,000 managers took management education programs at least once every year; 7,800 minicourses for executives were conducted at the University of Pennsylvania Wharton School in 1 year; and 14,000 managers were enrolled annually in management seminars at AT&T. In the new health care environment, a variety of creative and innovative agencies and programs are being developed. These entities serve to meet the ever-changing population and financial constraints they are increasingly facing. These organizations are no less complex than are hospitals and require cost controls and increased productivity to thrive. Unless nurses are educated to manage in these new environments, they will lose out to other professions or will manage poorly and be unhappy and unsuccessful.[25]

Nurses require preparation for their management work, including synthesis of nursing and management knowledge. The nurse manager is prepared to manage other nurses and health care professionals who will provide the clinical care. Education of nurses will provide human resource management skills, including preceptor and mentor assignments. A model of progression from nursing expertise to management expertise is illustrated in Exhibit 3-4.[26]

To prepare clinical nurses for beginning management roles, the Mount Sinai Medical Center of Greater Miami designed a voluntary 2-day taking-charge course. Goals included greater competence, confidence, and continuity; preparation for problem-solving; job satisfaction; and a positive leadership experience. A guidebook was prepared for use during the learning experience and for reference. Topics covered included communication, leadership styles, time management, managing stress, staffing, assignments, rounds, reports, ordering supplies, unit operations, position description, policies, patient care assessment, quality assurance, conflict management, and counseling. A posttest and 3-month follow-up showed the course to be successful. The clinical nurses were more effective, showing improved self-concept, self-esteem, and assertiveness. Their morale and the organizational climate both improved.[27]

Management development of nurses at Mount Sinai is taken seriously. Recognizing that nurse managers have onstage (on the scene) and backstage (behind the scene) roles to perform, one management program focused on communication skills required for onstage management, in which different "hats" are worn for each role: negotiator, counselor, director, delegator, collaborator, and controller. The nurse manager is a hands-on-the-organization person.

The communication course consists of one 2-hour session each week for 10 weeks. It covers topics such as communication style, nonverbal communication, listening, conflict management, verbal messages, rumors, committees, team building, and communication climate. The course helps prepare the nurse manager to respond to multiple issues from multiple sources. Backstage, it provides the nurse manager with the ability to communicate with other executives in the business world. These nurse managers should also be well versed in management theories, with knowledge of economics, finance, and accounting. They should be assertive, proactive, and collegial.[28]

A system for developing nurse administrators has been published by Fralic and O'Connor, who make frequent reference to the work of Katz and of Charns and Schaefer. Katz classifies management skills into three categories:

1. Conceptual skills, which are innate abilities, or thinking skills.
2. Technical skills, which include methods, processes, procedures, and techniques.
3. Human skills, which relate to leadership ability and intergroup relations.

In nursing, technical skills are divided into nursing management technology and nursing practice technology. Fralic and O'Connor relate the conceptual, human, and technical skills to three management levels, with the chief nurse executive needing the highest level of conceptual competence and the nurse manager needing the highest level of nursing practice technology. The needed staff development is evident in the role requirements.[29]

Spicer indicates that scientific management knowledge is at the base of the nurse manager's role, including knowledge of a model role and the ability to conceptualize it. Preparation for management and support during the transition are needed for the change from clinical nurse to nurse manager. The role model would demonstrate the relationships between politics and strategy and between power and influence.[30]

Preparation of nurse managers includes many things:

- Knowledge of legal labor practices and institutional policy in managing employees
- Preparation for continuing education and staff development, including principles of adult educa-

EXHIBIT 3-4
Management Progression for Nursing

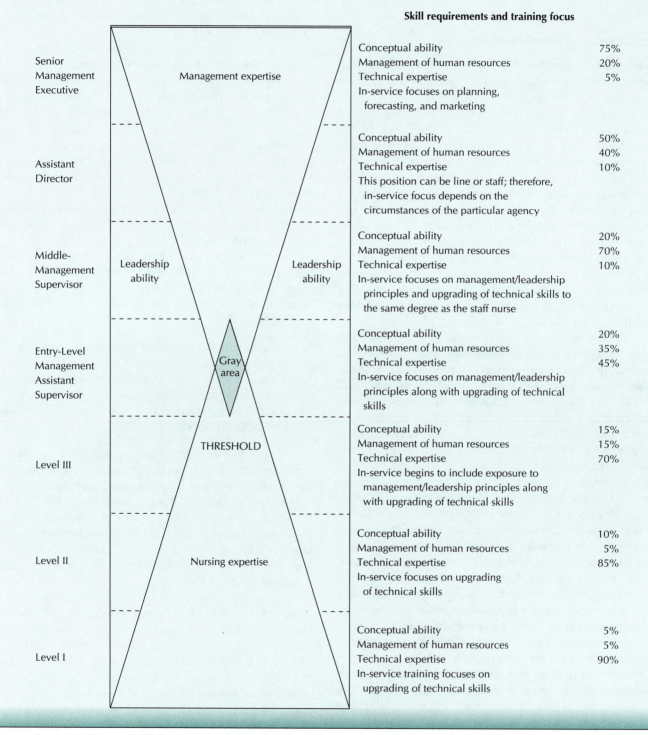

Skill requirements and training focus

Senior Management Executive	Management expertise

Conceptual ability — 75%
Management of human resources — 20%
Technical expertise — 5%
In-service focuses on planning, forecasting, and marketing

Conceptual ability — 50%
Management of human resources — 40%
Technical expertise — 10%
This position can be line or staff; therefore, in-service focus depends on the circumstances of the particular agency

Conceptual ability — 20%
Management of human resources — 70%
Technical expertise — 10%
In-service focuses on management/leadership principles and upgrading of technical skills to the same degree as the staff nurse

Conceptual ability — 20%
Management of human resources — 35%
Technical expertise — 45%
In-service focuses on management/leadership principles along with upgrading of technical skills

Conceptual ability — 15%
Management of human resources — 15%
Technical expertise — 70%
In-service begins to include exposure to management/leadership principles along with upgrading of technical skills

Conceptual ability — 10%
Management of human resources — 5%
Technical expertise — 85%
In-service focuses on upgrading of technical skills

Conceptual ability — 5%
Management of human resources — 5%
Technical expertise — 90%
In-service training focuses on upgrading of technical skills

Source: S. Gleason, O. W. Nestor, and A. J. Riddell. "Helping Nurses Through the Management Threshold." *Nursing Administration Quarterly* (winter 1983), 14. Reprinted with permission of Aspen Publishers, Inc., 1983.

tion; performing a needs survey; and preparing, presenting, and evaluating programs

- Knowledge of financial matters, including budgeting, managing cost and revenue centers, financing health care, and productivity

Nurse managers use performance appraisal as a continuum directed toward results. Preparation of nurse managers assists them in becoming self-directed.[31]

In the new management culture nurses will survive and prosper by updating skills. Entrepreneurial managers invest in their employees with adequate pay, fiscal quality in the workplace, and training.[32]

Leadership training is a huge industry. Content of leadership training includes feedback, personnel growth, skill building, and conceptual awareness. Values-based leadership is the goal of training, with values shared by leaders and constituents. Investing in training and technology will improve efficiencies.[33]

Roles and Nursing Management

Role Development

The nurse manager draws from the best and most applicable theories of management to create an individual management style and performance. This requires knowledge and the skill to use it. The nurse manager continues to acquire and use management knowledge to solve managerial problems, which requires a contingency approach because no single approach works for all situations. The nurse manager acts with the assumption that clinical nurses and other health care providers want to be competent and that with managerial support they will be motivated to achieve competence and greater levels of productivity. With achievement of competence and productivity goals, higher levels are set. Clinical nurses will seek out the organization that fits their needs.[34]

Adding to the nurse manager's ever-expanding role is the need to increase knowledge and sensitivity to other health care individuals providing clinical services. These services are integrated into the client's overall experience of health care, of which nursing is a critical component.

McClure vividly points out that nurse managers are managing a clinical discipline performed by professional nurses. Because most nurses are women, however, conflicts may arise between their professional and personal lives. The nurse manager devises strategies to deal with these conflicts. Some blue-collar nurses lack knowledge

of nursing research and do not read to keep up to date; they want nurse managers to do everything. White-collar nurses want to be treated differently; they want job enrichment, with primary nursing duties and professional autonomy. They want to be organized like the medical staff, with staff appointments and peer review. The nurse manager manages these two groups differently.[35]

Freund surveyed chief executive officers (CEOs) and directors of nursing (DONs) of 250 university-affiliated hospitals. The sample based the effectiveness of DONs on the following:

- General management-health-nursing knowledge, including finance, accounting, computer literacy, nursing, health care field, and productivity.
- Human management skills, including communication, interaction with people, sensitivity, and humor.
- Total view of the organization (theory and behavior), with nurses as part of the management team and nursing's interests blended with those of the entire organization.
- Support by CEOs. DONs did not think that CEOs viewed this as important.
- Medical staff relations. Smooth and peaceful nursing–medical staff relationships were important to CEOs, whereas DONs desired a collegial relationship.
- Flexibility, negotiation, and compromise. CEOs cited flexibility as being important in the effectiveness of DONs, whereas DONs cited negotiation and compromise.
- Political savvy. DONs thought that the political nature of their positions required political savvy, whereas CEOs did not view this as being crucial for DONs.
- Knowledge of advanced clinical practice. Neither CEOs nor DONs viewed this as being crucial to the effectiveness of DONs.

Of the DONs, 73.1% had graduate degrees, with 60.2% having Master of Science in Nursing degrees, 8.2% Master of Business Administration or Master of Hospital Administration degrees, and 4.7% doctoral or Doctor of Nursing Services degrees. Of CEOs, 92% had graduate degrees, with 81.6% being masters and 10.4% doctorates. Management experience averaged 19 years for CEOs and 13 years for DONs. DONs began in clinical practice.[36]

Cognitive Styles: Intuitive Thinking Versus Rational Thinking

Nugent states that management science is based on the assumption that reason or rational thinking is the only form of thought. Rational modes of thought are based on a cognitive style of learning, deciding, and solving problems that is systematic, analytic, reflective, and field-independent.

There is also thought that is based on a style of learning that is intuitive, global–relational, active, and field-dependent.[37]

Differences between rational and intuitive modes of thought are summarized in Exhibit 3-5.[38] These differences often are referred to as right- and left-brain thinking, in which both intuitive and rational modes of thinking are employed, thus enhancing creativity and problem-solving strategies.

Rational and intuitive modes alternate in real life. Intuitive thinkers are frequently blocked when confronted by rational thinkers. When intuitive thinkers have to think in causal terms rather than in terms of meaning and significance, they become stifled, and frustrated, which makes them inarticulate. Rational thinkers, in turn, can become frustrated and uncomfortable when confronted with intuitive thinkers. Many people are not aware that these different cognitive domains exist.[39]

How can knowledge of cognitive styles work for nurse managers? They should acknowledge that both rational and intuitive thinkers are needed in nursing to solve problems and make decisions. The nurse who thinks intuitively generates ideas; the nurse who thinks rationally orders and analyzes ideas. They complement each other.

Nurse managers and clinical nurses can benefit from having both intuitive and rational thinkers who set and evaluate goals. Intuitive thinkers will formulate goals that are flexible, generating ideas and images of hopes, desires, and expectations; they describe the future. The resulting Gestalt can then be translated by the rational thinkers into structure, with specific goals, objectives, means, and actions. The processes can alternate, with new ideas and goals emerging. Knowledge of intuitive and rational thinking should be applied to the job of managing nurses.[40]

Because the role of the nurse manager at evolving levels is complex, knowledge of cognitive styles can be important in selecting a balanced-ability management team that features both intuitive and rational cognitive skills. The ability to select and use such a team involves sound education that can be translated into skills. Didactic learning is combined with experiential learning. As the nurse manager progresses in the role, she or he learns to go to the source of new knowledge, synthesizing it with the old and eventually applying it to new situations. This evolution occurs as nurse managers progress through management levels.

Intuition is considered a characteristic of the right-brain thinker.[41]

Analysis of the concept of intuition by Rew shows the attributes of intuition as[42]:
1. "Knowledge of a fact or truth, as a whole;
2. Immediate possession of knowledge; and
3. Knowledge independent of the linear reasoning process."

Intuition has been observed in individuals and groups. It has been demonstrated to be basic to discovery, and its existence has been proven by means of

EXHIBIT 3-5
Characteristics of the Rational and Intuitive Modes of Thought

ASPECT	RATIONAL MODE	INTUITIVE MODE
Ordering of the mode	Linearity, sequence	Iteration, cycles
	Discrete steps	Simultaneity, interaction, association
Elements and their relationships	Discrete entities	Gestalts, integrated wholes
	Logically interrelated categories	Many experience forms (difficult to categorize)
		Integration through meaning and significance
Reliance on context	Little reliance on context	Strong reliance on context
	Assumption of boundaries	Unbounded or difficult to bound
	Explicitness	Large amount of implicitness
Movement and control of the process	Finalization of one step before passing to another	Emergence and evolution of gestalts
	Relative inflexibility	Relative flexibility
	Great control over process	Little control over the process

Source: P. S. Nugent. "Management and Modes of Thought." *Journal of Nursing Administration* (February 1982), 19–25. Reprinted with permission of J. B. Lippincott, Williams & Wilkins. © February 1982.

logic. Nurse managers can develop intuition through techniques such as group brainstorming sessions, group visualization, and quiet thinking time.[43] Nurse managers can also use the techniques of mediation, guided imagery, aromatherapy, and deep relaxation.

Whole-brain thinking, the combining of logical and intuitive thinking, may improve managerial ability and skills. Characteristics of left-brain thinking and right-brain thinking are listed in Exhibit 3-6. Techniques that assess whole-brain thinking are listed in Exhibit 3-7.[44]

Management Levels

Nurse managers perform at several levels in the health care organization. These include first-line patient care management at the unit level, middle management at the department level, and top management at the executive level. In some organizations decentralization has displaced the middle management level and redistributed department-level functions to staff functions under a matrix or other organizational structure. The roles of managers are developmental, building on knowledge and skills as the scope of the nurse manager's role increases in breadth and depth. Middle nurse manager roles are fast being eliminated, and clinical nurses are being empowered and given management education.

First-Line Nurse Managers

The following are some of the knowledge and skills needed by nurses in first-line management roles:

- Financial management knowledge and skills to prepare and defend a budget for expenses of unit personnel, supplies, capital equipment, and revenues to meet expenses. The ability to manage scarce and expensive resources for performance.
- The ability to match moral and ethical choices related to human needs, moral principles for behavior, and individual feelings in making decisions.
- Recognition of and advocacy for patients' rights.
- Active and assertive effort to share power within the organization, including shared power for nursing's practitioners. This includes nursing autonomy, which is threatened by authoritarian management. In turn, practicing nurses are involved in solving managerial problems.
- The ability to communicate and to promote effective communication and interpersonal relationships among nursing staff and others; presentation skills.
- Knowledge of internal factors related to purpose, tasks, people, technology, and structure.
- Knowledge of external factors related to economy, political pressures, legal aspects, sociocultural characteristics, and technology.
- The ability to study situations and use management concepts and techniques, analyze them, correctly make diagnoses of problems, and tie the process together to arrive at decisions.
- The ability to provide for staff development.
- The ability to provide a climate in which nurses clearly perceive that they are pursuing meaningful and worthwhile goals through their individual efforts.
- Knowledge of organizational culture and its impact on productivity and problem-solving.
- Ability to effect change through an orderly process.
- Commitment to maintain self-development by reading and attending workshops and other educational programs.

EXHIBIT 3-6
Accessing the Left and Right Hemispheres

LEFT	RIGHT
Writing: Words foster clear and effective left-brain thinking.	Brainstorming: Allows thinking to flow, free of critique.
Sorting thoughts: Outlining ideas in a logical sequence after classifying like thoughts into groups.	Relaxation techniques: Relaxation produces alpha brain waves which access the right brain.
Computer use: Input requires exact, sequential ordered data which stimulates the left hemisphere.	Music: Slow rhythmic musical pattern produces alpha brain waves, creating an internal cerebral atmosphere that allows for easy entry to "lateral thinking."
Stimulate left brain by note-taking, analyzing body language, tone of voice, organizing, prioritizing, writing, outlining, controlling the environment.	Functions that activate right brain: Visualizing; daydreaming; responding to body language; tone of voice; hugging; smiling; laughing; allowing events to happen; drawing; doodling; printing.

Source: D. C. Veehoff. "Whole Brain Thinking and the Nurse Manager," *Nursing Management* (August 1993), 34. Reprinted with permission of Springhouse.

EXHIBIT 3-7
Synchronization Techniques

SYNCHRONOUS FLASHING LIGHTS
Photodrive and synchronize both hemispheres of the brain by stimulating various brain wave frequencies. (Write to 21st Century Holdings, Inc., Sanlando Center Office Park, Suite 200, 2170 W. SR 434, Longwood, FL 32779.)

SYNCHRONOUS SOUNDS
Certain sound patterns create a frequency following response in the electrical activity of the brain wich leads the hemispheres to work together simultaneously. (Direct inquiries to: Robert Monroe, Monroe Institute, Route 1, Box 175, Faver, VA 22938.)

BIOGENICS®
Psychophysiological techniques that move body and mind toward a state of biochemical and electrical balance. (Write to C. Norman Shealy, Shealy Institute, 1328 E. Evergreen, Springfield, MO 65803.)

OPEN FOCUS
Emphasizes brain wave synchrony through attention training, utilizing electroencephalograph biofeedback. (Write to Lester Fehmi, Princeton Behavioral Medicine, 317 Mount Lucas Road, Princeton, NJ 08540.)

Source: D. C. Veehoff. "Whole Brain Thinking and the Nurse Manager." *Nursing Management* (August 1993), 34. Reprinted with permission of Springhouse.

- Knowledge of how to empower clinical nurses through committee assignments, quality circles, primary nursing, and even assigning titles.[45] At Mount Sinai Medical Center of Greater Miami, head nurses are department heads who write goals and objectives, prepare and manage the unit budget, and prepare plans. They are encouraged to be organized and unified, to network, and to be community leaders in the health care field, including working with legislators.[46]
- Knowledge of recruitment and retention strategies to promote and retain valued nursing and health care personnel.

To these could be added staffing and scheduling, management reports, hiring, performance appraisal, job productivity and satisfaction, constructive discipline dealing with stress and conflict, diversity, personnel management, culture, values, norms, and ways of doing things.[47] Although these skills and this knowledge may be obtained through staff development, master's level management preparation is essential.

In no way are these lists complete. They are a beginning, however, and will be built on in succeeding chapters.

Executive Nurse Managers

Executive nurse managers increase their knowledge and skills by building on what they learned as lower-level managers. Executive nurse managers should be able to:

- Apply financial management principles to costing and pricing nursing care and convey this knowledge to the nurses providing care.
- Coordinate the division budget.
- Empower lower-level nurse managers.
- Undertake corporate self-analysis of what nursing can do (skills, capabilities, weaknesses, the work of nursing) and assumptions about itself, its environment, and its beliefs and convey results to employees.
- Specify, weigh, interrelate, and simultaneously accomplish multiple goals.
- Abandon obsolete principles of standardization, centralization, specialization, and concentration.
- Decentralize and share authority and power through participatory management and transformational leadership, shared governance, professional nursing models, employee involvement, and programs on quality of work life.
- Establish a matrix organization using task forces and project teams with project leaders.
- Set the stage for clinical nursing practice, which does not necessarily require that the nurse executive be clinically competent.
- Promote application of a theory of nursing within a nursing care delivery system.
- Advise nursing educators on content of nursing administration programs.
- Set depth and breadth of nursing research programs.
- Anticipate the future of health care and of nursing.
- Manage strategic planning.
- Serve as mentor, role model, and preceptor to lower-level managers, graduate students, and others.
- Recognize and use authority and the potential for power.

Research data indicate that executive nurses prepared at the doctoral level need courses in ethical and accountable decision-making, including missions and goals, policies, human resources, financial and material resources, databases, and communication management. These courses would be organized under organizational structure and governance, resources, and information management.[48] (See Exhibit 3-8).

With major changes in business practices, lessons learned from Japan offer meaningful strategies to American business, including health care. For example, the Japanese have found that less variety is best when it comes to cutting costs and saving time. Consensus decision-making does not always work. With the help of high-tech information systems, lone decisions based on multiple data sources and data points may be the best decisions.[49]

EXHIBIT 3-8
Summary of Findings: Decision Making

ORGANIZATIONAL STRUCTURE AND GOVERNANCE		RESOURCES		INFORMATION MANAGEMENT	
MISSIONS AND GOALS*	**POLICIES AND POLITICS**	**HUMAN†**	**FINANCIAL AND MATERIAL**	**DATABASES**	**COMMUNICATION**
History	Environment ≈50%	Organizational	Acquire	Delimit	Processing
Philosophy	Administrative	behavior = 40%	Allocate	Establish	Managing
Purpose	process	Leadership	Budget	Utilize	Diplomacy
Objectives	Procedures/	Market	Monitor	Maintain	Interpersonal skills
Systems analysis	guidelines	Recruit	Manage	Evaluate	Team-building
Strategic planning/ forecasting	Legalities	Appoint/admit/hire	Cost analysis	Revise	Problem-solving
	Regulations	Assign work			Conflict resolution
Change agentry	Obstacles	Develop			Writing
	Bureaucratic/ professional conflict	Educate			
		Counsel/consult/ mentor			
	Power	Evaluate			
		Promote/progress			
		Retire/release/ graduate			
		Collective bargaining			

* Refers to the missions and goals either of the nursing school and the broader academic institution in which the school is a part, or of the nursing department and the broader health-care services institution in which the department is a part.
† Refers to faculty, students, staff.

Source: J. C. Princeton. "Education for Executive Nurse Administrators: A Databased Curricular Model for Doctoral (PhD) Programs." *Journal of Nursing Education* (February 1993), 62. Reprinted with permission.

Summary

A theory of nursing management evolves from a generic theory of management that governs effective use of human and material resources. The four major functions of management are planning, organizing, directing (or leading), and controlling (or evaluating). All management activities—cognitive, affective, and psychomotor—fall within one or more of these major functions, which operate simultaneously.

A main thrust of nursing management is a focus on human behavior. Nurse managers with knowledge and skills in human behavior manage professional nurses and nonprofessional assistive nursing workers to achieve the highest level of productivity of patient care services. To do this nurse managers must become competent leaders to stimulate motivation through relationships and interpersonal processes and communication with the workforce.

The primary role of the nurse manager is to manage a clinical practice discipline. To accomplish this requires numerous competencies supported by a theory of nursing management.

APPLICATION EXERCISES

EXERCISE 3-1   Define nursing management as it relates to your job. If you are a student, observe the work of a nurse manager and define management in terms of your observations.

EXERCISE 3-2   Describe a belief you have about nursing management in the organization in which you work or are doing clinical practice. Discuss your belief with your peers in clinical practice or students and with your nurse manager or instructor.

Summarize the conclusions. Is your belief valid? Totally? Partly? Not at all? Validity can be established by comparing your conclusions with viewpoints found in publications or by obtaining agreement from practicing nurse managers. You will codify selected theory of nursing management.

EXERCISE 3-3   Translate the management of time into nursing management theory with examples such as: "A nurse who practices good management will know how to use time effectively." The example may be one that applies to you as manager or to the observed behavior of another nurse manager. Keep a log for a day, making entries at 15-minute intervals on a separate sheet of paper and using the following format.

TIME	ACTIVITY	DELAYS AND BOTTLENECKS

Analyze your log. How much of your day was productive? How much was unproductive? What can be done to increase productive time? Using the following format, make a management plan to make better use of your time.

Management Plan

Goal:

ACTIONS	TARGET DATES	ASSIGNED TO	ACCOMPLISHMENTS

Based on your observations from this exercise, write a theory statement that describes management as the effective use of time.

EXERCISE 3-4   The following functions originate from a theory of the institution or organization and the division of nursing:

Plans for accomplishing objectives are made.
Strategies for accomplishing objectives are formulated.
Activities are organized by priority.
Work is assigned.
Managerial jobs are designed.
An organizational structure evolves.

Describe how each of these activities is evident in your place of practice as a student or a practicing professional nurse.

EXERCISE 3-5   Write a short theory of nursing management based on information presented in this chapter. Remember that a theory of nursing management is an accumulation of concepts, methods, and principles that can be or have been observed and verified to some degree when translated into the art or practice of nursing management.

EXERCISE 3-6   Examine the periodicals listed for the last 12-month period:

The Journal of Nursing Administration
Nursing Administration Quarterly
Nursing Management
Nursing Research

Note the following:

- The number of articles on nursing theory versus nursing management theory.
- Theories of nursing that could be incorporated into a theory of nursing management. Did the research indicate that the theory fulfilled its claim? Explain.
- According to these periodicals, what theory of nursing management is being used in the organization in which you are getting clinical experience as a student or in which you are employed?
- According to these periodicals, what theory of nursing management could be used in the organization in which you are gaining clinical experience as a student or in which you are employed? Consider the value the research has for meeting the goals of the organization, the division of nursing, and the nursing unit.
- Make a management plan for putting the research results into practice.

NOTES

1. H. Fayol, *General and Industrial Management*, trans. by C. Storrs (London: Pitman & Sons, 1949), 3.
2. Ibid., 5–6.
3. R. M. Hodgetts, *Management: Theory, Process, and Practice*, 5th ed. (Orlando, FL: Harcourt Brace, 1990), 38.
4. Fayol, op. cit., 8–9.
5. Ibid., 19–20.
6. L. Urwick, *The Elements of Administration* (New York: Harper & Row, 1944), 14–15.
7. L. C. Megginson, D. C. Mosley, and P. H. Pietri, Jr., *Management: Leadership in Action*, 5th ed. (New York: Harper & Row, 1996), 15–20.
8. V. White, "Nursing theory: A Viewpoint," *Journal of Nursing Administration* (July–August 1984), 6, 15.
9. P. F. Drucker, *Management Challenges for the 21st Century* (New York: HarperCollins, 1999), 9.
10. W. Skinner, "Big Hat, No Cattle: Managing Human Resources, Part I," *Journal of Nursing Administration* (July–August 1982), 27–29.
11. B. D. Steffy and A. J. Grimes, "A Critical Theory of Organizational Science," *Academy of Management Review* (April 1986), 322–336.
12. Ibid.
13. L. McKenzie, "Critical Thinking in Health Care Supervision," *Health Care Supervisor* (June 1992), 2.
14. K. E. Boulding, "General Systems Theory: The Skeleton of Science," *Management Science* (April 1956), 197–208.
15. Ibid.
16. F. E. Kast and J. E. Rosenzweig, "General Systems Theory: Application for Organization and Management," *Academy of Management Journal* (December 1972), 447–464.
17. P. F. Drucker, "The Emerging Theory of Manufacturing," *Harvard Business Review* (May–June 1990), 94–100.
18. Ibid.
19. S. E. Allison, K. McLaughlin, and D. Walker, "Nursing Theory: A Tool to Put Nursing Back into Nursing Administration," *Nursing Administration Quarterly* (spring 1991), 72–78.
20. Ibid.
21. D. L. Gardner, K. Kelly, M. Johnson, J. C. McClosky, and M. Maas, "Nursing Administration Model for Administrative Practice," *Journal of Nursing Administration* (March 1991), 37–41.
22. R. Anderson, "A Theory Development Role for Nurse Administrators," *Journal of Nursing Administration* (May 1989), 23–29.
23. V. Henderson, *The Nature of Nursing* (New York: MacMillan, 1966), 15.
24. P. F. Drucker, op. cit., 34.
25. S. Gleeson, D. W. Nestor, and A. J. Riddell, "Helping Nurses Through the Management Threshold," *Nursing Administration Quarterly* (winter 1983), 11–16.
26. Ibid.
27. B. A. Taylor and A. DeSimone, "Taking the First Steps to Becoming a Nurse Manager," *Nursing Administration Quarterly* (winter 1983), 17–22.
28. D. M. Reeves and N. Underly, "Nurse Managers and Mickey Mouse Marketing," *Nursing Administration Quarterly* (winter 1983), 22–27.
29. M. F. Fralic and A. O'Connor, "A Management System for Nurse Administrators, Part I," *Journal of Nursing Administration* (April 1983), 9–13; M. F. Fralic and A. O'Connor, "A Management Progression System for Nurse Administrators, Part 2," *Journal of Nursing Administration* (May 1983), 32–33; M. F. Fralic and A. O'Connor, "A Management Progression

System for Nurse Administrators Part 3," *Journal of Nursing Administration* (June 1983), 7–12.

30. J. G. Spicer, "Dispelling Illusions with Management Development," *Nursing Administration Quarterly* (winter 1983), 46–49.
31. Ibid.
32. D. Osborne and T. Gaebler, *Reinventing Government* (New York: Plume, 1992), 275–276.
33. J. Huey, "The Leadership Industry," *Fortune* (21 February 1994), 54–56; N. J. Perry, "How to Mine Human Resources," *Fortune* (21 February 1994), 96.
34. M. L. McClure, "Managing the Professional Nurse: Part I The Organizational Theories," *Journal of Nursing Administration* (February 1984), 15–21; M. L. McClure, "Managing the Professional Nurse: Part 11. Applying Management Theory to the Challenges," *Journal of Nursing Administration* (March 1984), 11–17.
35. Ibid.
36. C. M. Freund, "Director of Nursing Effectiveness: DON and CEO Perspectives and Implications for Education," *Journal of Nursing Administration* (June 1985), 25–30.
37. P. S. Nugent, "Management and Modes of Thought," *Journal of Nursing Administration* (February 1982), 19–25.
38. Ibid.
39. Ibid.
40. Ibid.
41. D. C. Veehoff, "Whole Brain Thinking and the Nurse Manager," *Nursing Management* (August 1993), 33–34.
42. L. Rew, "Intuition: Concept Analysis of a Group Phenomenon," *Advances in Nursing Science* (January 1986), 21–28.
43. Ibid.
44. D. C. Veehoff, op. cit.
45. J. O'Leary, "Do Nurse Administrators' Values Conflict with the Economic Trend?" *Nursing Administration Quarterly* (summer 1984), 1–9; M. L. McClure, "Managing the Professional Nurse: Part I. The Organizational Theories," *The Journal of Nursing Administration* (February, 1984), 15–21; M. A. Maidique, "Point of View: The New Management Thinkers," *California Management Review* (fall 1983), 151–160; M. A. Poulin, "Future Directions for Nursing Administration," *Journal of Nursing Administration* (March 1984), 37–41; M. A. Fralic and A. O'Connor, "A Management Progression System for Nurse Administrators, Part I," op. cit., 9–13; G. Gentleman, "Power at the Unit Level," *Nursing Administration Quarterly* (winter 1983), 27–31; M. A. Poulin, "The Nurse Executive Role: A Structural and Functional Analysis," *Journal of Nursing Administration* (February 1984), 9–14.
46. C. Gentleman, op. cit.
47. J. J. Mathews, "Designing a First Line Manager Development Program Using Organization-Appropriate Strategies," *The Journal of Continuing Education in the Health Professions*, (1988), 8(3), 181–188.
48. J. C. Princeton, "Education for Executive Nurse Administrators: A Databased Curricular Model for Doctoral (PhD) Programs," *Journal of Nursing Education* (February 1993), 59–63.
49. R. Henkoff, "New Management Secrets from Japan," *Fortune* (27 November 1995), 135–146.

REFERENCES

Blanchard, K. "Reaching Out to Others Through Simple Truths: Ken Blanchard's Theory of Good Managing and Fulfilled Living." *Caring* (October 1999), 20–24.

Cullum, N., and T. Sheldon. "Clinically Challenged." *Nursing Management* (July 1996), 14–16.

DeWeese, S. and D. Satecki. "Combining Management Education with an Assessment Center." *Nursing Management* (August 1986), 80–81.

Drucker, P. F. *Management: Tasks, Responsibilities, Practices* (New York: Harper & Row, 1973), 1974.

Hillestad, E. A. "Is It Lonely at the Top?" *Nursing Administration Quarterly* (spring 1984): 1–13.

Huey, J. "The New Post-Heroic Leadership." *Fortune* (21 February 1994), 42–44, 48, 50.

Marriner, A. "Development of Management Thought." *Journal of Nursing Administration* (September 1979), 21–31.

O'Reilly, B. "Reengineering the MBA." *Fortune* (24 January 1994), 38–40, 42, 44, 46–47.

Perra, B. M. "The Leader In You." *Nursing Management* (January 1999), 35–39.

Peters, T. *Thriving on Chaos: Handbook for a Management Revolution* (New York: Harper & Row, 1987), 615–617.

Pilette, P. C. and K. K. Kirby. "Expectations and Responsibilities of the Nursing Director Role." *Nursing Management* (March 1991), 77–80.

Pilon, B. A. "Outcomes and Surprises of Work Redesign." *Nursing Management* (August 1998), 44–45.

Price, V. "Counseling for Change." *Nursing Management* (September 1996), 22–23.

Roy, C. "The Interview—Calista Roy." *Nursing Management* (September 1997), 16–19.

Sowell, R. and J. W. Alexander. "A Model for Success in Nursing Administration." *Nursing & Health Care* (January 1988), 24–30.

Stahl, D. A. "Ethics in Subacute Care—Part I." *Nursing Management* (September 1996), 29–30.

Stewart, T. A. "Rate Your Readiness to Change." *Fortune* (27 February 1994), 106–107, 110.

Swansburg, R. C. *Management of Patient Care Services* (Saint Louis: Mosby), 1976.

Swansburg, R. C. *Nurses and Patients: An Introduction to Nursing Management* (Hattiesburg, MS: Impact 111), 1978.

Tumulty, G. "Head Nurse Role Redesign." *Journal of Nursing Administration* (February 1992), 41–48.

Van der Zalm, J. E., and V. Bergum. "Hermeneutic-Phenomenology: Providing Living Knowledge for Nursing Practice." *Journal of Advanced Nursing* (January 2000), 211–218.

Wagner, L., B. Henry, G. Giovinco, and C. Blanks. "Suggestions for Graduate Education in Nursing Administration." *Journal of Nursing Education* (May 1988), 210–218.

Theory of Human Resource Development

Russell C. Swansburg, PhD, RN

> The most exciting breakthroughs of the twenty-first century will occur not because of technology but because of an expanding concept of what it means to be human.
>
> John Naisbitt and Patricia Aburdene[1]

LEARNING OBJECTIVES AND ACTIVITIES

- Define the terms *human resource development, human resource autonomy*, and *human resource empowerment, andragogy*, and *human capital*.
- Give examples of the concept of human resource development (HRD).
- Give examples of the concepts of autonomy and empowerment.
- Illustrate the notion of self-help by applying it to nursing management.
- Give examples of the elements of HRD.
- Discuss the relevance of andragogy in HRD.
- Apply a typology of adult education to goals for an HRD program.
- Describe the relevance of human capital to HRD in nursing management.
- Project future changes in nursing HRD.

CONCEPTS: Human resource development (HRD), science of behavioral technology, autonomy, empowerment, self-help, HR planning, role theory, andragogy, strategic human resource management (SHRM), typologies and taxonomies of adult education and HRD, human capital.

MANAGER BEHAVIOR: Plans, organizes, directs, and controls all aspects of a human resource development program. Manages people.

LEADER BEHAVIOR: Establishes direction, aligns persons, stimulates motivation, and inspires people to cause drastic and useful change in performing their nursing roles. Uses research results to develop a model of HRD that leads people and makes them productive by putting to use their specific knowledge and strengths.

Introduction

Much of the voluminous theory of human resource development (HRD) comes from the generic fields of business and management. HRD is grounded in the theory of personnel or human resource management (HRM) and the science of behavioral technology. Nursing management is one process through which HRD is applied.

Because the success pattern of the industrial age is a liability to the current information age, corporations will have to reshape their policies and structures to recruit employees. The new millennium justifies coining a new term for it, such as "The Age of the Individual" or "The Age of the Human Being." We are already well into the information age, and during the next several decades, the following changes will continue to occur within the United States:

1. Agriculture will be reduced in manpower and productivity.
2. Only 10% of the population will be employed in manufacturing.
3. From 65% to 70% of the workforce will be employed in service industries.
4. The information–electronics industry will continue to create jobs at a rate of 4 to 4.5 million a year.
5. Education will be a dominant industry because services are education-intensive.
6. Training budgets will increase to $10 trillion per year.
7. The United States will be populated by 350 million people.
8. Income will average $40,000 per capita at a 2% per year compound model of growth in the gross national product (GNP).

9. A new accounting system will evolve to depreciate people as human capital, with education becoming the capital to replace losses.
10. There will be more organizations but fewer employees per organization.[2]

Nursing as a service industry will continue to grow, be education-intensive to develop new roles, and require increased capital for staff development and maintenance. More complex health care systems will require advanced nursing knowledge and skills.

Definition

Human resource development is the process by which corporate management stimulates the motivation of employees to perform productively. HRD provides the stimuli that motivate nursing personnel to provide nursing care services to clients at quality and quantity standards that keep the health care entity reputable and financially solvent, the nurses satisfied with their professional accomplishments and quality of work life, and the clients treated successfully.[3]

Nursing personnel generally want to earn a good living and live a good life, two goals that are inextricably linked. Both result from and are maintained by HRD programs that include professional or technical and liberal (general education, the liberal arts, and humanities) education. Maintenance education will enhance nurses' productivity when management recognizes that education and productivity are linked.

Human resource development practices the concepts of democracy. In HRD, people grow and prosper from learning to use the skills of problem-solving, application of logic, inquiry, critical thinking, and decision-making. HRD is a lifelong process, hence its relationship to adult education and lifelong learning. It is also a process of helping and sharing that leads to competence and satisfaction with both the process and outcomes. The HRD process facilitates self-direction, self-discipline, focus on immediate problems, and satisfaction related to employee participation in problem-solving and decision-making.[4]

Human resource development is not a function of personnel or labor relations. It is an internal process involving employees and HRD personnel who may be nurse managers, staff development personnel or in-service education personnel, among others. The HRD program may be administered at the corporate, division, or unit level. Although it is usually a staff function, HRD can be decentralized to the unit level as a function facilitated by the nurse manager.[5]

Obviously, nurse administrators and managers of today's work force must be well schooled in HRD. HRD theory includes the theory of change, problem-solving and decision-making, leadership, motivation, communication, participatory management, decentralization, and adult education. In nursing, HRD should be a proactive program as well as a part of strategic planning.

In recent years, HRD in many health care organizations has been strongly influenced by the following:

- A change in reimbursement systems from retrospective to prospective. These systems are cost-driven.
- A change in the structuring of health care organizations with the development of product lines, especially outpatient or ambulatory surgical centers, wellness programs, women's health programs, free-standing rehabilitation facilities, and many more.
- The decentralization of nursing organizations, which has made unit nurse managers department heads and eliminated intermediate levels of nursing management. Nursing staff governance and differentiated nursing practice are emerging. Case management and managed care are very evident.

Health care organization administrators and nurse managers at all levels are learning that efficiency and effectiveness result from advanced HRD programs. These advanced programs facilitate human relationships, reliability, initiative, autonomy, and talents. They do so through policies, procedures and leadership that are fair, promote trust, reduce stress, communicate through feedback, and increase productivity without undue emphasis on costs. Keeping employees satisfied with the work environment decreases turnover, an expensive aspect of HRM. Good HRD programs are therefore cost-effective.

Science of Behavioral Technology

The science of behavioral technology has as its basis the premise that consequences will influence behavior. This premise can be used to improve employee performance. People will work more willingly when supervisors or managers exercise concern for their feelings and needs. A basic question here is, What will the employee work for? Three applications of the science of behavioral technology are analyzing problems, influencing job behavior, and designing learning systems.

Analyzing Problems

The usual answer to identified problems is to give employees more training. Consider an example involving the writing of nursing notes. A nurse executive made scheduled unit rounds on a monthly basis. One announced activity that she performed was to evaluate the quality of nursing notes in relation to the nursing care plan. Because this facility was using the problem-oriented system, the nursing notes were to describe progress in relation to each nursing problem and the prescribed nursing approaches. Time after time, there were omissions in the recording system. The standard approach to the problem was to provide more in-service education to the personnel making the nursing notes. Finally the nurse executive met with key managers to analyze the problem. These were the questions they asked themselves:

What were the consequences of proper recordings?

- Financial: Salary had not been affected by writing satisfactory nursing notes. They were a requirement of the job description and the job standards.
- Supervision: Few comments by supervisors had related to satisfactory recordings.

What were the consequences of improper recordings?

- Financial: Salary had not been affected by writing unsatisfactory nursing notes. Salary increases had been approved regardless of the quality of the nursing notes.
- Supervision: There had been criticism by nurse managers of omissions and improper recordings by clinical nurses.

In further discussion, it was decided that more in-service education classes would not solve the problem. The approach was to be a positive one. A team of clinical nurses would be formed as a quality circle. They would be asked to solve the problem so that all nursing notes would reflect the quality of nursing care. The goal would be 100% quality nursing notes, reflecting 100% quality nursing care. A contract would be made to reward the team members with early raises and bonuses for accomplishing the goals. Management would facilitate the work of the team. In-service education would be used only for personnel who did not know how to write problem-oriented nursing notes.

Influencing Job Behavior

This approach is illustrated by the experience of Ms. Bins, a nurse executive who received daily written reports on selected patients. Much of this information was useless to her, since few comments related to the nursing diagnoses of patients or the prescribed nursing care. Progress was not usually indicated. The reports were composed mostly of trivia. Ms. Bins decided to reinforce the behavior she desired and ignore the undesirable behavior. Consequently she wrote positive comments on the reports that contained a nursing diagnosis

and prescription and described progress and returned these reports to the nurse managers. Within weeks progress was pronounced; nurses were writing reports that gave the nurse executive excellent knowledge of the patients' conditions as well as of the workload and performances of nursing personnel.

Designing Learning Systems

Where safety is involved, it is not enough to teach people skills that prevent injuries to themselves and to patients. Leaders should be taught to reinforce the correct behavior directly after the act. Verbal reinforcers are often as effective as monetary ones. They are particularly effective if followed by monetary rewards. When managers become skilled in the principles of behavioral technology, they know the amount of reinforcement needed by individual employees. The act should be identified with the reinforcement if the latter is to be effective. Reinforcement should be genuine so that the employee will recognize the correlation between the desired behavior and the reward.[6]

Human resource development programs have frequently competed with adult basic education and continuing education programs. An example is hospital chief executive officers having HRD departments organize and implement management development programs using external faculty while ignoring management faculty in the college of nursing. Some of the faculty have joint appointments in the service organization.

With the enormous future needs for employee education, HRD and adult continuing education (ACE) departments should cooperate. Before 1986, more than $210 billion was spent annually for adult education. In 1987, 40 million employees participated in 17 million courses paid for by employers. The biggest users were government and the communications, mining, insurance, and real estate industries. External sources provided 40% of HRD training. One reason has been that business leaders perceived that ACE personnel did not speak their language; that is, they were not practical. Business used consultants and still does.[7]

How can this perception be changed? ACE personnel should do the following[9]:

1. Market to business.

2. Market their expertise in restructuring.

3. Market their expertise in career development. Individuals want personal development: wellness, arts, humanities, personal finance, personal growth, family education, and hobbies. Education for life and living combined with technical education increases employee productivity.

4. Establish an effective and realistic political base with the corporate structure.

5. Develop programs for HRD for the entire organization.[8]

6. Attend to the trends in HRD, such as teamwork, flatter hierarchies, and decentralization.

7. Create staff development programs that address the three phases of HRD:

    a. Design product-driven training to teach skills specific to new products and services throughout the organization.

    b. Institute market-driven training when technology and services change rapidly and educational efforts become a more permanent, ongoing feature of the workplace. This is one of the niches where staff personnel should position themselves for managed competition in health care. The objective is to give the organization a competitive advantage.

    c. Integrate knowledge and skills as process-driven education and training.

Staff developers aligned with HRD need to decide which education and training strategies to follow to satisfy the needs of employees with broad educational backgrounds, those with high-level or specialized educational preparation, and all other categories of employees. Consensus building, collaboration, partnership, and mutually agreed-on objectives should support these decisions. See Exhibit 4-1 for differences between ACE and HRD.

Other applications of the science of behavioral technology can be found in Chapter 16, Decentralization and Participatory Management; Chapter 18, Leadership; Chapter 19, Motivation; and Chapter 20, Communication.

Autonomy and Empowerment

As part of HRD, health care corporations should increasingly develop programs to enlarge the authority of professional nurses, increase their voice in management of their clinical practice discipline, and improve their career development possibilities. The organization's administration and its employees want control over HRD events. As stakeholders in the health care system, clinical nurses and managers both have an obligation to keep the enterprise healthy. As economic stakeholders, nurses need security of income through wages and benefits while management's stake is profits and, in some cases, dividends for shareholders. Nurses have a psychological stake in their need for dignity. Nurses and managers have potential stakes related to rights and obligations, efficiency and controls, and the trend toward greater employee influence in decisions and subsequent outcomes. These stakes should be spelled out in policies. The leader who balances moti-

vation with control will manage effectively as "human beings strive to be involved and to gain influence over their lives to the extent that they are psychologically ready to do so and to the extent that economic organizational conditions allow them to do so."[10]

People want to work hard, perform well, learn new skills, and be involved in decisions about their work. They want to have input into placement and promotion. Managers who support the professional autonomy of nurses support empowerment of this group. Professional nurses thus gain control of their lives through feeling and using their own strength and power. Empowerment is therapeutic and spiritual; it is healthy for both employees and the organization. Empowerment stems from and gives support to useful experiential feelings or ideologies.[11]

Empowerment seeks to increase the power and influence of professional nurses.[12]

Nurses are empowered when administrators and managers share authority with them. Nurses seek community with other nurses as a form of empowerment. Their power is extended by new technologies and the ability to use them. They are empowered at work by computers with modems, cellular phones, fax machines, and access to e-mail systems. Nurses are empowered when society rewards their initiative as individuals.[13]

Empowerment motivates. Self-managed teams are empowered teams. One in five U.S. employers use these teams with resulting drops in labor costs, increases in morale, and signs of eased alienation. In 1986, the United Auto Workers (UAW) and Chrysler Corporation created self-managed teams at the rundown New Castle, Indiana, plant. Workers were renamed "technicians," and line supervisors became "team advisers." Seventy-seven teams were created to assign tools, confront sluggish performers, order repairs, talk with customers, hire new employees, and even alter work hours after consulting a labor–management steering committee. Team members are paid for extra training. As a result, absenteeism went from 7% to 2.9%, union grievances decreased from more than 1,000 a year to 33, and defects per million parts made fell from 300 a year to 20; production costs keep shrinking.[14]

Positive financial outcomes have resulted when transformational managers have developed and empowered their staff.[15]

Research: Graduate students enrolled in advanced practice nurse programs were empowered by learning that was driven by students' interests, respected and valued their experience, and guided them in defining and pursuing individual goals.[16]

EXHIBIT 4-1

The Differences Between Adult Continuing Education (ACE) and Human Resource Development (HRD)

ACE	HRD
PURPOSE AND MISSION	
Primary focus is on individual development and personal growth.	Primary focus is on organizational development and the role of employees in that development.
Education is the primary means for changing people, e.g., classes, courses, workshops, and individualized instruction.	Education is one dimension of organizational change. Others include job rotation/enrichment, organizational restructuring, and incentive plans.
PROGRAMMING	
Programming is primarily marketed for the general public.	Programs are for employees only. Some may be marketed, but on a space-available basis.
Program identification is community-wide, with needs analysis tapping a wide variety of groups and organizations.	Program identification is within the organization, with intensive needs analysis of management, employees, customers, competitors, and environment.
PARTICIPANTS (LEARNERS)	
The learners usually select the program to meet personal needs and goals.	The learner's performance is evaluated and training and development needs identified.
The learner is the primary client. The learner's employer is secondary to the learner's meeting his or her own goals.	The needs of the organization are primary. The employee's needs are met within the needs of the employer.
INSTRUCTIONAL RESOURCES	
Resources are primarily from education, because use of faculty is desired if not required.	Resources are from any source (expertise in or out of the organization) that meets the organization's needs and can be afforded (bought).
Certification is often required and ranges from a teaching certificate to approval by a faculty department.	The test of acceptance is, whether the person or program can meet the present needs of the organization? Accountability is driven by the bottom line.
FINANCES (PAYMENT OF FEES)	
Payment for the program is by the participant. Payment by participant's employer is usually through tuition reimbursement.	Payment is by the employer and usually includes salary while in training. Employee-selected courses must be approved by the employer.
MAJOR PLAYERS (ROLES)	
Directors/deans of ACE under a chief executive for instruction/academic affairs, coordinators, instructors (full/part-time).	Chief executive for human resources, director of HRD, instructional and content specialists, trainers, and consultants.
Prefer experience in ACE, with coursework in adult education desired. Increasingly, people with content expertise are being hired and trained in adult education. Terminal degree (master's/doctorate) preferred to relate with others in the school/college.	Prefer people from the organization or who have HRD experience in the base industry (banking, manufacturing, retailing, etc.). Coursework in adult education is not considered necessary, but coursework will be paid if desired. Performance is required; terminal degree is optional but increasingly becoming a plus.

Source: D. H. Smith. "Adult and Continuing Education and Human Resource Development—Present Competitors, Potential Partners." *Lifelong Learning: An Omnibus of Practice and Research*, 12(7), (1989). Used by permission of the author.

Autonomy and empowerment are achieved through collaboration and mutual planning leading to commitment, satisfaction, productivity, and identification and improvement of quality. Malcolm Knowles states that as adults mature, they move toward autonomy, activity, objectivity, enlightenment, increased abilities, increased responsibilities, altruism, focusing on principles, deep concerns, originality, and tolerance for ambiguity.[17] For more information, see Chapter 16 on Decentralization and Participatory Management.

Self-Help

A goal of HRD is the development of a self-reliant learner who remains a knowledgeable and skilled worker in the future. Another goal is the development of workers who learn and use the skills of self-help and of diagnosing their learning needs, being able to explore options in learning, thinking divergently, making decisions, and evaluating their role in cooperation at work and in the world.[18] The HRD program uses leadership, staff development, and the theory of adult education to accomplish these goals.

Self-help is a unique form of self-directed learning that spans the life cycle. A person does not necessarily help himself or herself independent of others. Self-help is also a process that occurs within small, voluntary, peer-run support groups, offering participants the opportunity to work together to overcome or cope with a common concern or problem.

According to Hammerman, the self-help movement began with Alcoholics Anonymous (AA). Participants tend to be white-collar and middle-class, with employment capability and the strong support of concerned spouses. As workers, professional nurses benefit from self-help groups that provide, among other things, a network of information, support, and help from peers. Authenticity being a strength of self-help, HRD programs can use the self-help process to validate the authenticity of the learning. Sometimes conflicts of peer versus management leadership and agency sponsorship arise. These conflicts can be prevented or resolved through a warm, supportive, accepting environment that lowers defenses and allows for open, trusting, authentic dialogue. Members learn things they can't learn anywhere else. Professionals put interests of group members first, and the group agrees on each professional person's tools for self-help.[19] As workers, professional nurses benefit from self-help groups.

Role theory supports the notion of self-help. Changing environments—between external forces and the organization and between the organization and its members—lead to role ambiguity, which increases with redesigned and new relationships. Role ambiguity can lead to role conflict as a result of competing role behaviors, particularly among members of multidisciplinary teams. Role conflict increases with increased interaction on new turf. Role overload occurs as added work crowds time allotments, particularly when new programs are added and old ones retained. HRD and staff development programs provide the organizational support employees need to cope with role changes and deal with role overload. These programs include learning the skills of priority setting and assertiveness.[20]

> A study of 253 self-help groups indicates that many have shared leadership, recruit group members, receive assistance from professionals, and receive guidance from national and local organizations. Self-help groups have great potential for assisting in managed care systems.[21] Other research results indicate that giving help to others predicts improvement in psychosocial adjustment.[22] Also, family physicians who were subjected to educational material specific to their concerns, changed their attitudes favorably toward self-help groups.[23]

Human Resource Planning

Human resource planning is undertaken as part of the strategic planning process and is essential to retain outstanding professional talent. It is not enough to address only the business activities of nursing such as management processes and functions, budgets, objectives, and staffing. The division's goals are accomplished through its people. Nurse managers serve in dual roles, as managers of human resources and as managers of nursing operations. Nurse managers need to enlist the support of the HR department. They also need to develop an understanding of the relationships between other operational departments and nursing.[24]

Strategic human resource planning takes into account how the full spectrum of human resources will affect the organization's strategic and operational plans. If the human resources do not fit the strategic plan, the nurse manager decides what actions to take. Options can include locating new people with special skills or upgrading the skills of senior personnel. A statement of objectives for the HR program should be included in the strategic plan, developed with input from clinical nurses[25] and executed by managers supported by staff development.

Other elements of strategic HR planning include the following:

1. Projection for future growth, changes in the employment market, external demographics, and balancing human resources against finances.
2. Development of a strategic HR planning approach that describes actions, roles, authorities, and responsibilities of the HR department, line management, and individual employees.
3. Inventory of HR planning skills that includes future issues, a system for translating business plans into HR requirements and programs, career development, two-way communication, attitude surveys, employee sensing, group feedback sessions, and exit interviews.
4. Analysis of current and future macro issues of major world influences that will affect the strategic business plan (SBP) and the human resources plan (HRP). These influences include factors such as the age of the population, productivity in U.S. industry, inflation, politics, unions, technology, and expectations of nurses.
5. Analysis of current and future micro issues of major organizational influences, including geographic location, availability of skills, potential in-house promotions, living costs, and unions.
6. Development of programs to support the SBP and HRP.
7. Provision for periodic and timely audits.
8. Support and commitment of all management levels.[26]

As part of strategic planning, nurse managers will develop goals and objectives that:

1. Address increased automation of nursing information systems.
2. Project changes that will occur in nursing products and services.
3. Project the organization and types of employees that will be needed for changed products and services.
4. Trace trends in the corporate culture related to values, cultural rituals, social processes, and learning patterns of clients and employees.
5. Address the retraining of employees who are in outmoded jobs.
6. Explore future leads through content analysis, trends extrapolation forecasting, simulation forecasting, modeling, scenario projection, and trend impact analysis. These complex techniques can improve forecasting.
7. Assess new management techniques that include open work systems, quality of work life programs, quality circles, and participatory management techniques.
8. Promote job security and career development, including management of nurses who are "fast burners" or stars, the top 5% to 10% of the nursing force.
9. Lower barriers to women, minorities, older workers, new workers, and immigrants.
10. Keep employee knowledge and skills updated, and provide more resources for learning and development.

11. Develop policies to deal with employees' dual careers, changing careers, and life values; changes in the work ethic related to personal and leisure activities; and downgrading and demoting employees.[27] The implications for those responsible for staff development are varied, comprehensive, and demanding.
12. Address the future. What services can nurses provide as product lines? Some examples are clinical nursing consultation service and services to customers desiring help with filing claims and appealing decisions of third-party payers.

Davis and Milbank indicate that laziness is not the reason for a fading work ethic. The work ethic is a psychological or spiritual state rather than an economic one. It wavers because of alienation between employer and employee. Sixty-five percent of U.S. families that are headed by married couples have two or more people at work. More than 6% of Americans hold down two jobs. U.S. managers are often unable to create a workplace suited to literate, independent-minded workers. Also, women and minorities are alienated by race and sex discrimination, sexual harassment, and pregnancy.[28] The implications for HRD and staff development are evident.

HRD planning should create a climate for the personal growth of learners, who should be included in the planning. The organizational structure should be planned to encourage member participation, goal understanding and acceptance, the seeking and sharing of information, disagreement and conflict management, participation in decision-making, an atmosphere that encourages expression of feelings, and leadership.[29]

Planning should provide for time to do the job because time is a precious human resource that must be protected.[30] In nursing, the HRD program should encourage nurse managers to understand and decide which programs will support the business strategy of the organization. Strategic plans will provide for the development of employees to maintain and upgrade competence, leading to increased productivity.

Exhibit 4-2 provides an example.

EXHIBIT 4-2
Example of a Strategic Plan

SCENARIO
HRD. To develop long-range (strategic) plans for the hospital, the administrator involved representatives of all levels and all departments in a series of meetings at which long-range goals were defined. Physicians were included. Top managers categorized these goals, and the organized list was integrated into a master plan that included budgetary projections and key personnel responsibilities. After ratification by the board of trustees, the plan was publicized and implementation begun.

Phases and stages in the process of strategic planning are summarized in Exhibit 5-4 in Chapter 5, The Planning Process.

Operational Human Resource Planning

Planning encompasses the writing of personnel policies that will assist in recruiting and maintaining a qualified staff. Data to help develop these policies will need to be collected and analyzed in cooperation with the human resource division and representatives of the entire nursing staff. Nursing management has an ethical responsibility to inform nurses about needed information compiled on them and to ensure that only needed information is retained. This information should be used to develop jobs and to recruit, select, assign, retain, and promote nursing personnel based on individual qualifications and capabilities and without regard to race, sex, creed, or color. The information will be used to develop personnel policies to classify personnel according to competence and to establish salary scales commensurate with qualifications and positions of comparable responsibility within the community and agency. Written copies of personnel policies, job descriptions, and job standards will be made available to all nursing personnel.

Models of Strategic Human Resource Management

Strategic human resource management (SHRM) is the process of building a human organization that makes a business successful. SHRM integrates HRM with the strategic needs of the firm. SHRM includes the components of policies, culture, values, and practices that are linked or integrated across levels of the organization. Schuler's 5-P Model of SHRM includes philosophy, politics, programs, practices, and processes systematically linked to the strategic needs of the organization (see Exhibit 4-3).

Human resource management is linked with the organization's strategic plan for survival, growth, adaptability, and profitability. To apply Schuler's 5-P Model of SHRM to nursing do the following[31]:

1. Take on the HR philosophy. Look at statements of business values of nursing. Also look at the culture of the organization regarding empowerment, training and education, teamwork, careers, and values. This culture includes all activities affecting the behavior of workers in their efforts to formulate and implement the strategic needs important to the success of the business, the participatory processes needed to link HR practices and strategy, a systematic and analytical mind-set, and opportunity for HR departments to impact through strategic initiatives.

2. Adopt HR policies. Link the HR philosophy with particular people-related business needs.

3. Follow HR programs. Make changes needed to effect strategic business needs. HR programs may be HR strategies.

4. Use HR practices. Provide leadership, managerial, and operational practices. Cue and reinforce role performance. Leadership involves establishing direction, aligning employees, motivating and inspiring individuals, and causing dramatic and useful change. Management involves planning, directing, delegating, organizing, and coordinating. Operational practices involve delivering services and making products.

5. Use HR processes. Combine the interaction of strategic education with line management. Promote empowerment, ownership, and participation.

In addition, nurse managers should view personnel as an expandable resource whose skills and capabilities are preserved, developed, and continuously improved through recruitment, training, and career progression. The human element is the key asset of any organization.[32] Research indicates that health care leaders should use marketing tools to attract HRM people from other industries, promote diversity in the workplace, promote employees from within, and cross-train people whenever possible.[33]

A SHRM system has two general responsibilities as follows:

1. Competence management. Skills needed to execute given organizational strategy, that is, competence acquisition, utilization, retention, and displacement.

2. Behavioral management. Activities to control employee behavior leading to organizational goals, that is, coordination across all personnel to support the organizational strategy.

According to Wright and McMahan, "A good theory enables one to both predict what will happen given a set of values for certain variables, and to understand why this predicted value should result." HRM has traditionally been viewed as the aggregate of practices of managing people in organizations: selection, training, appraisal, and rewards. SHRM is "the pattern of planned human resource deployments and activities intended to enable an organization to achieve its goals." SHRM links HRM practices, the strategic management process, and coordination or congruence among the various HRM practices. Theory of HRM models is a recent movement

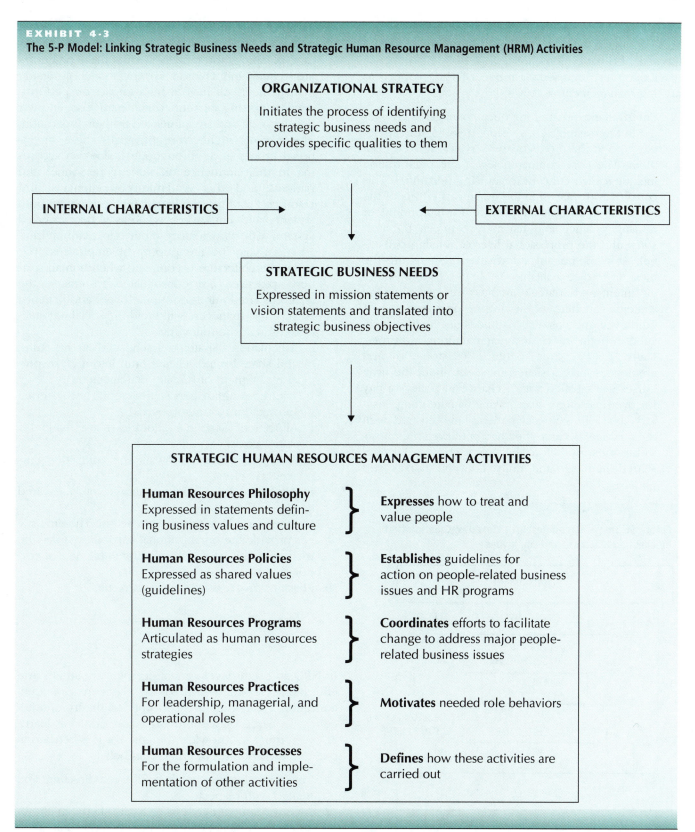

EXHIBIT 4-3
The 5-P Model: Linking Strategic Business Needs and Strategic Human Resource Management (HRM) Activities

ORGANIZATIONAL STRATEGY

Initiates the process of identifying strategic business needs and provides specific qualities to them

INTERNAL CHARACTERISTICS ⟶   ⟵ **EXTERNAL CHARACTERISTICS**

STRATEGIC BUSINESS NEEDS

Expressed in mission statements or vision statements and translated into strategic business objectives

STRATEGIC HUMAN RESOURCES MANAGEMENT ACTIVITIES

Human Resources Philosophy
Expressed in statements defining business values and culture
} **Expresses** how to treat and value people

Human Resources Policies
Expressed as shared values (guidelines)
} **Establishes** guidelines for action on people-related business issues and HR programs

Human Resources Programs
Articulated as human resources strategies
} **Coordinates** efforts to facilitate change to address major people-related business issues

Human Resources Practices
For leadership, managerial, and operational roles
} **Motivates** needed role behaviors

Human Resources Processes
For the formulation and implementation of other activities
} **Defines** how these activities are carried out

Source: Reprinted from *Organizational Dynamics*, R. S. Schuler, "Strategic Human Resources Management: Linking the People with the Strategic Needs of the Business," p. 20, Copyright 1992, with permission from Elsevier Science.

of the past 10 to 15 years. It is subject to consistent rigorous empirical tests. SHRM theory is grounded in the theories of organizations.[34]

Exhibit 4-4 represents a model of HRD applied to nursing management as follows[35]:

1. The strategic intent of the nurse manager is embodied in the organization's vision, mission, and strategies and in the products and services derived from them. The core competencies of the organization include a high concern for nursing personnel. This concern is displayed in the numerous efforts of the nurse administrator to provide for autonomy of nursing practice and harmony between the personal and the professional lives of nursing personnel. At work nursing information systems are the most up-to-date available. These two factors, strategic intent and strategic architecture, make up the strategic capability of the nursing organization.

2. Employee and customer attitudes are highly correlated in both service and manufacturing industries. Unity exists when patients (customers) and employees have a shared mind-set about the firm: nurses are satisfied with a change in policy to pay for overtime rather than having to take compensatory time off. Potential patients are satisfied with the outcome because they had perceived the nurses to be unhappy before the policy change. There is shared mind-set and unity between nurses and patients.

3. Systems architecture includes organizational processes such as staffing, rewards, training, structure, planning, and practices. All of these processes are strategic inputs into a systems model of nursing management. All have a high impact on performance of nursing personnel who participate in their development and are influenced by their application. The systems architecture privatizes these operational processes as throughput: It does so according to their influence on nursing personnel and patients and the available competencies and resources. Staffing may have a high priority for both patients and employees whereas a decentralized system with participatory input into planning and practices may be the priority of employees. The systems architecture is complete when human relations practices are consolidated to ensure the desired shared mind-set of employees and patients.

4. Next, nurse managers will build the social architecture through the following:
   a. Articulation. Strategic intent and architecture, and shared mind-set, are built into a clear, precise statement of nursing management.
   b. Awareness. Managers share internal and external information with employees.
   c. Allocation. Resource allocations are made for stated goals.
   d. Attention. Managers "walk the talk," doing as well as talking.
   e. Accountability. Progress should be measured and evaluated.

5. Put the social architecture into action. The employees provide the organizational capability. It may be tried on a unit basis before being implemented corporation-wide.

6. Measure progress and business results.

Andragogy

In HRD and staff development, learners are adults, and educational programs are based on theories of adult education. Andragogy is a concept and theory of adult education based on assumptions about adults as learners. According to Knowles, the concept is a behavioral one and incorporates the following beliefs[36]:

1. The adult learner needs to be self-directing and treated with respect.
2. An environment needs to be established that allows adults to participate in making decisions that affect their lives.
3. Because adults have experiences to share with others, experiential techniques should be a part of adult

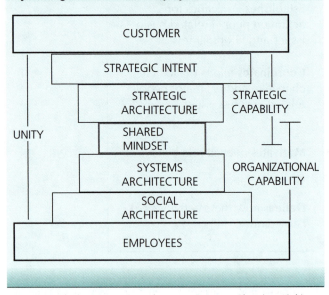

EXHIBIT 4-4
Future Strategy–Human Resource Linkages: Creating Unity by Linking Customers and Employees

Source: D. Ulrich. "Strategic and Human Resource Planning: Linking Customers and Employees." *Strategic and Human Resource Planning,* 15(2), (1992), 53.

education. Because adults are more closed to new concepts, they need to be "unfrozen."

4. Adults should be able to immediately apply what they have learned. Learning should relate to doing something or learning a skill.
5. Social role development determines an adult's readiness to learn.
6. Adults go through a sequence of learning from being a dependent personality to being self-directing, accumulating a reservoir of experience and shifting their orientation toward learning from that of being subject-centered to being performance-centered.

Knowles recommends the construction of a six-point process design for adult learners to produce a content design as follows:

1. Self-directed mutual planning by the adult learners.
2. Creation of a social climate that is an adult learning environment—informal, comfortable, friendly, and caring—one in which students are listened to and treated as unique persons.
3. Diagnosis of needs, that is, students' needs plus teachers' needs plus negotiation, leads to successful learning.
4. Sequential learning experiences, that is, follow the problem-solving process with sequence, with continuity, and with unity.
5. Construction of a training plan of self-directing activities that meet objectives for which the teacher acts as facilitator.
6. Evaluation to redirect learning, that is, identify competencies, assess levels of competence, identify gaps in competence as needs that motivate learners, then raise the level of competency to reduce gaps.[37]

Adult education reflects lifelong learning and is well established in our society and in nursing. Because staff development in nursing relates to adults, it should follow the precepts of adult learning, a humanistic educational process that values the individual. In nursing education, andragogy creates a horizontal power relationship between teacher and student.[38]

Teaching Adult Patients

Writing on the topic of teaching adult patients, Goodwin-Johansson notes the increasing number of adult patients. She states that education is an integral part of the health care of adult patients, the goals being achievement, maintenance, and protection of health. She describes patient education as "planned combinations of learning activities designed to help people who had experience with illness make changes in their behavior conducive to

good health."[39] The conduct of health care organizations affects application of the principles of andragogy.

Providers expect patients to be compliant rather than choose their own learning experiences. The patient has decreased energy and will for risk-taking, as opposed to being involved in solving problems, making immediate application of treatments, and participating voluntarily. Experts surround the patient, with staff controlling the patient's time schedule. The patient faces social barriers such as involuntary attendance, rules that limit freedom, decreased geographic boundaries, decreased privacy, and decreased personal identity. These conditions prevent the exercise of adult education principles such as taking into account life experiences, having a teacher who functions as a facilitator rather than as an authority, and individualization.[40]

> Many adults combine work and education. They may learn skills on the job such as writing. Drawing on such relevant experiences, they may bring writing skills to class. It is the facilitator's responsibility to determine whether the writing skills are appropriate and adequate. If so, they can be used. If not, the learners' input should be handled in a way that maintains their self-esteem.[41]

Facilitators of adult education should be technically proficient, effective leaders who engender images of interpersonal skills of caring, trust, and encouragement. Also, they need instructional planning skills that include needs assessment, context analysis, setting educational objectives, organizing learning activities, and evaluation. They also need teaching and learning skills that produce a favorable educational climate and offer teaching and learning interactions that provide challenge, closure, practice, feedback, and reinforcement. Facilitators should make learners think critically and reflectively.[42]

Adult educators respect learners. They mediate between information and individuals, organize opportunities, and stimulate learners. Adult educators exercise patience in coaching learners to take control of learning tasks. They may have to assist learners to unlearn. As educators relinquish control, they praise and communicate, motivate with deeds rather than words, avoid intimidating students, and are always concerned with what is right.[43]

Adult education enriches one's life because more education leads to better employment. To pursue higher education is a personal decision that can be advanced by management. Completion of the bachelor of science (BSN) by associate degree in nursing (ADN) or diploma graduates is an example. Research has validated that increased productivity comes from investing in people and their education.

Typologies and Taxonomies of Adult Education

Various typologies and taxonomies exist in education. The most commonly known taxonomies, or classifications, are those of educational objectives addressed to cognitive, affective, and psychomotor domains. Taxonomies and typologies help to connect the parts of an educational system, clarify the field, serve as a basis for allocating resources, design curricula, and eliminate duplication. Several taxonomies and typologies of adult education exist, including those of Houle, Boshier, Knowles, Bryson, and Grattan. Using these as background, Rachal has proposed his typology of adult education based on six major types and their subtypes (see Exhibit 4-5).[44]

1. Liberal. Individual- or group-structured study of the humanities, arts, and sciences in which there is free inquiry, curiosity, and intellectual growth. Such studies include university lecture series, Great Decisions programs, Great Books programs, reading circles, and writing clubs.
2. Occupational. Technological changes.
3. Self-help. Knowledge, information, skills, or recreational learning related to adjusting to the environment.
4. Compensatory. Knowledge to meet new standards and to combat illiteracy, including adult basic education and adult secondary education.
5. Scholastic. Graduate study and research.
6. Social action. Peace education, environmental education, drug education, and the fostering of understanding of major public issues. Because social action is, by definition, political, the adult educator would describe rather than prescribe and would focus on the educative aspect rather than the political orientation of the social action agents.

Other relevant typologies apply to life stages and "the question of the presence of underlying sequence in an adult's progression through working life."[45]

Sanderson dwells on the midcareer group of individuals (35 to 55 years of age) as the largest group in the organization. He indicates that the group has grief and confusion that leads to reassessment, which leads to further redefinition of values and goals and on to future commitment. It is during this period that self-fulfillment and self-actualization needs emerge.[46] An effective HRD program at this phase (or these phases) of work life could include the following:

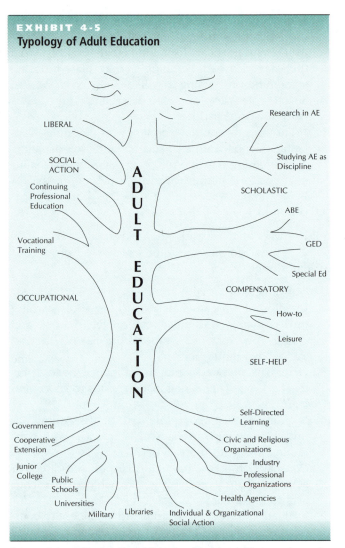

EXHIBIT 4-5
Typology of Adult Education

Source: John R. Rachal. Unpublished revision from "Taxonomies and Typologies of Adult Education." *Lifelong Learning*, 12(2), (1988), 20–23. Reprinted with permission of John R. Rachal.

- Providing mentorship activities.
- Assisting leaders to help employees to balance work, family, and self-development through programs promoting and supporting positive growth orientation.
- Assisting employees in making a fit with jobs within the organization by moving up, across, down, or out.
- Creating opportunities for staff to gain satisfaction from work.
- Providing variety and challenges in the job.
- Creating an aggressive organizational development (OD) program that values people; balances work, leisure, and learning; provides a climate for the whole person; redesigns positions to promote flexible hours, job sharing, pairing (teams), and permanent part-time positions; institutes self-managing

work teams; emphasizes on innovation; provides strong rewards and recognition; and creates a peer support program.

- Creating an aggressive staff development program that accomplishes all of the foregoing. It would include training in the skills of coaching, counseling, and mentoring; managing life transitions; retraining; expanded sabbaticals; providing opportunities for job exchanges outside the organization and in new fields; and creating a career subsidization fund.[47]

Human Capital

An emerging theory for HRD is that employees are human capital who can be treated as assets because they have high economic value. In a technological world, the assets of human beings are their knowledge and skills, which depreciate as new technology emerges. Employers invest in their human capital by providing HRD programs in the form of staff development and continuing education. Odiorne writes that "Human capital economics is a system of inputs, processes, outputs, and adjustments which individuals, firms, government agencies, institutions, and societies make toward the increases of potential and performance which the individual human or humans as groups may contribute to society, the economy, specific employers, or themselves."[48] In nursing, the inputs are newly employed nurses who come to organizations with a continuum of assets, such as specialty certification, graduate education, certification in life support systems, and skills in management, teaching, and research.

Processes provided by management include orientation, internships, preceptorships, staff development, certification, and continuing education. Self-directed continuing education, including courses and reading, add to the RN's assets. All of these processes lead to adaptation and growth, maintaining and increasing the value of the RN's assets.

Outputs of this system of management of human capital are competence, specialists, profits or return on equity, and value added to the human assets. Adjustments include retraining as new jobs emerge and rehabilitation after lapses in employment. Human capital—professional nurses—are kept valuable through HRD programs that promote motivation or job satisfaction. Their power should be unleashed by managers who bring them to the table to share the leadership role.[49]

Odiorne indicates that community colleges are a proven investment in human capital because their products increase the personal disposable income of people who complete college courses. Education promotes upward mobility. Educated citizens are informed citizens who make better citizenship decisions. Investment in education by minorities leads to increased social status. Investment in human capital increases capital promotion through increased earnings.[50]

Drucker observes that knowledge workers must know the task; manage themselves, that is, be autonomous; innovate continuously; learn continuously, produce quality work; and be seen and treated as assets. His observations apply to professional nurses.[51]

Human Capital Portfolio

There has been difficulty in placing a dollar value on human assets. The nursing skills that give the highest value to the nurse should be identified. If a nurse's value can be measured in terms of dollars, this value can be measured before and after HRD programs to ascertain the change in value. It can be measured annually to determine any increase or decrease in value. A number of models exist for treating human beings as assets, among which is the portfolio model.

Vocational education increases the value of human resources. The payoff comes with the fit of graduates into the economy and culture. This fit should be a goal of an effective HRD program.

Each employee is a human asset with current and contingent value, because he or she produces and will continue to produce salable goods and services. A nursing organization has a portfolio of people assets who can be managed to increase their value through expenditures for updated knowledge and skills. They thus maintain a return on equity called productivity.

Theoretically, a nurse researcher could study the effects of HRD as well as the interest on currently held assets by

1. Updating the skills or knowledge of one group but not another, and studying the income produced by each group.
2. Assigning nurses with one level of education to one group and those with a different level to another group (diploma-ADN versus BSN). The outcomes produced by each group would be measured and compared.

Default risk has been very high in nursing because of job availability. This high risk could be lowered by long-term employment contracts that spell out career development. Nursing has not always responded to market demands with greatly increased salaries. This lack of response may be partly due to the interchangeability of nurses with varying educational levels, with emphasis frequently being placed on technical rather than cognitive skills that include critical thinking. Nursing leadership can integrate technical skills with critical thinking by instituting differentiated practice, participative management, career development programs, and job enrichment.

Hiring and placement of nurses should have as an objective matching qualifications with need. Thus, the value of the nurse asset will correspond with market demand.

Forecasting changes in mission serves as a basis for forecasting needs for human assets. Although there may be some errors in the forecast, it should be done. The following are some of the factors that should be considered in forecasting nurse supply and demand:

- Population growth to approximately 291 million people by the year 2000, and aging of the population.
- Birth, death, and immigration rates.
- Migration (especially to the Sunbelt), urbanization, quantitative factors, differences in life span, changing values, new infrastructure, and new services.
- Status of formal investment in education as an investment in human capital.
- Student sources, faculty sources, and consumer characteristics.[52]

An "attractive human assets portfolio will produce a work force with high potential for contribution, versatility of skills, stability of tenure, long years of future services, and high quality of performance in relation to the goals of the firm."[53]

Many corporations have their own internal training organizations. They can retrain employees and plan for new business developments. This type of HRD leads to economic growth and reduction of human losses from the portfolio, although accountants do not readily accept the concept of treating human beings as assets.

Successful HRM programs are designed to do the following[54]:

1. Focus on behavior rather than personality; they want people to be productive, creative, and skilled.
2. Obtain results, rather than focus on the process. OD focuses on results, with successful programs that relate training to the organization's content, culture, and climate.
3. Recognize that not all management problems are behavioral problems.
4. Have specific objectives and criteria.
5. Produce agents of change and betterment.
6. Use simulations.
7. Break down the total training objectives in successive stages; job instruction training breaks training into steps for mastery.

8. Require the learner to take some action during training, making results easier to measure.
9. Give immediate feedback: simulated, fast, related to behavior, favorable or pleasant, and influencing behavior.
10. Measure results against goals. Define the desired behaviors in advance, break them down into small steps, simulate them, and measure mastery by percentage of success.

Typology for Human Resource Development of Personnel

Odiorne suggests a four-category typology for HRD of personnel: stars, workhorses, problems, and deadwood. He suggests training each group separately as follows[55]:

1. Stars. Stars are a small group of personnel with high potential whose performance lives up to that potential. Managers should educate stars to increase performance and develop their potential once they have been identified by the assessment center method, review board method, or staff analysis method.

   Top managers still pick successors like themselves with perceived star qualities, such as adaptability to change, company and career orientation, ability to manage self-expression, lateral and upward mobility, dedication, loyalty, adaptivity, quiet differentiation, early achievement, ability to work in a web of tensions, gamesmanship, flexibility, and ability to generalize.

   Stars of the future will be surrounded by technology, be comfortable with high-level decision-making and problem analysis, do less traveling, have more span of control over work, and be a collaborative group leader. Future stars will also be innovative. On their way to stardom, they will acquire a master's degree in business administration (MBA) or nursing administration (MSN), use skills, be creative, create new jobs, and be entrepreneurs in technology, engineers, and scientists. Stars will appreciate the liberal arts as the accumulated knowledge of civilization. Future stars will have skills of rational thought, decision-making, problem-solving, ethical evaluation, communication; knowledge of government; and special education and experiences. Future stars will be trained by stars as mentors who are goal oriented, are superior performers, behave to be imitated, support and help, delegate responsibility, give feedback, exhibit a positive attitude, mentor women and minorities, are sponsors, and provide support groups. Some nurses are stars inculcated with the success ethic. Nursing leaders can develop HRD programs that will provide the ingredients.

2. Workhorses. These persons can be trained to improve their performance. They can be motivated using theories of Maslow, McGregor, and Herzberg, among others. They should be well paid for their work, participate in decision-making by merging personal and organizational goals, and be provided with opportunities for job enrichment. Organizational development will motivate workhorses through job design, working conditions, increased variety of tools, development of higher skills, assignment of increased responsibility, job rotation, content change, and team competition. Workhorses thrive on HRD programs that provide for personal growth, self-fulfillment, and use of abilities to perform meaningful work in a pleasant workplace.

3. Problems. Problem employees exhibit undesirable behavior that can be corrected by remedial training. They may exhibit emotional outbursts or immaturity, ignore important things, be overcome by trivia, be slow to respond to change, retain obsolete ideas and procedures, treat people unfairly, enforce rules too rigidly, retain authority, fail to communicate, be too lax, and lack a sense of timing and the ability to anticipate. To avoid or remedy their poor performance, training should be preceded by specifying performance standards, removing obstacles to success, providing the needed training, providing favorable consequences for doing right, providing feedback, encouraging self-control, and helping them with their personal problems.

4. Deadwood. *Deadwood* is a term used to describe workers who do not respond to training or developmental discipline. They should be fired, using appropriate HR procedures. Not only are they nonproductive, they also negatively influence personnel who are workhorses and problems.

Nurse managers may want to turn workhorses into stars, which requires need and drive on the part of the workhorse. Bell Laboratories and Dupont Company have had considerable success in doing this. Stars say the most important skills include technical competence and taking initiative to go beyond basic job duties.[56]

The Future

Strategic HRD will envision future change so that the quality of work life and standard of living for nursing personnel will continue to improve in the twenty-first century. Change will include proactive involvement of nurses in the formulation of health care policy. Nursing leaders need to communicate the needs of the future, including skills and job requirements.[57]

Electronic technology is intrusive. As it becomes more intensive, it will increase time-based stress. This stress will be an area for further research, including reaction to demands on time and the social influences of electronic technology intrusion.[58]

Possible futures range from the very awful to the very wonderful. Although the threat that nuclear weapons will destroy human civilization has diminished, it still exists. Humankind has destabilized the environment with resource, food, energy, and population problems. HRD's goal is to avoid major deterioration of human life. The possibility of the utilization and settlement of space exists, as does that of contact with extraterrestrial intelligence. HRD programs will prepare for future interaction by developing a better understanding of our universe and our place in it. The future can be a highly positive one if adult educators, including nurse leaders, prepare people for it. HRD programs can help people regain a sense of social mission if the curricula and programs are designed accordingly. Adult education that prepares for the future would be studied and discussed in every community. HRD programs would train the leaders and help the helpers, conduct or encourage research in the field, and view nurse managers as learners themselves.[59]

Naisbitt and Aburdene, who view the future as providing more upward mobility for women and minorities as they gain credentials and tenure, echo the positive approach to the twenty-first century. An abundance of good jobs will be available for which people will be educated and trained. Two million new managerial, administrative, and technical jobs will be created annually. The entire work force must be upgraded constantly. More people will start their own businesses, or they will become highly skilled professionals who will not be managed authoritatively. "The dominant principle of organization has shifted, from management in order to control an enterprise to leadership in order to bring out the best in people and to respond quickly to change."[60]

The primary challenge of leadership today is to encourage the new, better-educated worker to be more entrepreneurial, self-managing, and oriented toward lifelong learning. Leaders will coach, inspire, and gain people's commitment. They will set personal examples of excellence. Leaders will manage to bring out the best in people and respond quickly to change. They will encourage self-management, autonomous teams, and entrepreneurial units. Leaders will move people in a direction without carrying them. They will inspire loyalty by giving it. Leaders will create vision and sell it to their constituents. They will be ethical, open, empowering, and inspiring as teachers, counselors, and facilitators who will keep employees excited by managing accelerated change.

In their book *Megatrends 2000*, Naisbitt and Aburdene proposed the following[61]:

1. "The booming global economy of the 1990s
2. A renaissance in the arts
3. The emergence of free-market socialism
4. Global lifestyles and cultural nationalism
5. The privatization of the welfare state
6. The rise of the Pacific rim
7. The decade of women in leadership
8. The age of biology
9. The religious revival of the new millennium
10. The triumph of the individual"

Naisbitt now says that society is a "technologically intoxicated zone" with these symptoms[62]:

1. "We favor the quick fix, from religion to nutrition.
2. We fear and worship technology.
3. We blur the distinction between real and fake.
4. We accept violence as normal.
5. We love technology as a toy.
6. We live our lives distanced and distracted."

Summary

As the clinical practice discipline of nursing evolves, so does the concept of wholeness. Staff development thus becomes a component of the larger domain of HRD. Business and industry leaders have found that productivity is positively influenced by a focus on development of personnel to their fullest potential. As a consequence, the assembly lines in factories have given way to self-directed work teams. Given responsibility for making decisions and accomplishing the organization's mission, employees rise to fulfill expectations.

The new management practice eliminates middle management and places trust in the worker. With this trust, workers are energized and empowered by autonomy, the control they have over the productive work of the enterprise.

Workers learn to work in teams and to rotate within the group roles, including being able to perform several jobs. They learn to support each other and to respect the varied talents of individual team members.

Adult education, or andragogy, is the process by which employees are kept updated to achieve both the goals of the organization and their own personal goals. Andragogy is also the process by which they develop their roles as citizens and benefit themselves, society, and the organization for which they work.

People are viewed and valued as human capital. As technology advances, they depreciate in knowledge capacity and ability to perform their jobs. Adult education as staff development is an investment that keeps human value from depreciating. This entire process represents the science of behavioral technology. Satisfied employees achieve organizational and personal objectives, satisfy customers, and make an organization successful. Included in the science of behavioral technology are theories such as decision-making, decentralization and participatory management, leadership, motivation, and the growing need for adult education that maintains the human capital and keeps the organization productive. The HRD theory will be developed further in subsequent chapters.

APPLICATION EXERCISES

Most of these exercises can be completed through individual or group work. If you desire, form a group of your peers and complete the exercises together.

EXERCISE 4-1   Identify a human resource problem from the area in which you work. How is this problem being resolved? How could it be resolved using the science of behavioral technology?

EXERCISE 4-2   Discuss the meanings of *autonomy* and *empowerment*. List working conditions in the organization in which you work that keep professional nurses from attaining autonomy and empowerment. Make management plans for resolving each condition using the following format.

OBJECTIVE:

ACTIVITIES	DATE TO BE COMPLETED	PERSONS RESPONSIBLE	ACCOMPLISHMENTS

EXERCISE 4-3

Describe learning activities in your life that are self-directed. Decide where you want to expand your self-directed learning and make a plan for doing so. List knowledge and skills you wish to acquire as a citizen, an employee, and an individual.

EXERCISE 4-4

Apply a brainstorming technique (see also Chapter 15, Committees and Other Groups). As a group technique, brainstorming seeks to develop creativity by free association of ideas. The object is to generate as many ideas as possible. All members of the group should respond positively. A member must never criticize the suggestions of another member because doing so stifles free expression of ideas.

1. Have available one poster pad (or chalkboard), one marker pen (or chalk), and masking tape.
2. Select any topic of current interest to the group that presents problems for which they can create solutions. If the group has no topic, they could discuss using one of the following: "Principles of adult learning (andragogy) as they are being practiced in the group workplace," "Middle management needs to be eliminated in health care organizations," or "There is no such thing as a lifetime job anymore."
3. Plan a 1-hour session. Elect a leader (facilitator) and a recorder for the group. The facilitator explains the process and the topic to the group and tells members to say whatever comes into their minds as quickly as possible. The facilitator prevents criticism of one member by another and encourages free expression of ideas throughout the process. Everyone is encouraged to participate—the wilder the ideas, the better.
4. The recorder writes the ideas on the poster pad. The goal is to come up with as many ideas as possible. If ideas fit together, the recorder combines them. When a page is filled, the recorder tears it off and tapes it to the wall or some other visible place.
5. After 45 minutes have elapsed, the facilitator uses the remaining time to evaluate all ideas. All ideas are evaluated positively, and the group decides how to proceed with the outcomes.

EXERCISE 4-5

Apply the nominal group technique (see also Chapter 15, Committees and Other Groups). The nominal group process is a method for structuring a group meeting to obtain a large number of ideas and to order and prioritize those ideas.

1. Supplies: pencils or pens and paper or 5 × 8 file cards, poster pad or chalkboard, marker pen or chalk, and masking tape.
2. Choose a topic of interest to the group, or discuss the following topic: "Professional nurses have limited autonomy and empowerment."
3. Time required: 1.5 to 2 hours.
4. Elect a leader or facilitator to define the process and assign the topic to the group.
5. Give each member a pencil or pen and a sheet of paper or a 5 × 8 file card. Ask them to write down all possible ideas about the assigned topic. Allow 5 to 10 minutes.
6. Have all group members present an idea to the group, one at a time, until all lists are exhausted. Do not allow discussion at this point. If an idea occurs to a group member as another is speaking, he or she can add it to the bottom of his or her list, to be shared later.
7. The leader or facilitator lists all ideas on the poster pad or chalkboard as they are shared, according to the following rules:
    7.1. No discussion or evaluation of ideas during the round-robin sharing and listing on the poster pad.
    7.2. No debate about equivalency of ideas. All are written on the chart, even if they appear to be the same or closely related to another on the chart.
    7.3. No rewording of an idea while it is being listed on the chart.
    7.4. No talking out of turn. If the process suggests a new idea to an individual, he or she can give it when his or her turn comes again.
8. As pad pages fill up, tear them off and tape them to the wall or other surface so they can be seen by group members.
9. Once all ideas are listed, each recorded idea is discussed for clarification, elaboration, defense, and evaluation. New items can be added or categories suggested for ideas.
10. After all ideas are discussed, the group votes on and gives priority to each.
11. The results are averaged and the final group decision is taken from the pool and prescribed to the appropriate entity for implementation.

NOTES

1. J. Naisbitt and P. Aburdene, *Megatrends 2000* (New York: William Morrow and Company, 1990), 16.

2. P. A. Strassman and S. Zuboff, "Conversation with Paul A. Strassman," *Organizational Dynamics* (fall 1985), 19–34; A. J. Rutigliano, "Naisbitt and Aburdene on 'Re-Inventing' the Workplace," *Management Review* (October 1985), 33–35.

3. M. Beer, B. Spector, P. R. Lawrence, D. Q. Mills, and R. E. Walton, *Managing Human Assets* (New York: The Free Press, 1984).

4. P. D. Carter, "Revitalizing Society: Practicing Human Resource Development Through the Life Span," *Lifelong Learning: An Omnibus of Practice and Research*, 11(6), (1988), 27–31.

5. M. Beer et al., op. cit.

6. D. M. Brethower and G. A Rummler, "For Improved Work Performance: Accentuate the Positive," *Personnel* (October 1966), 40–49; R. C. Swansburg, Management of Patient Care Services (St. Louis: C. V. Mosby, 1976), 232–234.

7. D. H. Smith, "Adult and Continuing Education and Human Resource Development: Present Competitors, Potential Partners," *Lifelong Learning: An Onmibus of Practice and Research*, 12(7), (1989), 13–17.

8. Ibid.

9. J. Bengtsson, "Education, Training and Labor Market Development," *Futures* (December 1991), 1085–1106.

10. M. Beer et al., 43.

11. M. L. Hammerman, "Adult Learning in Self-Help Mutual/Aid Support Groups," *Lifelong Learning: An Omnibus of Practice and Research*, 12(1), (1988), 25–27, 30.

12. L. Kuokkanen and H. Leino-Kilpi, "Power and Empowerment in Nursing: Three Theoretical Approaches," *Journal of Advanced Nursing* (January 2000), 235–241.

13. J. Naisbitt and P. Aburdene, op. cit.

14. J. S. Lublin, "Trying to Increase Worker Productivity, More Employers Alter Management Style," *The Wall Street Journal* (14 February 1992), B1, B7.

15. C. Zwingman-Bagley, "Transformational Management Style Positively Affects Financial Outcomes," *Nursing Administration Quarterly* (summer 1999), 29–34.

16. G. E. Chandler and S. J. Roberts, "Student Perceptions of Empowerment in Their Graduate Program," *Revolution* (summer 1998), 43–46.

17. P. D. Carter, op. cit.; M. S. Knowles, *The Modern Practice of Adult Education* (New York, NY: Association Press, 1980), L. H. Friedman and D. B. White, "What is Quality, Who Wants It and Why?" *Management Care Quarterly* (autumn 1999), 40–46.

18. D. Cassivi, "The Education of Adults: Maintaining a Legacy," *Lifelong Learning: An Omnibus of Practice and Research*, 12(5), (1989), 8–10.

19. M. L. Hammerman, op. cit.

20. B. L. Wells and S. C. Padgitt, "Timebinds: Mediating Organizational and Professional Role Expectations of the Adult Educator," *Lifelong Learning: An Omnibus of Practice and Research*, 12(7), (1989), 22–25.

21. S. Wituk, M. D. Shepherd, S. Slavich, M. L. Warren, and G. Meissen, "A Topography of Self-Help Groups: An Empirical Analysis," *Social Work* (March 2000), 157–165.

22. L. J. Roberts, D. Salem, J. Rappaport, P. A. Toro, D. A. Luke, and E. Seidman, "Giving and Receiving Help: Interpersonal Transactions in Mutual-Help Meetings and Psychosocial Adjustment of Members," *American Journal of Community Psychology* (December 1999), 841–868.

23. J. C. Carroll et al., "Changing Physicians' Attitudes Toward Self-Help Groups: An Educational Intervention," *Journal of Cancer Education* (spring 2000), 14–18.

24. E. J. Metz, "The Missing 'H' in Strategic Planning," *Managerial Planning* (May–June 1984), 19–23, 29.

25. E. C. Smith, "How to Tie Human Resource Planning to Strategic Business Planning," *Managerial Planning* (September–October 1983), 29–34.

26. Ibid.

27. E. J. Metz, op. cit.

28. J. S. Lublin, op. cit; B. Davis and D. Milbank, "If the U. S. Work Ethic is Fading, 'Laziness' may not be the Reason," *The Wall Street Journal* (7 February 1992), 1, A5.

29. D. Cassivi, op. cit.

30. B. L. Wells and S. C. Padgett, op. cit.

31. R. S. Shuler, "Strategic Human Resources Management: Linking the People with the Strategic Needs of the Business," *Organizational Dynamics* (summer 1992), 18–22.

32. M. Cameron and J. R. Snyder, "Strategic Human Resource Management: Redefining the Role of the Manager and the Worker," *Clinical Laboratory Management Review* (September–October 1999), 242–250.

33. J. Siddiqui and B. H. Kleiner, "Human Resource Management in the Health Care Industry," *Health Manpower Management*, 24(4–5), 143–147.

34. P. M. Wright and G. C. McMahan, "Theoretical Perspectives for Strategic Human Resource Management," *Journal of Management*, 18(2), (1992), 295–320.

35. D. Ulrich, Strategic and Human Resource Planning: Linking Customers to Employees," *Strategic and Human Resources Planning*, 15(2), (1992), 47–62.

36. M. S. Knowles, "Gearing Adult Education for the Seventies," *The Journal of Continuing Education in Nursing* (May 1970), 11–17, B. B. Nielsen, "Applying Andragogy in Nursing Continuing Education." *The Journal of Continuing Education in Nursing* (July–August 1992), 148–151.

37. Ibid.

38. F. Milligan, "In Defense of Andragogy. Part 2: An Educational Process Consistent with Modern Nursing's Aims," *Nurse Education Today* (December 1997), 487–493.

39. C. Goodwin-Johansson, "Educating the Adult Patient," *Lifelong Learning: An Onmibus of Practice and Research*, 11(7), (1988), 10–13.

40. Ibid.

41. T. M. Castaldi, "Adult Learning: Transferring Skills from the Workplace to the Classroom," *Lifelong Learning: An Omnibus of Practice and Research*, 12(6), (1989), 17–19.

42. M. W. Galbraith, "Essential Skills for the Facilitator of Adult Learning," *Lifelong Learning: An Omnibus of Practice and Research*, 12(6), (1989), 10–13.

43. D. Cassivi, op. cit.

44. J. Rachal, "Taxonomies and Typologies of Adult Education," *Lifelong Learning: An Omnibus of Adult Education*, 12(2), (1988), 20–23.

45. D. Riverin-Simard, "Phases of Working Life and Adult Education," *Lifelong Learning: An Omnibus of Practice and Research*, 12(2), (1988), 24–26.

46. D. R. Sanderson, "Mid-Career Support: An Approach to Lifelong Learning in an Organization," *Lifelong Learning: An Omnibus of Practice and Research*, 12(7), (1989), 7–10.

47. Ibid.

48. G. S. Odiorne, *Strategic Management of Human Resources*, (San Francisco: Jossey-Bass, 1984), 5.

49. L. F. Hepner and L. G. Hopkins, "Partnership 2000: A Journey to the 21st Century," *Nursing Administration Quarterly* (winter 2000), 34–44.

50. G. S. Odiorne, op. cit.

51. P. F. Drucker, *Management Challenges for the 21st Century* (New York: HarperCollins, 1999), 142.
52. G. S. Odiorne, op. cit.
53. Ibid, 46.
54. Ibid.
55. Ibid.
56. J. E. Rigdon, "Using New Kinds of Corporate Alchemy, Some Firms Turn Lesser Lights into Stars," *The Wall Street Journal* (3 May 1993), B1, B13.
57. M. Beer, B. Spector, P. R. Lawrence, D. Q. Mills, and R. E. Walton, op. cit.
58. M. L. Wells and S. C. Padgett, op. cit.
59. A. Tough, "Potential Futures: Implications for Adult Education," *Lifelong Learning: An Omnibus of Practice and Research*, 11(1), (1987), 10–12.
60. J. Naisbitt and P. Aburdene, op. cit., 218.
61. Ibid, 13.
62. J. Naisbitt, *High Tech High Touch* (New York: Broadway Books, 1999), 5.

REFERENCES

Cooper, J. M. "State of the Nation: Therapeutic Jurisprudence and the Evolution of the Right of Self-Determination in International Law." *Behavioral Science Law*, 17(5), (1999), 607–643.

Davenport, J. III. "Is There Any Way Out of the Andragogy Morass?" *Lifelong Learning: An Omnibus of Practice and Research*, 11(3), (1987), 17–20.

Hutchings, D. "Partnership in Education: An Example of Client and Educator Collaboration." *Journal of Continuing Education in Nursing* (May–June 1999), 128–131.

Johns, C. "Reflection as Empowerment." *Nursing Inquiry* (December 1999), 241–249.

Kelley, L. S. "Evaluating Change in Quality of Life from the Perspective of the Person: Advanced Practice Nursing and Parse's Goal of Nursing." *Holistic Nursing Practice* (July 1999), 61–70.

Kirsch, M. "The Myth of Informed Consent." *American Journal of Gastroenterology* (March 2000), 588–589.

Kreitlow, B. W., ed. *Examining Controversies in Adult Education* (San Francisco: Jossey Bass, 1981).

Kress, K. "Therapeutic Jurisprudence and the Resolution of Value Conflicts: What We Can Realistically Expect, in Practice, from Theory." *Behavioral Science Law*, 17(5), (1999), 555–588.

Lenz, R., R. Blaser, and K. A. Kuhn. "Hospital Information Systems: Chances and Obstacles on the Way to Integration." *Student Health Technology Information*, 68, (1999), 25–30.

Lloyd, P., J. Braithwaite, and G. Southon. "Empowerment and the Performance of Health Services." *Journal of Managerial Medicine*, 13(2–3), (1999), 83–94.

Morstain, B. R. and J. C. Smart. "A Motivational Typology of Adult Education." *Journal of Higher Education* (November–December 1977), 665–679.

Netten, A. and J. Knight. "Annuitizing the Human Capital Investment Costs of Health Care Professionals." *Health Economics* (May 1999), 245–255.

Platzer, H., D. Blake, and D. Ashford. "An Evaluation of Process and Outcomes from Learning Through Reflective Practice Groups on a Post-Registration Nursing Course." *Journal of Advanced Nursing* (March 2000), 689–695.

Podeschi, R. L. "Andragogy: Proofs or Premises?" *Lifelong Learning: An Omnibus of Practice and Research*, 11(3), (1987), 14–16, 20.

Strickland, D. and O. C. O'Connell. "Saving Your Career in the 21st Century." *Journal of Case Management* (Summer 1998), 47–51.

Sturt, J. "Placing Empowerment Research within an Action Research Typology." *Journal of Advanced Nursing* (November 1999), 1057–1063.

Snelgrove, S. and D. Hughes. "Interprofessional Relations Between Doctors and Nurses: Perspectives from South Wales." *Journal of Advanced Nursing* (March 2000), 661–667.

Zairi, M. "Building Human Resources Capability in Health Care: A Global Analysis of Best Practice—Part 1." *Health Manpower Management*, 24(2–3), (1998), 88–99.

Zairi, M. "Building Human Resources Capability in Health Care: A Global Analysis of Best Practice—Part II." *Health Manpower Management*, 24(4–5), (1998), 128–138.

Zairi, M. "Building Human Resources Capability in Healthcare: A Global Analysis of Best Practice." *Health Manpower Management*, 24(4–5), (1998), 166–169.

CHAPTER 5

The Planning Process

Russell C. Swansburg, PhD, RN

LEARNING OBJECTIVES AND ACTIVITIES

- Define planning.
- Differentiate among examples of the purposes of planning.
- Differentiate among examples of the characteristics of planning.
- Differentiate among examples of the elements of planning.
- Describe the strategic planning process.
- Describe operational planning.
- Differentiate among examples of strategic and tactical planning.
- Write a business plan.

CONCEPTS: Planning, strategic planning, functional planning, venture planning, operational planning, divisional planning, unit planning, business plan.

MANAGER BEHAVIOR: Does strategic and operational planning with key management personnel and uses on a daily basis.

LEADER BEHAVIOR: Develops a strategic plan with inputs from representative personnel of the entire organization. Coaches management staff in developing and implementing operational plans that support the strategic plan. With management staff, does periodic audits of results and the need for change.

What Is Planning?

Planning, a basic function of management, is a principal duty of all managers. It is a systematic process and requires knowledgeable activity based on sound managerial theory.

The first element of management defined by Fayol was planning, which he defined as making a plan of action to provide for the foreseeable future. This plan of action must have unity, continuity, flexibility, and precision. Fayol outlined the contents of a plan of action for his business, a large mining and metallurgical firm. The plan included annual and 10-year forecasts, taking advantage of input from others. Planning improves with experience, gives sequence in activity, and protects a business against undesirable changes. Fayol's concept was that planning facilitates wise use of resources and selection of the best approaches to achieving objectives. Planning facilitates the art of handling people. Because planning can fail, it requires moral courage. Effective planning requires continuity of tenure. Good planning is a sign of competence.[1]

Urwick wrote that research in administration provides needed information for forecasting. According to Urwick, investigations should be carried out and their results expressed in concrete terms. Planning should be based on objectives that should be framed in terms of making a product or providing a service for the community. Simplification and standardization are basic to sound planning procedures. The product or service should be of the right pattern. Planning provides information to coordinate work effectively and accurately. A good plan should be based on an objective; have standards; be simple, flexible, and balanced; and use available resources first.[2]

> Planning is a continuous process, beginning with the setting of goals and objectives and then laying out a plan of action to accomplish them, put them into play, review the process and the outcomes, provide feedback to personnel, and modify as needed. As planning is put into action, the management functions of organizing, leading, and evaluating are implemented, making all management functions interdependent.

Planning is a thinking or mental process of decision-making and forecasting. It is future oriented and ensures desirable probable outcomes. Planning involves determining objectives and strategies, programs, procedures, and rules to accomplish the objectives.[3] In nursing, planning helps to ensure that clients or patients will receive the nursing services they want and need and that these services are delivered by satisfied nursing workers.[4]

Ackoff describes four orientations to planning: reactivism, inactivism, preactivism, and interactivism.[5]

1. Reactivism. Reactivism looks to the past and considers technology an enemy. It supports the old organizational forms of an authoritarian, paternalistic hierarchy. Control operates from the top, with plans submitted from the bottom. Problems are addressed separately, with immediate supervisors adjusting, editing, and adding to plans as they proceed through the hierarchy to the top. Reactive planning is ritualistic; in such systems, planning is considered a prerogative of management. Experience is considered the best teacher and age gives knowledge, understanding, and wisdom. Technological advances of other organizations replace products and services of organizations oriented to reactive planning. Reactive oriented organizations support the arts and humanities, people and values, a sense of history, feelings of continuity, and preservation of traditions. Reactivists do tactical (short-range or operational) planning.

2. Inactivism. Inactivism as a planning orientation prevents change. It operates by crisis management, where the goal is to control discomfort without addressing its cause. Managers are kept busy with red tape and bureaucracy. The effective instrument is the committee, which operates to keep people busy until the work is outdated or success is thwarted by insufficient resources. Knowledge of current events plus connections is more important than is competency. Manners are valued. Inactivists do tactical or operational planning.

3. Preactivism. Dominant in U.S. organizations, preactivistic managers accelerate change to exploit the future. They believe technology causes change and is therefore a panacea. Values associated with preactivism include management by objectives, inventiveness, growth, permissiveness, decentralization, and informality. Planning is done from the top down, with objectives. The appeal of preactivism is that planning is associated with science and technology, the future. Because preactivism is based mainly on long-term forecasting, it is often full of errors.

4. Interactivism. Interactivists believe the future can be created, and therefore design a desirable future and invent ways to achieve it. In this view, technology is valued depending on how it is used; experience reveals problems, and experiment leads to their solutions. The focus is on development, learning, and adaptation. Interactivistic planners may establish a planning period for achieving goals, objectives, and ideals. Goals are considered ends to be attained within the planning period. Objectives are ends hoped for eventually, but progress is expected within the planning period. Ideals are ends that are not entirely attainable, but progress is expected within and after the planning period. Interactivists emphasize normative planning.

The present health care environment does not always support reactive planning by nurse managers. It is too competitive, both for patients and for scarce expert professional nurse providers. Nurse providers also resist authoritarianism and paternalism because they want to participate. Inactivism as a planning orientation is prevalent in subsidized government agencies, service departments of corporations, and universities. Nurse managers will participate in such planning in these institutions. Nurse managers fall into the technological traps of preactivism. Plans are frequently made; however, many never become operational. Preactivists concentrate on strategic (long-range) planning.

Ackoff's interactive planning–management model is a systems model that can be applied in nursing management to effect change. A planning board does interactive planning–management. In a decentralized organization the planning board would be the nurse manager of a unit, her or his boss, and the employees of the unit.[6]

The following are the five phases of Ackoff's interactive planning–management model[7]:

1. Formulation of the mess. The "mess" is the future we are now in—the future we are now creating. Formulation of the mess includes determination of what problems and opportunities the organization faces, how they interact, and what obstructs or constrains doing something about them. The output of this phase is a scenario of the future the organization would be likely to have if its behavior and that of its environment did not change in any significant way.

2. Ends planning (idealized redesign) is the design of the desired future. The output of this phase is the idealized design. This design is focused on the present, how it could be right now. The design must be technologically feasible and operationally viable and be capable of incorporating learning and adapting and being adapted.

3. Means planning is inventing ways to close the gaps between the idealized present and the mess. It involves identifying potential means, evaluating the alternatives, and selecting the best ones.

4. Resource planning includes determining when, where, and what resources will be required and how they will be generated. Resources include facilities, equipment, personnel, information, money, and other inputs.

5. Implementation and control involve translating the decisions made in the previous phases into a set of assignments and schedules that specify who will be responsible for doing what and when.

Exhibit 5-1 illustrates an interactive planning cycle.

Which type of planning is best for a nursing organization? Many nurse managers would opt for interactivism, because it is proactive. Some of the characteristics of reactivism, inactivism, and preactivism are also useful to present-day nurse managers. One could assess the working environment, decide which orientation to planning is most productive, and attempt to move in that direction. A nurse manager could select a style of planning that blends reactivism, inactivism, preactivism, and interactivism. Ackoff and others opt for the interactive planning–management model.

Purposes

The following are some reasons for planning[8]:

- It increases the chances of success by focusing on results, and not on activities.
- It forces analytic thinking and evaluation of alternatives, thereby improving decisions.
- It establishes a framework for decision-making that is consistent with top management objectives.
- It orients people to action rather than reaction.
- It includes day-to-day and future-focused managing.
- It helps to avoid crisis management and provides decision-making flexibility.
- It provides a basis for managing organizational and individual performance.
- It increases employee involvement and improves communication.
- It is cost-effective.

Among the activities of planning that Douglass addresses are assessment by collection, classification, analysis, interpretation, and translation of data; strategic planning; development of standards; identification of needs and priority setting; management by objectives; and formulation of policies, rules, regulations, methods, and procedures.[9]

Donovan wrote that planning has several benefits, among which are satisfactory outcomes of decisions;

improved functions in emergencies; assurance of economy of time, space, and materials; and the highest use of personnel. She included decision-making, philosophies, and objectives as key elements in planning.[10]

Several factors relative to successful planning should be known and put into action by successful managers, which are knowledge of the following:

- Characteristics of planning
- Elements of the planning process
- Strategic or long-range planning process
- Tactical or short-range planning process—functional versus operational
- Planning standards

A knowledge of and skill in applying the planning processes, including standards, to the work situation also is necessary as is skill in bringing the planning process up to the standard set when deficiencies exist.[11]

Characteristics

What is the nature of planning? What is so distinctive about it that requires a nurse administrator to have the knowledge and skills requisite to engage in planning? In an environment of changing technology, mounting costs, and multiple activities, there is a need for the chief nurse administrator and subordinate managers to plan. The forecasting of events and the laying out of a system of activities or actions for accomplishing the work of nursing and of the organization are prerequisites to success. Koontz and Weihrich define planning as "selecting missions and objectives and the actions to achieve them; it requires decision making, that is, choosing future courses of action from among alternatives."[12] They viewed planning as an elementary function of management. In their view of planning, nurse administrators avoid leaving events to chance; instead, they apply an intellectual process to consciously determine the course of action to take in accomplishing the work. Donovan stated that the planning process must be deliberate and analytic to produce carefully detailed programs of action that will achieve objectives.[13]

The nurse manager plans effectively to create an environment in which nursing personnel will provide the nursing care desired and needed by clients. In such an environment, clinical nurses will make decisions about the form or modality of practice, and nurse managers will work with nursing personnel to establish and meet their personal objectives while meeting the objectives of the organization.

According to Hodgetts, planning forces a firm to forecast the environment, gives direction in the form of objectives, provides the basis for teamwork, and helps management learn to live with ambiguity.[14] Planning

EXHIBIT 5-1
An Interactive Planning Cycle

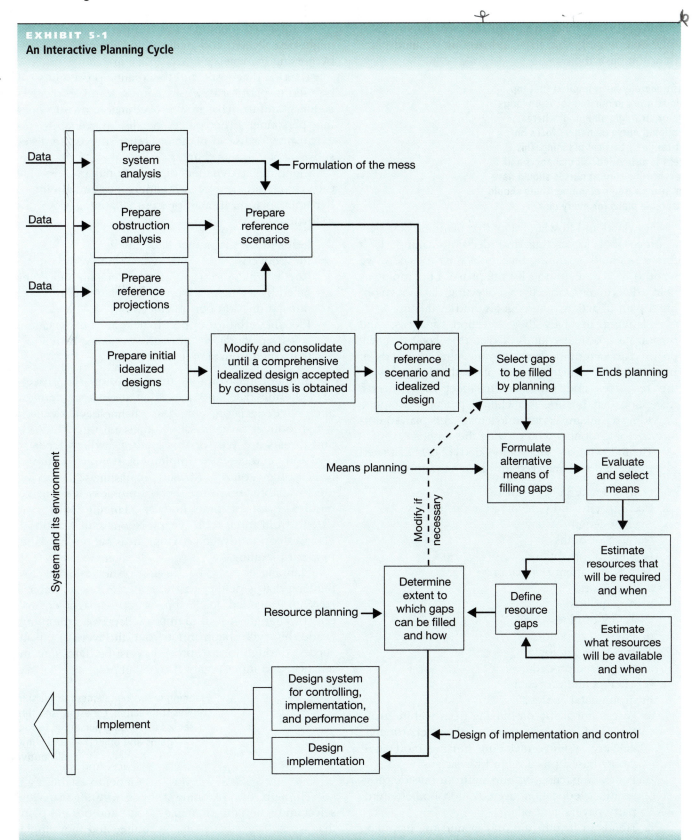

Source: R. L. Ackoff. "An Interactive Planning Cycle." *Creating the Corporate Future*, p. 75. © 1981 John Wiley & Sons, Inc. Reprinted by permission of John Wiley & Sons, Inc.

should be comprehensive, with nurse managers carefully determining objectives and making detailed plans to accomplish them.

It has generally been implied that top administrators in nursing focus on long-range or strategic planning, whereas operational nurse managers focus on short-range or tactical planning. This process is outmoded. All managers and representative clinical nurses should have input into strategic planning. There should be strategic plans for every unit.

Rowland and Rowland state that planning is largely a process of forecasting and decision-making. It is future oriented, spanning time from now to where we want to be. These authors list the phases of planning as being determining objectives, collecting data, developing a plan of action, setting goals, and evaluating.[15]

Planning involves the collection, analysis, and organization of many kinds of data (the *how*) that will be used to determine both the nursing care needs of patients and the management plans that will provide the resources and processes to meet those needs. Accepting that nursing is a clinical practice discipline providing a human service, nurse managers plan to nurture the practitioners who provide the service.

The following are some of the kinds of data that need to be collected and analyzed for planning purposes:

1. Daily average patient census
2. Bed capacity and percentage of occupancy
3. Average length of stay
4. Number of births
5. Number of operations
6. Trends in patient populations
   a. Diagnoses
   b. Age groups
   c. Acuity of illness
   d. Physical dependency
7. Trends in technology
   a. Diagnostic procedures
   b. Therapeutic procedures
8. Environmental analysis
   a. Forces impacting on nursing from within: availability of nurses; turnover; other departments; delivery systems, including nursing modalities; theory-based practice; and physicians
   b. Forces impacting on nursing from outside: government, education, accreditation bodies, third-party payers, and others
   c. Trends in health care and in nursing, including changes in characteristics
   d. Threats to the nursing profession
   e. Opportunities for the nursing profession

Exhibit 5-2 demonstrates examples of data that might be collected and analyzed for planning purposes by nursing managers.

Data on diagnostic and therapeutic procedures will be used to plan for new procedures, to revise old procedures, and to make new procedures known to nursing personnel. The preceding list is certainly not exhaustive for use in planning; other sources are listed subsequently in this chapter.

Planning, a dynamic organizational process, has the characteristics of an open system, being a dynamic, organizational process. Planning does the following:

- Leads to success rather than failure.
- Prevents crisis and panic, which are costly, unrealistic, chaotic, distorting of achievement, and dominated by a single person. Thus, planning improves nursing division performance.
- Identifies future opportunities and expectations based on conditions through forecasting techniques that range from simple to complex.

Simple forecasting techniques follow the process of gathering data and analyzing them to determine alternative decisions and the effects each decision will produce. Strengths, weaknesses, opportunities, and threats are part of this analysis, which leads to decision, choice, and implementation. In complex forecasting, computer-based mathematical models are available that are becoming less expensive, require a lot of time and specialized skills, and extend from three to 15 years. New simulation models are constantly improving and are essential to modern planning.

Planning is viewed as resting on logical, reflective thinking that is neither cast in concrete nor all encompassing. If needed, leadership or top management will effect change to undertake effective planning. Leadership will obtain input from all levels to ensure success through format, procedures, time frames, maintenance, and input review.

Planning is the key element of nursing that gives it direction, cohesion, and thrust. It causes all nursing personnel to focus on goals and objectives and stimulates their motivation.

Through the planning process, nurse managers select and retain the elements of past and present plans that work. They focus on the future, and they implement and evaluate. Thus, they successfully manage nursing personnel and material resources to achieve the objectives of the nursing enterprise.

EXHIBIT 5-2
Planning Data for Nurse Managers

- Live births have decreased 30% in the 3 years since the institution of a family planning program.
- Sixty-three percent of live births are discharged within a 24-hour period.
- The number of deliveries with complications has increased from 210 to 257 in 1 year.
- A new cardiac catheterization laboratory has been completed.
- The hospital planning board has decided to coordinate with other hospitals in the area to consolidate specialty services for newborn care, cardiovascular surgery, and neuroscience services.
- Enrollment of students for clinical nursing affiliation has increased from 450 to 792 in 1 year.
- Enrollment of students in the nursing cooperative education program has increased from 102 to 187 students.
- Medicare reimbursement pays $__ per patient for a day of home care.
- Early discharge has decreased average daily census from 381 to 304.
- Patient acuity has increased by 10.6 percentage points overall.

Elements

Although planning is characterized as being a conceptual or thinking process, it produces readily identifiable specific elements or constituents, including written statements of mission or purpose, philosophy, objectives, and detailed management or operational plans. Operational plans are the blueprints by which the purpose, philosophy, and objectives are put into measurable actions. Management or operational plans include decision-making and problem-solving processes that include strategies, policies, and procedures.

The nursing division's strategic and operational plans are road maps that describe the business by name and location. Nurse managers will make them informative by including a description that is a summary of the work of the division.

The summary describing the nursing division will include enough information to give outsiders a bird's-eye view of its totality. This information will include the nursing products and services provided (by quantity), which can be admissions, discharges, patient days, number of patients by acuity categories, research projects, educational programs, students, outpatient visits, and other products and services. The description will summarize marketing activities of the nursing division, including total revenues and expenses, and will describe the managerial style of the division and its impact on employees, which will be related to the organizational plan of the division of nursing.

Planning is the assessment of the nursing division's strengths and weaknesses, covering factors that affect performance and facilitate or inhibit the achievement of objectives. This assessment process will have both long- and short-range objectives of its own. For example, if the clinical promotion ladder is a strength in nurse retention but is weakly applied by selective nurse managers, the problem will be addressed by written objectives.

Planning entails formulation of planning premises by extrapolating assumptions from the information analyzed.[16] If data indicate that nurses will be in increased supply because of increased enrollments in schools of nursing or in short supply as a result of increased opportunities for women to enter other fields, these findings should be translated into a premise. Other premises evolve related to increased salaries and fringe benefits and improved working conditions. These premises will lead to further premises for marketing a career in nursing to high-school students and persons changing careers.

Planning entails writing specific, useful, realistic objectives (the *why*) that will reflect both strategic and operational goals for the division of nursing and its personnel. Objectives become the reasons for an operational nursing management plan (the *what*) that will detail the activities to be performed, the target dates or time frames for their accomplishment (the *when*), the persons responsible for accomplishing the activities (the *who*), and strategies for dealing with technical, economic, social, and political aspects. These operational plans will have control systems for monitoring performance and providing feedback. They will address the budget.

In addition to the foregoing elements of planning, Meier indicates that good management begins "with a coordinated purposeful organization of people who collectively on a functional responsibility basis"[17]:

- Plan the organization
- Provide personnel
- Provide facilities
- Provide capital
- Set performance standards
- Develop management information systems
- Activate people

Good management keeps the nursing agency successful, ensuring its growth, success, and direction and a return on investment in the future. Objectives and operational plans are discussed in detail in Chapter 6, Mission Philosophy, Objectives, and Management Plans.

Strategic Planning

Nursing administrators can increase effectiveness through strategic planning, which can promote professional nursing practice and the long-range goals of the organization and the division of nursing. Drucker defines strategic planning as "a continuous, systematic process of making risk-taking decisions today with the greatest possible knowledge of their effects on the future; organizing efforts necessary to carry out these decisions and evaluating results of these decisions against expected outcome through reliable feedback mechanisms."[18]

Strategic planning in nursing is concerned with what nursing should be doing. Its purpose is to improve allocation of scarce resources, including time and money, and to manage the agency for performance. Strategic planning provides strategic forecasting from one year to more than 20 years. It should involve top nurse managers and representatives of all levels of nursing management and practice. It will include analysis of factors such as projected technological advances, the internal and external environments, the nursing and health care market and industry, the economics of nursing and health care, availability of human and material resources, and judgments of top management.[19]

In today's world, the strategic planning process is used to acquire and develop new health care services and product lines, including new nursing services and products. Strategic planning is also used to divest outdated services and products. Both activities present moral and ethical dilemmas for the managers and practitioners of nursing. Strategic planning can foster better goals, better corporate values, and better communication about corporate direction. It can lead to changes in operating management and organization. Strategic planning can produce better management strategy and analysis and can forecast and mute external threats.

The process of strategic planning is more important than the plan itself. The process serves to give planners a sense of direction, involves everyone, and enables unexpected opportunities to be seized and unexpected crises dealt with.[20]

"Environmental scans" are tools of the strategic planning process. These scans include identification of future trends, risks, and opportunities. Environmental scans also identify projected governmental, demographic, and social changes that will affect nursing strategic planning in an era of health care reform, aging population, single parenthood, drug use, crime and violence, and the education system.[21]

Odiorne recommends the following process for crafting strategic plans[22]:

1. Identify the major problems of your organization to determine where you are headed and where you want to be, which is called *gap analysis*. This technique examines markets, products, customers, employees, finances, technology, and community relations. Cabinets or task forces from each area may be helpful in performing gap analysis and identifying major problems.
2. Examine outside influences that relate to the key problems of your organization. Focus on the few major issues.
3. List the critical issues, that is, those that affect the entire organization, have long-term impact, and are based on irrefutable evidence rather than media hype.
4. Rank the critical issues according to their importance to your organization, and plan accordingly: "must do," "to do," and "important, but not urgent." Then divide these critical issues into "success producers" and "failure preventers."
5. Decide the critical issues to all organization managers.
6. Include time in the budget.

Exhibit 5-3 lists ways in which strategic planning can be used to improve management. The process of strategic planning has several phases, as summarized in Exhibit 5-4.

EXHIBIT 5-3

How Strategic Planning Can Be Used to Improve Nursing Management

- To provide accountability and monitoring of performance; to tie merit to performance.
- To set up more formal planning programs and require divisional and unit planning.
- To integrate strategic plans with operational and financial plans.
- To think and concentrate more on strategic issues.
- To improve knowledge of and training in strategic planning.
- To increase top management involvement and commitment.
- To improve focus on competition, market segments, and external factors.
- To improve communication from top administration and nursing management.
- To allow better execution of plans.
- To be more realistic and less rationalizing and vacillating.
- To improve the development of nursing management strategies.
- To improve the development and communication of nursing management goals.
- To put less emphasis on raw numbers.
- To anticipate the future and plan for it.
- To develop the annual budget.
- To focus on quality outputs that will improve nurse performance and productivity, decrease losses, and increase return on equity.

EXHIBIT 5-4
Summary of Phases of Strategic Planning Process

PHASE 1
THE MISSION AND THE CREED

Develop statements that define the work, the aims, and the character of the division of nursing. These include idea statements of shared values and beliefs. They are called mission (or purpose) and creed (or philosophy) statements, and relate to personnel, patients, community, and all other potential customers.

PHASE 2
DATA COLLECTION AND ANALYSIS

Collect and analyze data about the health care industry and nursing. Such data should include internal forces that define the work and affect employees, clients, stockholders, and creditors; technological advances; threats; opportunities to improve growth and productivity; external forces such as competition, communities, government and political issues, and legal requirements; marketing and public relations or image; trends in the physical and social work environments; and communication. Use simple and complex forecasting techniques including trend lines, group consensus, nominal group process, and a qualitative decision matrix that uses probabilities based on conditions of certainty, risk, and uncertainty.

PHASE 3
ASSESS STRENGTHS AND WEAKNESSES

Define those factors from the data analysis that influence management of the division of nursing. List them as strengths or opportunities that will facilitate effectiveness and achievement of goals and objectives or as weaknesses or threats that will impede achieving goals and objectives. Define the current position and strength of the unit.

PHASE 4
GOALS AND OBJECTIVES

Write realistic and general statements of goals. Break the goals down into concrete written statements of objectives the division of nursing intends to accomplish in the next 3 to 5 years.

PHASE 5
STRATEGIES

Identify untoward conditions that could develop in achieving each objective. Note administrative actions to avoid or manage them. Use this information to modify goals and objectives, making contingency plans for alternative actions. Define the organization needed for doing and implementing strategic plans. It should be interactive if cross-functional activities are involved—a matrix organization.

PHASE 6
TIMETABLE

Develop a timetable for accomplishing each objective. Identify by geographic units as well. This phase will produce or become part of the plans.

PHASE 7
OPERATIONAL AND FUNCTIONAL PLANS

Provide guidelines or general instructions that lead functional and operational nurse managers to develop action plans to implement the goals and objectives. These will include detailed actions, policies, practices, communication and feedback, controlling and evaluation plans, budgets, timetables, and persons to be held accountable.

PHASE 8
IMPLEMENTATION

Put the plans to work.

PHASE 9
EVALUATION

Provide for formative evaluation reports before, during, and after the operational plan is implemented. Provide for summative evaluation that is quantified. Report actual versus expected results. Evaluate the strategic mission, and plan frequently. Provide continuous feedback that can be used to modify and update the plan. Use people who implement the plan to evaluate it.

Strategic planning includes both planning of the process and strategy for implementing the plan. During the strategic planning process, analysis of the business environment and the internal capabilities of the organization for producing a product or service suited to success in the business environment are analyzed. Goals and strategies are also set during the planning process.[23]

Peters believes that strategic planning should be a line exercise rather than a staff one. Also, the focus should be on building a work force that is well trained, flexible, and quality conscious.[24] Strategic plans should be developed from the bottom up, the front line where

business occurs. The written plan should be shared with everyone and should not be slavishly followed since it will be constantly affected by change and should be modified every year.[25]

Obviously, with constant, quick changes in markets and operations, time management is vital to strategic planning. Strategic plans should be capable of being quickly made and changed.

Implementation of strategic plans includes strategies related to proper activities, organizational structure, company resources, and support systems. The various strategic plans of the organization should be linked to avoid internal conflicts. These links include operations, finance, human relations, marketing, budgeting, and personal action. All the elements of a strategic plan make up a system, and these elements of a system need constant monitoring for their success.[26]

Strategic, or long-range, planning came into vogue after World War II and is widely used in business and industry. It is becoming prevalent in the health care world because of technological change, modernization of the industry, increased government roles, and increased complexity of nursing management. In strategic planning, nurse managers are required to manage in the future tense by defining the future of nursing in areas such as setting objectives; developing an organization to achieve the objectives; allocating resources; implementing objectives through specific policies and plans; evaluating and providing feedback for accomplishing these objectives; and finally developing a new strategic plan with new objectives that includes planning for research use in nursing practice.[27]

A strategic plan is coldly objective in evaluating what the nursing business is and what it will be. It does not leave success to chance and prevents the status quo from paralyzing nursing progress. Strategic planning leads to strategic management and becomes an integral part of thinking in all management operations, including budgeting, information, compensation, organization, leadership development, patient education, and decision support systems.[28]

Critical thinking about the past, present, and future state of affairs helps in developing, implementing, and evaluating a well-formulated strategic plan. During this process, sensitivity to the needs of the institution, its personnel, and its clientele is required. The plan will be flexible and adaptable to environmental changes. Quantifiable outcomes increase the accuracy of a strategic plan. Each day, the nurse manager makes sound decisions that can range from the simple to the complex and should be positively related to advanced planning.

Participants in the strategic planning process will range from top nursing management to a cross-section of all levels of management. Including input from clinical nursing personnel promotes professional satisfaction throughout the nursing department.

One of the benefits of strategic planning is that it gives a sense of direction to all managers and practitioners of nursing within the organization. The strategic plan becomes a flexible control mechanism that can be modified to deal with variables, conserve resources, and provide professional satisfaction. The strategic plan deals concretely with complex projects or programs in multistage time sequences.[29]

Conclusions About the Strategic Planning Process

Strategic planning is considered to be a goal-setting process that is largely carried out by top management. There are many instances of long-range plans being made but fewer instances of their having been put to use. In truth, operating nurse managers have needed to be trained in the strategic planning process. This training should include techniques to involve operational managers and thereby commit them to decisions. Development of global goals and strategies broaden the identification and solution of problems, reducing threats to and unveiling opportunities for the organization.

The demonstrated usefulness of scientific planning will influence the behavior of operating managers. Rewards, in the form of both pay and praise, will motivate these operating managers.

Strategic planning has many benefits. It provides for objective consideration of strategic choices or options that are better matched with organizational goals and objectives. With strategic planning the outlook becomes futuristic, resources are allocated systematically, and rapid change is accommodated.[30] Strategic plans must be dynamic to take advantage of these benefits, projecting trends and directions. These plans are the blueprints that are to be updated as the environment changes phases and stages in the process of strategic planning, as summarized in Exhibit 5-4.

A cyclic model of strategic planning provides for continuous assessment of an organization's mission, values, vision, and primary strategies. This assessment is based on feedback from benchmark analysis, shareholder impact, and progress in implementation of strategies.[31]

If they are to survive, urban health care organizations will have to do strategic planning similar to that done by some rural hospitals. This will include the following[32]:

- Involvement of outside organizations in fostering community change.
- A high degree of community commitment and investment in all stages of the process.
- Comprehensive identification of problems in the health care system by outside consultants.
- The use of periodic meetings of communities confronting similar issues.
- Identification and development of local leadership.
- Enhancing teamwork among local health care providers.
- Development of conflict-resolution mechanisms within health care organizations.

Health care institutions have to make global competitiveness a strategic goal. With the world awash in "virtual money" in portfolios of investments, health care leaders have responsibility for institutional investments of endowment funds. For-profit institutions are a part of people's investment portfolios.[33] Nurse leaders should take advantage of this situation through the strategic planning process.

Functional and Operational Planning

Operational management is the organization and directing of the delivery of nursing care. It includes planning such as creating a budget; creating an effective organizational structure that encompasses a quality monitoring process; and directing nurse leaders, an administrative staff, and new programs.[34]

Nursing planning performed at a service or departmental level is referred to as functional planning. It generally relates to a specialty service within a nursing division. For example, the staff development director would be included in development of the strategic plan but would develop operational plans for staff development as a whole and for specific services or units. Likewise, the director of a home health care agency would assist in developing the strategic plan for the company but would develop agency mission, philosophy, goals, objectives, and operational plans. With decentralization each nurse manager would develop a strategic plan for his or her unit to be integrated into the organization's strategic plan.

Operational plans are everyday working management plans developed from both long-range objectives and the strategic planning process and short-range or tactical plans. In development of operational objectives, new strategic objectives can emerge or old ones can be modified or discarded. Strategic and tactical plans are made into operational plans and carried out at all levels of nursing management, not just at the patient-care level.

Operational managers develop goals, objectives, strategies, and targets to set the strategic plan in motion. They match each unit goal or objective to a strategic goal or objective. Their objectives can be much more detailed and specific than the strategic objectives. Numerous operational objectives can support one strategic objective.

All aspects of an operational plan are based on goals and on their achievement. The individual leadership style determines whether goal setting will be of the top-down or bottom-up variety. Bottom-up goal setting is participatory, using guidelines from the operational manager.[35] Participatory goal setting is believed to increase

workers' commitment and achievement. Increased participation leads to greater group cohesiveness, which in turn fosters increased morale, increased motivation, and increased achievement and productivity. Individuals, including nurse managers, can ensure greater relative success in achievement of goals by building additional resources and time into their plans. Nurse managers who reject goals of participating staff should explain reasons for rejection. Participation in goal setting alone will not ensure success. Exhibit 5-5 suggests a timetable for strategic and operational planning. Like the plan itself, such planning should be flexible.

The concept of goals being global in nature and objectives being detailed is confusing to some participants in the planning process, particularly nurse managers. In nursing, written organizational goals have seldom been used and probably did not exist in many agencies. More attention is being given to this aspect of management today. External influences create a

---

EXHIBIT 5-5
Timetable for Strategic and Operational Planning

1. Organization
   Mondays 7–9 A.M. Conference room. Breakfast.
   Attendees: Chief executive officer (CEO), assistants (including for division of nursing), and understudies.
   Agenda: CEO, with input from all others, relates each item to strategic plan. CEO updates and develops written operational plans at meeting or immediately following, then reviews them for next agenda for progress and for strategic plan development.
   Minutes: Prepared and distributed to attendees.

2. Division of Nursing
   Monday 3–4 P.M. Nursing conference room.
   Attendees: Chief nurse executive (CNE), associates, department heads, chairs of clinical consultants, nursing management, and staff nurse committees.
   Agenda: Chairs, with input from CNE and all others, relate each item to strategic plan of division of nursing. These goals and objectives have already been coordinated with the organizational strategic plan. CNE and others update operational plans of division and departments during meeting or immediately following, then review them for next agenda for progress and nursing strategic plan development.
   Minutes: Prepared and distributed to attendees, to CEO, and to selected others.

3. Service and Unit
   CNE and/or associates meet with their nurse managers and representative clinical nurses at mutually determined times and places. The groups have agendas, keep minutes, update written operational plans, and provide feedback to top nurse managers and clinical nurse staff.

demand for a strategic plan, and more nurse managers have had management education and training.[36]

Some organizations do not develop separate goals and objectives. Instead, they develop objectives and from them create management plans. In actual practice, as organizational objectives are developed into operational plans, specific goals and objectives are written for each major activity.

The goal is to plan, assess progress toward goals and objectives at all levels, and provide feedback to all levels of management. Efficiency is also a goal; all levels of management should guard against unnecessary time spent in meetings. As organizing changes are occurring, controlling activities are in operation and activities are being evaluated.

Planning New Ventures

In an era of competitiveness, each nurse manager can be called on to develop ideas for new ventures, be they nursing products or services. For example, continuing education courses can be packaged, marketed, and presented within the organization or taken on the road. Hospitals have moved into home health care, durable medical goods, wellness and fitness programs, and many other ventures. The basic rule for undertaking new ventures is to do sound planning.

Any new venture should have a separate marketing plan. The nurse manger will consult with marketing department personnel and develop a marketing operation plan that will[37]:

- Define problems and opportunities that may confront the new enterprise and product.
- Define the competitive position of the product and set objectives to meet anticipated problems and opportunities.
- Detail work steps, schedules, assignment of responsibility, budgets, and other elements of implementation.
- Describe the monitoring (control) plan.

The marketing plan should be separate from a primary operational plan and should include gathering and analysis of data related to the product or service as it already exists in the area. For example, if the product is continuing education, who will the customers be? They could be nurse managers, nurse educators, RNs, or LPNs. What is the competition in the market area? Is it local or imported from educational institutions and for-profit companies? Who will pay for the course—employers and/or individuals?

In addition, the operational plan will gather and analyze data that pinpoint possible strengths and weak-nesses, problems, and opportunities. It will identify strategies for taking competitive advantages. Each opportunity, problem, strength, and weakness should be addressed by definitive objectives developed into operational plans for advertising, product development, and even personal selling.

Before any new venture is launched, a control plan is made. This plan will include measures of performance, such as numbers or amounts of products or services to be sold within specific time frames. Managers will be assigned responsibility for comparing expected results with actual results and for making corrections in all elements of the plan and its implementation. This plan can be achieved with marketing and operational plan checklists.[38] Exhibit 5-6 illustrates an operational plan for development of an intermediate cardiac rehabilitation program.

Nursing service planning supports the mission and objectives of the institution. For this reason the nurse administrator needs to know the plans and programs of the health facility administrator and of other departments where personnel contribute to the joint effort of providing health care services. The nurse administrator should be a voting member of all important committees of the institution and should give input into the planning done by these committees. These committees include those dealing with budgets, planning, credentialing, auditing, utilization, infection control, patient care improvement, the library, and all others concerned in any way with nursing service, nursing activities, and nursing personnel.

The nurse administrator who participates in institutional committee work achieves an overall view of agency problems and activities and is in a position to interpret problems, policies, and plans of the agency to nursing personnel. He or she can also interpret nursing needs and problems to personnel of other departments. This planning integrates the nursing care program into the total program of the health care institution.

Business Plans

Business plans are detailed descriptions of the process for ensuring launching of a new product or product line, project, unit, or service. Business plans meet many of the standards for strategic planning as they are projected over an extended time period of months or years. Their purpose is to provide sources of information for investors and decision-makers within and external to the organization, motivation, and measurement of performance.[39] Business plans are the blueprints for ventures. A clinical nurse specialist who decides to enter private practice as a consultant should write a business plan to solidify ideas and prepare for the unexpected.[40]

Division of Nursing–Cardiac Rehabilitation Program

STRATEGIC OBJECTIVE

The patient is provided with an effective patient and patient–family teaching program, which includes guidance and assistance in the use of medical center resources and community agencies that can contribute support to the patient's total needs.

OPERATIONAL OBJECTIVES	ACTIONS	TARGET DATES AND PERSONS RESPONSIBLE	ACCOMPLISHMENTS
Determine cardiologist's perception of the program: goals, resources to be used, breadth of services to be provided, etc.	1. Prepare an agenda for meeting with cardiologist.	Do by July 1, 200x. Swansburg (S) and Perry (P)	The following agenda was developed: • Need for new services. • What will they be? • What will they cost? • What will be charged? • Who will pay? • Where will they be done? • Who will do them? • How many patients? • What equipment and supplies are needed?
	2. Make appointment with cardiologist.	May 3, 200x, at 11 A.M. in Dr. C's office; S and P	May 3, 200x: Had a meeting with Dr. C, the cardiologist. The purpose of this program is to rehabilitate patients following open-heart surgery, angioplasty, and post-MI. It is the intermediate phase between acute care and when they enter "bounce back." The following decision evolved from the meeting: 1. This program will be limited because no other such services are available. 2. Services will include physical exercises, monitoring, progress report by patient, counseling as indicated. 3. Only patients with insurance or ability to pay will be accepted. 4. It will be done in PT on Mon., Wed., and Fri. from 7 to 9 A.M. 5. Equipment and supplies will be in-house. 6. The CV clinical nurse specialist will be the project director.

(continued)

EXHIBIT 5-6 (continued)

OPERATIONAL OBJECTIVES	ACTIONS	TARGET DATES AND PERSONS RESPONSIBLE	ACCOMPLISHMENTS
Meet with the CV clinical nurse specialist and plan the program.	3. Make appointment with nurse D to plan the program.	May 4, 200x, 8 A.M.; S and P with D.	Plan: 1. D will coordinate with PT director. 2. P will figure cost of program by the hour and set charges with accounting office. 3. D will borrow equipment to run the program until the next capital budget. 4. Accomplish this by May 12, 200x.
Have plan completed by May 31, 200x.	4. Set up a control chart to identify when each phase of project will be completed.	May 12, 200x; P.	May 10, 200x: Done. Posted.
	5. Write policy and procedure for the program. Include admission and discharge procedures and emergency plan.	May 31, 200x; D.	May 29, 200x: Draft presented; minor changes needed. May 31, 200x: Done.
	6. Obtain equipment and supplies.	May 31, 200x; D.	May 17, 200x: Done.
	7. Coordinate with PT director.	May 12, 200x; D.	May 17, 200x: Done.
	8. Meet with cardiologist when all this is done.	June 1, 200x; P, S, and D.	June 2, 200x: Met with cardiologist. Dr. C is happy with plan and will be ready to start on July 1, 200x.
Provide for third-party reimbursement.	9. Discuss with insurance companies.	June 15, 200x; P.	June 15, 200x: Insurance reps will visit the program and make decision. Appointment made.
Develop marketing plan.	10. Prepare detailed marketing plan.		Marketing plan is already in operation with announcements mailed to all area cardiologists. D has a good evaluation plan.
Develop evaluation plan.	11. Prepare evaluation plan.	June 30, 200x; P and D.	
	12. Implement program.	July 1, 200x; D.	July 1, 200x: Had our first patient today. Cardiologist was there as required by insurance companies. All went well.
	13. Evaluate the program weekly until stabilized.	D, beginning July 8, 200x.	

The following are key elements of a business plan as described by Johnson and others[41]:

1. Introduction: the nature, goals, objectives, and desired outcomes of the proposed business.
2. Description of the business: the goals, nature, and history of the sponsoring institution, nature and history of the product, and industry trends.
3. Market and competition analyses: these include the target audience, pricing, promotion, placement, and positioning; data from solid market research are used.
4. Product development: product description, resources, time frames for development, and quality control plan.
5. Operational plan: the location, facilities, labor force, and equipment.
6. Marketing plan to market services or products: the mission, marketing research, measurable goals, strategies, and staffing and financial plans.
7. Organizational plan to recruit qualified employees: an organizational chart and job descriptions.
8. Developmental schedule that includes planning for growth.
9. Financial plan to secure capital.
10. Executive summary.

Business plans are often categorized as strategic plans. Many of the key elements are the same, although a business plan would be more detailed than a strategic plan. Actually, a business plan would be developed for each new venture emerging from a strategic plan. Exhibit 5-6 illustrates an operational plan for development of an intermediate cardiac rehabilitation program. The plan was made and carried out by a team led by a cardiovascular clinical nurse specialist.

Practical Planning Actions

Practical day-to-day planning actions of value to the nurse administrator include the following exercises:

1. At the beginning of each day, make a list of actions to be accomplished for the day. Cross off the actions as they are accomplished or at the end of the day. At the beginning of the next workday, carry over actions not accomplished. Either do them first or decide if they are actions that really need to be done. Do not hold tasks over from one day to the next indefinitely.
2. Plan ahead for meetings. If the meeting is a nursing responsibility, prepare and distribute the agenda in advance. Have a secretary call members for their items to be listed on the agenda. Forward nursing items for the agenda of organizational meetings to the appropriate chair in advance. Prepare for the presentation.
3. Identify developing problems and put them in the appropriate portion of the division's operational or management plans.
4. Review the operational or management plan on a scheduled basis. Do this with key managers so that each knows his or her responsibilities for accomplishment of activities.
5. Review the appropriate portions of the division operational or management plan with other nurse managers when they are being counseled.
6. Plan for discussion of ideas gleaned from professional publications. This activity can be part of a job standard, with different managers assigned specific topics or journals. Doing so may help to integrate research results into practice.
7. Suggest similar practical planning actions to other nurse managers.

Planning will also be necessary to provide programs for orientation and continued learning of nursing personnel so that all will have current knowledge and be current in practice methods. Improvement of patient care and of other administrative and hospital services necessitates initiation and utilization of and participation in studies or research projects in the health care field. Two additional important areas for planning are (1) educational programs that include student experience in the division of nursing and (2) evaluation of clinical and administrative practices to determine whether the objectives of the division are being achieved.

Why Divisional Planning?

There are many good reasons for planning, and avoiding duplicated efforts is one of them. Planning will also improve communication throughout the division and the institution and will reduce fragmentation by helping to keep functional units headed in the same direction. Planning is good management training for all nurse managers. During its initial phases, planning will use an objective analysis of the division to determine its current status. The mission, strengths, weaknesses, and environment will be analyzed and a survey performed of how all employees feel about the division. The analysis also will assess the future of the division and the major threats and opportunities it will face during the next year and the next 5 to 10 years. Planning will engineer a design for monitoring and evaluating divisional performance. This design will involve as many people as possible in planning and managing their areas of responsibility.

Once managers and employees have agreed on objectives, programs and projects, and schedules, employees can control their own jobs and report only when things turn out better or worse than planned.

Planning is such a primary and essential element of management that managers cannot be effective without it.

Problems with Divisional Planning

All planning requires discipline and organization on the part of managers. Being human, managers usually prefer short-range solutions to problems. They prefer to shoot from the hip, and some may enjoy management by crisis. Many managers are threatened by the change produced by planning and may resist it even to the point of sabotage.

Planning should be approached logically and calmly. Planning will threaten the insecure and may even threaten the nurse administrator, who must provide total support in terms of giving or obtaining the resources to accomplish divisional planning. Strategies are developed to address these problems and to ensure that representative nurse managers participate on all planning teams.

Provision of nursing care to patients is the purpose of a division of nursing. Nursing standards indicate that there will be qualified nursing personnel who will collect data and make nursing diagnoses based on patients' needs and according to patient care standards. Nursing standards further indicate that cooperation among disciplines is expected.

Successful Planning

Keeping the responsibility for planning as a line management function is better than creating a separate planning staff of nurses. Because nurses who use plans make them effective and productive, they should be the ones to write the plans. Nurse managers should be sure the plans are based on data from all sections and not biased by a few. Some people see planning as a management style; planning is a tool as well. Plan for what the health care of the future will be: With inflation and recession, the impact of the local economy on health care needs will become greater than it is today. Economics is forcing us to teach people to do more for themselves and their families. Nurse managers will certainly have to plan for changes in value systems.

Nurse managers should make decisions about the kind of planning to be undertaken and which management level should perform specific aspects of the planning. Involve personnel in planning activities they will carry out. Teach and combine the elements of planning with other management functions. Ensure that all managers are involved. Accept outcomes that are different from those originally planned because activities may quickly become outdated and require modified plans.

Unit Planning

Planning extends to the operational units of any health care agency. The processes involved are the same. It is here that the work for which nursing exists takes place. Planning should be done on a daily, weekly, and long-term basis. Daily planning is related to patient care and includes history taking, assessment, and nursing diagnosis and prescription. It involves matching people to jobs, developing policies and procedures specific to the types of clients cared for, identifying training needs, preparing and conducting training programs, coordinating all patient care activities, supervising personnel, and evaluating the planning process and its results as summarized in Exhibit 5-8. Also included in unit planning are implementing a theory of nursing into the management and practice of nursing, an effective and efficient nursing care delivery system, and a system of statistical process control.

Unit objectives should be clearly defined and a sound management or operational plan made to achieve them. An operating instruction from one nursing agency states, "The division of nursing has a stated philosophy and objectives. Personnel of each unit within the division will have their own philosophy and will set up their own objectives. The objectives will be continuously evaluated, and a written statement as to progress will be sent to the chair's office each August and February."

Exhibit 5-7 is a modified business plan for accomplishing objectives related to management improvement and resource management for an intensive care unit.

Relationships to Organization

Planning within the nursing organization is intended to assist in fulfilling the mission of the health care facility. Planning supports the organization's objectives and meshes

Operational Plan—Intensive Care Unit

MANAGEMENT IMPROVEMENT: UNIT OBJECTIVES, FEBRUARY 1, 200X

1. Precipitate imaginative thinking to improve existing procedures, capitalize on time expenditure, and introduce modern concepts and materials that directly enhance unit accomplishment.
2. Promote creativity in improving the existing patient environment.
3. Provide more modern concepts of total patient care by constant review and revision of unit administrative/managerial policies.

PLANS FOR ACHIEVEMENT OF OBJECTIVES	ACTIONS	TARGET DATES	ACCOMPLISHMENTS
Plan and implement a continuing unit improvement program.	1. Conduct a continuous review and analysis of unit improvement efforts through:	February	Reviewed and found current for following reasons: Turnover in personnel is fast. Not all objectives were adequately met; need to establish a better way of accomplishing them.
	a. Monthly unit conferences to review and update philosophy and objectives. Strive to accomplish more in each objective area.	February–July	
	b. Patient suggestions	Review each month	
	c. Suggestions of superiors	Daily	
	d. Revise unit procedures	April	Done
	e. Brief all personnel. Discuss philosophy, objectives, job descriptions, performance standards, hospital and nursing service policies and procedures, and unit procedures.	February	Done. In addition, all nurses were counseled by the charge nurse. Nursing technicians are presently receiving counseling, and all is being documented. Counseling had not been documented in 6 years, except for remarks such as "Things went well and we did our job, so no counseling was needed."
	2. Review equipment and supplies for improvement by addition or deletion.		
	a. Submit work order to alter a locker as a drying cabinet for respirator parts, since moisture provides a growth medium for *Pseudomonas* bacteria.		Disapproved. Disposable tubing was approved, ordered, and in use by June.
	b. Check on status of new floor, piped-in compressed air system, and cardiac monitors.	February–April	New floor to be done by August 1. Compressed air started by March 15. Cardiac monitors arrived April 3. Patient units 1, 3, and 4 were equipped. Unit 4 was designated the maximum monitoring site and is to be used to monitor patients with Swan-Ganz arterial lines and questionable cardiac conditions.

(continued)

EXHIBIT 5-7 (continued)

PLANS FOR ACHIEVEMENT OF OBJECTIVES	ACTIONS	TARGET DATES	ACCOMPLISHMENTS
Review standardized policies and procedures for implementation of more current concepts of improved care accomplishments.	3. Evaluate all areas of management for current standardized efficiency. a. Check all areas of infection sources.		This was done, and cleaning procedures were looked at and improved when they appeared poor. HEPA filters were replaced in February. Wall suction valves were replaced. Pipelines were found to be clogged with secretions, and system had to be purged. Shelves were mounted on wall by four units to replace bedside stands. Respirators, nebulizers, and blenders were mounted on wall above each patient unit. Suction bottles were relocated and outlets changed in an effort to isolate them from the oxygen nebulization units. Swan-Ganz catheters were standardized, and requisitioning was transferred from the unit to central supply. Ambu bags were equipped with corrugated tubing to serve as an oxygen reservoir and deliver a maximum concentration of 99% to 100%. The disposable Aqua-pack nebulizer was deleted, resulting in a $40 per case saving.
	(i) Air exchange and pressure checked quarterly.	February	
	(ii) HEPA filters changed quarterly.	February	
	(iii) Check wall suction, since filters do not appear to be doing the job.	February	
	(iv) Eliminate messy bedside stands.	February	
	b. Improve safety.		
	(i) Secure equipment.	April	
	(ii) Isolate oxygen nebulization units from suction.	April	
	(iii) Send all equipment to central supply for processing.	April	
	(iv) Improve efficiency of Ambu resuscitators.	April	
	4. Projected: An anesthesiologist will be assigned to the intensive care unit. All bronchoscopies will be done here. Open heart surgery is still an open and current topic.		

(continued)

EXHIBIT 5-7 *(continued)*

RESOURCE MANAGEMENT

1. Provide, secure, and maintain the appropriate and economical use of supplies and equipment that will permit unit personnel to devote maximum time and care to patient activities.
2. Provide the unit with adequate tools for safe and effective patient care.
3. Provide the unit with conservative utilization and centralization of unit supplies and equipment, thus promoting peak efficiency in meeting patients' needs.

PLANS FOR ACHIEVEMENT OF OBJECTIVES	ACTIONS	TARGET DATES	ACCOMPLISHMENTS
Plan, evaluate, and project needed supplies and equipment that will enhance effective and safe nursing care.	Identify projected needs with unit manager through review of: 1. Unit inventories of equipment and budgetary estimate. 2. Standards for supplies. 3. Availability of supplies and equipment. 4. Economical use of supplies and equipment.	February	Items ordered (projected replacements for 200x–200x): 1 electronic thermometer 1 IV pump 5 transducers 1 ventilator 1 sphygmomanometer 1 Wright respirometer 4 metal storage cabinets 4 Ambu bags 1 blood gas analyzer New cubicle curtains Items replaced: ECG and defibrillator portable ECG machine spirometers suction regulators Items deleted: 1 electronic thermometer 1 internal/external defibrillator (to dog lab) 2 compressor units
Plan and execute appropriate utilization of materials.	1. Economical use of expendable supplies and adequate safeguards to prevent misuse and loss. 2. Knowledge of principles of operation of appropriate mechanical equipment and procedures for effecting prompt servicing and repairs.		Miscellaneous: file card supply system revamped shelving obtained for lower doors Personnel turnover: Projected losses: Ms. Speich, RN, June Ms. Ullman, RN, August Ms. Urbom, RN, May Ms. Malloy, RN, June Mr. Falco, ward clerk, April Projected gains: Ms. Tishoff, RN, May Mr. Robertshaw, RN, May Mr. Angelus, RN, April Mrs. Figuera, unit secretary, April

Myra C. Breck, R.N.
Nurse Manager, ICU

with the plans of all other departments contributing to provision of total health care needs. Planning includes delineation of the responsibilities of nurse managers in relation to activities in other departments with which nursing interrelates. The organizational chart will show the relationship of the division of nursing to the board of control, the administrator, and other departments.

Plans will provide for optimum support of the nursing agency by other departments providing services, supplies, and equipment used by the nursing service. There will be plans for regular meetings with the hospital administrator for participation on all agency committees concerned with general administrative policies and activities and the total program of the organization. Plans will also exist for periodic reports to the board of control (through administrators) concerning the programs, major plans, and problems of the division of nursing. Exhibit 5-8, Standards for Planning Process, outlines activity for evaluating the plans of a nursing unit, division, and department.

Summary

Planning is a mental process by which nurse managers use valid and reliable data to develop objectives and determine the resources needed and a blueprint for their use in achieving the objectives. The major purpose of planning is to make the best possible use of personnel, supplies, and equipment.

Strategic planning sets objectives for long-range nursing activities of one to five years, or longer. Although traditionally done by top managers, strategic planning is an important skill for all nurse managers to develop. It ensures survival. Human resource planning will ensure effective use of a scarce commodity, the professional nurse. Strategic planning has a mission, collects and analyzes data, assesses strengths and weaknesses, sets goals and objectives, uses strategies, operates on a timetable, gives operational and functional guidance to nurse managers, and includes evaluation.

Tactical planning is short-range planning. Operational planning is synergistic, putting strategic and tactical planning in motion. It includes goals, objectives, strategies, actions, a timetable, identification of responsible persons, and note of accomplishments. Operational planning is daily, weekly, and monthly planning and can provide data for further strategic and tactical planning.

EXHIBIT 5-8
Standards for Planning Process

	YES	NO
1. The plan is written.		
2. It defines the nursing business.		
3. It contains objectives (general and specific goals).		
4. It defines strategies.		
5. It supports the mission.		
6. It details forecasted activities for one year.		
7. It details forecasted activities for longer than one year.		
8. It has been developed with input from clinical nurses and line managers.		
9. It addresses resources (personnel and facilities).		
10. Changes are evident.		
11. Financial plans are included.		
12. Needs are identified and supported.		
13. Priorities are listed.		
14. Timetables are listed.		
15. It is based on current data analysis.		
16. It assesses both strengths and weaknesses.		
17. It derives from a good nursing management information plan.		
18. It is used and modified consistently.		

APPLICATION EXERCISES

EXERCISE 5-1 From materials in this chapter, prepare a checklist and use it to determine the length of the planning process for a unit, service, department, or division of nursing. From your survey, summarize the effectiveness of the planning process. How can it be improved? Can you initiate this improvement? If not, who can?

EXERCISE 5-2 Write a summary of a nursing unit, service, department, or division that describes its work, the volume of products and services, marketing activities, trends, financial summary, and impact on employees.

EXERCISE 5-3 Interview a chief executive officer and a chief nurse executive officer of an organization. Determine their orientation to strategic planning. Compare the results. Prepare a list of questions to ask from exhibits in this chapter before doing the interview.

EXERCISE 5-4 Make a management plan for your work for a day.

EXERCISE 5-5 Make a management plan for a meeting.

EXERCISE 5-6 List some threats to nursing, their severity, and the probability that they will occur. Consider technological, economic, demographic, politicolegal, and sociocultural forecasting.

EXERCISE 5-7 List some opportunities for nursing, their attractiveness, and the probability that they will occur. Consider technological, economic, demographic, politicolegal, and sociocultural forecasting.

NOTES

1. H. Fayol, trans. by C. Storrs, *General and Industrial Management* (London: Isaac Pitman & Sons, 1949), 43–50.
2. L. Urwick, *The Elements of Administration* (New York: Harper & Row, 1944), 26–34.
3. H. S. Rowland and B. L. Rowland, *Nursing Administration Handbook*, 4th Ed. (Gaithersburg, MD: Aspen, 1997), 13, 32–36.
4. M. Beyers and C. Phillips, *Nursing Management for Patient Care*, 2nd Ed. (Boston: Little, Brown, 1979), 41–48.
5. R. L. Ackoff, "Our Changing Concept of Planning," *The Journal of Nursing Administration* (October 1986), 35–40.
6. W. H. Schmeling, J. R. Futch, D. Moore, and J. W. MacDonald, "The Interactive Planning/Management Model," *Nursing Administration Quarterly* (fall 1991), 14, 31.
7. Ibid.
8. L. Curtin, "Learning for the Future," *Nursing Management*, 25, (1) (1994), 7–9.
9. L. M. Douglass, *The Effective Nurse: Leader and Manager*, 5th Ed. (St. Louis: Mosby, 1996), 125–151.
10. H. M. Donovan, *Nursing Service Administration: Managing the Enterprise* (Saint Louis: C. V. Mosby, 1975), 50–64.
11. P. F. Drucker, *Management: Tasks, Responsibilities, Practices* (New York: Harper & Row, 1973), 121–129.
12. H. Koontz and H. Weihrich, *Management*, 9th Ed. (New York: McGraw-Hill, 1988), 16.
13. H. M. Donovan, op. cit., 63–64.
14. R. M. Hodgetts, *Management: Theory, Process, and Practice*, 5th Ed. (Orlando, FL: Harcourt, Brace, Jovanovich 1990), 123–124.

15. H. S. Rowland and B. L. Rowland, op. cit.
16. W. E. Reif and J. L. Webster, "The Strategic Planning Process," *Arizona Business* (April 1976), 14–20.
17. A. P. Meier, "The Planning Process," *Managerial Planning* (July–August 1974), 1–5, 9.
18. P. F. Drucker, op. cit., 125.
19. D. H. Fox and R. T. Fox, "Strategic Planning for Nursing," *The Journal of Nursing Administration* (May 1983), 11–16; R. N. Paul and J. W. Taylor, "The State of Strategic Planning," *Business* (January–March 1986), 37–43.
20. D. Osborne and T. Gaebler, *Reinventing Government* (New York: Plume, 1992), 233–234.
21. G. S. Odiorne, "The Art of Crafting Strategic Plans," *Training* (October 1987), 94–96, 98.
22. Ibid.
23. S. R. Baldwin and M. McConnell, "Strategic Planning: Process and Plan Go Hand in Hand," *Management Solutions* (June 1988), 29–36.
24. T. Peters, *Thriving on Chaos* (New York: Harper & Row, 1987), 477; D. N. Sull, "Why Good Companies Go Bad," *Harvard Business Review* (July–August, 1999), 42–48, 50–52, 183; A. Campbell, "Tailored, Not Benchmarked: A Fresh Look at Corporate Planning," *Harvard Business Review* (March–April 1999), 41–48. 50, 189.
25. T. Peters, op. cit., 615–617.
26. S. R. Baldwin and McConnell, op. cit.
27. Z. C. Mercer, "Personal Planning: An Overlooked Application of the Corporate Planning Process," *Managerial Planning* (January–February 1980), 32–35; C. Van Mullem et al., "Strategic Planning for Research Use in Nursing Practice," *Journal of Nursing Administration* (December 1999), 38–45.
28. Ibid.; Mercy Health Services Nurses' Council. "Mercy Health Services: Systemwide Redesign of Patient Care Services," *Nursing Administration Quarterly* (fall 1991), 38–45.
29. D. H. Fox and R. T. Fox, op. cit.
30. D. Jones and V. Crane, "Development of an Organizational Strategic Planning Process for a Hospital Department," *Health Care Supervisor*, 9, 1 (1990), 1–20.
31. J. Begun and K. B. Heatwole, "Strategic Cycling: Shaking Complacency in Healthcare Strategic Planning," *Journal of Healthcare Management* (September–October 1999), 339–352.
32. B. A. Amudson and R. A. Rosenblatt, "The WAMI Rural Hospital Project. Part 6: Overview and Conclusions," *Journal of Rural Health* (fall 1991), 560–574.
33. P. F. Drucker, *Management Challenges for the 21st Century* (New York: HarperCollins, 1999).
34. L. J. Johnson, "Strategic Management: A New Dimension of the Nurse Executive's Role," *Journal of Nursing Administration* (September 1990), 7–10.
35. R. Cushman, "Norton's Top Down, Bottom-Up Planning Process," *Planning Review* (November 1979), 3–8, 48.
36. When the terms *goals* and *objectives* are used, their meaning should be defined. Some references cite goals as being strategic and objectives as being tactical or operational; others, vice versa.
37. D. W. Nylen, "Making Your Business Plan an Action Plan," *Business* (October–December 1985), 12–16.
38. E. K. Singleton and F. C. Nail, "Guidelines for Establishing a New Service," *Journal of Nursing Administration* (October 1985), 22–26.
39. K. W. Vestal, "Writing a Business Plan," *Nursing Economics* (May–June 1988), 121–124.
40. L. Schulmeister, "Starting a Nursing Consultation Practice," *Clinical Nurse Specialist* (March 1999), 94–100.
41. J. E. Johnson, "Developing an Effective Business Plan," *Nursing Economics* (May–June 1990), 152–154; J. E. Johnson, D. G. Sparks, and C. Humphreys, "Writing a Winning Business Plan," *Journal of Nursing Administration* (October 1988), 15–19; J. M. Reiboldt, "Writing a Group Practice Business Plan," *Healthcare Financial Management* (July 1999), 58–61.

REFERENCES

Anderson, M., J. Cosby, B. Swan, H. Moore, and M. Broekhoven. "The Use of Research in Local Health Service Agencies." *Social Science Medicine* (October 1999), 1007–1019.

"'Balanced Scorecard.' Helps Fix Overlake Strategic Plan." *Healthcare Benchmarks* (September 1999), 103–105.

Brendtro, M. and M. Hegge. "Nursing Faculty: One Generation Away from Extinction." *Journal of Professional Nursing* (March–April 2000), 97–103.

Bryan, E. L. and R. E. Welton. "Let Your Business Plan be a Road Map to Credit." *Business* (July–September 1986), 44–47.

Chrispin, P. "Decisions, Decisions." *Journal of Managerial Medicine*, 10(6), (1996), 42–49, 3.

"Development of an Organizational Strategic Planning Process for a Hospital Department." *Health Care Supervisor* (September 1990), 1–20.

Edsel, W. M. "How to Develop a Business Plan for Your Medical Group." *Medical Group Management Journal* (November–December 1999), 36–39.

Forman, L. "Which Comes First, the Planning Process or the Planning Model?" *Business Economics* (September 1979), 42–47.

Gray, D. H. "Uses and Misuses of Strategic Planning." *Harvard Business Review* (January–February 1986), 89–97.

Hansen, R. D. "Strategic Planning: The Basics and Benefits." *Medical Group Management Journal* (May–June 1999), 28–35.

Kelly, K. J. "Administrators' Forum." *Journal of Nursing Staff Development* (March–April 1992), 90–91.

Kotler, P. and P. E. Murphy. "Strategic Planning for Higher Education." *Journal of Higher Education* (May 1981), 470–489.

Matthews, P. "Planning for Successful Outcomes in the New Millennium." *Topics in Health Information Management* (February 2000), 55–64.

McNeese-Smith, D. K. "Job Stages of Entry, Mastery, and Disengagement Among Nurses." *Journal of Nursing Administration* (March 2000), 140–147.

Moller-Tiger, D. "Long-Range Strategic Planning: A Case Study." *Healthcare Financial Management* (May 1999), 33–35.

Nadler, D. A. and M. L. Tushman. "A Model for Diagnosing Organizational Behavior." *Organizational Dynamics*, 9(2) (1980), 35–51.

Norris, J. E. S. "Eight Steps to Strategic Planning." *Nursing Management* (March 1992), 78–79.

Palesy, S. R. "Motivating Line Management Using the Planning Process." *Planning Review* (March 1980), 3–8, 44–48.

Paul, R. N. and J. W Taylor. "The State of Strategic Planning." *Business* (January–March 1986), 37–43.

Pearce, W. H. "I Thought I Knew What Good Management Was." *Harvard Business Review* (March–April 1986), 59–65.

Pender, N. J. "The NIH Strategic Plan. How Will It Affect the Future of Nursing Science and Practice?" *Nursing Outlook* (March–April 1992), 55–56.

Redman, L. N. "The Planning Process." *Managerial Planning* (May–June 1983), 24–30, 40.

Sechrist, K. R., E. M. Lewis, and D. N. Rutledge. "Data Collection for Nursing Work Force Strategic Planning in California." *Journal of Nursing Administration* (June 1999), 9–11, 29.

Siwicki, B. "What's the CEO's Role? Why More Chief Executives Are Playing Pivotal Roles in I.T. Strategic Planning." *Health Data Management* (February 1999), 76–78, 80–82, 84–85.

Taft, S. H., P. K. Jones, and E. L. Minch. "Strengthening Hospital Nursing, Part 2: Characteristics of Effective Plannine Processes." *Journal of Nursing Administration* (June 1992), 36–46.

S. Taft and J. Stearns. "Organizational Change with a Nursing Agenda: Lessons from the Strengthening Hospital Nursing Program." *Journal of Nursing Administration*, 21(2) (1991), 12–21.

Thunhurst, C. and C. Barker. "Using Problem Structuring Methods in Strategic Planning." *Health Policy Planning* (June 1999), 127–134.

CHAPTER 6

Mission, Philosophy, Objectives, and Management Plans

Russell C. Swansburg, PhD, RN

LEARNING OBJECTIVES AND ACTIVITIES

- Define the mission or purpose statement as it pertains to nursing services.
- Use a set of standards to evaluate a purpose or mission statement for a nursing agency.
- Write a purpose or mission statement for a nursing agency. Identify the vision and values to be imparted to customers.
- Define *philosophy* as it pertains to nursing services.
- Use a set of standards to evaluate the philosophy statement of a nursing agency.
- Write a philosophy statement for a nursing agency.
- Define objectives as they pertain to nursing services.
- Use a set of standards to evaluate the objectives statements of a nursing agency.
- Write objectives for a nursing agency.
- Define the operational plan (management plan) as it pertains to nursing services.
- Use a set of standards to evaluate an operational plan of a nursing agency.
- Describe strategy as it relates to the planning function of nursing services.

CONCEPTS: Mission, purpose, vision, values, philosophy, objectives, operational plan, strategy.

MANAGER BEHAVIOR: Directs senior managers in developing statements of mission (purpose), vision, values, philosophy, objectives, and operational plans. Gives the human resource department the task of disseminating these statements.

LEADER BEHAVIOR: Involves representatives of all units of the organization in developing and implementing statements of mission (purpose), vision, values, philosophy, objectives, and operational plans. Includes a system for evaluation, feedback, and update of these statements.

Introduction

Statements of mission or purpose, vision and values, philosophy or beliefs, and objectives and an operational or management plan have been addressed in previous chapters. This chapter discusses these basic tools of management in greater detail. Knowledge of their use is part of the theory of nursing management. The tools are part of the planning function of nursing management, and skill in using them successfully is part of the strategy of nursing management planning.

Written statements of purpose, vision and values, philosophy, objectives, and written operational plans are the blueprints for effective management of any enterprise, including a health care institution. These components of planning exist at each management level. Statements at the corporate level serve the top managers of the organization. Statements at the division level serve the managers and personnel of major divisions, such as nursing, operations, or finance. These statements evolve from and support those of the institution. Services, departments, and units each have written statements of purpose, vision and values, philosophy, objectives, and written operational plans that are developed from and support the documents at division and corporate levels (see Exhibit 6-1).[1]

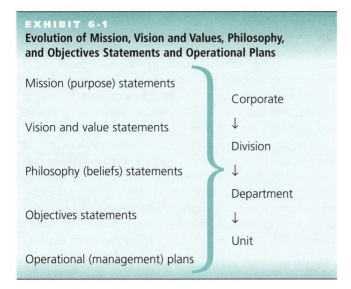

EXHIBIT 6-1
Evolution of Mission, Vision and Values, Philosophy, and Objectives Statements and Operational Plans

Mission (purpose) statements

Vision and value statements

Philosophy (beliefs) statements

Objectives statements

Operational (management) plans

Corporate
↓
Division
↓
Department
↓
Unit

Mission or Purpose, Vision, and Values

Mission or Purpose

The mission of an organization describes the purpose for which that organization exists. Mission statements provide information and inspiration that clearly and explicitly outline the way ahead for the organization. Mission statements provide vision.[2]

The purpose of any organization is to provide individuals with the means to lead productive and meaningful lives. Therefore, the purpose of the organization and each unit should be defined, a teamwork approach should prevail, constituents should be properly trained, and all individuals should be treated with respect.[3]

Organizational purpose moves, guides, and delivers the organization to a perceived goal. Many writers indicate that the purpose or mission statement should be created from a vision statement that describes the things the company stands for. The vision statement is created with the customer's needs in mind. To determine these needs, one must ask and listen to the customer. External customers who purchase the products or services may be given a tour of the organization. In nursing, external customers are prospective patients and families, accreditation and licensing officials, faculty and students, and even taxpayers and shareholders. Internal customers include employees, both departmental and intradepartmental. The mission or purpose statement incorporates the culture of the organization, including strong leadership, rules and regulations, achievement of goals, and the notion that people are more important than work.[4]

Vision

Employees who participate in developing the vision statement believe in their own abilities and are more committed to the organization than employees who do not participate. The vision statement is shared company-wide so that employees may live the vision. It is updated to keep pace with technology and trends.[5] A vision statement is sometimes considered more strategic than a mission statement. The mental exercise of creating one is more meaningful than are the contents of the statement itself.

Vision, values, mission, or purpose statements are meaningful only to the creators.[6] Translated for the community, these statements place value on the way nurses care for people. It follows that ethnic populations are considered in developing vision and values statements for nursing entities. Nursing education teaches the meaning of values such as tolerance and compromise.

Nurse managers must find both the vision and the courage to move nursing forward as a knowledge-intensive profession.

Values

Examples of values are informality, creativity, honesty, quality, courtesy, and caring. Values are the moral rationale for business. Values statements make employees feel proud and managers feel committed. They give meaning to the right way to do things; they give employees enthusiasm and energy. Values bond people and set the behavior standards of employees.[7] Half of U.S. corporations have a values statement. Agreement on values eliminates managers and provides built-in quality. Adherence to values makes companies successful.[8]

Each institution and organization exists for specific purposes or missions and to fulfill specific social functions. For health care organizations, this means providing health care services to maintain health, cure illness, and allay pain and suffering. Business enterprises and government agencies provide most of the economic resources to pay for these services. Although nursing has not been considered a profit-making enterprise, this condition is changing, as third-party payers require better cost-accounting procedures.

Nursing Mission or Purpose

Defining a mission or purpose allows nursing to be managed for performance. It describes what nursing should and will be. The mission or purpose describes the constituencies to be satisfied. It is the professional nurse manager's commitment to a specific definition of purpose or mission.

One purpose of a nursing entity is to provide nursing care to clients, which can include promotion of self-care concepts. Thus, the statement should include definitions of nursing and self-care as defined by professional nurses.

Virginia Henderson has defined nursing as follows[9]:

The unique function of the nurse is to assist the individual, sick or well, in the performance of those activities contributing to health or its recovery (or to peaceful death) that he would perform unaided if he had the necessary strength, will or knowledge. And to do this in such a way as to help him gain independence as rapidly as possible.

Yura and Walsh describe the nursing process as follows[10]:

. . . an orderly, systematic manner of determining the client's health status, specifying problems defined as alterations in human need fulfillment, making plans to solve them, initiating and implementing the plan, and evaluating the extent to which the plan was effective in promoting the optimum wellness and resolving the problems identified.

King defined nursing as[11]:

. . . a process of action, reaction, interaction, and transaction whereby nurses assist individuals of any age group to meet their basic human needs in coping with their health status at some particular point in their life cycle. Nurses perform their functions within social institutions and they interact with individuals and groups. Therefore, three distinct levels of operation exist: (1) the individual; (2) the group; and (3) society.

Orem defined nursing as follows[12]:

Nursing is an art through which the nurse, the practitioner of nursing, gives specialized assistance to persons with disabilities of such character that more than ordinary assistance is needed to meet daily needs for self-care and to intelligently participate in the medical care they are receiving from the physician. The art of nursing is practiced by "doing for" the person with the disability, by "helping him to do for himself," and/or by "helping him to learn how to do for himself." Nursing is also practiced by helping a capable person from the patient's family or a friend of the patient to learn how "to do for" the patient. Nursing is thus a practical and didactic art.

Kinlein suggested that "nursing is assisting the person in his self-care practices in regard to his state of health."[13]

Emerging from these and other theories of nursing is a commonality of terms central to the definition of nursing: nurse, patient or client, individual, group, society, nursing process, self-care, and health.

A further mission of nursing is to provide a public good. This purpose should be indicated in the statement of mission that explains why the nursing entity exists. Because it gives the reason for their employment, the mission statement is written so that all people working within the organizational entity can know it. An ultimate strategy is to have nursing personnel participate in developing mission statements and in keeping them updated so that they will know, understand, and support them.

The mission should be known and understood by other health care practitioners, by clients and their families, and by the community. A statement of purpose must be dynamic, giving action and strength to evolving statements of philosophy, objectives, and management plans. Statements of purpose can be made dynamic by indicating the relationship between the nursing unit and patients, personnel, community, health, illness, and self-care. Exhibits 6-2, 6-3, and 6-4 are examples of mission statements of an organization, the division, and the unit, respectively. Exhibit 6-5 lists the standards for evaluation of the mission statements of an organization.

Mission statements are used in successful business and industrial organizations to provide a clearly defined reason for being. These simple statements move the organization forward and are formulated for performance, products, and services. They contain statements of ethics, principles, and standards that are understood by workers. Workers who clearly perceive that they are pursuing meaningful and worthwhile goals through their individual efforts are more committed and dedicated than those who do not.[14]

Proprietary changes have brought change and competition to the health care industry. They have also brought business techniques that have moved the hospital industry from being facilities dominated to being market driven. The corporate structures of for-profit hospitals consider product line and function and focus on mission. This focus has been adopted by not-for-profit hospitals that now look at mission statements relative to new markets, market share, and diversification. The organization of these new not-for-profit corporate structures can be compared with a chain, with regionalization and integration as links. The leadership of these organizations is dynamic and future oriented rather than being focused on maintenance.[15]

Good mission statements express the organization's vision and values, evoking passion in the employees. Good mission statements delineate the organization's uniqueness. Effective nurse leaders make sure that employees see, feel, and think the mission by following it themselves. They expect and accept resistance.[16]

EXHIBIT 6-2
Mission Statement of an Organization

SUBJECT: MISSION STATEMENT

It is the mission of the University of South Alabama Hospitals & Clinics to:

1. Provide high-quality and continually improving acute and long-term health care services and resources to the people of the community and region without regard to race, creed, color, age, sex, national origin, or handicapping condition, and to provide a high-quality setting conducive to the education and research activities of the University and the community.
2. Provide a dynamic and innovative setting for clinical experiences and postgraduate education of health care professionals.
3. Establish and maintain sound financial practices and procedures while providing cost-effective care, recognizing that patient care and education missions will only be achieved through the protection and growth of the system's assets. Health care for the medically indigent is the responsibility of society and the community. Our obligation for providing this care is limited to what the community supports.
4. Recognize that our future success is dependent on developing and utilizing our most important asset—people. Toward that end, we will provide an environment for professional employee growth through career opportunity and continuing education.
5. Work cooperatively with physicians and other health care providers to improve the standards of health care delivery in our community.

Source: Reprinted with permission of the University of South Alabama Medical Center, Mobile, Alabama.

EXHIBIT 6-3
Mission Statement of a Division

SUBJECT: STATEMENT OF MISSION AND PURPOSE FOR THE DIVISION OF NURSING

The mission and purpose of the Division of Nursing is consistent with the mission and purpose of the University of South Alabama Medical Center. The mission and purpose of the Division of Nursing is fourfold:

1. To provide the patient, at a reasonable cost, a quality of nursing care that can be measured and evaluated.
2. To provide an environment that facilitates nursing research and education and its application to patients under nursing practice.
3. To create a working milieu that encourages professional growth and personal satisfaction for all levels of nursing practice.
4. To foster a positive, professional image of nursing to the public through community involvement and guest relations.

Source: Reprinted with permission of the University of South Alabama Medical Center, Mobile, Alabama.

EXHIBIT 6-4
Mission Statement of a Unit

SUBJECT: PURPOSE: SIXTH FLOOR

The purpose of the sixth floor is consistent with the purpose of the Division of Nursing.

1. To assess the physical, emotional, and spiritual needs of patients, their families, and/or significant others so as to provide optimal care.
2. To provide patients with an individualized plan of care, in regard to their needs, in a cost-effective manner to the patient and the hospital.
3. To serve as the patient's, family's, and/or significant other's advocate to assure complete care with regard to the patient's, family's, and/or significant other's needs.
4. To provide and promote continuing education through in-services, research projects, and patient-care conferences to improve the quality of our health care.
5. To incorporate all disciplines related to patient's care in evaluating the needs of the patient, family, and/or significant others.
6. To assess and evaluate our quality of nursing care on an ongoing basis through quality assurance and monthly audits.

Source: Reprinted with permission of the University of South Alabama Medical Center, Mobile, Alabama.

EXHIBIT 6-5
Standards for the Evaluation of Mission Statements of the Nursing Division and Its Departments, Services, and Units

1. The mission statement tells the reason for the existence of the nursing division, department, service, or unit in relation to the practice of nursing and of self-care as defined by the nursing staff and in relation to the service being provided to the community of clients. Once definitions of nursing and self-care have been developed by the nursing staff and ratified by the nursing administration, they may be quoted in the mission statement.
2. The nursing division mission statement supports the mission of the organization. Unit mission statements are customized by line personnel.
3. The statement indicates that the nursing organization exists to provide a public good.
4. The mission statement is developed by the people who will live by it.
5. It includes a set of core values held by the people who will live by it.
6. It is short, clear, and unambiguous; it has a clear meaning.
7. The mission statement describes the organization's uniqueness.

A mission statement is the first step in the strategic planning process. Business and industry leaders have learned that customers are the most critical stakeholders and frequently note this fact in their mission statements.[17] In today's world professional nurses use their mission, vision, and values statements to give impetus to mergers of several home health care organizations into one effective and focused organization. Such mergers benefit patients, families, payers, and providers.[18]

Philosophy

A written statement of philosophy sets out values, concepts, and beliefs that pertain to nursing administration and nursing practice within the organization. It verbalizes the visions of both nurse managers and nurse practitioners regarding what they believe nursing management and practice to be. It states their beliefs as to how the mission or purpose will be achieved, giving direction toward this end. Statements of philosophy are abstract and contain value statements about human beings as clients or patients and as workers, about work that will be performed by nursing workers for clients or patients, about self-care, about nursing as a profession, about education as it pertains to competence of nursing workers, and about the setting or community in which nursing services are provided.

The character and tone of service are set by planning that evolves purpose and philosophy statements, one from the other, for the organization and each of its units.

Hodgetts indicates that "all managers bring a set of values to the workplace." Managers have economic, theoretical, political, religious, aesthetic, and social values. During recent years managers have been much more oriented to social responsibility than in the past. Values are inherent in a management philosophy.[19] Predictions of future values for the twenty-first century will reflect the future values of society. Nurse managers will be involved and will reflect the values of the times in their statements of philosophy. The philosophy of organizations is very often implicit and is not written down.

Contents

Among the contents of a philosophy statement are the core values related to a nursing modality; the need for advanced preparation, continuing education, students, research, nursing management; and nursing's role in the organization. Philosophy statements pertain to patients' involvement in their care and to their extended families.

Philosophy statements also pertain to nurses' rights, including commitment to staff promotion, and nurses' responsibility to the profession.[20]

From a business aspect, the philosophy statement is an outgrowth of the culture. Most Fortune 500 companies have a philosophy statement, and all better performing companies have one. It is evident on posters or plastic cards, in brochures, articles, annual reports, speeches, and books. People who believe in a company philosophy perform ethically, help employees make correct decisions, speak with one voice, have a sense of corporate purpose, and work more productively.[21]

Concerns prevalent in a business philosophy are customers, quality, excellence, growth, profits, shareholders, society, employees, decentralization, and fun. The philosophy statement supports the mission statement as the glue that binds the separate parts together as a cohesive, productive whole. It motivates employees to accomplish complex tasks in an intimate, relatively simple work environment.[22]

As with the mission statement, the philosophy statement is most effective when developed by those who will live by it. Unit statements of philosophy support the organizational philosophy. Philosophy that is communicated zealously and totally supported by top management is most effective. Unlike mission and objectives statements, the philosophy statement remains constant. As with mission statements, philosophy statements evolve from higher levels of management and practice.

Exhibits 6-6, 6-7, and 6-8 are examples of the philosophy statement of an organization, division, and unit, respectively.

Exhibit 6-9 lists the standards for evaluation of philosophy statements of an organization.

Objectives

Objectives are concrete and specific statements of the goals that nurse managers seek to accomplish. They are action commitments through which the key elements of the mission will be achieved and the philosophy or beliefs sustained. Objectives are used to establish priorities. They are stated in terms of results to be achieved, and focus on the provision of health care services to clients. Like the statements of mission and philosophy, they must be meaningful, relevant, and functional. They must be alive. Moore has stated, "If objectives are presented in terms of what can be observed, they can serve as useful tools for evaluation of nursing care and personnel performance, and as a basis for planning educational programs, staffing, requisition of supplies and equipment, and other functions associated with the nursing department."[23]

EXHIBIT 6-6
Organizational Philosophy Statement

SUBJECT: PHILOSOPHY OF THE UNIVERSITY OF SOUTH ALABAMA MEDICAL CENTER

We believe that:

- The University of South Alabama Medical Center is dedicated to excellence in the fields of patient care, teaching, and research.
- We are dedicated to providing the most effective and efficient patient care.
- We are committed to providing services for patients requiring highly specialized and unique medical treatment.
- We are committed to providing the same level of health care to all patients with the same health problem within the hospital.
- We are committed to providing a safe environment for patients, staff, and guests. We assure the rights of patients to confidentiality, full disclosure of risks involved in care, and involvement in decision making.
- The University of South Alabama Board of Trustees, the Medical Executive Committee, the medical staff at large, and the University of South Alabama Medical Center Administration support both in concept and by resource allocation the implementation and ongoing activities of the Risk Management program designed to reduce risks and losses and promote safety in the hospital setting.
- Continuing education is essential to competence of staff. Professional growth and development is both a personal and organizational responsibility.
- Research should be fostered to the extent possible and should follow acceptable guidelines for protection of human subjects.

- We have an obligation to monitor and continuously improve all activities through quality assessment and improvement as an integral part of Quality Assurance.
- Everyone should be treated with dignity.
- There are fiscal limits to what we can do, and every employee must market the hospital to obtain revenues to maintain financial stability.
- Health care for the medically indigent is the responsibility of society and the community from which they come. Our capacity and obligation for providing indigent care is limited to what the community supports.
- We have an obligation to use our finances and limited resources responsibly and to maintain and improve the fiscal integrity of our institution.
- Health care should focus on prevention and wellness in addition to illness. We promote and plan for patients to care for themselves from time of admission.
- We are the leaders in health care in this community. We believe in supporting laws and regulations and in working to make changes that benefit our mission.
- Our staff are our best asset and they will be treated with respect.
- Our staff have a responsibility to serve this Medical Center with total commitment to our philosophy, goals, policies, and procedures to assure a successful organization.
- We have a responsibility to provide learning experience for all students in the health care field, including providing appropriate clinical settings and role models.

Source: Reprinted with permission of the University of South Alabama Medical Center, Mobile, Alabama.

EXHIBIT 6-7
Philosophy Statement for a Division

SUBJECT: PHILOSOPHY OF THE DIVISION OF NURSING

We believe that:

- The philosophy of the Division of Nursing is consistent with the philosophy of the University of South Alabama Medical Center.
- We are dedicated to excellence in patient care, teaching, and research and to providing the most effective and efficient care.
- Everyone should be treated with dignity.
- Health is not merely the absence of disease or infirmity but a state of optimum physical, mental, and social well-being.
- Nursing care promotes self-care concepts, enabling patients to meet their basic human needs in coping with their health status throughout their life cycles. Nursing involves a broad approach of health care aimed at a healthy society through education of the public.
- Professional nursing care at University of South Alabama Medical Center is provided equally to all patients accepted for treatment.
- Patients and their families have a right to be kept informed about all aspects of their health status and to participate in decisions affecting their care to the fullest extent possible.

- The physical, mental, spiritual, and social needs of our patients can be achieved by striving to maintain goal-directed multidisciplinary plans of care.
- The highly specialized care offered at the Medical Center requires qualified staff for all positions. The most important assets of the institution are the staff and they will be treated with respect.
- We have an obligation to manage personnel and finances to achieve maximum productivity.
- Improvement of the quality of nursing is assured by the continuous evaluation of nursing care and positive modifications to nursing techniques and activities.
- Continuing education is essential to the delivery of quality professional nursing and is both a personal and organizational responsibility.
- We have a responsibility to provide appropriate learning experiences and role models for all students in the health care field.
- We accept the responsibility of being involved in nursing research.

Source: Reprinted with permission of the University of South Alabama Medical Center, Mobile, Alabama.

EXHIBIT 6-8
Philosophy Statement of a Unit

SUBJECT: PHILOSOPHY OF SIXTH FLOOR

- We believe that all patients should be given equal, individualized care by all nursing staff and that such care should incorporate physical, emotional, and spiritual needs.
- We believe the goal of health care should be to assist the patient to progress toward a level of optimal health.
- We believe that the patient should be encouraged by all nursing staff to progress toward self-care and independence.
- We believe that it is the responsibility of all nursing staff to act as a patient advocate to provide quality care according to the wishes of the patient, family, and/or significant others.
- We believe that continuing education is a necessary component of continuing improvement in health care.
- We believe that nursing is an integral part of health care and that the nurse is an important member of the health care team.
- We believe that patients, their families, and/or significant others have the right to be well informed about the patient's state of health, prognosis, and care.

Source: Reprinted with permission of the University of South Alabama Medical Center, Mobile, Alabama.

EXHIBIT 6-9
Standards for Evaluation of Philosophy Statements of the Nursing Division, Department, Service, or Unit

1. A written statement of philosophy should exist for the nursing division and each of its units.
2. A written statement of philosophy should be developed in collaboration with nursing employees, the consumers, and other health care workers.
3. Nursing personnel should share in an annual (or more frequent) review and revision of the written statement of philosophy.
4. The written statement of philosophy should reflect these beliefs or values:
   (a) The meaning of the clinical practice of nursing.
   (b) Recognition of rights of individuals and of the responsibility of nursing personnel to serve as advocates for those rights.
   (c) Selective other statements about humanity, society, health, nursing, nursing process, and self-care relevant to external forces (community, laws, etc.) and internal forces (personnel, clients, material resources, etc.), research, education, and family as are deemed appropriate to accomplishing the mission of the division and each of its units.
5. The nursing philosophy should support the philosophy of the organization as expressed at all levels above the nursing division.
6. The statement of philosophy should give direction to the achievement of the mission.

According to Moore, nursing organizations should have objectives for evaluation of patient care, evaluation of personnel performance, planning of educational programs, staffing, and requisition of supplies and equipment.

Drucker indicates that mission and purpose, as well as the basic definition of a business, must be translated into objectives if they are to become more than insight, good intentions, and brilliant epigrams never to be achieved.[24]

Objectives are concrete statements that become the standards against which performance can be measured. Objectives are the basic tactics of any business, including the business of nursing management. Objectives must be selective rather than global, and they must be multiple rather than single to balance a wide range of needs and goals related to nursing services for clients or patients: productive use of people, money, and material resources; updating through innovation; and the discharge of a social responsibility to the community. Objectives must be used, and one way to use them is to develop them into specific management and operational plans.

The nursing staff, and specifically the nurse manager, must decide where efforts will be concentrated to achieve results. Some areas of concentration have already been mentioned. Others may be similar to those related to business and industry. They include marketing and the development of health care services in areas of need. As an example, there has recently been increased activity in the area of physical and mental wellness or fitness. Great potential exists in the area of prevention of disease and injury. Another area for objectives is innovation, which includes the introduction of new methods and particularly the application of new knowledge.

Areas for objectives are organization of and use of all resources: human, financial, and physical. Objectives address the need to develop managers; the needs of major groups within the division, including nonmanagerial workers, labor relations, the development of positive employee attitudes, and maintenance and upgrading of employee skills. Objectives provide for attractive job and career opportunities and for activities to control worker assignment and productivity. They are the means by which productivity in nursing is measured.

Objectives are also needed in the areas of social responsibility, innovation, and wellness. Society must believe that nursing is useful and productive and that it does a desired job (see Exhibit 6-10).

Management balances objectives. There are short-range objectives with their accomplishment in easy

---

EXHIBIT 6-10
Examples of Categorical Areas for Writing Objectives

- *Evaluation of patient care.* To develop methods of measuring the quality of patient care.
- *Evaluation of personnel performance.* The patient benefits from close nursing supervision of all nonprofessional personnel who give patient care and from continuous appraisal of the nursing care given and the performance of all nursing personnel based on professional standards.
- *Planning educational programs.* The patient benefits from a continuous, flexible program of in-service education for all divisions of nursing personnel adapted to orientation, skill training, continuous education, and leadership development.
- *Staffing.* To establish a systematic staffing pattern for patient care so that all members of each department can function in accordance with their skill levels for the maintenance of continuity of nursing care and management of nursing service.
- *Requisition of supplies and equipment.* To supply nursing personnel with adequate resources to facili-

tate patient care; to anticipate future nursing needs and plan for the acquisition of needed resources.
- *Marketing.* To collaborate and consult with intradepartmental health team members for maximal effectiveness in promoting health care and disease prevention. New programs will be developed to meet identified needs.
- *Innovation.* To influence progressive nursing practices and research training programs in supporting changing trends that improve the quality of patient care.
- *Organization and use of all resources (human, financial, and physical).* To apply standards for decentralization of decision-making, and to increase efficiency and effectiveness of staffing and budgeting.
- *Social responsibility.* To support, publicize, and sustain service to the community in health endeavors.
- *Research and development.* To sustain the nursing profession and the organization.

---

view or reach; long-range objectives, and some objectives in the "hope to accomplish" category. The budget is the mechanical expression of setting and balancing objectives. The nurse manager plans two budgets, one for operations and one for future capital expenditures. Some priorities will be set with the budget, as illustrated in Exhibit 6-11.

Objectives are the fundamental strategy of nursing, because they specify the end product of all nursing activities. They must be capable of being converted into specific targets and specific assignments so that nurses will know what they have to do to accomplish them. Objectives become the basis and motivation for the nursing work necessary to accomplish them and for measuring nursing achievement. They make possible the concentration of human and material resources and

of human efforts. Objectives are needed in all areas on which the survival of nursing and health care services depends. In nursing, all objectives should be performance objectives that provide for existing nursing services for existing patient groups. They should provide for abandonment of unneeded and outmoded nursing services and health care products and provide for new services and products for existing patients. Objectives should provide for new groups of patients, for the distributive organization, and for standards of nursing service and performance.

Objectives are the basis for work and assignments. They determine the organizational structure, key activities, and allocation of personnel to tasks. Objectives make the work of nursing clear and unambiguous, with measurable results, deadlines, and specific assignments of accountability. They give direction and make commitments that mobilize the resources and energies of nursing for the making of the future. Objectives are needed for the organization, division, and all units. They should be changed as necessary, particularly when a change of mission occurs or when the objectives no longer are functional.[25] Last but not least, objectives should exist for research and development of new nursing services and products. Refer to Exhibit 6-12 for a breakdown of the elements of objectives.

Exhibits 6-13, 6-14, and 6-15 are examples of objectives for an organization, a nursing division, and a nursing unit, respectively. Exhibit 6-16 contains standards for evaluating the objectives of an organization.

EXHIBIT 6-11
Examples of Balanced Objectives

- *Long-range objective.* Write a plan to develop patient teaching guides for all areas.
- *Short-range objective.* Establish procedures for safe nursing care by having fire department personnel hold classes on fire evacuation procedures for all nursing personnel on all three shifts.
- *Future budget.* Plan with the budget director to have funds allocated to repaint patients' rooms and replace worn and torn furniture.
- *Current budget.* Implement the classes for expectant parents for which funds have been allocated.

EXHIBIT 6-12

The Elements of Objectives

- *A performance objective.* The patient receives individualized care in a safe environment to meet total therapeutic nursing needs—physical, emotional, spiritual, environmental, social, economic, and rehabilitative (also illustrates next provision).
- *Existing nursing services for existing patients.* Nurse consultants have been made available from medical nursing, surgical nursing, mental health nursing, and maternal and child health nursing. Their services can be requested by any professional nurse or physician.
- *Abandonment of outmoded nursing services and products.* Universal precautions have been implemented and the old handwashing basins have been discarded.

- *New nursing services for new groups of patients.* Plans are being made to offer consultative nursing services from the general hospital to nursing homes in the area. In the future this will be extended to retirement homes. Both actions are the result of market surveys.
- *Organization for new nursing services.* The nurse manager has evaluated the necessity of restructuring the organization of the division of nursing to provide new nursing services.
- *Standards of nursing service and performance.* The nurse manager has decided to use the Standards of Nursing Practice developed by the ANA Congress for Nursing Practice for all nurses within the division.

EXHIBIT 6-13

Goals of the University of South Alabama Medical Center

GLOBAL GOALS

Increase number of paying patients

Increase awareness of resources among public

Short-term plan of what we sell

Long-term plan of what we sell

Increase in services

Educate the staff to sell the formal hospital plan to build hospital on campus

Research provision of differently priced services

Market hospital to university employees

Improve access to hospital

Improve sources of intelligence within community

Residents to use Medical Center for private practice

Improve management of patients for maximum reimbursement

Create new markets

Improve efficiency

Recognize hospital as a business

Reconcile difference in goals between Foundation and hospital

DEFINITIVE GOALS

1. Increase number of paying patients
   (1) Plan for incentive for M.D.'s (Steve)
   (2) Who are private M.D.'s using hospital? (Pat)
   (3) Survey private M.D.'s in town (John)
   (4) Market HMO (internal) (Susie and John)
   (5) Input from department heads (Brookley meeting)
   (6) Create new markets and identify opportunities through money arrangements
      (i) Where are they? (Dept. Heads)
      (ii) Maintain ROA
      (iii) Maintain Keesler arrangement

      (iv) Surrounding counties
      (v) HHC
      (vi) Public service (plan for industry) (Pat)
      (vii) Organizations and involvement (clinic and campus)
      (viii) Student organizations on campus
   (7) Market hospital to university employees
2. Increase awareness of resources among public
   (1) PR plan
   (2) Short-term marketing plan of what we sell (identifying what we are selling now)
3. Long-term marketing plan of what we sell
   (1) What new products can we sell (or divert)?
   (2) Formal plan to build hospital on campus
4. Educate the staff to sell the hospital
   (1) Just for the pride of it
   (2) Management people in civic organizations
   (3) Reference 1(4)
   (4) Employees identify with PR and marketing people
   (5) Recognize hospital as a business
5. Research provision of differently priced services
   (1) Innovative ways to bill for services
6. Improve access to hospital
   (1) Parking
   (2) Waiting areas
   (3) Emergency Department
7. Improve sources of intelligence (above board)
   (1) Professional groups
   (2) Reference 4(2)
   (3) Internal network
8. Residents to use Medical Center for private practice
9. Improve efficiency
   (1) Improve management of patients for maximum reimbursement
      (i) Audit bills with charts
10. Improve cooperative relationship between Foundation (College of Medicine) and Medical Center (hospital)

Source: Reprinted with permission of the University of South Alabama Medical Center, Mobile, Alabama.

EXHIBIT 6-14
Objectives of the Department of Nursing

SUBJECT: OBJECTIVES OF THE DIVISION OF NURSING

The objectives of this Division of Nursing shall be to provide the patient:

1. Individualized care in a safe environment to meet the patient's total needs as assessed by the professional nurse and utilizing the nursing process. This care covers physical, emotional, spiritual, environmental, social, economic, and rehabilitational needs involved in planning total patient care.
2. An effective teaching program which will include guidance and assistance in the use of medical resources and community agencies.
3. Benefits of effective communication, cooperation, and coordination with all professional and administrative services involved in the planning of total patient care.
4. Benefits of a continuous, flexible program of in-service education for all department of nursing personnel adapted to orientation, in-service, continuing education and leadership development.
5. Benefits from Nursing Services' participation in education of students.
6. With cost-effective care by the timely procurement, effective utilization, and proper handling of equipment and supplies.
7. Benefits through a positive work atmosphere in which nurses' job satisfaction is attained.
8. Benefits from a close association between Division of Nursing personnel and community nursing organizations and groups to keep abreast of current trends and advancements in nursing.
9. Maximum nursing care hours by relieving nursing personnel of non-nursing duties.
10. Benefits from the development of a cost-effective balanced budget for the Division of Nursing.
11. Benefits from close supervision by an RN of all personnel who give patient care, and from continuous evaluation of the care given.
12. Benefits from implementation of the results of nursing research.

Source: Reprinted with permission of the University of South Alabama Medical Center, Mobile, Alabama.

EXHIBIT 6-15
Objectives of a Nursing Unit

SUBJECT: OBJECTIVES OF SIXTH FLOOR

The objectives of the Sixth Floor shall be to provide the patient, family, and/or significant others:

1. Individualized total patient care based on an assessment by an RN, considering all needs, physical, emotional, and spiritual, of the patient, family, and/or significant others.
2. The nursing process will be the basis of all care given by the professional nurse.
3. To provide quality care in a cost-effective manner to patient and hospital.
4. To coordinate information from all disciplines, to plan for optimum care while hospitalized and after discharge.
5. To involve the patient's family and/or significant others in caring for the patient to meet their needs.
6. To identify problem areas in nursing care through monthly audits to ensure the quality of our nursing care.
7. To increase knowledge and improve nursing care by providing a variety of in-service [training] from all departments involved in the care of the patient.

Source: Reprinted with permission of the University of South Alabama Medical Center, Mobile, Alabama.

EXHIBIT 6-16
Standards for Evaluation of Statements of Objectives for a Nursing Division, Department, Service, or Unit

1. The objectives for the nursing division, department, service, or unit should be in written form.
2. The objectives should be developed in collaboration with the nursing personnel who will assist in achieving them.
3. Nursing personnel should share in an annual (or more frequent) review and revision of the written statements of objectives.
4. The written statement of objectives should meet these qualitative and quantitative criteria:
   (a) They operationalize the statements of mission and philosophy; they can be translated into actions.
   (b) They can be measured or verified.
   (c) They exist in a hierarchy or prioritized sequence.
   (d) They are clearly stated.
   (e) They are realistic in terms of human and physical resources and capabilities.
   (f) They direct the use of resources.
   (g) They are achievable (practical).
   (h) They are specific.
   (i) They indicate results expected from nursing efforts and activities; the ends of management programs.
   (j) They show a network of desired events and results.
   (k) They are flexible and allow for adjustment.
   (l) They are known to the nursing personnel who will use them.
   (m) They are quantified wherever possible.
   (n) They exist for all positions.

Operational Plan

Objectives must be converted into actions, that is, activities, assignments, and deadlines, all with clear accountability. The action level is where nurse managers eliminate the old and plan for the new. It is where time dimensions are put into perspective and new and different methods can be tried. The action level is where nurse managers answer these questions over and over again: What is it? What will it be? What should it be?

An operational plan is the written blueprint for achieving objectives. The operational plan does the following:

- Specifies the activities and procedures that will be used.
- Sets timetables for the achievement of objectives.
- Tells who the responsible persons are for each activity and procedure.
- Describes ways of preparing personnel for jobs and procedures for evaluating patient care.

- Specifies the records that will be kept and the policies needed.
- Gives individual mangers freedom to accomplish their objectives and those of the institution, division, department, or unit.

The operational plan is sometimes called a management plan (see Exhibits 6-17 and 6-18).

Strategy

A theory of the business is its objectives, results, customers, and what customers value and pay for. Strategy converts theory into performance. In the twenty-first century strategy is based on five certainties[26]:

1. "The collapsing birthrate in the developed world.
2. Shifts in the distribution of disposable income.
3. Defining performance.
4. Global competitiveness.
5. The growing incongruence between economic globalization and political splintering."

Planning is the strategy of an organization and is essential to all businesses, including those providing health care. Planning techniques used in business and industry increasingly are being used in health care organizations. Strategy is the process by which an organization achieves success in a changing environment. Nursing has only tapped the surface of a business strategy.[27] Myriad services are available that can be offered to potential clients, such as telephone and e-mail access to information on drug prices, durable medical equipment prices, educational services, research briefs, and a host of therapeutic nursing products. A nursing strategy will outline how the firm achieves its strategic goals and objectives in a competitive marketplace.

Top management has to answer planning questions like these:

- Where do we go and what do we want to become? Such questions seek to define the organization's mission and objectives.
- What and where are we now? The purpose here is to examine and define the organization's philosophy and objectives.
- How can we best get there? The answer to this question will take the form of ongoing plans that include organizing, directing, and controlling concepts.

Such activities constitute the strategy of top management. They are developed into the strategy of the nursing division's top management and subsequently into the strategy of nursing and other business units of the organization. Planning is neither a top-down nor

EXHIBIT 6-17

OBJECTIVE

The Clients receive skilled nursing services to meet their total individual needs as diagnosed by professional nurses. This process is systematic, beginning with the gathering of base data, and it is planned, implemented, evaluated, and revised on a continual basis. It covers physical, emotional, spiritual, environmental, social, economic, and rehabilitational needs and includes health teaching involved in the planning of total client care. Its ultimate goal is to assist clients to, or return them to, optimal health status and independence as quickly as possible.

ACTIONS	TARGET DATES	ACCOMPLISHMENTS
Institute primary care nursing	January 1–June 30	Assigned to Ms. Scott. Decision made to attempt to use self-care concepts of Orem: (1) definition, and (2) nursing systems.
1. Assign problem of overall development of a plan	January 31	
2. Assign development of a self-care concept for application using Orem and Kinlein as references	February 15	January 19: Assigned to Ms. Longez. In a discussion with Ms. Scott and Ms. Longez, the decision was made to investigate application of self-care using the nursing process as described by Kinlein. The nursing staff were particularly interested in the nursing history process described by Kinlein. Ms. Longez has added this dimension to her assignment. She has requested Mr. Jarmann be assigned to assist her, and he has agreed.
3. Organize resources	February 28	February 5: Ms. Scott has just updated me on the project. A good portion of her plan has been developed. They are now doing a staffing plan, including job descriptions and job standards.
		February 27: The plan is completed and has been discussed with me. A few minor adjustments are being made.
4. Coordinate plan (a) Nursing personnel (b) Administrator (c) Public relations (d) Physicians (e) Other as needed	March 31	Done. All want to participate. Done. Announcements made to community through news media. Done and well received. Presented to board per request of administrator. They want progress reports.
5. Select and train staff	April 30	Assigned to Ms. Finch for training. Will be assisted by Ms. Scott and Ms. Longez. I will select staff with their recommendation.
6. Implement	June 30	Ms. Scott wants to direct implementation and I have concurred.

bottom-up proposition. Each level must harmonize its strategies with those below and above.[28]

Focusing on development and use of planning strategies is a key element that gives direction, cohesion, and thrust to the nursing division. Nurse employees involved in achieving objectives and goals are motivated. They should be clearly defined and focus on the future without losing sight of the present. Successful implementation of management plans to achieve mission objectives and goals while sustaining philosophy results in productivity, profitability, and achievement. This process is managing, and managers perform it.[29]

Cavanaugh relates strategy to power, indicating that organizational power gives nurse managers the power to do their jobs better. Her suggestions for nurse managers to strategize are summarized as follows[30]:

1. Use the political system to turn personal power into organizational power.
2. Recognize the self-interests of others in the organization and use them in a win-win manner.
3. Diagnose, plan, and execute an effective political campaign to achieve a well-thought-out, purposeful goal.
4. Define ways to achieve objectives while helping others. Know people and their goals.
5. Disengage from losing issues and from issues in which you have to defend yourself on someone else's turf. A technique for doing this is placing it at the end of an agenda or omitting it from the minutes.
6. Defend your territory.
7. Plan and carry out an offense on issues of your own choosing and commitment.

EXHIBIT 6-18

Standards for Evaluation of Management Plan of Nursing Division, Department, Service, or Unit

1. The written management plan should operationalize the strategic goals of the organization as well as the objectives of the nursing division, department, service, or unit. It should specify activities or actions, persons responsible for accomplishing them, and target dates or time frames, as well as providing for evaluation of progress. Each activity or action should be listed in problem-solving or decision-making format, as appropriate.

2. The management plan is personal to the incumbent, who should select the standards for developing, maintaining, and evaluating it. The nurse manager should solicit desired input from appropriate nursing persons and others.

3. The actions listed should reflect planning for:
   (a) Nursing care programs to ensure safe and competent nursing services to clients.
       (i) The nursing process, including data gathering, assessment, diagnosis, goal setting and prescription, intervention and application, evaluation, feedback, change, and accountability to the consumer.
       (ii) A process and outcome audit.
       (iii) Promotion of self-care practices.
   (b) Establishment of policies and procedures for employing competent nursing personnel: recruitment, selection, assignment, retention, and promotion based on individual qualifications and capabilities without regard to race, national origin, creed, color, sex, or age.
   (c) Integration of nursing care programs into the total program of the health care organization and community through committee participation in professional and service activities, and credentialing of individuals in organizations, including nursing organizations.
   (d) A budget that is evaluated and revised as necessary.
   (e) Job descriptions that include standards stated as objectives, outcomes, or results, and that are known to the incumbents.
   (f) Specific utilization of personnel. This part of the plan should:
       (i) Conform to a staffing plan that is based on timing nursing activities and rating of patients.
       (ii) Match competencies of people to total job requirements.
       (iii) Place prepared people in practice.
       (iv) Place prepared people in administration.
       (v) Place prepared people in education.
       (vi) Place prepared people in research.
       (vii) Foster identification of non-nursing tasks and their assignment to appropriate other departments or non-nursing personnel.
       (viii) Recognize excellence in all fields: administration, education, research, and practice.
   (g) Provision of needed supplies and equipment for nursing activities.
   (h) Provision of input into remodeling and establishing required physical facilities.
   (i) Orientation and continuing education of all nursing personnel.
   (j) Education of students in the health care field according to a written agreement and collaborative implementation between faculty of the educational institutions and personnel of the service organization.
   (k) Development of nursing research staff, research activities, and application of the research findings of others.
   (l) Evaluation of all objectives—organizational, divisional, departmental, and at the service and unit level, as well as those stated in the individual's job description and standards.

4. The management plans should have mileposts that are reasonable and attainable, with deadlines included.

5. Management plans should be based on complete information.

---

8. Build coalitions.
9. Exploit opportunities, using situations to your advantage. Go after winning issues.
10. Set up situations to benefit persons who can benefit you. Then deliver the goods at a cost-effective price.

A political climate exists in any organization, and its democratic nature requires compromise, trade-offs, favors, and negotiation. Nurse managers must be political to gain their goals and objectives in such a climate. Ehrat identifies four considerations of political strategy[31]:

1. Structure considerations. The first major political concept is to learn the history of the organization, including its past struggles and their outcomes.

Budgets reflect one of these political outcomes. What is valued by the organization? The successful nurse manager identifies these valued data and operates within their constraints and boundaries.

2. Economic considerations. What are the costs versus the benefits? Give something in return for gaining something better. All departments expect to gain a fair share of an increased budget. To ensure that nursing has equity, nurse managers develop clientele, confidence, a meaningful network, administrative support, and effective platform skills. Nurse managers also exploit their opportunities. In gaining and sustaining this influence, they do not go beyond tolerated limits.

3. Process considerations. Timing is important and is learned from managerial experience and maturation. Resolution is needed to prepare for and carry out negotiation and compromise. Impact must be considered from the viewpoint of opposition, support, risks, price, and trade-offs, all of which require strategies.

4. Outcome considerations. The outcome must meet minimum standards of satisfaction and avoid problems. It must meet some of the needs of everyone. (*Consensus* means 70% to 80% approval, agreement, and support.)

Resources in the health care field are scarce, causing political conflicts and power struggles. Nurse managers should learn the strategy associated with political knowledge and skills.[32]

The nurse manager moving into a new nursing management position plans strategies for success. From day one, this person arrives early, listens, is polite, and does not criticize the predecessor. This nurse manager makes friends with the boss, assumes authority, eliminates nonessentials, trains subordinates, and delegates decision-making to them. She or he establishes a psychological distance, avoids gripers, treats all employees as adults, maintains an open mind, and follows good communication skills by keeping people informed and accepting their input.

When conflicts occur, the nurse manager does not take sides. This individual attends to actions that produce quick results, impact the organization, are favorable to employees, and require a small investment. Giving a sense of nursing's mission, its importance, its relevance, and the meaningfulness of nursing work provides vision. This is done by listening, sharing, developing mutual ideas, and enlisting the support of informal leaders.

Clear, complete plans are developed in seven areas of key results:

1. Client satisfaction
2. Productivity
3. Innovation
4. Staff development
5. Budget goals
6. Quality
7. Organizational climate

These plans will include standards of performance that challenge and inspire. The nurse manager follows the rules. Rewards are given, including praise to relieve anxiety and to recognize accomplishments, and the best pay possible. Employees who talk back, disobey, are insubordinate, and are malcontents are not tolerated;

they are won over or neutralized. Decisions are made based on test data and judgment.[33]

Research

Research could be considered as a key results area under innovation, as discussed previously. However, it is good strategy to separate research into an eighth key results area. Research studies show that 20% of small businesses that did *not* perform strategic planning failed, wheras only 8% of small businesses that performed strategic planning failed.[34]

A research study of the relationship between nursing department purpose, philosophy, and objectives and evidence of their implementation examined documents in 35 nursing departments. Specific indicators used were patient classification systems and staffing patterns, standards of patient care, and cost containment activity. Implementation rates of desired nursing activity varied from 9% to 25%, indicating a "low rate of implementation negates a causal relationship between references in the documents to desired nursing activity and actual nursing activity." The researchers suggest that purpose statements are sometimes unrealistic and unachievable. The framework for this study should be used to expand the research in this area.[35]

Summary

The basic tools of planning are statements of mission or purpose, vision and values, philosophy or beliefs, and objectives and an active operational or management plan. All managers use such documents to accomplish the work of nursing.

The statement of mission or purpose gives the reasons an entity exists, whether it is an organization, division, department, or unit. The nursing mission statement pertains to the clinical practice of nursing supported by research, education, and management.

The statement of philosophy reflects the values and beliefs of the organizational entity. It is translated into action by nursing personnel.

Objectives are concrete statements describing the major accomplishments nurses desire to achieve. Major categorical areas for objectives include:

- Organization and use of all resources: human, financial and physical
- Social responsibility
- Staffing
- Requisition of supplies and equipment
- Planning of educational programs

- Innovation
- Marketing
- Evaluation of patient care
- Evaluation of personnel performance

Operational or management plans convert objectives into action and include activities, assignments, deadlines, and provision for accountability. A major strategy of an organization is the planning process; the formulation and use of statements of mission, philosophy, and objectives; and the formulation of organizational plans developed with the broadest possible input.

Statements of mission, philosophy, and objectives support each other at different agency levels, from the unit to the service or department and then to the division and finally to the organization.

APPLICATION EXERCISES

EXERCISE 6-1   Use Exhibit 6-5, Standards for the Evaluation of Mission Statements of the Nursing Division and Its Departments, Services, and Units, to

1. Evaluate a mission statement.
2. Develop a mission statement.

EXERCISE 6-2   Use Exhibit 6-9, Standards for Evaluation of Philosophy Statements of the Nursing Division, Department, Service, or Unit, to

1. Evaluate a philosophy statement.
2. Develop a philosophy statement.

EXERCISE 6-3   Use Exhibit 6-16, Standards for Evaluation of Statements of Objectives for a Nursing Division, Department, Service, or Unit, to

1. Evaluate objectives.
2. Develop objectives.

EXERCISE 6-4   Use Exhibit 6-18, Standards for Evaluation of Management Plan of Nursing Division, Department, Service, or Unit, to

1. Evaluate management plans.
2. Develop a management plan.

EXERCISE 6-5   Identify and develop a statement of the planning strategy for a nursing organization or unit.

EXERCISE 6-6   Examine the statements in Exhibit 6-19 of a new economy organization called Earthlink, Inc. Discuss whether these core values would have meaning for nursing management in terms of personnel and clients. How can these values be used to prevent insensitivity to people in an era in which profits are emphasized and nursing workers are rushed?

EXHIBIT 6-19
Standards of Operation: Earthlink, Inc.

OUR MISSION

To become the leading Internet service provider in the world, as measured by number of members, member satisfaction, and profitability.

OUR PURPOSE

To change the way the world does business by demonstrating what a company based on integrity and respect for the individual can accomplish.

To improve people's lives by giving them the ability to communicate better than ever before.

To enable our employees and shareholders to flourish and prosper.

CORE VALUES AND BELIEFS

We respect the individual, and believe that individuals who are treated with respect and given responsibility respond by giving their best.

We require complete honesty and integrity in everything we do.

We make commitments with care, and then live up to them. In all things, we do what we say we are going to do.

Work is an important part of life, and it should be fun. Being a good businessperson does not mean being stuffy and boring.

We love to compete, and we believe that competition brings out the best in us.

We are frugal. We guard and conserve the company's resources with at least the same vigilance that we would use to guard and conserve our own personal resources.

We insist on giving our best effort in everything we undertake. Furthermore, we see a huge difference between "good mistakes" (best effort, bad result) and "bad mistakes" (sloppiness or lack of effort).

Clarity in understanding our mission, our goals, and what we expect from each other is critical to our success.

We are believers in the Golden Rule. In all our dealings, we will strive to be friendly and courteous, as well as fair and compassionate.

We feel a sense of urgency on all matters related to our customers. We own problems and we are always responsive. We are customer-driven.

Permission requested from Earthlink, Inc.

NOTES

1. For a classic article on purpose, philosophy, and objectives, refer to M. A. Moore, "Philosophy, Purpose, and Objectives: Why Do We Have Them?" *Journal of Nursing Administration* (May–June 1971), 9–14.
2. D. L. Calfee, "Get Your Mission Statement Working!" *Management Review* (January 1993), 54–57.
3. P. Crosby, *Running Things: The Art of Making Things Happen* (New York: NAL-Dutton, 1989).
4. J. R. Reyes and B. H. Kleiner, "How to Establish an Organizational Purpose," *Management Decision: Quarterly Review of Management Technology*, 28(7), (1990), 51–54.
5. Ibid.
6. E. E. Spragins, "Resource—Constructing a Vision Statement," *Inc.* (October 1992), 33.
7. A. Campbell, "The Power of Mission: Aligning Strategy and Culture," *Planning Review* (September–October 1992), 10–12, 63.
8. A. Farnham, "State Your Values, Hold the Hot Air," *Fortune* (19 April 1993), 117–124.
9. V. Henderson, *The Nature of Nursing* (New York: Macmillan, 1966), 15.
10. H. Yura and M. B. Walsh, *The Nursing Process*, 5th Ed. (New York: Appleton-Century-Crofts, 1988), 1.
11. I. M. King, "A Conceptual Frame of Reference in Nursing," *Nursing Research* (January–February 1968), 27–31.
12. D. E. Orem, *Nursing: Concepts of Practice*, 5th Ed. (New York: McGraw-Hill, 1995), 7.
13. M. L. Kinlein, *Independent Nursing Practice with Clients* (Philadelphia: J. B. Lippincott, 1977), 23.
14. S. D. Truskie, "The Driving Force of Successful Organizations," *Business Horizons* (May–June 1984), 43–48.
15. G. E. Sussman, "CEO Perspectives on Mission, Healthcare Systems, and the Environment," *Hospital & Health Services Administration* (March–April 1985), 21–34.
16. A. Farnham, op. cit.; J. R. Reyes and B. H. Kleiner, op. cit.
17. R. D. Ireland and M. A. Hitt, "Mission Statements: Importance, Challenge, and Recommendations for Development," *Business Horizons* (May–June 1992), 34–42.
18. J. K. Hoelscher and W. Sprick, "Integrating Home Care into a Community Healthcare System: One Agency's Experience," *Home Healthcare Nurse Management* (July–August 1999), 11–17.
19. R. M. Hodgetts, *Management: Theory, Process, and Practice*, 5th Ed. (Orlando, FL: Harcourt, Brace, Jovanovich, 1990), 73–74.
20. G. W. Poteet and A. S. Hill, "Identifying the Components of a Nursing Service Philosophy," *Journal of Nursing Administration* (October 1988), 29–33.
21. "Corporate Philosophies," *Compressed Air Magazine* (August 1988), 31–34.
22. Ibid.
23. M. A. Moore, op. cit.; 13; D. L. Calfee, op. cit.
24. P. F. Drucker, *Management: Tasks, Responsibilities, Practice* (New York: Harper & Row, 1978), 99–102.
25. *Report on the Project for the Evaluation of the Quality of Nursing Service* (Ottawa, Ontario: The Canadian Nurses' Association, 1966), 47–48.
26. P. F. Drucker, *Management Challenges for the 21st Century* (New York: HarperCollins, 1999), 43–44.
27. D. E. Morris and S. E. Rau, "Strategic Competition: The Application of Business Planning Techniques to the Hospital Marketplace," *Health Care Strategic Management* (January 1985), 17–20.

28. R. Cushman, "Norton's Top-Down, Bottom-Up Planning Process," *Planning Review* (November 1979), 3–8, 48.

29. A. P. Meier, "The Planning Process," *Managerial Planning* (July–August 1974), 1–5, 9.

30. D. E. Cavanaugh, "Gamesmanship: The Art of Strategizing," *Journal of Nursing Administration* (April 1985), 38–41.

31. K. S. Ehrat, "A Model for Politically Astute Planning and Decision Making," *Journal of Nursing Administration* (September 1983), 29–35.

32. Ibid.

33. V. C. Sherman, "Taking Over: Notes to the New Executive," *Journal of Nursing Administration* (May 1982), 21–23.

34. R. D. Ireland and M. A. Hitt, op. cit.

35. B. J. Trexler, "Nursing Department Purpose, Philosophy, and Objectives: Their Use and Effectiveness," *Journal of Nursing Administration* (March 1987), 8–12.

REFERENCES

Cohen, M. "Tools for the Practice Manager." *New England Journal of Medicine* (January 2000), 49–50.

Glen, S. "Educating for Interprofessional Collaboration: Teaching about Values." *Nursing Ethics* (May 1999), 202–213.

Mendes, I. A., M. A. Trevizan, M. S. Nogueira, and N. O. Sawada. "Humanizing Nurse-Patient Communication: A Challenge and a Commitment." *Medical Law*, 18(4), (1999), 639–644.

Moller-Tiger, D. "Long-Range Strategic Planning: A Case Study." *Healthcare Financial Management* (May 1999), 33–35.

Molloy, J. and A. Cribb. "Changing Values for Nursing and Health Promotion: Exploring the Policy Context of Professional Ethics." *Nursing Ethics* (September 1999), 411–422.

Sabatino, C. J. "Reflections On the Meaning of Care." *Nursing Ethics* (September 1999), 374–382.

Schmieding, N. J. "Reflective Inquiry Framework for Nurse Administrators." *Journal of Advanced Nursing* (September 1999), 631–639.

Sorrells-Jones, J. and D. Weaver. "Knowledge Workers and Knowledge-Intense Organizations, Part 3. Implications for Preparing Healthcare Professionals." *Journal of Nursing Administration* (October 1999), 14–21.

Weaver, H. N. "Transcultural Nursing with Native Americans: Critical Knowledge, Skills, and Attitudes." *Journal of Transcultural Nursing* (July 1999), 197–202.

CHAPTER 7

Staffing and Scheduling

Russell C. Swansburg, PhD, RN

Russell C. Swansburg, PhD, RN

LEARNING OBJECTIVES AND ACTIVITIES

- Describe the components of the staffing process.
- Do a work sampling study covering a specific period of time.
- Determine the responsibility for staffing activities.
- Determine the core staff and the complementary staff for nursing unit.
- Prepare a staffing plan for a nursing unit.
- Describe the components of a patient classification system (PCS).
- Use a PCS to classify patients on a nursing unit.
- Analyze the staffing problems on a nursing unit.
- Determine the modified approaches to nurse staffing and scheduling used by a health care organization.
- Identify methods for improving productivity in a health care agency.
- Measure the productivity of the nursing staff on a nursing unit.

CONCEPTS: Staffing philosophy, staffing process, staffing activities, work contract, staffing modules, cyclic staffing, self-scheduling, patient classification systems, modified workweeks, temporary workers, productivity.

MANAGER BEHAVIOR: Oversees staffing activities through human resource management that includes use of a patient classification system and provision of qualified nursing personnel in adequate numbers to meet patient care needs.

LEADER BEHAVIOR: Uses input from employees to develop and implement a staffing philosophy and staffing policies that inspire personnel to work to their maximum level of productivity.

Staffing Philosophy

Staffing is certainly one of the major problems of any nursing organization, whether it is a hospital, nursing home, home health care agency, ambulatory care agency, or another type of facility. Aydelotte has stated that[1]

> Nurse staffing methodology should be an orderly, systematic process, based upon sound rationale, applied to determine the number and kind of nursing personnel required to provide nursing care of a predetermined standard to a group of patients in a particular setting. The end result is prediction of the kind and number of staff required to give care to patients.

Components of the staffing process as a control system include a staffing study, a master staffing plan, a scheduling plan, and a nursing management information system (NMIS). The NMIS includes these five elements[2]:

1. Quality of patient care to be delivered and its measurement.
2. Characteristics and care requirements of patients.
3. Prediction of the supply of nurse power required for components 1 and 2.
4. Logistics of the staffing program pattern and its control.
5. Evaluation of the quality of care desired, thereby measuring the success of the staffing itself.

West adds a position control plan and a budgeting plan (see Exhibit 7-1).[3]

Nurse staffing must meet certain regulatory requirements, among which are legal requirements of Medicare. (Medicare and Medicaid regulations are excerpted in Exhibit 7-2). This legal standard is further supported by, for example, the standards of the Joint Commission on Accreditation of Healthcare Organizations

EXHIBIT 7-1
Components of the Staffing Process

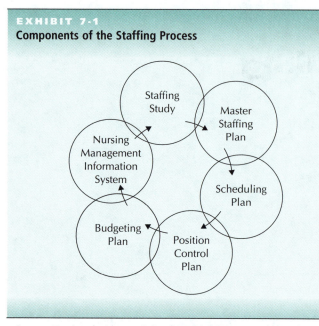

Source: Reprinted with permission from M. E. West. "Implementing Effective Nurse Staffing Systems in Managed Hospitals." *Topics in Health Care Financing*, 6(4), 1980, 15. © 1980, Aspen Publishers, Inc.

(JCAHO). Some other standards include the American Nurses Association (ANA) Scope and Standards for Nurse Administrators, the ANA Standards of Clinical Nursing Practice, and state licensing requirements.

From all of these standards and from the expectations of the community, of nurses, and of physicians, the nurse administrator will develop a staffing philosophy as a basis for a staffing methodology. Community expectations will be related to economic status, local value and belief systems, and local standards of culture. Nurses' expectations will be related to the same community standards, their perceptions of the practice of nursing and its components, desired results, and tolerated workload. See Appendix 7-1 on staffing and assignment guidelines.

Nurse managers can discern various values related to staffing from the nursing division's existing statements of purpose, philosophy, and objectives. A staffing philosophy may encompass beliefs about using a patient classification system (PCS) for identifying patient care needs. The PCS may cover beliefs about the use of skilled personnel as a core staff, with a float pool of nurses for supplemental staffing. The PCS may also specify who will be responsible for hiring.[4]

Objectives of nurse staffing are excellent care and high productivity. Professional nurses can develop a statement of purpose that is comprehensive in stating the quality and quantity of performance it is intended to motivate. Purpose statements should be quantified.[5]

Current and future trends indicate extensive structural changes in the health care system, including downsizing, mergers, closures, and increased ambulatory care services. Managers and clinical nurses will be faced with making staffing decisions to increase productivity. These decisions should be based on lessons learned in the 1980s and 1990s about management of human resources (HR) or human capital.

Staffing Study

A staffing study should gather data about environmental factors within and outside the organization that affect staffing requirements. Aydelotte listed four techniques drawn from engineering to measure the work of nurses, all of which involve the concept of time required for performance[6]:

1. Time study and task frequency:
   a. Tasks and task elements (procedures).
   b. Point and time started.
   c. Point and time ended.
   d. Sample size.
   e. Average time.
   f. Allowance for fatigue, personal variations, and unavoidable standby.
   g. Standard time = step 1.5 + step 1.6.
   h. Frequency of task × standard time = the measurement of nursing activity.
   i. Total of all tasks × standard time = volume of nursing work.
2. Work sampling (variation of task frequency and time); the procedure is as follows:
   a. Identify major and minor categories of nursing activities.
   b. Determine number of observations to be made.
   c. Observe random sample of nursing personnel performing activities.
   d. Analyze observations. Frequency occurring in a specific category = percentage of total time spent in that activity. Most work sampling studies sample direct care and indirect care to determine ratio.
3. Continuous sampling (variation of task frequency and time). Technique is the same as for work sampling except that,
   a. Observer follows one individual in the performance of a task.
   b. Observer may observe work performed for one or more patients if they can be observed concurrently.
4. Self-reporting (variation of task frequency and time):
   a. The individual records the work sampling or continuous sampling on himself or herself.
   b. Tasks are logged using time intervals or time tasks start and end.
   c. Logs are analyzed.

EXHIBIT 7-2
Medicare and Medicaid Regulations

482.23   Condition of participation: Nursing services.
The hospital must have an organized nursing service that provides 24-hour nursing services. The nursing services must be furnished or supervised by a registered nurse.

(a) *Standard: Organization.* The hospital must have a well-organized service with a plan of administrative authority and delineation of responsibilities for patient care. The director of nursing service must be a licensed registered nurse. He or she is responsible for the operation of the service, including determining the types and numbers of nursing personnel and staff necessary to provide nursing care for all areas of the hospital.

(b) *Standard: Staffing and delivery of care.* The nursing service must have adequate numbers of licensed registered nurses, licensed practical nurses (vocational), and other personnel to provide nursing care to all patients as needed. There must be supervisory and staff personnel for each department or nursing unit to ensure, when needed, the immediate availability of a registered nurse for bedside care of any patient.

(1) The hospital must provide 24-hour nursing service furnished or supervised by a registered nurse, and have a licensed practical nurse or registered nurse on duty at all times, except for rural hospitals that have in effect a 24-hour nursing waiver granted under §405.1910(c) of this chapter.

(2) The nursing service must have a procedure to ensure that hospital nursing personnel for whom licensure is required have valid and current licensure.

(3) A registered nurse must supervise and evaluate the nursing care for each patient.

(4) The hospital must ensure that the nursing staff develops, and keeps current, a nursing care plan for each patient.

(5) A registered nurse must assign the nursing care of each patient to other nursing personnel in accordance with the patient's needs and the specialized qualifications and competence of the nursing staff available.

(6) Non-employee licensed nurses who are working in the hospital must adhere to the policies and procedures of the hospital. The director of nursing service must provide for adequate supervision and evaluation of the clinical activities of non-employee nursing personnel which occur within the responsibility of the nursing service.

(c) *Standard: Preparation and administration of drugs.* Drugs and biologicals must be prepared and administered in accordance with Federal and State laws, the orders of the practitioner or practitioners responsible for the patient's care as specified under §482.12(c), and accepted standards of practice.

(1) All drugs and biologicals must be administered by, or under supervision of, nursing or other personnel in accordance with Federal and State laws and regulations, including applicable licensing requirements and in accordance with the approved medical staff policies and procedures.

(2) All orders for drugs and biologicals must be in writing and signed by the practitioner or practitioners responsible for the care of the patient as specified under §482.12(c). When telephone or oral orders must be used, they must be

(i) Accepted only by personnel who are authorized to do so by the medical staff policies and procedures, consistent with Federal and State law;

(ii) Signed or initialed by the prescribing practitioner as soon as possible; and

(iii) Used infrequently.

(3) Blood transfusions and intravenous medications must be administered in accordance with State law and approved medical staff policies and procedures. If blood transfusions and intravenous medications are administered by personnel other than doctors of medicine or osteopathy, the personnel must have special training for this duty.

(4) There must be a hospital procedure for reporting transfusion reactions, adverse drug reactions, and errors in administration of drugs.

Source: Reprinted from CCH's *Medicare and Medicaid Regulations*, with permission of CCH Incorporated, Riverwoods, IL, © 1986.

Many work-sampling studies focus on procedures, ignore standards, and are lacking in objectivity, reliability, and accuracy. The techniques themselves, however, are sound. (See Exhibit 7-3.)[7]

According to West, "There are three cardinal rules for forecasting staffing requirements."[8] The first is to base staffing projections on past staffing history; Exhibit 7-4 is designed as a data sheet for this purpose. The data can be collected from the PCS reports and census reports. Such data are readily available in most hospitals. Some NMISs, such as Medicus, provide numbers of personnel required, including the mix of RNs, LPNs and NAs. Other data needed are sick time, overtime, holidays, and vacation time. The attrition rate is also important and is discussed in Chapter 8, Human Resource Management Activities. In some PCS, these data are built into the staffing formula.

The second cardinal rule for staffing is to review current staffing levels. Review of future plans for the institution is the third cardinal rule.[9] Clinical nurses who are involved in staffing plans will have confidence in the plans. These staffing studies can be made with electronic spreadsheets.

EXHIBIT 7-3
Work Sampling Study

RN, LPN, NA (CIRCLE ONE)

TASK OR PROCEDURE	TIME STARTED	TIME ENDED	MINUTES
1. _____			
2. _____			
3. _____			
4. _____			
5. _____			
6. _____			
7. _____			
8. _____			
9. _____			
10. _____			

(A) Total number of tasks and procedures = _____

(B) Total minutes = _____

AVERAGE TIME

Total minutes	÷	Total number of tasks and procedures	=	Average time per procedure or task
(B) _____	÷	(A) _____	=	(C) _____

STANDARD TIME

Average time	+	Time allowed for fatigue, personal variation, and unavoidable standby	=	Standard time in minutes
(C) _____	+	(D) _____	=	(E) _____

MEASUREMENT OF NURSING ACTIVITY

Standard time	×	Frequency of an individual task or procedure	=	Measurement of nursing activity
(E) _____	×	(F) _____	=	(G) _____

VOLUME OF NURSING WORK

Standard time	×	Total number of tasks and procedures	=	Volume of nursing work
(E) _____	×	(A) _____	=	(H) _____

Source: Adapted from: M. K. Aydelotte. *Nurse Staffing Methodology: A Review and Critique of Selected Literature* (Washington, DC: U.S. Government Printing Office, January 1973.)

Staffing requires much planning on the part of the nurse administrator. Data must be collected and analyzed. These data include facts about the following:

- The product, that is, patient care.
- Diagnostic and therapeutic procedures performed by physicians and nurses.
- The knowledge elements of professional nursing translated into professional nursing skills of taking a medical history, performing an assessment, providing a nursing diagnosis and prescription, applying care, evaluating, keeping records, and all other actions related to primary health care of patients.

EXHIBIT 7-4
Staffing History Data Sheet

Year _____   Month _____   Cost Center _____

Day	Average Daily Census	Patient Acuity	Personnel				
			Sick Hours	Overtime Hours	Holiday Hours	Vacation Hours	Other
1							
2							
31							
Average							

Source: Adapted with permission from M. E. West. "Implementing Effective Nurse Staffing Systems in the Managed Hospitals." *Topics in Health Care Financing*, © 1980, Aspen Publishers, Inc.

Basic to planning for staffing of a division of nursing is the fact that qualified nursing personnel must be provided in sufficient numbers to ensure adequate, safe nursing care for all patients 24 hours a day, 7 days a week, 52 weeks a year. Each staffing plan must be tailored to the needs of the agency and cannot be determined with a simple worker-patient ratio or formula.

Planning for staffing requires judgment, experience, and thorough knowledge of the requirements of the organization in which the individual nurse administrator is employed. It requires the support of hospital administration, physicians in charge of clinical services, and nursing staff.

The basic requirement is unchanging, regardless of the type or size of the institution: plan for the kinds and numbers of nursing personnel that will give safe, adequate care to all patients and will ensure the work of nursing is productive and satisfying.

Changing, expanding knowledge and technology in the physical and social sciences, the medical field, and economics influence planning for staffing. Health-care institutions are treating more clients on an outpatient basis than ever before. New drugs, improved diagnostic and therapeutic procedures, and reimbursement changes have decreased the lengths of hospitalization.

Standards of the JCAHO, ANA, and other professional and governmental organizations have required upgrading of health care.

The following influence planning for staffing[10]:

1. Changing concepts of nursing roles for clinical nursing practitioners and specialists.
2. Patient populations that are changing as birth rates decline and longevity increases.
3. Institutional missions and objectives related to research, training, and many specialties.
4. Personnel policies and practices.
5. Policies and practices related to admission and discharge times of patients, assignment of patients to units, and intensive and progressive care practices.
6. The degree to which other departments carry out their supporting services. Plans should be made to furnish staffing requirements for nursing personnel to perform nonnursing duties such as dietary functions, clerical work, messenger and escort activities, and housekeeping. Whether these services should or should not be carried out by nursing personnel is not the point; the relevance is that the degree to which the situation exists must be considered in any planning. Nurse managers should avoid assuming responsibility for nonnursing services and encourage the appropriate departments to perform such

services. When departments do not do so, nurse managers should have a system of charging the provided services to the appropriate cost center other than the nursing cost center. The services will then become revenue of the nursing cost center.

7. The number and composition of the medical staff and the medical services offered. Nursing requirements will be affected by characteristics of patient populations determined by the size and capability of the medical staff. Factors that affect the quality and quantity of nursing personnel required and influence their placement are special requirements of individual physicians and the time and length of physicians' rounds; time, complexity, and number of tests, medications, and treatments; and kind and amount of surgical procedures.

8. Arrangement of the physical plant has a large impact on staffing requirements. Fewer personnel are needed for a modern, compact facility equipped with laborsaving devices and efficient working arrangements than for one that is spread out and has few or no laborsaving devices. Different staffing is required for a facility that is arranged functionally than for one that is not. If, for example, the surgical suite is not next to the birthing rooms, recovery room, and intensive care units, more staff will be needed to meet acceptable standards of quality and safety. Many other architectural features must be considered, such as locations of specialized units, patient rooms in relation to nursing stations, work rooms, and storage space; and the time required to transport patients to other sections of the hospital for diagnostic or therapeutic services such as radiography and nuclear medicine.

9. The organization of the division of nursing. Plans should be reviewed and revised to organize the department to operate efficiently and economically with written statements of mission, philosophy, and objectives; sound organizational structure; clearly defined functions and responsibilities; written policies and procedures; effective staff development programs; and planned periodic systems evaluation. Staffing plans for such a department will be different from those for one that is loosely organized, with overlapping functions and responsibilities, vague or conflicting policies, and poorly defined standards of nursing practice.

10. Data to be analyzed will include number of admissions, discharges, and transfers; amount of supervision needed for assistive personnel; patient teaching; emergency responses; mode of care delivery; and staff mix.

Staffing Activities

Price identified 17 staffing activities and suggested that the nurse administrator identify by name the persons responsible for each activity. Price made four additional suggestions[11]:

1. The one person ultimately responsible for each activity should be identified.
2. The category and position of the person who should be responsible for each activity should be identified.
3. The activity should be specified as requiring nursing or nonnursing personnel.
4. The review should be performed for the day, evening, night, weekend, and holiday shifts.

A modified format by Price for gathering data and analyzing responsibility for staffing activities would cover the following: recruitment; interviewing, screening, and hiring RNs, LPNs, and NAs; assignment to clinical units and shifts; preparing work schedules in advance; maintaining daily schedules; adjusting for staff absences and patients' needs; calculating turnover and hours of care; checking time cards and payroll; policy development; telephone communication; and contract compliance.

Orientation Plan

A main purpose of orientation is to help the nursing worker adjust to a new work situation. Orientation should be a planned program that includes a buddy system, a special orientation unit, or other method. Those nursing tasks and skills required of each nursing worker who is not proficient in them should be the focus of this program. Productivity is increased because fewer personnel are needed when they are fully oriented to the work situation. Exhibit 7-5 is an example of an orientation plan.

Staffing Policies

Written staffing policies should be readily available for at least the following areas:

1. Vacations
2. Holidays
3. Sick leave
4. Weekends off
5. Consecutive days off
6. Shift rotation
7. Overtime
8. Part-time and temporary personnel
9. Use of float personnel
10. Exchangeability of staff

EXHIBIT 7-5
Nursing Orientation—Week 1

MONDAY	TUESDAY	WEDNESDAY	THURSDAY	FRIDAY
8:00–4:30 Personnel Orientation 　Benefits 　Quality assurance 　Employee health 　Infection control 　Fire & safety	8:00–10:00 Introduction 　Philosophy 　Dress code 　Staffing 　Time/attendance 　Skills Assessment 10:00–10:15 Break 10:15–12:15 Documentation 12:15–1:15 Lunch 1:15–4:30 MAR Medical Policies Medical Exam	8:00–8:15 Computer Class Assignment 8:15–12:00 Code 1 CPR 12:00–1:00 Lunch 1:00–4:30 Clinical Skills RN/LPN 　BGM 　Emergency trach R. 　TPN dressing C. NA 　BGM 　Vital signs 　Body mechanics 　Infection control 　Legal	8:00–4:30 RN IV Therapy	8:00–8:45 Alabama Eye Center 8:45–9:30 Alabama Organ Center 9:30–9:45 Break 9:45–10:00 Nutrition Service 10:00–11:00 Telephone System 11:00–12:00 Lunch 12:00–4:30 Team Building

Source: Reprinted courtesy of The University of South Alabama Medical Center, Mobile, Alabama.

11. Use of special abilities of individual staff members
12. Exchanging hours
13. Requests of personnel
14. Requests of management
15. The workweek

Work Contracts

A work contract should be set up between each employee and the institution. The contract should state the date employment is to commence, job classification, work hours, pay rate, full-time or part-time designation, and all other specific points agreed on between the employee and institutional representative. Both parties should sign the contract. Work contracts may be superseded by union contracts.

Staffing Function

The staffing function should probably be centralized to remove a clerical burden from first-line nurse managers and provide more time for their attention to direct patient care and nursing practice activities. All of the activities related to staffing should be developed into policies and procedures that reflect the thinking of nursing administration and can be performed by nonnurse employees. Obviously, nurse managers will remain involved in hiring, firing, and promotions, and in consultation with top nurse managers and HR specialists.

A sign of maladministration in nursing is too many levels of supervision. Often, a professional nurse is employed at the department or division level to perform the function of scheduling. Scheduling is time-consuming and can be done by nonnursing personnel. Price recommends that a nonnurse perform the staffing function, advised by professional nurses as needed. The staffing employee should be a very competent person: "a good business person, mature, effective in interpersonal relations, objective in dealing with personnel, fair and firm; one who can communicate effectively orally, by phone, and in writing, and finally, one who has above average mathematical ability."[12]

Staffing the Units

Each patient care unit should have a master staffing plan that includes the basic staff needed to cover the unit for each shift. *Basic staff* is the minimum or lowest number of personnel needed to staff a unit and includes fully oriented full- and part-time employees. The number may be based on examination of previous staff records and expert opinion of nurse managers. *Basic staff* includes all categories: RNs, LPNs, and assistive personnel for each shift. Exhibit 7-6 shows a formula for determining a core staff per shift.

The number of complementary personnel is determined next. *Complementary personnel* are scheduled as additions to the basic group. Financial resources and the availability of personnel will control the total number in both groups. Complementary personnel provide the flexibility needed to meet short-range and unexpected changes. These personnel are not ensured a permanent pattern and are usually scheduled for 4-week periods.

Float personnel are not permanently assigned to a station. They provide flexibility to meet increased patient loads and unexpected personnel absences. The number and kinds of float personnel can be accurately determined from general monthly records that show absence rates, personnel turnover, and fluctuations in patient care workloads. Float personnel may be assigned to a pool or by unit.

Some nurse administrators do not hire part-time nursing personnel, who may be an economic or cost-control factor in staffing, because they usually do not receive the same benefits as full-time personnel. Part-time personnel will be better motivated if they receive some benefits, such as a number of paid holidays and vacation days proportionate to days worked and pay increases when they complete the aggregate days worked by full-time personnel.

Their total hours worked can be controlled to fill actual shortfalls.

Whatever the staffing policy, it should be arrived at through consultation with clinical nurses. The nursing department personnel budget is also a master staffing plan. The process for developing a master

---

EXHIBIT 7-6
Formula for Estimating a Core Staff per Shift

The average daily census for a 25-bed medical-surgical unit over a 6-month period is 19 patients. The basic average daily hours of care to be provided are 5 hours per patient per 24 hours. How many total hours of care will be needed on the average day to meet these standards? $19 \times 5 = 95$ hours. If the workday is 8 hours, this means $95 \div 8 = 11.9$ or 12 full-time-equivalent (FTE) staff are needed to staff the unit for 24 hours. An FTE is one person working full time (40 hours a week) or several persons who together work a total of 40 hours a week. A total of 12 FTE $\times$ 7 days per week = 84 shifts per week, if the staffing is to be the same each day. If each employee works five 8-hour shifts per week, $84 \div 5 = 16.8$ is the number of FTEs needed as basic staff for this unit.

The number of nursing personnel to cover sick leave, vacations, and holidays or other absences can also be determined and added to the basic staff. This information is determined from a study of personnel policies and use. It is frequently included in patient classification system formulas. Such additional staff may be provided from a float pool.

The next determination to be made is the ratio of RNs to other nursing personnel. If the ratio is determined as 1:1,

how many of the basic staff of 16.8 should be RNs? One-half of the total, which would be 8.4 RNs and 8.4 others (LPNs, nurse's aides, orderlies, or nursing assistants). A study of staffing patterns in 80 med/surg, pediatrics, and postpartum units in 12 Salt Lake City community hospitals recommends a mix of 58% RNs, 26% LPNs, and 16% aides.[13]

The final determination is how many personnel are needed for each shift. Warstler recommends proportions of: day, 47%; evening, 35%; and night, 17%.[14] This means that for a total staff of 16.8 personnel, 8 would be assigned to days, 6 to evenings, and 2.8 to nights. Obviously, this is an approximation; other patterns could also be chosen by the nurse administrator.

The number of complementary nursing personnel would be added to this basic staff. They could be a group of one RN, one LPN, and one other and assigned accordingly. The staff is entered into the following table as numbers in parenthesis added to the figure for basic staff.

In today's reimbursement environment, complementary personnel may be budgeted as a pool, and may exist as only a portion of basic personnel assigned to a pool.

Basic Staffing Plan for a 25-Bed Medical-Surgical Unit

CATEGORY	DAY	EVENING	NIGHT	TOTAL
RNs	4 + (1)	3	1.4	8.4 + (1)
LPNs	2	2 + (1)	1.4	5.4 + (1)
Others	2	1	0 + (1)	3 + (1)
Totals	8 + (1)	6 + (1)	2.8 + (1)	16.8 + (3)

staffing plan is depicted in Exhibits 7-6, 7-7, and 7-8. The basic staff for a unit may be determined by using Exhibit 7-6. It may be translated to a staffing board, using Exhibit 7-7. Exhibit 7-8 may be used for self-scheduling.

Staffing Modules

Cyclic Scheduling

Cyclic scheduling is one of the best ways of staffing to meet the requirements of equitable distribution of hours of

EXHIBIT 7-7
Staffing Board Showing the Number of Personnel Needed for 6 Weeks

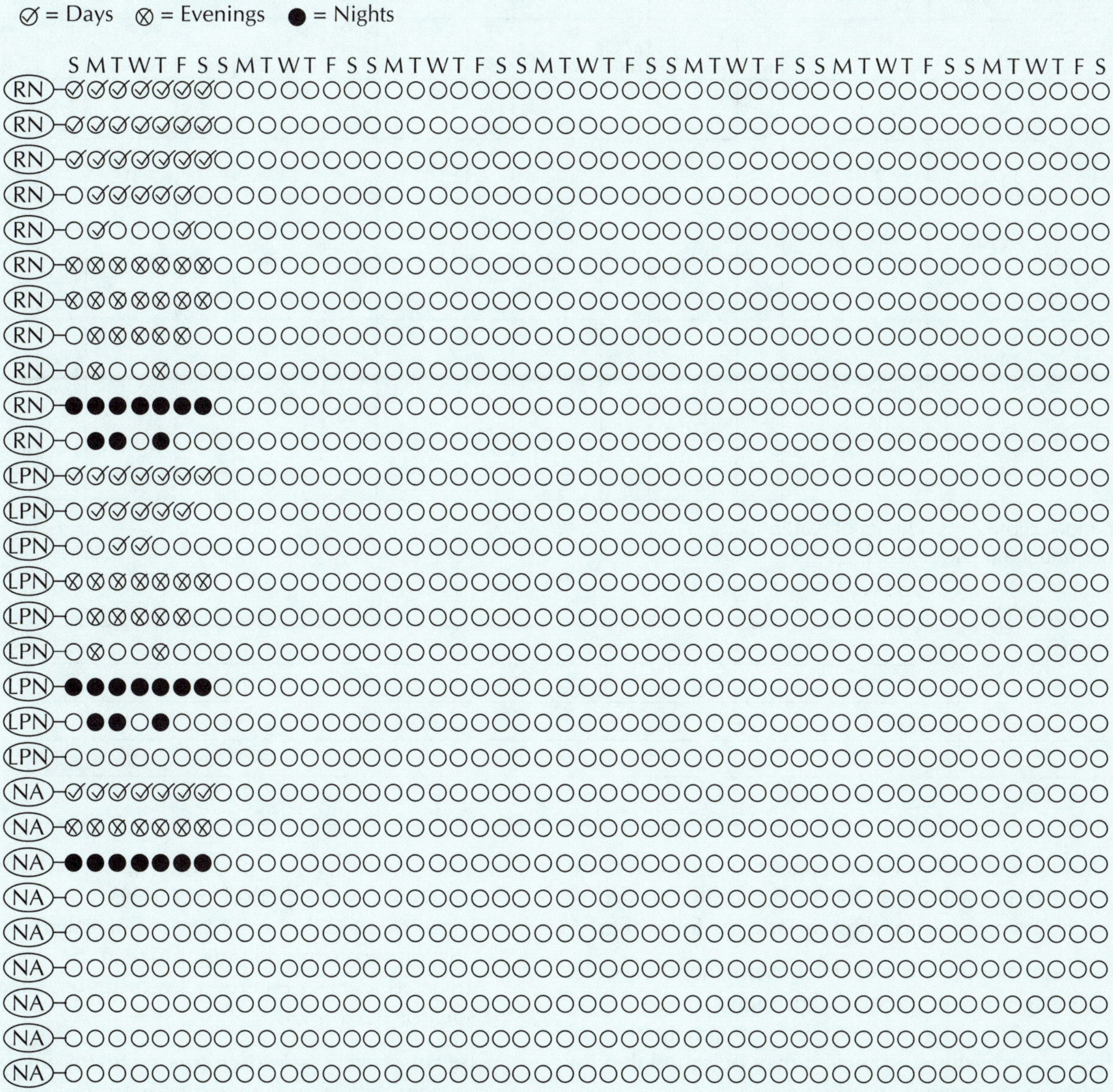

Left row of pegs is coded by category of personnel: RN, LPN, NA (nursing assistant). There are peg holes on the board for 29 persons for 7 weeks. Larger boards can be used. Pegs for scheduling would be color-coded for shifts: day, evening, night, weekend, off, etc.

EXHIBIT 7-8
Self-Scheduling Format

	S	INITIALS	M	INITIALS	T	INITIALS	W	INITIALS	TH	INITIALS	F	INITIALS	S	INITIALS
Week *Jan 15* 11 A.M.	3RNs 1LPN 1NA	JH	5RNs 2LPNs 1NA		4RNs 3LPNs 1NA		4RNs 3LPNs 1NA		4RNs 2LPNs 1NA		5RNs 2LPNs 1NA		3RNs 1LPN 1NA	
3 P.M.	3RNs 1LPN 1NA	JH	5RNs 2LPNs 1NA		4RNs 3LPNs 1NA		4RNs 3LPNs 1NA		4RNs 2LPNs 1NA		5RNs 2LPNs 1NA		3RNs 1LPN 1NA	
7 P.M.	2RNs 1LPN 1NA		4RNs 3LPNs 1NA		3RNs 2LPNs 1NA		3RNs 2LPNs 1NA		4RNs 3LPNs 1NA		3RNs 2LPNs 1NA		2RNs 1LPN 1NA	
11 P.M.	2RNs 1LPN 1NA		4RNs 3LPNs 1NA		3RNs 2LPNs 1NA		3RNs 2LPNs 1NA		4RNs 3LPNs 1NA		3RNs 2LPNs 1NA		2RNs 1LPN 1NA	
3 A.M.	1RN 1LPN 1NA		2RNs 2LPNs 1NA	JH	2RN 2LPN 1NA	JH	1RN 1LPN 1NA	JH	2RNs 2LPNs 1NA	JH	1RN 1LPN 1NA		1RN 1LPN 1NA	
7 A.M.	1RN 1LPN 1NA		2RNs 2LPNs 1NA	JH	2RN 2LPN 1NA	JH	1RN 1LPN 1NA	JH	2RNs 2LPNs 1NA	JH	1RN 1LPN 1NA		1RN 1LPN 1NA	
Week 11 A.M.														
3 P.M.														
7 P.M.														
11 P.M.														
3 A.M.														
7 A.M.														

Each block represents 4 hours of staffing.
Names and Initials:

RN Jane Hatfield JH _____ _____ _____ _____

_____ _____ _____ _____ _____

_____ _____ _____ _____ _____

_____ _____ _____ _____ _____

_____ _____ _____ _____ _____

work and time off. A basic time pattern for a certain number of weeks is established and then repeated in cycles. Advantages of cyclic scheduling include the following:

- Once developed, it is a relatively permanent schedule, requiring only temporary adjustments.
- Nurses no longer have to live in anticipation of their time off-duty, because it may be scheduled for as long as 6 months in advance.
- Personal plans may be made in advance with a reasonable degree of reliability.
- Requests for special time off are kept to a minimum.
- It can be used with rotating, permanent, or mixed shifts and can be modified to allow fixed days off

and uneven work periods, based on personnel needs and work period preferences.

- It can be modified to fit known or anticipated periods of heavy workloads and can be temporarily adjusted to meet emergencies or unexpected shortages of personnel.

Because cyclic scheduling is relatively inflexible, it works only with a staff that rotates by policy and personal choice. Personnel who need flexible staffing to meet their personal needs, such as those related to family and educational pursuits, do not generally accept it.

An infinite number of basic cyclic patterns can be developed and tailored to suit the needs of each unit.

(Samples are shown in Exhibit 7-9.) Patterns should reflect policy, workload factors, and staff preferences. Nursing personnel may use a staffing board (Exhibit 7-7) to develop a pattern and cycle satisfactory to them. The staffing board is used to show the number of nursing personnel required for each day of the week for 6 weeks. Using the numbers from the basic staffing plan, the nurse manager and staff determined the following:

- One fewer RN was needed on weekdays, Saturdays, and Sundays.

EXHIBIT 7-9
Cyclic Schedules

Minimum Basic Schedule

week		1							2							3							4					
	S	M	T	W	T	F	S	S	M	T	W	T	F	S	S	M	T	W	T	F	S	S	M	T	W	T	F	S
1	N	N	N	N	N	—	—	—	—	—	E	E	E	E	E	E	—	—	D	D	D	D	D	D	—	—	N	N
2	D	D	D	—	—	N	N	N	N	N	N	—	—	—	—	E	E	E	E	E	E	—	—	D	D	D		
3	E	E	—	—	D	D	D	D	D	D	—	—	N	N	N	N	N	N	—	—	—	—	E	E	E	E	E	
4	—	—	E	E	E	E	E	E	—	—	D	D	D	D	D	D	—	—	N	N	N	N	N	N	—	—		
charge	—	D	D	D	D	D	—	—	D	D	D	D	D	—	—	D	D	D	D	D	—	—	D	D	D	D	D	—
N	1	1	1	1	1	1	1	1	1	1	1	1	1	1	1	1	1	1	1	1	1	1	1	1	1	1	1	1
D	1	2	2	1	2	2	1	1	2	2	1	2	2	1	1	2	2	1	2	2	1	1	2	2	1	2	2	1
E	1	1	1	1	1	1	1	1	1	1	1	1	1	1	1	1	1	1	1	1	1	1	1	1	1	1	1	1

Eight-Week Cycle—Mixed Shifts

	week		1							2							3							4					
		S	M	T	W	T	F	S	S	M	T	W	T	F	S	S	M	T	W	T	F	S	S	M	T	W	T	F	S
Permanent shifts	1	N	N	N	—	—	N	N	N	N	N	—	—	N	N	N	N	N	—	—	N	N	N	N	N	—	—	N	N
	2	N	N	N	N	—	—	—	—	N	N	N	N	N	N	N	N	N	N	—	—	—	—	N	N	N	N	N	
	3	E	E	E	E	—	—	E	E	E	E	E	—	—	E	E	E	E	E	—	—	E	E	E	E	E	—	—	
	4	—	—	E	E	E	E	E	—	—	E	E	E	E	E	—	—	E	E	E	E	E	—	—	E	E	E	E	E
	5	E	E	—	—	D	E	E	E	E	—	—	D	E	E	E	E	—	—	D	E	E	E	E	—	—	D	E	E
	6	D	—	—	N	N	N	N	N	N	N	—	—	D	D	D	D	D	D	—	—	—	D	D	D	D	D	—	
Rotate	7	—	D	D	D	D	D	—	—	D	D	D	—	D	D	D	—	—	N	N	N	N	N	N	N	—	—	D	
	8	—	D	D	D	—	D	D	D	D	D	D	D	—	—	—	D	D	D	D	D	—	—	D	D	D	—	D	D
Leave relief	9	D	D	D	D	D	—	—	—	D	D	D	D	D	—	—	D	D	D	—	D	D	D	D	D	D	D	—	—
	10	—	—	D	D	D	D	D	D	D	D	—	D	D	D	—	—	D	D	D	D	D	D	D	D	—	D	D	D
Assistant	11																												
Charge	12																												

		5							6							7							8					
	1	N	N	N	—	—	N	N	N	N	N	—	—	N	N	N	N	N	—	—	N	N	N	N	N	—	—	N	N
	2	N	N	N	N	—	—	—	—	N	N	N	N	N	N	N	N	N	N	—	—	—	—	N	N	N	N	N	
	3	E	E	E	E	—	—	E	E	E	E	E	—	—	E	E	E	E	E	—	—	E	E	E	E	E	—	—	
	4	—	—	E	E	E	E	E	—	—	E	E	E	E	E	—	—	E	E	E	E	E	—	—	E	E	E	E	E
	5	E	E	—	—	D	E	E	E	E	—	—	D	E	E	E	E	—	—	D	E	E	E	E	—	—	D	E	E
	6	—	D	D	D	—	D	D	D	D	D	D	—	—	—	D	D	D	D	D	—	—	—	D	D	D	—	D	D
	7	D	D	D	D	D	—	—	—	D	D	D	D	D	—	—	D	D	D	—	D	D	D	D	D	D	D	—	—
	8	D	—	—	N	N	N	N	N	N	N	—	—	D	D	D	D	D	D	—	—	—	D	D	D	D	D	—	
	9	—	D	D	D	D	—	—	—	D	D	D	—	D	D	D	—	—	N	N	N	N	N	N	N	—	—	D	
	10	—	—	D	D	D	D	D	D	D	D	—	D	D	D	—	—	D	D	D	D	D	D	D	D	—	D	D	D
	11																												
	12																												

Source: Department of the Air Force. *USAF Hospital Nursing Service Manual* (Washington, DC: U.S. Government Printing Office, 1971), 4-4–4-14.

- One more RN could best be used on Mondays and Fridays because these were high-volume work days as determined by the standards.
- Only two RNs were needed on Saturday and Sunday evenings.
- Four RNs were needed on Monday and Thursday evenings.
- One RN was needed on night shifts, except on Monday, Tuesday, and Thursday nights when two RNs were needed.

Similar basic staffing for LPNs and others is shown on the staffing board in Exhibit 7-7. These numbers are then transferred to the self-scheduling format shown in Exhibit 7-8.

In Exhibit 7-8, the nurse manager notes the numbers of staff for each 4 hours of staffing. Nursing personnel insert their initials in each block according to the givens of staffing policies. Additional pages can be used for self-scheduling for 4, 6, or any other number of weeks. Exhibit 7-8 illustrates full-time equivalent nurses needed for one week and a blank for one week. Signature and initials indicate that employees have scheduled themselves for specific days and hours of work.

Patterns should be reviewed periodically to determine whether they are meeting the purpose, philosophy, and objectives of the organization and the division of nursing; practical regarding the numbers and qualifications of personnel; satisfactory to nursing personnel; that they are meeting patients' needs; and using personnel effectively.

Scheduling records should be retained for a specific time, usually a year. They provide valuable statistical information for planning staffing as well as historical information for questions related to personnel on duty when specific events occurred.

It has been stated previously that staffing policies should be established in specific areas. The following are some policies that might be considered:

- Personnel are scheduled to work their preferred shift as much as possible.
- Personnel choices are balanced to meet the needs of the unit and other employees.
- Each employee is allowed to make her or his own arrangements for special time off to exchange within specific personnel policies.
- Policies have been established for making schedule changes.
- Each employee has a copy of his or her work schedule.
- Consideration has been given to staffing during hours of clinical experience for students.
- A weekend and holiday schedule policy is in place. It is a common practice in many U.S. organizations to plan alternate weekends off for nursing person-

nel. Weekend coverage can be by "weekends only" employees. Staffing levels needed can be influenced by agency policies on admissions, discharges, and weekend staffing policy.

Self-Scheduling

Self-scheduling is an activity that may make a staff happier, more cohesive, and more committed. It should be planned carefully on a unit (cost center) basis. Planning may use either a self-directed work team or a quality circle technique approach. Self-scheduling matches staff to individual preferences. It has been found to shorten scheduling time; increase retention and job satisfaction; and reduce conflicts, illness time, voluntary absenteeism, and turnover.

> A nurse manager who had 12 RNs with absentee problems asked a nurse administrator how she could reduce these absences. A discussion followed about self-scheduling and the procedures to use to implement it. Several months later, the nurse manager reported to the nurse administrator that she had implemented self-scheduling and found that only one of the twelve employees still posed an absentee problem. The problems were solved with self-scheduling. The nurse manager then successfully proceeded to use self-scheduling with all other employees who requested it.

Self-scheduling leads to more responsible employees. It meets personal goals such as family, social life, education, childcare, and commuting. It is an example of participatory management with decentralized decision-making. The planning must include the givens, or rules, to be followed. These rules should be minimal to meet legal and professional standards.[15]

Patient Classification Systems

A patient classification system (PCS), which quantifies the quality of nursing care, is essential to staffing nursing units of hospitals and nursing homes. In selecting or implementing a PCS, a representative committee of nurse managers and clinical nurses should be used. The committee can include a representative of hospital administration, which would decrease skepticism about the PCS.

> The primary aim of patient classification is to be able to respond to the constant variation in the care needs of patients.[16]

Purposes

The committee will identify the purposes of the PCS to be purchased or developed. Among other purposes are the following[17]:

- Staffing. The system will establish a unit of measure for nursing, that is, *time*, which will be used to determine numbers and kinds of staff needed. Perceived patient needs can be matched with available nursing resources.
- Program costing and formulation of the nursing budget. A prescribed unit of time will be used to determine the actual costs of nursing services. Profits and losses of nursing can then be determined.
- Tracking changes in patient care needs. A PCS gives nurse managers the ability to moderate and control delivery of care services, adjusting intensity and cost.
- Determining values for the productivity equation: output divided by input. Reducing input costs reduces the cost of each output (time unit). In the prospective payment system (PPS), this output measure has been the discharged patient. Outputs become the criteria for measuring nursing productivity, regardless of quality. PCSs provide workload indices as productivity measures.
- Determining quality. Once a standard time element has been established, staffing is adjusted to meet the aggregate times. A nurse manager can elect to staff below the standard time to reduce costs. Thus, the nurse manager makes a decision to reduce quality by reducing times and costs. It is best to do this in collaboration with clinical nurses, the personnel who are continually present. Clinical nurses can assist with developing and applying more efficient procedures and protocols, which can involve rearrangement of the physical setting and the assembling of equipment and supplies. Involvement by clinical nurses will increase their trust and respect, improve their attendance and work habits, improve work force stability, and reduce errors. Input from clinical nurses into decision-making can be through product evaluation and selection, identification of nonnursing tasks to be done by lower-paid workers, increased mechanization, and job evaluation.

Nursing Management Information Systems

Nursing management information systems are described in more detail in Chapter 21, eNursing. A good system is basic to a sound PCS. It will provide shift reports of personnel needed and assigned, by type; staffing and productivity data, by unit and area; average data on the intensity of care needed, by class of patient; and the cost per time unit of patient care, by class of patient.[18]

Desired Characteristics

The following characteristics are desirable in PCSs, which should[19]:

1. Differentiate intensity of care among definitive classes.
2. Measure and quantify care to develop a management engineering standard.
3. Match nursing resources to patient care requirements.
4. Relate to time and effort spent on the associated activity.
5. Be economical and convenient to report and use.
6. Be mutually exclusive, counting no item under more than one work unit.
7. Be open to audit.
8. Be understood by those who plan, schedule, and control the work.
9. Be individually standardized as to the procedures needed for accomplishment.
10. Separate requirements for registered nurses from those of other staff.

Components

The first component of a PCS is a method for grouping patients or patient categories. Johnson indicates two methods of categorizing patients. Using factor evaluation, each patient is rated on independent elements of care, each element is scored (weighted), scores are summarized, and the patient is placed in a category based on the total numerical value obtained. Using prototype evaluation, each patient is categorized to a broad description of care requirements.[20]

Johnson describes a prototype evaluation with four basic categories and one category for a typical patient requiring one-on-one care. Each category addresses activities of daily living, general health, teaching and emotional support, and treatments and medications. Data are collected on average time spent on direct and indirect care (see Exhibit 7-10).

A second component of a PCS is a set of guidelines describing the way in which patients will be classified, the frequency of classification, and the method of reporting the data (see Exhibit 7-11). The third component of a PCS is the average amount of time required for care of a patient in each category (see Exhibit 7-12).

A method for calculating required staffing and required nursing care hours is the fourth and final component of a PCS. The formula is "the sum of the standard times for each category multiplied by the number of patients in that category plus the indirect care time equals required hours of patient care. Dividing this value by 7.0 (number of hours staff actually work each shift) results in the number of staff required to work each shift."[21]

EXHIBIT 7-10
Classification Categories—Medical Surgical Units

CATEGORY I—SELF-CARE

1. Activities of daily living.
   a. Eating—feeds self or needs little assistance.
   b. Grooming—almost entirely self-sufficient.
   c. Excretion—goes to bathroom alone or almost alone. Not incontinent.
   d. Comfort—self-sufficient.
2. General health—good. Admitted for a diagnostic procedure, simple procedure, or surgery that is simple or minor.
3. Teaching and emotional support—routine teaching for simple procedures, follow-up teaching or discharge teaching. No unusual or adverse emotional reactions. Patient may require orientation to time, place, and person once a shift.
4. Treatments and medications—none or simple medications or treatment.

CATEGORY II—MINIMAL CARE

1. Activities of daily living.
   a. Eating—needs help in preparing food, positioning, or encouragement to eat. Can feed self.
   b. Grooming—can do majority of care unassisted or with minimal assistance.
   c. Excretion—needs help getting to bathroom or using urinal. Not incontinent or experiences occasional stress incontinence or dribbling.
   d. Comfort—turns self or turns with minimal encouragement or assistance
2. General health—mild symptoms including more than one mild illness. Requires monitoring of vital signs, diabetic urines, uncomplicated drainage, or infusion.
3. Teaching and emotional support—needs 5–10 minutes per shift for teaching or emotional support. Patient may be mildly confused, belligerent, or agitated, but is well-controlled by medications, frequent orientation, or restraints.
4. Treatments and medications—requires 20–30 minutes a shift. Needs evaluation of effectiveness of medication or treatment frequently. May require observation q2h for mental status.

CATEGORY III—MODERATE CARE

1. Activities of daily living.
   a. Eating—needs to be fed but can chew and swallow.
   b. Grooming—unable to do much for self.
   c. Excretion—needs bedpan or urinal placed or removed. Can only partially turn or lift self. Incontinent two times each shift.
   d. Comfort—completely dependent and needs turning but can be turned by one person.
2. General health—acute symptoms may be impending or subsiding. Requires monitoring and evaluation of physiological or emotional state q2-4h. Has continuous drainage or infusion that requires monitoring q1h.
3. Teaching and emotional support—requires 10–30 minutes a shift. Very apprehensive or mildly resistive to teaching. Patient may be confused, agitated, or belligerent but is fairly well controlled by medications, frequent orientation, or restraints.
4. Treatments and medications—requires 30–60 minutes a shift. Requires frequent observation for side effects or allergic reaction. May require observation q1h for mental status.

CATEGORY IV—EXTENSIVE CARE

1. Activities of daily living.
   a. Eating—cannot feed self. Difficulty chewing and swallowing. May require tube feeding.
   b. Grooming—complete bath, hair care, oral care. Patient cannot assist at all.
   c. Excretion—incontinent more than two times a shift.
   d. Comfort—cannot turn self or assist with turning. May require two people to turn.
2. General health—seriously ill. Exhibits acute symptoms such as bleeding and/or fluid loss, acute respiratory episodes, or other episodes requiring frequent monitoring and evaluation.
3. Teaching and emotional support—requires more than 30 minutes a shift. Teaching of very resistive patients or care and support of patients with severe emotional reactions. Patient may be confused, belligerent, or agitated and is not controlled by medications, frequent orientation, or restraints.
4. Treatment and medication—requires more than 60 minutes a shift. Elaborate treatments done more than once per shift or requiring two persons. May require observation more frequently than q1h for mental status.

CATEGORY V—INTENSIVE CARE

Requires one-to-one observation or continuous monitoring each shift.

Source: K. Johnson. "A Practical Approach to Patient Classification." *Nursing Management* (June 1984), 40. Reproduced by permission.

The Commission for Administration Services in Hospitals (CASH) system of patient classification appears to be of the prototype evaluation type. CASH rates patients by intensity of care and establishes a category relating to nursing hours required based on patients' ability to feed and bathe themselves with supervision; mobility status; special procedures and treatments; and observational, institutional, and emotional needs. The

EXHIBIT 7-11
Directions for Classifying Patients

1. Patient classification will be reviewed one time each shift by the charge nurse or her designee on the 7–3 and 3–11 shifts.
2. Classification is made by comparing the individual patient with each of the categories. If a charge nurse is unsure as to what category a patient belongs, she should refer to the ADL indicator only and classify by those guidelines.
3. The cue sheet is only a guideline. It is not expected that every patient will be classified in the same category by disease entity alone.
4. After the category is selected, the charge nurse will place a number on the Kardex to denote that patient's classification.

Self-Care	—I
Minimal Care	—II
Moderate Care	—III
Extensive Care	—IV
Intensive Care	—V

5. The charge nurse (or designee, i.e., secretary) will tally the number of patients in each category. The nursing office will call for the tallies at approximately 1 p.m.–9 p.m.
6. Patients who have private duty nurses and sitters are classified according to the level of care the staff on the unit must provide to the patients.

Source: K. Johnson. "A Practical Approach to Patient Classification." *Nursing Management* (June 1984). Reprinted with permission.

EXHIBIT 7-12
Data Collection—Standard Care Hours per Patient Category

Directions: Consider a patient whom you have cared for today in each of the following categories. Indicate, to the best of your ability, the amount of time that was required to care for the patient. If you did not care for a patient in one of the categories this shift, please leave that category blank. Your cooperation in completing these forms is appreciated.

Category I	—Self-Care	_____Minutes
Category II	—Minimal Care	_____Minutes
Category III	—Moderate Care	_____Minutes
Category IV	—Extensive Care	_____Minutes

Check one:

		Fill in blank:
RN	_____	_____Shift
LPN	_____	_____Unit
Aide/Attendant	_____	_____Date

Please leave this form in the area designated for that purpose on the nursing unit.

Source: K. Johnson. "A Practical Approach to Patient Classification." *Nursing Management* (June 1984). Reprinted with permission.

CASH design is quantified by determining the nursing care time associated with the critical indicators.

The GRASP® PCS uses a workload measurement design to evaluate the categories of tasks that nurses perform in providing patient care and identifies how much nursing time is required for each task. The time is then totaled.[22] GRASP® is a factor evaluation design, as is Medicus.

Only general agreement exists that three to five categories of patient acuity are sufficient for a PCS. Alward argues that four categories are best to reduce variance and statistical probability of error. She also states that the factor evaluation instrument is better than the prototype system because it prevents ambiguity and overlap among the categories.[23] Some PCSs are based on models of nursing developed in-house and on microcomputer models.

Examples

Nursing Models
PCSs based on a model of nursing are rare. Auger and Dee describe one based on the Johnson Behavioral System Model, which has eight behavioral subsystems: ingestive, eliminative, affiliative, dependency, sexual, aggressive-protective, achievement, and restorative. (See Exhibit 7-13.) Patient behaviors and nursing interventions were rank-ordered for four categories of patient acuity (see Exhibit 7-14). Patient behaviors and nursing intervention criteria by category for eliminative and affiliative subsystems are given in Exhibit 7-15.

Fourteen pairs of observers were used to rate each subsystem of behavior for all patients present on the unit during the shift. Observers agreed on independent ratings of patient behavior for the eight subsystems. Employees were trained to perform patient ratings. New employees rate patients differently, indicating a need to develop a common frame of reference for all observer-raters. This system applies to psychiatric patients but indicates the need to rate psychosocial factors for all patients.[24]

Auger and Dee list four advantages to relating nursing models to PCSs[25]:

1. Providing a frame of reference for the systematic assessment of patient behaviors and the development of nursing intervention.

EXHIBIT 7-13

Definitions and Behavioral Characteristics of Behavioral Subsystems

SUBSYSTEM	DEFINITION	CRITICAL BEHAVIORAL CHARACTERISTICS
Ingestive	Behaviors associated with the intake of needed resources from the external environment, including food, information, and objects, for the purpose of establishing an effective relationship with the environment	Food/fluid intake; sensory perception; mental status
Eliminative	Behaviors associated with the release of physical waste products	Bowel/bladder patterns; hygiene
Affiliative	Behaviors associated with the development and maintenance of interpersonal relationships with parents, peers, authority figures; establishes a sense of relatedness and belonging with others	Attachment behaviors; interpersonal relationships; communication skills
Dependency	Behaviors associated with obtaining assistance from others in the environment for completing tasks and/or emotional support; includes seeking of attention, approval, and recognition	Basic self-care skills; emotional security
Sexual	Behaviors associated with a specific gender identity for the purpose of pleasure and procreation	Knowledge and behavior congruent with biological sex
Aggressive-Protective	Behaviors associated with real or potential threat in the environment for the purpose of ensuring survival	Protection of self through direct or indirect acts; identification of potential danger
Achievement	Behaviors associated with mastery of oneself and one's environment for the purpose of producing a desired effect	Problem-solving activities; knowledge of personal strengths and weaknesses
Restorative	Behaviors associated with maintaining or restoring energy equilibrium; relief from fatigue, recovery from illness, and so on	Sleep behavior; leisure/recreational activities; sick-role behavior

Source: J. A. Auger and V. Dee. "A Patient Classification System Based on the Behavioral System Model of Nursing: Part 1." *Journal of Nursing Administration* (April 1983), 40. Reprinted with permission of J. B. Lippincott.

2. Providing a frame of reference for all practitioners in the clinical setting.
3. Providing a theoretical framework of knowledge and behavior.
4. Providing for consistency and continuity of care.

Dee and Auger emphasize orientation and teaching of all new personnel so the system will be used effectively. This is true of all PCSs, including their use to make decisions about admissions.

Research

A research study was conducted at a 1,000-bed acute care, urban, university-affiliated hospital in Canada. The purpose of the research study was to examine whether three methods of patient classification estimate the same hours of care when applied to the same patient population. The three PCSs used were GRASP®, Project Research in Nursing (PRN), and Medicus, all factor evaluation designs.

Developed in Canada, PRN includes 154 care activities organized within a needs approach model, which was adapted from the Henderson model. GRASP®

assumes that 15% of activities in which nurses are involved take up 85% of their time. Classification instruments are developed around these activities and are hospital-specific. The Medicus tool has its origins in operations research with approximately 37 condition indicators rated daily. PRN and Medicus require modification to account for layout and other physical modifications of individual workplaces.

The mean hours of care estimated by each PCS are presented in Exhibit 7-16. Exhibit 7-16 shows that for the average patient on the average day, PRN predicted more care (9.06 hr) than Medicus or GRASP® (6.63 and 6.57, respectively). No significant difference existed between the GRASP® and Medicus systems in mean estimates of total care (t = 1.05, P = 0.30).

From Exhibit 7-17 it can be noted that PRN predicted, on the average, more direct care time (4.51 hr per patient) than did GRASP® or Medicus (3.35 and 3.22, respectively). GRASP® estimated an average of 0.13 hr more of direct care than did Medicus. All three systems demonstrated significant differences in time estimates for direct care (P < 0.0001). PRN fairly consistently estimated more hours of direct care than did the other two systems.

EXHIBIT 7-14
General Framework for Categorization of Nursing Care Requirements

PATIENT BEHAVIORS	NURSING INTERVENTIONS

Behaviors that are
  a. Healthy
  b. Appropriate to developmental stage
  c. Adaptive to environment
Behavioral subsystems that are currently inactive
Physical health status: normal
	I Maintain and support healthy, developmentally appropriate behaviors.
	Reinforce independent behaviors in adaptive areas.
	Provide general supervision.

Behaviors that are
  a. Inconsistent
  b. In process of being learned
  c. May or may not be appropriate to developmental stage
  d. Maladaptive to the environment
Physical health status: chronic or acute health problem of minor significance, such as a cold
	II Provide moderate/periodic supervision.
	Maintain behavioral programs designed to modify maladaptive behaviors and maintain new adaptive behaviors.
	Structure environment as needed to provide limits on behaviors.
	Provide care in the context of group setting.
	Provide nursing care appropriate to illness and handicaps.
	Implement medical regimen.

Behaviors that are
  a. Severely maladaptive to the environment
  b. Not appropriate to developmental stage
Physical health status: chronic or acute health problem of major significance, such as seizures
	III Provide direct supervision.
	Implement behavioral programs designed to modify maladaptive behaviors.
	Initiate teaching of new behaviors.
	Reinforce healthy adaptive behaviors.
	Structure environment to provide limits on behaviors.
	Provide intensive nursing care appropriate to illness and handicaps.
	Critical activities: new admissions, seclusions and restraint, electroconvulsive therapy.

Category III and IV behavior in one or more subsystems of acute intensity and/or frequency: includes self destructive acts and aggression toward others	IV Care provided on a one-to-one basis for eight hours per shift—that is, suicide observation.

Source: J. A. Auger and V. Dee. "A Patient Classification System Based on the Behavioral System Model of Nursing: Part 1." *Journal of Nursing Administration* (April 1983), 40. Reprinted with permission of J. B. Lippincott.

Medicus tended to estimate more hours than did GRASP® in ICU settings but fewer in non-ICU settings.

The following are the results of the study[26]:

- Different PCSs generate different estimates of hours of care and related nursing workload.
- PRN predicts more hours of care than does Medicus or GRASP®.
- The GRASP® PCS will estimate fewer hours of care than will the Medicus or PRN PCS and therefore is the least costly of the three.
- The Medicus PCS will estimate fewer hours of care than will the PRN PCS and therefore is less costly than is PRN; however, Medicus is more costly than is GRASP®.
- PRN has construct validity.

In-House Versus Purchased

Purchased PCSs are very expensive and must be modified for specific hospitals. An in-house PCS can be developed using work analysis techniques. Methods for developing such systems are described in several references; most use observation or self-reporting techniques. In the self-reporting techniques, personnel are trained to list activities they perform at timed intervals. Observation on a continuous or internal basis can be costly in time and money. Self-reporting is cheaper, but employees must be trained.[27]

Alward states that it is more realistic to use the budget to determine staffing. She suggests selecting a prototype or factor-evaluation classification instrument and revising it to conform to the division's nursing practice.[28]

EXHIBIT 7-15
Samples of Level III Categorization Criteria for Two Behavioral Subsystems

PATIENT BEHAVIORS

ELIMINATIVE SUBSYSTEM

1. Absence of bowel control.

2. Absence of bladder control.

3. Absence of established pattern of elimination or disruption of established pattern resulting in dehydration.
4. Failure to dispose of body wastes in sanitary manner: for example, fecal smearing.
5. Excessive diaphoresis.

AFFILIATIVE SUBSYSTEM

1. Absence of emotional attachment to others or excessive intense attachments.
2. Failure to establish or maintain relationships on an individual basis.
3. Failure to establish or maintain relationships in group interactions.
4. Failure to initiate/maintain effective communication: verbal, nonverbal, and written.
5. Indiscriminate attachment to others.

6. Resistant to change in milieu or daily routine.

7. Lack of awareness of personal space.

8. Unable to express positive/negative feelings in direct way; denial of feelings.

NURSING INTERVENTIONS

1. Implement behavioral program for toilet training, bed-wetting, and encopresis.
2. Total care of eliminative needs: diapers, colostomy care, drains, and so on.
3. Teach self-care, independent skills related to hygiene/eliminative tasks.
4. Direct supervision of hygiene care.

5. Attend closely to changes in elimination pattern for signs and symptoms of physical problems.
6. Provide medications, as ordered by physician.

1. Provide regular, intensive one-to-one interactions to establish relationship.
2. Implement behavioral program to increase frequency of interactions with staff/family/peers.
3. Implement behavioral program to increase participation in group activities.
4. Promote adaptation to change by planning and limiting number of changes.
5. Limit contact with family when indicated; provide information regarding denial of rights.
6. Implement behavioral program to develop basic communication skills and role model interactional techniques.
7. Assist in identification and expression of positive/negative feelings.

Source: J. A. Auger and V. Dee. "A Patient Classification System Based on the Behavioral System Model of Nursing: Part I." The *Journal of Nursing Administration* (April 1983), 41. Reprinted with permission.

EXHIBIT 7-16
Means of Total Nursing Care Hours by Different Classification Systems[*][†]

	X	SD	MIN	MAX	SEM	CV
Medicus	6.63	6.18	1.75	31.9	0.14	0.93
PRN	9.06	7.04	0	36.0	0.15	0.77
GRASP	6.57	5.21	1.4	22.5	0.12	0.79

*Result of Paired *t*-tests:

PRN—Medicus	$t = 35.50$	$p = 0.0001$
Medicus-GRASP	$t = 1.05$	$p = 0.30$
PRN—GRASP	$t = 32.40$	$p = 0.0001$

†N = 2002

Source: Reprinted from L. O'Brien-Pallas, P. Leatt, R. Deber, and J. Till. "A Comparison of Workload Estimates Using Three Methods of Patient Classification." *Canadian Journal of Nursing Leadership* (September–October 1989), 20, with permission, © 1989.

EXHIBIT 7-17
Means of Direct Nursing Care Hours by Different Classification Systems[*][†]

	X	SD	MIN	MAX	SEM	CV
Medicus	3.22	3.36	0.79	17.9	0.08	1.04
PRN	4.51	3.77	0	18.29	0.08	0.84
GRASP	3.35	2.66	0	13.81	0.06	0.79

[*]Result of Paired t-tests:

PRN—Medicus	$t = 38.16$	$p < 0.0001$
Medicus-GRASP	$t = -4.08$	$p < 0.0001$
PRN—GRASP	$t = 32.14$	$p < 0.0001$

[†]N = 2002

Source: Reprinted from L. O'Brien-Pallas, P. Leatt, R. Deber, and J. Till. "A Comparison of Workload Estimates Using Three Methods of Patient Classification." *Canadian Journal of Nursing Leadership* (September–October 1989), 20, with permission, © 1989.

Nyberg and Wolff describe a PCS that calculates the total time, direct and indirect, needed to care for each patient by unit, shift, and job classification. The required time is compared with actual and budgeted nursing time per patient. This system has been used for several years and has been found to identify patient care trends, improve efficiency of staffing, and justify budgeting changes. It is used for utilization review: using access to admitting and working diagnoses, surgical procedures, physician-consultants, patient classification categories, and a list of all daily nursing care activities. When hospitalization is not justified, a chart review is done. This computerized system determines nursing costs per patient by unit, Medicare patients and non-Medicare patients by diagnosis, and average and total costs of Medicare and non-Medicare patients. In one 2-week period, Medicare patients required 10% more nursing resources per day and 40% more nursing time for their entire hospitalization.[29]

Microcomputer Models

Microcomputer models of PCSs exist. One of these, described by Grazman, has modules for planning nursing care and dealing with the budget. This system projects the number of hours of care, for each of four patient levels, that will meet budgetary and program delivery constraints of the staffing parameters. It is a staffing system that addresses the "demand" function based on planning and the "management" function based on a blending of planning and actual situations. Thus, the input variables can be changed and the budget renegotiated. This model plans nursing time and resource allocation daily, based on patient case mix and census. It gives the nurse manager control over resource use.[30]

Adams and Duchene describe a PCS that includes nursing diagnosis with related cause, nursing care goals, and potential patient outcomes. It is an in-house system, the advantages of which include[31]:

- Knowledge of the data tool
- Capability for altering the system to accommodate changes in procedural time standards
- Ability to make changes in staffing levels
- Ability to make percentage alterations of time given to indirect activities

This PCS produces a plan of care, with acuity used as the basis of determining nurse staffing needs.

Problems

One of the major problems of PCSs is to maintain reliability and validity. This can be done through continuing education and quality checks. A calendar can be established to have external personnel from staff development or another nursing department or unit perform a classification following that done by unit personnel (interacter reliability). This classification can be done monthly or more or less often, depending on the results. Patients can be monitored on different days and different shifts, with a stratified random sample of about 15% or 20% of the patient census. Simple percentage agreement of 90% or higher indicates satisfactory reliability. If agreement is below 80%, the system should be reviewed and adjusted.

A calendar can also be established to take a unit rotation work sample to determine whether procedures or tasks change with time and technology. The calendar can be used as an annual spot-check. Validation of PCSs varies. A questionnaire can be used to evaluate nursing staff's satisfaction with hours of care. Validity can also be tested using an expert panel of nurses. Patient category descriptions or critical indicators of nursing intervention and patient requirement lists should be reviewed annually by using standards. The PCSs must be altered when results of quality checks or work samples so indicate.

Orientation and continuing education are the best methods of ensuring reliability and validity. The nursing staff must find the PCS credible. If nurses believe that the classifications are accurate and useful, they will try to rate patients accurately. They need periodic classes to be updated and kept well informed. Managers must support the use of a valid and reliable PCS, because it indicates the institution's commitment to quality patient care.

Nursing should orient other department heads and physicians to the use of PCSs. Admission and placement of patients are related to PCS outcomes.[32]

Practicing nurses want the PCS to provide more staff. Managing nurses want to use it to validate staffing and scheduling and permit variable staffing. These objectives must be kept in harmony.

Modified Approaches to Nurse Staffing and Scheduling

Many different approaches to nurse staffing and scheduling are being tried in an effort to satisfy the needs of employees and meet workload demands for patient care. These include game theory, modified workweeks (10- or 12-hour shifts), team rotation, "premium day" weekend nurse staffing, and "premium vacation" night staffing. Such approaches should support the underlying purpose, mission, philosophy, and objectives of the organization and the division of nursing and should be well defined in a staffing philosophy statement and policies. Nurses are like other workers in one respect: They would like to live as normal a home life as possible. In addition, shifts must be staffed and patient care needs met. The successful nurse executive will try to accommodate both by using the best available administrative staffing methodology, which must be considered from the economic or cost-benefit viewpoint.

Staffing and scheduling are reasons for turnover and job retention. Understaffing has a negative effect on staff morale, delivery of quality care, and the nursing practice modality. It can close beds. It causes absenteeism resulting from staff fatigue, burnout, and professional dissatisfaction. Conversely, nurse managers want to receive value for their money. Economic constraints exist that are further limited by the costs of recruiting, hiring, and orienting new nurses and for overtime and temporary personnel when the environment creates turnover and absenteeism. Overstaffing is expensive and has a negative effect on staff morale and productivity. Staffing and scheduling must balance the personal needs of nurses with the economic and productivity needs of organization.[33]

Modified Workweek

Modified workweek schedules using 10- and 12-hour shifts and other methods are commonplace. A nurse administrator should be sure work schedules are fulfilling the staffing philosophy and policies, particularly with regard to efficiency. Also, such schedules should not be imposed on the nursing staff but should show a mutual benefit to employer, employees, and the clients served.

The 10-Hour Day

One modification of the workweek is four 10-hour shifts per week in organized time increments. One problem with this model is time overlaps of 6 hours per 24-hour day. The overlaps can be used for patient-centered conferences, nursing care assessment and planning, and staff development. Also, the overlap can be scheduled to cover peak workload demands, which can be identified by observation, consensus, or self-recording by professional nurses. It can be done by hour or by a block of 3 to 4 hours. Starting and ending times for the 10-hour shifts can be modified to provide minimal overlaps, the 4-hour gap being staffed by part-time or temporary workers. The staffing board shown in Exhibit 7-7 can be used to solve these problems.

Longer workdays can decrease overtime because of overlapping shifts, and absenteeism and turnover are decreased because nurses have more days off. All of these factors decrease costs. Such a system can increase staffing needs, however, when mechanisms are not used to maintain productivity. Some organizations use a 7-days-on, 7-days-off schedule but pay for 70 hours of work for the 2-week period.[34]

The 4-day, 10-hour work schedule for night nurses was studied in a hospital that had difficulty recruiting qualified nurses for the night shift. It had been perceived that 10-hour shifts had stabilized staffing in intensive care, with increased productivity and decreased turnover.

Turnover on the night shift had been 70% for an 8-month period. Positions stayed vacant longer than for other shifts and sick time was higher, which increased recruitment and orientation time. Nurses were involved in planning the 4-day 10-hour night shift schedule. Night nurses agreed to use overlapping hours to assist with day shift care. The day shift agreed to reduce staff by one FTE. Plans were discussed with and accepted by the union. Making assignments of personnel and meeting schedules were addressed and resolved through participatory management. The results of these changes included reduced sick time on the 10-hour shift, reduced turnover, increased incentive, increased requests for night shift, and decreased labor hours.[35] (See Exhibit 7-18.)

EXHIBIT 7-18
A Graph Comparing Casual Absenteeism on One Unit with Different Schedules

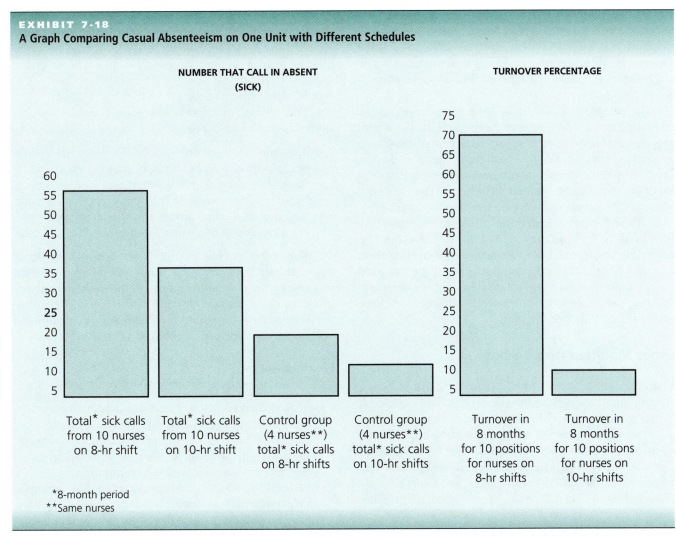

Source: J. A. Ricci. "10-Hour Night Shift: Cost vs. Savings." *Nursing Management* (January 1984), 38. Reprinted with permission.

The 12-Hour Shift

A second scheduling modification is the 12-hour shift, on which nurses work seven shifts in 2 weeks: three on, four off; four on, three off. They work a total of 84 hours and are paid 4 hours of overtime. Twelve-hour shifts and flexible staffing have been reported to have improved care and saved money because nurses can better manage their home and personal lives.[36]

Vik and MacKay report a study of the quality of care by nurses who worked 12-hour versus 8-hour shifts. It was a matched study of three units each. The Quality Patient-Care Scale was used as the measuring instrument. The "quality of care received by patients on the 8-hour shift units was significantly higher than that received by patients on the 12-hour shift units."[37] Shift patterns worked by nurses do affect the care received by patients. Recruitment and retention of nurses, however, can balance out reduced quality of care when vacancies are high. This study was limited and needs to be replicated.

A research study was done to measure the effect of fatigue from 12-hour shifts on critical thinking. The findings are that there were "no significant differences between levels of fatigue and critical thinking ability in nurses working 8 and 12 hours."[38]

There is a break-even point for costs. It is the point at which recruiting, absenteeism, retention, and overtime cost savings equal the shift losses from 12-hour scheduling.[39]

The Weekend Alternative

Another variation of flexible scheduling is the weekend alternative. Nurses work two 12-hour shifts and are paid for 40 hours plus benefits. They can use the weekdays for continued education or other personal needs. The weekend schedule has several variations. Nurses working Monday through Friday have all weekends off.

Metcalf reports a test of the 12-hour weekend plan of two shifts on Saturday and Sunday, 7:00 A.M. to 7:00 P.M., and 7:00 P.M. to 7:00 A.M. The day shift was paid at the rate of 36 hours of pay for 24 hours worked. The night shift was paid at the rate of 40 hours of pay for 24 hours worked.

The sample included RNs, LPNs, and nurses' aides. Employed staff could volunteer for the shift, and new staff was required to work it, because the schedule was not a weekends-only one. Full-time staff participating in the test had two of three weekends off. Results showed that only 3% of the total sample wanted the schedule discontinued, whereas 75% perceived weekend staffing as better.

Although illness and other absences increased by 19%, positive findings outweighed this negative finding. Recruiting improved, with vacancy rates dropping from 13% to 7% of budgeted positions. Use of agency personnel was cut in half and salary costs did not increase. Staffing and morale improved. Problems were addressed to improve the plan.[40]

Other Modified Approaches

Team rotation is a method of cyclic staffing in which a nursing team is scheduled as a unit. It would be used if the team nursing modality were a team practice.[41]

"Premium day weekend" nurse staffing is a scheduling pattern that gives a nurse an extra day off duty, called a premium day, when he or she volunteers to work one additional weekend within a 4-week scheduling block. This staffing technique could be modified to give the nurse a premium day off for every additional weekend worked beyond those required by nurse staffing policy. This technique does not add directly to hospital costs.[42]

"Premium vacation night" staffing follows the same principle as does premium day weekend staffing. An example would be the policy of giving extra 5 working days of vacation to every nurse who works a permanent night shift for a specific period of time, say, 3, 4, or 6 months.

A study by Imig, Powell, and Thorman indicated that flexible staffing filled vacant positions, but it did not increase payroll costs, hours per patient day, or overtime, and it decreased absenteeism by 60%. The hospital in this study returned to 8-hour shifts because primary nursing was threatened. In this particular study, there was no change in incidence of medication errors, patient and staff injuries, quality of care plans, complaints, recruitment, or staff attitudes from before to 6 months after flexible staffing. Also, use of agency nurses was not reduced.[43]

A Flexible Role: Resource Acuity Nurse

At West Virginia University Hospital, top nurse executives established a resource acuity nurse position to provide greater flexibility and ensure adequate staffing during peak workload periods. The executives envisioned having nurses in positions who would be available to provide immediate relief to units whenever the greatest care needs arose. The resource acuity nurse would stay at the agency for as long as needed.

The nurse managers developed guidelines for undertaking the resource acuity nurse responsibilities:

- Assisting with special procedures such as central line placement and extensive dressing changes.
- Supporting nursing staff whenever an increased number of patients were returning from the operating room.
- Assisting in cardiac arrests or other emergencies.
- Transferring unstable patients to the intensive care units.

This program has enabled the hospital to better meet the staffing needs of units whenever workload increases. Since establishment of the resource acuity nurse position, nurses' morale has improved because they know short-term help is more readily available and will be more equitably distributed among units.[44]

Flexible Hours

Other flexible hours programs are used at the following[45]:

- Metropolitan Life: 90% of 28,000 administrative employees can begin work between 7:30 A.M. and 10:00 A.M.
- American Express's travel group: employees benefit from job sharing, a shorter workweek, compressed workweeks, and telecommuting.
- Federal Express's treasury and credit departments: one-third work at home.
- Clerical personnel tend to opt for working at home, whereas professionals fear it will make their job less critical.

Positive Aspects

Nurses of the new millennium want flexible scheduling to better accommodate their personal lives. Flexible time (frequently called flextime) schedules have become an increasingly important aspect of employment practices since 1980, when 11.9% of all nonfarm wage and salary workers were reported to be on flextime schedules. They have resulted in improved attitudes and increased productivity as employees have gained more control over their work environment. Employees have been able to adjust to their own bioclocks. Transportation has become more efficient and flexible. Employees have better control of work activities.[46]

A study of staggered work hours compared with fixed work hours done by the New York State government to control for weaknesses of previous studies, showed that[47]:

1. The greatest level of satisfaction and the least dissatisfaction with the workday was expressed by

employees in agencies with the greatest flexibility in scheduling.

2. Those in agencies with fixed schedules expressed the strongest dissatisfaction and lowest level of satisfaction.
3. Decreased commuting time may improve satisfaction with flextime.

Flexible scheduling improves recruiting, reduces absenteeism, and increases retention by boosting morale.

Many flexible scheduling variations are available. Before using them, nurse managers should establish a philosophy and set objectives.

Negative Aspects

The following are some of the disadvantages of 10- and 12-hour days[48]:

- Minimum weekend staffing (or excess staff on weekends).
- Unsafe travel times versus fewer travel times.
- Shift overlaps that decrease total number of personnel on duty.
- Costs for overtime.
- Sleep deficit and fatigue may result in more cognitive problems.
- Strain on family life versus markedly improved domestic and social life of worker.
- Increased staffing if the schedule is not carefully planned to avoid loss of shifts.
- Possible requirement by state law to pay overtime wages for hours worked in excess of 8 in a day and 40 in a week.
- Less continuity of care, although continuity of care may improve when there are only two shifts per day.
- Less communication among staff.
- Need to develop, maintain, and explain the master schedule.
- Need to modify primary assessing.
- More problems managing longer shifts for older nurses.
- Absent days result in greater loss of pay or paid days off.

Working night shifts, split shifts, or extended shifts may create problems such as sleeping on the job, conflicts with family members on other shifts, muddy thinking, and poor memory. Experts suggest the following ways to better handle late or rotating shifts[49]:

- Use consistency in working shifts. If possible, work one shift all the time.
- Rotate shifts clockwise, one shift for a week, 48 hours between changing shifts.

- Use caffeine drinks judiciously at work.
- Get enough sleep. Avoid caffeine, alcohol, nicotine, and other sleep-disturbing chemicals for several hours before bedtime.
- Follow the workday routine on days off as much as possible. Change the workday routine if you find yourself feeling as if you are on autopilot.
- Prepare for a new shift by splitting time between sleep and wakefulness.
- Eat healthy snacks such as carrots or apples, rather than heavy foods.
- Drink liquids such as water or fruit juice to stay hydrated.
- Take exercise breaks.
- Talk to coworkers.
- Alter dress and environment to stay comfortable.
- Shade eyesight on long drives to and from work.

Cross-Training

Cross-training of nursing personnel can improve flexible scheduling. Nurses can be prepared through cross-training to function effectively in more than one area of expertise. They can be kept in similar clinical specialty or in families of clinical specialties. To prevent errors and increase job satisfaction during cross-training, nurses assigned to units and in pools require complete orientation and ongoing staff development. Nurses should be provided with policies, job descriptions, and performance evaluations. Nurse pools can be in-house supplemental staffing agencies that use full- and part-time nurses. Benefits can be prorated, or employees can chose between increased pay and benefits.

Temporary Workers

Nurses have been doing work as temporary employees for several decades. They have gone to staffing agencies because they wanted control over their lives, personal and professional. Temporary work was the only way they could get such control until nurse managers and hospital administrators realized the need to apply the science of behavioral technology, including HR management, to nursing. Many organizations are downsizing to make themselves more productive by decreasing overhead, and one result of downsizing is the use of contract or external workers.

The number of temporary jobs, professional and nonprofessional, has increased annually and is now in the millions. In many instances temporary employment has caused workers to experience downward mobility. The lesson for nursing personnel is to gain a reputation for competence in more than one clinical area or in more than one of the areas of clinical practice, teaching, research, and management.

Some analysts predict that half of all working Americans, some 60 million people, will soon have joined the ranks of freelance providers of skills and services. Others say their jobs will be reduced to part-time ones. Today, more than 21 million Americans work part-time; more than 6.4 million of them would rather have full-time jobs.

Part-timers fill slots at every level of organizations. Of 18 million jobs created since 1983, 20% are part-time jobs. Part-time employees provide security for full-time employees because they work for lower pay. Nurse leaders should consider whether a part-time or disposable work force that is not empowered would continue to be motivated, creative, and independent. Contingent workers have less authority than do tenured workers.[50]

Work forces in today's organizations are leaner and meaner. Temporary employees prevent hiring mistakes by employers and employees. Nearly half of hospitals use temporary workers.

Temporary employees include engineers, chemists, and systems analysts. Of 75,000 temporary employees working for Uniforce Temporary Services, one-third have elected to make a career of it. They like to try out new companies and new locations. Many employees work as temporaries because of conflicts between work and personal life. This has been true of nurses for years.

Trial work periods are effective in hiring the right person for the job. A trial work period allows both employer and the temporary employee to decide whether to make the position permanent. On the negative side, trial employees receive few fringe benefits.

Potential temporary employees should become informed about the temporary agency they will use. They can ask other nurses who have used it about it, screen the agency by telephone to determine customer treatment, visit the agency on a busy Monday morning, and then interview with the agency.[51]

Strategic Staffing

Accounting firms have developed strategic staffing as an approach to downsizing. Strategic staffing analyzes a unit's staffing needs, based on long-term objectives for the unit and organization, to find a combination of permanent and temporary employees with the best skills to meet these needs. Temporary staffing may protect the jobs of permanent or core employees when the temporary employee is used to cover a vacancy while the position or job is analyzed.

Temporary employees may want to sample the work. A variety of professional occupations are represented in the temporary work force. Temporary workers provide relief for overworked permanent employees; many do one-time projects, including internal audits

and forensic accounting. They work as trainers of permanent employees. Using temporary employees controls personnel expenses related to benefits, rehiring, and training.

To make strategic staffing work, managers should study staffing once annually, analyzing workload peaks and valleys, looking at the financial blueprint, and communicating with providers and staff.

The warning signs that strategic staffing is required include excessive overtime, high turnover, excessive absenteeism, employees whose skills do not match job requirements, absence of regular staffing planning, missed deadlines, last-minute staffing using temporary employees, lack of a budget line for temporary employees, absence of communication with the HR department, and low employee morale. Obtaining the best temporary workers may require consultation with specialized temporary firms.[52]

Temporary workers are cost effective for small businesses, because they eliminate the expense of an HR department. For large businesses, temporary workers are cost-effective for the flexibility attendant with seasonal and short-term work. Also, using temporary employees enables employers to evaluate them for permanent jobs.[53]

Transfer Fair

One hospital used a "transfer fair" to place staff quickly and fairly when downsizing. The key participants were

- Managers with vacancies
- Recruitment staff with a list of vacancies
- Employee relations staff to answer personnel policy questions
- Staff affected by downsizing

Each affected staff member made three choices. Seniority then determined placement, with decisions being made within 48 to 72 hours.

The atmosphere and tone of a transfer fair is gracious, welcoming, professional, relaxed, and supportive. Planners prepare well and make the fair convenient for all shifts. Refreshments are served and top nursing administrators attend.[54]

Scheduling with Nursing Management Information Systems

Planning the duty schedule does not always match personnel with preferences. This is one major dissatisfaction among clinical nurses. Posting the number of nurses needed by time slot and allowing nurses to put colored pins in slots to select their own times can improve satisfaction with the schedule. (Refer to the staffing board in Exhibit 7-7.)

Staffing is a major reason for having an NMIS. A microcomputer can be used to show, via menus and printouts, the number of nurses required by time slot, restrictions, off-duty policy, continuous or other than intermittent days off, cyclical schedules, and single rotations.[55]

Hanson defines a management information system as "an array of components designed to transform a collective set of data into knowledge that is directly useful and applicable in the process of directing and controlling resources and their application to the achievement of specific objectives."[56]

Information stimulates action through management decision-making. Data do not; they must be processed to be useful. Information must be timely to be useful. The following is the process for establishing any MIS[57]:

1. State the management objective clearly.
2. Identify the actions required to meet the objective.
3. Identify the responsible position in the organization.
4. Identify the information required to meet the objective.
5. Determine the data required to produce the needed information.
6. Determine the system's requirement for processing the data.
7. Develop a flowchart.

Refer to Chapter 21, eNursing, for a more detailed discussion.

Productivity

"The most valuable asset of the twenty-first century institution, whether business or nonbusiness, will be its knowledge workers and their productivity." Frederick Winslow Taylor set the stage for scientific management. He developed a method for job analysis and eliminating unneeded motions. Scientific management makes the worker productive.[58]

Definition

Productivity is commonly defined as output divided by input. Hanson translates this definition into the following:

$$\frac{\text{Required staff hours}}{\text{Provided staff hours}} \times 100 = \text{Percent productivity.}$$

To illustrate,

$$\frac{380.50 \text{ Required staff hours}}{402.00 \text{ Provided staff hours}} \times 100 = 94.7\% \text{ productivity.}$$

Productivity can be increased by decreasing the provided staff hours while holding the required staff hours constant or increasing them. These data become information when related to an objective that indicates variances.[59] Because health care resources are limited, the nurse manager is faced with the task of motivating clinical nurses to increase productivity.

Productivity in nursing is related to both efficiency of use of clinical nursing in delivering nursing care to avoid waste and the effectiveness of that care relative to its quality and appropriateness. Brown indicates that U.S. productivity can decline with increased labor costs without corresponding increases in performance. This decline can be due to factors such as inexperienced workers, technological slowdown from outdated equipment and decreased research and development, government regulations, a diminished work ethic, increased size and bureaucracy in business and industry, and erosion of the managerial ethic.[60]

Measurement

In developing a model for an MIS, Hanson indicates several formulas for translating data into information. He indicates that in addition to the productivity formula, hours per patient day (HPPD) are a data element that can provide meaningful information when provided for an extended period of time. HPPD is determined by the formula

$$\frac{\text{Staff hours}}{\text{Patient days}} = \text{HPPD.}$$

For example,

$$\frac{52{,}000 \text{ Staff hours}}{2883.5 \text{ Patient days}} = 18.03 \text{ HPPD,}$$

Staff hours are calculated as:

52,000 Staff hours = 25 FTEs $\times$ 2,080 work hours per year

2883.5 Patient days = 7.9 Average daily census (ADC) $\times$ 365 days per year.

No allowance is made for personal time such as coffee breaks, meals, vacations, holidays, sick time, and decreased census time. The figure of 18.03 HPPD may be a high provision of HPPD even for intensive care.

Another useful formula is

$$\frac{\text{Provided HPPD}}{\text{Budgeted HPPD}} \times 100 = \text{Budget utilization.}$$

$$\frac{18.03 \text{ Provided HPPD}}{16.0 \text{ Budgeted HPPD}} \times 100 = 112.7\% \text{ Budget utilization.}$$

The result would be over budget if the provided hours had been the net of personal time. Because they were not, the HPPD provided may be highly productive. The adequacy of the budget is determined as:

$$\frac{\text{Budgeted HPPD}}{\text{Required HPPD}} \times 100 = \text{Budget adequacy,}$$

or,

$$\frac{16.0 \text{ Budgeted HPPD}}{18.03 \text{ Required HPPD}} \times 100 = 88.74\% \text{ Budget adequacy.}$$

Obviously, if the required HPPD is equal to the provided HPPD and exceeds the budgeted HPPD, productivity is high because of budget inadequacy. According to Hanson, all data become information when related to the objective.[61] Staffing should be defined in terms of the goal of HPPD to be provided. This will relate to productivity, budget utilization, and budget adequacy. Whether it will be effective or not depends on measurement of quality of outcomes.

Artinian, O'Connor, and Brock measured nursing productivity by using the number of physicians' orders written during a specific period as an estimate of nursing services provided for a particular patient. They counted the number of patient contacts generated by each physician order and separated by need for licensed or unlicensed nursing personnel. Nurses were asked to summarize and enumerate changes in nursing care during the preceding 5 years, and changes related to physicians' orders were selected. They did not measure independent nursing functions or indirect care, assuming the latter to be similar to direct care. A pilot study to show whether the sickest patients generated the most nursing contacts indicated these results[62]:

1. Three patients who were not acutely ill had 59.5 licensed nurse contacts and 47.5 nonlicensed nurse contacts in 5 days.
2. Three acutely ill patients had 302.7 licensed nurse contacts and 58.3 nonlicensed nurse contacts in 5 days.
3. There was a 103% increase in licensed nurse–patient contact from 1975–76 to 1981–82, a statistically significant result. It converted to a 27% increase in the nursing productivity index.

One could conclude that the more acutely ill patients are, the more licensed nurse contacts they require.

Davis indicates that productivity in nursing is the volume and quality of products divided by the cost of producing and delivering them. It is directly related to what nurses do and how they do it. Systems have been developed to determine nursing cost per patient per shift. For example, at University Hospitals of Cleveland, the following formula is used:

Nurse competence rank
$\times$ Hourly salary rate
$\times$ Required nursing hours
$\times$ Care acuity
= Nursing cost per patient.

For example,[63]

Clinician III $\times$ \$25.00
$\times$ 3 hr
$\times$ 5
= \$1,125.00 per shift.

Smith, Mackey, and Markham developed a productivity monitoring system for the recovery room. The performance ratio was the required FTEs divided by worked FTEs. The data were used to decide whether to fill vacant positions and to develop a budget.[64]

Mailhot reported an analysis of problems in an operating room: poor physical environment, inadequate financial support, poor systems, and low morale. The department was overstaffed by 10 FTEs. Task forces used brainstorming and open forums to solve the problems. They used Lewin's force field analysis, putting complex decision alternatives through an outcome matrix, developing needed evaluation tools, and using pilot projects to test all changes. The task force made 87 changes in one year (see Exhibit 7-19).

In addition the task forces marketed services to patients and surgeons, provided management training for operating room managers, analyzed operating room procedures, and held an open day between director and staff once every 6 weeks during which each person could see the director. They reduced the staffing by 38 FTE positions and the budget by \$1.5 million in 3 years. Job satisfaction surveys indicated improvement.[65]

High input for low output produces low productivity and high output for low input produces high productivity. Thus, the objective of a nursing productivity model is low input for high output.

The first step toward improving productivity is to study or measure it, as it exists. The personnel of the education department at one hospital decided to improve their productivity. They considered using a time-based method versus a value-based method in developing the productivity system.

A time-based method of productivity considers the length of time required to do each task. The first steps of a time-based method are to review the literature, do a time study, and then compare the results with those in the literature. This is done for activities unique to the unit. Units are then assigned to activities according to the estimated time for completing each. The time-based method does not give priority to activities.

EXHIBIT 7-19

Examples of Major Operating Room Department Changes

RENOVATION	RESTRUCTURING OF DEPARTMENT	COMMUNICATION	SYSTEMS	STRATEGIC PLAN
Instrument room	Reorganized management team	Nurse-physician committee	Materials management (established 5–7 day inventory)	Attained voting privileges on OR medical committee
Lounge locker room	Implemented RN specialization	OR delay reporting form	Equipment preventive maintenance program	Reallocated block time
Office space	Developed clinical ladder for RNs	House-wide staff exchange program	Established consignment program	Developed satellite ORs for same-day surgery
Fail-safe electrical project	Reclassified eight positions	Provide internal external consultation	Held vendor fairs	Developed five-year goals
Storage area	Revised job descriptions for all staff	Publish in OR and general nursing journals	Resolved phantom scheduling	Developed PERT chart for 1 1/2-year master plan
Hospital modernization plan	Redesigned staff nurse orientation	Staff development programs	OR computer scheduling	Marketed new procedures/equipment
	Developed and implemented management education series	Sought and attained medical director	Computerized utilization statistic program	Attained treatment room
	Assessed and modified all policies and procedures	Brought perfusionists under OR management	Computerized room-delay program	Established health fairs
	Hired staff specialists	Developed patient teaching tools	Restructured pricing	Initiated annual department/get-together
	Evaluated and purchased new scrubs	Developed staff teaching tools	Modified billing process	
	Initiated "open door" policy	Developed audiovisual modules for basic programs	Color coded scrub clothes	
	Implemented director's "open days" with staff every 6 weeks	Initiated monthly meetings with staff and assistant head nurses	Established cost containment committee	
	Supported 11 managers in their return to school		Established quality assurance committee	
	Initiated written commendations		Developed FTE control mechanism	
			Restructured for DRGs	
			Developed equipment education plan	
			Began instrument repair, replacement program	
			Initiated environment rounds	

Source: C. B. Mailhot. "Setting OR's Course Toward Greater Productivity." *Nursing Management* (October 1985). Reprinted with permission.

A value-based system considers the value of activities to the institution. Steps for developing a value-based system of productivity include listing activities, grouping them by their value to the institution, and assigning units of productivity. The HR department should be involved in developing a productivity system.

Exhibits 7-20 and 7-21 demonstrate tools for collecting data for a value-based productivity system used by the McKay-Dee education department at McKay-Dee Hospital Center, Ogden, Utah.[66]

Productivity Model Differences

Producers of services do not fit the same productivity models as do producers of material goods. Marked discretion exists in determining both expected and actual role performances of nurses who do not produce phys-

EXHIBIT 7-20
Value-Based Productivity Form

NAME _____   DATE _____

REQUIRED CLASSES	SUNDAY			MONDAY			TUESDAY			WEDNESDAY			THURSDAY			FRIDAY			SATURDAY		
	HRS	UNITS	#PRT	HRS	UNITS	#PRT	HRS	UNITS	#PRT	HRS	UNITS	#PRT	HRS	UNITS	#PRT	HRS	UNITS	#PRT	HRS	UNITS	#PRT
4 units x Hrs / 3 units x Hrs <5 part																					
Orientation																					
Fire, Safety, Disaster																					
Hazardous Material																					
Infection Control																					
AIDS																					
NECESSARY TO FUNCTION 4 units x Hrs / 3 units x Hrs <5 Part / +2 units per Station																					
ACLS																					
EKG																					
Critical Care																					
CPR Lecture																					
Computer																					
Management																					
Glucoscan																					
CEU .5 extra unit x Hrs																					
CPR CHECK OFF 2 units x Hrs																					
UPDATE CLASSES 3 units x Hrs / 2 units x Hrs <5 Part																					
Departments																					
Clinical Instruction (one-to-one) 2 units x Hrs																					
Skill Lab 3 units x Hrs plus / 2 units per station																					
PROJECTS High value 2 units x Hrs																					
Lower value 1 unit x Hrs																					
COMMITTEES Meeting (1 unit x Hrs)																					
Work (2 units x Hrs)																					
ROUNDS (1 unit x Hrs)																					
PT/COMMUNITY EDUC. 4 units x Hrs / 3 units x Hrs <5 Part																					
Units																					
PARTICIPANTS																					
PARTICIPANT HOURS																					

COMMENTS _____

GRAND TOTAL

UNITS _____

NO. OF PARTS _____

PART. HRS _____

*PRODUCTIVITY % _____

HOURS   APL   VAC   HOLIDAY

*Average is based on a 40-hr week; divide hours worked into value productivity to determine percent

Source: C. R. Waterstadt and T. L. Phillips. "A Productivity System for a Hospital Education Department." *Journal of Nursing Staff Development* (May-June 1990), 142. Reprinted with permission.

ical outputs. For this reason, nursing prescriptions such as "emotional support" are difficult to measure. Patient outputs or outcomes can be measured by client satisfaction and client condition on discharge.

Greater emphasis has been placed on the nursing process rather than nursing outcome. Haas defines efficiency as the relationship of personnel assigned and time spent to materials expended, as well as capital and man-

EXHIBIT 7-21
Value-Based Productivity

DATE	CLASS TITLE	SPEAKER	HRS. TAUGHT	NO. OF PARTICIPANTS	VALUE OF CLASS	COST TO PARTIC.
_____	Childbirth					
_____	Refresher					
_____	Early Bird					
_____	C-Section					
_____	Repeat Childbirth					
_____	Children's Workshop					
_____	Diabetic Series					
_____	Coronary Artery Disease					
_____						
_____						
_____						

PROFESSIONAL COMMUNITY

DATE	CLASS TITLE	SPEAKER	HRS. TAUGHT	NO. OF PARTICIPANTS	VALUE OF CLASS	COST TO PARTIC.
_____	Diabetic Workshop					
_____	Collaborative Nursing Practice					
_____	Medical Technology					
_____						

DATE	PATIENT'S NAME	HRS	NO. OF PARTIC.	PATIENT EDUCATION COST

Source: C. R. Waterstadt and T. L. Phillips. "A Productivity System for a Hospital Education Department." *Journal of Nursing Staff Development* (May-June 1990), 143. Reprinted with permission

agement employed, for the greatest economy in use. Productive nurses must balance their personal energies and their institution's resources with their own effectiveness.[67]

Curtin proposes that productivity in nursing is related to the application of knowledge. Professional productivity must be measured by means of efficacy, effectiveness, and efficiency in applying knowledge. Curtin indicates that these processes can be objectively measured by using the following[68]:

1. Objective measures of efficacy: years of formal education, levels of academic achievement, evidence of

continuing education and skill development, and years of experience.
2. Objective measures of effectiveness: demonstrated ability to execute job-related procedures, correctly prioritized activities, perform according to professional and legal standards, record appropriate information clearly and concisely, and cooperate with others.
3. Objective measures of efficiency: promptitude, attendance, reliability, precision, adaptability, and economical disposition of resources.

Curtin and Zurlage acknowledge that human services such as nursing are difficult to test, return, or exchange if they are unsatisfactory. They propose a system for measuring nursing productivity that includes a nursing productivity equation, an equation relating nursing productivity ratio to hospital revenue, and a nursing productivity index.[69]

A nursing intensity index has been developed and tested in all departments at The Johns Hopkins Hospital. A pilot study was done in which records of eight major services were examined. These records were scored by three raters each for average agreement, which varied from 82% to 95%. Modifications were made in the index as a result of the pilot study. A full study was then done using 784 records, each scored by two nurses. The results are as follows[70]:

- Nursing intensity levels varied widely within every clinical department and nursing unit.
- The full study sample included 239 diagnosis-related groups (DRGs). Of these, 64% consist of only one level of nursing intensity, 31% contain two levels, 4% contain three levels, and 1% contains four levels.
- A weighted average coefficient of variation for total charges across all clinical departments was computed.
- Average interraters' agreement across all clinical departments was 84%.
- The nursing intensity index is both a valid and reliable instrument for patient classification.
- The nursing intensity index correlates strongly (0.61) with the severity of illness index.
- The nursing intensity index can be used to systematize cost allocation for nursing and do variable billing, establish sound nurse staffing systems, monitor quality of patient care delivery, trace patient population trends, and do case mix analysis.

Improving Nursing Productivity

Nursing productivity is being improved, and the reported knowledge and skills are adding to the theory of nursing management. Rabin indicates that professionals can impose productivity values on themselves. Managers should develop managerial goals and values. They need a standard of performance for themselves. Professionals can commit themselves to fostering innovative attitudes and technologies, stimulating performance by commitment to constructive action and follow-ups, living up to standards of practice, keeping up-to-date, and being receptive to public review. Most professions can develop measurable standards of performance and productivity.[71] This may be done using computer online spreadsheets and software programs such as Lotus or Excel.

Employers should measure nursing output objectively and pay for it accordingly in salary, benefits, and promotions. Some progress has been made in nursing in the form of standards of practice, clinical ladders, and models of peer review, among others. These areas, along with respect for the individual dignity of nurses, support for their personal commitment to professional goals, and support for the integrity of their professional judgments, need to be supported in the workplace.[72]

Productivity can be managed and improved through the following[73]:

1. Planning that increases the variations between inputs and outputs by:
   a. Outputs increasing, inputs decreasing.
   b. Outputs increasing, inputs remaining constant.
   c. Outputs increasing faster than inputs.
   d. Outputs remaining constant, inputs decreasing.
   e. Outputs decreasing more slowly than inputs.
2. Soliciting staff's ideas and recommendations.
3. Creating challenges.
4. Showing interest in the staff's achievement and concerns.
5. Praising and rewarding good performance.
6. Involving staff.
7. Having a meaningful set or family of easily understood outcome measures for which data are available or easy to gather and over which workers have some control.
8. Selecting measures compatible with white-collar functions and corporate measures.
9. Monitoring workload changes in staffing requirements with established standards.
10. Combining support with employees' understanding, motivation, and recognition.
11. Increasing the ratio of professional to nonprofessional staff.
12. Placing admitted patients based on resource availability.
13. Improving skills, energy, and motivation through incentives such as staff development, books, and tuition reimbursement; paid meals; yoga lessons; bonuses; and vacation days.
14. Using approaches such as work simplification, work flow analysis, and others.
15. Making an organizational diagnosis of problems, resources, and realities.
16. Setting the climate for productivity by asking nurses what makes them productive, acting on their suggestions, and measuring the results.
17. Decreasing waiting and standby time, coffee klatches, social breaks, and meal times.

18. Stimulating nurse managers and clinical nurses to want to achieve excellence.
19. Setting targets for increasing output annually without additional capital or employees.
20. Having personnel keep and analyze time diaries to determine personal improvement actions.
21. Setting personal objectives, and measuring performance against them.
22. Making a commitment to improved productivity, effectiveness (doing the right things), and efficiency (doing things right).
23. Seeking new products and services and new methods and ways of producing them.
24. Seeking new and useful approaches to old problems.
25. Improving quality of nursing products, emphasizing ideas such as consistency, longevity, riskiness, perfectibility, and value.
26. Maintaining concern about the process and method of producing nursing care.
27. Improving use of time.
28. Reducing the costs of what nurses do by returning unused budgeted funds.
29. Improving esthetics: the quality of work life and the pleasantness and beauty of the environment.
30. Applying the ethical policy statements of professional nursing organizations.
31. Gaining the confidence of peers.
32. Recognizing the need to do better.

Personnel working in service areas can improve productivity by doing the following[74]:

- Focusing on organizational strategy, customer service, mission, and results rather than methodology.
- Using self-directed work teams to break jobs into observable tasks and responsibilities. Possible breakdowns are step to step, person to person, machine to person, and unit to client or division and then to organization.
- Observing and then making changes or providing training to correct deficiencies.
- Watching for problems such as repetition, duplication, recurring delays, and waste of resources.
- Observing the outcome of the person's work by splitting the job into four main areas: managing self, resources, and activities and working with others. Suggestions for the key skills required are analytical thinking, ability to learn, adaptability, positive self-image, emphasis on results, good time management, concern for standards, ability to influence others, and independence.
- Providing feedback that is specific, constructive, and frequent.

Case Study. At the Presbyterian Hospital of Dallas, a study revealed that more time was spent on clerical functions, telephone calls, and reporting patient conditions to other caregivers than on direct patient care. Several actions were taken that changed this and greatly improved productivity[75]:

- A fax machine network was instituted between nursing units and the pharmacy, reducing the number of telephone calls and medication errors.
- A keyless narcotic system was installed that included personnel pass codes. The main control system was in pharmacy, but nurses could enter their personal pass code at the narcotics cabinet. This reduced time wasted to search for keys and produced an audit trail.
- A unit beeper system with eight beepers was purchased at a local store for $375. Beepers given to every staff member at the beginning of each shift made nursing assistants feel valued.

Summary

Staffing and scheduling are major components of nursing management. Traditional patterns have been slavishly adhered to until recent years. A nursing division needs a practical and written philosophy that guides all staffing and scheduling activities and that is acceptable to the staff.

Staffing studies can be used to determine staffing needs related to personnel skills, numbers of personnel, and time and workload requirements. Staffing can be planned by using computer models that calculate workload requirements from patient classification data or PCSs. Many modified approaches can be taken to nurse staffing and scheduling, including game theory, modified workweeks, team rotation, permanent shifts, and permanent weekends. Some consultants advise against mixing modified workweeks, but in practice such workweeks are frequently mixed.

Productivity, the unit of output of nursing, is a focus of increasing interest to nurse managers. It must include quality care indicators that can be observed and measured.

Research needs to be undertaken to determine the key to increased productivity by professional nurses. Is it salary or some other aspect of job satisfaction? One theory is that a combination of work, environment, and rewards will maintain or increase productivity.

Productivity is commonly defined as the outputs of production divided by the inputs of production.

APPLICATION EXERCISES

EXERCISE 7-1

Based on the information listed below, use Exhibit 7-6, Formula for Estimating a Core Staff per Shift, to do the following exercise.

1. The average daily census (ADC) of a unit is 29 patients.
2. The basic average daily hours of care to be provided are 6 hours per patient per 24 hours.
3. The workday is 8 hours.
4. Determine the following:
   4.1. The total hours of care needed on the average day to meet these standards.
   4.2. The total number of FTEs needed to staff the unit for 24 hours.
   4.3. The number of 8-hour shifts needed per week.
   4.4. The number of FTEs needed as basic staff for this unit.
5. Using the Salt Lake City Community Hospital recommendation of staff mix, determine the mix of RNs, LPNs, and aides.
6. Using Warsler's proportion for staffing shifts, determine the number of FTEs for days, evenings, and nights.
7. Create a table for basic staffing for this unit. Do not add complementary staff unless there is some rationale for doing so.

EXERCISE 7-2

Group Exercise:

1. Form groups of five to eight persons, which can be your permanent seminar group. You may want to consult with a larger representative group of nursing personnel to gain their insights and ideas and to incorporate their beliefs and values into the staffing philosophy.
2. Elect a leader to move the group to completion.
3. Elect a recorder to keep a written record of the group's accomplishments.
4. Prepare to write a staffing philosophy, a statement of beliefs about staffing. It should be representative of the beliefs professional nurses hold about staffing and scheduling. Refer to the exhibits in Chapter 6, Mission, Philosophy, Objectives, and Management Plans; Appendix 7-1; and Appendix 8-2, Identification of Factors Causing Job Dissatisfaction.
   4.1. Make a list of key words or statements that you believe should be addressed in a staffing philosophy.
   4.2. Prepare an outline.
   4.3. Write a staffing philosophy.

Remember that a hospital or other health care institution exists to provide health care to people—to patients or clients. Also, an institution has to make a profit to stay in business. Profits also apply to not-for-profit institutions, in which all profits go toward improving the facility and its human and material resources. Patients must be cared for 24 hours a day by nurses satisfied with their conditions of work. Prepare a rationale for your final document.

EXERCISE 7-3

Use Hanson's formula to determine productivity on each nursing unit for a division or department of nursing:

$$\frac{\text{Required staff hours}}{\text{Provided staff hours}} \times 100 = \text{Percent productivity}$$

EXERCISE 7-4

Identify at least 12 activities that can be done to improve productivity in a division or department of nursing in which you work.

NOTES

1. M. K. Aydelotte, *Nurse Staffing Methodology: A Review and Critique of Selected Literature* (Washington, DC: U.S. Government Printing Office, January 1973), 3.
2. Ibid., 26.
3. M. E. West, "Implementing Effective Nurse Staffing Systems in the Managed Hospital," *Topics in Health Care Financing* (summer 1980), 11–25.
4. J. N. Althaus, N. M. Hardyck, P. B. Pierce, and M. S. Rodgers, "Nurse Staffing in a Decentralized Organization: Part I," *The Journal of Nursing Administration* (March 1982), 34–39.
5. R. C. Minetti, "Computerized Nurse Staffing," *Hospitals* (16 July 1983), 90, 92; P. P. Shaheen, "Staffing and Scheduling: Reconcile Practical Means with the Real Goal," *Nursing Management* (October 1985), 64–69.
6. M. K. Aydelotte, op. cit., 26–31.
7. H. M. Bell, J. C. McElnay, and C. M. Hughes, "A Self-Reported Work Sampling Study in Community Pharmacy Practice," *Pharmacy World Science* (October 1999), 210–216; V. V. Upenieks, "Work Sampling. Assessing Nursing Efficiency," *Nursing Management* (April 1998), 27–29; L. D. Urden and J. I. Roode, "Work Sampling. A Decision-Making Tool for Determining Resources and Work Redesign," *Journal of Nursing Administration* (September 1997), 34–41; P. Cardona, R. M. Tappen, M. Terrill, M. Acosta, and M. I. Eusebe, "Nursing Staff Time Allocation in Long-Term Care: A Work Sampling Study," *Journal of Nursing Administration* (February 1997), 28–36; M. E. Miller, M. K. James, C. D. Langefeld, M. A. Espeland, J. A. Freedman, D. K. Martin, and D. M. Smith, "Some Techniques for the Analysis of Work Sampling Data," *Statistical Medicine* (March 1996), 607–618.
8. M. E. West, op. cit., 16.
9. Ibid., 17.
10. P. J. Schroder and K. L. McKeon, "What is a Safe Staffing Pattern for Locked Long-Term and Acute Care Units for Adults?" *Journal of Psychosocial Nursing*, 28(12), (1990), 36–37.
11. E. M. Price, *Staffing for Patient Care* (New York: Springer, 1970), 12.
12. Ibid., 21–22.
13. "Study Questions All-RN Staffing," *RN* (November 1983), 15–16.
14. M. E. Warstler, "Some Management Techniques for Nursing Service Administrators," *Journal of Nursing Administration* (November–December 1972), 25–34.
15. K. V. Rondeau, "Self-Scheduling Can Increase Job Satisfaction," *Medical Laboratory Observer* (November 1990), 22–24; B. Teahan, "Implementation of a Self-Scheduling System: A Solution to More Than Just Schedules," *Journal of Nursing Management* (November 1998), 361–368; S. A. Irvin and H. N. Brown, "Self-Scheduling with Microsoft Excel," *Nursing Economics* (July–August 1999), 201–206.
16. L. Fagerstrom and A. K. Rainio, "Professional Assessment of Optimal Nursing Care Intensity Level: A New Method of Assessing Personnel Resources for Nursing Care," *Journal of Clinical Nursing* (July 1999), 369–379.
17. T. P. Herzog, "Productivity: Fighting the Battle of the Budget," *Nursing Management* (January 1985), 30–34; T. Porter-O'Grady, "Strategic Planning: Nursing Practice in the PPS," *Nursing Management* (October 1985), 53–56; K. Johnson, "A Practical Approach to Patient Classification," *Nursing Management* (June 1984), 39–41, 44, 46; R. E. Schroeder, A. M. Rhodes, and R. E. Shields, "Nurse Acuity Systems: CASH vs. GRASP," *Nursing Forum* (February 1984), 72–77; R. R. Alward, "Patient Classification Systems: The Ideal vs. Reality," *The Journal of Nursing Administration* (February 1983), 14–18; J. Nyberg and N. Wolff, "DRG Panic," *The Journal of Nursing Administration* (April 1984), 17–21.

18. E. J. Halloran and M. Kiley, "Case Mix Management," *Nursing Management* (February 1984), 39–41, 44–45.
19. R. E. Schroeder, A. M. Rhodes, and R. E. Shields, op. cit.
20. K. Johnson, op. cit.
21. Ibid., 41.
22. R. E. Schroeder, A. M. Rhodes, and R. E. Shields, op. cit.
23. R. R. Alward, op. cit.
24. J. A. Auger and V. Dee, "A Patient Classification System Based on the Behavioral System Model of Nursing: Part I," *The Journal of Nursing Administration* (April 1983), 38–43.
25. V. Dee and J. A. Auger, "A Patient Classification System Based on the Behavioral System Model of Nursing: Part 2," *The Journal of Nursing Administration* (May 1983), 18–23.
26. L. O'Brien-Pallas, P. Leatt, R. Deber, and J. Till, "A Comparison of Workload Estimates Using Three Methods of Patient Classification," *Canadian Journal of Nursing Administration* (September–October 1989), 16–23.
27. R. R. Alward, op. cit.
28. Ibid.
29. J. Nyberg and N. Wolff, op. cit.
30. T. E. Grazman, "Managing Unit Human Resources: A Microcomputer Model," *Nursing Management* (July 1983), 18–22.
31. R. Adams and P. Duchene, "Computerization of Patient Acuity and Nursing Care Planning," *The Journal of Nursing Administration* (April 1985), 11–17.
32. P. Giovannetti and G. G. Mayer, "Building Confidence in Patient Classification Systems," *Nursing Management* (August 1984), 31–34; R. R. Alward, op. cit.
33. American Hospital Association, "Strategies: Flexible Scheduling," 1985.
34. Ibid.
35. J. A. Ricci, "10 Hour Night Shift: Cost vs. Savings," *Nursing Management* (January 1984), 34–35, 38–42.
36. C. M. Fagin, "The Economic Value of Nursing Research," *American Journal of Nursing* (December 1982), 1844–1849.
37. A. G. Vik and R. C. MacKay, "How Does the 12-Hour Shift Affect Patient Care?" *Journal of Nursing Administration* (January 1982), 12.
38. M. S. Washburn, "Fatigue and Critical Thinking on Eight- and Twelve-Hour Shifts," *Nursing Management* (September 1991), 80A-CC, 80D-CC, 80 F-H-CC.
39. T. W. Lant and D. Gregory, "The Impact of 12-Hour Shift: An Analysis," *Nursing Management* (October 1984), 38A–38B, 38D–38F, 38H.
40. M. L. Metcalf, "The 12-Hour Weekend Plan: Does the Nursing Staff Really Like It?" *The Journal of Nursing Administration* (October 1982), 16–19.
41. D. Froebe, "Scheduling: By Team or Individually," *Staffing: A Journal of Nursing Administration Reader* (Wakefield, MA: Contemporary Publishing, 1975).
42. D. W. Fisher and E. Thomas, "A 'Premium Day' Approach to Weekend Nurse Staffing," *Staffing: A Journal of Nursing Administration Reader* (Wakefield, MA: Contemporary Publishing, 1975).
43. S. I. Imig, J. A. Powell, and K. Thorman, "Primary Nursing and Flexi-Staffing: Do They Mix?" *Nursing Management* (August 1984), 39–42.
44. K. O'Donnell, "A Flexible Role: Resource Acuity Nurse," *Nursing Management* (March 1992), 75–76.
45. K. B. Salwea, "Flexible Work Arrangements," *The Wall Street Journal* (19 January 1993), A1.
46. J. B. McGuire and J. R. Liro, "Flexible Work Schedules, Work Attitudes, and Perceptions of Productivity," *Public Personnel Management* (Spring 1986), 65–73.
47. Ibid.

48. American Hospital Association, op. cit., B. Arnold and E. Mills, "Care-12: Implementation of Flexible Scheduling," *The Journal of Nursing Administration* (July–August 1983), 9–14; A. Mech, M. E. Mills, and B. Arnold, "Wage and Hour Laws: Their Impact on 12-hour Scheduling," *The Journal of Nursing Administration* (March 1984), 24–25; M. L. Metcalf, op. cit.; R. J. Mitchell and A. M. Williamson, "Evaluation of an 8 Hour Versus a 12 Hour Shift Roster on Employees at a Power Station," *Applied Ergonomics* (February 2000), 83–93; M. A Bourdouxhe, Y. Queinnec, D. Granger, R. H. Baril, S. C. Guertin, P. R. Massicotte, M. Levy, and F. L. Lemay, "Aging and Shift Work: The Effects of 20 Years of Rotating 12-Hour Shifts Among Petroleum Refinery Operators," *Exp Aging Research* (October–December 1999), 323–329; A. Federwisch, "Shift Priorities," *HealthWeek* (23 November 1998); J. Erwin, "Staying Alert," *HealthWeek* (9 November 1998), 20.

49. P. Ancona, "Working Shifts Can Be Dangerous to Your Health, Experts Say," *San Antonio Express-News* (19 February 1994), 1F–2F.

50. J. Fierman, "The Contingency Work Force," *Fortune* (24 January 1994), 30–34, 36; K. M. Edwards, "Productive Working Relationships in the Midst of Change in Health Care," *Journal of Health Administrative Education* (Spring 1999), 139–150; B. Tone, "What Works?" *HealthWeek* (24 May 1999), 1, 26.

51. A. Bruzzese, "Companies Turning to Temps to Fill Voids in Workplace," *San Antonio Express-News* (19 April 1994), 1C, 7C.

52. M. Messmer, "Strategic Staffing," *Management Accounting* (June 1992), 28–30.

53. L. Hicks, "The Rise in Temps," *San Antonio Express-News* (12 December 1993), 1-H, 6-H.

54. D. M. Tuttle, "A 'Transfer Fair' Approach to Staffing," *Nursing Management* (December 1992), 72–74.

55. B. Moores and A. Murphy, "Planning the Duty Rota, One, Computerized Duty Rotas," *Nursing Times* (4 July 1984), 47–48; D. Canter, "Planning the Duty Rota, Two, Back to Basics," *Nursing Times* (4 July 1984), 49–50.

56. R. L. Hanson, "Applying Management Information Systems to Staffing," *The Journal of Nursing Administration* (October 1982), 5–9.

57. Ibid.

58. P. F. Drucker, Management Challenges for the 21st Century (New York: HarperCollins 1999), 135–140.

59. R. L. Hanson, "Staffing Statistics: Their Use and Usefulness," *Journal of Nursing Administration* (November 1982), 29–35.

60. D. S. Brown, "The Managerial Ethic and Productivity Improvement," *Public Productivity Review* (September 1983), 223–250.

61. R. L. Hanson, "Staffing Statistics: Their Use and Usefulness," op. cit.; the formulas are Hanson's; applications are the author's.

62. B. M. Artinian, F. D. O'Connor, and R. Brock, "Comparing Past and Present Nursing Productivity," *Nursing Management* (October 1984), 50–53.

63. D. L. Davis, "Assessing and Improving Productivity in the Operating Room," *AORN Journal* (October 1984), 630, 632, 634.

64. J. L. Smith, M. K. V. Mackey, and J. Markham, "Productivity Monitoring: A Recovery Room System for Economizing Operations," *Nursing Management* (May 1985), 34A-D, K-M.

65. C. B. Mailhot, "Setting OR's Course Toward Greater Productivity," *Nursing Management* (October 1985), 42I, J, L, M, P.

66. C. R. Waterstradt and T. L. Phillips, "A Productivity System for a Hospital Education Department," *Journal of Nursing Staff Development* (May-June 1990), 139–144.

67. S. A. W. Haas, "Sorting Out Nursing Productivity," *Nursing Management* (April 1984), 37–40.

68. L. Curtin, "Reconciling Pay with Productivity," *Nursing Management* (February 1984), 7–8.

69. L. L. Curtin and C. L. Zurlage, "Nursing Productivity: From Data to Definition," *Nursing Management* (June 1986), 32–34, 38–41.

70. J. A. Reitz, "Toward a Comprehensive Nursing Intensity Index: Part I, Development," *Nursing Management* (August 1985), 21–24, 26, 28–30; J. A. Reitz, "Toward a Comprehensive Intensity Index: Part II, Testing," *Nursing Management* (September 1985), 31–32, 34, 36–40, 42.

71. J. Rabin, "Professionalism and Productivity," *Public Productivity Review* (September 1983), 217–222; L. DiJerome, J. Dunham-Taylor, D. Ash, and R. Brown, "Evaluating Cost Center Productivity," *Nursing Economics* (November–December 1999), 334–340.

72. L. Curtin, op. cit.

73. M. F. Fralic, "The Modern Professional and Productivity," Annual Meeting of the Alabama Society for Nursing Service Administrators, Huntsville, AL, 1982; R. L. Hanson, "Managing Human Resources," *The Journal of Nursing Administration* (December 1982), 17–23; G. H. Kaye and J. Utenner, "Productivity: Managing for the Long Term," *Nursing Management* (September 1985), 12–13, 15; S. A. W. Haas, op. cit.; D. L. Davis, op. cit.; D. S. Brown, op. cit.

74. P. Ancona, "How to Measure Productivity and Improve Effectiveness Among Workers," *San Antonio Express-News* (24 July 1993), 1 B.

75. M. Gilliland, V. S. Crane, and D. G. Jones, "Productivity: Electronics Saves Steps—and Builds Networks," *Nursing Management* (July 1991), 56–59.

REFERENCES

Althaus, J. N., N. M. Hardyck, P. B. Pierce and M. S. Rodgers. "Nurse Staffing in a Decentralized Organization: Part II." *The Journal of Nursing Administration* (April 1982), 18–22.

Bermas, N. F. and A. Van Slyck. "Patient Classification Systems and the Nursing Department." *Hospitals* (16 November 1984), 99–100.

Domrose, C. "A Good Day's Sleep." *HealthWeek* (10 January 2000), 22.

Evans, C. L. S. "A Practical Staffing Calculator." *Nursing Management* (April 1984), 68–69.

Flynn, E., M. M. Heinzer, and M. Radwanski. "A Collaborative Assessment of Workload and Patient Care Needs." *Rehabilitation Nursing* (May–June 1999), 103–108.

Gebhardt, A. N. "Computers and Staff Allocation Made Easy." *Nursing Times* (September 1982), 1471–1473.

Harrington, C., C. Kovner, M. Mezey, J. Kayser-Jones, S. Burger, M. Mohler, R. Burke, and D. Zimmerman. "Experts Recommend Minimum Nurse Staffing Standards for Nursing Facilities in the United States." *Gerontologist* (February 2000), 5–16.

Henney, C. R. and R. N. Bosworth. "A Computer-Based System for the Automatic Production of Nursing Workload Data." *Nursing Times* (10 July 1980), 1212–1217.

Jecmen, C. and N. M. Stuerke. "Computerization Helps Solve Staff Scheduling Problems." *Nursing Economics* (November–December 1983), 209–211.

Jelinek, R. C., T. K. Zinn, and J. R. Brya. "Tell the Computer How Sick the Patients are and It Will Tell How Many Nurses They Need." *Modern Hospital* (December 1973), 81–85.

Linna, M. "Health Care Financing Reform and the Productivity Change in Finnish Hospitals." *Journal of Health Care Finance* (spring 2000), 83–100.

Lloyd, R. and J. Goulding. "Nursing Rotas. Shift Up." *Health Service Journal* (14 October 1999), 28.

"Nurse Staffing Law May Herald Benchmarks." *Healthcare Benchmarks* (December 1999), 137–138.

Purdum, T. S. "New California Law Sets Fixed Nurse-to-Patient Ratios." *San Antonio Express-News* (13 October 1999), 6A.

Robertson, R. H. and M. Hassan. "Staffing Intensity, Skill Mix and Mortality Outcomes: The Case of Chronic Obstructive Lung Disease." *Health Service Management Research* (November 1999), 258–268.

Snyder, J. and D. Nethersole-Chong. "Is Cross-Training Medical/Surgical RNs to ICU the Answer?" *Nursing Management* (February 1999), 58–60.

Sochalski, J., C. A. Estabrooks, and C. K. Humphrey. "Nurse Staffing Outcomes: Evolution of an International Study." *Canadian Journal of Nursing Research* (December 1999), 69–88.

Spetz, J. "The Effects of Managed Care and Prospective Payment on the Demand for Hospital Nurses: Evidence from California." *Health Service Research* (December 1999), 993–1010.

Stuerke, N. "Computers Can Advance Nursing Practice." *Nursing Management* (July 1984), 27–28.

APPENDIX 7-1

University of South Alabama Medical Center Hospital Department of Nursing Staffing and Assignment Guidelines

SUBJECT: STAFFING AND ASSIGNMENT

I. Policy Statement

II. Purpose

To provide a uniform system for:

1. Adequate staffing mix to meet acuity needs of patients.
2. Maintain equitable and consistent staffing for all professional and support groups within nursing.

III. General Information

A. Appropriate resources are provided to meet patient needs. Indicators for patient outcomes are monitored on an ongoing basis through the Quality Assessment and Improvement Plan. These results are reviewed as part of the budget review process to determine if the same patient care needs are being met throughout the hospital. If outcomes are not acceptable and/or do not demonstrate improvement and if insufficient information exists related to staffing, further investigation may be required.

B. Staffing requirements are projected by each Nurse Manager and weekly schedules are submitted to the Staffing Office. If there are vacancies, the Staffing Coordinators utilize in-house PRN personnel as well as other staff to provide coverage.

C. Daily staffing needs are determined by the skill level of employee, acuity measurement, census and anticipated changes in activity. Adjustments are made each shift to meet the staffing requirement, as well as during the shift.

D. The staffing office is staffed by Staffing Coordinators on the 7–3 and 3–11 shifts, 7 days a week. Staffing for the 11–7 shift is provided by the 3–11 Shift Coordinator. Adjustments to increased acuity of patients or census variations are made by the Staffing Coordinator or Clinical Administrator providing house supervision.

E. Staffing is individualized and the acuity of patients is the primary concern when assignments are made. Consideration is given to the special needs of selected patients.

F. Support personnel, which includes ward clerks, telemetry technicians, wound care technicians, guest relation aides, and students are considered when staffing the unit.

G. The staffing is adjusted to meet patient needs as effectively as possible. At times it is necessary to reassign nursing personnel on a daily or temporary basis to meet these needs. Whenever possible nursing personnel will be reassigned to a unit within their nursing division, or to a like unit. PRN staff are expected to work where assigned. If scheduled for any Med/Surg Unit, they may be required to work any Med/Surg Unit.

H. Personnel will be clinically cross-oriented within each division to the individual nursing units.

I. If staff are reassigned to a unit outside of their division they are assigned as support working with regular unit staff. Licensed personnel reassigned out of their division are not assigned charge duties.

J. Nursing personnel will be floated based on their qualifications. Refusal to accept reassignment will be handled individually by the Director of Nursing or Assistant Administrator for Nursing. Negotiations between personnel is encouraged.

K. Regular scheduled staff members cannot be floated in lieu of overtime, PRN, or float staff. Regular staff may be only floated when no other (overtime, PRN, or float) staff is available.

L. When personnel are requested to work overtime, they can be offered the option to work overtime only within their division, e.g., Med/Surg or Critical Care. No agreement for overtime will be made that specifies one particular unit.

M. All scheduled overtime work will be approved by the Nurse Manager or Director of Nursing. Directors and Nurse Managers are ultimately responsible for monitoring overtime.

N. Mandatory meetings of nursing personnel are an extreme inconvenience to off-duty personnel. Personnel will be paid for hours worked when mandated to return for a meeting. Meetings must be approved by the Assistant Administrator prior to announcement.

Source: Courtesy of the University of South Alabama Medical Center, Mobile, Alabama.

CHAPTER 8

Human Resource Management Activities

Russell C. Swansburg, PhD, RN

- Discuss demographic implications for recruitment of students into nursing.
- Develop a list of strategies to use in recruiting students into nursing education programs.
- Develop an effective nurse recruitment advertisement.
- Conduct an effective simulated interview *of* a nurse applicant.
- Conduct an effective simulated interview *as* a nurse applicant.
- Discuss the nurse credentialing process of an employing agency.
- Determine turnover rates for an agency.
- Make a career development plan for yourself.
- Discuss the promotion and termination policies of an employing organization.
- Describe the assessment center process.
- Design a plan for the development of an assessment center process.

CONCEPTS: Human resource management, recruiting, selecting, credentialing, assigning, assessment center, retaining, turnover, career planning, promoting, terminating.

MANAGER BEHAVIOR: Directs the development of a human resource management program that meets all legal requirements governing personnel employment. HRM policies and procedures reflect industry standards.

LEADER BEHAVIOR: Uses input from employees to identify those factors that will recruit and retain the best personnel available. Promotes human resource management activities reflecting the cutting edge of advancements in the field.

The theory of nursing management includes knowledge of personnel management related to recruiting, selecting, credentialing, assigning, retaining, promoting, and terminating personnel. Recruiting has two facets, recruiting students into generic programs and recruiting registered nurses (RNs) into service institutions and agencies. Credentialing includes licensing.

Recruiting

Recruiting Students into Nursing

In 1980, there was a national shortage of 100,000 hospital nurses.[1] A flood of publicity on this shortage led to the formation of a National Commission on Nursing. This commission listed "eight top themes in descending order of importance" that it considered significant in reducing the shortage[2]:

1. Nursing leadership should be an integral part of senior management.
2. Nursing should be more involved in all levels of hospital decision-making.
3. Nurses' management skills should be developed, and nurses should be provided more opportunities for leadership positions.
4. The organizational structure should be decentralized to facilitate communication and decision-making.
5. Collaborative or joint practice programs between nurses and physicians should be established.
6. The nursing educational system needs to be rationalized in terms of entry-level requirements and clinical practice preparation.

7. Career development programs for clinical practice and administrative positions should continue to be developed and implemented.

8. Nursing leaders should be appointed to key committees to foster and strengthen nurses' interaction with medical staff and the board of directors of the agency.

During the next 20 years the supply of nurses ebbed and flowed with changes in reimbursement systems and restructuring of the entire health care system. We are currently experiencing shortages, with at least one publication editor writing a wish list for National Nurses Week as follows[3]:

1. I wish the federal and state government funded nursing education to the same extent it funds medical education.

2. I wish that all nursing education programs could accept all academically qualified applicants, and that the number of graduate and doctoral students was a function of the BSN students graduated.

3. I wish that nursing deans, directors, and faculty salaries had some relationship to the market of similarly educated and prepared nurses.

4. I wish that all nursing curricula were fully articulated so that nurses could continue their education in a logical and efficient manner.

5. I wish every nurse were proud and happy that they chose nursing and eagerly encouraging their children to follow in their footsteps.

6. I wish every high school career event included nursing and promoted health professions as honorable and worthy career choices that offer flexibility and access to many industries.

7. I wish every public or private school had a full-time, on-site nurse for their students, teaching a health curriculum addressing all health care concerns.

8. I wish every hospital executive spent an entire 12-hour shift with a registered nurse to better understand the work environment and resource issues from a patient care perspective.

9. I wish the salary differential between the novice and expert nurse was similar to that of other professions and recognized differing educational levels.

10. I wish every health care organization recognized the value and importance of having visible nursing leadership representation at its executive table.

Job Market

Nationally, more jobs are being created and filled at levels that are keeping the unemployment rate low. Whether this will translate into more jobs in the health care system and the nursing profession depends on whether health insurance benefits are a part of the benefits package of these workers. The health care system has been an "enormous job-generating machine." More than 10 million people, almost 10% of employed Americans, work in the health care system. Further increasing the demand for health care are a growing U.S. population and baby boomers becoming eligible for Medicare. The work force of nurses also is aging.[4]

One of the new strategies of employment is job expansion. Predictions are that "advanced practice nurses will be increasingly called upon to perform physical exams and treat minor illnesses," a strategy to increase access to health care while containing costs. Nurse practitioners are in demand in hospitals and ambulatory care settings including managed care organizations.[5] Richman indicated that the greatest demand would be for managers of health care networks, nurses, home health aides, and outpatient therapists. He goes on to state[6]:

> Leading the growth will be demand for so-called "nurse practitioners," diagnostic specialists—in HMOs, inner cities, and rural areas. The training they need to serve as patient care managers lasts six years—half as long as it takes to train a doctor and at just one-fifth the cost. More than 100,000 nurses now provide some form of primary care and another 300,000 could join them with a couple of years of training. Salaries for experienced specialists reach $80,000 a year."

A study of 1,300 people during a 6-month period indicates that overall patient satisfaction with nurse practitioners is equal to overall patient satisfaction with physicians. Patients in the study group were equally healthy.[7] Woods projects that the number of jobs for RNs will increase (from 1,727,000 in 1990) by 35% or more between 1990 and 2005. RNs head the list of professionals for projected job growth.[8]

Another positive job indicator is that earnings increase for employees with degrees. Although workers who are not college graduates experienced an earnings decrease during the past 15 years, college-educated workers' earnings rose. During the next decade, 25 million of 26 million jobs created will be in service industries. "Of the 10 occupations expected to add the most jobs in the next 20 years, only two require a college degree; registered nurses and systems analysts." Exhibit 8-1 illustrates the earnings differences among full-time workers with a high school diploma versus those with a college degree.[9]

> Nurse practitioners will be competing with physician assistants, whose growth will expand in the next decade. Physician assistant jobs are predicted to grow 44% between 1990 and 2005.[10]

Coping Without a College Degree

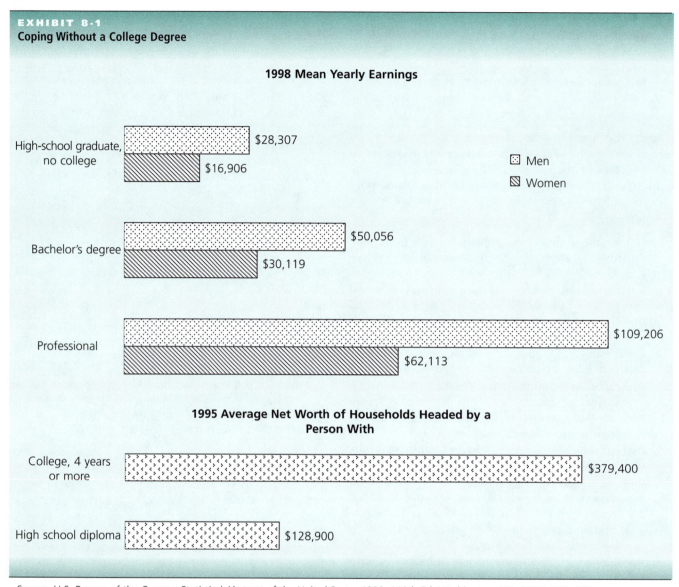

1998 Mean Yearly Earnings

High-school graduate, no college
$28,307
$16,906

☐ Men
☒ Women

Bachelor's degree
$50,056
$30,119

Professional
$109,206
$62,113

1995 Average Net Worth of Households Headed by a Person With

College, 4 years or more
$379,400

High school diploma
$128,900

Source: U.S. Bureau of the Census. *Statistical Abstract of the United States 1999*, 119th Ed. Washington, DC: 1999: 170, 488.

Progress and job destruction go hand in hand; every week, 400,000 U.S. workers lose jobs and another 400,000 gain jobs. This process is called *churning*. It advances the quality of life. For example, in 1900 it took 40 of every 100 Americans to feed the country. Today it takes three workers. The other 37 Americans are producing new homes, appliances, computers, and a whole array of goods and services.[11]

Workers are this country's national resource. They have or obtain the advanced education and training to work in technically advanced industries with better jobs as less-skilled jobs migrate to other countries. Workers in those jobs remaining produce goods and services of higher value. Emerging new jobs will relate to technologies associated with discoveries in the areas of DNA, lasers, fiber optics, high-tech ceramics, hard

plastics, holography, photonics, micro-machines, and genomics. American workers displaced from eliminated jobs will be retrained and learn to enter the new job market.[12]

Companies shedding workers to stay competitive are cutting fringe benefits. Four-fifths of companies increased employee copayments for health insurance from an average of $69 a month for family coverage in 1981 to $107 a month in 1993. Also companies are reducing employer-paid pension plans and trimming or eliminating health insurance for retirees. Increased labor costs result in fewer employees being hired.[13] Half of bankruptcies are the result of unmanageable medical bills. Some companies have insurance but are vulnerable to employee long-term illness or injury.[14]

The number of programs for registered nursing students increased from 1,387 in 1980 to 1,508 in 1997. Of these, baccalaureate programs increased from 377 to 523 and associate degree programs from 697 to 876, while the number of diploma programs decreased from 311 to 109. Nursing enrollment in registered nursing preparation programs decreased from 270,228 in 1994 to 268,350 in 1995, 261,219 in 1996, and 238,244 in 1997. The number of graduates decreased from 97,052 in 1995 to 94,757 in 1996. Enrollment in all nursing programs, including baccalaureate, associate degree, and diploma programs, decreased in 1997.[15] In 1998, approximately 9,904,000 persons were employed in the health services industry.[16] In 1996, there were 2,162,000 active RNs in the United States, up from 1,273,000 in 1980. The rate per 100,000 population increased from 560 to 815 during this period.[17]

Since 1995, enrollment in all basic nursing education programs (baccalaureate, associate degree, or diploma) has fallen each year by approximately 5%. A study by Buerhaus predicts that by the year 2020, the RN workforce will be nearly 20% below projected requirements. The Bureau of Labor Statistics estimates the number of nurses needed by 2008 will increase by 450,864.[18]

Students entering the nursing profession need to meet academic standards as rigid as do those entering medicine, law, or other professions. An effort that promotes qualification of more American high-school students for competition and upward mobility is good for the profession and the nation.

Job Sharing

An option for nursing is *job sharing*, that is, two persons filling one full-time equivalent job at a ratio of work agreed on by them. This option is convenient for nurses who want and can afford to work part-time and need the personal time. Less acceptable to nurses has been mandatory sharing of available work in a world in which high-tech and organizational restructuring has reduced the amount of available labor for pay.[19] One outcome has been lower enrollments in registered nurse programs.

Job and Employee Retention

To retain their jobs, employees can make themselves more valuable by gaining new skills and experiences and taking on new responsibilities, including volunteering for interdepartmental project teams. Employees also can maintain their reputations as helpful, resourceful coworkers, and keep a folder or journal of their suc-

cesses and use it to build a résumé of major accomplishments or new skills.[20]

Here are several suggestions for recruiting students into registered nurse programs[21]:

1. Schools of nursing should now begin to profile their students. Who are they? Where do they come from? What is their level of achievement in high school?
2. More adults should be recruited into nursing. These include both men and women seeking second careers and women entering a career field after their children have begun school.
3. Nurse educators, managers, researchers, and clinical practitioners should collaborate with the public schools and should be proactive in the recruitment effort. Nurses in these positions can advise school counselors about program requirements and support the schools to meet these requirements. Such measures might include financial assistance to keep students in school through graduation and to enable them to enter nursing programs after graduation.
4. Potential students in the African-American, Hispanic, and Asian communities should be given support to help them graduate from high-school qualified to enter college. Some students will require assistance with language, culture, and finances.
5. Nurses should give proactive support to public education at all levels. The future of nursing and of our society depends on it.
6. With millions of immigrants requiring socialization into U.S. culture, nurses should become a part of the process. Again, nurses must be proactive in encouraging students to take elective courses in liberal arts that reflect the cultures of members of minority groups.
7. Higher education needs to be adapted to assimilate minority group members, which is a challenge for nurse educators. The process will have to begin at the high-school level with programs of study that prepare numbers of minority groups to enter nursing programs, including supplemental and remedial programs. Such efforts will need to be continued throughout the nursing education program.
8. High-school graduates of lower ability must receive support.
9. Attention to the retention of college and university students can be valuable to schools of nursing. A plan should be made to recruit the more than 50% of 4-year-degree candidates who do not graduate. These candidates include students in 24 fields of study, with 1,300 different undergraduate academic majors.
10. Male students can be recruited by dispelling the notion that nursing is a woman's occupation.

11. Employers need to prepare members of minority groups—including nurses—for promotion, thus making them visibile to potential nursing students. The military services have been doing a better job of this. One has only to look at the hierarchy of educational institutions, health care institutions, and business and industrial institutions to discern this.

12. Community colleges educate most students who are considered to be outside the mainstream because of their ethnicity, age, and cultural background; however, this can be changed. Baccalaureate faculty can initiate the changes. Otherwise, the number of nursing graduates with associate degrees will continue to increase faster than will the number of baccalaureate nursing graduates. Both need to be maintained at levels that meet market demand.

13. Emphasis on research and publication should not diminish. However, faculty also should be promoted and tenured based on teaching excellence.

14. Teaching methodology should focus on wide use of teaching strategies and less on lectures, which keep students passive.

Of late, women have been entering career fields such as medicine, law, business administration, and dentistry that traditionally have been predominated by males with higher pay and better working conditions than those in nursing. Although numerous studies exist showing dissatisfaction among nurses, there appears to be sporadic progress in improving nurses' pay and working conditions.

Nurse managers are not the only people who can change the work environment. An all-RN staff may not appear to be financially possible. The professional nurse practitioner is highly qualified in terms of knowledge and skills and is the decision maker in the nursing field. She or he can direct the work of others without continual direct involvement in procedures such as bathing, making beds, and feeding patients. The professional nurse should take the history, make the nursing diagnosis, direct the application of nursing care, evaluate the results, and make changes as needed. The debate on entry into practice needs to be redesigned and realigned to focus on the professional nurse as the clinical decision maker. Requirements of the baccalaureate degree in nursing for certification programs will advance this notion.

Every major agency or institution employing nurses should have a committee that focuses on the recruitment of students into nursing education programs. Small organizations can form recruitment consortiums. Clinical nurses should be well represented because

their ideas will give an authentic and positive image of professional nursing practice. The focus should be realistic but positive for men and women, for minorities, and for a cross section of high-school students. The latter will come from backgrounds in which the number[22]:

- Of individuals below the poverty line decreased.
- Of white, suburban, middle-class decreased.
- Of nonwhites increased.
- Of single parents increased.
- Of non–English-speaking or bilingual individuals increased.
- Of persons with physical and emotional disabilities increased.
- Of working mothers increased.

Exhibit 8-2 lists activities to pursue in recruiting students into nursing education programs.

The business of recruiting students into nursing requires long-term strategies for all educators and providers. Recruitment will be more effective if potential consumers of nursing services are involved. Professional nurses can work through community organizations to involve the community in changing the image of nursing and in the recruitment effort. The image of nursing should include information about qualifications and credentials of caregivers who provide safe, effective care to individuals and communities.

Efforts should be made to provide education at times convenient to students, most of whom have to work. More is being done to provide evening and weekend courses for basic or generic students, which could be a major area of breakthrough in recruitment, particularly for older adults. RN completion programs are now available through the Internet, as are required general education programs. These programs are being expanded to include generic nursing programs and graduate nursing education.[23]

Research Study

The number of new entrants into baccalaureate nursing programs needs to be increased to keep pace with the demand for professional nurses. Using a descriptive design, 641 college-bound high-school seniors were surveyed to determine why nursing is not selected more frequently as a career. The survey was taken to obtain data helpful to nurse educators in developing strategies to increase the number of high-school seniors who choose a career in nursing. Although a majority of those sampled had grade point averages between 3.00 and 3.99, 92.3% did not choose nursing as a career.

Questions measuring knowledge regarding nursing education, hours, salaries, and work settings indicated that the overall knowledge of these areas of nursing among respondents was fairly accurate. Students were

---

EXHIBIT 8-2

Strategies for Recruiting Students into Nursing Education Programs

1. Form a committee to create a plan.
   a. Include clinical nurses
   b. Set goals
   c. Create a management plan for each goal
2. Obtain recruitment materials from organizations.
   a. National League for Nursing (NLN)
   b. American Nurses Association (ANA)
   c. American Organization of Nurse Executives (AONE)/American Hospital Association (AHA)
   d. National Student Nurses Association (NSNA)
   e. American Association of Colleges of Nursing (AACN)
   f. State
   g. Local
3. Prepare additional recruitment materials.
   a. News stories for newspapers, TV, and radio
   b. Posters for schools
   c. Speakers' bureau
   d. Model speeches
   e. Tours
4. Coordinate with other nurse education programs and prospective employers of nurses.
   a. Associate degree programs
   b. Diploma programs
   c. BSN programs
   d. Hospitals
   e. Public health
   f. Staffing agencies
   g. Ambulatory care facilities
   h. Nursing homes
   i. LPN programs
   j. Other
5. Prepare and offer consultation programs for junior and senior high schools.
   a. Administrators
   b. Teachers
   c. Guidance counselors
   d. Students, including potential dropouts
   e. Financial advisers
   f. Language and cultural resource advisers
6. Coordinate activities of recruiters in schools of nursing.
   a. Sources of information by telephone and mail
   b. Target adults seeking second careers, men, minorities, and immigrants
7. Involve community agencies in recruitment efforts.
   a. Professional organizations
   b. Social organizations
   c. Service organizations
   d. Others
8. Evaluate results accomplished.
   a. Number and locations of programs presented
   b. Number of students counseled
   c. Number of follow-ups
   d. Number of applicants to local or other programs
   e. Homerooms visited
   f. Career days held by high schools, schools of nursing, and employers
   g. Inquiries to source persons by telephone or letter
9. Do work-study programs.
   a. High schools with employer
   b. High schools with schools of nursing
   c. Schools of nursing with employers
   d. Cooperative education

---

relatively uninformed, however, about the roles and tasks of nurses, and 91.8% were unaware that nurses worked with computers.

The overall opinion about nursing was favorable. A large percentage (86%) of students believed that nurses mainly followed doctors' orders, but many students (72.5%) believed that nurses make a lot of money and many (81.1%) also believed that nursing is a career only for smart people. Very few students believed that nurses do important work (5.4%); that nursing is challenging (9.4%), a real profession (9.3%), or an important profession (5.4%); or that it provides a good opportunity to help people (3%).

Neither knowledge nor opinion of nursing was significantly associated with students choosing or not choosing nursing as a career. Significant differences in gender, ethnicity, and age existed between students who chose nursing and those who did not. Students who chose nursing as a career were significantly more likely to be African-American, female, and 16 to 17 years of age. No significant differences in religion, socioeconomic status, or grade point average existed between those who chose nursing and those who did not.

Knowing a nurse personally, caring for a seriously ill person, having a family member who is a nurse, and living with someone who is seriously ill were significantly associated with the decision to become a nurse. The reason cited most frequently for choosing nursing was the desire to help people. Those who did not choose nursing indicated a dislike for being near dying people and insufficient salary as the main reasons. These findings are important to nurse educators as they plan recruitment strategies aimed at increasing the enrollment of high-school students in baccalaureate nursing programs.[24]

Recruiting Nurses into Employment

Employers of RNs are competing for available personnel through channels such as newspaper and journal ads, professional placement agencies, placement bureaus at universities, special publications, and the Internet. Professional nurses seeking jobs may have personal contacts and can obtain information at job fairs, career days, professional meetings, and conventions. The business of recruiting clinical nurses into jobs should be managed using planning, an organization, direction, and a method of evaluating its effectiveness.

The Recruiter

Many large organizations employ a nursing recruiter, who may be a professional nurse or a personnel recruitment specialist. Either employee should work from a management plan that includes input from clinical nurses working within the organization.

The objective of the recruiter is to attract qualified professional nurses to apply for jobs. First, information about the organization's job openings is made known to the target population through advertisements in Sunday newspapers, in nursing journals, and on the Internet. The ads should be broad enough to give potential applicants knowledge of particular positions, salaries, and fringe benefits and the organizational climate. Results of studies of factors that attract nurses can be used as a basis for developing job ads.

In 1983, an American Academy of Nursing study depicted both nurse administrators and staff nurses as agreeing on which factors attracted nurses to become and remain employees of hospitals. Among those factors were "adequate and competent colleagues, flexibility in scheduling, educational programs that allow for professional growth, and recognition as individuals."[25] These institutions were labeled *magnet hospitals*.

During 1985–86, Kramer and Schmalenberg resurveyed 16 of the magnet hospitals, comparing them with the best-run corporate communities as described by Peters and Waterman in their book *In Search of Excellence*. They found many similarities: Magnet hospitals "are infused with values of quality care, nurse autonomy, informal, nonrigid verbal communication, innovation, bringing out the best in each individual, value of education, respect and caring for the individual, and striving for excellence."[26]

A well-thought-out ad can be a successful method for recruiting nurses. It is better to spend money to develop an effective advertisement than to save money on an ineffective one. A successful ad will get attention when it focuses on its subject: the professional nurse. It will obtain results when it piques the interest of the professional nurse to seek more information. Exhibit 8-3 lists criteria for developing an effective newspaper, nursing journal, or Internet advertisement.

Professional nurses should be recruited as are other professional persons. Clinical nursing is important, and clinical nurses should be recruited in the same way as nursing

---

EXHIBIT 8-3

Criteria for Developing an Effective Nurse Recruitment Advertisement

1. Target the population.
2. Catch the reader's attention.
3. Consider a picture that depicts a professional nurse in action, the kind of action nurses say they want.
4. List several factors that attract nurses. These may include:
   a. Opportunity for self-fulfillment
   b. Knowledge of helping others
   c. Intellectual stimulation
   d. Educational opportunity
   e. Fellowship with colleagues
   f. Adequate income
   g. Opportunity for innovation
   h. Opportunity to choose hours
   i. Opportunity for advancement
   j. Chance to be a leader
   k. Adequate support systems
   l. Child-care facilities
   m. Good fringe benefits
   n. Entrepreneural opportunities
5. Involve clinical nurses in developing the advertisement.
6. Test the advertisement on the clinical nurse staff.
7. Run the ad in the Sunday newspapers, selecting those that are read by the target population.
8. Run the ad in nursing journals that are read by the target population.
9. Establish a web site.
10. Provide for telephone and mail replies from applicants.
    a. Free telephone numbers
    b. Specific address
    c. Fax number and e-mail address
11. Provide for effective telephone and mail replies to be returned from the organization.
    a. The phone should be answered with positive responses that elicit interviews. Clinical nurses making immediate follow-up calls to prospective applicants can be effective.
    b. Effective packages of recruitment materials mailed to prospective applicants. (Depict and detail factors listed under number 4.)
12. Arrange for interview, including a visit to the organization.
    a. Contact person and sponsor
    b. Travel reimbursement
    c. Paid room and meals
    d. Interviews with person doing hiring; personnel specialists, including recruiter; and clinical nurses
13. Make a follow-up offer in writing.
14. Form a cadre of retired nurses (over 65 years of age)
    a. Establish with an appealing name
    b. Use a specific identification (a uniform or patch)
    c. Identify specialties needed
    d. Identify shifts needed
    e. Reward with good pay and continuing education

managers, educators, and researchers are. To recruit nurses from outside the local community efforts should be directed toward factors that would attract professional nurses to move, which might include geographic attractions such as winter sports, or sunshine and beaches. They also might include cultural attractions, such as museums, symphony orchestras, and operas or educational opportunities.

A formal nurse recruitment plan is suggested for each fiscal year, because objectives will be influenced by factors such as structural reorganization, turnover and retention, and vacant positions. The following are six steps of a formal plan[27]:

1. Gathering a database through situational scanning, forecasting, and variance audits comparing demand with supply data.
2. Setting desirable objectives.
3. Designing strategies to accomplish the objectives.
4. Establishing the annual nurse recruitment budget.
5. Implementing the strategies through operational plans.
6. Evaluating and using feedback to take corrective action.

Marketing

Several authors recommend a marketing approach to recruitment of nurses. Such an approach would focus on the nurse as the consumer of employment. Connelly and Strauser advocate a marketing audit of the nursing environment. Exhibit 8-4 presents a scheme for a marketing survey for recruiting and retaining nurses that includes some of these ideas. The marketing plan would be a management plan that would determine what needs to be done to sell employment to prospective professional nurses. Data would be analyzed, objectives set and evaluated, and a plan made and promoted.[28]

The primary focus of the selling approach to nurse recruitment is the needs of the employer. This approach is more effective when nurses are plentiful. Marketing focuses on many things: the needs of the prospective employee as customer; factors such as job profile, organizational culture, working location and conditions, the reputation of the institution, and compensation; and the institution as a superior place to work.[29]

Long-range management plans can include increasing the productivity of local schools. Will they increase production? What support do they need? Will other organizations cooperate to provide that support, including a marketing survey, recruitment program, and financial assistance for students?

Selecting, Credentialing, and Assigning

Selecting, credentialing, and assigning are all part of the hiring process. Assigning has sometimes been done

after the professional nurse is hired; however, applicants find this system unsatisfactory. They want to know where they will work before reporting for duty and orientation. New employees do not want surprises and will begin work dissatisfied if they occur.

Selecting

Selecting includes the interviewing, the employer's offer, the applicant's acceptance, and the signing of a contract or written offer. Although the chief nurse executive may interview and hire prospective applicants, it is best for the nurse manager who will directly supervise the employee to do the hiring. This person should elicit the input and support of clinical nurses with whom the prospective employee will be working.

The Interview

The nurse recruiter or an HR specialist will have completed a personnel folder that contains a completed application form; a résumé or curriculum vitae; references; and any documents that are required by policy or law, such as a current, valid license to practice nursing and school transcripts. The interviewer should prepare for the interview by reading the information in the applicant's folder. Exhibit 8-5 is a checklist to use in reviewing the folder. The interviewer should make notes of questions to ask about the information contained in the folder.

Adequate time should be set aside for the interview, which should take place in a private office where there will be no interruptions. An interview guide will be helpful in conducting an interview satisfactory to both the nurse manager and the applicant (see Exhibit 8-6).

Thompson defines an interview as "an equal level, face-to-face discussion between a job seeker and a person with full authority to fill the position under discussion."[30] Nurses, as the job seekers, want a face-to-face discussion with the person who has hiring authority. They may be considering several jobs, having narrowed the field down to those that specifically fit their career goals. Nurses know how to make contacts and now want interviews to create opportunities to sell themselves.

Introductions

The interviewer should step out from behind the desk, shake hands with the applicant, call the applicant by name, and introduce himself or herself. The interviewer should then seat the applicant so that she or he will not be blinded by sunlight and will be facing the interviewer. All these things are done to put the applicant at ease.

Questions

Questions, which should be prepared beforehand, may include those listed in Exhibit 8-6. Any others specifically

EXHIBIT 8-4
Marketing Survey for Recruiting and Retaining Nurses

1. Number of vacant positions.
   a. Current
   b. Previous month
   c. Percentage increase (or decrease)
2. Turnover rate by month and unit.
3. Exit interview results.
   a. Number of interviews performed
   b. Number of negative comments (list separately) (See Appendix 8–3)
4. New hire demographics.
   a. Diploma graduates
   b. AD graduates
   c. BSN graduates
   d. MSN graduates
   e. Doctoral graduates
   f. Average years of experience
   g. Males
   h. Females
   i. Average age
   j. Percent married
   k. Percent with children of preschool age
   l. Percent with children in school
   m. Percent minorities
   n. Other
5. Demographics of employed nurses. Profile the "stayers" and target similar recruits.
   a. Diploma graduates
   b. AD graduates.
   c. BSN graduates
   d. MSN graduates
   e. Doctoral graduates
   f. Average years of experience
   g. Males
   h. Females
   i. Average age
   j. Percent married
   k. Percent with children of preschool age
   l. Percent with children in school
   m. Percent minorities
   n. Other
6. Attitude survey (list results separately).
7. Audit of meeting minutes.
   a. Staff nurses
   b. Others (list results separately)
8. Audit of performance evaluations (list results separately). Include variations by education, specialty, and longevity.
9. Salary levels (list by clinical level and longevity).
10. Overtime.
    a. Hours by month and unit
    b. Costs
    c. Include variations by education, specialty, and longevity
11. Absenteeism data.
    a. Daily average
    b. Cause
    c. Monthly total
    d. Include variations by education, specialty, and longevity
12. Agency nurse use.
    a. Hours by month and unit
    b. Costs
    c. Include variations by education, specialty, and longevity
13. Monthly budget variances by unit.
14. Utilization of productivity reports (refer to Chapter 7).
15. Acuity data by category and unit.
16. Average daily census by day of week and by month (report trends).
17. Recruiting expenses.
18. Major competitors for prospective hires.
19. Analysis of professional literature on recruitment and availability.
20. Analysis of patient relations reports.
21. Reputation and visibility of the organization and division.
    a. Community
    b. Employees
    c. Organizational culture
    d. Location of employment
22. Factors causing nurses to avoid organization.
23. Factors that would attract nurses to organization because it is a superior place to work.
24. Sources for recruiting nurses.

desired by the interviewer should be added to the list. The answers should not be written down, because doing so is distracting and time-consuming. Written notes should be made immediately after the interview.

All candidates for nurse jobs should be treated as professionals. It is illegal to ask them certain questions, such as those listed in Exhibit 8-7. Because information about age and date of birth may be necessary for insurance or other fringe benefits, it can be obtained after the candidate is hired.

Candidates will have questions they want answered. When complete information cannot be given, the interviewer should make a note, get the information, and communicate it to the candidate as quickly as possible. Exhibit 8-8 lists questions that candidates may ask and that the interviewer should be prepared to answer.

The objective of both interviewer and candidate at the outset of an interview is to create a positive, amicable relationship that results in a job offer. The interview is the most important factor in obtaining this result, because it allows expression of personal ideas, abilities, and accomplishments. It adds individual personality to the résumé and completed application forms.

To prepare for a job interview, nurse managers should do the following:

EXHIBIT 8-5

Checklist for Reviewing Job Applicant's Folder

1. The application form
   a. Completed as directed
   b. Written statements are positive
   c. Contains no blanks
   d. Contains no gaps in employment data
2. References
   a. Listed
   b. Have been checked
   c. Are satisfactory
   d. Need further checking
3. Registered Nurse licensure
   a. Has been verified
   b. Is current and valid
   c. No legal suits pending
4. Transcripts
   a. Have been verified
   b. Are available
5. Forms signed
6. Curriculum vitae or resume
   a. Up to date
   b. Lists career goals
7. Job description provided, including blank performance contract
   a. Clinical level established as_____
   b. Years of longevity established as_____
8. Salary information available
   a. Base salary: $_____
   b. Clinical level pay: $_____
   c. Longevity pay: $_____
   d. Differential: $_____
   e. Credentialing (certification): $_____
   f. Total pay: $_____
   g. Paydays made known

EXHIBIT 8-6

Interview Guide

CANDIDATE:
DATE AND TIME OF INTERVIEW:

1. Arrange seating.
2. Make introductions and establish rapport.
3. Ask prepared questions.
   a. Tell me about yourself.
   b. What is your present job?
   c. What are your three most outstanding accomplishments?
   d. What is the extent of your formal education?
   e. What three things are most important to you in your job?
   f. What is your strongest qualification for this job?
   g. What other jobs have you held in this or a similar field?
   h. What were your responsibilities?
   i. Do you mind irregular working hours? Explain.
   j. Would you be willing to relocate? To travel?
   k. What minimum salary are you willing to accept?
   l. Are you more comfortable working alone or with other people?
4. Answer candidate's questions.
5. Note the following: Candidate was
   a. On time
   b. Well-dressed
   c. Well-mannered
   d. Positive about self
6. Maintain eye contact.
7. Note candidate's personal values.
8. Close the interview.
   a. Make an offer
   b. Obtain acceptance
   c. Set timetable for making offer or receiving response to offer

EXHIBIT 8-7

Questions That Are Illegal

Employment interviewers are forbidden by law to ask the following questions:

1. Age
2. Date of birth
3. The length of time residing at present address
4. Previous address
5. Religion; church attended; spiritual adviser's name
6. Father's surname
7. Maiden name (of women)
8. Marital status
9. Residence mates
10. Number and ages of children; who will care for them while applicant works
11. Transportation to work, unless a car is a job requirement
12. Residence of spouse or parent
13. Whether residence is owned or rented
14. Name of bank; information on outstanding loans
15. Whether wages were ever garnished
16. Whether bankruptcy was ever declared
17. Whether ever arrested
18. Hobbies, off-duty interests, clubs

EXHIBIT 8-8
Possible Questions from Candidates and Tips for Interviewing

QUESTIONS

1. How much job security does this job have?
2. What previous experience does this type of job require?
3. What is the future of this type of job?
4. What is the growth potential for this particular job?
5. Where will the most significant growth for this type of job in the health care industry occur?
6. What is the starting salary for this job?
7. How do pay raises occur?
8. How does one find out when other job openings occur?
9. What are the fringe benefits of this job?
10. What are the requirements for working shifts and weekends?
11. What is the floating policy?
12. What are the opportunities for continuing education?
13. What are the opportunities for promotion?
14. What child care facilities are available?
15. What are the staffing and scheduling policies?

TIPS

1. Keep the atmosphere positive, pleasant, and businesslike.
2. Focus on the essential goals.
3. Provide answers in a brief, factual, and friendly manner; use a soft and clear tone of voice; maintain a relaxed posture; and keep hands still.
4. Do not attempt to bluff answers to questions.
5. Review information sent to you before the interview.
6. Be prepared for questions related to personal philosophy and style, community relations, professional goals, clinical and administrative style, decision-making ability, flexibility in working with diverse groups, fiscal issues, personnel management, and group relationships.
7. Avoid controversial issues of religion, abortion, and politics; do not discuss confidential matters.
8. Do not identify problems or offer solutions unless asked, and then indicate the need to have more information and time to study the issue.

- Decide beforehand that they want the interview to end in a job offer.
- Know the specific qualifications needed by the organization. Relating them to the candidate will help to identify a fit between candidate and job.
- Decide to win the candidate's favor. The interviewer should come across as someone who respects and values employees. It is important for both interviewer and interviewee to have self-confidence, optimism, good manners, charm, and enthusiasm.
- Gain a feeling for the values of the candidate. Are they compatible with the organization's mission, philosophy, and objectives?
- Have expectations about the dress, mannerisms, and other personal characteristics of the candidate. (These will, of course, be objective.) A serious candidate will dress conservatively for the interview. If the applicant is a man, he should be clean-shaven, have neatly cut and styled hair, be dressed in a business suit and tie, and have appropriate footwear. A beard is acceptable but should be neatly trimmed. If the applicant is a woman, she should have a neat hairdo, be dressed in a business suit or dress, wear hosiery, and wear appropriate jewelry. Makeup should be in good taste, and perfume or cologne, if worn, should be discreet. Appearance should be interpreted as an indication of a person's good judgment and impeccable taste. Candidates thus tell the prospective employer they regard the interview as important. Likewise, the

interviewer should dress, act, and look like the right person to be the candidate's manager.

The applicant should come across as a thoroughly pleasant, cooperative, and competent person who can tactfully, objectively, and successfully deal with the most difficult people problems. The applicant should be neither blustery or flamboyant nor mouselike and servile. The interviewer should meet the same personal standards as those of the person being interviewed. Candidates who disagree with the interviewer's tastes or values should not be rejected unless the disagreement is related to the welfare of the organization. Candidates should not be made to feel intimidated. Exhibit 8-9 summarizes what happens during an interview.

Eye Contact

It is important to maintain good eye contact during an interview. Following some simple rules can help the interviewer do this. The interviewer should look at the applicant's eyes for about eight seconds, then look away, shifting the body position at the same time. Doing so avoids being thought of as having "shifty" eyes. When the interviewer is uncomfortable with eye contact, however, the focus can be shifted to the bridge of the applicant's nose at a spot between the eyes. Eye contact tells the applicant the interviewer has trust and credibility.

Rapport

Rapport can be established with the candidate at the outset of the interview by talking about common

---

EXHIBIT 8-9
What Happens During an Interview

THE HIRING EXECUTIVE

1. Gives information about job and institution.
2. Assesses the competencies the candidate possesses in relation to the job opening.
3. Evaluates the candidate's personal characteristics in relation to the staff members with whom candidate will work (fit to staff).
4. Assesses candidate's potential to move organization toward its goals.
5. Assesses candidate's enthusiasm and state of health.
6. Forms impressions about candidate based on behavior, appearance, ability to communicate, confidence, intelligence, personality.
7. Assesses candidate's ability to do the job.
8. Determines facts about candidate.

THE CANDIDATE

1. Gives information about self.
2. Assesses the opportunity for developing and using competencies on the job.
3. Assesses ability to relate to the employees with whom candidate will work.
4. Assesses potential for achieving personal career goals.
5. Assesses the institution's climate and the morale of the employees.
6. Assesses opportunities for promotion and success.
7. Assesses own ability to do the job.
8. Determines facts about the organization and working conditions.

---

friends or interests. This friendly chat should be kept short, because time is important to both parties.

Closing the Interview

Closing the interview means that the session is at a point at which the interviewer is ready to make an offer or has all the information needed to evaluate the applicant. When ready to make an offer, the interviewer should have all of the information related to salary, fringe benefits, assignment, and scheduling ready for presentation and discussion. If the applicant wants the information in writing or wants time to consider the offer, a definite time schedule should be set: "I want you for this position. I will mail you an offer tomorrow," or, alternately, "I want you for this position. Please call me and give me your decision between 8 and 10 A.M. on Monday."

If the interviewer needs more information, the applicant should be so advised and told they will be informed of the results of the interview as soon as the information is provided. When there are several candidates for a specific job, all will have to be interviewed before a selection is made. Applicants should be notified of their rejection. If possible, reasons for rejection should be stated but in terms that will not destroy candidate's self-esteem or cause legal problems for the employer.

The Assessment Center Process

An assessment center is a method for screening candidates for jobs. It is specific to the job for which candidates are applying. Sullivan, Decker, and Hailstone describe an assessment center for the selection of a nurse manager that has the following 17 job dimensions, each of which is subdivided into abilities that are observed and scored[31]:

1. Clinical nursing background
2. Development of subordinates
3. Delegation/management control
4. Planning and organization
5. Perception/sensitivity
6. Problem analysis
7. Problem-solving/decision-making
8. Risk taking
9. Initiation/leadership
10. Communication skills
11. Listening skills
12. Energy level
13. Stress tolerance
14. Resilience
15. Assertiveness
16. Behavioral flexibility
17. Accessibility

The following are some other characteristics of this process[32]:

1. Exercises are developed to measure job dimensions.
2. Assessors from the supervisor group are selected and trained to rate the candidates.
3. The Head Nurse Assessment Center (HNAC) is conducted for one day. Each candidate is assessed by at least two persons.
4. Reliability and validity of assessment centers are high. The HNAC has many benefits, including selection of competent nurse managers, objectivity, broader

applicant support, consistency, selection of qualified applicants, nurse manager development, and improved management reputation.

5. Among the drawbacks of the HNAC are that it is stressful, time-consuming, and tiring for assessors; it favors outsiders; and it causes intimidation.
6. The process is job specific.
7. The process is equitable to minorities and women.
8. Supervisors who will work with applicants select them.
9. The process has self-development value for participants.
10. The process is expensive, is stressful, may favor conformists, and may create self-fulfilling prophecies.
11. The process diminishes the risk for hiring or promoting inappropriate candidates.
12. The process is used in more than 2,000 companies.

In a similar process, a master interview tool has been developed that categorizes content such as documented clinical and administrative expertise, research, education, and other significant factors Points are assigned according to the weight of each rating category for various positions. A pool of interview questions is developed to determine the applicant's ability to communicate, organize thoughts, solve problems, and relate to others; to assess the applicant's knowledge, philosophy, experience, and personality traits; and to reveal the applicant's frame of reference, level of expectation, attitudes, feelings, and management style. Interview panels consist of three members, the chair being appointed by the chief nurse executive. The tool is claimed to have fairly high interrater reliability, to decrease interview time, and to assist in selecting the most qualified applicant.[33]

Hiring is an investment in the right and best-qualified person. Interviewing techniques are often cursory and do not result in hiring the right person. Assessment center techniques should be considered for the hiring of all categories of nursing personnel. delBueno, Weeks, and Brown-Stewart define the assessment center as "a comprehensive, standardized process by which multiple sampling techniques are used to determine an individual's actual or potential ability to perform skills and activities vital to success on the job." The assessment center process pools information from total sources and for noted performance dimensions. It may be used to plan orientation programs, for promotions, and for placement in clinical and career ladders. It is a cost-effective process because it avoids the unneeded orientation and turnover costs of hiring the wrong applicant.[34]

As a result of a research project involving six assessment centers serving a variety of persons with disabilities, the recommendation was made that evaluators develop policies and procedures for ensuring the rights of clients as consumers of assessment services. Clients should be fully informed of the process and its purpose, including dissemination of information.[35]

Peters's recommendations support the principles underlying the assessment center process[36]:

- Applicants should have multiple lengthy interviews over one to two days.
- Senior line people should interview applicants, peers, and potential subordinates.
- Interviews should unequivocally stress the attitudes and skills necessary to thrive in an ever more ambiguous and fast-changing world.

The Search Committee

A job opportunity having a large impact on the organization will result in the appointment of a search committee. The objective is to obtain input into the hiring process from the people who will be affected by the appointment. Such committees are widely used in higher education, where faculty members expect to share in the governance of the institution and particularly in the area of curriculum. The following is an outline of search committee procedures:

1. A search committee is appointed by the chief executive officer (CEO) with input from the population to be affected.
2. A chair will be appointed by administration or elected by the search committee to serve as the liaison between the two.
3. The search committee's responsibilities will be clearly laid out by policy or by the committee itself. Most committees will recruit, screen, interview, and recommend applicants. Administrators generally make final decisions about appointments. Members of search committees are committed to their tasks and responsibilities. They may be committing themselves to five or six months of arduous work. The search committee usually agrees at the outset to consider all information about applicants as confidential. It will not discuss any individual candidate outside the committee, except in general terms of progress reports to staff or faculty.
4. The search committee decides on a strategy for recruiting candidates and implements it.
5. Applications are screened after references and credentials have been obtained.
6. Applicants are scheduled for interviews and visits to the institution. Exhibit 8-10 contains a list of possible search committee interview questions.
7. After all applicants have been interviewed the committee meets to analyze the information and rank-order the candidates.
8. A list of recommended applicants is sent to the CEO.

9. The CEO invites an applicant for a return visit and decides whether to make a job offer.

Credentialing

Credentialing is the process by which selected professionals are granted privileges to practice within an organization. In health care organizations this process has been largely confined to physicians. Limited privileges have been granted to psychologists, social workers, and selected categories of nurses such as nurse anesthetists, surgical nurses, and midwives. These categories generally have been restricted by physician credentialing policies and fall into the category of allied professional staff. The purpose of credentialing is to provide one mechanism by which nurses and other health care professionals can ensure that they possess the level of knowledge and skill required to perform the advanced activities required of them and consequently avoid negative legal repercussions. This process is considered to be especially true of advanced practice nurses.[37]

The Joint Commission on Accreditation of Healthcare Organizations (JCAHO) requires that hospitals investigate, develop recommendations, reach conclusions, and be responsible for their actions in credentialing the medical staff. Licensing and certification provide data to consider in the process.

Components

As for physicians, the components of a credentialing system for nurses would be as follows:

- Appointment. Evaluation and selection for nursing staff membership.
- Clinical privileges. Delineation of the specific nursing specialties that may be performed and the types of illnesses or patients that may be managed within the institution for each member of the nursing staff.
- Periodic reappraisal. Continuing review and evaluation of each member of the nursing staff to ensure that competence is maintained and is consistent with privileges.[38]

Criteria for Appointment

Criteria for appointments include proof of licensure, education and training, specialty board certification, previous experience, and recommendations. Clinical privileges criteria include proof of specialty training and of performance of nursing procedures or specialty care during training and previous appointments.

During the credentialing process the committee should look for red flags of high mobility, graduation from foreign schools, professional liability suits, and professional disciplinary actions. Each red flag is a reason for exercising extra care in reviewing the applicant.

EXHIBIT 8-10
Preparatory Questions for Search Committee

1. What style of management do you follow?
2. What are your personal weaknesses and strengths?
3. What are your perceptions of the role the person in this job will perform?
4. How can this organization benefit your career?
5. What are your ideas of what the relationship should be between nurses and physicians?
6. What job in nursing would you like most to have?
7. What do you view as the role of nursing in this organization?
8. What do you view as the role of nursing in the community?
9. What do you think of collective bargaining?
10. How would you go about determining that your department operates efficiently and effectively?
11. Why should I (we) hire you?
12. How would you go about meeting the goals of the organization?
13. How would your family adapt to this area?
14. What are your career goals?

Professional nurses have mostly been hired through HR offices, but nurse managers should give consideration to increasing the professional status of nursing through the credentialing process. (See Appendix 8-1.)

The American Nurses Association

A report of the Committee for the Study of Credentialing in Nursing, undertaken in 1979, included 14 principles of credentialing related to the following[39]:

1. Those credentialed
2. Legitimate interests of involved occupation, institution, and the general public
3. Accountability
4. A system of checks and balances
5. Periodic assessments
6. Objective standards and criteria and persons competent in their use
7. Representation of the community of interests
8. Professional identity and responsibility
9. An effective system of role delineation
10. An effective system of program identification
11. Coordination of credentialing mechanisms
12. Geographic mobility
13. Definitions and terminology
14. Communications and understanding

Credentialing in a hospital relates to appointing health professionals to the staff. Credentialing by professional organizations, such as ANA certification-recertification programs, can be a qualification for such appointments[40]:

The American Nurses Association, Inc. established the ANA Certification Program in 1973 to provide tangible recognition of professional achievement in a defined functional or clinical area of nursing. Based on the 1989 recommendation from the ANA Commission on Organizational Assessment and Renewal (COAR), the American Nurses Credentialing Center (ANCC) has been established as a separately incorporated center through which ANA would serve its own credentialing programs. The ANCC bases its credentialing programs on the standards set by the ANA Congress for Nursing Practice. Goals of the ANCC include promoting and enhancing public health by certifying nurses and accrediting organizations using ANA standards of nursing practice, nursing services, and continuing education. Primary responsibility for the ANCC certification and recertification programs rests with the Boards on Certification whose members are nominated by the respective peer group. These Boards are: Community Health Nursing Practice, Maternal-Child Nursing Practice, Medical-Surgical Nursing Practice, Primary Care in Adult and Family/Health Nursing Practice, Gerontological Nursing Practice, Nursing Administration Practice, General Nursing Practice, and Nursing Continuation Education/Staff Development Nursing Practice.

More than 90,000 RNs have been certified by the ANCC. Beginning in 1998, all generalist programs were required to have a baccalaureate in nursing for the initial certification process.

Credentialing at Carondelet St. Mary's Hospital and Health Center in Tucson, Arizona, focuses on patient care, leadership, and education. Benefits to the nurses include clinical ladder promotions, compensation, paid education time, tuition reimbursement, and a paid day monthly for meetings and research. Patients benefit from improved infection control, reduced numbers and increased healing of pressure ulcers, new product introduction, and improved teaching. The employer benefits from retention of satisfied customers, nurses, and patients.[41]

Assigning

Assigning professional nurses to jobs is the third part of the hiring process. During the assignment period the new nurse is oriented to the job description and its use. Although assignment to a specific position may not be possible during the selecting and credentialing processes, candidates should have a choice of the possible units to which they will be assigned.

Where can a candidate who wants to work in the operating room (OR) be assigned when there are no vacancies in the OR? The candidate can be offered a choice of vacant positions. Make a verbal or written contract to transfer the individual to a vacated OR position when one becomes available. If others are waiting for a similar assignment, indicate the order in which they will be assigned to the OR.

Candidates should not receive assignment surprises when they arrive for orientation. When assignment policies are fair, reasonable, and acceptable, candidates will start work with a positive attitude. A principle for a nurse manager to follow is to provide necessary orientation and training to nursing employees to ensure competency, job satisfaction, and high productivity in the particular assignments they are accepting.

> **Leadership requires that nurse managers be absolutely truthful in dealing with assignment of personnel, including reassignment by floating to other units.**

Retaining

The retention of competent professional nurses in jobs is a major problem of the U.S. health care industry, particularly for hospitals and long-term care facilities. Most Americans change jobs about 15 times by the age of 35, and nurses are no exception. Nurses change and achieve major career goals four or five times in their lifetime, including changing their specialty or the role they play in the profession.[42] Many do both. Some even retire from two or more systems.

Career Dissatisfaction Versus Job Dissatisfaction

There is a difference between career dissatisfaction and job dissatisfaction. A nurse may make a job change because of job dissatisfaction. If dissatisfied with several jobs, a professional nurse looks at the work itself, the tasks involved, and the purposes to be served. If all are distasteful, a professional nurse may make a decision to leave the profession. (See Appendix 8-2.)

Turnover

The annual national turnover rate among hospital nurses is between 20% and 70%. An organization should determine its turnover rate by unit and by organization. Such determinations should be done monthly to keep abreast of trends. Nurses who leave should be profiled and defined by average age, marital status, type of program from which they graduated, additional education, years of experience, specialty, sex, race, and any other characteristic that will give clues that could decrease turnover and increase retention of competent nurses. Nurse managers should also review the performance of nurses who leave and do exit interviews.

The crude turnover rate depicts the volume of turnover and is not a very selective index. An example is given in Exhibit 8-11. Other data that provide information about turnover and retention are the mean and median service of nurses who stay. These data provide the average tenure of employees. Examples of these data are also illustrated in Exhibit 8-11, as are mean and median service of those who leave, instability rate, wastage rate, and survival curve of those who leave.[43] The sum of the number of months of employment of each nurse as well as other data can be determined by having a good nursing management information system (NMIS), which will accumulate the data on electronic spread sheets.

The Leadership, Evaluation and Awareness Process (LEAP), was developed by DeBerry. The outcome of LEAP has been an 80% reduction in turnover of first-line managers at an average turnover cost of $125,000 each and a positive cost-benefit analysis. LEAP is a common preselection process for first-line managers that consists of the following[44]:

- A one-day program called "Is Management for Me?" covering the realities of management; 60% of attendees self-selected out of competition.
- A developmental session with current managers covering skills such as charisma, individual consideration, intellectual stimulation, courage, dependability, flexibility, integrity, judgment, and respect for others.
- A three-way evaluation of manager as coach, peers, and self-profile of leadership on nine skills.
- A panel of executives using "in-basket" exercises and oral and written tests on nine skills; 75% of candidates were endorsed.
- Application.

Spitzer-Lehmann indicates that it is better to retain nurses than to recruit them. These benefits include cost benefits, high morale, and high-quality care. A study indicated that nurses stayed in their jobs when they received peer support, participated in a professional practice model, received tuition reimbursement, had input into decision-making, and communication was open and medical staff was supportive.[45] The policy of floating to other units should be discontinued or modified to provide nurses with confidence and comfort in the workplace. Other retention strategies provide for assistance when needed, recognition of the private lives of employees, and matching skills and abilities to jobs. Employees want meaningful work assignments; equal, not subordinate, treatment; opportunities for development and use of knowledge and skills; and flexibility and independence on the job. Employees' perceptions of the work environment should be evaluated frequently. Feedback should be frequent and include the institution's financial position, strategy, market position, and future plans.[46]

Because 70% of families are headed by a single working parent or by two wage earners, vanguard companies are changing their corporate culture to accomplish goals of work force dedication, focus, and productivity. Vanguard companies consider it good business to make coming to work easier for employees; the outcomes have been loyalty, dedication, and team spirit. Vanguard companies are changing corporate culture to[47]:

- Make it family friendly.
- Provide childcare around the clock.
- Foster candor, assertiveness, and commitment.
- Focus on managers bringing about cultural change through a common collaborative management style and a HR philosophy, the bedrocks of which are equity and flexibility.
- Provide elder care referral.
- Provide professional counseling for coping with stress.
- Provide paid days off for taking care of personal obligations.
- Empower managers and the work force.
- Provide resources.
- Tailor the culture to the individual's needs.

Because nursing is a work force with many of the same characteristics of working parents, the objective of staffing should be staff retention by making it easier for nursing personnel to come to work.

An insurance company adopted a service strategy to retain its employees and its customers. Through a problem-solving process called DOME (*d*iagnosis, *o*bjectives, *m*ethod, and *e*valuation), the company determined that service was a commodity as well as a product line. The service strategy was identified as "an organizing principle that directs people to provide services that benefit the customers." To accomplish this end, the fragile elements of motivation and staff commitment require that a motivational environment be created and maintained. This environment should address quality of work life, morale, energy levels, and optimism. This kind of environment creates new promotional and training opportunities.[48]

Turnover causes increased costs for hiring and orienting as well as staff instability and decreased quality of care. Exhibit 8-11 presents a conceptual framework for nursing turnover. Among the causes of turnover are job stress, lack of autonomy, job dissatisfaction and a poor overall health care environment (regulatory, political, economic, and social factors). These factors include political ones, such as resource allocation; economic ones, such as profit margins; policy; and organizational diagnosis involving structures, interaction, and competition.

EXHIBIT 8-11
Turnover Data

1.

$$\text{Crude turnover rate} = \left[\frac{\text{Number } (N) \text{ of Leavers}}{\left(\dfrac{N \text{ at start} + n \text{ at end}}{2} \right)} \right] \times 100$$

Number (N) of leavers = number of nurses who left during a year
N at start = number of nurses employed at beginning of year
n at end = number of nurses employed at end of year

Example: (N) = 189
        N = 543
        n = 529

$$\frac{189}{\dfrac{543 + 529}{2}} \times 100 = \frac{189}{536} \times 100 = 35.3\%$$

2.

$$\text{Mean service of stayers} = \frac{\text{Sum of the number of months of employment of each nurse}}{\text{Number of nurses employed}}$$

Example:

$$\frac{10,563 \text{ months}}{529 \text{ nurses}} = 19.97 \text{ months}$$

3. Median service of stayers
Rank currently employed nurses by the number of months of employment from the shortest to the longest and choose the middle ranking value.

Example:

Months	1–6	7–12	13–18	19–24	25–30	31–36	37–42	43–48	49–54	55–60+
No. of Employees	73	61	55	50	41	39	40	27	39	104
Total	73	134	189	239	280	319	359	386	425	529

Total nurses (stayers) = 529

$$\text{Median} = \frac{529}{2} = 264.5$$

Median occurs at 25 to 30 months, indicating that more than one-half of the nurses have been employed 30 months or less. The median is considered a better measure of central tendency than the mean.

4.

$$\text{Mean service of leavers} = \frac{\text{Sum of the number of months of employment of each nurse who left}}{\text{Number of nurses who left}}$$

Example:

$$\frac{2,417 \text{ months}}{189 \text{ nurses}} = 12.79 \text{ months}$$

(continued)

EXHIBIT 8-11 (continued)

5. Median service of leavers

Example:

Months	1–6	7–12	13–18	19–24	25–30	31–36	37–42	43–48	49–54	55–60+	61+
No. of Employees	49	35	27	19	14	9	9	10	7	6	4
Total	49	84	111	130	144	153	162	172	179	185	189

Total nurses (leavers) = 189

$$\text{Median} = \frac{189}{2} = 94.5$$

The median occurs at 13 to 18 months. Because both the mean and median of leavers are low, short-term employees are leaving.

6.

$$\text{Instability rate} = \frac{\text{Number of leavers who had been employed at beginning of year}}{\text{Number of nurses employed at beginning of year}} \times 100$$

Example:

$$\frac{151}{529} \times 100 = 28.54\%$$

Of nurses employed at the beginning of the year, 28.54% left during the year.

7.

$$\text{Wastage rate} = \frac{\text{Number of newly hired nurses who leave during first year}}{\text{Number of nurses newly hired during year}} \times 100$$

Example:

$$\frac{40}{113} \times 100 = 35.4\%$$

Of newly hired nurses, over one-third, or 35.4%, leave before the end of 1 year.

(continued)

Turnover includes both replacement and transfer employees. The direct costs of turnover are attributed to recruitment of replacements. The costs of turnover range from $1,280 to $50,000 per RN turnover. Turnover benefits include savings on salaries and benefits and infusion of new knowledge and ideas. Incentives for retention include financial ones, flexible scheduling, participative management, job expansion, job enrichment, job reframing (looking at a job in a new way), and preventive career maintenance.[49]

Job Expectations and Satisfaction

Ginsberg and co-authors contend that the high turnover rate in nursing is a result of job dissatisfaction (see Appendix 8-2). In a survey of nurse job and career sat-isfaction and dissatisfaction, 6,277 surveys were mailed to nurses in a five-county area around Jacksonville, Florida. There were 1,921 responses, with the following rank-order results[50]:

1. Money was the number one concern and the pre-ferred remedy.
2. Recognition.
3. Hours and scheduling.
4. Too much responsibility for the money.
5. Stress.

A study to determine why new graduates select particular settings and why many leave in a short time surveyed 279 nursing seniors in five schools in northern Alabama. The new graduates had the following expectations[51]:

EXHIBIT 8-11 (continued)

8. Survival curve of leavers

Example:

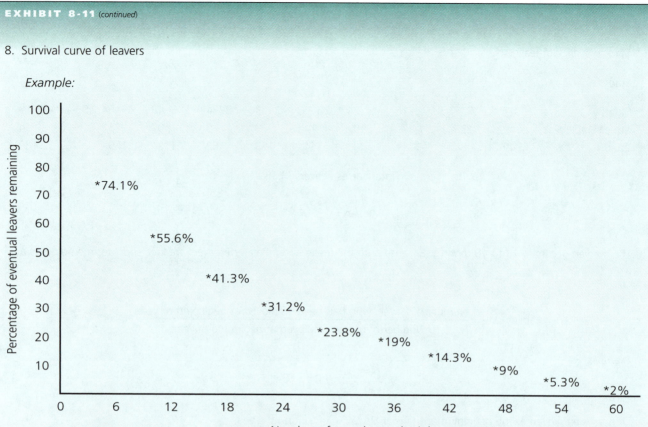

Number of months on the job

Using the data from item 5, 100% of 189 leavers were employed at the beginning of the 12-month period.

$$\frac{189 - 49}{189} \times 100 = \frac{140}{189} \times 100 = 74.1\% \text{ of leavers were employed 6–12 months.}$$

$$\frac{140 - 35}{189} \times 100 = \frac{105}{189} \times 100 = 55.6\% \text{ of leavers were employed 13–18 months.}$$

Because the curve drops sharply and then gradually, it shows that the turnover concentration is among new employees. A straight line would indicate turnover to be independent of length of service.

Source: Adapted from M. L. Duxbury and G. D. Armstrong. "Calculating Nurse Turnover Indices." *The Journal of Nursing Administration* (March 1982), 18–24. Reprinted with permission of J. B. Lippincott.

1. Full-time work
2. Day work or a desired shift (46% of single nurses and 36.5% of married nurses would work evenings)
3. Work in a medium-sized to large hospital
4. Good salary
5. Pleasant working conditions
6. Self-fulfillment and a sense of achievement from giving adequate and complete care
7. Educational opportunities, intellectual stimulation, and opportunity to develop new skills
8. Satisfactory supervision by nurse managers
9. Recognition and encouragement
10. Professional autonomy and power
11. Work in a community that offers higher education opportunities and a good place to raise a family; factors considered important included good schools, a low crime rate, an economically stable region, a low tax structure, and a low cost of living

In addition, more baccalaureate degree nurses expected to become head nurses, supervisors, and public health nurses than did associate degree nurses. Many would *not* consider working in small hospitals (17.2%), veteran's administration or federally owned hospitals (19.5%), investor-owned hospitals (18.8 percent), nursing homes (65.7%), doctor's office or clinic (18.6%), temporary or private-duty agency (41%), or psychiatric or mental health clinic (45.5%).[52]

Drucker states that salaries are not the basic problem with nurse retention and recruitment, a position in opposition to most surveys. He states:

> The basic problem is that nurses aren't allowed to do nursing. I've been saying that now for 20 years. The doctors still treat nurses as if they were scullery maids, and that's just not going to work any longer.

Drucker believes that hospital administrators must change the attitudes of doctors. Also, focusing nurses' responsibilities on their professional role and increasing their salaries will improve retention.[53]

A study of nurse manager satisfaction in Massachusetts hospitals indicated that this group was dissatisfied with educational reimbursements received (50%), inadequate role orientation (52%), support from other hospital departments (59%), the lack of control over budget process (12%), salary (53%), added duties of expanded role (60%), staffing issues (73%), information received (40%), and negative effects of stress (67%). A plan was developed to alleviate these dissatisfactions and was to be implemented by nurse executives.[54]

Career Planning

Nurse managers must recognize the results of nurse satisfaction surveys. They must learn to manage professional nurses so that they will achieve career and job satisfaction. The first step is to establish a career plan for them within the nursing organization.

To be successful in their careers, professional nurses need a sense of personal fulfillment and job significance, indicating that they are growing as persons. Nurse managers create these conditions by determining and correcting the causes of the following[55]:

- Anxiety and uncertainty
- Inability to meet personal and organizational goals
- Lack of clarity about roles played
- Contradictory demands
- Dissatisfaction with human relations
- Rebellion against rules, policies, and regulations
- Inherent nature of the tasks of the job
- Competition
- Overwork and underutilization
- Lack of personal and professional growth
- Dissatisfaction with the quality of associates

> **A professional nurse is a reasonable person, and reasonable people can accommodate to reality, accept themselves, be interested in others, learn from experience, and be self-actualized.[56]**

Nurse managers should restructure nursing services to link assignments and responsibilities to education, experience, and competence. Doing so should be a part of a career program for professional nurses that[57]:

- Provides more promotions and pay for clinical nurses.
- Provides higher pay for increased competence, and increased participation.
- Provides for continuing education to upgrade knowledge and skills.
- Provides clinical rotation policies that prevent burnout.
- Meets scheduling and salary preferences.

When a career structure has been established, it will provide for upward mobility for clinical nurses, nurse managers, nursing teachers, and nursing researchers. Professional nurses will decide to take advantage of career advancement opportunities. Jobs for those advancing will be identified and will require advanced knowledge and skills, particularly those related to decision-making. RNs who do not want promotions will be rewarded with merit pay increases for doing their jobs well. Advancing nurses will be rewarded for increased responsibility and accountability. Nurses will finally have a career rather than just a job.

Career Counselor

A career counselor should be part of the grand strategy for establishing a nursing career program. Even though an organization may not have a career counselor, every nurse should have one in the person of a superior. This person helps nurses clarify their career goals and make a plan for achieving them. The plan also includes work experiences related to off-duty time, such as courses, workshops, community service, professional activities, and other activities specifically related to goals. It is a total plan that develops individuals professionally to meet their career aspirations. The career counselor facilitates that program. A supervisor who is not the career counselor can be asked to become one or to provide the opportunity to use someone else as a mentor.

The counselor should be able to help nurses advance their careers in nursing and not just within the organization. At least one counselor should be available to help nurses assess their interests, skills, and values; to assist with analyzing all the open options; and to aid in making the career plans that will lead to achieving career goals. That individual could be a supervisor, a nurse administrator, a staff development person, or an expert in the chosen field of nursing. In the final analysis, only the individual nurse can develop and direct a career toward achievement of life goals. All others, whether employers, colleagues, peers, or counselors, can form only a support group.

Staff Development Career Counselor

One group to contact about career opportunities is the staff development department. There is an awakening notion that staff development can advance the career opportunities of professional nurses. Because such counselors traditionally serve in an organizational relationship that provides a staff service to line management of the nursing hierarchy, nursing administration should identify their role. Traditionally, the staff development department fulfills functions of initial orientation and conducts classes in cardiopulmonary resuscitation, intravenous therapy, and the like. In contrast, some departments are moving toward a career development orientation by becoming involved in functions such as specialty orientation and training and in implementing the process of planning, organizing, directing, and evaluating the development of nurses through levels of competency in clinical practice, management, teaching, and research.

Sovie labels the career development functions of the staff development department as professional identification, professional maturation, and professional mastery. These areas can be related to a career ladder program in which competencies have been identified for the nurse practicing at several rungs of the ladder. The competencies are stated in the form of job descriptions and increase in complexity. Policies and procedures exist for the process of climbing the ladder. A program of staff development for career advancement facilitates the process.

Sovie's model could educate nurses to gain advanced specialized knowledge and skills through individual plans, with staff development educators acting as counselors and teachers. Nurses could learn to provide the leadership in solving the health care problems of patients and families. They could develop materials for patient and family education. They could learn to be a primary nurse in practicing the nursing process, not just within the nursing modality. They could learn to engage in professional nursing dialogue with colleagues. Training for nurses could include the competencies of consulting, participation in quality assurance activities, processing and applying reports of research findings, participation in research, and involvement in committee functions. This learning could be part of a personal career plan.[58]

Efforts Outside the Department

In many organizations maturation skills are shaped outside the staff development department. Professional nurses who select the management ladder enter into a continuous program of staff development. As clinical nurses develop the credentials of mastery in a specialty area, they are assigned to that level of practice. They could be encouraged to produce their own staff development functions (e.g., conducting workshops) for which they would earn a fee that, in turn, could be used to pay for their own continuing education outside the organization. They could provide nurse-to-nurse consultation in their areas of specialization. They could participate on unit, divisional, and organizational committees. Their mastery is rewarded by higher salaries and additional perquisites because with professional mastery they produce more at the same cost.

Nurses working in an organization that has a career development program should be moving up the ladder of their choice. The career development program should also provide an opportunity for moving laterally into clinical practice, management, teaching, or research. It should provide job satisfaction and a salary that increases with development and mastery.

If such a career development program does not exist in the organization, nurses can stimulate it. First they can learn about career development through research and study; then they master the knowledge of career development; and finally, they present it to and gain the support of their supervisors. When attempts to move up fail, nurses may want to move out, but they should not give up easily.

Career Ladders

Clinical nursing offers the most diverse kinds of opportunities. Clinical nursing was largely a nonpromotable area until recent years. Numerous interesting clinical areas had been expanded with advanced technology, but nurses seldom could be promoted within a clinical area. This is changing fast with the development of clinical career ladders and levels of increasing competence to mastery.

A career ladder requires individual effort, assisted by organizational support and reward. When appropriately conceived and implemented, a career ladder program results in career satisfaction for the nurse and increased productivity for the employer. More results must occur than title changes and increased wages.

Among the opportunities to be considered are clinical coordinator, clinical specialist, nurse practitioner, primary nurse, patient health educator, case manager, and flight nurse. Advertisements in nursing journals and local newspapers identify these and many more opportunities.

Nurses who want to stay in clinical nursing and advance (in terms of all rewards, including salary, fringe benefits, professional achievement, and satisfaction) will need to be prepared at the highest level of clinical practice. Clinical nurse specialists are professionals with education and experience at the level of the most complicated patient care problems and needs. Examples are clinical nurse specialists in ostomy care, oncology, or cardiovascular care. They should have the experience and education to perform in a consultative nurse capacity. Most clinical nurse specialists have education beyond the bachelor's level and hold an advanced degree or certificate. They also have the advanced clinical experience to match the knowledge.

A clinical career ladder is a horizontal development system based on specific criteria used to develop, evaluate, and promote nurses who desire and intend to remain at the bedside. Clinical ladders apply to nurses who want to remain in the clinical setting, whereas career ladders are for those who leave the clinical realm in pursuit of a future in administration, teaching, or research.

A clinical career ladder should:

1. Improve the quality of patient care.
2. Motivate staff in terms of
   a. Job proficiency and expertise, that is, motivate nurses to reach their highest level of professional competence.
   b. Pursuit of education, which is an important factor in mobility.
   c. Development of career goals.
3. Provide methods of objective and measurable performance evaluation, and reward clinical competence for the purpose of advancement.
4. Promote retention within the clinical area, and reduce the turnover rate.

Nurses who are interested in working under this type of system should understand several points. First, most health care organizations have a promotion system of some kind, but only a few are of the clinical ladder type. Unfortunately, many are based on a seniority system or include seniority as the primary criterion for advancement. Some administrators adopt a form of clinical ladder to help alleviate their recruitment and retention problems. Their ladder may look good on paper, but the question is whether it provides administrative advantages rather than the advantages nurses want. If the system in which a nurse is working promotes to the next higher level according to a time frame, without regard for educational status or job performance, then the individual is at a disadvantage. There is no competition or motivation to improve. Everyone will be promoted when they have "served their time," both average and above-average nurses.

Small pay differentials between levels also will impede motivation to change. Salary increases should be enough to further motivate nurses to improve their skills (competence). Responsibility should increase with promotion. If nurses are still performing the same tasks with the same supervision and no additional responsibility after advancement, they cannot be said to have really advanced professionally.

Performance criteria in any clinical ladder system should be clearly differentiated and specific at each level. The evaluation process must be measurable. Salary differentials must be significant enough to provide motivation. Any system should involve evaluation of educational and leadership criteria as well as skill performance.

Finally, the evaluation of each individual should include input from the direct supervisor and the individual nurse. A board or panel of three or more nurses may be assembled to review all eligible personnel for promotion. The advantages of such a system are that it increases job satisfaction, improves clinical skills, offers positive motivation for acceptance of continued leadership and educational responsibility, and provides an opportunity for career advancement while remaining in clinical nursing. The disadvantage is that positions may not always be available at higher levels.

Management promotes the system to the end that productivity will be increased. Also, management must ensure the maintenance of quality of nursing care.

Exhibit 8-12 is a basic clinical ladder model that can be added to or fleshed out by management. Because salary and benefits are the most concrete method of recognizing outstanding performance, valid career ladders should not be undermined by the practice of higher pay for nurses who work in certain areas, such as critical care. Rewards should be given for levels of responsibility, preparation, experience, and performance. General duty nurses share equal responsibility and greater work load variety than do specialty care nurses.

Spitzer and Bolton report the results of a staff survey of 956 career-track RNs. There were 583 respondents who strongly agreed to the following statements about salary and salary equity[59]:

1. "When first hired, staff nurses should be paid according to years of experience, acute care experience, and education.
2. Salary adjustments (raises) should be based on clinical performance, additional acquired education, and additional clinical experience (regardless of specialty)."

When redesigning a wage and salary structure, nurse managers need input from the staff. Clinical ladders should be related to productivity. They can be

EXHIBIT 8-12
Basic Clinical Ladder Model

A. CLINICAL/STAFF NURSE I (BEGINNER/NOVICE)

1. Experience and Education
   Current state licensure with less than one year of experience.
2. Description
   a. Needs close supervision.
   b. Performs basic nursing skills/routine patient care.
   c. Begins to develop patient assessment skills/communication skills.

B. CLINICAL/STAFF NURSE II (ADVANCED BEGINNER)

1. Experience and Education
   a. Current state licensure with more than one year of experience.
   b. BSN with more than 6 months of experience.
   c. MSN without experience.
2. Description
   a. Demonstrates adequate/acceptable performance.
   b. Can differentiate importance of situations and set priorities.
   c. Requires less supervision.
   d. Demonstrates interest in continuing education.

C. CLINICAL/STAFF NURSE III (COMPETENT)

1. Experience and Education
   a. Current licensure with two or more years of experience.
   b. BSN with more than one year of experience.
   c. MSN with more than 6 months of experience.
2. Description
   a. Demonstrates unsupervised competency using the nursing process.

b. Is able to plan and organize in terms of short-range and long-range goals.
c. Demonstrates direction in actions.
d. Accepts leadership responsibility readily.
e. Demonstrates well-developed communication skills.
f. Shares ideas and knowledge with peers.

D. CLINICAL/STAFF NURSE IV (PROFICIENT)

1. Experience and Education
   a. Current licensure with 3 years of clinical experience and pursuit of BSN.
   b. BSN with more than 2 years of experience.
   c. MSN with more than one year of experience.
2. Description
   a. Demonstrates specialized knowledge and skills.
   b. Continues professional education.
   c. Assumes leadership/supervisory responsibility.
   d. Recognizes and adjusts to situations that vary from the norm.
   e. Delegates responsibility appropriately; uses wide range of alternatives in solving problems.

E. CLINICAL/STAFF NURSE V (EXPERT)

1. Experience and Education
   a. MSN with more than 2 years of appropriate clinical experience.
   b. BSN required with more than 3 years of experience; pursuing MSN.
2. Description
   a. Demonstrates expertise in clinical practice.
   b. Assumes/delegates personnel and management responsibility.

---

based on a professional practice model and can reward competence, knowledge, and performance. The essential components are[60]:

1. A number of practice levels
2. Differentiation among practice levels
3. Job description for performance evaluation
4. Criteria for placement of new hires
5. Communication methods
6. Identification of the development needs of staff
7. Criteria for measuring the effectiveness of the ladder relative to quality of care, staff satisfaction and retention, and cost-effectiveness.

To these could be added:

8. Keep the process simple and easy to manage with concise criteria for promotion and for the management process involved.

Master Plan

A master plan for career development should be created for the nursing organization and for each unit within the organization. It should include objectives, policies on posting of jobs, development of résumés and curricula vitae, and strategies for moving up in the organization. It should consider lateral transfers, specialty training and cross training, and plans for nurses who become physically unable to perform the rigors of acute care nursing, particularly due to aging.

Promoting

Promotions are becoming more competitive across all sectors of the economy because of increased numbers of qualified competitors and because downsizing has eliminated tens of thousands of middle-management jobs. This lack of a future causes great stress for the individual employee.

Employees are starting their own businesses by buying franchises and turning hobbies that are special skills into profitable ventures. Some employees make lateral moves within a company to learn new skills. Others return to school, retire early, or do community work to increase their self-satisfaction. Employers are granting long-term, unpaid sabbaticals to employees to return to school or work for noncompetitive organizations. Some loan out executives to charitable organizations. Many have moved authority to lower levels to increase autonomy and job satisfaction.[61]

Professional nurses have had to turn to management, education, or research for promotion. The development of professional nurse clinical ladders is making some headway, albeit not quickly enough. Many professional nurses want to stay in clinical nursing and will do so if they can be rewarded with promotions that increase their pay and standing within the organization.

One way for nurse managers to ensure that all professional nurses have promotion opportunities is to develop a promotion system that indicates all promotion categories within the organization (see Exhibit 8-13).

Nurse managers should develop specific promotion policies with input from all categories of professional

nurses and the HR department. These policies should include the following[62]:

1. All vacant positions will be posted even if change in pay and rank does not occur. Some nurses will want to change units, specialty, shifts, and so on.
2. All interested applicants should file applications for promotion in the HR department.
3. Personnel in the HR department should prepare promotion rosters that rank all candidates by education, experience, and performance. The best-qualified candidate should be at the top of the list.
4. Applicants should be interviewed and rated by the same set of criteria, a process described previously in this chapter in the section under Selecting.
5. The best-qualified candidates should be selected for promotion.
6. The results of the promotion process should be announced. Those not selected should be notified and counseled individually rather than learn that they were passed over from a third party or by seeing the list of those promoted.
7. The promotion system must be fair and be perceived as fair by professional nurses.

An effective promotion policy provides the same opportunity for people of equal ability to apply and

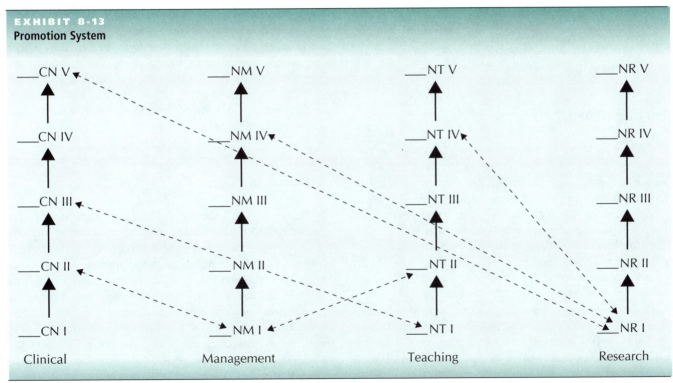

EXHIBIT 8-13
Promotion System

This is a model. Each level would require specific and increasing education, experience, and performance accomplishments. The arrows indicate the levels at which nurses from each group could advance. The clinical nurse II (CN II) could advance to nurse manager (NM I), or vice versa. The nurse teacher IV (NT IV) could advance to nurse researcher I (NR I), or vice versa. The number of budgeted positions would be entered in the blanks in front of each group. For nurse researchers, this could be only one position but would allow for appointment at, or promotion to, higher levels.

treats such people equitably during interviews. Employees who are not promoted should be allowed to discuss their disappointment. Managers may expect a temporary decrease in performance from them.[63]

Darling and McGrath write that nurses experience much trauma when moving upward from clinical to managerial nursing. They are unaware of the transition process involved in a promotion, including the fact that their social and professional ties with other clinical nurses are cut. They take on more responsibilities and burdens and soon feel isolated and alone. They gain visibility and prestige but also receive complaints instead of appreciation from their staff.[64]

To prevent promotion trauma, supervisors of promotees can plan a transition program that will alert promotees to the changes in relationships that will occur. Such a program will help keep them from blaming their difficulties on personal failings. A transition program should include clear role descriptions and expectations, clear job descriptions, and classes in management to help them gain the needed knowledge and skills. Staff development is as essential for nurses promoted to management as it is for those who stay in the clinical domain. They should know what to expect and how to deal with Darling and McGrath's five stages of promotion: uninformed optimism, informed pessimism, hopeful realism, informed optimism, and rewarding completion. A management development program will keep clinical nurses who are promoted to manager positions from bailing out at the second stage.[65]

Terminating

Employees cannot be terminated at will. They are protected by public policy set forth in the National Labor Relations Act, the Civil Rights Act of 1964, the Discrimination in Employment Act, the Vocational Rehabilitation Act, and the Occupational Safety and Health Act. Also, laws protect whistle-blowers.

Employees should be terminated only after all efforts to retain them have been exhausted. The theory of management includes concepts and principles that, when learned and applied by nurse managers, will assist employees to be competent and productive. Punishment or disciplinary action should be a last resort and should be progressive, moving from verbal conference, to a recorded conference, to suspension, to discharge. Such action should be covered by written policies and procedures.

First-line nurse managers should have authority to fire employees. They should consult with superior managers and HR personnel when terminating staff to make sure the action will stand up in court. All policies must be legal, and they must be consistently and correctly enforced. All employees are entitled to a fair hearing and review. The process allows for appropriate representatives for employees at investigating interviews. Terminated employees should be paid all benefits they have accrued.[66]

Firing an employee is an unpleasant job. It is done for the following reasons:

- Economic downturns when employees are in surplus
- Personality mismatches occur, that is, everything has been tried, including transfers, but the employee does not fit anywhere
- Progressive discipline in which the employee fails to meet previously agreed on performance expectations
- Incorrigibility, that is, the employee has made serious mistakes, has stolen, or has had other gross failures

The nurse manager needs to plan the session well ahead and be well prepared to do the following:

- Coordinate with the personnel office, superiors, unions, outplacement people, and others.
- Keep the firing from the grapevine.
- Time the session for the end of the day and middle of the week to keep it confidential and to rebuild the organization.
- Be straightforward and up-front.
- Have all documentation ready.
- Deal with four stages of employee reaction: shock with physical symptoms, rejection, emotion, and withdrawal. Be quiet during the shock and emotion stages. Confirm the message during rejection. Provide information during the withdrawal stage and terminate the meeting.[67]

Summary

A major focus of a theory of nursing management is that personnel should be managed for productivity, that is, for achieving the mission and objectives of the organization. Management of nursing personnel involves recruiting, selecting, credentialing, and assigning nurses, first into the educational program and then into the division or department of nursing.

Because nursing, a predominantly female occupation, must now compete with all other professions for students, nurse managers should create conditions of work that will be attractive, including competitive salaries and fringe benefits, optional schedules, and satisfying conditions of work such as autonomy and recognition.

The population from which all occupations will recruit will change greatly in the first decade of the twenty-first century. The demographic makeup of this population will shift, causing recruitment goals to change. Nurse managers should plan student recruitment at early stages of the secondary education process. The poor, minorities, children of single parents, and those with physical and emotional disabilities must be prepared now for careers, including careers in nursing. Equal opportunity is the promise of America.

Each nurse manager should work with other health care system managers and with secondary school teachers and counselors to prepare young men and women for careers in nursing. Once nurses are recruited, selected, credentialed, and assigned, nurse managers should develop strategies to retain them. For high-level positions, search committees are frequently used for recruiting. The implication is that professional workers will have input into selecting those with whom they will work and who will provide leadership.

Nurse managers should consider a credentialing process for professional nurses similar to that used for physicians. It is essential that career planning be a major personnel management program within each nursing organization. Employees are not motivated by dead-end jobs. They desire the opportunity to qualify for promotion in clinical, management, education, and research positions. Communication should be clear about job vacancies, which should be filled by the best-qualified individuals.

Personnel who do not meet acceptable standards of performance should be counseled, warned in writing, and suspended without pay. When all else fails, they should be terminated.

APPLICATION EXERCISES

EXERCISE 8-1   Design a questionnaire and perform a random survey of clinical and management personnel in your organization to identify problems in the areas of recruitment, selection, credentialing, assignment, staffing, retention, promotion, and termination.

1. Tabulate and analyze the results.
2. What are the problems?
3. What are the possible solutions to these problems?
4. How would an assessment center improve nurse selection or promotion? Support your decision.
5. How can the productivity of professional nurses be improved in this setting?

EXERCISE 8-2   Using Exhibit 8-2, Strategies for Recruiting Students into Nursing Education Programs, prepare a management plan to accomplish the strategies you select. This may be done as a group exercise. You may use the following format for management plans.

MANAGEMENT PLAN

OBJECTIVE:

ACTIONS	TARGET DATES	ASSIGNED TO	ACCOMPLISHMENTS

EXERCISE 8-3   Using Exhibit 8-3, Criteria for Developing an Effective Nurse Recruitment Advertisement, prepare a management plan. Prepare the advertisement. Make it a marketing rather than a selling ad. This may be done as a group exercise.

EXERCISE 8-4   Using Exhibit 8-6, Interview Guide, simulate interviewing a job applicant by interviewing one of your group members. Discuss the results with your group.

EXERCISE 8-5   Review Appendix 8-1, University of South Alabama Medical Center Department of Nursing Credentialing Process. Credentialing is a process requiring top management decisions and support for implementation. What changes would you make in the exhibit? Note them. Make an appointment to explore this process with the chief nurse executive. Plan your interview.

EXERCISE 8-6   Using Exhibit 8-11, Turnover Data, collect turnover data to establish the following for a nursing unit, department, or division.

1. Crude turnover rate.
2. Mean service of "stayers."
3. Median service of "stayers."
4. Mean service of "leavers."
5. Median service of "leavers."
6. Instability rate.
7. Wastage rate.
8. Survival curve of "leavers."

EXERCISE 8-7   Do an exit interview using the format in Appendix 8-3. Discuss the results with your peer group.

NOTES

1. American Hospital Association, "Background on the National Nursing Shortage," *Hospital Nurse Recruitment and Retention: A Source Book for Executive Management* (Chicago: American Hospital Association, November 1980).
2. National Commission on Nursing, *Nursing in Transition: Models for Successful Organizational Change* (Chicago: American Hospital Association, Hospital Research and Educational Trust and American Hospital Supply Corporation, 1982), 41–42.
3. C. Bradley, "My Wish List for National Nurses Week," *HealthWeek* (17 May 2000), 4.
4. B. B. Gray, "Another Shortage? Bet on It," *HealthWeek* (5 May 1997), 20.
5. Associated Press, "Health-Care Job Machine May Shift into Low Gear," *Mobile Register* (19 September 1993), 4F; M. A. Hellinghauser, "Retaining Good Nurses," *HealthWeek* (17 April 2000), 18; American Academy of Pediatrics Committee on Hospital Care, "The Role of the Nurse Practitioner and Physician Assistant in the Care of Hospitalized Children," *Pediatrics* (May 1999), 1050–1052.
6. L. S. Richman, "Jobs That Are Growing and Slowing," *Fortune* (12 July 1993), 52–53.
7. Reuters Health, "NPs, Physicians Equal in Patients' Eyes," *HealthWeek* (10 January 2000), 9.
8. W. Woods, "The Jobs Americans Hold," *Fortune* (12 July 1993), 54–55.
9. U.S. Bureau of the Census, *Statistical Abstract of the United States 1999*, 119th Ed. (Washington, DC: 1999) 170, 488.
10. Knight-Ridder Service, "Physician-Assistant Training Draws Many," *San Antonio Express-News* (15 August 1993), 3J.
11. D. Hendricks, "Jobs Don't Die; They Move Up," *San Antonio Express-News* (4 June 1993), 1B; A. Federwisch, "Designer Genes: How Genomics Could Change Your Life," *HealthWeek* (13 September '1999), 1.

12. Ibid.
13. R. J. Samuelson, "R.I.P.: The Good Corporation," *Newsweek* (5 July 1993), 41.
14. R. A. Marini, "Half of Bankruptcies due to Medical Bills," *HealthWeek* (15 May 2000), 9.
15. U. S. Bureau of the Census, *Statistical Abstract of the United States, 1999*, 132.
16. Ibid., 131.
17. Ibid.
18. "State of the Nursing Shortage," *American Journal of Nursing* (20 December 2000); P. I. Buerhous, D. O. Staiger, and D. I. Auerbach, "Policy Responses to an Aging Registered Nurse Workforce," *Nursing Economic$* (November–December 2000) 278–284.
19. Editorial, *Times-Colonist* (Victoria, British Columbia, Canada, (12 July 1993), A4.
20. P. Ancona, "Make Yourself More Valuable at Work," *San Antonio Express-News* (4 September 1993), 1 B; M. A. Hellinghausen, "Interview Ace," *HealthWeek* (31 August 1998), 1, 24; M. Flaherty, "New Horizons," *HealthWeek* (7 June 1999), 1, 26; A. Federwisch, "Career Shaping," *HealthWeek*, 4(17), (1999), 1, 9.
21. "Online Courses," *Excellence*, Sigma Theta Tau International Society of Nursing Post Convention Wrapup Issue, (January 2000), 1, 2.
22. H. L. Hodgkinson, "Reform? Higher Education? Don't Be Absurd!" *Phi Delta Kappan* (December 1986), 271–274.
23. Ibid.
24. K. A. Stevens and E. A. Walker, "Choosing a Career: Why Not Nursing for More High School Seniors?" *Journal of Nursing Education* (January 1993), 13–17.
25. American Academy of Nursing Task Force on Nursing Practice In Hospitals, *Magnet Hospitals: Attraction and Retention of Professional Nurses* (Kansas City, MO: American Nurses'

Association, 1983), 99; T. Stein, "Respect Breeds Contentment," *HealthWeek* (1 May 2000), 10.

26. M. Kramer and C. Schmalenberg, "Magnet Hospitals: Part II Institutions of Excellence," *Journal of Nursing Administration* (February 1988), 17.

27. J. E. Pattan, "Developing a Nurse Recruitment Plan," *Journal of Nursing Administration* (January 1992), 33–39.

28. J. A. Connelly and K. S. Strauser, "Managing Recruitment and Retention Problems: An Application of the Marketing Process," *The Journal of Nursing Administration* (October 1983), 17–22.

29. J. E. Pattan, "Nurse Recruitment: From Selling to Marketing," *Journal of Nursing Administration* (September 1991), 16–20.

30. M. R. Thompson, *Why Should I Hire You?* (New York: Jove Publications, 1975), 94.

31. E. J. Sullivan, P. J. Decker, and S. Hailstone, "Assessment Center Technology: Selecting Head Nurses," *The Journal of Nursing Administration* (May 1985), 14.

32. Ibid.

33. E. H. Battle, S. Bragg, J. Delaney, S. Gilbert, and D. Roesler, "Developing a Rating Interview Guide," *Journal of Nursing Administration* (October 1985), 39–45.

34. D. J. delBueno, L. Weeks, and P. Brown-Stewart, "Clinical Assessment Centers: A Cost-Effective Alternative for Competency Development," *Nursing Economics* (January–February 1987), 21–26.

35. S. T. Murphy and D. C. Hagner, "Evaluating Assessment Settings: Ecological Influences on Vocational Evaluation," *Journal of Rehabilitation* (January–February–March 1988), 53–58.

36. T. Peters, *Thriving on Chaos* (New York: Harper & Row, 1987), 378–385.

37. W. Chaboyer, K. Forrester, and D. Harris, "The Expanded Role of Acute Care Nurses: The Issue of Liability," *Australian Health Review*, 22(3), 1999, 110–117; M. F. Kamajian, S. A. Mitchell, and R. A. Fruth, "Credentialing and Privileging of Advanced Practice Nurses," *AACN Clinical Issues* (August 1999), 316–336.

38. H. S. Rowland and B. L. Rowland, *Hospital Legal Forms, Checklists, & Guidelines* (Rockville, MD: Aspen, 1987), 17:1.

39. Committee for the Study of Credentialing in Nursing, "Credentialing in Nursing: A New Approach," *American Journal of Nursing* (April 1979), 674–683.

40. American Nurses Credentialing Center, *Recertification Catalog* (Washington, DC: American Nurses Credentialing Center, 1994).

41. C. Richelson, "Update on Credentialing," *Nursing Management* (October 1991), 101–102.

42. P. E. Norris, *How to Find a Job* (Fairhope, AL: National Job Search Training Laboratories, 1982), 1.

43. M. L. Duxbury and G. D. Armstrong, "Calculating Nurse Turnover Indices," *The Journal of Nursing Administration* (March 1982), 18–24.

44. L. DeBerry, "Preselection Process for First Line Managers Cuts Turnover," *Training* (July 1992), 80.

45. R. Spitzer-Lehmann, "Recruitment and Retention of Our Greatest Asset," *Nursing Administration Quarterly* (summer 1990), 66–69.

46. Ibid.

47. P. Berns and J. Berns, "Good for Business: Corporations Adopt the Family," *Management Review*, 81(9), (1992), 34–38.

48. W. Osler, "Retention Through a Service Strategy," *Manager's Magazine* (April 1992), 18–23.

49. C. B. Jones, "Staff Nurse Turnover Costs: Part 1, A Conceptual Model," *Journal of Nursing Administration* (April 1990), 18–23; T. Butler and J. Waldroop, "Job Sculpting: The Art of Retaining Your Best People," *Harvard Business Review* (September–October 1999), 144–152, 186; D. Mass, "Staff Retention: A Major Key to Management's Success," *Clinical Laboratory Management Review* (September–October 1999), 266-274; A. Federwisch, "Career Shaping," op. cit; B. B. Gray, "Get a Tuneup," *HealthWeek* (31 August 1998), 4.

50. E. Ginsberg, J. Patray, M. Ostow, and E. A. Brann, "Nurse Discontent: The Search for Realistic Solutions," *The Journal of Nursing Administration* (November 1982), 7–11.

51. C. E. Burton and D. T. Burton, "Job Expectations of Senior Nursing Students," *The Journal of Nursing Administration* (March 1982), 11–17.

52. Ibid.

53. "P. F. Drucker and D. Karl Bays Discuss the Toughest Job: Running a Hospital, Part 2," *HMQ* (summer 1982), 2–5.

54. S. S. Stengrevics, K. K. Kirby, and E. R. Ollis, "Nurse Manager Job Satisfaction: The Massachusetts Perspective," *Nursing Management* (April 1991), 60–64.

55. A. Levenstein, "Career Dissatisfaction," *Nursing Management* (November 1985), 61–62.

56. Ibid.

57. E. Ginsberg, J. Patray, M. Ostow, and E. A. Brann, op. cit; P. S. Crose, "Job Characteristics Related to Job Satisfaction in Rehabilitation Nursing," *Rehabilitation Nursing* (May–June 1999), 95–102.

58. M. D. Sovie, "Fostering Professional Nursing Careers in Hospitals: The Role of Staff Development, Part 1," *The Journal of Nursing Administration* (December 1982), 5–10.

59. R. B. Spitzer and L. B. Bolton, "Attitudes Toward Equitable Pay," *Nursing Management* (June 1984), 32, 36–38.

60. Ibid.

61. Cox News Service, "Chances for Moving Up at Work Going Down," *San Antonio Express-News* (12 December 1993), 6H.

62. "Who Gets the Promotion?" *Small Business Reports*, 17(10), (1992), 28; B. Pfister, "Good Timing, Attitude, Key to Pay Boost," *San Antonio Express-News* (28 March 1999), 25K, 31K.

63. Ibid.

64. L. A. W. Darling and L. G. McGrath, "The Causes and Costs of Promotion Trauma," *The Journal of Nursing Administration* (April 1983), 29–33.

65. Ibid.

66. B. C. Rutkowski and A. D. Rutkowski, "Employee Discharge: It Depends . . . ," *Nursing Management* (December, 1984) 39–42.

67. J. C. Dumville, "Delivering the Mortal Blow," *Supervision*, 54(4), (1993), 6–7.

REFERENCES

Bradley, C. "Building a Workforce." *HealthWeek* (17 April 2000), 4.

Bradley, C. "Taking Our Data to the Street." *HealthWeek* (12 June 2000), 4.

Buerhaus, P. I., D. O. Staiger, and D. I. Auerbach. "Implications of an Aging Registered Nurse Workforce." *Journal of the American Medical Association*. 2000; 283: 2948–2954.

Chaudhuri, S. and B. Tabrizi. "Capturing the Real Value in High-Tech Acquisitions." *Harvard Business Review* (September–October 1999), 123–130, 185.

Chalfant, A. "Money Isn't Everything." *HealthWeek* (31 August 1998), 14.

Coffman, J. and J. Spetz. "Maintaining an Adequate Supply of RNs in California." *Image* (Fourth Quarter 1999), 389–393.

Colavecchio, R. "Direct Patient Care: A Viable Career Choice." *The Journal of Nursing Administration* (July–August 1982), 17–22.

Derstine, J. B. "Planning for Career Flexibility." *Gastroenterology Nursing*, 18(6), (1995), 215–218.

Domrose, C. "Foreign Aid." *HealthWeek* (6 December 1999), 23.

Drucker, P. F. *Management Challenges for the 21st Century* (New York: HarperCollins 1999).

Fitzgerald, T. "Nurse Appeal." *HealthWeek* (10 January 2000), 15.

Flaherty, M. "Steps to Success." *HealthWeek* (16 August 1999), 20–21.

Flaherty, M. "A Nurse is a Nurse." *HealthWeek* (31 August 1998), 6–7.

Fuszard, B., E. Green, E. Kujala, and B. Talley. "Rural Magnet Hospitals of Excellence: Part 1." *Journal of Nursing Administration* (January 1994), 21–26.

Gray, B. B. "Future Work." *HealthWeek* (31 August 1998), 10–11.

Hellinghausen, M. A. "Looking Good on Paper." *HealthWeek* (16 August 1999), 16–17.

Hellinghausen, M. A. "Finding Their Way." *HealthWeek* (6 December 1999), 1, 28.

Kiechel, W. "A Manager's Career." *Fortune* (4 April 1994), 68–72.

Kurec, A. S. "Recruiting, Interviewing, and Hiring the Right Person." *Clinical Laboratory Management Review* (September–October 1999), 251–261.

Landers, A. "Nurses Sick of Long Hours and Paltry Pay." *San Antonio Express-News* (11 October 1998), 12H.

Mangan, K. S. "Nursing Schools Perplexed by Falling Enrollments." *The Chronicle of Higher Education* (12 March 1999), A41–A42.

McGinn, D. and J. McCormick. "Your Next Job." *Newsweek* (1 February 1999), 43–45,48–51.

Mitchell, S. "Raising the Bar: Green Light for Accreditation Agencies Signals Better Nursing Education." *HealthWeek* (1 May 2000), 12.

Morgan, L. "Look Before You Leap." *HealthWeek* (31 August 1998), 15.

Pedersen, D. "How We Work Now." *Newsweek* (1 February 1999), 46–47.

"Recruitment and Retention: A Positive Approach." *Nursing Management* (April 1984), 15–17.

Sloan, F. A., C. J. Conover, and D. Provenzale. "Hospital Credentialing and Quality of Care." *Social Science Medicine* (January 2000), 77–88.

Swansburg, R. C. and P. W. Swansburg, *Strategic Career Planning and Development for Nurses* (Rockville, MD: Aspen 1984), 160–162.

"Workplace Trends: Who Gets the Promotion?" *Small Business Reports*, 17(10), (1992), 28.

APPENDIX 8-1
USAMC Department of Nursing Credentialing Process

DEFINITIONS

Credentialing: Those degrees, licenses, skill checklists, and certificates that allow a nurse to practice nursing at USAMC.

Clinical Privileges: Permission given to an individual professional nurse by USAMC to practice specific skills based on credentials, experience, and demonstrated competence/performance.

Clinical privileges will be delineated for each member of the professional registered nursing staff. According to this standard, privileges are granted based on demonstrated competence, performance, and results of care.

When patient-care problems arise in areas that require qualification or certification, the nurse's credentials are checked first. If the nurse is credentialed for that activity, counseling may reveal the need for remediation; if the nurse is not credentialed, immediate steps are taken to correct the deficiency.

1. The first step is to complete application for entry. In completing this form, please do not leave *any* blanks. Indicate information that does not apply as N/A. Submit this completed form to the Nurse Manager of the designated area for which application is made.
2. Secondly, general nursing orientation must be completed as scheduled. Demonstrating entry-level requirements at 6 months credentials nurses to practice as nurses at this institution.
3. The third step, meeting the requirements criteria for distinct specialty areas, allows nurses working in these specialty areas to practice advanced skills. These nurses must complete critical care or other specialty care skills and a preceptorship with a senior staff member. We identify skills on particular specialty units that require training beyond that encompassed in the basic orientation.

Review of departmental and/or individual practice and results of care will be an ongoing process through the hospitals' Quality Assessment & Improvement Program. Professional Nursing Practice is expected to assist the Department of Nursing in meeting Standards of Practice. It is further expected that results of nursing care reveal patients' attaining desirable outcomes and without any adverse effects related to individual performance.

In summary, prior to privileges, professional nurses must meet all credentialing requirements for their designated level of expected practice. Advanced practice at USAMC requires completion of orientation, appropriate courses, demonstrated skills, and preceptorship.

Successful performance of required skills will be verified annually for recredentialing by the Clinical Nurse Specialist, Clinical Coordinator, Clinical Consultant, or a preceptor. This process is the responsibility of the Nurse Manager, CNS, and individual involved.

(continued)

APPLICATION FOR ENTRY

Area for which you are applying

I. DEMOGRAPHICS

Name _____   SSN _____

Address _____   Phone(s) _____

_____   _____

Emergency notification (Name) _____   Phone _____

Languages spoken (other than English/include sign language) _____

_____

Military Status _____   Branch _____   Rank _____

II. PROFESSIONAL EDUCATION

ADN/YR _____   Diploma/YR _____   BSN/YR _____   MSN/YR _____   PHD/YR _____

Other Degrees _____

III. PRACTICE

Have you ever been on probation with a State Board of Nursing? YES/NO (Circle)

CERTIFICATION TYPE	ORGANIZATION	EXPIRATION	CERT. INITIALS
1. _____	_____	_____	_____
2. _____	_____	_____	_____
3. _____	_____	_____	_____

Areas of nursing experience beginning with most current: Date From   To

_____	_____	_____
_____	_____	_____
_____	_____	_____
_____	_____	_____
_____	_____	_____

IV. VERIFICATION

I have read the credentialing process information.   ____Yes   ____No

I have read the standards of practice expected of me.   ____Yes   ____No

I have read standards of care that my patients expect.   ____Yes   ____No

SIGNATURE _____   Date _____
                            Applicant

ACCEPTED _____   Date _____
                         Nurse Manager

Source: Courtesy of the University of South Alabama Medical center, Mobile, Alabama.

APPENDIX 8-2
Identification of Factors Causing Job Dissatisfaction

ITEM	NOT AT ALL ⟶ A GREAT DEAL				

1. Factor: Salaries and fringe benefits

(1) Pay is satisfactory.	1	2	3	4	5
(2) Education and experience are recognized and used.	1	2	3	4	5
(3) Opportunities exist for career advancement.	1	2	3	4	5
(4) The pay system rewards my years of experience.	1	2	3	4	5
(5) The pay is adequate for shifts, weekends, and holidays.	1	2	3	4	5
(6) Fringe benefits are known.	1	2	3	4	5
(7) Employees are satisfied with fringe benefits.	1	2	3	4	5
(8) Child-care services are satisfactory.	1	2	3	4	5
(9) The retirement program is a strong one.	1	2	3	4	5

2. Factor: Staffing philosophy; clerical work; floating; rotating shifts

(1) The staffing philosophy is fair.	1	2	3	4	5
(2) A float pool covers absences and supplemental staffing.	1	2	3	4	5
(3) Clinical nurses have input into staffing policies and procedures.	1	2	3	4	5
(4) Opportunities exist for flexible work schedules.	1	2	3	4	5
(5) Clerical duties are performed by clerical personnel.	1	2	3	4	5
(6) Appropriate activities are performed by other departments, such as pharmacy, medical laboratory, and dietary.	1	2	3	4	5

3. Factor: Professionalism; interdisciplinary relationships; public relations

(1) Clinical nurses serve on all organizational committees.	1	2	3	4	5
(2) Administrators promote cooperative interdisciplinary relationships.	1	2	3	4	5
(3) Clinical nurses spend their time giving care to patients.	1	2	3	4	5
(4) Clinical nurses make decisions about patient care.	1	2	3	4	5
(5) Clinical nurses participate in nursing management.	1	2	3	4	5
(6) Clinical nurses are recognized and rewarded for nursing excellence.	1	2	3	4	5
(7) Clinical nurses participate in quality assurance.	1	2	3	4	5
(8) Clinical nurses receive awards for merit.	1	2	3	4	5
(9) The communication system is informative, provides for clinical nursing input, and gives feedback.	1	2	3	4	5
(10) Job vacancies are posted.	1	2	3	4	5
(11) Clinical nurses participate in public relations functions.	1	2	3	4	5

4. Factor: Staff development

(1) A career development program exists.	1	2	3	4	5
(2) Good opportunities for continuing education are available.	1	2	3	4	5
(3) A good orientation program is in force.	1	2	3	4	5
(4) Personnel are reimbursed for staff development activities.	1	2	3	4	5
(5) Refresher courses are available.	1	2	3	4	5
(6) Staff development programs are marketed.	1	2	3	4	5
(7) Incompetent nurses are identified and handled appropriately.	1	2	3	4	5
(8) Good leadership training courses are available.	1	2	3	4	5
(9) Clinical nurses participate in staff development planning.	1	2	3	4	5

(continued)

APPENDIX 8-2 (continued)

ITEM	NOT AT ALL ──────▶ A GREAT DEAL				
5. Factor: Administration support					
(1) Clinical nurses can follow through on beliefs and values.	1	2	3	4	5
(2) Clinical nurses are not subjected to punitive action by supervisors.	1	2	3	4	5
(3) Productivity standards are known.	1	2	3	4	5
(4) Employees have access to senior management.	1	2	3	4	5
(5) Nursing service and nursing education are in harmony.	1	2	3	4	5
(6) Patient safety is emphasized.	1	2	3	4	5
(7) An up-to-date nursing management information system is available.	1	2	3	4	5
(8) Managers are visible to nursing staff and patients.	1	2	3	4	5

Compiled from: Mabel A. Wandelt et al., "Why Nurses Leave Nursing and What Can Be Done About It," *American Journal of Nursing* (January 1981), 72–77; Alabama Hospital Association, *Report from the Task Force to Study Nurse Shortage Situation in State of Alabama* (December 1981), (Mobile, AL); National Commission on Nursing, *Summary of the Public Hearings,* 1981; and *Nursing in Transition: Models for Successful Organizational Change* (August 1982), (Chicago: American Hospital Association, Hospital Research and Educational Trust, and American Hospital Supply Corporation); American Academy of Nursing, Task Force on Nursing Practice in Hospitals, *Magnet Hospitals: Attraction and Retention of Professional Nurses* (Kansas City: American Nurses Association, 1983); Alabama Hospital Association, *The Alabama Nurse Study: A Survey of Registered Nurses' Attitudes About Their Profession* (Montgomery, AL, 1983); Committee on Nursing and Nursing Education, Institute of Medicine, *"Recommendations: Meeting Current and Future Needs for Nurses"* (Washington, DC), 1983.

APPENDIX 8-3
University of South Alabama Medical Center Employee Exit Interview

Date _____

Name _____ Date Hired _____ Shift _____

Position Title _____ Department _____

Supervisor's Name _____ Date Separated _____

CHECKLIST:

_____ ID card returned to personnel department
_____ Final payroll check form completed
_____ State retirement refund form completed
_____ Received insurance conversion information
_____ Locker keys returned

I. REASON FOR SEPARATION (CHECK APPROPRIATE BOX)

VOLUNTARY RESIGNATION

_____ New position
_____ Retirement (voluntary)
_____ Relocation
_____ Illness
_____ Pregnancy
_____ Job dissatisfaction
_____ Return to school
_____ Other (specify)
_____

INVOLUNTARY TERMINATION

_____ Retirement (mandatory)
_____ Reduction of staff
_____ Other (specify)
_____
_____

(continued)

II. INTERVIEW

    A. SELECTION

What kind of work have you been doing in our hospital? _____

_____

_____

_____

What kind of work did you do prior to joining our hospital? _____

_____

_____

_____

What type of work do you like best? _____

_____

_____

What type of work do you like least? _____

_____

Why? _____

_____

    B. ORIENTATION

Who explained your job to you? _____

Describe your orientation. _____

_____

_____

Length of time? _____

What did your orientation lack? _____

_____

_____

Were in-service education programs sufficient for your needs? _____

If not, how could programs be improved? _____

_____

    C. SUPERVISION

How do you feel about your supervisor? _____

_____

_____

_____

Did you take any complaints to your supervisor? _____ Yes _____ No

If yes, how were they handled? _____

_____

_____

Have you had any problems with your supervisor? _____ Yes _____ No

If yes, describe.   _____

_____

_____

_____

What kind of working relationship did you have with the staff in your department? _____

_____

_____

Was there ample opportunity for communication with co-workers, your supervisor, and your department head?

_____

_____

_____

How could communication be improved? _____

_____

_____

Have you felt administrative support by hospital administrators? _____

_____

_____

D. FINANCIAL

How do you feel about your pay? _____

_____

_____

How do you feel about your progress within this hospital? _____

_____

_____

(continued)

E. FOR NURSES

Was your unit adequately staffed? _____

_____

How do you feel about being pulled to other units? _____

_____

How often were you pulled? _____

_____

F. SUMMARY

What did you like best about your job? _____

_____

_____

What did you like least about your job? _____

_____

_____

What did you like best about our hospital? _____

_____

_____

What did you like least about our hospital? _____

_____

_____

Why are you really leaving? _____

_____

_____

Would you be willing to stay with our hospital under a more satisfactory arrangement? _____ Yes _____ No

What changes would be required? _____

Would you return to this hospital if the opportunity existed? _____

_____

III. INTERVIEWER COMMENTS

_____

_____

_____

Source: Courtesy of the University of South Alabama Medical Center, Mobile, Alabama.

CHAPTER 9

Collective Bargaining

Phillip Kendrick, PhD, CRNA

- Discuss the meaning of *collective bargaining*.
- Discuss the history of collective bargaining in nursing.
- Identify the characteristics of a profession and their relationship to collective bargaining.
- Identify and discuss the issues that lead to unions and collective bargaining.
- Describe the process of collective bargaining.
- Describe a grievance procedure and illustrate how it should work.
- Discuss the processes of arbitration and mediation.
- Discuss the benefits of collective bargaining.
- Discuss the ills of collective bargaining.

CONCEPTS: Collective bargaining, professional employee, grievance, arbitration, supervisory influence, strike.

MANAGER BEHAVIOR: Designs human resource management policies to prevent possible union organizing activities.

LEADER BEHAVIOR: Designs human resource management policies to make employment satisfying to employees and facilitate open communication among employees and managers.

Introduction

Collective bargaining is the "process by which organized employees participate with their employers in decisions about their rates of pay, hours of work, and other terms and conditions of employment."[1] Collective bargaining is the process through which the representatives of the employers and employees meet at reasonable times; confer in good faith about wages, hours, and other matters; and put into writing any agreements reached. The duty to bargain is required of both the employer and union.[2]

Collective bargaining is the means by which professional nurses can influence hospital nursing care delivery systems and labor–management relations through a united voice.[3] Collective bargaining is often viewed as a power relationship, either adversarial or cooperative.[4] During recent years executives of firms have learned that employee empowerment and autonomy is good for business. As productivity increases, this knowledge has led to increased training of employees at the production level, elimination of middle management, decentralization of decision making with participatory management at the production level, and an upsurge in the success of the firm. This commitment to sharing power gives employees less reason to resort to collective bargaining.

History in Nursing

Laws

The following is a chronology of collective bargaining laws related to nursing in the United States:

1935 The National Labor Relations Act (NLRA), which is sometimes called the Wagner Act, noted that hospitals were "employers." Thus, it protected employees of private, for-profit health care institutions.

1947 Under the amendment to the NLRA (called the Taft–Hartley Act), Congress excepted not-for-profit hospitals from coverage, and from the right to organize and from the right to bargain collectively.

1960 The National Labor Relations Board (NLRB) excepted proprietary hospitals from coverage by the NLRA.

1974 The NLRA amendments repealed exceptions and subjected all acute care hospitals to coverage by the act. These amendments made no change in the NLRB's authority to determine the appropriate bargaining unit in each case.

1989 The NLRB ruled that eight bargaining units were appropriate for each hospital. One such unit would be solely for registered nurses. The ruling was challenged by the American Hospital Association.

1991 The U.S. Supreme Court upheld the ruling for eight bargaining units, which included separate units for RNs, physicians, other professionals, technical employees, skilled maintenance employees, clerical employees, guards, and other nonprofessional employees. The exception is units with fewer than six employees.[5]

1994 Supreme Court decision indicates that in any business in which supervisory duties are necessary to the provision of services, personnel who use independent judgments to direct the work of less-skilled employees are supervisors and are not protected by the NLRA. Today employers of nurses are using this decision to challenge unions, decrease licensed personnel, and increase assistive, nonlicensed personnel.[6]

1995 With the support of the American Nurses Association (ANA), the Michigan Nurses Association argued successfully before the NLRB that nurses are not supervisors, as claimed by the Michigan Hospital Medical Center, and are, therefore, eligible to bargain collectively.[7]

The National Labor Relations Act of 1947 defines a professional employee as:

(a) any employee engaged in work (i) predominantly intellectual and varied in character as opposed to routine mental, manual, mechanical, or physical work; (ii) involving the consistent exercise of discretion and judgment in its performance; (iii) of such a character that the output produced or result accomplished cannot be standardized in relation to a given period of time; (iv) requiring knowledge of an advanced type in a field of science or learning customarily acquired by a prolonged course of specialized intellectual instruction and study in an institution of higher learning or a hospital, as distinguished from a general academic education or from an apprenticeship or from training in the performance of routine mental, manual, or physical processes; or (b) any employee who (i) has completed the courses of specialized intellectual instruction and study described in clause (iv) of paragraph (a), and (ii) is performing related work under the supervision of a professional person to qualify himself to become a professional employee as defined in paragraph (a).[8]

Strauss summarizes the following characteristics of professional behavior as[9]:

- Specialized education and expertise
- Autonomy
- Commitment
- Societal responsibility for maintenance of standards of work.

Pavalko differentiates between professionals and other workers by stating that professionals have[10]:

- A systematic body of knowledge and theory as a basis for work and expertise
- Social ability in times of crisis; are sought out by the public
- Specified training, including transmission of ideas, symbols, and skills
- Motivation for service to clients
- Autonomy, self-regulation, and control by individual practitioners
- A sense of long-term commitment
- A need for common identity and destiny, with shared values and norms
- A code of ethics

Nurses have noted these characteristics through the actions of professionals. Their profession organizations have supported the development of nursing theory and the goal of self-regulation and have long had a code for nurses. (See Exhibit 9-1.) When unable as individuals to attain their goals, professional nurses pursue them through collective bargaining.

Nursing Organizations and Unions

The American Nurses Association (ANA) historically views itself as the professional organization for nurses. The history of collective bargaining by nursing organizations is outlined as follows[11]:

1946 ANA became active.

1970 One-third of U.S. workforce is organized.

1977 Twenty percent of hospital workers are represented by labor unions.

1980 Twenty-three percent of U.S. workforce is organized.

1982 ANA represented 110,000 nurses, the goal being the control and protection of nursing practice.

1985 Ohio Nurses' Association represented nurses in 29 facilities. The Michigan Nurses' Association represented 4,000 nurses in 60 bargaining units.

1989 Seventeen percent of U.S. workforce is organized, a decline of six percent since 1980.

1990 SNAs represented 139,000 registered nurses, with 841 bargaining units in 27 states. Other unions represented 102,000 RNs. Twelve percent of U.S. workforce is organized (according to T. Porter-O'Grady).

EXHIBIT 9-1
ANA Code for Nurses

1. The nurse provides services with respect for human dignity and the uniqueness of the client, unrestricted by considerations of social or economic status, personal attributes, or the nature of health problems.
2. The nurse safeguards the client's right to privacy by judiciously protecting information of a confidential nature.
3. The nurse acts to safeguard the client and the public when health care and safety are affected by the incompetent, unethical, or illegal practice of any person.
4. The nurse assumes responsibility and accountability for individual nursing judgments and actions.
5. The nurse maintains competence in nursing.
6. The nurse exercises informed judgment and uses individual competence and qualifications as criteria in seeking consultation, accepting responsibilities, and delegating nursing activities to others.
7. The nurse participates in activities that contribute to the ongoing development of the profession's body of knowledge.
8. The nurse participates in the profession's efforts to implement and improve standards of nursing.
9. The nurse participates in the profession's efforts to establish and maintain conditions of employment conducive to high-quality nursing care.
10. The nurse participates in the profession's efforts to protect the public from misinformation and misrepresentation and to maintain the integrity of nursing.
11. The nurse collaborates with members of the health professions and other citizens in promoting community and national efforts to meet the health needs of the public.

Source: Reprinted with permission from *Code for Nurses with Interpretative Statements*, © 1985, American Nurses Association, Washington, DC.

1991 Within three months of the Supreme Court decision allowing all-RN bargaining units, 20 petitions for union elections were filed by nurses in seven states. An estimated 1.12 million nurses do not belong to unions.

1992 According to Joel, 20% of health care workers are now organized, an increase of 6% of health care workers since 1980. Approximately 3.6 million hospital employees are protected by collective bargaining.

The difference between the 1977 version and the 1992 version of percentages may relate to hospital workers versus the entire health care industry. An additional 10 petitions for RN bargaining units brought the total to 30 petitions, 23 of which were filed by constituent members of the ANA.

Of more than 1.6 million practicing registered nurses, with approximately 67.9% working in hospitals, about 250,000 are represented by collective bargaining. Collective bargaining by the California Nurses Association is more than 50 years old. The pioneers were Shirley Titus, RN, a nurse leader, and J. St. Sure, a labor lawyer, who together built a good public relations image and a solid database. Their work promoted a sense of self-confidence among nurses. Their interest preceded that of the ANA.[12]

In 1999, the ANA House of Delegates passed historic changes in bylaws to better support SNAs in their organizing and collective bargaining efforts. The United American Nurses (UAN) replaced the Institute of Constituent Member Collective Bargaining Programs. The UAN focuses on existing work to organize and represent RNs who want support through collective bargaining to deal with issues such as staffing levels and workplace safety.[13]

The National Labor Assembly of the UAN will elect the seven-member Executive Council. The Council will be composed of a chairperson, vice-chairperson, secretary, treasurer, and four directors-at-large. The first Council will be members of the Executive Board of the Institute for Constituent Member Collective Bargaining.[14]

Many nurses are represented by trade unions; the ANA would rather that the ANA represent them. Of the 2.6 million RNs in the United States, 190,000 are members of the ANA. Through the ANA, the SNAs represent 102,000 nurses in collective bargaining.[15]

Issues

Issues that lead to petition for unions develop between employers and employees, usually because employers do not want to share power with employees. Historically, the chief executive officers of firms built bureaucratic organizations to retain power in the management structure. This has been costly for firms and has resulted in their restructuring to eliminate layers of management, empower employees with management knowledge and skills, and improve productivity and profits.

Among the major issues leading to unions and collective bargaining are the following[16]:

- Absence of procedures for reporting unsafe or poor patient care. Quality of patient care is the number one issue
- Short staffing and improper skills mix to complement patient acuity
- Floating without orientation and training
- Use of temporary personnel and unlicensed assistive personnel

- Resistance of employers to accept joint decision-making
- Adversarial relationships between nurses and management and exploitation of nurses by management
- Lack of respect for employees
- Lack of autonomy, that is, incursion by management into the scope of practice
- Lack of promotional opportunities
- Lack of professional practice committees
- Lack of staff development and continuing education opportunities
- Lack of child care and elder care
- Lack of involvement
- Poor differentials for shift work, education, and experience
- Low wages and limited benefits
- No pension portability
- Lack of employee assistance programs
- Poor on-call arrangements and lack of flexible schedules
- Overwork, mandatory overtime, and shift rotation
- Low morale
- Performance of nonnursing duties
- Poor management and poor communication
- Being able to take sufficient breaks
- Having and implementing fair policies and practices for discipline and dismissal
- Assurance that patient classification systems have practicing nurse inputs
- Fair and consistent standards, policies, and practices
- Adequate health insurance
- Assurance that competence and qualification are considered with seniority
- Vacancy posting so that all nurses have an opportunity
- Lack of a system to apply peer review
- Lack of career ladders

The professional nurse works in an environment where human resources are not always valued but are viewed as a commodity. To do their jobs as taught, professional nurses might get fired for such actions as questioning physician authority or refusing to work where they feel they are not qualified. Thus, they often work in a climate of fear that results in poor morale, poor productivity, stifling of creativity, reluctance to take risks, ineffective communication, and reduced motivation.[17] Ultimately, these factors lead to an unbearable level of job stress, which culminates with a letter of resignation.

Kleingartner believes the ANA is working on too many issues simultaneously. She also states that nurses lack economic sophistication, as well as financial resources.[18]

Process

Once nurses have decided to pursue collective bargaining because they believe they have no alternative, the general process is as follows:

1. An organization committee is formed. It should be broad based in structure and representative of the major issues so as to represent all prospective members on all shifts and in all practice areas. Members should be well known and respected.
2. The major campaign issues are identified and discussed.
3. The organizing committee does research to obtain extensive knowledge of all facets of the institution, including history, structure, organization, finances, administration, and culture.
4. A timetable is prepared, delineating the specific organizing activities.
5. Possible employer tactics are identified and discussed, and specific strategies are developed to manage them.
6. A system is established for keeping in constant communication with nurses.
7. A structural plan is made, including adoption of a set of bylaws and election of officers.
8. Recognition occurs by the employer or NLRB certification. Voluntary recognition requires authorization cards signed by a majority of nurses. If the employer will not recognize the action, NLRB certification requires that at least 30% of the nurses sign cards. A majority is best.
9. An election is held in which nurses vote for or against a collective bargaining unit. The NLRB sets the election date by mutual agreement. Notices posted on employee bulletin boards include the date, hours, and places of election; payroll period for voter eligibility; description of the voting unit; a sample of the ballot; and general rules for conduct of the election. With a majority of voting nurses (50% plus one) voting for it, the NLRB certifies the petitioners as the exclusive bargaining unit. If there is no majority, the NLRB will not accept another petition for 1 year.
10. A bargaining committee is elected by the nurses to negotiate a contract.[19]
11. A contract is negotiated. Members of the bargaining committee should survey the membership to gather data for contract proposals. At the first bargaining meeting proposals are made. The easiest ones should be settled first. Management strategy will be to try to set the tone of the sessions and to package proposals so that they can slip some past the nurses. Their strategies will include flattery, conciliation, anger, astonishment, and total silence. For

this reason, nurse members should track all proposals using minutes of the meetings and make index cards listing the proposals of each side. Debriefings at the end of each session are helpful. The nurse team should respond to management with care, spirit, and no unconditional concessions.[20]

12. When all proposals have been fully discussed and agreed on, the contract is written.

13. The contract is then presented to union members who vote to ratify or reject it. If ratified, it is signed by both sides.

14. The contract is enforced through grievance and arbitration procedures. It is reviewed or amended on a regular basis.[21]

Grievance Procedures

A strong grievance procedure increases employee satisfaction, so it is a good human resource management tool, with or without a union. Potential trouble spots are identified early and may include claims for higher wages when jobs are modified. Grievance procedures must be perceived as fair. Their contents should be told to all employees, and managers should be trained to follow them. This training allays managers' fears.[22]

The grievance policy should be communicated as an employee benefit and included in the personnel handbook (see Exhibit 9-2). Peer review should be used in employee appraisals involving grievances and final decisions. Some courts have equated peer review to due process. Peer review builds values of conflict resolution, teamwork, decision-making at lower levels, employee empowerment, and ownership.[23]

Eldridge suggests the following points for effective settlement of grievances[24]:

1. Accurate definition of the problem: Does it violate the contract or the law? Is it timely? Documented?

2. Timely presentation: Follows the time limits and steps of the grievance procedure and for notifying appropriate persons.

3. Documentation: Facts; claim adjustment desired; form signed, dated, and given to appropriate persons.

4. Done with a businesslike attitude to facilitate objectivity and communication.

Nursing is difficult, complex, and requires specialized knowledge. All nurses should commit to a written employment agreement with a grievance procedure. This should be done whether they are representing themselves or are represented by a union. When nurses use a labor organization, they should use one with a large membership and a long and successful history.[25] The ANA and some SNAs fall into this category.

Mediation

> **Mediation is a process under which an impartial person, the mediator, facilitates communication between the parties to promote reconciliation, settlement, or under standing among them. The mediator may suggest better ways of resolving the dispute, but may not impose his own judgment on the issues for that of the parties.[26]**

Mediation is assisted negotiation. When the negotiating parties cannot reach agreement on an issue during contract negotiations or during a labor dispute unresolved by grievance procedures, the issue is referred to a mediator trained to resolve such disputes. The mediator assists the parties in defining the issues, dissolving obstacles to communication, exploring alternatives, facilitating the negotiations, and reaching an agreement. In law cases, mediation works 80% of the time or better.

The mechanics of mediation are good faith; all parties present during the entire mediation session; adequate time; mediator lays ground rules, describes the process, and answers questions; session is private; parties are separated into "caucuses" where their conversations are private; and the mediator shuttles between parties until a settlement is reached. The parties negotiate the settlement.[27]

Arbitration

Whereas the mediator works with the parties in a dispute to get them to resolve their differences, the arbitrator examines the facts and makes a decision that is binding. Arbitration uses as the source of law the express provisions of the contract, past practices of the industry, and the shop (health care and nursing). Past practices must[28]:

- Be unequivocal (clear, consistent, acceptable); be accepted by the people involved as the normal and proper response to the underlying circumstances presented.
- Have longevity; have existed for a sufficient length of time to have developed a pattern.
- Have mutuality; both parties regard the conduct as correct and customary in handling the situation.

Practices that have been long-standing and accepted by both parties are as binding as if written. Subjects not covered in the agreement remain the residual rights of management, including the methods of operation and direction of the work force. Union rights include areas of benefits, wages, and working conditions. Unchallenged customs and practices are considered accepted as part of the agreement by both parties. Arbitrators should effectuate the agreement and contain conflict.[29]

EXHIBIT 9-2
Sample Employee Grievance Procedure

GRIEVANCES AND DISCIPLINARY ACTIONS

6.1 GRIEVANCE AND APPEAL PROCESS

The University of South Alabama provides a means for you, as a regular employee who has completed the probationary period, to appeal disciplinary actions, including dismissal, suspension, or demotion when used as a disciplinary action, that you feel are unjust or to submit a grievance for any working condition that results in inequities or other situations which have a negative effect on morale. The University, in its sole discretion, reserves the right to determine whether an action is a management right as outlined in Section 2.2 of this Handbook and, therefore, not subject to grievance and/or appeal. Layoffs and written warnings may not be appealed.

This process may be used in a situation where there are allegations that an individual has been discriminated against based on race, sex, religion, color, national origin, age, disability, disabled veteran or Vietnam Era veteran status. In such event, if the individual against whom such allegations have been made is either in the first or second step of the grievance and appeal process, the employee should contact the Office of Personnel Relations to institute a grievance. This process is available to an employee who alleges such discrimination is related to the issue of sexual harassment.

Employees in their probationary period may only appeal if they feel they have been discriminated against based on race, sex, religion, color, national origin, age, disability, disabled veteran, or Vietnam Era veteran status. Additionally, this process is available to a probationary employee who alleges such discrimination is related to the issue of sexual harassment.

6.1.1 FIRST STEP

If you are considering initiating a grievance or appeal, you should first discuss the matter with your Department Head. You should state your case, in writing, to your Department Head and state the adjustment desired. This should be done within 10 working days of the occurrence.

6.1.2 SECOND STEP

If your grievance is not settled to your satisfaction with your Department Head, you may appeal, in writing, to your Dean or Assistant Hospital Administrator within 10 working days of the response to step one.

6.1.3 THIRD STEP

If your grievance is not handled to your satisfaction in step two, you may appeal, in writing, to your Division Head within 10 working days of the response to step two.

6.1.4 FINAL STEP

If your grievance is not handled to your satisfaction in step three, you may request, in writing, the Assistant Vice President of Personnel Relations to schedule a hearing before the Staff Grievance and Appeal Committee.

A hearing before the committee is a non-adversarial proceeding and attorneys are not allowed to participate on either side. You may select another university employee who is both willing and able to arrange his/her work schedule accordingly to represent you in the grievance/appeal hearing.

The committee's recommendations are presented to the Vice President for Financial Affairs for a final decision. The Assistant Vice President of Personnel Relations will advise the concerned parties of the decision and assist in any personnel action required.

6.2 DISCIPLINARY GUIDELINES

Disciplinary guidelines have been established by the University of South Alabama so that you and other employees will be accorded a process of progressive discipline as set forth in these guidelines. The guidelines on the following pages show example violations and the degree of disciplinary action that may be required for each.

Your supervisor has the authority to determine an appropriate corrective measure through disciplinary action for any other violation of conduct not listed in the guidelines. The University reserves the right to change the particular type of discipline noted on the listed guidelines, due to the extent and severity of a particular offense. In some instances, even though previous violation of policy has not occurred, the severity of the offense may result in disciplinary action, up to and including dismissal.

(continued)

EXHIBIT 9-2 *(continued)*

So that the safety and productivity of all employees of the University is insured, a progressive disciplinary program has been established. If you fail to observe the accepted norm of behavior, your supervisor may issue either a verbal or written warning. Written warnings will be made a part of your permanent personnel file. Oral and written warnings may not be appealed. A layoff may not be appealed as it is not a disciplinary action.

6.2.1 FELONY CHARGES

If you, as a regular or temporary employee of the University, are charged with a felony offense, you shall be suspended without pay pending the outcome of your trial. A temporary or grant-funded employee who is charged with a felony offense shall be suspended without pay pending the outcome of the trial or the ending date of the employee's temporary appointment or grant funding, whichever is earlier. You are responsible for notifying your supervisor if you are charged with a felony offense.

If you are suspended without pay because of a felony charge, and are otherwise eligible for benefits, you may continue to participate in the group medical and life insurance programs. You are responsible for making arrangements with the Payroll Office to pay the total monthly premium costs for these benefits.

If you are convicted of a felony offense, you shall be immediately dismissed.

If you are found not guilty of the felony offense as charged, you shall be reinstated with back pay for the period during which you were suspended without pay pending outcome of your trial with no break in service and you shall retain accrued vacation and sick leave benefits. A temporary or grant funded employee shall be reinstated with back pay until the ending date of the employee's temporary appointment or grant funding, whichever is earlier.

Source: Courtesy of the University of South Alabama, Mobile, Alabama. Reprinted with permission.

Supervisory Influence

With the power of unions generally declining, goals for unions of professional nurses are best met by multipurpose organizations that can respond and adapt to the particular concerns of nurses, such as "supervisory influence." Generally, employers raise these concerns relative to whom will represent professional nurses. Rank-and-file nurses may be concerned that nurse managers will dominate the bargaining unit through membership in the SNA. The bargaining unit needs some insulation from SNA members who are managers. The issue usually extends beyond legal characterizations to political overtones of power and control within the organization. The California Nurses Association established the legal standard on the issue of "supervisory influence" in the Sierra Vista case in 1979. This standard is best met by an integrated, multipurpose professional association as a bargaining agent.[30] This agent would include and meet the needs of clinical nurses of all specialties along with nurse managers, educators, and researchers who are members of the SNA.

Benefits

Unions view the health care field as a potential pool for membership, which is a threat to hospital leaders. Concrete evidence shows "that collective bargaining,

when used effectively, actually facilities delivery of the best care and services."[31]

Collective bargaining has contributed to the high standard of living for the working people of Western countries. Employee compensation levels are higher when they are determined at the bargaining table.[32]

Collective bargaining is viewed by employees as an enforceable way to secure justice in the workplace, and a way for them to share power with employers. It provides fundamental protection against arbitrary or unfair treatment in the matter of promotions, remuneration, dismissal, and retirement. The bargaining agreement or contract balances management power with the combined might of all the employees. Protection under collective bargaining is greater than the contract itself. Unfair management authority can be challenged through a grievance system.[33] Contracts with nurses frequently include reference to the ANA code for nurses and standards of nursing practice.[34]

Research indicates that nurses have been reluctant to exercise collective power. Involvement peaks during organizing activity and in times of crisis or conflict. Nurses are more involved with committees related to the nursing product than those related to bargaining unit affairs.[35]

The Michigan Nurses' Association views nurses who choose this association as their exclusive labor representative as having combined the philosophies of professional nursing care and collective bargaining. The goal of this association is protection of patients through protection of nurses' professional and economic rights.[36] Contracts give nurses input on nursing care standards, policies, and procedures. Unions improve working conditions related to shift rotation, floating, nonnursing duties, flexible staffing, meal breaks, rest periods, time away from work, continuing education, tuition reimbursement, educational leave, grievance and arbitration procedures, maternity-paternity leave, discipline, posting of vacancies, recall from layoffs, peer review, career ladders, joint committees to improve safety and quality of patient care, and adherence to the Code for Nurses. (See Exhibit 9-1.)[37]

The success of unions depends on the quality of the work environment and the credibility and effectiveness of the organization as a bargaining agent and workplace advocate.[38] Outcomes of labor negotiations will depend on employee and employer relationships, attitudes, and philosophies.[39] Estimates are that union members average 6% higher salaries than do nonunion workers.[40]

Hannah and Shamian state that the foundation of modern nursing is a professional practice model of nursing. This model can be achieved through collective bargaining and nursing information.

The characteristics of a professional practice model of nursing are[41]:

- Multidisciplinary and interdisciplinary collaboration
- Accountability
- Practice based on a sound and discipline-specific foundation scholarship, that is, knowledge, theory, and inquiry
- Autonomy rooted in a clear understanding of the scope and boundaries of the discipline of nursing
- Awareness of the social-political context of practice
- Self-motivated professional development, including self and peer evaluation, aimed at maintaining currency of practice knowledge

The professional practice model of nursing care can be achieved through functional, team, primary, or case management methodologies. The best environment is a decentralized organizational structure using self-governance.

Collective bargaining environments can be suitable for a professional practice model of nursing that provides for career mobility, advancement, and wage increases using criteria beyond mere seniority.[42]

The purposes of collective bargaining include "facilitating communication between the parties to the contract; establishing and maintaining mutually satisfactory salaries, hours of work, and working conditions; prompt disposition of differences of opinion or grievances; and resolution of disputes."[43] The goal is collaboration. A fully implemented nursing information system provides clinical data quickly; improves nurses' work; and coordinates management activities, physician-delegated

tasks, and professional nursing practice. Decision-support systems are information systems designed to provide the information needed to make clinical decisions about patient care. Inputted data (such as history and test results) are processed against stored data to give decision outputs such as differential nursing diagnosis and suggested therapeutic recommendations.

Source data entry should be from bedside terminals or through two-way radio transmission. Patient discharge abstracts should be expanded to include nursing care delivery information. A nursing minimum data set is available. The collective bargaining unit can be a powerful ally to nursing management in integration of a professional practice model of nursing informatics.[44]

Ills

Unions cost money and create adversarial relationships. They focus on seniority rather than merit. Before joining a union, the nurse should study its experience or history and its track record. The nurse should talk to union members, tally the annual costs for dues and fees, and read the financial statement.[45]

A former union member claims that unionism is a lopsided religion with management as the devil.

Because they are elected as are politicians, union officials have a vested interest in maintaining a combative relationship with management. Unions discourage hard work and personal ambition while encouraging dependence.[46]

Once nurses gain collective bargaining status they exhibit low participation in related activities. A survey of 261 registered nurses employed in voluntary hospitals in New York State and represented by the New York State Nurses' Association for collective bargaining indicated[47]:

1. Few nurses attended union meetings regularly, although more did than do blue-collar workers.
2. Only 10.3% of respondents attended union conventions. Excuses included family responsibilities, location, expense, time off, and lack of interest.
3. Members read literature from the bargaining agent.
4. Few nurses submit bargaining demands.
5. Of respondents, 45% voted in local bargaining unit elections and 35% in statewide elections.
6. About two-thirds read the bargaining agreement.
7. Few file formal grievances. Of those who did file, 65% filed for professional concerns and 37.5% for economic concerns. One-third knew little about the grievance procedure. They handled grievances informally first.

assume leader-

re militant about

urses who have
o fail to exercise
for the abridge-
ccess or failure of
ons."[48]

a last resort. Striking
n a negative way by
893 articles on strikes
ented a more negative
image of the nurse than did newspaper articles on other nursing subjects. There were more negative headlines, criticism of nurses, and negative relationships reported. A desire for higher salaries was the major strike issue reported by newspapers, conveying the message that nurses were more interested in personal economic gain than in quality of patient care.[49]

Causal factors contributing to a strike vote include the following[50]:

1. Perceived lack of responsiveness by nurse administrators in solving everyday problems experienced by nursing staff
2. Fear of change experienced by nursing staff
3. Resistance by nurses to the national trend of using unlicensed, assistive personnel to reduce operating costs
4. Perceived reduction in benefits for the nursing staff
5. Environmental and workplace health and safety concerns
6. Perceived inequities in salaries between the nursing staff and senior executives

Firing striking workers is illegal, but it is standard management strategy for companies to threaten to hire permanent replacements. Companies are then obligated to hire former strikers only as future openings occur. In 1989, approximately 21,000 workers in U.S. companies lost their jobs through permanent replacement policies. Organized labor has been unable to obtain federal legislation banning replacement of employees who strike. The Supreme Court ruled permanent replacements legal in 1938.[51]

Vulnerability

There has been increased interest in collective bargaining among health care workers since the Supreme Court

decision of 1991. The long-term goal of the ANA is to "enable the country's two million nurses to achieve control over their own practice and work environment."[52] If nurse administrators wish to avoid dealing with collective bargaining units, they should create the conditions under which nurses have equivalent control.

The signs and symptoms of increased vulnerability to collective bargaining activity are those of an unhealthy environment[53]:

1. Increased nursing staff turnover
2. Increased employee-generated incidents
3. Increased grievances filed
4. Breakdown in communication
5. Sudden changes in staff behavior
6. Increased inquiries about personnel policies and practices
7. Changes in behavior of "problem children"
8. Pro-union, collective bargaining, or professional organization literature, posters, or graffiti
9. Organization of and invitation to off-site meetings for staff members only
10. Formation and submission of petitions
11. Managers' "gut" feelings

Nurse administrators should do a formal assessment of collective bargaining and make a plan for action that prevents it. Some of the activities to consider in this plan of action are training of front-line management in communications, counseling, mentoring, participatory management, shared governance, and addressing quality-of-care issues immediately.[54] Other actions to take include the following:

- Make the nurses feel like stakeholders. This is especially important with advanced, technically trained nurse specialists.
- Make nurses feel connected and invested in their work so they will be creative and productive.
- Prepare nurses to increase their role functions as members of interdisciplinary teams.
- Examine the possibility of new partnership models with nurses: shared ownership, gainsharing, bonusing, pay for performance, outcome pay, per diem contracting, caseload payment structures, benefit smorgasbords, increased autonomy of work, participation, and self-managed teams.
- Work can be redesigned as a result of union leadership and management partnership, with mutually formed mission, goals, and planning for the future.[55]

Collective bargaining is unnecessary when nurses and management communicate well and participate in decision-making. It is unnecessary when nurses receive adequate support and appropriate recognition. Nurses should be provided with a voice in decision-making, resources to do the job, safeguarding of standards of nursing practice, protection of employment rights, and attractive terms and conditions of employment.[56] These are all aspects of a model of HRM that works, that keeps nurse employees happy.

One of the most important benefits of collective bargaining is increased job security. Nurses can be fired for economic reasons and for incompetence, but management should be sure terminations are done only for good and just causes. Laws prevent discrimination on the basis of sex, race, religion, national origin, age, handicap, and for some types of whistle-blowing. The NLRA prevents discrimination because of union activity. Termination should never be related to acts violating public policy or for refusal to perform an illegal practice.[57]

The employer is considered to have the absolute right to determine staffing patterns, ratios, and other personnel requirements. Employers should consider input from nurses in formulating standards of nursing practice; providing education benefits; ridding nurses of nonnursing work; and input into hiring, promotions, and transfers.[58]

Good management prevents the need for collective bargaining by nurses. Poor management promotes collective bargaining (see Exhibit 9-3).

Summary

Collective bargaining through unionization is a process whereby employees join together to gain collective power that somewhat neutralizes the power of management. The collective bargaining process has been used in the nursing profession for approximately 50 years. In 1991, the U.S. Supreme Court affirmed the ruling of the NLRB that professional nurses could form a distinctly separate bargaining unit within hospitals.

Issues related to collective bargaining include pay, fringe benefits, and conditions of work related to provision of quality care to patients. Many professional nurses are reluctant to use the process of collective bargaining. Those who do put the safety of patients above their own concerns.

The theory of human resource management that puts trust in employees by training them to manage themselves is the best management strategy to deter collective bargaining. Nursing and health care leaders who work collaboratively with practicing clinical nurses through decentralization and participatory management prevent collective bargaining. It has been proved time and time again that people who manage their own work, who make professional decisions about their practice, increase the productivity and profitability of the firm.

EXHIBIT 9-3
Case Study of Events Leading to Formation of a Collective Bargaining Unit

Nurses at the county-owned University Hospital were unilaterally told they would no longer be paid time-and-a-half for overtime. In the past, they had been subjected to other unfavorable "adjustments."

The American Federation of State, County, and Municipal Employees, Local No. 2399, took out a large ad in the *Medical Gazette*, a weekly newspaper distributed free at area hospitals. The ad announced three union organization meetings at a hotel near the hospital. Nurses reported rumors of newspapers being confiscated and nurses being told they would be fired if caught reading the paper while on duty. A personnel director at one of the larger nonprofit hospitals called the *Medical Gazette* editor to complain about the ad, saying, "This is Texas, and we don't have much use for unions here."[1]

A subsequent column in the city newspaper, written by a registered nurse (RN) who was president of AFGE Local 4032, stated that registered nurses were burdened by low wages, understaffing, and increasing work load. The nurse further stated that RNs are routinely excluded from hospital policy decisions that directly affect their care of patients.

This nurse went on to state that "since 1978, Texas Nurses' Association has refused to support collective bargaining for registered nurses."[2]

The problem issues that led to an attempt at unionization at the University/Medical Center Hospital were:

- Elimination of time-and-a-half overtime pay for RNs
- A 50% reduction in merit-pay scales for RNs
- No rollover of merit pay into base pay, resulting in a de facto salary cap
- No change in mandatory overtime policy
- Implementation of policy before additional staff were brought on-line[3]

A series of additional letters to the editor supported the formation of a union and indicated that nurses were told to take compensatory time off rather than be paid time-and-a-half for overtime. This occurred even though nurses could not get vacation requests honored.[4]

The overtime pay was restored at $8 per hour in excess of their regular pay for overtime.[5] Apparently, this action terminated efforts to establish the union.

1. R. Casey. "Indicted by SAC Prof, My Plea Is 'Not Innocent.'" *San Antonio Express-News* (15 February 1994), 2A.
2. V. C. Barrera. "Besieged Nurses Opted to Unionize." *San Antonio Express-News* (25 February 1994), 5C.
3. Ibid.
4. M. Barrera. "Hospital Can't Run Without Nurses." *San Antonio Express-News* (28 April 1994), 5B.
5. "Nurses' Overtime Pay Restored." *San Antonio Express-News* (30 April 1994), 3C.

APPLICATION EXERCISES

EXERCISE 9-1 Interview a professional nurse who is a member of a union. Determine his or her perceptions of the benefits of collective bargaining. What are perceived as the weaknesses of collective bargaining?

EXERCISE 9-2 Prepare a plan to evaluate the vulnerability of a health care organization to collective bargaining. Use it to assess the organization. Prepare a list of recommendations for decreasing the vulnerability of the organization to collective bargaining. Present the results to the nurse administrator. This exercise may be done by a small group of nurse managers or students.

NOTES

1. B. White, "An Introduction to Collective Bargaining," *Oregon Nurse* (May 1984), 23, 27.
2. "Common Questions about Union Organizing and Representation," *Michigan Nurse* (March–April 1985), 3; W. E. Fulmer, *Union Organizing: Management and Labor Conflicts* (New York: Praeger, 1982).
3. K. J. Hannah and J. Shamian, "Integrating a Nursing Professional Model and Nursing Informatics in a Collective Bargaining Environment," *Nursing Clinics of North America* (March 1992), 31–45.
4. E. E. Beletz, "Nurses' Participation in Bargaining Units," *Nursing Management* (October 1982), 48–50, 52–53, 56–58.
5. V. S. Cleland, "A New Model of Collective Bargaining," *Nursing Outlook* (September–October 1988), 228–230; "Supreme Court Affirms Eight Bargaining Units per Hospital," *The Regan Report on Nursing Law* (June 1991), 1; J. F. Easterling, "Autonomy, Professionals, and Collective Bargaining," *Michigan Nurse* (March–April 1983), 86–87; L. G. Acord, "Protection of Nursing Practice Through Collective Bargaining," *International Nursing Review*, 29(5), (1982), 150–152; K. B. Stickler, "Union Organizing Will Be Divisive and Costly," *Hospitals* (5 July 1990), 68–70; P. S. Brenner, "Labor Relations in Nursing," *Michigan Nurse* (July–August 1983), 2–4; L. Flanagan, "How the Bargaining Process Works," *The American Nurse* (October 1991), 11–12; H. Lippman, "Expect to Hear About Unions," *RN* (October 1991), 57–72; "Nurses Hail Crucial Supreme Court Ruling," *California Nurse* (June 1991), 1.
6. K. Markus, "Ruling May Change Labor Relations," *NURSEWeek* (2 December 1994), 5, 12.
7. Anonymous, "ANA Supports MNA in Lansing NLRB Case," *Michigan Nurse* (April 1995), 13.
8. P. S. Brenner, op. cit., 2–4.
9. G. Strauss, "Professionalism and Occupational Associations," *Industrial Relations*, 2(3), (1968), 7–31.
10. R. Pavalko, *Sociology of Occupations and Professions* (Itasca, IL: Peacock, 1971).
11. J. F. Easterling, op. cit.; P. S. Brenner, op. cit.; L. G. Acord, op. cit.; L. D. MacLachlan, "Meeting the Challenges of Collective Bargaining," *California Nurse* (March 1990), 1, 4–5; T. Porter-O'Grady, "Of Rabbits and Turtles: A Time of Change for Unions," *Nursing Ecomonic$* (May–June 1992), 177–182; L. Joel, "Collective Bargaining: A Positive Force in the Workplace," *The Missouri Nurse* (September–October 1992), 18–20; H. Lippman, op. cit.; L. J. Shinn, "NLRB Rulemaking Upheld: What's Next for Hospitals?" *Aspen's Advisor for Nurse Executives* (March 1992), 7–8; "Nurses Hail Crucial Supreme Court Ruling," op. cit.; "Beyond Collective Action: Individuals Can Protect Their Jobs," *Ohio Nurses Review* (March 1985), 5–6; "Steps to Organize and Obtain a Collective Bargaining Contract," *Michigan Nurse* (March–April 1985), 2; J. O. Hepner and S. E. Zinner, "Nurses and the New NLRB Rules," *Health Progress* (October 1991), 20–22; J. Stanley, "Collective Bargaining Turns 40," *California Nurse* (December 1986–January 1987), 1, 3.
12. Ibid.
13. Anonymous, "News From ANA: ANA House of Delegates Approves Significant Reshaping of the Association," *Nevada Rnformation* (November 1999), 14–15.
14. Anonymous, "ANA Creates New Labor Entity," *Oregon Nurse* (September 1999), 8.
15. Ibid.
16. P. S. Brenner, op. cit.; H. Lippman, op. cit.; L. J. Shinn, op. cit.; K. M. Fenner, "Unionization: Boon or Bane?" *Journal of Nursing Administration* (June 1991), 7–8; "Nurses Hail Crucial Supreme Court Ruling," op. cit.; J. O. Hepner and S. E. Zinner, op. cit.; T. Benton, "Union Negotiating," *Nursing Management*, 23(3), (1992), 70, 72; J. A. Krasnansky, "Time to Stop the Debate," *RN* (May 1992), 116; L. Holmsted, "E & GW Annual Business Meeting," *The Maine Nurse* (winter 1991), 5.
17. D. Wheaton, "Collective Bargaining: Confronting the Conflicts," *The Maine Nurse* (winter 1991), 10.
18. A. Kleingartner, "Professional Association: An Alternative to Unions?" In R. Woodworth and R. Peterson, eds., *Collective Negotiations for Public and Professional Employees* (Glenview, IL: Scott, Foresman, 1969), 241–245.
19. "Steps to Organize and Obtain a Collective Bargaining Contract," op. cit.; E. E. Beletz, op. cit.
20. M. K. Friedheim, "Negotiating a Union Contract," *Medical Laboratory Observer* (December 1982), 58–63.
21. "Steps to Organize and Obtain a Collective Bargaining Contract," op. cit.
22. P. Eubanks, "Employee Grievance Policy: Don't Discourage Complaints," *Hospitals* (20 December 1990), 36–37.
23. Ibid.
24. I. Eldridge, "Some Techniques and Strategies of Collective Bargaining," *Washington Nurse* (April 1986), 13.
25. J. A. Krasnansky, op. cit.
26. S. Brutsche, "Mediation Cross-Examined," *Texas Bar Journal* (June 1990), 584.
27. Ibid.

50. P. R. Pointe, M. S. Fay, P. Brown, M. Doyle, J. Perron, L. Zizzi, and C. Barrett, "Factors Leading to a Strike Vote and Strategies for Reestablishing Relationships," *Journal of Nursing Administration* (February 1998), 35–43.
51. M. Levinson and F. Chideya, "One for the Rank and File," *Newsweek* (19 July 1993), 38–39.
52. "Sparks of Union Activity," *Journal of Nursing Administration* (September 1991), 4.
    K. M. Fenner, op. cit.
    ?id.
    ?ter-O'Grady, op. cit.
    ?p. cit.
    ?ond Collective Action: Individuals Can Protect Their Jobs,"
    ?p. cit.
    A. Cohen, "The Management Rights Clause in Collective Bargaining," *Nursing Management* (November 1989), 24–26, 28–30.

?4. ?bid.
45. H. Lippman, op. cit.
46. R. Worsler, "Still Fighting Yesterday's Battle," *Newsweek* (27 September 1993), 12.
47. E. E. Beletz, op. cit.
48. Ibid.
49. P. A. Kalisch and B. J. Kalisch, "Policy and Perspectives on Newspaper Reports of Nurse Strikes," *Research in Nursing and Health* (August 1985), 243–251.

REFERENCES

Fay, M. S. and A. K. Morrill. "The Grievance-Arbitration Process: The Experience of One Nursing Administration." *The Journal of Nursing Administration* (June 1985), 11–16.

Reynolds, A. "ANA Institute Makes Great Strides for Collective Bargaining." *Pennsylvania Nurse* (May 1992), 17.

CHAPTER 10

Principles of Budgeting

Russell C. Swansburg, PhD, RN

Introduction

Because the amount and quality of nursing services depend on budgetary plans, nurses should become proficient in related procedures. This proficiency will provide the resources necessary for safe and effective nursing care. With limited resources and a competitive market, personnel and material resources need to be used wisely and efficiently. The enlightened nurse knows that the person who controls the budget is the person who controls nursing services. The costs of nursing services have been identified for many years, but the income earned from nursing services has been included in "bed and board" on the budget sheets. Achieving reimbursement for nursing services means that many government regulations and third-party payer policies must change to allow for direct payment to nursing providers, based on the amount of care given and the skills of the persons giving it.

Budgeting is an ongoing activity in which revenues and expenses are managed to maintain fiscal responsibility and fiscal health. The nurse manager has financial responsibility; is accountable for managing the nursing budget; and makes all of the decisions about how to adjust the nursing budget to manage programs and costs, including those related to adding and dropping programs, expanding and contracting programs, and all modifications of revenues and expenses within the nursing unit.

Basic Planning

Planning yields forecasts for 1 year and for several years. The budget is an annual plan, intended to guide effective use of human and material resources, products or services, and managing the environment to improve productivity. Budgetary planning ensures that the best methods are used to achieve financial objectives. It should be based on valid objectives to provide a product or service that the community needs and for which it will pay. In nursing, budgetary planning helps ensure that clients or patients receive the nursing services they want and need from satisfied nursing workers. A good budget is based on objectives; is simple, flexible, and balanced; has standards; and uses available resources first to avoid increasing costs.

There is no formula for the form, detail, or periods covered by budgets. Each budget system is designed for the situation at hand, bearing in mind the character of the company, the company's position, and the nature of the plans involved. Ordinarily, the budget system is most detailed in aspects of operations most important to the firm's success. Furthermore, the period covered by the budget varies with the nature of the plans and with the degree of accuracy possible in the preparation of estimates.[1]

A nursing budget is a systematic plan that is an informed best estimate by nurse administrators of revenues and nursing expenses. It projects how revenues will meet expenses and projects a return on equity, that is, profit. The budget should be stated in terms of attainable objectives to maintain motivation of nurses at the unit or cost-center level. The nursing budget serves three purposes:

1. To plan the objectives, programs, and activities of nursing services and the fiscal resources needed to accomplish them.
2. To motivate nursing workers through analysis of actual experiences.
3. To serve as a standard to evaluate the performance of nurse administrators and managers and increase awareness of costs.

These purposes should include the group's mission, strategic plans, new programs or projects, and goals.

Managing the financial end of nursing through an operational budget obviously can create a new dimension for nurses. The budget can be a strong support for developing written objectives for the nursing division

and for each of its units. It can provide strong motivation for effective planning, and it can certainly provide standards by which to evaluate the performance of nurse managers.[2] Effective planning provides for contingencies by indicating which programs or activities can be reduced or eliminated if budget goals are not met.

> Revenues and costs, or expenses, and operating and capital budgets should all be projected for the long term. Possible problems in future years should be flagged. Every planning decision, whether for the long or short term, should be accounted for in the budget.[3]

Procedures

Decentralized budgeting involves the nursing unit managers and their staff in the process. Nursing service is labor-intensive, which is reflected in the fact that the first six budget-planning steps pertain to labor. Note that only steps 7 and 8 are concerned with nonlabor expenses. The steps are as follows[4]:

1. Determine the productivity goal. The director of nursing services and the nurse manager determine the unit's productivity goal for the coming fiscal year.
2. Forecast the work load. The number of patient days expected on each nursing unit for the coming fiscal year are calculated.
3. Budget patient care hours. The expected number of hours devoted to patient care for the forecasted patient days are calculated.
4. Budget patient care hours and staffing schedules. The budgeted patient care hours are reflected in recommended staffing schedules by shift and by day of the week.
5. Plan nonproductive hours. Vacation, holiday, education leave, sick leave, and similar hours are budgeted for the coming year.
6. Chart productive and nonproductive time. To aid in the planning process, a graph is used to show nurses how the level of forecasted patient days, and therefore the staffing requirements, are expected to increase and decrease during the year. Productive time is the time spent on the job in patient care, administration of the unit, conferences, educational activities, and orientation.
7. Estimate costs of supplies and services. The supplies and services to be purchased for the year are budgeted.
8. Anticipate capital expenses. The expected capital investments for the coming year are included in the budget.

These eight steps result in a proposed budget that goes to the nursing administrator for review. After preliminary acceptance, this budget is sent to the accounting department, where the forecasted patient days are translated into expected revenue. The budgeted productive and nonproductive times are converted into dollars, as are the costs for supplies, services, and other operating expenses that will be allocated to a given nursing unit for the coming year. A pro forma operating statement is then returned to the director of nursing for review with the nurse manager. When the director of nursing and the nurse manager accept the budget, it is returned to the accounting department and forwarded with the rest of the agency manager's budgets to administration and the board of directors.[5]

People who pay high prices for health care want accountability of both costs and quality of service. The nursing budget can be a shared responsibility, with unit budgets being prepared with staff involvement at the clinical level. The planning and controlling processes are ongoing. Through their participation, clinical nurses enhance their professional stature. A budget prepared and executed as a shared experience becomes an object of ownership to a staff that will put forth effort to work within its framework.

According to Osborne and Gaebler, budgets should be developed without line items, based on the idea that funds can be moved around to fit shifting needs. Many health care organizations follow this policy. In one instance, a new cardiac rehabilitation program was developed and budgeted based on this policy. Cost-center managers agreed to shift funds because they could see the advantages of the program and had been led to believe that they owned their budgets. A policy should be developed that motivates managers to accumulate unused funds. This policy reduces the wasteful practice of spending money to keep budgets constant or to prevent reduction.[6]

Managing Cost Centers

A *cost center* is a given area of assigned accountability for both direct and indirect expenditures. A department of nursing is a cost center, as are each of its units, each clinic, in-service education, surgical suites, long-term care, home health care, and any other section with a nursing mission in which nurses provide services to clients. Each cost center is assigned a code. A reference (Seawell) is available for a uniform accounting and reporting system for hospitals. An organization may use this coding system, usually referred to as the patient care system. Work load measurements, sometimes referred to as performance classifications or units of measure, are necessary. The *unit of measure* for each cost center is identified as a specific, quantitative statistic, such as inpatient days or relative value units (RVUs).

The number of RVUs defines the tangible things done as evidence of production and to measure quantity, quality, and cost.

Each cost center is an internal department dealing with distribution of services and products. The cost-center manager is responsible for determining the cost of such services or products and how they are distributed within the organization. Two types of cost centers are mission, or revenue-producing, and service cost centers. Examples of mission, or revenue-producing, centers are radiology and laboratory departments. These centers have monetary income related to the purpose of the organization. A *service center* is a support center that provides a service to other units and charges for that service; no exchange of revenue takes place. The unit served adds the costs of these support services to its costs of output.[7] Examples of support centers are communications, purchasing, and laundry.

Each cost center has a manager, called the cost-center manager or the responsibility-center manager, who is responsible for identifying needs for equipment and programs to maintain progress at the current level of technology in the unit.

Budgeted costs within the cost center are broken down into subcodes. This promotes better budgetary planning and control because items are specifically identified during the budget planning process. Also, each item purchased is charged to (deleted from) the balance shown for that specific subcode.

Relationship of Budget and Objectives

One of the chief planning activities is to identify the objectives of the nursing division and each of its units, including developing a management plan with a budget for each objective. One of the first sources of budgetary information is the nursing objectives. By using these objectives, nurse managers see the benefit of developing pertinent, specific, practical budgeting objectives.

Budget Stages

For practical purposes, the nursing budget follows three stages of development: formulation, review and enactment, and execution. The entire budgeting process is given a specific time frame, and a target date is assigned for each step. (See Exhibit 10-1.) During the fiscal year of the execution stage of budgeting, the formulation and review and enactment stages for the next fiscal year are being carried out. The budget stages are sometimes labeled forecasting, preparation, and control, respectively.[8]

EXHIBIT 10-1
The Budget Calendar

FORMULATION STAGE

1. Develop objectives and management plans.
2. Gather all financial, historical, and statistical data and distribute to cost-center managers.
3. Analyze data.

REVIEW AND ENACTMENT STAGE

4. Prepare unit budgets.
5. Present unit budgets for approval.
6. Revise and combine into organizational budget.
7. Present to budget council.
8. Revise and present to governing board.
9. Revise and distribute to cost-center managers.

EXECUTION STAGE

10. Direct and evaluate expenses and receipts.
11. Revise budget if indicated.

Formulation Stage

The formulation stage is usually a set number of months (6 or 7) before the beginning of the fiscal year for the budget. During this period, procedures are used to obtain an estimate of the funds needed, funds available, expenses, and revenues. Financial reports of expenses and revenues of the previous fiscal year and the year to date will be analyzed by the chief nurse executive, department heads, and cost-center managers.

One of the first steps in writing a budget is gathering data for accurate prediction of expenses (costs) and revenues (income). This task can be developed into a system. Primary sources of data are the objectives for the division of nursing and for each cost center. Each program and activity needs to have an estimated cost placed on it. If in-service educators want new audiovisual equipment, they should not walk into the nurse administrator's office and expect to have it next week or next month. Purchasing this equipment should be planned for 6 to 7 months before the next fiscal year begins, and it may be budgeted for any quarter or month within that fiscal year. In surveying the objectives, nurse administrators and managers evaluate the previous year, review the philosophy, and rewrite the objectives for the future.

Other data include programs from other departments that will require use or expansion of nursing resources, expansion of nursing clinics and client teaching programs, travel costs for attendance at professional and educational meetings, incentive awards, library requirements, clinical and office supplies and equipment, investment equipment and facilities modification on a 5-year plan, and contracts for items such as intravenous pumps and oxygen equipment. Data

can be obtained from historical financial records of the organization.

Among the cost-center reports that will assist the nurse manager are the following:

- Daily staffing reports
- Monthly staffing reports
- Payroll summaries
- Daily lists of financial categories of patients
- Biometric reports of occupancy
- Biometric reports of work load
- Monthly financial summaries of revenues and expenses

Review and Enactment Stage

Review and enactment are budget development processes that put all the pieces together for approval of a final budget. Once the cost-center managers present their budgets to the budget council, the chief nurse executive will consolidate the nursing budget. The budget officer will then further consolidate the budget into an organizational budget. The chief executive officer of the organization and the governing board will then give their approval. Throughout this process, conferences will be held at which budget adjustments are made. Nurses can sell a budget by using a marketing strategy, anticipating challenges, being persuasive without being emotional, and working toward win-win situation.[9]

Execution Stage

The formulation stage and the review and enactment stage of the budget are planning activities. Execution of the budget involves directing and evaluating activities. The nurse administrators and managers who planned the budget execute it. Revisions in execution of the budget are scheduled at stated intervals, frequently once or twice during the fiscal year. Certain procedures are followed for evaluating the budget at cost-center levels. Budgets are prepared for either fiscal years that coincide with government budgets or calendar (fiscal) years, depending on the policy of the organization.

Cost Factors

Cost is money expended for all resources used, including personnel, supplies, and equipment. The volume of service provided is the greatest factor affecting costs. Others factors include length of patient stays, salaries, prices of material, case mix, seasonal factors, and efficiencies such as simplification of procedures and quality management to prevent errors that increase patient complications (morbidities and mortalities) and increase costs. Still other factors that have an impact on costs are regulation and competition for market share; third-party payers; the age and size of the agency; type and amount of services provided; the agency's mission; and relationships among nurses, physicians, and other personnel.

Fixed, Variable, and Sunk Costs

Fixed costs are not related to volume. They remain constant as volume increases and decreases over a period of time. Among fixed costs are depreciation of equipment and buildings, salaries, fringe benefits, utilities, interest on loans or bonds, and taxes.

Variable costs do relate to volume and census (patient days). They include items such as meals and linen. Supplies are usually volume-responsive, meaning that total costs increase or decrease according to use. The cost of supplies varies by patient census, physician orders, and diagnosis. For example, the cost of surgical dressings increases when a patient's wound has drainage and dressings must be changed frequently. Also, the cost of supplies increases or decreases with the census. For this reason, every cost center should have an established unit of measure for productivity. This unit may be numbers of tests, procedures, patients of a specific acuity type, hours or minutes of service, discharges, or RVUs. Most activities include elements of both fixed and variable costs. For example, personnel costs and utility costs can be both fixed and variable because a minimum is required for each.

Sunk costs are fixed expenses that cannot be recovered even if a program is canceled. Advertising is a good example.[10]

Direct and Indirect Costs

Direct costs are the costs of providing the product or service and are often considered to be those directly related to patient care, such as personnel costs and the variable cost of supplies. The definition of direct costs varies by department. In areas not involved in direct patient care, each department incurs its own category of direct costs.

Indirect costs are those incurred in supporting the provision of the product or service, are not directly related to patient care, and include utilities, administration, housekeeping, and building maintenance. As previously mentioned, however, they are direct costs for the source department. Some indirect costs are fixed, such as depreciation and administration. Others, such as laundry and accounting, are variable. All indirect costs are allocated or transferred by a specific method to the departments that use the service.

Every hospital has a method to establish costs, including the Hospital and Hospital Health Care Complex Cost Report Certification and Settlement Summary, commonly known as the Medicare Cost Report. In a few agencies the method is more refined. Nurse administrators should become informed about this activity.

Cost Accounting

A cost-accounting system assigns all costs to cost centers. Periodically, usually monthly, reports of costs are provided to cost-center managers, but they do not reflect all costs. Many indirect costs are allocated only once a year in the Medicare Cost Report. Included are costs of items such as utilities, accounting, administration, data processing, and admitting. Informed and influential nurse managers use these cost allocations when preparing budgets. Such allocations are usually hidden in the operational budget under the category of "room costs."

Cost assignments to cost centers are made on the basis of direct costing if they are direct costs of patient care. Otherwise, they are made by transfer costing from a patient care support department or by cost allocation if not related to direct patient care or support. Job order sheets are used to account for all services to patients. Direct overhead costs that cannot be identified with specific services rendered are allocated based on some other measurement, such as square feet of floor space.

Service Units

Service units are measurable units of productivity or volume for identifying and counting costs. They must be measurable, known to managers, and affected by volume. The number of service units produced measures productivity.

Unit of Service

The *unit of service* is a measurement of the output of agency services consumed by the patient. In the surgical suite and recovery room, it is measured in minutes or hours; in the emergency room, it is the number of visits or time and procedures; and in the nursing units, it is based on the acuity category of patients and hours per day expressed in RVUs. Types of measurement include procedures, patient days, patient visits, and cases.

With the increased sophistication of information systems, it is easier for nurse managers to become involved in identifying and costing service units, which can be quantified by hours of nursing care per category of acuity of illness. To make this an RVU, all other direct and indirect costs must be allocated on the basis of hours of nursing care per category of acuity of illness.

Chart of Accounts

A chart of accounts that includes a number and table for each cost center (see Seawell in references section) is subdivided into major classifications and subcodes. Examples are salaries and wages, employee benefits, medical and surgical supplies, professional fees, nonmedical and nonsurgical supplies, purchased services, utilities, other direct expenses, depreciation, and rent. These classifications are further subclassified.

To be assigned to the correct cost center, all movement of labor and materials between cost centers must be recorded. All fringe benefits must be charged to the appropriate cost center by some established method, and so must all purchases, including shared ones. This is usually done using allocated shares of service units.

Amortized expenses are deferred charges allocated to units over a specified period of time. They include depreciation charges for aging plant and equipment in addition to prepaid items. Prepaid items usually are charged monthly as service units. Other deferred expenses include unamortized borrowing costs and costs incurred for capital expansion or renovation programs.

Inventory and Cost Transfer

Identifying actual costs of any service unit is improved through an accurate system of inventory control. Based on the number of orders or requisitions for any item, the appropriate proportion of its costs can be transferred to the cost center that ordered the items.

Financial Accountability

In being assigned and accepting financial accountability, nurses' first duty is to their patients, who have given them their trust. Nurses should be accountable to themselves for their work, to their professional peers, to their employers, and to taxpayers in publicly funded institutions.

In one way or another, patients pay the costs of health care. They may do so through insurance premiums, taxes, or fringe benefits or from their own pockets. Financial accountability means that nurses and others can account for the efficient spending of the money paid for health care.

Nurse managers need information on the costs of all services provided by their own and competing institutions. This information, in turn, can be provided to clinical nurses, who should know what it costs to do their work. Cost consciousness leads to waste reduction and effective cost management.

Some managers mistakenly believe that controlling nursing labor power and expenditures can control overspending. Holding nurses accountable for their budgets, including both revenues and expenses, can rectify this misconception.

> **Nurse managers have to justify the cost-benefit ratio of services provided and devise new methods to increase cost-effectiveness.**

The Cost of Nursing Care

To determine the cost of nursing care, several factors should be considered. Nursing charges should be quantifiable. A patient acuity system serves this purpose. The patient acuity system usually separates patients into four or five levels of nursing care and enumerates nursing requirements for each level. Charges could be set by level and negotiated with third-party payers. These costs could be separated from the cost of nonnursing requirements. Nonnursing tasks would be reassigned to ensure that the charges for nursing care reflect the actual cost of providing such care.

A second method of costing nursing services is determining what share of total agency cost is attributable to nursing. This will vary by diagnosis-related group (DRG) or patient acuity. An industrywide effort for each region could produce standards for nursing costs and charges. Otherwise, a majority of the health care institutions in the United States would need to undertake research to determine nursing costs and charges on an agency-specific basis. Multinational corporations, of course, can apply research studies across member institutions.

Activity-Based Costing

Drucker recommends activity-based costing that accounts for the total process of doing business from personnel, supplies, material, and parts to installation and service of products. Health care organizations will know and manage the costs of the entire economic chain, tying the costs to all sources of payment. To do this requires foundation, productivity, competence, and resource allocation information. Personnel are placed to perform specific expectations and evaluated accordingly. Old organizational structures are replaced with new cost centers that support activity-based costing in which managers turn data into information through analysis and interpretation that lead to action.[11]

Definitions

Budget

According to *Webster's New Twentieth Century Dictionary, Unabridged, Second Edition*, a budget is "a plan or schedule adjusting expenses during a certain period to the estimated or fixed income for that period." Herkimer stated, "An effective budget is the systematic documentation of one or more carefully developed plans for all individually supervised activities, programs, or sections. . . . The budget is a tool which can aid decision-makers in evaluating operating performance and projecting what future operations might produce."[12]

A *budget* is an operational management plan, stated in terms of income and expenses, covering all phases of activity for a future division of time. It is a financial document that expresses an operations plan of action. In the division of nursing, it sets the limits of financial support, thereby controlling the extent and quality of nursing programs. The budget determines the number of kinds of personnel, materials, and financial resources available to care for patients and to achieve the stated nursing objectives. It is a financial policy statement. Budgeting is the process whereby objectives and plans are translated into financial terms and evaluated using financial and statistical criteria.

Revenue

Revenue is the income from sale of products and services. Nursing revenue traditionally has been included with room charges. Increasingly, it is being unbundled from the room rate as a separate charge per patient acuity category and per visit, day, or procedure.

Revenue can include assets, such as accounts receivable and income-producing endowments. The latter can be restricted to specific purposes. Buildings, land, and other items can be assets if they produce income or are capable of producing income. Total income is frequently termed *gross income*; the excess of revenues over expenses is known as *net income* or *profit*.

Revenues also come from research grants, gift shops, donations, gifts, rentals of cots and televisions, parking fees, telephone charges, and vending machines. Revenues may be elements of product lines such as orthopedic services that include orthopedic nursing, traction equipment, and prostheses.

Columbia Advanced Practice Nurse Associates (CAPNA), the brainchild of Columbia University School of Nursing dean Mary Mundinger, DrPH, RN, FAAN, has persuaded several New York insurers to list CAPNA in their directories and to reimburse participating nurse practitioners at the same rate as physicians.[13]

Revenue Budgeting

Revenue budgeting, or *rate setting*, is the process by which an agency determines revenues required to cover anticipated costs and to establish prices sufficient

to generate these revenues. Not all patients (purchasers) pay an equal, fair share of an agency's costs, which complicates the process.

To remain viable, any business must generate sufficient revenues to cover operating costs and make a profit. These revenues include increases in working capital, capital replacements, and inflation adjustments.

Nonprofit agencies are identified as such for tax status only.

Nonprofits use profits to improve plants and services; profits do not go to stockholders or owners. Profit appears as a positive balance on account ledgers.

Fundamental to the rate-setting process are adequate statistical data, historical and projected, for implementing the rate-setting method to be employed. On a departmental basis, these data include volume of services, current rate, allocated costs, and rate increase constraints. The goal is to obtain the greatest impact from a minimum cumulative rate increase in today's cost-management environment. Increasing rates in high-profit departments while instituting rate reductions in low-profit departments so that they offset each other does this.

In today's reimbursement milieu, revenues are often budgeted before expenses. Doing so is necessary to determine how much revenue will be available.

Expenses

Expenses are the costs of providing services to patients. They are frequently called *overhead*, and include wages and salaries, fringe benefits, supplies, food service, utilities, and office and medical supplies. As part of the budget, expenses are a collection or summary of forecasts for each cost center's account.

Full costs include both direct and indirect expenses. Although direct costs such as nursing can be traced to the source, indirect costs such as utilities, telephones, or purchasing services are allocated to the source department by a standard formula.

Expense Budgeting

Expense budgeting is the "process of forecasting, recording, and monitoring the manpower, materials and supplies, and monetary needs of an organization in such a manner that the operation of the various components of the organization can be controlled."[14] The components of expense budgeting are cost centers. Purposes of expense budgeting include the following:

- To predict labor hours, material, supplies, and cash flow needs for future time periods

- To establish procedures for making comparative studies
- To provide a mechanism for determining when changes in procedures need to be made, providing gross information on the kinds of changes needed, and providing evidence that control has been established or reestablished

Historical trends are the single best inexpensive indicator available to the institution. They are valid for prediction of present and future trends.

Patient Days

Patient days are used to project revenues. They are commonly used as units of service to compute staffing. Patient day statistics are usually derived from census reports that are done daily at midnight and summarized monthly for the year to date and annually. A patient admitted on May 2 and discharged May 10 is charged for nine patient days. Exhibit 10-2 illustrates the number of patient days per unit for one month.

Fiscal Year

The *fiscal year* (FY) is the budgetary or financial year. It may be the calendar year in some organizations, beginning on January 1 and ending on December 31. Many organizations use October 1 to September 30 as the fiscal year. Some use July 1 to June 30 to coincide with budget decisions of state legislatures and the U. S. Congress. In the latter examples, the fiscal year obviously overlaps two calendar years.

Year to Date

The term *year to date* (YTD) describes the accumulated units of service at a particular point in the fiscal year. If the fiscal year begins October 1, the year-to-date patient days for December 31 would be the summary for 92 days. Exhibit 10-3 illustrates year-to-date statistics.

Average Daily Census

The census is summarized for a specific number of days and divided by that number of days. For example, the average daily census (ADC) for the month of June would be the total patient days for June divided by 30. In Exhibit 10-2, the number of patient days for June was 7,436. When this is divided by 30, the average daily census is 248.

Hours of Care

From the nursing viewpoint, hours of care have traditionally been the number of hours of care allocated per patient per day (24 hours) on a unit. With the use of patient acuity rating systems, hours of care can be determined to the hour or even fraction of an hour. Patients usually fall into one of four or five patient acuity categories, each of which is assigned a specific number of hours of care per patient day.

Caregiver

Each nurse who works with patients is labeled a *caregiver*. In nursing, the three common types of caregivers are registered nurses (RNs), licensed practical nurses (LPNs), and nurse aides (NAs) or extenders. Most personnel budgets have a ratio of RNs to other caregivers. Considerable research supports an all-RN caregiver staff. The current cost-management environment often alters this goal.

Operating Budget

The *operating budget* is the overall plan identifying expected revenues and expenses, both fixed and variable, for the forthcoming fiscal year. It is an annual budget that includes the cash budget and the capital budget. In addition, the operating budget identifies the source and nature of expected revenues and expenses. The operating budget determines the per diem and other charges to be made to the patient. A cost-to-charge ratio is used.

Cost-to-Charge Ratios

Cost-to-charge ratios are convenient tools for computing the cost of providing a service. For example, if the charge to a patient for fiber optic laboratory services were $1,000 and the cost-to-charge ratio 0.815626, one would know that the cost to the hospital for these services was approximately $815.63 (see Exhibit 10-3). This cost includes the expense of running the fiber optic laboratory and a portion of the hospital's overhead cost. In some instances, the cost-to-charge ratio is greater than one, which means the cost of operating these cost centers is greater than the charges.

The hospital has two types of cost centers. The first is the revenue-producing cost center, such as the fiber optic laboratory, which bills patients for services provided. The second type is the overhead cost center, such as the accounting department, which exists to support the revenue-producing centers. The cost of the overhead cost centers is allocated to the revenue-producing centers by various statistical methods. For example, utility costs are allocated to revenue-producing departments based on the square footage of space they occupy. However, accounting department costs are allocated based on the size of the operating budget of

EXHIBIT 10-2

A Patient Day Census

NURSING STATION	CURRENT YEAR			YEAR TO DATE		
	JULY	OCC (%)	JUNE	CURRENT YEAR	OCC (%)	PREVIOUS YEAR
3rd Floor	1,014	79.8	833	9,792	78.6	8,650
4th Floor	811	76.9	718	7,834	75.8	7,255
5th Floor North	526	65.3	524	5,300	67.1	4,838
5th Floor South	622	77.2	592	5,587	70.7	5,603
6th Floor	792	71.0	866	8,730	79.8	8,176
7th Floor	850	68.5	895	9,086	74.7	8,885
8th Floor	0	0.0	0	0	0.0	4,403
8th Floor North	376	60.6	383	4,624	76.1	2,393
8th Floor South	303	69.8	274	3,253	76.4	1,729
9th Floor	0	0.0	0	0	0.0	5,138
9th Floor North	526	84.8	501	5,332	87.7	2,690
9th Floor South	481	77.6	506	5,118	84.2	2,617
MINU	104	83.9	89	1,041	85.6	432
SINU	73	58.9	84	964	79.3	471
Burn Unit	173	79.7	188	1,723	81.0	1,912
Labor and Delivery	138	37.1	99	1,228	33.7	1,258
CCU	206	83.1	148	1,848	76.0	1,937
Clinical Research Unit	137	73.7	132	1,342	73.6	1,361
EAU	23	0.0	7	390	0.0	634
MICU	213	85.9	191	2,099	86.3	2,291
PICU	169	54.5	112	1,612	53.0	1,834
SICU	229	92.3	207	2,175	89.4	2,302
NTICU	209	84.3	87	1,891	77.8	2,277
Total	7,975	73.2	7,436	80,969	75.3	79,086
NURSERY						
Newborn	832	103.2	632	7,666	97.0	7,307
Intermediate	577	103.4	457	4,761	87.0	3,991
Intensive Care	955	110.0	716	8,526	100.2	7,022
Total	2,364	105.5	1,805	20,953	94.7	18,320

Source: Reprinted with permission of the University of South Alabama Medical Center, Mobile, Alabama.

each revenue-producing cost center. The cost-to-charge ratio is computed by dividing the total cost of the cost center, both direct and overhead, by the total charges for the same department.

Cost-Benefit Analysis

Cost-benefit analysis is a planning technique[15] that answers the following questions: What are the costs of pursuing a goal, an objective, a program, or a specific nursing intervention? How do costs compare with the benefits? Is the project worthwhile? Comparison of different nursing interventions for the same nursing diagnosis or problem results in using the least costly interaction to achieve similar or better results. The intervention used is then cost-effective.

Zero-Base Budgeting

Zero-base budgeting is a method of budgeting used to control costs. In a zero-base budget, the budgeting process starts from zero, and everything must be justified by each new budget cycle. A previous activity can be included in the budget, but its relation to the current organizational objectives must justify funding for it. In theory, each function in a zero-base budget must stand on its own merits, and the merits of each function are reviewed annually. All labor power and costs are recalculated, and decisions are made about whether to continue the function and at what levels.

When using zero-base budgeting it is important to have a policy in place to motivate cost-center managers to accumulate unused funds.

EXHIBIT 10-3
Cost-to-Charge Ratios

COST CENTER	COST-TO-CHARGE RATIO
Operating room	1.072993
Recovery room	0.731813
Delivery room	0.920547
Radiology	0.846045
Laboratory	0.502010
Respiratory therapy	0.288370
Physical therapy	1.261435
EKG-EEG-CVL	0.698327
Fiber optic lab	0.815626
Medical supplies	0.303416
Drugs	0.275234
Cast room	0.238285
Emergency room	1.131543
Routine inpatient	1.321196
Surgical ICU	1.044988
Coronary care	0.892522
Burn unit	2.054106
Pediatric ICU	1.153027
Medical ICU	1.038597
Nursery ICU	0.756198
Nursery	1.138131

Source: Reprinted with permission of the University of South Alabama Medical Center, Mobile, Alabama.

Program Budgeting

Program budgeting is a part of budget planning. Items such as continuing education programs, employee benefits fairs, and health promotion programs should be incorporated into the annual budget. The budget for each program should enumerate fixed expenses, such as rent, advertising, fixed speaker fees, and department overhead, and variable expenses, such as for food, handouts, and per-person honorarium speaker fees. Some costs, such as those for advertising, are unrecoverable even if the program is canceled. They are *sunk costs* and should be in the cost center budget as well as in the individual program's budget.

Program budgets should include a break-even analysis. If the cost of the program is $2,000 and the reasonable charge is $50 per participant, the break-even point is 40 participants. A break-even chart can be made for each program (see Exhibit 10-4). Income above the break-even point is profit; below it is loss.

The point at which the cost to carry out a program is equal to the cost to cancel it is called the *least-loss point*. If enough people have registered to pay the sunk costs, the net loss will be the same whether the program is canceled or held. It may be good public relations to carry out a program at the least-loss point.[16]

Operating or Cash Budget

The *cash budget* is the actual operating budget in detail, usually excluding the capital budget. A cash budget indicates whether cash flow will be adequate to meet anticipated payments, such as debt obligations, including replacement and expansion of facilities; unanticipated requirements; payroll; payment for supplies and services; and a prudent investment program. Cash receipts come from third-party payers, tuition, endowment fund earnings, and sales of food, gifts, and services.

The cash budget is the day-to-day budget and represents money coming in and going out. It is advisable to have cash reserves so that *cash flow*—the money coming in—will pay the bills. Otherwise, revenues must be speeded up or payment of bills slowed down. Cash reserves should not be excessive; they may represent money that should be working for the organization. Cash budgets show revenues and expenses, whereas operating budgets show plans. They are usually considered integrated entities.[17]

Negative Cash Flow

The four major factors that influence negative cash flow are:

1. Time lag between delivery of services and collection of payments.
2. The difference in cycles between the timing of net income and flow of cash.
3. Lag created by the large up and down cycles of volume during different seasons (cash deficit during a busy census cycle or surplus during a low census cycle).
4. Labor expense (60% to 70% of operating expense) paid out in salary and wages does not cycle concurrently with collections.

To maintain solvency, cash flow must be managed carefully and cycles of cash shortage planned for appropriately. The cash budget should plan for the ability to borrow cash during shortfalls, investment of excess cash, and *strict* monitoring and reporting of lost charges and of the billing and collecting process. The cash budget is a part of the total budget and is apportioned to departments based on individual cost-center activity.

Developing the Operating Budget

Operating budget information supplied to the chief nurse executive, department heads, and cost-center managers includes a budget worksheet and a worksheet that explains budget adjustments (see Exhibits 10-5 and 10-6). The budget worksheet depicts information by the

EXHIBIT 10-4
Break-Even Analysis

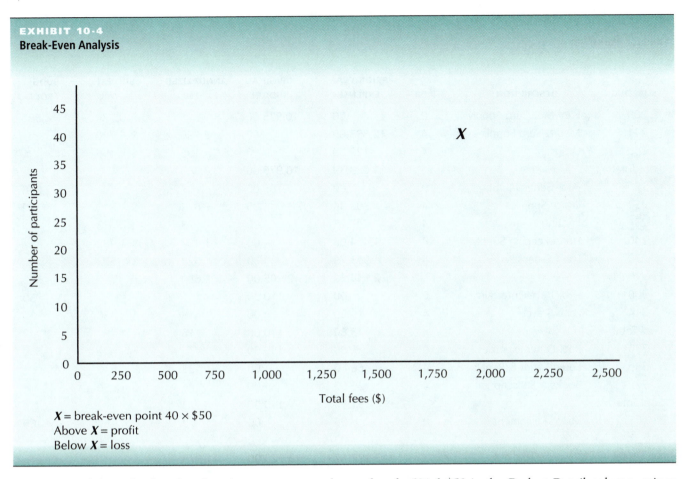

X = break-even point 40 × $50
Above X = profit
Below X = loss

account number and subcode of each cost center and lists prior-year expense, original budget, and annualized expense. This form usually is provided during the new budget formulation stage, and the *annualized expense* is the projected total expense if current rates continue to the end of the fiscal year. The columns headed Budget Detail and Budget Pool are empty so that the cost-center manager can fill in the budget expenses for the projected fiscal year. Note in Exhibit 10-5 that the cost-center manager had projected an increased budget of $10,975 for subcode 200, the pool for medical and surgical supplies and drugs. This amount was reduced to an annualized projection of $8,985 (subcodes 211 and 213, Budget Detail and Budget Pool columns) at the budget council hearings when hospital administration decided *not* to project inflation.

Also in Exhibit 10-5, note that subcode 232, office supplies, was increased by $138 (from $672 to $810). This increase was justified on the adjustment explanation (Exhibit 10-6). Information available to the administrator, however, indicated that $320 had been budgeted and expended in the current year for new chart holders. Because this was a one-time expense, it was taken out of the budget (–$320 in the Budget Pool column). A similar transaction for $53 was taken out of

subcode 501 (–$53 in the Budget Detail column, minor equipment). Overall, increases were approved for subcodes 501 and 372 (books and subscriptions). A total budget for supplies and minor equipment for this cost center was approved for $14,595. Exhibit 10-6 shows the adjustment explanation for subcodes 232 and 372. In the formulation stage described here, the assistant administrator for finance distributes the worksheets to the other assistant administrators and department heads, who develop budgets with their cost-center managers and defend them before the budget council.

Osborne and Gaebler refer to the operational budget as the expenditure control budget. It sets up accounts for various major expenditures. These authors recommend shifting among accounts as needed, and allowing departments to carry over into the new budget what they do not spend. A recommended formula for establishing an expenditure control budget is: same as previous year plus account for inflation and growth or decline plus any carryover funds. Management should apply additional money for the new initiatives. The strengths of such a mission-driven budget are[18]:

- Every employee has an incentive to save money.
- Resources are freed up to test new ideas.

EXHIBIT 10-5
Budget Worksheet

SUBCODE	DESCRIPTION	ABR	PRIOR-YEAR EXPENSE	ORIGINAL BUDGET	ANNUALIZED EXPENSE	BUDGET DETAIL	BUDGET POOL
200	Pool-Med/Surg Supply	0	.00	10,975.00		$10,780	$ 8,985
211	Med & Surg Supplies	4	10,893.80	.00	8,790	$ 8,790	
213	Drugs	4	129.59	.00	195	$ 195	
Pool Total			11,023.39	10,975.00	8,985		
220	Pool-General Supply	0	.00	2,705.00			$ 2,848
232	Office Supplies	4	303.34	.00	672	$ 810	−320
234	Printing	4	37.75	.00	3	$ 3	
240	Housekeeping Supply	4	1,404.06	.00	1,482	$ 1,482	
270	Food Expense	4	913.73	.00	523	$ 523	
Pool Total			2,658.88	2,705.00	2,680		
300	Pool-Travel/Entertain	0	.00	110.00			$ 50
314	Local Travel	4	13.80	.00	18	$ 50	
Pool Total			13.80	110.00	18		
320	Pool-Other Expenses	0	.00	130.00			$ 660
336	Equip Maint & Repair	4	66.60	.00	123	$ 610	
372	Books & Subscription	4	25.00	.00		$ 50	
Pool Total			91.60	130.00	123		
501	Minor Equipment	0	.00	.00	72	−53	$ 465
Pool Total			.00	.00	72		
Acct Total			13,787.67	13,920.00	11,878		
						Total	$14,968
							−373
							$14,595

Source: Reprinted with permission of the University of South Alabama Medical Center, Mobile, Alabama.

- Managers have the autonomy they need to respond to changing circumstances.
- A predictable environment is created.
- The budget process is enormously simplified.
- Much money can be saved on auditors and a budget office.
- Management can focus on other important issues.

Personnel Budgeting

Most budgets for nursing personnel are based on quantitative work load measurements, such as a patient acuity system. A computer software program usually produces staffing requirements by shift and day. It produces an acuity index for each patient, and the formula indicates needed staff by qualification level (RN, LPN, NA) and by shift. It also compares actual staffing with that required and a summary can be provided by month and year. Each day at a given time, a clerk enters each patient's acuity rating, as determined by an RN, into a computer terminal. To promote objectivity of the ratings, nurses should be trained to use the same procedures when evaluating each patient. Quality checks can compare the trainer's ratings with those made by RNs.

Exhibit 10-7 is a nursing personnel budget based on a patient-acuity rating system. The ADC is obtained from records produced in the admissions office. It is the result of dividing the total patient days for a unit for 1 year by 365 days. Census reports are computer-generated daily, monthly, and annually.

Acuity is the result of the sum of all acuities for 1 year divided by 365 days. This figure is also computer-generated daily, monthly, and annually. The nursing hours are generated from the acuity standard listed in item 1 of Exhibit 10-7. Application of a staffing formula for preparing the personnel budget for a specific unit is illustrated in Exhibit 10-8.

EXHIBIT 10-6
Adjustment Explanation, for calendar year _____

DEPARTMENT NAME _____ 9th floor

DEPARTMENT NUMBER _____ 60686

SUBCODE NUMBER	SUBCODE DESCRIPTION	ADJUSTMENT AMOUNT	ADJUSTMENT EXPLANATION
		$ 30.00	2 lg blue policy binders 15.00 ea
		6.00	1 sm blue policy binder
		32.00	2 large red 4" (8 1/2 x 11) 3-ring binders— normal wear and tear, 2 yrs old
232	Office Supplies	$ 25.00	4 black 3-ring binders (MAR & Kardex)— normal wear and tear
		28.00	48" x 36" cork and wood-frame bulletin boards— ↑ appearance ↓ clutter
		17.00	25" x 25" 1/4" thick Plexiglas— ↑appearance
		$138	
		$ 30.00	Tabers Medical Dictionary—ref. book needed to ↑ professionalism
372	Books	$ 20.00	Websters Ninth New Collegiate Dictonary— ↑ learning
		$ 50.00	

Source: Reprinted with permission of the University of South Alabama Medical Center, Mobile, Alabama.

In planning the personnel budget, the nurse has quantitative information related to staffing and can accurately predict the number of full-time equivalents (FTEs) needed for patient care. Other considerations must be weighed at the same time: Will there be a pay increase next year? If so, it must be calculated and budgeted. Will fringe benefits increase or decrease? They must also be budgeted. If new programs are being implemented, do they require additional labor power? Will this labor power come from cutbacks in other programs, or from added FTEs? See Exhibit 10-9 for adding new positions to the budget.

In the budgeting process, personnel account for the largest portion of the nursing budget. When one is preparing budgets for clinics, emergency departments, recovery rooms, operating rooms, delivery rooms, and home care, it is important to have quantitative data, such as numbers of visits, procedures, and deliveries. Records of length of time required for each activity can be obtained by using management-engineering techniques in which visits, procedures, or other activities are charted over a period of time.

Data should be collected over a representative period to show the actual hours worked by shift and by

EXHIBIT 10-7
Nursing Personnel Budget

NURSING BUDGET

1. The attached personnel budget for all nursing units is based on a patient-acuity rating system purchased from Medicus Systems. The standard is

	Nursing Hours per Patient Needed
Acuity	During 24-hour Period
0.5	0–2 hours
1.0	2–4 hours
2.5	4–10 hours
5.0	10–24 hours

2. The staffing formula is

$$\frac{\text{Average census} \times \text{nursing hours} \times 1.4 \times 1.14}{7.5}$$

3. The total nursing personnel needed includes ward clerks and units not using a patient-acuity rating system:

MATERNAL CHILD

UNIT	ADC	ACUITY	NSG/HRS	RN	LPN	NA	OTHER	TOTAL
3rd	31.8	0.9	4.0	14	9	4	5	32
Peds	22.0	1.3	4.5	16	5	0	4	25
PICU	4.4	3.4	12.0	11	0	0	2	13
ICN	21.7	2.9	12.0	41	7	6	4	58
Inter.	11.9	2.3	4.5	6	4	1	1	12
NBN	19.7	1.0	4.0	9	6	1	3	19
Del. Rm.	—	—	—	20	3	1	4	28
Play Rm.	—	—	—	—	—	—	1	1
Total				117	34	13	24	188

MEDICAL

UNIT	ADC	ACUITY	NSG/HRS	RN	LPN	NA	OTHER	TOTAL
5 No.	14.3	1.3	4.5	11	3	0	3	17
5 So.	22.1	1.3	4.5	12	5	4	3	24
CRU	3.6	—	4.5	6	—	1	1	8
8th	25.1	1.7	4.5	15	7	2	3	27
MICU	7.2	4.0	12.0	18	0	0	3.5	21.5
CCU	6.5	3.0	12.0	16	0	0	1	17
Telemetry	—	—	—	—	1	5	0	6
Total				78	16	12	14.5	120.5

SURGICAL

UNIT	ADC	ACUITY	NSG/HRS	RN	LPN	NA	OTHER	TOTAL
9th	16.2	1.2	4.5	11	2	2	3	18
6 Surg.	26.5	1.6	4.5	16	6	3	3	28
6 Ortho.	23.5	1.5	4.5	15	4	4	3	26
SICU	6.4	3.8	12.0	17	0	0	2	19
B.U.	3.7	2.8	12.0	8	2	0	1	11
Ortho Tech	—	—	—	—	—	—	1	1
Total				67	14	9	13	103

(continued)

EXHIBIT 10-7 *(continued)*

UNIT	ADC	ACUITY	NSG/HRS	PSYCHIATRY RN	LPN	NA	OTHER	TOTAL
7th	23.5	—	5.5	11	4	11	6	32

UNIT	ADC	ACUITY	NSG/HRS	OR/RR/EAU/ED RN	LPN	NA	OTHER	TOTAL
OR	—	—	—	21	13	4	2	40
RR/EAU	—	—	—	16	0	1	2	19
ED	—	—	—	25	0	7	8	40

UNIT	ADC	ACUITY	NSG/HRS	ADMINISTRATION RN	LPN	NA	OTHER	TOTAL
N/S Adm.	—	—	—	13.0	0	0	3.5	16.5
Staff Dev.	—	—	—	8.5	0	0	1.0	9.5
Health Nurse	—	—	—	1.0	—	—	—	1
CVICU								
Pool	—	—	—	4.5	12	18	2	36.5
Total				362	93	75	76	606

Note: The formulary budget is based on actual ADC for 12 months (July–June). All positions above formula calculations are placed in CVICU budgeted cost center and held vacant.

Source: Reprinted with permission of the University of South Alabama Medical Center, Mobile, Alabama.

EXHIBIT 10-8
Calculating the Nursing Personnel Budget

The staffing formula is

$$\frac{\text{Average daily census} \times \text{nursing hours} \times 1.4 \times 1.14}{75}$$

Example: 3rd Floor
Average daily census = 31.8
Nursing hours = 4 (per 24 hours)
1.4 is a constant representing 7 days in a week with a full-time worker working 5 days in a week:
$7 \div 5 = 1.4$
1.14 is a constant representing an allowance of 0.14 FTE for vacation, illness, etc. for
each 1.0 FTE
7.5 represents one workday

$$\frac{31.8 \times 4 \times 1.4 \times 1.14}{7.5} = 27 \text{ FTEs}$$

There are 14 RNs, 9 LPNs, and 4 NAs (27 FTEs) budgeted for 3rd floor. The Others column in Exhibit 10-7 represents unit clerks or other nonnursing personnel not included in the formula. While quantitative measurements justify a full complement of nursing personnel, the budget committee can reduce this number. Note in Exhibit 10-7 that ICN has been reduced from the formula calculation by 1.0 FTE.

day. These data will indicate fluctuations in the work load by shift and by day of the week. Use a second data sheet to determine the total number of patients in the emergency department area at any one time, including patients in a holding status. Conversion of these data into graphs provides information to compare staffing with work load. These data will provide the following information[19]:

- Current nursing hours available per patient visit
- Fluctuations in available hours by shift and by day.
- Fluctuations in work load by time of day.
- Fluctuations in ratio of staffing levels to patient load.

EXHIBIT 10-9
New Position Questionnaire, Budget Year _____

1. Department _____ Department number _____

2. Position class, title _____ Position FTE _____

3. Minimum starting salary _____ Expected starting date _____

4. Permanent _____ Temporary _____ If temporary, ending date _____

5. Describe briefly the new position responsibilities:

_____

_____

_____

_____

NEED FOR NEW POSITION

6. New service _____ Increased volume _____
   If new service, complete question 7.
   If increased volume, complete question 8.

7. Describe the new service to be provided and estimate new revenues.

_____

_____

_____

_____

_____

8. Document increased volume and provide staffing analysis for your department.

_____

_____

_____

_____

(Attach additional pages if necessary)

_____

_____

Source: Reprinted with permission of the University of South Alabama Medical Center, Mobile, Alabama.

Piper indicates that the basic staffing of an emergency room should be calculated to handle a *critical mass*, the staffing level required to handle an unexpected emergency. In addition to quantitative data, the nurse administrator should collect qualitative data from the staff to assist in containing stress, determining mix of staff, and improving support services. Data can be compared with those from other institutions. The result will then be translated into personnel dollars.[20]

In the process of budgeting, the nurse manager knows how much each decision will cost and whether it involves numbers and kinds of personnel or amounts and kinds of supplies and equipment. Few nurse managers have the luxury of a budget that provides all of the resources that can be used. Hard decisions must be made. These decisions are easier to substantiate when work loads are quantified. In the personnel area if the patient dependency or acuity system is reliable and valid and has quality checks on the raters, it will provide data that justify the personnel budget. When the number of adult patients of the highest acuity level increases from 24 to 32 per shift and day, the budget must be adjusted. Comparisons must be made to determine whether other levels have decreased. Estimates must be made as to whether the increases and decreases are permanent or temporary. Then the budget decisions are made.

Nurse managers study fluctuation trends in patient census and use these data for minimum staffing requirements to determine the percentage of time to staff one nurse less and the percentage of time to staff one nurse more per shift. The salary expense for the one time that one nurse less per shift is needed should be subtracted from the budget. The salary expense for the one time that one nurse more per shift is needed should be added to the budget. The result is an improved salary expense budget result. (See Exhibit 10-10.)

Strategies to reduce budget overages include[21]:

- Maintain good staff retention.
- Use nurse extenders to perform non-RN functions.
- Monitor and control unscheduled absenteeism.
- Implement an effective on-call system.
- Institute a "flex-team" in related clinical areas to avoid overtime and agency nurse expenses.
- Create a large pool of part-time casual nurses.
- Budget according to trends.
- Negotiate for a reasonable budget that considers turnover and orientation.

Nonproductive Full-Time Equivalents

Nonproductive FTEs are hours for which an employee is paid but does not work. Nonproductive FTEs include vacation days, holidays, sick days, education and training time, jury duty, leave for funerals, and military leave. These nonproductive hours must be determined and added to personnel expenditures as replacement FTEs. An FTE is based on 2,080 hours per year. If the nonproductive FTE average is to be used for personnel budgeting, the human resource (HR) department payroll section will provide it. For example:

Average vacation FTE	12.5 days
Average holiday FTE	7.0 days
Average sick days FTE	3.5 days
Average training and education FTE	3.0 days
Average other leave FTE	1.5 days
Total	27.5 days, or 220.0 hours

The total work time is 2,080 hours less 220 hours; the actual work time is 1,860 hours. The percentage of nonworked to total hours paid is 10.6%. The percentage of nonworked to worked hours is 11.8%.

A cost-center manager prepares the budget according to management rules. The budget should include a line item for replacement FTEs to cover nonproductive FTEs by assigning a fixed amount to each person's paid time off. An option is to determine percentage of nonproductive FTEs and add this total to the budget. This information is then used for staffing determination, taking into consideration seasonal fluctuations for vacations, census, and other pertinent factors.[22]

Supplies and Equipment Budget

The supplies and equipment budget is part of the operating or cash budget. It includes all supplies and equipment used in provision of services, except capital equipment and supplies charged directly to patients. Examples of supplies to be budgeted are office supplies, medical and surgical supplies, and pharmaceutical supplies. (See Exhibits 10-5 and 10-6.)

Minor equipment includes items such as sphygmomanometers, otoscopes, and ophthalmoscopes. Minor equipment costs less than the base amount set for capital equipment. If the base amount is $500, all equipment under $500 appears as minor equipment in the supplies and equipment budget.

EXHIBIT 10-10

Budgeting for Fluctuating Census

STAFFING	CENSUS	%	TOTAL DAYS	REQUIRED HOURS/DAY	TOTAL HOURS REQUIRED	BUDGETED LABOR RATE	SALARY EXPENSE BUDGET
Minimum staffing	9	100.00%	365	12	39,420	$17	$670,140
1 less nurse/shift	<6	4.98%	(18)	24	(432)	$17	($7,344)
1 more nurse/shift	>9	39.99%	146	24	3,504	$30	$105,120
Total					42,492		$767,916

Source: E. Tzirides, V. Waterstraat, and W. Chamberlin. "Managing the Budget with a Fluctuating Census." *Nursing Management* (March 1991), 80H. Reprinted with permission of Springhouse Corp.

Generally, the director of materials management furnishes the total cost of supplies and equipment per cost center to the accounting office, which generates a cost per patient day. This cost is used for budgeting purposes, and increases for inflation are a decision of top management. Based on projected patient days and revenues, decisions can be made to increase or decrease the supplies and equipment budget.

Controlling the amounts of supplies can decrease costs and equipment kept in inventory. Nurse managers should look at the inventories they control and reduce them according to usage.

Factors that might influence the supply and equipment aspects of the budget include new program development in the institution, new physicians, and product upgrades. A product evaluation committee may be very cost effective.

Product Evaluation

Product Evaluation Committee

A product evaluation committee usually has as its members representatives of nursing, medical staff, central supply, and purchasing (see Exhibit 10-11). The committee is headed by a products and equipment specialist or medical materials manager, who can be a nurse. This committee is responsible for evaluation and purchase of supplies and equipment. The following are among its goals:

- Standardization, with all units using the same products
- Lower prices through higher volume
- Removal of contract negotiations between vendors and individual nursing units, allowing valuable time to be spent on nursing functions
- Addition of a clinical perspective to purchase of all products

The purchasing department does not just make changes in products or purchases without appropriate assessment. All clinical implications are considered.

Thus, systematic control of the introduction of patient care products into the institution is achieved. Exhibits 10-12 and 10-13 present a product information and justification checklist and minutes from a product evaluation and standardization committee meeting, respectively.

The following is a suggested process for product evaluation by a committee[23]:

1. Determine objectives of product evaluation.
2. Define use of the product with input from potential users.
3. Define objectives for each evaluation project.
4. Do initial review of various products: features, techniques for use, and prices.
5. Select products for evaluation and evaluate techniques for use, staff acceptance, and problems.
6. Conduct in-service tests to use products.
7. Use simple closed-ended questions, open-ended questions, and rating scales to evaluate the product.
8. Compile and analyze data, including costs, cost savings, conversion cost, and reimbursement potential. The Deming theory of working with one supplier to improve products is noted in Chapter 25.
9. Make a decision for purchase.

Capital Budget

A capital budget is usually separate from the operating budget (see Exhibit 10-14). A capital budget projects the planned costs of major purchases. Each capital budget item is defined in terms of dollar value and is an item of equipment that is used over a period of time. The budget provides for depreciation of each item in the capital budget, sets aside the amount of depreciation in an escrow account, and uses this account to finance new capital budgets (see Exhibit 10-15). Depreciation records the declining value of a physical asset. In addition, department heads are required to justify and set priorities on capital budget items (see Exhibit 10-16). The exact definition of what constitutes a capital budget item with regard to dollar amount and life expectancy varies among hospitals.

Capital budgets also deal with maintenance, renovations, remodeling, improvements, expansion, land acquisition, and new buildings (see Exhibits 10-15 and 10-17). The financial manager for nursing is the nurse manager, who should evaluate past decisions and advise the nurse administrator whether they were good or bad.

All proposals for capital equipment must be fully evaluated for amount of use, method of payment, safety, replacement, duplication of service, and every other conceivable factor, including the need for space, personnel, and facility renovation. The needs and desires of the medical staff should be considered. Staff involvement in planning helps ensure wise purchases of capital equipment.

A strategic capital-budgeting method based on principles of decision analysis can help health care organizations allocate capital effectively when meeting requests for capital expenditures. The eight steps of the strategic capital-budgeting method are establishing evaluation criteria, classifying proposals by area of investment, ensuring that proposals are complete and easy to understand, determining costs of proposals, rating proposals with respect to individual criteria, setting priority weights for criteria, calculating weighted value

EXHIBIT 10-11
Product Evaluation and Standardization Committee

I. *Purpose*
  1. To bring about cost containment in supply and equipment utilization through the review of the quality and cost of products utilized.
  2. To review product utilization or special problems in order to maintain standards on the products throughout the hospital system and eliminate needless duplication.
  3. To maintain communication among Hospitals, Nursing Service Departments, Medical Staff, and the Purchasing Department concerning product utilization and quality.
  4. To evaluate items presented to Purchasing on which formal bids will be obtained.
  5. To evaluate items not on bid as recommended by the Purchasing Department, a member of the committee, Administration, or individual departments through requests for evaluation or for addition to inventory.
  6. To review performance of in-house products to determine if they fit present needs.

II. *Membership.* Membership of the committee shall consist of
  1. Manager of Hospital Resource Analysis
  2. Hospital Resource Analyst
  3. Budget Director
  4. Purchasing Agent
  5. Nursing representative from each hospital
  6. Ancillary representative from each hospital

  Nursing and Ancillary representatives from each hospital shall be appointed by the Administrator on a rotating basis. The infection control nurses will serve in an ex-officio capacity when a product has infection control implications. Additional representatives from a facility will be used when a product is to be evaluated that has a distinctive group involved (e.g., OR representatives when OR equipment is involved).

III. *Operations/Meetings.* The Manager of Hospital Resource Analysis shall call and conduct the meeting and shall have voting privileges only in the case of a tie. The Committee shall meet on the third Friday of each month with the location rotating among the facilities. Meetings will usually be one hour long and shall not exceed two hours. A written agenda will be issued to each member prior to the meeting. The agenda will be strictly adhered to unless the committee votes to change it. The chairperson will provide time at the end of each meeting to discuss general information. If a problem arises, the Chairperson may appoint a subcommittee or member to investigate and resolve the problem and to report back to the committee at the next meeting.

Everyone will be given a chance to express his or her ideas before voting. The majority vote shall rule in all cases unless otherwise overridden by Administration. Visiting guests shall have no voting power.

Routine minutes shall be taken at each meeting and will be distributed at the following meeting.

Established July _____, Policy 949-14, by authority of _____.

Reviewed: July _____, July _____.
Revised: August _____, October _____.

Source: Courtesy University of South Alabama Medical Center, Mobile, Alabama.

scores for each proposal, and ranking proposals by cost-benefit ratios. The results provide a reliable basis for optimal capital allocation.[24]

The capital budget must address increased forms of competition, dwindling financial resources, and regulatory constraints. Management should enhance conditions under which effective planning and capital budgeting increase the agency's chance of long-term survival. Capital budgeting is a part of the overall budget planning process for the organization and not an entity unto itself.

When each entry or item in the capital budget list has been analyzed and reduced to the amount available, the budget is again tabulated. It is now ready to present to the board of directors (see Exhibit 10-14). With the board's approval, the list is distributed to cost-center managers, who prepare requisitions for purchase. The purchasing department prepares bid specifications, with input from cost-center managers. Purchases are finalized based on results of bids submitted by vendors who meet the required specifications. Exhibit 10-18 is a status report of a capital budget in which all remaining dollars are committed. Finally, purchases are entered into the depreciation budget schedule. The latter is published by American Hospital Publishing and is considered the standard for the industry. The following are a few examples of the composite estimated useful lives of depreciable hospital assets: boiler house (30 years), masonry building, wood/metal frame (25 years), bed, electric (12 years), and otoscope (7 years). For budgetary purposes, the nurse manager should have access to the entire publication.[25]

Capital equipment accounts for approximately 10.4% of a hospital's annual expenditures.[26]

EXHIBIT 10-12
Product Information and Justification Checklist

The goal of product evaluation is to provide optimal patient care while managing costs. Therefore, please provide all information requested on this checklist to the department of Hospital Resource Analysis for consideration by the Product Evaluation and Standardization Committee. This report must be reviewed and signed by your Assistant Administrator before it can be evaluated by the committee.

1. Name and function of the product.
2. Is this a new product or a replacement?
3. How will the product be paid for (departmental budget, patient chargeable, etc.)?
4. Why is this product necessary or preferable to the current or other products, in your own words? Please discuss at least two other similar products.
5. What products are currently being used to perform this function in other departments and at all three hospitals?
6. What is the expected utilization of this product throughout the USA System?
7. What is the current utilization of the products that are performing this or a similar function throughout the USA System?
8. If this product is used to treat or prevent a specific ailment or range of ailments, what is the incidence of this ailment that is seen in the USA System?

9. What are the following costs, if applicable, for this product as compared to other similar products and how can these costs be justified?

   - purchase price
   - installation
   - training
   - personnel
   - support
   - maintenance (Also include who is responsible for maintenance.)

10. If cost savings are anticipated with the use of this product, how will those "savings" be utilized?
11. Who will control the use of the product?
12. If applicable, please provide a sample protocol for the use of this product that will be used to ensure proper use of this product.
13. What are the long-term implications of this product?

If you need assistance, please contact _____ or _____ at _____.

Source: Courtesy University of South Alabama Medical Center, Mobile, Alabama.

When evaluating capital equipment, one should evaluate similar products one at a time. When purchasing capital equipment, one should determine whether it can be upgraded or must be replaced when the technology improves. One should consider construction, durability, modularity, warranty, availability of parts, and service agreements as part of the total cost of equipment. Consider leasing versus buying.[27]

Part of the capital equipment budgeting process includes estimating the use of each item. For revenue budgeting purposes, a price or charge should be assigned to the use of each item. The cost-center manager can then determine the break-even point at which the item will be paid for.

Performance Budgeting

Performance budgeting focuses on the activities of a cost center such as indirect care, direct care, and quality monitoring. Each activity has objectives with specific financial resources, and the focus is on what is expected to be accomplished. Performance is evaluated based on a variety of outputs. Flexible budgeting that evaluates actual costs based on actual work load is an improvement over traditional budgeting but is a limited evaluation of nursing performance. Performance budgeting is an improvement over flexible budgeting because it ties performance to financial resource consumption. The steps involved are[28]:

1. Define the performance activities or area of accomplishment for the cost center, which may include providing direct care, improving quality of care, nursing staff satisfaction, patient satisfaction, productivity, and innovation. (See Exhibit 10-19.)
2. Identify the line item operating budget costs for the cost center being evaluated. These costs will be manager and clinical salaries, education costs, supplies, and overhead. (See Exhibit 10-19.)
3. Define how much of the resources represented by each line item are to be devoted to each of the performance areas. Exhibit 10-20 indicates percentages, and Exhibit 10-21 shows dollar allocations.
4. Choose measures of performance for each performance area, budget an amount of work for each area, and determine the budgeted cost per unit of work based on these measures. For an example of an actual performance budget, see Exhibit 10-21.

The performance budget evolves or is converted from the operating budget. Potential output measures are proxies and consist of both process and outcome measures. These output measures may include[29]:

EXHIBIT 10-13
Product Evaluation and Standardization Committee Meeting

December 9, _____
8:30 A.M., Board Room, USA Knollwood

MEMBERS PRESENT
Chairman, Hospital Resource Analyst, USAMC
Director of Nursing, USAKPH
Director of Respiratory Therapy, USADH
Nurse Manager, Surgical Services, USADH
Director of Radiology, USAMC
SPD Supervisor, USAKPH
Nurse Manager, High Risk/Antenatal Obstetrics, USAMC
Director of Budgets, USAMC

MEMBERS ABSENT
Purchasing Agent, USAMC
Hospital Resource Analyst, USAMC

GUESTS
Trauma Coordinator, USAMC

PRODUCT EVALUATION

Closed Arterial Line System
The Director of Respiratory Therapy and the Trauma Coordinator presented their findings from the evaluation of the closed arterial line system. In their discussion with Nursing and Respiratory Care providers, there were many issues raised regarding the practicality of such a system. These issues revolved around tubing size, heparinization and sampling through the ports available on the SafeSite system. In general, they concluded that the issue of blood waste could be solved without purchasing such a system and that there was no documentation present which could prove that contamination with the current stopcock system was a problem. They therefore recommended that we not pursue this system any further at this time. However, they did recommend that we evaluate such systems again when it is time to bid our current system again.

The committee unanimously agreed to not recommend the addition of a Closed Arterial Line System.

OLD BUSINESS

Gloves
The data provided regarding glove usage was determined to have been helpful to managers in evaluating their departments. _____ requested that _____ provide comparable information for the current fiscal year to date.

_____ addressed the quality issue with our current stock gloves. None of the other committee members have been made aware of a major quality problem with the gloves. It is unclear whether the problem has not been apparent in other departments or is just not being reported. _____ was not present at the meeting to answer how the company has responded to his inquiry regarding the quality issue.

After much discussion, it was decided that _____ would send a memo to all managers asking them to address specific quality issues to the committee representatives in their respective facilities.

Communication Issues
_____ brought up the problem that managers have in being informed of bid item changes in advance. Although it may not be possible to evaluate every item that is on bid, the committee determined that it would be helpful if the Purchasing Department could announce upcoming bids 3 to 6 months ahead of time. This would allow managers the opportunity to provide information regarding specific products. It was also suggested that bids be posted in all three facilities, rather than just at USAMC; this problem seems to be most apparent at USADH and USAKPH. _____ will discuss this with _____.

Presentation of Committee's Purpose to Managers
This presentation has not yet been accomplished. _____ agreed to have a proposal for this purpose ready for the January meeting. It was suggested that it might be helpful to have each facility's representatives make the presentation at their facility.

NEW BUSINESS

None.

The next regularly scheduled meeting will be held at USAMC on Friday, January 20, _____ at 8:30 A.M. in the USAMC Board Room.

The meeting was adjourned at 9:30 A.M.

Respectfully submitted,

Chairman

Source: Courtesy of University of South Alabama Medical Center, Mobile, Alabama.

EXHIBIT 10-14
Capital Budget Requested Fiscal Year 200x–200x: University of South Alabama Medical Center

DEPT.	ITEM	QUANTITY	AMOUNT
7th & 8th	Beds & misc. pat. furn.	85	$ 200,000.00
Admin	Pneumatic tube system	1	75,000.00
Anest	Capnograph-portable	1	4,200.00
Anest	Trans. Mon.- inc NIPB & O_2 Sat	1	9,200.00
Anest	Ventilators	2	5,050.00
Aero Med	Pro Pac 106	1	13,790.00
Bio Med	Safety tester	1	1,695.00
Blood Bk	Table top centrifuge	1	2,000.00
Blood Bk	Automated cell washer	1	6,250.00
Cath Lab	Pulse oximetry	1	2,600.00
Cath Lab	Dynamap	1	3,800.00
Clin. Lab	Miscellaneous equipment	1	250,000.00
Dialysis	Dialysis machine	1	25,000.00
Dietary	Refrigerator-bakery	1	3,500.00
Dietary	Refrigerator-bakery	1	6,950.00
Dietary	Refrigerator-cook area	1	3,500.00
Dietary	Refrigerator-PFS	1	3,100.00
Dietary	Meat slicer	1	3,500.00
ED	New monitoring system	1	160,000.00
ED	Propak monitor	1	3,500.00
Envir	High-speed burnisher	4	8,000.00
Envir	Slow-speed buffers	2	1,600.00
GI Lab	Video processor CV-100	1	20,000.00
HStation	Blood pressure monitor	1	4,500.00
HStation	Stress test system	1	20,000.00
HStation	ECG management system	1	70,000.00
MICU/CCU	Faceplates-central monitors	12	4,920.00
Nursing	Medication carts	17	25,000.00
Nutri	Computer & printer	1	2,011.00
OR	Laparoscopic video system	1	30,165.00
OR	Electrosurgical cautery	2	17,200.00
PACU	RR stretchers	10	20,000.00
Plant Op	4000-watt portable generator	1	1,495.00
Plant Op	8 ch. OPS card for telephone swi	1	1,337.00
Radio	Rebuilt film processor	1	12,000.00
Res. Th	Sterile pass-through drier	1	12,567.00
SPD	Washer decontaminator	1	75,000.00
Staff Dev	Overhead projector	1	700.00
Staff Dev	CPR mannikin	1	5,641.00
Total requested USA Medical Center			$1,114,771.00

Source: Courtesy University of South Alabama Medical Center, Mobile, Alabama.

EXHIBIT 10-15
Investment in Plant Assets for the 10 Months Ended July 31, _____

Plant assets consisting of land, buildings, and equipment are stated at cost or, if contributed, at fair market value at date of gift. No provision is made in the accounts for depreciation of plant assets. Investment in plant is reduced for disposal of plant assets.

All Hospital equipment purchases are funded by the renewals and replacements fund. The hospital also uses plant assets purchased by the University. These assets are not presented in the Hospital's financial statements.

Depreciation expense is included in Medicare, Medicaid, and Blue Cross cost reports. This information is presented below.

	COST	DEPRECIATION EXPENSE 07-31-XX	ACCUM. DEPRECIATION 07-31-XX	NET BOOK VALUE 07-31-XX
HOSPITAL-DESIGNATED FUNDS				
Land	$ 186,096	$ 0	$ 0	$ 186,096
Buildings	8,070,647	184,063	3,942,812	4,127,835
Fixed Equipment	10,386,318	605,671	5,878,008	4,508,310
Major Movable Equipment	15,079,892	1,235,052	8,971,493	6,108,399
Minor Equipment	186,757	0	186,757	0
Construction in Progress	762,874	0	0	762,874
Total	$34,672,584	$2,024,786	$18,979,070	$15,693,514
UNIVERSITY-DESIGNATED FUNDS				
Buildings	$ 1,544,927	$ 39,481	$ 581,958	$ 962,969
Fixed Equipment	2,564,683	158,533	1,914,366	650,317
Major Movable Equipment	5,315,499	0	5,315,499	0
Total	$ 9,425,109	$ 198,014	$ 7,811,823	$ 1,613,286
Total equipment used for patient care	$44,097,693	$2,222,800	$26,790,893	$17,306,800

Source: Reprinted with permission of the University of South Alabama Medical Center, Mobile, Alabama.

- Compliance with patient care plan procedures, with the goal of a percentage reduction in errors
- Improved compliance costs money to provide the fix, which is usually additional resources of some kind
- Staffing decisions using reduced management time
- Cost reduction
- Increased productivity
- Increased patient and staff satisfaction
- Innovation and planning
- Direct care
- Indirect care

Multiple measures can be developed for each performance area.

Revenues

The sources of nursing revenue or for securing a financial base for nursing include grants, continuing education, private practice, community visibility, health care for students and staff, health maintenance organizations, city health departments, industry, unions, third-party payments, professional corporations, and nurse-managed centers.

Operating room nursing is an example of a cost that can be billed as a source of revenue. Determining the level of care needed for different procedures and the room charges, based on use of supplies and equipment, and billing the services separately can do this. In computing the nursing charges, the cost of nursing personnel per case can be determined from the records. To this can be added the cost of preparation time for assembling supplies and equipment and setting up the room, preoperative and postoperative patient visits, nursing administration, and staff development. Room costs include environmental services and maintenance.[30] Using product-line strategy, nursing divisions can sell a number of product lines, such as staff development programs, consultation services, home health care, wellness programs, and computer software.

EXHIBIT 10-16
Capital Equipment Request Form

Hospital: ___USA Medical Center___

Dept: ___Department of Nursing___   **Dept no.** ___60601___

Equipment requested: ___85 electric beds/7th–8th floor___

Equipment description: Give a simple description of the device and its use.

85 electric beds with high-low features, ability for trendelenburg/reverse trendelenburg positions; instant CPR

emergency lever; head of bed frame removable to facilitate cervical traction and emergency procedures; side

arm control for patient use.

_____

_____

_____

$210,000.00	**Equipment costs**	None	**Training costs**
Minimal	**Maintenance costs**	Incl in Eqpt.	**Shipping costs**
None	**Personnel costs**	None	**Supply costs**
None	**Installation/renovation costs**		

Expected useful life: __15__ **yrs**

___1___   List priority (1-2-3-4) of equipment with regard to the other requests submitted by your department.

     (Y/N) Will this item be a replacement for an existing piece of equipment? If "Y," what is to become
___Yes___   of the existing equipment? Equipment to be evaluated by the Hospital Committee to determine.

     (Y/N) Is this new technology or a new procedure? If "Y," how will the expense be recuperated
___No___   (e.g., through revenue)?

Manager: _____, RN, MSN Director, Nursing Resources _____

Assistant administrator: _____

Apr # _____

Source: Courtesy of The University of South Alabama Medical Center, Mobile, Alabama. Reprinted with permission.

Many items and services have been used to generate revenues for hospitals, including drugs, supplies, respiratory therapy, and physical therapy. In most instances, the charges have been excessive, and areas exist where cost shifting has accounted for revenues (and profits) to cover services delivered and charged at a price below costs. As the hospital bill is unbundled, charges will eventually reduce to costs at a 1:1 ratio.

Because a not-for-profit hospital is not allowed a return on equity or credit for bad debts as a cost of doing business, the hospital must carry these items as cash or ledger balances.[31]

In business and industry, technology is used to reduce costs by increasing output; the opposite has been encouraged in the health care industry by charge-based reimbursement schemes. Third-party payers

EXHIBIT 10-17

Statement of Changes in Fund Balance
Renewals and Replacements Fund for the 10 Months Ended July 31, _____

ACCOUNT NUMBER	DESCRIPTION	BALANCES PRIOR YEAR	FUNDED DEPRECIATION	OTHER ADDITIONS DEDUCTIONS	EXPENDED FOR PLANT FACILITIES	INTRAFUND TRANSFERS	BALANCES CURRENT YEAR
79008	Unallocated—USAMC	$ 9,915,392.38	$ 2,222,800.29	$ 78,134.71	$ .00	$ 159,538.18–	$ 12,056,789.20
79030	Defects—Joint Commis	65,818.19	.00	.00	.00	65,818.19–	.00
79039	Information System	92,709.68	.00	.00	.00	.00	92,709.68
79050	Helicopter—USAMC	712,120.33	.00	127,667.94	.00	.00	839,788.27
79057	USAMC Emer Generator	48,562.09	.00	.00	.00	.00	48,562.09
79063	Donated Eq—Others	2,313.49	.00	153.00	1,928.70–	384.79–	153.00
79064	USAMC Aux Purch Eq	.00	.00	688.08–	538.08	150.00	.00
79068	Hosp Adm Purch Eq	.00	.00	33,809.52	33,809.52–	.00	.00
79075	HVAC System—Surgery	74,475.00	.00	.00	.00	74,475.00–	.00
79077	Labor Deliv Unit 3FL	291,990.72	.00	.00	.00	.00	291,990.72
79083	H.A.S. Telephone Sym	13,007.00	.00	.00	.00	13,007.00–	.00
79092	Capital Budget previous	364,110.78	.00	5,208.00–	334,654.47–	.00	24,248.31
79093	Xray Silver Recovery	49,944.03	.00	12,678.45	.00	.00	62,622.48
79095	Capital Exp <$10,000	75,414.38	.00	.00	146,864.18–	150,000.00	78,550.20
79097	Linear Accelerator	.00	.00	.00	45,994.26	45,994.26–	.00
79098	Mini Van	1,606.48	.00	2,847.51	.00	.00	4,453.99
79099	O/P Surg Cap Equip	161,720.27	.00	.00	225,718.54–	64,324.93	326.66
79101	O/P Surg Renov	37,425.00	.00	.00	1,316.60–	.00	36,108.40
79102	Angiograph Lab Eqmnt	1,000,000.00	.00	.00	189,259.00–	.00	810,741.00
79103	Nuclear Medical Eqmnt	284,000.00	.00	.00	246,035.68–	.00	37,964.32
79104	Telethon Purch Equip	.00	.00	40,185.00	40,185.00–	.00	.00
79105	Medical Rec Dict Sys	.00	.00	.00	.00	86,288.00	86,288.00
79106	Renal Transplant Prg	.00	.00	.00	.00	96,000.00	96,000.00
79110	ELENA-USAMC Damage	31,916.36	.00	5,629.15	.00	37,545.51–	.00
	Final Totals	$13,222,526.18	$ 2,222,800.29	$295,209.20	$1,173,239.35–	$ .00	$14,567,296.32

Source: Courtesy of The University of South Alabama Medical Center, Mobile, Alabama. Reprinted with permission.

EXHIBIT 10-18

Capital Budget, as of June 30, _____

DEPARTMENT	DEPT. NO.	ITEM DESCRIPTION	BUDGET	PAID 06-30-XX	ENCUMBRANCES	TOTAL COMMITTED	BUDGET BALANCE
NURSING SERVICES							
Nursing Services—Admin	60601	Software License	$ 0.00	$ 18,135.00	$2,000.00	$ 0.00	$0.00
		External Modem		527.12			
		Electric & Manual Beds—6		31,704.72			
		Cardio System Special Care Beds		13,725.00			
		Telemetry Monitoring System		113,080.12			
		COMPAQ Computer		9,842.70			
		Department Total	$189,014.66	$187,014.66	$2,000.00	$189,014.66	$0.00
Private U. 6th Floor	60609	Lifepack 7 Defibrillator		5,500.00			
		Facsimile Machine		1,600.00			
		Lifepack 7 Defibrillator		5,208.00			
		Department Total	$ 12,308.00	$ 12,308.00	0.00	$ 12,308.00	0.00
Coronary Care	60615	Lifepack 6 Defibrillator		7,621.32			
		Department Total	$ 7,621.32	$ 7,621.32	0.00	$ 7,621.32	0.00
5th Fl—Shared Supplies	60619	Facsimile Machine		1,550.00			
		Department Total	$ 1,550.00	$ 1,550.00	0.00	$ 1,550.00	0.00
Fifth Floor—North	60622	Lifepack 7 Defibrillator		5,500.00			
		Department Total	$ 5,500.00	$ 5,500.00	0.00	$ 5,500.00	0.00
CCU	60626	Telemetry Transmitters		3,300.00			
		Department Total	$ 3,300.00	$ 3,300.00	0.00	$ 3,300.00	0.00
Pediatric Unit	60630	Lifepack 7 Defibrillator		5,500.00			
		Facsimile Machine		1,550.00			
		Department Total	$ 7,050.00	$ 7,050.00	0.00	$ 7,050.00	$0.00

Source: Courtesy University of South Alabama Medical Center, Mobile, Alabama. Reprinted with permission.

EXHIBIT 10-19
Summary of Percentage Allocation to Performance Areas

COST ITEM	QUALITY	STAFFING	COST CONTROL	PRODUCTIVITY	PATIENT SATISFACTION	STAFF SATISFACTION	INNOVATION	DIRECT CARE	INDIRECT CARE	OTHER	TOTALS
Nurse											
Manager	15%	15%	20%	20%	10%	5%	15%	0%	0%	0%	100%
Staff Salary	5	0	5	2	5	0	0	30	30	23	100
Education	20	0	20	20	10	10	20	0	0	0	100
Supplies	0	2	2	0	0	0	0	90	5	1	100
Overhead	0	0	0	0	0	0	0	100	0	0	100

Source: S. A. Finkler. "Performance Budgeting." Reprinted with permission of Jannetti Publications, Inc., publisher, *Nursing Economic$*, vol. 9, No. 6 (November/December 1991), 405.

EXHIBIT 10-20
Allocation of Expenditures to Performance Areas

COST ITEM	TOTAL	QUALITY	STAFFING	COST CONTROL	PRODUCTIVITY	PATIENT SATISFACTION	STAFF SATISFACTION	INNOVATION	DIRECT CARE	INDIRECT CARE	OTHER
Nurse											
Manager	$50,000	$7,500	$7,500	$10,000	$10,000	$5,000	$2,500	$7,500	0	0	0
Staff Salary	800,000	40,000	0	40,000	16,000	40,000	0	0	$240,000	$240,000	$184,000
Education	20,000	4,000	0	4,000	4,000	2,000	2,000	4,000	0	0	0
Supplies	40,000	0	800	800	0	0	0	0	36,000	2,000	400
Overhead	90,000	0	0	0	0	0	0	0	90,000	0	0
Totals	**$1,000,000**	**$51,500**	**$8,300**	**$54,800**	**$30,000**	**$47,000**	**$4,500**	**$11,500**	**$366,000**	**$242,000**	**$184,400**

Source: S. A. Finkler. "Performance Budgeting." Reprinted with permission of Jannetti Publications, Inc., publisher, *Nursing Economic$*, vol. 9, No. 6 (November/December 1991), 405.

have paid for increases in equipment costs and types and numbers of procedures. That has changed somewhat with the prospective payment system. With control of reimbursement, less expense is best. The old revenue producers such as drugs, respiratory therapies, laboratory tests, and x-rays, are being reimbursed at their true costs. Nursing care is the source of revenue for the future. Nurses must identify the relative value units of care by which they will be reimbursed. They must learn to use information systems to process data and to select and use the supply item that does the best job for the least money. Nurses must standardize procedures and practices and review and revise jobs.

Because of relatively high fixed costs, hospitals must maintain high productivity. If productivity declines, costs must be decreased. Decreasing staff level and the amount of supplies used does this by making other reductions in use of resources.

The Controlling Process

Now that the nursing budget has been viewed from its planning and directing aspects, we turn to its controlling or evaluating aspects. The budget establishes financial standards for the division of nursing and through the division's cost center for each nursing unit. Daily, weekly, monthly, and quarterly feedback supplies information to compare managerial performance with the established standards. The results are used to make adjustments. What kind of feedback do nurses need relative to their budgets and cost control? Nurses need information to determine whether their goals are being met. Are they exceeding the budget? Is the excess both for costs and for revenues? Are the supplies and expenses of the quantity and quality planned? Is the equipment being purchased and installed as scheduled? Are employees being recruited and used effectively to produce the expected quality and quantity of nursing

EXHIBIT 10-21
Performance Budget

	TYPE OF ACTIVITY	DESCRIPTION OF OUTPUT MEASURE	AMOUNT OF OUTPUT BUDGETED	TOTAL COST OF ACTIVITY	AVERAGE COST
Quality Improvement	Patient care planning	Patient-care plan compliance	10% reduction in failure rate	$ 51,500	$5,150/Percent drop in failure rate
Staffing	Daily staff calculations	Number of daily calculations Reduction in paid hours per patient day over staff guide minimum	365 daily calculations 0.2 paid hours per patient day	8,300	$22.74/Daily calculation $4,150/0.1 Hour reduction
Cost Control	Reduce	Reduction in cost/patient day	$8/patient day	54,800	$6,850/ $ reduction
Increase Productivity	Revise procedures Work more efficiently	Reduction in total unit cost per direct care hour	$3 reduction per direct care hour	30,000	$10,000/ $ reduction
Increase Patient Satisfaction	Respond to needs	Complaints	10% reduction in complaints	47,000	$4,700/1% reduction in complaints
Increase Staff Satisfaction	Respond to needs	Turnover	25% reduction in staff turnover	4,500	$180/1% reduction in turnover
Innovation & Planning	Planning sessions	Number of meetings	12 meetings	11,500	$958.33/meeting
Direct Care	Direct patient care	Hours of care	10,000 hours	366,000	$36.66/direct care hour
Indirect Care	Patient charting	Number of patient days	7,300 patient days	242,000	$33.15/patient day
Other				184,400	
Total				$1,000,000	

Source: S. A. Finkler. "Performance Budgeting." Reprinted with permission of Jannetti Publications, Inc., publisher, *Nursing Economic$*, vol. 9, No. 6 (November/December 1991), 405.

services? Is employee morale good? What adjustments need to be made? Where are the problems, and who is responsible for them?

Budget processes should be flexible to allow for increased and decreased volume of business. The hospital's business office provides cost-center managers with needed biometric information to make adjustments in staffing and in use of supplies.

A budget is a plan based on the best estimates of the costs of running an organization. It cannot be inflexible, but neither can it hide waste and inefficiency.

The nurse administrator should be sure that nurses are not penalized when budgetary objectives are not met as a result of events beyond their control. Nurses are working within the confines of an organizational environment that is affected by both internal and exter-

nal constraints. One of the external constraints is federally mandated cost control or cost containment, which is seen by some administrators as reimbursement control.

The colossal mistakes of budgeting are made in the control area. Top management should view variations in budget as a tool for decision-making, and not as an instance to make arbitrary cuts that result in unrealistic operating budgets for line managers. One way to overcome this problem is through employee education about the budget process. Such knowledge helps employees view the budget as an aid rather than an obstacle.[32]

Decentralizing the Budget

Cost-center managers, usually nurse managers and unit supervisors, are capable of planning and controlling their own budgets. The nurse administrator, assisted by financial managers, should prepare them to do so.

Through decentralized budgeting, cost-center managers propose innovative objectives and gather data to defend their objectives and operating plans. The unit budget becomes their responsibility, and they zealously guard its integrity. They sense when adaptations have to be made because of increased costs or decreased revenues, and they make or recommend immediate remedies. Decentralized budgeting provides for internal controls.

Monitoring the Budget

Various techniques have been described and defined for monitoring the budget; however, all budget objectives should contain procedures for quality review, including identification of a team to perform such a review. If a program is not successful—that is, if it is not meeting objectives or is running above predicted costs and below predicted revenues—a decision should be made about whether to rework or cancel it. Although very difficult, making this decision is essential to good control. The technique of canceling budgeted programs is sometimes referred to as *sun setting*. A nurse manager should accept the responsibility for sun setting programs that are costly and unprofitable.

In developing the nursing budget, it is necessary that the unit structures for nursing administration are comparable in type and quantity of work load. Developing and providing financial policies and guidelines can ensure this. Developing these policies and guidelines is most successful when the top administrative team works with the budget monitor in doing so. The nurse administrator is part of this team and brings to its meetings standards of service that are defensible, such as data on work load, including numbers and types of procedures, patients, surgical operations, and visits. These policies should reflect the long-range plans of the governing board.

Part of the information furnished to nurse administrators and managers is in the form of reports, which include statistical reports of revenues and expenditures for the current year. Exhibit 10-22 illustrates financial information that is needed by the cost-center manager and the nursing service administrator.

Note that the account number at the head of the table in Exhibit 10-22 is 4-60680. The prefix 4 denotes that the account balance *does not* turn over at the end of the fiscal year. The cost center or department is 60680. Financial transactions, including purchase orders for supplies and minor equipment, as well as the payroll, are identified with this cost center number and are charged by the purchasing and accounting departments to this number and to the appropriate subcodes 100 through 501. Table columns indicate the operational budget, the actual expenditures for the current month and for the

fiscal year, open encumbrances, and the balance available. Because 83% of the fiscal year (which begins October 1) has elapsed, this has some relationship to the Percent Used column. Although 103% of the budgeted salary has been used, indicating a variance of 20%, only 78% of employee benefits have been used, which indicates a use of overtime plus part-time employees working less than the 0.5 FTE required to qualify for fringe benefits. Zero percent of the budgeted money for minor equipment has been spent to date. Total budget expenses were 96% indicating a variance of 13% overspending. This report serves as a control for nurse managers, but the expenditure of budgeted money for any one subcode could cause the total expenses to date to be greater than the percentage of fiscal year elapsed without creating an alarm. In this instance, overspending should be related to increased census and revenue.

Exhibit 10-23 informs the nurse managers of the specific financial transactions that took place during the month of July. These transactions can be checked against Exhibit 10-22.

Information on revenues is reported in a similar manner. Exhibit 10-24 illustrates the inpatient revenue for the Medical Intensive Care Unit, which includes nursing and hotel services. All the revenue is credited to nursing. The revenue account is 4-30815, and the cost center is the same as for expenses, 60680. The budgeted revenues for the year are listed, as are the revenues for the month and for the fiscal year. Note that although 83% of the fiscal year has elapsed, only 76% of the budgeted revenues have been charged, a variance of −7%. Also, Exhibit 10-25 indicates that 76% of budgeted equipment revenues have been billed.

Because the amount billed (that is, the unit's revenues), 76%, is less than the 83% of fiscal year elapsed, the nurse managers can note that revenues are currently lower than expenses, which is a negative financial report. The manager's goal is to improve this financial status by the end of the fiscal year.

Additional financial information can be furnished to each nurse manager, including summary reports in whole dollars and for all cost centers supervised. This can be done by subcode, by subcode and cost center, or by any unit or department (see Exhibits 10-26 to 10-29).

Rollover funds, designated by prefix 3, are also included in the financial reports that can be provided to the chief nurse executive and nurse managers. Balances in these funds are carried over into the next fiscal year to be spent at any future date. An example of a rollover fund is account 3-64155, the Maternal Child Health Education Fund. Exhibit 10-30 shows activities for this fund for the month, and Exhibit 10-31 shows how the debits were spent. The chief nurse executive, a department head, or a cost-center manager can manage rollover funds.

EXHIBIT 10–22
Accounting System Report

Account statement in whole dollars for fiscal year ending _____

Computer Date _____
Time of Day _____
Acct: 4-60680
Dept: 60680

83% of fiscal year elapsed
Distribution code = 700
Medical Intensive Care Unit—Expense

| | | BUDGET | | ACTUAL | | | | |
| | | | | CURRENT | FISCAL | OPEN | BALANCE | PERCENT |
SUBCODE	DESCRIPTION	ORIGINAL	REVISED	MONTH	YEAR	ENCUMBRANCES	AVAILABLE	USED
100	Pool—Salary & Wages	948,742	901,053				901,053	0
130	Professional Salry			72,533	775,790		775,790–	***
135	Tech Salry & Wages			4,085	50,947		50,947–	***
140	Office Salaries			4,347	53,168		53,168–	***
155	Service Empl Wages			3,936	52,195		52,195–	***
160	Student Wages		14,898	1,518	14,898			100
166	Accrued Salaries		32,791	11,462	32,791			100
	Salaries	948,742	948,742	97,880	979,789		31,047–	103
170	Pool—Empl Benefits	254,683	55,722				55,722	0
182	Employers FICA		112		112			100
183	Group Life Ins		2,569	264	2,569			100
184	Disability Ins		4,869	526	4,869			100
185	Teachers Retirement		134		134			100
188	Group Health Ins		59,973	5,887	59,973			100
198	State Paid Retiremnt		62,158	5,591	62,158			100
199	State Paid FICA		69,146	6,313	69,146			100
	Employee Benefits	254,683	254,683	18,581	198,961		55,722	78
200	Pool—Med/Surg Supply	75,000	23,920				23,920	0
211	Med & Surg Supplies		128,235	14,846	128,235			100
213	Drugs		1,317	140	1,317			100
214	Solutions		36,091	4,389	36,091			100
	Med/Surg Supplies	75,000	189,563	19,375	165,643		23,920	87
220	Pool—General Supply	5,789	2,553–				2,553–	0
232	Office Supplies		1,070	19	1,069	1		100
233	Copying & Binding		36	30	36			100
234	Printing		1,494	115	1,494			100
235	Printing Paper		633	83	633			100
240	Housekeeping Supply		1,880	323	1,880			100
243	Housekeeping Furnish		1,395		1,395			100
244	Linen Replacement		214		214			100
250	Maintenance Supplies		1,001		1,001			100
270	Food Expense		619	49	619			100
	General Supplies	5,789	5,789	620	8,341	1	2,553–	144
300	Pool—Travel/Entrtain	1,430	1,005		425		1,005	0
316	Workshop & Training		425					100
	Travel/Entertainment	1,430	1,430		425		1,005	30
320	Pool—Other Expenses	157,000	12,624				12,624	0
324	Contract Service		140,390	16,720	140,390			100

(continued)

EXHIBIT 10–22 (continued)

SUBCODE	DESCRIPTION	BUDGET		ACTUAL		OPEN ENCUMBRANCES	BALANCE AVAILABLE	PERCENT USED
		ORIGINAL	REVISED	CURRENT MONTH	FISCAL YEAR			
336	Equip Maint & Repair		3,700		2,950	750		100
372	Books & Subscription		286		286			100
	Other Expenses	157,000	157,000	16,720	143,626	750	12,624	92
501	Minor Equipment	4,000	4,000				4,000	0
	Total Expenses	1,446,644	1,561,207	153,176	1,496,785	751	63,671	96
	Account Total	1,446,644	1,561,207	153,176	1,496,785	751	63,671	96

OPEN ENCUMBRANCE STATUS

ACCOUNT	P.O. NUMBER	P.O. DATE	DESCRIPTION	ORIGINAL ENCUM.	LIQUIDATING EXPENDITURES	ADJUSTMENTS	CURRENT ENCUM.	LAST ACT DATE
4-60680-232	H01764	10/06/xx	Waller Brothers	.85			.85	10/18
4-60680-336	H07584	07/24/xx	Scaletronix Inc	750.00			750.00	08/01
			Account Total	750.85			750.85	

Source: Courtesy of the University of South Alabama Medical Center, Mobile, Alabama. Reprinted with permission.

Motivational Aspects of Budgeting

Budgeting can be a motivating force for personnel if current programs must increase in effectiveness and efficiency to remain, if decentralization and staff involvement provide an increased sense of responsibility and satisfaction, and if merit increases, promotions, and bonuses are tied or linked to budgetary performance.

Budgeting facilitates communication within interdependent departments, thus increasing knowledge and understanding of other areas. It provides learning opportunities for future nurse managers.

Cutting the Budget

When the budget must be cut, planning is a vital aspect of the process. Budget cuts are happening today as hospital admissions and stays decrease and reimbursement takes on a new character. The form and the process of nursing management can determine the course of events when the budget has to be cut.

A nursing administration that delegates decision-making to the lowest level and encourages participative management is an effective administration. When clinical nurses are informed at the unit level and invited to give their input, they can help with suggestions for cutting costs. They will gladly implement and support the activities they recognize as resulting partly from their input. A nursing organization that promotes self-direction at the levels of clinical nurse, nurse manager, clinical

consultant, and executive nurse will support direction to reduce costs and to increase productivity and profits. As an example, when a hospital CEO discovered that self-pay patient care was the only category not reviewed for use of resources, a clinical nurse established a review process. Physicians and other health care professionals supported this process.

Nursing budgets are enormous, and budgets for a single unit can run into hundreds of thousands of dollars per year. Pay awards or increases must be met by budget cuts (personnel cutbacks), use of less expensive supplies and techniques, or increased productivity. The latter requires more paying patients, shorter stays, and increased sales of all paying services. When personnel cuts are to be made, numbers make nursing vulnerable. Some cuts can come from all services, but nursing has greater numbers. The nurse manager who controls these numbers daily, weekly, and yearly has greater credibility. Many sources indicate that turnover is costly. The cost of turnover of personnel low on the salary scale is sometimes weighed against the higher cost of employees who are at the top of the salary scale. An assumption is made that long-time employees are better satisfied with their jobs and do better work, an assumption that needs to be validated through research.

As work load data indicate shifts from one unit to another, resources also must be shifted. Asking for volunteers, moving vacated positions, and using PRN pools can do this. Inpatient procedures in hospitals have shifted to outpatient procedures either in hospitals or at ambulatory surgery centers. New reimbursement rates, which are a system of ambulatory patient classifications, have been issued by the Health Care Financing Administration and

EXHIBIT 10-23
Accounting System Report

Computer Date _____
Time of Day _____
Acct: 4-60680
Dept: 60680

Report of transactions for fiscal year ending _____

Distribution code = 700
Medical Intensive Care Unit—Expense

SUBCODE	DESCRIPTION	DATE	EC	REF.	2ND REF.	J.E. OFFSET ACCOUNT	BUDGET ENTRIES	CURRENT REV/EXP	ENCUMBRANCES	BATCH REF.	DATE
130	Payroll Expense	07/07	64	900001		0-10080-118CR		35,017.03		PPS584	07/07
130	Payroll Expenses	07/21	64	900001		0-10080-118CR		37,516.33		PPS588	07/21
130	CM Total Professional Salry							72,533.36			
135	Payroll Expense	07/07	64	900001		0-10080-118CR		1,630.89		PPS584	07/07
135	Payroll Expense	07/21	64	900001		0-10080-118CR		2,454.11		PPS588	07/21
135	CM Total Tech Salry & Wages							4,085.00			
140	Payroll Expense	07/07	64	900001		0-10080-118CR		2,082.44		PPS584	07/07
140	Payroll Expense	07/21	64	900001		0-10080-118CR		2,264.26		PPS588	07/21
140	CM Total Office Salaries							4,346.70			
155	Payroll Expense	07/07	64	900001		0-10080-118CR		1,884.26		PPS584	07/07
155	Payroll Expense	07/21	64	900001		0-10080-118CR		2,051.29		PPS588	07/21
155	CM Total Service Empl Wages							3,935.55			
160	Payroll Expense	07/07	64	900001		0-10080-118CR		494.83		PPS584	07/07
160	Payroll Expense	07/21	64	900001		0-10080-118CR		1,022.81		PPS588	07/21
160	CM Total Student Wages							1,517.64			
166	Susp Corr/Accr Sal	06/30	60		S01544	0-13000-160CR		65.00		HJV002	07/10
166	Susp Corr/Accr Sal	06/30	60		S01543	0-13000-160CR		45.00		HJV002	07/10
166	RVS Accrd Sal & Wage	07/01	60		075101	0-15300-220DR		40,318.00—		HJV001	07/10
166	RVS Accrd Sal & Wage	07/01	60		075101	0-15300-220DR		65.00—		HJV001	07/10
166	RVS Accrd Sal & Wage	07/01	60		075100	0-15300-220DR		45.00—		HJV001	07/10
166	Accrued Sal & Wages	07/31	60		075100	0-15300-220CR		51,780.00		HJV019	07/31
166	CM Total Accrued Salaries							11,462.00			
183	Payroll Expense	07/21	64	900001		2-77000-180CR		264.04		PPS588	07/21
183	CM Total Group Life Ins							264.04			
184	Payroll Expense	07/21	64	900001		2-77000-180CR		526.48		PPS588	07/21
184	CM Total Disability Ins							526.48			
188	Payroll Expense	07/07	64	900001		2-77000-180CR		65.81		PPS584	07/07
188	Payroll Expense	07/21	64	900001		2-77000-180CR		5,821.12		PPS588	07/21
188	CM Total Group Health Ins							5,886.93			
198	Payroll Expense	07/07	64	900001		2-77000-180CR		2,659.96		PPS584	07/07
198	Payroll Expense	07/21	64	900001		2-77000-180CR		2,930.66		PPS588	07/21

(continued)

EXHIBIT 10-23 (continued)

SUBCODE	DESCRIPTION	DATE	EC	REF.	2ND REF.	J.E. OFFSET ACCOUNT	BUDGET ENTRIES	CURRENT REV/EXP	ENCUMBRANCES	BATCH REF.	DATE
198	CM Total State Paid Retiremnt										
199	Payroll Expense	07/07	64	900001		2-77000-180CR		5,590.62		PPS584	07/07
199	Payroll Expense	07/21	64	900001		2-77000-180CR		3,019.55		PPS588	07/21
199	CM Total State Paid FICA							3,293.55			
211	Inventory Exp Alloc	07/31	60		075264	0-12100-140CR		6,313.10		HJV027	07/31
211	CM Total Med & Surg Supplies							14,845.75			
213	Pharmacy Distrib—Jul	07/31	60		075006	4-60730-213CR		14,845.75		HJV033	07/31
213	CM Total Drugs							140.34			
214	Inventory Exp Alloc	07/31	60		075264	0-12100-140CR		140.34		HJV027	07/31
214	CM Total Solutions							4,389.27			
232	Inventory Exp Alloc	07/31	60		075264	0-12100-140CR		4,389.27		HJV027	07/31
232	CM Total Office Supplies							19.49			
233	Xerox Expense—J/l 89	07/31	60		075008	4-60960-965CR		19.49		HJV026	07/31
233	CM Total Copying & Binding							30.21			
234	Print Shop Chrgs—Jul	07/26	60		075011	4-60960-960CR		30.21		HJV013	07/27
234	CM Total Printing							115.20			
235	Inventory Exp Alloc	07/31	60		075264	0-12100-140CR		115.20		HJV027	07/31
235	CM Total Printing Paper							82.69			
240	Inventory Exp Alloc	07/31	60		075264	0-12100-140CR		82.69		HJV027	07/31
240	CM Total Housekeeping Supply							323.42			
270	Inventory Exp Alloc	07/31	60		075264	0-12100-140CR		323.42		HJV027	07/31
270	CM Total Food Expense							48.61			
324	Nephrology Applicati	07/26	68		563631	0-15030-211CR		48.61		HPD850	07/26
	Accure Jly	07/31	60		075259	0-15030-210CR		3,520.00		HJV024	07/31
324	CM Total Contract Service							13,200.00			
336	Scaletronix Inc	07/24	50	H07584				16,720.00	750.00	HEN010	07/31
336	CM Total Equip Maint & Repair								750.00		
	Account Total							153,176.40	750.00		

Source: Courtesy University of South Alabama Medical Center, Mobile, Alabama. Reprinted with permission.

EXHIBIT 10-24
Accounting System Report

Account statement in whole dollars for fiscal year ending _____
83% of fiscal year elapsed
Distribution code = 700

Medical Intensive Care Unit—Revenue

Computer Date _____
Time of Day _____
PGM = AM090-B1

Acct: 4-30815
Dept: 60680

TAB CODE	DESCRIPTION	BUDGETS		ACTUAL		OPEN ENCUMBRANCES	BALANCE AVAILABLE	PERCENT USED
		ORIGINAL	REVISED	CURRENT MONTH	FISCAL YEAR			
040								
0/0	Inpatient Revenue	1,511,400–	1,511,400–	115,500–	1,146,600–		364,800–	76
	Total Revenues	1,511,400–	1,511,400–	115,500–	1,146,600–		364,800–	76
	Account Total	1,511,400–	1,511,400–	115,500–	1,146,600–		364,800–	76

Source: Courtesy of the University of South Alabama Medical Center, Mobile, Alabama. Reprinted with permission.

EXHIBIT 10-25
Accounting System Report

Account statement in whole dollars for fiscal year ending _____
83% of fiscal year elapsed
Distribution code = 700

Medical Intensive Care Unit—SP&D—Revenue

Computer Date _____
Time of Day _____
PGM = AM090-B1

Acct: 4-30818
Dept: 60680

SUBCODE	DESCRIPTION	BUDGETS		ACTUAL		OPEN ENCUMBRANCES	BALANCE AVAILABLE	PERCENT USED
		ORIGINAL	REVISED	CURRENT MONTH	FISCAL YEAR			
040								
	Inpatient Revenue		1,080,088–	101,637–	818,031–		262,057 –	76
	Total Revenues		1,080,088–	101,637–	818,031–		262,057 –	76
	Account Total		1,080,088–	101,637–	818,031–		262,057 –	76

Source: Courtesy of the University of South Alabama Medical Center, Mobile, Alabama. Reprinted with permission.

EXHIBIT 10-26
Accounting System Report

Computer Date _____
Time of Day _____
PGM = AM095-B1

Summary report in whole dollars for fiscal year ending _____
Distribution code = 750

SUBCODE	DESCRIPTION	BUDGETS		ACTUAL		PROJECT YEAR	OPEN COMMITMENTS	BALANCE AVAILABLE	PERCENT USED
		ORIGINAL	REVISED	CURRENT MONTH	FISCAL YEAR				
001	Prior Year Balance		302,976					302,978	0
002	Transfers								0
010	Income	16,419,272–	16,419,272–	1,342,529–	13,782,618–	13,782,618–		2,636,654–	84
020	Income			13,078–	127,981–	127,981–		127,981	0
023	Interest Income			1,353–	11,022–	11,022–		11,022	0
025	Original Budget	600,000–	600,000–	77,740–	1,236,565–	1,236,565–		636,565	206
026				191–	210–	210–		210	0
028	Bad Debt Recovery				169,932	169,932		169,932–	0
030									0
040	Inpatient Revenue			1,852–	29,682–	29,682–		29,682	0
041	Outpatient RF								0
042	Outpatient ED								0
050	Ded/Gross Revenue	75,009,000	75,009,000	8,904,127	72,586,402	72,586,402		2,422,598	97
099	State Paid Benefits	57,989,728	58,292,706	7,467,383	57,568,256	57,568,256		724,450	99
	Total Revenues								
100	Pool—Salary & Wages	1,416,748	82,157					82,157	0
110	Exec & Adm Salaries		170,518	23,443	170,518	170,518			100
120	Instruction Salaries								0
130	Professional Salary		210,392	15,839	210,592	210,592		200–	100
131	Interns Salaries								0
135	Tech Salary & Wages		11,906	1,195	11,906	11,906			100

(continued)

EXHIBIT 10-26 *(continued)*
Accounting System Report

		BUDGETS		ACTUAL					
SUBCODE	DESCRIPTION	ORIGINAL	REVISED	CURRENT MONTH	FISCAL YEAR	PROJECT YEAR	OPEN COMMITMENTS	BALANCE AVAILABLE	PERCENT USED
140	Office Salaries		840,893	79,028	840,893	843,866		2,973–	100
150	Craft/Trade Wages				143	808		808–	0
155	Service Empl Wages					154		154–	0
159	Temp Craft/Trade Wge					2,431		2,431–	0
160	Student Wages		20,975	2,678	20,975	20,975			100
164									
166	Accrued Salaries		41,158	10,264	41,158	41,158			100
167									0
168	Tuition Reimbursement		6,971	2,756	6,971	6,971			100
169	Budget Correction Salaries	1,416,748	1,384,969	135,202	1,303,156	1,309,378		75,591	95
170	Pool—Empl Benefits	340,007	116,982					116,982	0
180	Employee Benefits	187,747	205,413	3,318	421,300	421,300		215,888–	205
181	Unemployment Ins	41,307	41,307	7,722	22,717	22,717		18,590	55
182	Employers FICA	266	266	54	266	1,871		1,605–	703
183	Group Life Ins	91,969–	91,969–	435	91,969–	91,967–		3–	100
184	Disability Ins	9,090	9,090	1,015	9,106	9,110		20–	100
185	Teachers Retirement	4	4		4	4			100
186	Meal Books								0
187	TIAA–CREF Retirement	2,068	2,068	259	2,068	2,068			100
188	Group Health Ins	96,262	96,262	12,650	116,322	116,342		20,080–	121
190	Tuition Reimbursement	56,911	56,911	7,955	49,916	49,916		6,996	88

Source: Courtesy of the University of South Alabama Medical Center, Mobile, Alabama. Reprinted with permission.

EXHIBIT 10-27
Accounting System Report

Subcode summary audit report for fiscal year ending _____

Computer Date _____
Time of Day _____
PGM = AM095-B1

Distribution code = 750

SUBCODE	SUBCODE DESCRIPTION	ORIGINAL BUDGET	REVISED BUDGET	CURRENT MONTH	YEAR TO DATE	PROJECT TO DATE	OPEN COMMITMENTS	BALANCE AVAILABLE
001								
364100	General Hospital Fnd	0.00	30,653.57	0.00	0.00	0.00	0.00	30,653.57
364105	Burn Unit	0.00	22,495.81	0.00	0.00	0.00	0.00	22,495.81
364110	Intensv Care Nursery	0.00	4,438.37	0.00	0.00	0.00	0.00	4,438.37
364120	J Erwin Ped Surgery	0.00	942.96—	0.00	0.00	0.00	0.00	942.96—
364127	Heart Statn—Holters	0.00	14,205.00	0.00	0.00	0.00	0.00	14,205.00
364173	Helping Hands/3&4 Fl	0.00	3,618.70	0.00	0.00	0.00	0.00	3,618.70
364174	Telethon—C&W USAMC	0.00	32,797.51	0.00	0.00	0.00	0.00	32,797.51
364175	Heart Fund Donations	0.00	864.10	0.00	0.00	0.00	0.00	864.10
364176	Telethon—C&W	0.00	71,327.96	0.00	0.00	0.00	0.00	71,827.96
364178	WOCD/Palmer Mem Fund	0.00	1,403.81	0.00	0.00	0.00	0.00	1,403.81
364179	Telethon—C&W	0.00	122,923.92	0.00	0.00	0.00	0.00	122,923.92
364197	Payroll Inserter	0.00	1,308.00—	0.00	0.00	0.00	0.00	1,308.00—
	Subcode Total	0.00	302,977.79	0.00	0.00	0.00	0.00	302,977.79

Source: University of South Alabama Medical Center, Mobile, Alabama. Reprinted with permission.

EXHIBIT 10-28
Accounting System Report

Time of Day _____
PGM = AM047-H1

Responsibility roll-up report as of fiscal year ending _____

Revenue

Cost-Center 9-82301
Reports to: 9-81000

RESPONSIBILITY UNITS	BUDGETS		ACTUAL			OPEN COMMITMENTS C	BALANCE AVAILABLE A-B-C	PERCENT USED (B + C)/A
	ORIGINAL	REVISED A	CURRENT MONTH	FISCAL YEAR	PROJECT YEAR B			
Cardiovas Rehab	790–	790–		869–	869–		79	110
Revenue–Enter Thpy	3,968–	3,968–	2,960–	39,582–	39,582–		35,614	997
Chemotherapy–O/P Revn	90,729–	90,729–	15,107–	110,452–	110,452–		19,723	121
Clinical Research Un	268,800–	482,051–	34,340–	346,521–	346,521–		135,530–	71
Cardiac ICU	1,524,600–	3,254,816–	252,996–	2,426,084–	2,426,084–		828,732–	74
Orthopedic Cast Room	108,459–	108,459–	8,128–	91,765–	91,765–		16,696–	84
5th Floor North/Reve	31,592–	31,592–	4,013–	39,076–	39,076–		7,484	123
5th Floor South/Reve	2,054,000–	2,977,320–	236,359–	2,331,656–	2,331,656–		645,664	78
Psychiatric Unit/Rev	1,701,300–	1,725,507–	137,906–	1,463,792–	1,463,792–		261,715–	84
8th Flr Medical/Reve	2,315,220–	2,959,584–	216,324–	2,456,181–	2,456,181–		503,403–	82
Medical ICU/Revenue	1,773,840–	2,853,928–	244,778–	2,232,035–	2,232,035–		621,893–	78
Coronary Care/Revenu	2,148,888–	2,148,888–	167,130–	1,801,879–	1,801,879–		347,010–	83
6th Flr Surgical/Rev	1,787,100–	2,409,563–	172,079–	1,930,916–	1,930,916–		478,648–	80
Burn Center/Revenue	1,254,000–	3,090,809–	193,436–	2,155,646–	2,155,646–		935,163–	69
9th Flr Surgical/Rev	2,029,260–	3,122,028–	230,728–	2,446,790–	2,446,790–		675,238–	78
Neuro/Trauma ICU/Rev	1,504,800–	1,504,800–	111,100–	1,035,650–	1,035,650–		469,150–	68
Newborn Nursery/Reve	804,600–	896,817–	87,603–	794,535–	794,535–		102,282–	88
Premature Nursy/Reve	615,672–	615,672–	71,803–	596,432–	596,432–		19,240–	96
Neonatal Nursy/Reven	4,692,600–	5,468,373–	580,112–	5,178,067–	5,178,067–		290,306–	94
Obstetric Unit/Reven	1,930,440–	2,379,997–	217,489–	2,091,217–	2,091,217–		288,781–	87
Pediatric Unit/Reven	1,438,080–	2,013,282–	171,673–	1,658,513–	1,658,513–		354,769–	82
Pediatric ICU/Revenu	1,141,800–	1,915,268–	115,489–	1,208,778–	1,208,778–		706,490–	63
Delivery Room/Reven	3,396,552–	3,396,552–	410,192–	3,553,291–	3,553,291–		156,738	104
Emergency Room	4,922,867–	4,922,867–	446,310–	4,716,353–	4,716,353–		206,514–	95
Total	37,539,957–	48,373,660–	4,128,055–	40,706,080–	40,706,080–		7,667,586–	84

(continued)

216

EXHIBIT 10-28 *(continued)*

Time of Day _____
PGM = AM047-H1

Cost-Center 9-82301
Reports to: 9-81000

Responsibility roll-up report as of fiscal year ending _____

Revenue

	BUDGETS		ACTUAL			OPEN COMMITMENTS	BALANCE AVAILABLE	PERCENT USED
	ORIGINAL	REVISED A	CURRENT MONTH	FISCAL YEAR	PROJECT YEAR B	C	A–B–C	(B + C)/A
REV/EXP BY FUND								
Operating Revenues	37,539,957–	48,373,660–	4,128,055–	40,706,080–	40,706,080–		7,667,586–	84
Total	37,539,957–	48,373,660–	4,128,055–	40,706,080–	40,706,080–		7,667,586–	84
REV/EXP BY TYPE								
Revenues	37,539,957	48,373,660	4,128,055	40,706,080	40,706,080		7,667,586	84
EXPENSES								
Salaries								
Employee Benefits								
Med/Sur Supply								
Office/Other Suply								
Travel/Entertain								
Other Expenses								
Minor Equipment								
Cost Offsets								
Total Expenses								

Source: Courtesy of the University of South Alabama Medical Center, Mobile, Alabama. Reprinted with permission.

EXHIBIT 10-29
Accounting System Report

Computer Date _____
Time of Day _____
PGM = AM047-H1
Cost-Center 9-823010
Reports to: 9-81000

Responsibility roll-up report as of fiscal year ending _____
Expenses

| RESPONSIBILITY UNITS | BUDGETS | | ACTUAL | | | OPEN COMMITMENTS C | BALANCE AVAILABLE A – B – C | PERCENT USED (B + C)/A |
	ORIGINAL	REVISED A	CURRENT MONTH	FISCAL YEAR	PROJECT YEAR B			
Medical Nursing	1,446,644	1,561,207	153,176	1,496,785	1,496,785	751	63,671	95
Psychiatric Nursing	659,186	661,552	63,520	590,664	590,664	566	70,323	89
Staff Development	274,449	274,748	17,680	295,828	295,828	2	21,082–	107
Nursing Svcs-Admin	869,036	880,078	91,347	779,791	779,791	6,242	94,044	89
Clinical Resch Unit	211,846	222,854	17,962	250,545	250,545	16	27,707–	112
Cardiac ICU	429,808	429,807	3,424	53,440	53,440		376,367	12
Float Nurses Pool			110	2,589	2,589		2,589–	
Orthopedic Cast Room	27,195	27,196		12,461	12,461	1,172	13,563	50
Employee Health Nurs	155,423	155,423	18,779	149,601	149,601	5	5,817	96
9th Floor-North	527,221	527,222	46,442	496,133	496,133	98	30,991	94
9th Floor-South	521,411	521,412	40,785	461,240	461,240	2	60,170	88
8th Floor-Medical	810,508	894,965	109,696	1,131,504	1,131,504	1,557	238,095–	126
5th Floor-Shrd Supp	66,529	157,455	25,770	185,295	185,295	862	28,702–	118
Burn Center	546,449	940,030	77,567	836,022	836,022	3,353	100,656	89
6th Floor-Surgical	1,222,187	1,363,087	117,908	1,278,709	1,278,709	2,101	82,276	93
Surgical ICU	1,074,332	1,332,394	138,564	1,309,157	1,309,157	338	22,899	98
7th Floor-Shrd Supp	626,522	696,032	72,802	833,026	833,026	787	137,781–	119
Newborn Nursery	667,925	939,910	81,197	892,992	892,992	868	46,051	95
Intermediate Nursery	236,612							
Intensive Care Nursy	1,810,927	1,944,960	202,179	1,749,864	1,749,864	1,241	193,856	90
Obstetric Unit	628,047	668,254	64,748	632,055	632,055	226	35,974	94
Pediatric Unit	923,577	998,643	91,105	895,375	895,375	263	103,005	89
Pediatric ICU	560,288	645,410	48,874	568,314	568,314	50	77,045	88
Delivery Room	1,113,286	1,208,604	134,770	1,107,944	1,107,944	20,154	80,506	93
Emergency Room	1,613,253	1,691,149	160,935	1,524,713	1,524,713	13,885	152,550	90
Patient Transport	220,377	220,377	18,889	186,146	186,146	40	34,191	84
Total	17,243,038	18,962,769	1,798,229	17,720,193	17,720,193	54,579	1,187,999	93

(continued)

EXHIBIT 10-29 *(continued)*

| | BUDGETS | | ACTUAL | | | OPEN | BALANCE AVAILABLE | PERCENT USED |
	ORIGINAL	REVISED A	CURRENT MONTH	FISCAL YEAR	PROJECT YEAR B	COMMITMENTS C	A – B – C	(B + C)/A
REV/EXP BY FUND								
Nursing Division	17,060,420	18,750,317	1,771,862	17,527,171	17,527,171	53,402	1,169,746	93
Professional Division	27,195	57,029	7,588	43,421	43,421	1,172	12,436	78
Administrative Divis	155,423	155,423	18,779	149,601	149,601	5	5,817	96
Total	17,243,038	18,962,769	1,798,229	17,720,193	17,720,193	54,579	1,187,999	93
REV/EXP BY TYPE								
Revenues								
Expenses								
Salaries	12,382,495	12,461,654	1,256,095	12,391,869	12,391,869		69,785	99
Employee Benefits	3,031,241	3,033,250	239,363	2,487,863	2,487,863		545,387	82
Med/Sur Supply	1,502,492	3,020,154	262,420	2,447,985	2,447,985	30,781	541,387	82
Office/Other Suply		109,306	9,788	107,656	107,656	1,652		100
Travel/Entertain	43,989	45,788	2,209	27,555	27,555		18,233	60
Other Expenses	212,976	211,676	19,555	196,765	196,765	4,019	10,891	94
Minor Equipment	55,585	66,681	7,590	21,443	21,443	18,127	27,113	59
Cost Offsets	14,060	14,060	1,209	39,057	39,057		24,797–	273
Total Expenses	17,243,038	18,962,769	1,798,229	17,720,193	17,720,193	54,579	1,187,999	93
Net Revenue/Expense	17,243,038	18,962,769	1,798,229	17,720,193	17,720,193	54,579	1,187,999	93
Total	17,243,038	18,962,769	1,798,229	17,720,193	17,720,193	54,579	1,187,999	93

Source: Courtesy of the University of South Alabama Medical Center, Mobile, Alabama. Reprinted with permission.

EXHIBIT 10-30
Accounting System Report

Account statement in whole dollars for fiscal year ending _____

Computer Date _____
Time of Day _____
PGM = AM090-B1

83% of fiscal year elapsed
Distribution code = 700
Maternal Child Health
Education Fund

Acct: 3-64155
Dept: 64155

| SUBCODE | DESCRIPTION | BUDGETS | | ACTUAL | | | BALANCE AVAILABLE | PERCENT USED |
		ORIGINAL	REVISED	CURRENT MONTH	FISCAL YEAR	OPEN ENCUMBRANCES		
001	Prior Year Balance		3,624				3,624	0
020	Income				5,285–		5,285	***
021	Refunds				55–		55–	***
	Total Revenues		3,624		5,230–		8,854	144–
224	Recreation Supplies				60		60–	***
231	Postage				60		60–	***
234	Printing				257		257–	***
	General Supplies				377		377–	***
311	Travel			459	1,463		1,463–	***
314	Local Travel				27		27–	***
316	Workshop & Training			3,338	3,498	2,500	5,998–	***
	Travel/Entertainment		3,796	4,989	2,500	7,489–		***
422	Honorarium				425		425–	***
450	Expense Offset				1,000–		1,000	***
	Total Expenses			3,796	4,790	2,500	7,290–	***
	Account Total		3,624	3,796	440–	2,500	1,563	57

OPEN ENCUMBRANCE STATUS

ACCOUNT	P.O. NUMBER	P.O. DATE	DESCRIPTION	ORIGINAL ENC	LIQUIDATING EXPENDITURES	ADJUSTMENTS	CURRENT ENC	LAST ACT DATE
3-64155-316	H04118	01/26/XX	Perdido Hilton Hotel	2,500			2,500	03/22/XX
		Account Total		2,500			2,500	

Source: Reprinted with permission of University of South Alabama Medical Center, Mobile, Alabama.

will affect revenues from ambulatory services. Many more diagnostic procedures also are now being done on an outpatient basis; as a result, inpatients are often a sicker group, requiring more nursing care.

Because nurse administrators control multimillion-dollar budgets, they are powerful people. They are also vulnerable to personnel cuts. Much of this vulnerability stems from external controls imposed by state and federal governments and health insurance companies. Power comes from the ability of nurse administrators to use knowledge and skills in defending, directing, and controlling their budgets. They learn to hold the line on staffing and overtime and monitor for the appropriate use of supplies and equipment.

Legitimate Budget Activities

Health care organizations should be managed like other businesses. Charges should be determined from costs and should include allowance for profits or return on equity and for bad debts. The practice of cost shifting to make certain services revenue producers should be stopped.

Oszustowicz suggests the following seven-step system by which total financial requirements eventually determine the gross patient revenue equal to meet the financial needs of a department[33]:

1. Detail demand for nursing services and equipment needs.

EXHIBIT 10-31

Accounting System Report

Computer Date _____
Time of Day _____
PGM = AM090

Report of transactions for fiscal year ending _____
Distribution code = 700
Maternal Child Health Education Fund

Acct: 3-64155
Dept: 64155

| | | | | | | | | | | | | BATCH | |
SUBCODE	DESCRIPTION	DATE	EC	REF.	2ND REF.	J.E. OFFSET ACCOUNT	BUDGET ENTRIES	CURRENT REV/EXP	ENCUMBRANCES	REF.	DATE
311	Dorothy May	07/11	48		218418			458.65		HPC804	07/11
311	CM Total Travel							458.65			
316	Perdido Beach Hilton	07/19	48		220893			3,337.73		HPC832	07/19
316	CM Total Workshop & Training							3,337.73			
	Account Total							3,796.38			

Source: Courtesy of the University of South Alabama Medical Center, Mobile, Alabama. Reprinted with permission.

2. Detail direct expenses.
3. Detail indirect expenses.
4. Detail working capital requirements.
5. Detail capital requirements.
6. Detail earnings (profit) requirements.
7. Detail deductions from patient revenues.

Summary

It is important for nurses to have a working knowledge of the objectives of budgeting and of component costs. Every activity that takes place in a health care agency costs money. A standard must exist for assigning costs to user departments. The nursing department should pay its user share, and no more. Knowledge of the cost-accounting system will provide accurate information for budgeting and for cost management.

Efficient nurse managers use a budget calendar that covers formulation, review and enactment, and execution stages of the total budget process.

The major elements of nursing budgets are personnel, supplies and equipment (minor), and capital equipment. Generally, equipment that costs less than a fixed dollar amount is included in the supplies and equipment budget. A product evaluation committee is a useful process for ensuring that supplies and equipment will promote effective and efficient patient care. The capital equipment budget includes equipment that costs more than a fixed dollar amount; it is prepared separately from the supplies and equipment budget.

Evaluation is an administrative aspect of budgeting that in itself serves as a controlling process. Decentralization vests control at the lowest competent level of decision-making. Good budget feedback is essential if the budget is to be an effective controlling process. Good feedback includes information about revenues and expenses as well as internal comparisons of projected and actual budgets. The budget can motivate professional nurses to facilitate their development of innovations.

The belief of nurses that budgets are beyond comprehension can effectively sabotage the nurse's effectiveness. Spiraling health care costs, cost-management efforts, and increasing accountability from individual cost centers should serve as an impetus for nurses to learn at least the fundamentals of budgets and the budget process. Assuming the responsibility for budget work increases the nurse's potential realm of planning, predicting, and reviewing programs within the nurse's jurisdiction.

Similar to a nursing care plan, the budget is an activity guidance tool. It is a plan expressed in monetary terms and carried out within a time frame. To be an effective caregiver, the nurse knows how to develop and use a nursing care plan. Similarly, to be most effective as a manager, the nurse manager knows how to develop and use a budget.

APPLICATION EXERCISES

EXERCISE 10-1   Develop a performance budget for a cost center to be used as a model for a health care organization.

EXERCISE 10-2
1. Every hospital prepares the Hospital and Hospital Health Care Complex Cost Report Certification and Settlement Summary, commonly known as the Medicare Cost Report. Obtain the latest one for your employing or clinical experience hospital. Select a nursing cost center and complete Exhibit 10-32, Preparing a Budget for a Unit or Project.

This exercise has acquainted you with the Medicare Cost Report. You can use projected medical inflation rates to prepare a budget for the following year. If the inflation rates are projected to be 8%, multiply all costs by 1.08 to project and budget costs. You will note that intensive care units are budgeted separately. All other inpatient units are grouped as Adults and Pediatrics (General and Routine Care). To separate these units for revenue and expenditures, make the following calculations:

EXERCISE 10-2
(continued)

1. Select a patient care unit of a hospital: _____
2. Determine the number of patient days of occupancy for this unit (from the biometric records): _____

3. From the Medicare Cost Report determine:
    3.1. Total direct and indirect costs: $_____
    3.2. Total patient days: _____
    3.3. Divide the total direct and indirect costs $_____ by total patient days_____ = $_____ cost per patient day.
    3.4. Patient days for unit (from 3.2) _____ × cost per patient day (from 3.2) _____ = $_____, or approximate expenses for the nursing unit for this year.

For help, refer to Russell C. Swansburg and Richard L. Sowell. "A Model for Costing and Pricing Nursing Service." *Nursing Management* (February 1992), 33–36; Russell C. Swansburg. *Budgeting and Financial Management for Nurse Managers* (Sudbury, MA: Jones and Bartlett, 1997).

EXHIBIT 10-32
Preparing a Budget for a Unit or Project

Unit _____ Revenue Center Number _____

Direct Expenses (Directly Assigned)		
Salaries (attach position questionnaire for new ones)	$_____.___	
Employee benefits	$_____.___	
Personnel services	$_____.___	
Supplies	$_____.___	
Other	$_____.___	
Total Direct	$_____.___	
Indirect Expenses		
Depreciation of capital buildings and fixtures	$_____.___	
Capital equipment (movable) (attach requests for new items)	$_____.___	
Worker's compensation	$_____.___	
Life insurance	$_____.___	
Communications	$_____.___	
Data processing	$_____.___	
Purchasing	$_____.___	
Admitting	$_____.___	
Patient accounts	$_____.___	
General administration	$_____.___	

Plant operations	$_____.___
Biomedical	$_____.___
Laundry	$_____.___
Housekeeping	$_____.___
Nursing administration	$_____.___
Patient transport	$_____.___
Preparation	$_____.___
Central supply	$_____.___
Pharmacy	$_____.___
College of nursing (or other college)	$_____.___
Interns and residents	$_____.___
Other	$_____.___
Total Indirect	$_____.___
Total Costs (Direct + Indirect)	$_____.___
Total Charges or Revenues	$_____.___
Cost-to-Charge Ratio (Divide total costs by total charges or revenues.)	$_____.___
divided by	$_____.___
minus	$_____.___
or _____ %	

EXHIBIT 10-33
Management Plan

UNIVERSITY OF SOUTH ALABAMA MEDICAL CENTER
MANAGEMENT ACTION PROGRAM
FISCAL YEAR
TO: Russell C. Swansburg, Administrator
FROM: Gail C. Lee, Director of Social Services
SUBJECT: Objectives for Social Service Department, 1989–90

OBJECTIVE	AS MEASURED BY	RESOURCES		INTERIM REVIEW
		ADMIN. COST	OTHER COST	JAN./JUNE
4.3 Active membership on hospital committees by all professional staff	A. Participation on one committee by each social worker			
4.4 Increased involvement in patient education	A. Lectures given by professional staff for families and patients			
	B. Staff involvement in support groups			
	C. Distribution of literature to patients and families		$50/yr	
4.5 Involvement in staff development	A. Lectures for hospital staff in areas such as coping with stress, understanding hostility, etc.			

Management Plan

OBJECTIVE	AS MEASURED BY	RESOURCES		INTERIM REVIEW
		ADMIN. COST	OTHER COST	JAN./JUNE

Source: Reprinted with permission of the University of South Alabama Medical Center, Mobile, Alabama.

NOTES

1. R. W. Johnson and R. W. Melicher, *Financial Planning* (Boston: Allyn & Bacon, 1982).
2. J. D. Baker, "The Operating Expense Budget, One Part of a Manager's Arsenal," *AORN Journal*, 54(4), (1991), 837–841; S. Klann, "Mastering the OR Budgeting Process is Key to Success," *OR Manager* (October 1989), 10–11.
3. D. Osborne and T. Gaebler, *Reinventing Government* (New York: Plume, 1992), 237, 241.
4. J. N. Althaus, N. M. Hardyck, P. B. Pierce, and M. S. Rodgers, *Nursing Decentralization: The El Camino Experience* (Gaithersburg, MD: 1981); G. R. Whitman, "Analyzing and Forecasting Budgets," in C. Birdsall, ed. *Management Issues in Critical Care* (St. Louis: Mosby, 1991), 287–307.
5. Ibid.
6. D. Osborne and T. Gaebler, op. cit., 3.
7. R. N. Anthony and D. W. Young, *Management Control in Nonprofit Organizations*, 4th. Ed. (Chicago: Irwin, 1988).
8. S. Klann, op. cit.
9. B. Huttman, "Taking Charge: Selling Your Budget," *RN* (April 1964), 25–26.
10. G. J. Talbot, "Key for Successful Program Budgeting," *The Journal of Continuing Education in Nursing*, 14(3), (1983), 8–10.
11. P. F. Drucker, *Management Challenges for the 21st Century* (New York: HarperCollins 1999), 111–129.
12. A. G. Herkimer, Jr., *Understanding Hospital Financial Management* (Rockville, MD: Aspen, 1978), 132.
13. C. Sponselli, "Equal Footing," *Healthweek* (28 September 1998), 12–13.

14. R. P. Covert, "Expense Budgeting," in William O. Cleverly, ed. *Handbook of Health Care Accounting and Finance* (Rockville, MD: Aspen, 1982), 261–278.

15. J. Buchan, "Cost-Effective Caring," *International Nursing Review*, 39(4), 1992, 117–120.

16. G. J. Talbot, op. cit.

17. R. K. Campbell, "Understanding the Management Process and Financial and Managerial Accounting," Part IV. "Cash Flow Analysis and Budgeting," *Diabetes Education* (February–March 1989), 126–127, 129.

18. D. Osborne and T. Gaebler, op. cit., 119–124.

19. L. R. Piper, "Basic Budgeting for ED Nursing Personnel," *Journal of Emergency Nursing* (November–December 1982), 285–287.

20. Ibid.

21. E. Tzividies, V. Waterstraat, and W. Chamberlin, "Managing the Budget with a Fluctuating Census," *Nursing Management* (March 1991), 80B, 80F, 80H.

22. "Planning Your Replacement Budget," *Journal of Nursing Administration* (November 1990), 3, 17, 24.

23. M. Dickerson, "Product Evaluation: A Strategy for Controlling a Supply and Equipment Budget," in H. C. Scherubel, ed. *Patients and Purse Strings* (New York, National League for Nursing, 1988 NLN Publication # 20–2192), 2, 465–468.

24. C. E. Kleinmuntz and D. N. Kleinmuntz, "A Strategic Approach to Allocating Capital in Healthcare Organizations," *Healthcare Financial Management* (April 1999), 52–58.

25. G. S. Arges, *Estimated Useful Lives of Depreciable Hospital Assets* (Chicago, IL: American Hospital Publishing, 1998).

26. C. Tokarsi, "Creative Proposal Plays to Tough Crowd," *Modern Health Care* (4 March 1991), 53–56.

27. B. Aronsohn and N. Deal, "Navigating the Maze of Capital Equipment Acquisition," *Nursing Management* (November 1992), 46–48.

28. S. A. Finkler, "Performance Budgeting," *Nursing Economic$* (November–December 1991), 404–408.

29. Ibid.

30. P. N. Palmer, "Why Hide the Revenue Produced by Perioperative Nursing Care?" *AORN Journal* (June 1984), 1122–1123.

31. In business and industry, bad debts are considered an expense of doing business. In hospitals, bad debt is subtracted from revenue. It becomes a reduction of revenue rather than a cost of doing business. Medicare or Medicaid does not allow profit or return on equity except for profit hospitals. A few third-party payers allow a return on equity.

32. G. R. McGrail, "Budgets: An Underused Resource," *Journal of Nursing Administration* (November 1988), 25–31.

33. R. J. Oszustowicz, "Financial Management of Department of Nursing Services," NLN Publication 20-1798, (New York National League for Nursing, 1979), 1–10.

REFERENCES

American Hospital Association. *Managerial Cost Accounting for Hospitals*. Chicago: American Hospital Publishing, 1980.

Applegeet, C. J. "AORN's Budget: Planning and Forecasting Uncover Future Needs." *AORN Journal* (August 1989), 212, 214.

"Benchmark Data, Improved Productivity Help Team Save $6.9 Million in Labor Costs." *Data Strategic Benchmarks* (November 1998), 18–170, 161.

Borgelt, B. B., and C. Stone. "Ambulatory Patient Classifications and the Regressive Nature of Medicare Reform: Is the Reduction in Outpatient Health Care Reimbursement Worth the Price?" *International Journal of Radiation Oncology and Biological Physics* (October 1999), 729–734.

Brown, B. "How to Develop a Unit Personnel Budget." *Nursing Management* (June 1999), 34–35.

Cochran, J. Sr. "Refining a Patient-Acuity System Over Four Years." *Hospital Progress* (February 1979), 56–60.

Cokins, G. "Why Is Traditional Accounting Failing Managers." *Hospital Materials Management Quarterly* (November 1998), 72–80.

Drucker, P. F. "The Emerging Theory of Manufacturing." *Harvard Business Review* (May–June 1990), 94–100.

Esmond, T. H., Jr. *Budgeting Procedures for Hospitals 1982 Edition* (Chicago: American Hospital Publishing), 1982.

Esterhuysen, P. "Budgeting: A Serious Matter." *Nursing News* (May 1993), 8.

Finkler, S. A. *Budgeting Concepts for Nurse Managers*, 2nd. Ed. (Philadelphia: W. B. Saunders, 1992).

Goetz, J. F. and Smith, H. L. "Zero Base Budgeting for Nursing Services: An Opportunity for Cost Containment." *Nursing Forum* (February 1980), 122–137.

Hahn, A. D. "Payment Reform Will Shift Home Care Agency Valuation Parameters." *Healthcare Financial Management* (December 1998), 31–34.

Hallows, D. A. "Budget Processes and Budgeting in the New Authorities." *Nursing Times* (4 August 1982), 1309–1311.

Hancock, C. "The Nursing Budget." *Nursing Mirror* (20 October 1982), 47–48.

Hauser, R. C., D. E. Edwards, and J. T. Edwards. "Cash Budgeting: An Underutilized Resource Management Tool in Not-for-Profit Health Care Entities." *Hospital Health Services Administration* (fall 1991), 439–446.

Hicks, L. L. and Boles, K. E. "Why Health Economics?" *Nursing Economics* (May–June 1984), 175–180.

Hutton, J., and Moss, D. "Budgetary Control: The Role of the Director of Nursing Services and Treasurers." *Nursing Times* (11 August 1982), 1364–1365.

Johnson, K. P. "Revenue Budgeting/Rate Setting." in William O. Cleverly, ed. *Handbook of Health Care Accounting and Finance* (Rockville, MD: Aspen, 1982), 279–311

Kaden, R. J. "Ensuring Adequate Payment for the Use of New Technology." *Healthcare Financial Management* (February 1998), 46–52.

Kilty, G. L. "Baseline Budgeting for Continuous Improvement." *Hospitals Materials Management Quarterly* (May 1999), 29–32.

La Violette, S. "Classification Systems Remedy Billing Inequity." *Modern Healthcare* (September 1979), 32–33.

Lyne, M. "Grasping the Challenge." *Nursing Times* (November 23, 1983), 11–12.

Marriner, A. "Budgetary Management." *The Journal of Continuing Education in Nursing* (November–December 1980), 11–14.

McCarty, P. "Nursing Administrators Control Millions." *The American Nurse* (20 September 1979), 1, 8, 19.

Matson, T. and J. Georgoulakis. "Outpatient PPS Will Create Hospitals' Greatest Challenge." *Health Care Strategic Management* (November 1999), 10–13.

Department of Health and Human Services (HHS), Health Care Financing Administration (HCFA). "Medicare Program; Changes to the Hospital Inpatient Prospective Payment Systems and Fiscal Year 2000 Rates. Final Rule." *Federal Register* (30 July 1999), 41489–41641.

Narayanasamy, A. "Evaluation of the Budgeting Process in Nurse Education." *Nurse Education Today* (August 1990), 245–252.

Orem, D. E. *Nursing Concepts of Practice*, 5th Ed. (New York: McGraw-Hill, 1995).

Rowsell, G. "Economics of Health Care." *AARN Newsletter*, 37(7) (July–August 1981), 6–8.

Ruskowski, U. "A Budget Orientation Tool for Nurse Managers." *Dimensions in Health Service* (December 1980), 30–31.

Schirm, V., T. Albanese, and T. N. Garland. "Understanding Nursing Home Quality of Care: Incorporating Caregivers' Perceptions Through Structure, Process, and Outcome." *Quality Management Health Care* (fall 1999), 55–63.

Seawell, V. L. 1994. *Chart of Accounts for Hospitals: An Accounting and Reporting Reference Guide* (Burr Ridge, IL: Probus, 1994).

Shmueli, A., and J. Glazer. "Addressing the Inequity of Capitation by Variable Soft Contracts." *Health Economics* (June 1999), 335–343.

Sonberg, V. and Vestal, K. E. "Nursing as a Business." *Nursing Clinics of North America*, 18(3) (September 1983), 491–498.

Starck, P. L., and B. Bailes. "The Budget Process in Schools of Nursing: A Primer for the Novice Administrator." *Journal of Professional Nursing* (March–April 1996), 69–75.

Suver, J. D. "Zero Base Budgeting." In William O. Cleverly, ed. *Handbook of Health Care Accounting and Finance* (Rockville, MD: Aspen, 1982), 353–391.

Swansburg, R. C., and Swansburg, P. W. *The Nurse Manager's Guide to Financial Management* (Rockville, MD: Aspen, 1988).

Thurgood, J. "Definitions and Explanations of the New Financial Vocabulary." *British Journal of Nursing* (March 1993), 295–296.

Trofino, J. "Managing the Budget Crunch." *Nursing Management* (October 1984), 42–47.

Vracin, R. A. "Capital Budgeting." In W. O. Cleverly, ed. *Handbook of Health Care Accounting and Finance*. (Gaithersburg, MD: Aspen, 1982), 323–351.

Ward, D. L. "Operational Finance and Budgeting." In P. R. Kongstvedt, ed. *The Managed Care Handbook*, 2nd. Ed. (Gaithersberg, MD: Aspen, 1993): 281–298.

Wild, J., and L. Imbrogno. "Market Changes Create Need for Practice Budgets." *Healthcare Financial Management* (July 1996), 77–78.

Willock, M. and C. Motley. "Financial and Material Management." *International Anesthesiology Clinic* (winter 1998), 41–57.

Zachry, B. R. and R. L. Gilbert. "Director of Nursing Planning and Finance: A New Role." *Nursing Management* (February 1992).

CHAPTER 11

Managing a Clinical Practice Discipline

Russell C. Swansburg, PhD, RN

LEARNING OBJECTIVES AND ACTIVITIES

- Discuss the use of nursing theory.
- Discuss differences among the modalities of nursing practice, including functional nursing, team nursing, primary nursing, case method, joint practice, and case management.
- Identify selected ethical concerns and ethical issues and make plans for resolving them.
- Confirm the assessment of cultural needs in patient assessment.
- Discuss the responsibility of the nurse manager for managing a clinical practice discipline.

As the twenty-first century begins, the excitement of applying results of the advancement of nursing research and theory to effect positive patient outcomes is within the control of nurse leaders.

CONCEPTS: Nursing theory, modalities of nursing practice, functional nursing, team nursing, primary nursing, case method, joint practice, case management, managed care, ethical concerns, advance directives.

MANAGER BEHAVIOR: Manager behavior uses effective human resource policies and procedures to manage a group of clinical nursing personnel to achieve the outcomes of the nursing process.

LEADER BEHAVIOR: Leader behavior supports the application of a theory of nursing by a group of nursing personnel. It provides a conduit for ethical deliberations by nursing personnel and furthers the inclusion of cultural needs assessment of individual patients.

Introduction

Nursing is a clinical practice discipline. Professional nurses want autonomy in their own practice. They want to apply their nursing knowledge and skills without interference from nurse managers, physicians, or persons in other disciplines. The effective nurse manager trusts the professional nurse to apply knowledge and skills correctly in caring for a group of patients. In turn, the clinical nurse trusts the nurse manager to coordinate supplies, equipment, and support systems with personnel in other departments. Clinical nurses trust a human relations management in which they participate rather than one in which they have rules and regulations imposed on them. They use the body of nursing knowledge (theory) gained in nursing school and maintained through continuing education and staff development to practice nursing as they determine it should be practiced. In doing so, they adhere to management policies regarding such things as documentation or quality improvement, because these requirements are also part of clinical nursing practice.

Use of Nursing Theory

In developing nursing as a scientific discipline, nursing educators and researchers have developed theoretical frameworks for the clinical practice of nursing that are used by clinical nurses as models for testing and validating applications of nursing knowledge and skills. The results are added to the body of knowledge commonly called the theory of nursing. Theory gives practicing nurses professional identity. It is based on scientific inquiry: nursing research. Each result of nursing research adds tested facts to nursing theory that can be learned by nursing students and active practitioners.

Models and Examples

Models are frequently used in the development of nursing theory. A model usually communicates in graphic format an abstract entity, structure, or process that cannot be observed directly. Models depict behavioral processes that cannot be observed directly except as indirect behaviors of those engaged in the process. They order, clarify, and systematize selected components of the phenomena they serve to depict. Models illustrate and clarify theories. Because nursing theories have not been applied widely, they are frequently described as models.[1]

Orem's and Kinlein's Theories

Dickson and Lee-Villasenor report testing of Orem's self-care nursing theory as modified by Kinlein. As independent generalist nurses, they did their research in a private nursing practice setting. They used grounded theory methodology to systematically obtain and analyze data from clients. As the clients spoke, the researchers recorded data, identifying self-care assets, self-care demand, and self-care measures with their clients.

In performing a content analysis, Dickson and Lee-Villasenor classified events as expressions of need, self-care assets, self-care demands, and self-care measures. They catalogued events by numbers of expressions of need—a perception of self, an action taken, a want, a wish, or a question—and by perception of self according to mind–body combinations. Events were also catalogued according to evidence of patterns of self-care actions that contributed positively to the client's state of health and number of self-care assets: action, motivation, knowledge, and potential.[2] Orem's general theory of nursing is used as a frame of reference in many instances.[3]

Roy's Theory

Roy advocates adaptation level theory to nursing intervention. She notes that a person adapts to the environment through four modes: physiologic needs and processes, self-concept (beliefs and feelings about oneself), role mastery (behavior among people who occupy different positions within society), and interdependence (giving and receiving nurturance).[4] Just as the individual patient adapts to changes in the environment, so does the nursing worker.

According to Roy, the goal of nursing is to assist the patient to adapt to illness so as to be able to respond to other stimuli. The patient is assessed for positive or negative behavior in the four adaptive modes. Once the assessment is made at the necessary (first or second) level, intervention is established by a nursing care plan of goals and approaches. The approach is selected to match the goal.[5] According to Mastal and Hammond, Roy's views are "that the developing body of nursing knowledge now contains verifiable theories and general laws related to: (1) persons as holistic beings, and (2) the role of nursing in promoting the person's maximum potential health and harmonious interaction with the environment."[6]

Frederickson illustrates application of the Roy adaptation model to the nursing diagnosis of anxiety. He describes or defines anxiety from the nursing perspective as exhibited by "poor nutritional status, reduction in unusual physical activity, and lowered self-esteem, in addition to concern for job security." The nurse diagnoses the symptoms of anxiety through assessment via the four modes and then designs and implements intervention that promotes client adaptation.[7]

Evaluation criteria for empirical testing of nursing theory were developed by Silva and expanded by others. Theory testing includes processes to verify whether what was purported or experienced is true or solves problems in one's discipline or practice. Silva and Sorrell define nursing theory as "a tentative body of diverse but purposeful, creative, and logically interrelated perspectives that help nurses to redefine nursing and to understand, explain, raise questions about, and seek clarification of nursing phenomena in their research and practice."[8] They list three alternative approaches of testing to verify nursing theory:

1. Through critical reasoning.
2. Through description of personal experiences.
3. Through application to nursing practice. (This concept has been applied at the National Hospital for Orthopedics and Rehabilitation, Arlington, Virginia, where the Roy adaptation model has been implemented throughout the hospital.)

Newman's Theory

Engle tested Margaret Newman's conceptual framework of health in a sample of older women. She indicates that Newman uses Rogers' concept of the life process and the relationship of the individual within the environment. In this model, aging is considered a natural process, the person's individual state being a fusion of health and disease. Movement is a correlation of health measured by a basic time factor and tempo.[9] Engle indicates tempo to be the characteristic rate of performing a task. Time is the second correlation of health. Tempo and time occur in a succession of events, rhythmic patterns of temperatures and movement, and patterns within the environment. Time perception and tempo are hypothesized to be altered by age and illness. The patient does self-assessment of his or her health as a criterion measure. Self-assessment and physician assessment of health have been shown to correlate. Self-assessment of health is altered by one's ability to perform everyday activities, by one's age self-concept, and by movement and time.[10]

In her study, Engle measured personal tempo, time perception, and self-assessment of health by using the Cantril ladder in 114 women age 60 or older. She found no age effect for time perception in this study, nor did Newman and Tompkins in similar studies. Nor was there any age effect for personal tempo.[11]

A significant relationship existed between time perception and personal tempo that could have significance for the patient and the clinical nurse. The patient or nurse with a physical or mental condition that alters personal tempo may have an altered perception of time. This could be true in older nurses in whom physical and mental states are more often altered. Further research in this area is needed, particularly as the population ages.

Levine's Theory

Levine indicates that nursing practice has mirrored prevailing theories of health and disease. Nursing has created an environment for healing: cleanliness, safety, and physical and emotional comfort. Nursing enhances the reparative process. Nursing became disease-oriented when diseases, rather than patients, were the focus of treatment. As nurses became concerned with the multiple factors impacting the course of disease, they developed the total-patient-care concept.[12]

People respond to illness in individual ways. Nursing intervention should match the individual response, which is identified from observation and data analysis. Assessment reveals unique needs requiring unique nursing measures. Nursing supports repair and maintenance of a person's integrated self-homeostasis and equilibrium. Equilibrium is maintained by adaptation. The nurse intervenes to support successful adaptation to achieve a therapeutic or supportive role.[13]

Johnson's Theory

The Johnson behavioral system model is a theory of nursing practice. Johnson incorporated the nursing process (assessment, diagnosis-planning, intervention, and evaluation) into a general systems model. Rawls applied it to care of a patient for the purpose of testing, evaluating, and determining its utility for predicting the effect of nursing care on a patient. Rawls indicates that the model has disadvantages but is a tool that can be used "to accurately predict the results of nursing interventions prior to care, formulate standards of care, and most importantly administer truly holistic empathic nursing care."[14]

Derdiarian sampled 223 cancer patients to verify the relationship among the eight subsystems of Johnson's behavioral system model. These eight subsystems (achievement, affiliative, aggressive/protective, dependence, eliminative, ingestive, sexual, and restorative) function through behavior to meet a person's demands (see Exhibit 11-1). Illness disrupts and changes behavior sustained in the subsystems, resulting in negative effects on the behavioral systems. Changes in one subsystem initiate changes in others. Findings of this research indicated "fairly large, statistically significant (P<.001) direct relationships between the aggressive/protective subsystems and each of the other subsystems." The research presents a model for continued research of Johnson's behavioral system model with "implications for comprehensive assessment, early intervention, prevention of patients' potential problems, and ultimately for efficient care."[15]

Peplau's Theory

Peplau's theory defines nursing as a "significant, therapeutic, interpersonal process."[16] Peplau's theory involves such concepts as communication techniques, assessment, definition of problems and goals, direction, and role clarification.

Peplau states that four components make up the main elements of the nurse–patient relationship: nurse, patient, professional expertise, and client need. The nurse–patient relationship has three phases: the orientation phase, the working phase, and the resolution phase. During encounters with patients, the nurse observes, interprets what she or he observes, and then decides what needs to be done. Interpersonal relations

---

EXHIBIT 11-1
Elements of the Eight Subsystems

DRIVES	GOALS
Aggressive/ Protective	Protection of person, property, ideas, beliefs, and emotional and cognitive well-being
Sexual	Demand for libido, relief of sexual tension, and procreation
Eliminative	Expulsion of biologic wastes
Ingestive	Satisfaction of hunger, thirst
Achievement	Ego gratification, mastery
Dependence	Succor
Affiliative	Belonging
Restorative	Relief of fatigue

Source: Compiled from A. K. Derdiarian, "The Relationships Among the Subsystems of Johnson's Behavioral System Model," *Image* (winter 1990), 219–225. Reprinted with permission.

uses the theoretical constructs of concepts, processes, and patterns:

- †A *concept* is a small, circumscribed set of behaviors pertaining to a particular phenomenon such as conflict.
- †A process is more complicated—it is more comprehensive and longer lasting.
- †A pattern is made up of separate acts that may have variations but share the same theme, aim, or intention.

Interpersonal theory is especially useful in psychiatric nursing and is useful in relation to psychosocial problems and nurse–patient relationships in all clinical areas of nursing. The joint effort of the nurse–patient relationship "includes identification of the presenting problems, understanding the problems and their variation in pattern, and appreciating, applying, and testing remedial measures in order to produce beneficial outcomes for patients."[17]

Orlando's Theory

Orlando's theory of nursing develops three basic concepts:

1. Professional nursing has as its function the identification and meeting of patients' immediate needs for help.
2. Professional nursing has as its intended outcome or product both verbal and nonverbal improvement in the patient's behavior.

3. Regardless of its form, the patient's presenting or initial behavior may be a plea for help.

Schmieding applied Orlando's theory to solving problems in managing the behavior of clinical nurses. She recommends that the work of one theorist be used as the practice model within a given organization. This application of Orlando's model has helped nurses apply common concepts and a framework for nursing. The model could be adapted if the nursing staff synthesized the concepts of several theories.[18]

Other Theories

Wiens presents Meyer's model of patient autonomy in care as a theoretical framework for nursing (see Exhibit 11-2). With laws for advance directives and increased emphasis on patient's rights, the right to patient self-determination has greater implications for care providers. Historically, patients have been perceived by providers to be dependent and compliant. Autonomy competency includes a repertory of skills or abilities that contribute to an individual's life plan of value, emotional ties, and personal ideals:

- Self-reference, where a person recognizes his or her response to life situations.
- Self-direction, where a person expresses himself or herself in ways considered fitting and worthy of self.

EXHIBIT 11-2
Patient Control in the Nurse–Patient Relationship

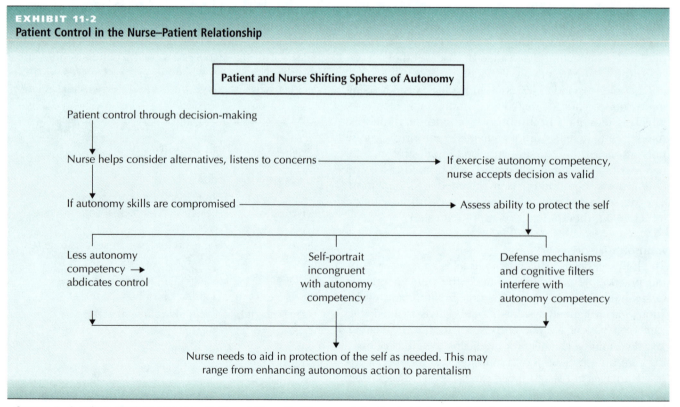

Source: A. G. Wiens. "Patient Autonomy in Care: A Theoretical Framework for Nursing." *Journal of Professional Nursing* (March–April 1993), 102. Reprinted with permission.

- Self-definition, where a person knows and acts as his or her true self.
- Self-discovery, where a person examines his or her socialization for self-understanding and future self-control.
- Self-portrait or self-concept.

Patients need to be encouraged to be autonomous and to ask questions and make decisions about their care. Nurses will have to change their nurse–patient relationships to accommodate autonomy competency in patients.

Illness decreases the patient's autonomy competency. To accomplish autonomy competency requires that patients be encouraged to make decisions regarding their care. Frequently, as patients become increasingly autonomy-competent, they are viewed as noncompliant troublemakers. Informed consent requires decision-making and truth telling. In the case of truth telling, providers need to be kind and caring.[19]

Sociotechnical systems theory views an organization as an open and living system interacting with the environment. The components of this system are social, technological, physical design, and work setting. The system produces products or services. Employers participate in designing and redesigning work and jobs to achieve a high-quality work life. More studies are needed to test the assumption that the work environment is important to care delivery.[20]

Modalities of Nursing Practice

Several modalities or methods of nursing practice have evolved during the past 50 years. These include functional nursing, team nursing, primary nursing, case method, and joint practice. All are practiced in various forms in health care institutions in the United States and all may be practiced with case management and managed care.

Functional Nursing

Functional nursing is the oldest nursing practice modality. It can best be described as a task-oriented method in which a particular nursing function is assigned to each staff member. One registered nurse is responsible for administering medications, one for providing treatments, and one for managing intravenous administration; one licensed nurse is assigned admissions and discharges, and another gives bed baths; a nurse's aide makes beds and passes meal trays. No nurse is responsible for total care of any patient. The method divides the tasks to be done, with each person being responsible to the nurse manager, who coordinates and over-

sees the care. It is efficient and the best system for a nursing staff confronted with a large patient load and a shortage of professional nurses.

The advantage of functional nursing is that it accomplishes the most work in the shortest amount of time. Its disadvantages are that:

- It fragments nursing care.
- It decreases the nurse's accountability and responsibility.
- It makes the nurse–client relationship difficult to establish, if it is ever achieved.
- It gives professional nursing low status in terms of responsibility for patient care.

Functional nursing was largely a development of the World War II era, when large numbers of nurses entered military service and ancillary personnel were trained to staff many nursing functions in hospitals. It is still alive and well in many institutions.

Team Nursing

Team nursing developed in the early 1950s when various nursing leaders decided that a team approach could unify the different categories of nursing workers. Under the leadership of a professional nurse, a group of nurses work together to fulfill the full functions of professional nurses. Patients are assigned to a team consisting of a registered nurse as a team leader and other staff—RNs, LPNs, and aides—as team members. The team leader is responsible for coordinating the total care of a block of patients and is the leadership figure.

The intent of team nursing is to provide patient-centered care. The patient's nursing care needs are identified and met through nursing diagnosis and prescription. Ward clerks and unit managers perform the nonnursing functions of the unit. The process requires planning, with the objective of taking nursing personnel to the bedside so that they can focus on nursing care of patients.

Implementing team nursing requires study of the literature on the team plan, development of a philosophy of team nursing, planning for appropriate utilization of all categories of nursing workers, and planning for team conferences, nursing care plans, and development of team leadership. Exhibit 11-3 depicts schema for a team nursing organization, with team members performing different but coordinated roles in self-managed work teams. The following is a summary of the team plan:

> The team plan gives priorities to the development of leadership potential—leadership in the practice of nursing—leadership that is creative and that encourages improvement of communications among team members, patients, and leaders. It gives priority to emphasis on

EXHIBIT 11-3
Team Nursing Organization

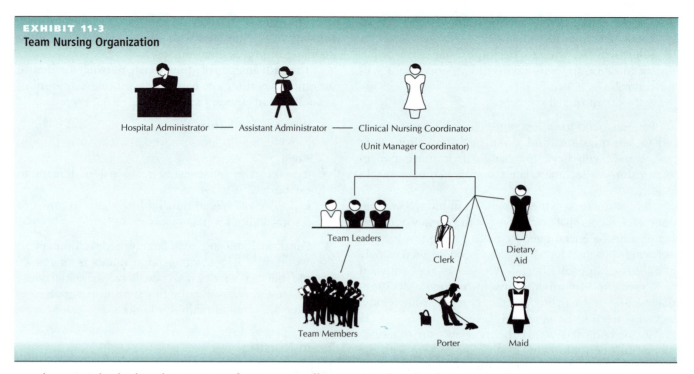

Hospital Administrator — Assistant Administrator — Clinical Nursing Coordinator
(Unit Manager Coordinator)

Team Leaders

Clerk

Dietary Aid

Team Members

Porter

Maid

democratic leadership, the nurturing of cooperative effort and free expression of ideas of all team members. It gives priority to motivation of people to grow to this self-approved or maximum level of performance. Through the team plan the contributions of all team members in improving patient care are recognized. Priority is given to the strengthening of their weaknesses.

Patient-centered care employs effective supervision and recognizes that personnel are the media by which the objectives are met in a cooperative effort between team leaders and team members. Through supervision the team leader identifies nursing care goals; identifies team members' needs; focuses on fulfilling goals and needs; motivates team members to grow as workers and citizens; guides team members to help set and meet high standards of patient care and job performance—all of them supporting the priority of practicing nursing.[21]

The advantages of team nursing are as follows:

- It involves all team members in planning patients' nursing care through team conferences and written nursing care plans.
- It provides the best care at the lowest cost, according to some advocates.

Disadvantages of team nursing include the following:

- It can lead to fragmentation of care if the concept is not implemented totally.
- It can be difficult to find time for team conferences and care plans.
- It allows the registered nurse who is the team leader to have the only significant responsibility and authority.

The disadvantages of team nursing can be overcome by educating competent team leaders in the principles of nursing team leadership.

Primary Nursing

Primary nursing is an extension of the principle of decentralization of authority, with the primary authority for all decisions about the nursing process being centered in the person of the professional nurse. The primary nurse is assigned to care for the patient's total needs for the duration of the hospital stay. Responsibility covers a 24-hour period, with associate nurses providing care when the primary nurse is not available. The care given is planned and prescribed totally by the primary nurse.

Marram, Schlegel, and Bevis state that "primary nursing . . . is the distribution of nursing so that the total care of an individual is the responsibility of one nurse, not many nurses."[22] They indicate autonomy to be the key to the development of professional nursing. The following are characteristics of the primary nursing modality:

1. The primary nurse has responsibility for the nursing care of the patient 24 hours a day, from hospital admission through discharge.
2. Assessment of nursing care needs, collaboration with the patient and other health professionals, and formulation of the plan of care are all in the hands of the primary nurse.

3. Execution of the nursing care plan is delegated by the primary nurse to a secondary nurse during other shifts.
4. The primary nurse consults with nurse managers.
5. Authority, accountability, and autonomy rest with the primary nurse.[23]

Fagin states that research studies on primary nursing showed that it reduced hospital stays and complications of renal transplant patients at the University of Michigan Medical Center in Ann Arbor, where the savings were $51,000 in one year. Primary nursing at Evanston (Illinois) Hospital near Chicago resulted in fewer nursing hours and less salary expense per patient during a 5-year period. Nurses aides had 27% unoccupied time per day, whereas registered nurses had 8% unoccupied time at Rush Presbyterian. Also, turnover was decreased in the operating room, with an increased registered nurse-to-operating room technician ratio. Other studies indicate that primary nursing saves money; increases job satisfaction, group adhesion, and patient satisfaction; and decreases costs of overtime, sick time, and compensatory time.[24]

The following are advantages of primary nursing:

- It provides for increased autonomy on the part of the nurse, thus increasing motivation, responsibility, and accountability.
- It ensures more continuity of care as the primary nurse gives or directs care throughout hospitalization.
- It makes available increased knowledge of the patient's psychosocial and physical needs, because the primary nurse does the history and physical assessment, develops the care plan, and acts as liaison between the patient and other health workers.
- It leads to increased rapport and trust between nurse and patient that will allow formation of a therapeutic relationship.
- It improves communication of information to physicians.
- It eliminates nurses aides from the administration of direct patient care.
- It frees the charge nurse to assume the role of operational manager to deal with staff problems and assignments and to motivate and support the staff.

The main disadvantage of primary nursing is that it is said to require that the entire staff consist of registered nurses, which increases staffing costs. This has been disputed in cost studies, however. For example, money is saved when nonnursing duties are performed by other categories of personnel and are not taken over by registered nurses.[25]

In recent years primary nursing has been modified to employ nurse extenders as technical assistants to registered nurses. The registered nurses assess the patients, develop care plans, and direct others. Modifications of team nursing and primary nursing to merge the advantages of each will result in more efficient and effective outcomes. This is particularly true in the new health care environment.

Case Method

The case method of nursing provides for a registered nurse-to-client ratio of 1:1 and constant care for a specified period of time. Examples are private duty, intensive care, and community health nurses. This method is similar to that of primary nursing, except that relief nurses on other shifts are not associate registered nurses.

Joint Practice

Joint practice is more than a modality. It entails nurses and physicians collaborating as colleagues to provide patient care. Nurses and physicians work together to define their roles within the joint practice setting, such goals being reciprocal and complementary rather than mutually exclusive. They may use mutually agreed on protocols to manage care within a primary setting.[26]

The primary nursing modality is preferred for joint practice, or collaborative practice. There must be an adequate number of professional nurses who are freed from nonnursing tasks. Decision-making is decentralized, and in-service education and certification are used to upgrade the nurse's scope of practice. Compensation is increased to match increased responsibility and accountability.

Physicians are required to accept responsibility for their part in joint collaborative practice. Administration includes joint practice nurses on every committee within the hospital. It takes as long as a year to establish truly functional relationships, because both physicians and nurses have to modify their behaviors.

The following elements are needed to establish successful joint practice in a hospital setting:

1. A committee of physicians and nurses with equal representation and equal voice in establishing the objectives and ground rules of operation.
2. An integrated patient record system.
3. Primary nursing and case management.
4. Collaborative practice with honest communication and encouragement of clinical decision-making by nurses.
5. Joint education of physicians and nurses.
6. Joint nurse–physician evaluation of patient care.
7. Trust.

Results of a joint practice demonstration project at four hospitals concluded the following:

- Patients receive better nursing care and are highly satisfied with their care.
- Physician–nurse communications are better, and there is increased mutual respect and trust between nurses and physicians.
- Both physicians' and nurses' job satisfaction is increased.[27]

Joint practice has developed rapidly in managed care organizations. This has led to issues and changes in licensure, clinical autonomy, prescriptive authority, and third-party insurance payments.[28] Nurse practitioners emerge as a group of highly educated and competent providers of patient care.[29]

Case Management

Case management is more than a modality of nursing. It has been described as:

> A clinical system that focuses on the accountability of an identified individual or group for conditioning a patient's care (or care for a group of patients) across a continuum of care; insuring and facilitating the achievement of quality, and clinical and cost outcomes; negotiating, procuring, and coordinating services and resources needed by the patient/family; intervening at busy points (and/or when significant variance occurs) for individual patients; addressing and resolving patterns in aggregate variances that have a negative quality–cost impact; and creating opportunities and systems to enhance outcomes.[30]

Simply stated, case management is a process of coordinating services and the case manager is the person who does the coordinating.[31]

The Center for Case Management's model of case management was designed as a clinical one. The model's underlying assumption was that caregivers of each discipline needed to have management skills, better patient care management tools, and more responsible administrative support to create quality clinical outcomes within a new cost-conscious milieu. The organizational structure is flat, with attending-level physician and "selected primary care nurses expanded into case managers to produce the integration of processes, aided by critical paths."[32] Critical paths have been integrated into CareMaps® (see Exhibit 11-4). It should be noted that the *CareMap® is used as the nursing care plan and for documentation.*

EXHIBIT 11-4
CareMaps®: The Core of Cost/Quality Care

CareMaps® are the newest breakthrough in cost/quality outcomes management. They have evolved from their longer version, Case Management Plans, and their condensed version, Critical Paths, into "user friendly" documents, which:

- *replace nursing care plans* as patient care plans[1]
- describe the contributions of every department
- show standards of care and standards of practice, and the timed, sequenced relationship between the two for a given case type, DRG, ICD9, or *constellation of problems*
- individualize care through analyzing and acting on variances
- provide a data base for Continuous Quality Improvement (CQI)
- integrate with *acuity* systems, *costing* systems, and *research*.

CareMaps® are cause-and-effect grids; i.e., staff actions should result in patient/family reactions or responses, which over time are "transformed" into desired outcomes. Staff actions are equivalent to Standards of Practice; patient reactions are equivalent to Standards of Care. CareMaps® are built on a basic formula:

Patient/Family
Problems ——————————————→ Outcomes
                    ↑
            Staff Actions

This basic formula describes very complex practice patterns, which themselves have many sources. *To build a CareMap® requires deep respect for the knowledge, concern, and tradition that the clinicians of each discipline use in the care of their patients.* They reflect good practice and can never replace good judgement.

FORMAT
CareMaps®, like their Critical Path predecessors, are simplistic charts that graph phenomena associated with a homogeneous patient population on two axes: action vs. time. Critical Paths graph multidisciplinary staffs' actions in terms of interventions against the timeline most appropriate for the phase of treatment of a specific population. CareMaps® go an additional step by including patient/family actions in terms of responses to staffs' interventions.

Classic Critical Path		Time →
Patient/Family Actions	problems	
Multidisciplinary Staff Actions	categories	

Patient/Family actions are categorized by problem statements, which transform into intermediate goals and, by the last time frame, outcomes. Patient/Family actions are measurable and behavioral and may include responses in the

(continued)

EXHIBIT 11-4 *(continued)*

realms of physiological, self-care, activities of daily living, fol-low-up plans, psychological, and absence of complications often related to their medical diagnoses. In 1987, Stetler and DeZell suggested four generic categories that should always be considered for inclusion in problem outcome statements:[2]

1. **Potential for Complications Self-care.** Presence of risk factors that may limit a patient's ability to manage his or her own disease and/or engage in health-promoting activities in the home environment.

2. **Potential for Injury Unrelated to Treatment.** Presence of risk factors related primarily to the person's general state of health and/or to the specific disease symptom that could lead to physical injury within the institutional setting.

3. **Potential for Complications Related to Treatment.** Presence of risk factors, at times inherent in the inhospital treatment, that endanger the health and safety of the patient if (a) appropriate preventive measures are not instituted and maintained, and/or (b) on-going observations and monitoring are not instituted.

4. **Potential for Extension of the Disease Process.** Presence of a specific condition or pathological process that carries with it a risk that endangers the recovery of the patient; i.e., presence of a risk that will be increased if a treatable extension or sequela are undetected. Multidisciplinary staff actions can be categorized in a variety of ways. Over the past five years, eight classic categories have emerged:
   1. Consults/Assessments
   2. Treatments
   3. Nutrition
   4. Meds (IV, other)
   5. Activity/Safety
   6. Teaching (Patient, Significant Other)
   7. Discharge Planning/Coordination
   8. Specimens/Tests

Additional Categories such as "Chest-Tube Management" or "Psychosocial" may be desired depending on the case type. Some institutions have incorporated their intermediate patient/family goals and outcomes into the traditional (staff action) Critical Path. Others have written the staff's actions into the patient/family outcomes section. Yet others have integrated actions and outcomes into their current data flow sheets. *Anytime both the staff's and patient/families' behaviors are graphed against a timeline, the concept of a CareMap®—by whatever name—is being used.*

A CAREMAP® SYSTEM

A CareMap® System includes the use of CareMaps® 24 hours a day. The heart of the system is the written CareMap® and the variances that arise from the standard interventions and outcomes. In a CareMap® System, variances are not bad, they are real and reflect the way staff are responding to individual patient needs. Variances can be categorized

per patient using standard codes, and when aggregated retrospectively for groups of similar patient populations, form a data base for continuous quality improvement.

The ultimate result of a CareMap® system is that unnecessary variance is reduced to a minimum because of an increasingly accurate learning curve that helps clinicians predict, prevent, and manage. It is not unusual for collaborative groups to begin developing CareMaps® for the more straightforward diagnoses, proceed to several varieties of that map, then combine constellations of problems, and finally map care for the patient populations that were initially felt to be totally unpredictable.

Currently, CareMaps® are used either on paper as references only, on paper as permanent documentation, on personal computers, or on mainframes. As institutions and clinicians become increasingly comfortable with CareMap® development, and as computer systems convert to CareMap® systems, higher percentages of patients will be managed by them (with daily or per visit screens). Similarly, variances are presently being handled differently depending on each agency's goals for implementing the system in the first place. Minimally, patient/family and community variances are recorded in the medical record. A few institutions have decided to also include clinician and hospital-generated variances in the chart as well.

SUMMARY

A complete CareMap® System includes variance analysis, use of CareMaps® in change-of-shift report, case consultation, and health care team meetings for patients at more-than-acceptable variance, and continuous quality improvement. The challenge, of course, is creating a dynamic system of complex care management from a static piece of paper. This can be accomplished with a series of CareMaps® for different phases of treatment (i.e., Acute Myelogenous Leukemia: AML—induction, AML—consolidation, AML—fever and neutropenia, etc.) and the use of blank CareMaps® for anecdotal documentation or for those patients who require a totally individualized map. Any individualized outcomes and interventions written on a CareMap® are generally outside the variance field. When a patient's reason for remaining in the hospital changes in a major way (such as a patient having a craniotomy who remains on a vent), the CareMap® changes as well.

All professional disciplines should be involved in the formation of CareMaps® and education as to their use. Secretaries, computer and medical records department members, and the "forms" department are all integral to the implementation of a CareMap® System. Our future issues will address physician involvement in CareMap® Systems and Case Management, as well as other key development and maintenance factors.

NOTES

1. P. Brider, "Who Killed the Nursing Care Plan?" *American Journal of Nursing* (May 1991), 35–39.
2. C. Stetler, and A. DeZell, *Case Management Plans: Designs for Transformation* (Boston: New England Medical Center Hospitals, 1987), 26–32.

(continued)

EXHIBIT 11-4 (continued)

CAREMAP®: CONGESTIVE HEART FAILURE

LOCATION	DAY 1 ER 1–4 HOURS	DAY 1 FLOOR TELEMETRY OR CCU 6–24 HOURS	DAY 2 FLOOR	DAY 3 FLOOR	DAY 4 FLOOR	DAY 5 FLOOR	DAY 6 FLOOR
			BENCHMARK QUALITY CRITERIA				
PROBLEM							
1) Alteration in gas exchange/profusion and fluid balance due to decreased cardiac output, excess fluid volume	Reduced pain from admission or pain free; Uses pain scale; O$_2$ sat. improved over admission baseline on O$_2$ therapy	Respirations equal to or less than on admission	O$_2$ sat = 90; Resp 20–22; Vital signs stable; Crackles at lung bases; Mild shortness of breath with activity	Does not require O$_2$; Vital signs stable; Crackles at base; Respirations 20–22; Mild shortness of breath with activity	Does not require O$_2$ (O$_2$ sat. on room air 90%); Vital signs stable; Crackles at base; Respirations 20–22; Completes activities with no increase in respirations; No edema	Can lie in bed at baseline position; Chest X-ray clear or at baseline	No dyspnea
2) Potential for shock	No signs/symptoms of shock	No signs/symptoms of shock	No signs/symptoms of shock	No signs/symptoms of shock; Normal lab values	No signs/symptoms of shock	No signs/symptoms of shock	No signs/symptoms of shock
3) Potential for consequences of immobility and decreased activity: skin breakdown, DVT	No redness at pressure points; No falls	No redness at pressure points; No falls	Tolerates chair, washing, eating, and toileting	Has bowel movement; Up in room and bathroom with assist	Up ad lib for short periods	Activity increased to level used at home without shortness of breath	Activity increased to level used at home without shortness of breath
4) Alteration in nutritional intake due to nausea and vomiting, labored	No c/o nausea; No vomiting; Taking liquids as offered		Eating solids; Takes in 50% each meal	Taking 50% each meal	Taking 50% each meal; Weight 2 lb from patient's normal baseline	Taking 75% each meal	Taking 75% each meal
5) Potential for arrhythmias due to decreased cardiac output: decreased irritable foci, valve problems, decreased gas exchange	No evidence of life-threatening dysrhythmias	Normal sinus rhythm with benign ectopy	K(WNL); Benign or no arrhythmias	Digoxin level DNL; Benign or no arrhythmias	Digoxin level WNL; Benign or no arrhythmias	Digoxin level WNL; Benign or no arrhythmias	Digoxin level WNL; Benign or no arrhythmias

(continued)

EXHIBIT 11-4 (continued)

CAREMAP*: CONGESTIVE HEART FAILURE

BENCHMARK QUALITY CRITERIA

LOCATION	DAY 1 ER 1–4 HOURS	DAY 1 FLOOR TELEMETRY OR CCU 6–24 HOURS	DAY 2 FLOOR	DAY 3 FLOOR	DAY 4 FLOOR	DAY 5 FLOOR	DAY 6 FLOOR
PROBLEM							
6) Patient/family response to future treatment & hospitalization	Patient/family expressing concerns Following directions of staff	Patient/family expressing concerns Following directions of staff	Patient/family expressing concerns Following directions of staff	States reasons for and cooperates with rest periods Patient begins to assess own knowledge and ability to care for CHF at home	Patient decides whether he/she wants discussion with physician about advanced directives	States plan for 1–2 days postdischarge as to meds., diet, activity, follow-up appointments Expresses reaction to having CHF	Repeats plans States signs and symptoms to notify physician/ER Signs discharge consent
7) Individual problem							
Staff Tasks							
Assessments/ Consults	Vital signs q 15 min Nursing assessments focus on lung sounds, edema, color, skin integrity, jugular vein distention Cardiac monitor Arterial line if needed Swan Ganz Intake & output	Vital signs q 15 min–1 hr Repeat nursing assessments Cardiac monitor Arterial line Swan Ganz Daily weight Intake & output	Vital signs q 4 hr Repeat nursing assessments D/C cardiac monitor 24 hr D/C arterial and Swan Ganz Daily weight Intake & output	Vital signs q 6 hr Repeat nursing assessments Daily weight Intake & output	Vital signs q 6 hr Repeat nursing assessments Daily weight Intake & output Nutrition consult	Vital signs q 6 hr Repeat nursing assessments Daily weight Intake & output	Vital signs q 6 hr Repeat nursing assessments Daily weight Intake & output
Specimens/Tests	Consider TSH studies Chest X-ray EKG CPK q 8 hr × 3 ABG if pulse Ox: (range) Lytes, Na, K, Cl, CO_2 Glucose, BUN, creatinine Digoxin: (range)	B/G	Evaluate for ECHO Lytes, BUN, creatinine			Chest X-ray Lytes, BUN, creatinine	
Treatments	O_2 or intubate IV or Heparin lock	O_2 IV or Heparin lock	IV or Heparin lock	DC pulse Ox if stable D/C IV or Heparin lock			

(continued)

EXHIBIT 11-4 (continued)

CAREMAP*: CONGESTIVE HEART FAILURE

BENCHMARK QUALITY CRITERIA

LOCATION / PROBLEM	DAY 1 — ER 1–4 HOURS	DAY 1 — FLOOR TELEMETRY OR CCU 6–24 HOURS	DAY 2 FLOOR	DAY 3 FLOOR	DAY 4 FLOOR	DAY 5 FLOOR	DAY 6 FLOOR
Medications	Evaluate for Digoxin Nitrodrip or paste Diuretics IV Evaluate for antiemetics Evaluate for antiarrhythmics	Evaluate for Digoxin Nitrodrip or paste Diuretics IV Evaluate for pre-load after-load reducers K supplements Stool softeners	D/C Nitrodrip or paste Diuretics IV or PO K supplements Stool softeners Evaluate for nicotine patch	Change to PO Digoxin PO diuretics K supplements Stool softeners Nicotine patch if consent	PO diuretics K supplement Stool softeners Nicotine patch if consent	PO diuretics K supplement Stool softeners Nicotine patch if consent	PO diuretics K supplement Stool softeners Nicotine patch if consent
Nutrition	None	Clear liquids	Cardiac, low-salt diet	Cardiac, low-salt diet	Cardiac, low-salt diet	Cardiac, low-salt diet	Cardiac, low-salt diet
Safety/Activity	Commode Bedrest with head elevated Reposition patient q 2 hr Bedrails up Call light available	Commode Bedrest with head elevated Dangle Reposition patient q 2 hr Enforce rest periods Bedrails up Call light available	Commode Enforce rest periods Chair with assist ½ hr with feet elevated Bedrails up Call light available	Bathroom privileges Chair × 3 Bedrails up Call light available	Ambulate in hall × 2 Up ad lib between rest periods Bedrails up Call light available	Encourage ADLs that approximate activities at home Bedrails up Call light available	Encourage ADLs that approximate activities at home Bedrails up Call light available
Teaching	Explain procedures Teach chest pain scale and importance of reporting	Explain course, need for energy conservation Orient to unit and routine	Clarify CHF Dx and future teaching needs Orient to unit and routine Schedule rest periods Begin medication teaching	Importance of weighing self every day Provide smoking cessation information Review energy conservation schedule	Cardiac rehab level as indicated by consult Provide smoking cessation support Begin medication teaching Dietary teaching	Review CHF education material with patient	Reinforce CHF teaching
Transfer/Discharge Coordination	Assess home situation; notify significant other If no arrhythmias or chest pain transfer to floor Otherwise transfer to ICU	Screen for discharge needs Transfer to floor	Consider Home Health Care referral		Evaluate needs for diet and anti-smoking classes Physician offers discussion opportunities for advanced directives	Appointment and arrangement for follow-up care with Home Health Care nurses Contact VNA	Reinforce follow-up appointments

Source: The Center for Case Management, South Natick, MA. CareMap is a registered trademark of the Center for Case Management. Reprinted with permission.

A collaborative team approach is used when integration of care occurs across geographic care units such as the emergency room, coronary care unit, step down unit, and ambulatory clinic. Formally oriented primary nurses from these units join the team.[33]

Personnel at the Center for Case Management believe that 100% of patients need their care managed by a CareMap®. Approximately 20% of patients need a case manager in addition to or instead of a CareMap® system.[34]

In the restructuring of nursing care, Zander places increased emphasis on accountability, demonstrated in Exhibit 11-5. It should be noted that case management is not a care delivery system.

Quality improvement is an integral part of the case management system. Quality management is operationalized by the use of critical paths, CareMaps®, and case management, all of which provide the tools for accomplishing the nursing process.[35] When interventions and goals are recorded that are different than planned, they are termed *variances*. Variances show how the CareMap® and reality differ, both positively and negatively. CareMaps® present problems by defining quality as a product.[36] A variance indicates deviations from a norm or standard. Variance indicates intervention that works or does not work. Variances alter discharge dates, expected costs, and expected outcomes[37] (see Exhibits 11-6 and 11-7).

Variance that shows negative outcomes requires action to improve quality. Variance data are collected, totaled, analyzed, and reported and then result in

EXHIBIT 11-5
Expanding Scope of Accountability

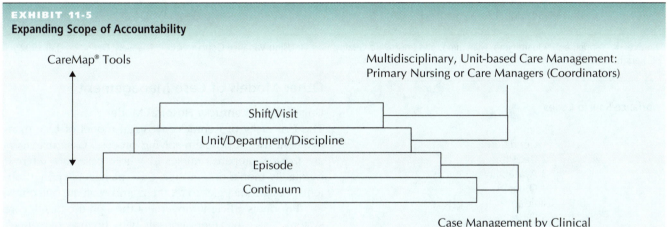

GLOSSARY

Shift or Visit: A typical 8-, 10-, 12-hour nursing shift, consult, outpatient, or home health visit by any discipline, etc. A "billable" amount of service.

Unit, Department, Discipline: The classic ways in which services are organized, i.e., nursing units, satellite pharmacies, dietary departments, GYN services.

Episode: All services given to a patient and family from the first contact to the last contact for that specific set of symptoms or procedures; i.e., chest pain to cardiac rehab, diagnosis through hospice, MD office through surgery and recuperation.

Continuum: An infinite time frame, which includes a person's health and life-style. May include chronic but stable states, such as well-maintained diabetes or handicaps.

Primary Nursing: A unit-based model for the decentralization of accountability for the outcomes of nursing care from the head nurse to designated staff nurses. Usually all staff nurses who work 4–5 shift equivalents per week are included as primary nurses, making a caseload (not shift assignment) number of 2 to 6.

Accountability: The answerability for outcomes and results. Accountability assumes that the necessary underlying authority to act has been acquired.

Care Management: A unit-based model for the decentralization of accountability for the outcomes of nursing care and an acknowledgment of the authority to coordinate all outcomes important to the treatment team. Nurses serve as care coordinators, sometimes in tandem with other professional disciplines. Only several nurses (avg. 1 to 4) are care managers.

Case Management: A clinical system that focuses on the accountability of an identified individual or group for coordinating a patient's care across a continuum of care; ensuring and facilitating the achievement of quality, clinical and cost outcomes; negotiating, procuring and coordinating services and resources needed by the patient/family; intervening at key points for individual patients; addressing and resolving patterns in aggregate variances that have a negative quality–cost impact; and creating opportunities and systems to enhance outcomes.

Responsibility: The fulfillment of distinct behaviors and expectations.

Source: Center for Case Management, 1993. Developed by K. Bower; adapted by K. Zander, 1994. Reprinted with permission.

EXHIBIT 11-6
Sample Variance Sheet

DATE	DESCRIPTION	PROB	PATH	SOURCE	ACTION	INITIALS
1-Feb	Son unavailable: out of town on business	8		A3	Ask ICU to call 2/2	AB
1-Feb	Afib	5	•	A1	Transfer to ICU	CD
	O$_2$ sat + 85%	1	•	A1	Lasix, O$_2$ 6L	
	glucose 250		•	A1	Diabetic regimen	
	no Swan Ganz	1		B6		
2-Feb	Unable to transfer to floor	•		C9	Order to drop pt. to general care rate	EF
	•	5		•		
	Afib—benign			A1	No action needed	
2-Feb	Echo not done		2	C9	Schedule for Monday	EF
	Hct 34, Hgb 13				Begin FeSO4	

Source: K. Zander, ed. "Quantifying, Managing, and Improving Quality. Part III: Using Variance Concurrently." *The New Definition* (fall 1992), 3. Reprinted with permission.

EXHIBIT 11-7
Variance Source Codes

A Patient/Family
   1 Condition
   2 Decision
   3 Availability
   4 Other
B Clinician
   5 Order
   6 Decision
   7 Response Time
   8 Other
C Hospital
   9 Bed/Appt. Availability
   10 Info/Data Availability
   11 Other
D Community
   12 Placement/Home Care
   13 Transportation
   14 Other

Source: K. Zander, ed. "Quantifying, Managing, and Improving Quality. Part III: Using Variance Concurrently." *The New Definition* (fall 1992), 3. Reprinted with permission.

decisions that revise CareMaps® critical paths, procedures, and other elements of the Plan-Do-Check-Act (PDCA) cycle (see Exhibit 11-8). Since CareMaps® can be used to document nursing care, are outcome-based, and have been found to be effective and efficient, nurses may want to use a computerized version for documentation.

Other Models of Case Management

University of Kentucky Hospital Model

The University of Kentucky Hospital model of case management uses a problem-solving process. Case managers are masters-prepared nurses to whom cases are referred by quality-monitoring groups. Case managers verify problems, design strategies to fix them, and evaluate outcomes.

Priority is efficient movement through the health care system. Case managers consult with finance personnel, administrators, and health care providers. They collaborate with physicians, primary nurses, and other health care providers. They establish therapeutic relationships with patients and families. A case management advisory board meeting takes place quarterly. Members do prospective or retrospective survey for clinical problems. Case managers follow up with diagnoses and procedure codes specific to the cases with verified problems. Sample problems of outcomes include poor continuity in patient's care, inadequate discharge planning, inadequate patient teaching, extended preoperative and postoperative stays, and poor nutritional status of patients.

Among the results were:

- Reduced glucose levels in diabetic, adult open-heart surgery patients (saved $11,585 in room charges during a six-month period).
- Decreased arterial blood gas charges in cardiovascular patients.
- Intensive care newborn patients home 218 days earlier than comparable patients during the previous year (saved $82,731 for Medicaid patients alone).

Management will pay for performance when hiring case managers in the future.[38]

EXHIBIT 11-8
Comparison of Generic Steps in Clinical Decision-Making

SCIENTIFIC METHOD	CAREMAP® SYSTEM CONCURRENT USE	CAREMAP® SYSTEM RETROSPECTIVE USE	CQI TECHNIQUE (PDCA)*
1. Assess	Assess		
2. Plan; using problem/ approach statements	Plan; using a CareMap® tool with collaboratively determined outcome measures	CareMap® tool	Plan
3. Intervene	Intervene		Do
4. Evaluate	Evaluate; using variance	Aggregate Variance	Check
	Compare		
	Consult		
	Analyze		
	Document		
5.		Inform	Act
		Discuss	
		Revise CareMap® if needed	
		Make other changes	

* PDCA Control circle: K. Ishikawa. *What Is Total Quality Control? The Japanese Way* (Englewood Cliffs, NJ: Prentice-Hall, 1985), 59.

Source: K. Zander, ed. "Quantifying, Managing, and Improving Quality. Part III: Using Variance Concurrently." *The New Definition* (South Natick, MA: Center for Case Management, fall 1992). Reprinted with permission.

Carondelet–St. Mary's Hospital and Health Center Model
Another model of case management is the Carondelet–St. Mary's Hospital and Health Center in Tucson, Arizona. In this model, nurse case managers work in partnership with high-risk individuals in the hospital (30%) and in the community (70%). Reports of application of this model of nursing case management indicate that it results in financial savings and liability defenses. It has been described as both a hospital-based and a community-based model of case management. It is case management in which the nurse manages and coordinates the entire spectrum of a patient's care in all settings, hospital and community. Effective case management wins the confidence of all team members, including social workers and physicians. Nursing case management supports the highest use of clinical nursing skills. In this report case management reduced total admissions, mean admissions per patient, mean length of stay per patient, and net reimbursement. The authors recommend mandating Bachelor of Science in Nursing qualifications for case managers, and five years of clinical experience. They worked out comparable arrangements with social workers.[39]

Lyon summarizes case management models as including such hospital-based models as the Center for Case Management model, the discharge planner and arbitration model, and the geriatric clinical nurse specialist model, and models such as the Arizona model that stretch across the health care continuum. Community case management models include the Denver and Indianapolis models. Lyon would call case management in hospitals managed care, as it does not make maximum use of community health services.[40]

Other Factors Related to Case Management

Bower reported case managers at Hennepin County Medical Center in Minneapolis responsible for[41]:

1. In excess of $1 million of direct cost savings.
2. Readmission rates for patients having major bowel procedures reduced from 67% to 26%.
3. Readmission rates for patients with cerebrovascular disorders (except transitory ischemic attacks) reduced from 43% to 31%.
4. Compliance with antibiotic protocols in patients having hip and femur procedures increased from 38% to 89%.

Nurses have been at the forefront of case management as it relates to moving patients through the hospital efficiently. There may be conflicts between nurse case managers and other providers within the community. Professional nurses should become educated about case management programs, interagency groups, use of interdisciplinary teams, and legal issues, with respect for clients' wishes and rights continually in mind.[42]

Strong indicates that clinical nurse specialists have the expert clinical and management skills to enhance planning, clinical decision-making, and evaluation of resource use. The case management system has been applied to promote cost-effective, long-term wellness in migrant children by addressing cultural, nutritional, and dental care needs and using available resources. This has also been done with homeless families. Case management identifies the clients' needs and makes and implements plans to meet those needs efficiently and effectively. Case management may be performed by a group practice of primary nurses.[43]

Referring to people with learning disabilities, Thomas describes case management applied to a client in his or her local community as managing a team of field workers who assess clients' needs and make action plans with them.[44] These plans address assessment, action planning, package development, and financial management. Case managers draw up a contract for clients' services. Contracts involving groups of clients may obtain discounts. Third-party payers usually approve contracts.

The package includes an estimate of hours required for one month's care and residential versus home care costs, and it breaks down costs into those for such workers as community care assistant, respite care home outreach worker, physiotherapist, and occupational therapist, and for transportation.

Thomas states that caseworkers are frequently social workers, and case management may develop into a new autonomous profession.

Dowling states that nursing case management makes the patient's nurse the central decision hub for the entire spectrum of patient care requirements and services.[45] It is matrix management. The common results of nursing case management fall into five primary areas:

1. Early, or appropriate, patient discharges.
2. Expected, or standardized, clinical outcomes.
3. Promotion of collaborative practice, coordinated patient care, and true continuity of care.
4. Promotion of nurses' professional development and job satisfaction.
5. Use of appropriate, or reduced, resources.

The model is the "critical path" forecasting physician intervention, diagnostic testing, ancillary department patient care, support department input, and supply and equipment requirements. The individual critical path is a communication tool for all care given. It is a production schedule. The critical path provides the hospital material manager with a dynamic distribution of patient care supplies and equipment needed in advance of any requests.

Hospital information supplements provide the information needed for supplies and equipment planning to be case specific. Just-in-time programs can provide patient-specific supplies for multiple-supply-retention locations on a nursing unit.

Research indicates that using the critical path technique for assessing the postoperative recovery of coronary artery bypass graph patients prevents complications, reduces lengths of stay, and reduces hospital costs. Nursing interventions such as use of inspirometers, resumption of activity, and patient education support this finding. Critical paths may be used by nurses to identify appropriate nursing interventions and their costs.[46]

Case management is outcome based. Outcome-based nursing practice was used at the Medical Center of Central Georgia in Macon. The population studied consisted of stable cardiovascular patients receiving specialty infusions. By treating them on the telemetry unit rather than in the coronary care unit, a cost avoidance of $46,121.83 was realized in one year. Patient classification systems estimate caregiver time and caregiver costs. Weighted salary of caregivers was $14.34/hr. in the coronary care unit versus $10.00/hr in the telemetry unit. Cost per patient day was $102.45 versus $49.23, for a cost avoidance of $53.22 per patient day.[47]

Zander states that the complete results of case management must include length of stay statistics, readmission rates, and some tally of patient satisfaction.[48]

Bower catalogues the reasons for implementing case management to be[49]:

1. A client–family focus on the full spectrum of needs.
2. Outcome orientation to care.
3. Coordination of care by team collaboration.
4. Cost management through facilitation through the health care system.
5. Response to insurers and payers.
6. A merger of clinical and financial interests, systems, and outcomes.
7. Inclusion for marketing strategies.

Patient Outcomes

Outcomes have been a major topic related to productivity in human relations management. At the University of Iowa College of Nursing, nurse researchers and practitioners have developed the Nursing Outcomes Classification (NOC). At the University of Iowa College of Nursing, the NOC has been integrated with the Nursing Diagnoses Classification, the Nursing Interventions Classification, and the Nursing Management Minimum Data Set.[50] Patient outcomes are the outcomes resulting from care of patients by nurses or an interdisciplinary care team. Patient outcomes include those related to patient satisfaction and health status, nosocomial infection control, and risk events and adverse outcomes. Activities related to patient outcomes are directed toward improving organizational performance continually over time.[51]

Ethical Concerns

Many ethical issues are directly related to the providing of patient care services. These have become more important during the past decade because of the increased sophistication of medical science and technology, interprofessional relationships, organ donations and transplants, AIDS, the uninsured, the aged, high-risk neonates, concern about practical limits on financial resources for health care, changes in society, and growing emphasis on the autonomy of the individual.[52]

Professional nurses implement the employer's policy concerning the moral responsibility of health care. They have responsibility for supervising and reviewing patient care, meeting quality standards, making certain that decisions about patients are based on sound ethical principles, developing policies and mechanisms that address questions of human values, and responding to social problems and dilemmas that affect the need for health care services.[53]

To fulfill this responsibility, professional nurses support nurses confronted with ethical dilemmas and help them think through situations by open dialogue. Nurse managers establish the climate for this. Davis recommends ethics rounds as a means of discussing ethical dilemmas. Such discussions can stem from hypothetical cases, case histories, or a case based on a current patient. Ethical reasoning requires participation by a knowledgeable person. Davis describes four ethical principles[54]:

1. *Autonomy.* Personal freedom of action is an ethical principle to be applied by nurse managers toward professional nurses, who in turn apply the principle in the care of their patients. The professional nurse is given autonomy to deliberate about nursing actions and has the capacity to take nursing actions based on this deliberation.

   Hospitalized or ambulatory patients may have diminished autonomy, and the professional nurse becomes an advocate or autonomous agent for these patients' rights. The patient is responsible for making decisions about his or her care, and the family may be involved with the patient's consent.

2. *Nonmalficence.* Avoidance of intentional harm or the risk of inflicting harm on someone is termed *nonmalficence.* The use of restraints is an area that pits the principle of autonomy and self-determination against that of nonmalficence. When risks outweigh costs, one must protect the patient. Side rails, safety vests, tranquilizers, and wrist restraints all have the potential for abuse.

   Discharge planning can prevent negative outcomes and potential errors. When errors occur, the nurse should acknowledge them to the patient or a surrogate, with full and immediate disclosure to the physician and the institution's administration. Nurses can protect patients from incompetent practitioners but yet protect their own rights at the same time.

3. *Beneficence.* Beneficence is the principle of viewing persons as autonomous and not harming them, contributing to their health and welfare.

4. *Justice.* Justice involves giving people what is due or owed, deserved, or legitimately claimed.

The four ethical principles of autonomy, nonmalficence, beneficence, and justice are being studied and debated as they relate to nursing research and practice, to drug trials including the use of placebo controls, and to cost-cutting in provider organizations.[55]

Many ethical issues relate to nursing and health care, including the issue of the right to health care. However, we do not have a law that says society is obliged to provide health care. The following are some other ethical issues:

1. The rights of individuals and their surrogates versus the rights of the state or society. This issue creates confrontations among consumers and practitioners and may lead to management efforts to cut costs by cutting services (staff) or closing treatment centers. A survey of the Association of Community Cancer Centers indicated that 84% of them staff oncology units higher than other medical/surgical units.[56]

2. The rights of patients unable to make their own decisions versus the rights of their family versus the rights of institutions.

3. The rights of patients to forgo treatment versus the rights of society.

4. Issues related to:
   a. Reproductive technology—preselection of desired physical characteristics of children, genetic screening.
   b. Organ harvesting and transplants.
   c. Research subjects.
   d. Confidentiality.
   e. Restraints.
   f. Disclosure.
   g. Informed consent.
   h. Patient incapacity.
   i. Court intervention.

5. Reporting of ethical abuse of patients and staff.

The American Nurses Association Committee on Ethics has published several position statements and guidelines that seek to assist nurses in making ethical decisions in their practice. These guidelines are based on ethical theory and the ANA Code for Nurses, an expression of "nursing's moral concerns, goals, and values." They are designed to provide nurses with guidance on a range of ethical issues, including the withdrawing or withholding of food or fluid; risk versus responsibility in providing care; safeguarding client health and safety from illegal, incompetent, or unethical practices; nurses' participation in capital punishment; and nurses' participation and leadership in ethical review practices.[57]

Nurse managers need to know the legal framework for their actions. They should help clinical nurses to balance teaching, research, clinical investigation, and patient care. All should work for social justice to ensure a desirable quality of life and health care services. Nurses may promote compassion and sensitivity through protest of public policies that reduce quality of or access to health care for the poor. They pursue human values, wholeness, and health values.[58] This does not mean that nurses must subsidize health care by working for lower salaries; rather they should work to have the cost shared by all of society.

A study of ethical issues and problems encountered by 52 nurses in their work in one hospital used a 32-item ethical-issues-in-nursing instrument. Results indicated that nurses encountered few ethical issues. The five most common issues were inadequate staffing patterns, prolonging life with heroic measures, inappropriate resource allocations, dealing with situations where patients were being discussed inappropriately, and dealing with irresponsible activity of colleagues. Ethical issues were more frequent in critical care units than in medical or surgical units. Since the frequency was not increasing, the study group recommended institutional ethics committees and nursing ethics rounds to sensitize nurses to ethical issues.[59]

A 1988 survey of institutions in the metropolitan New York area was done to determine how nurses were addressing ethical concerns in their practice. In this survey, 71 of 116 hospitals responded. Topics addressed by hospital ethics committees are listed in Exhibit 11-9; the

formats for addressing these issues are listed in Exhibit 11-10; and the ethical issues in nursing practice are listed in Exhibit 11-11. All ethics committees had nursing representatives, mostly from administrative and management positions. It was concluded that a majority of institutions do not adequately address nursing issues and concerns.[60]

Among the ethical dilemmas seldom addressed by nurse managers are ethical boundaries, particularly those involving sex. Nurse managers and administrators should provide continuing education to increase nurses' awareness of improper nurse–patient relationships, including accepting gifts and favors, doing business with patients and their families, being coerced or manipulated by patients, visiting patients at home while off duty, and making nontherapeutic disclosures. Risk environments include inpatient psychiatric services and chemical dependency treatment programs.[61]

Patients are still being denied pain relief by lazy or policy-adamant providers. Although letters to Ann Landers are not scientific, they are revealing. One writer wrote that a physician would not give her father pain medication the night before he died of terminal cancer. Reason: The physician would have had to walk to another unit for a small needle. In another letter, the wife of a terminal cancer patient requesting relief of intense pain was told by a nurse, "He has to wait another 30 minutes." The ethical and professional answer to such incidents is for assertive nurses to obtain adequate pain medication orders and implement them.[62]

One of the leading experts in nursing ethics, Leah Curtin, advocates creation of moral space for nurses to preserve their integrity. A nurse who believes an action to be wrong should not be forced to take that action.[63] Curtin states that since ethics deals with values as well as with facts and interests, answers to ethical questions do not fall strictly within the bounds of any one discipline. Because ethical questions are complex, they are puzzling, even bewildering. Since any answer we frame

EXHIBIT 11-9
Topics Addressed By Ethics Committees (N = 41)

TOPIC	NUMBER	%
Do-not-resuscitate (DNR)	29	70
Withholding/withdrawing treatment	10	24
AIDS	9	22
Allocation of resources	9	22
Patient's rights	8	19
Death and dying	7	17
Minors	4	9
Professional practice issues	3	7
Abortion	1	2
Prison health	1	2
Institutional issues	1	2

Source: C. Scanlon and C. Fleming. "Confronting Ethical Issues: A Nursing Survey." *Nursing Management* (May 1990), 64. Reprinted with permission.

EXHIBIT 11-10
Formats for Addressing Ethics Issues (N = 44)

FORMAT	NUMBER	%
Nursing meetings	29	66
In-service education	8	18
Hospital committees	4	9
Individual discussion/consultation	4	9
Hospital ethics committee	4	9
Interdisciplinary rounds	2	4

Source: C. Scanlon and C. Fleming. "Confronting Ethical Issues: A Nursing Survey." *Nursing Management* (May 1990), 64. Reprinted with permission.

EXHIBIT 11-11
Ethical Issues in Nursing Practice

FORMAT	NUMBER	%
Do-not-resuscitate (DNR)	31	44
Patient's rights	25	35
Professional practice issues	22	31
AIDS	15	21
Death and dying	14	20
Allocation of resources	14	20
Withholding/withdrawing treatment	7	10
Institutional issues	6	8
Abortion	3	4
Minors	3	4
Prison health	0	

Source: C. Scanlon and C. Fleming. "Confronting Ethical Issues:
A Nursing Survey." *Nursing Management* (May 1990), 64.
Reprinted with permission.

has inflections that touch many areas of concern, we cannot foresee all the consequences of the answers we choose. To solve an ethical problem, Curtin recommends that we:

1. Gather as much information as possible to understand precisely what the problem is.
2. Determine as many possible ways to resolve the problem as present themselves.
3. Consider the arguments for and against each alternative we can discover or imagine.

The nurse has an obligation to protect the welfare of patients and clients by virtue of his or her legal duties, the code for nurses, and nurses' social role. From a moral perspective, one cannot knowingly harm another person. Any freely chosen human act is right insofar as it protects and promotes the human rights of individual nurses. Professionals have duties to guide their young members, and nurses on all levels have mutual duties to support and guide one another.[64]

Values-based management stems from the actions of CEOs who set the stage for using a values credo of shared beliefs that govern the decisions and actions of top management. Two companies that do this are Levi Strauss & Company and Holt Companies. Their values include openness, teamwork, diversity, ethical behavior, and honest communication. Their priority is on ethics, human dignity, and self-fulfillment. The employees believe they make important contributions to the company, customers, and the community. Such companies find that productivity and products increase.[65]

Ethics committees should be established to prevent burnout. Their goals would include being a forum for expressing concerns, promotion of awareness and education, participation in clinical decision-making, policy and procedure development, professional identity, and linkage to other committees.[66]

Advance Directives

An advance directive is "a written instruction, such as a living will or a durable power of attorney for health care, recognized under state law (whether statutory or as recognized by the courts of the state) and relating to the provision of such care when the individual is incapacitated." Advance directives are mandated by the Patient Self-Determination Act (a provision of the Omnibus Budget Reconciliation Act of 1990).[67] Advance directives are considered necessary because people are living longer and have to face choices about procedures to prolong life. Studies related to advance directives indicate the following[68]:

1. Use of proxies for persons with serious mental illness is neither meaningful nor beneficial.
2. Increased use of advance directives reduces use of health care services without affecting satisfaction or mortality of persons in nursing homes.
3. Elderly persons can use an interactive multimedia CD-ROM program to learn about advance directives.

The advance directive is a directive to physicians and other health care providers given in advance of incapacity without regard to a person's wishes about medical treatment. As an example, the Texas Natural Death Act gives a person the right to provide instructions about care when faced with a terminal condition. It covers such procedures as cardiopulmonary resuscitation (CPR), tube feeding, respirators, intravenous therapy, and kidney dialysis. A durable power of attorney for health care allows a person to name another person to make medical decisions for an incapacitated person.

A directive to physicians may be called a living will. The attending physician and another physician certify that a person has a terminal condition that will result in death in a relatively short time and that the person is comatose, incompetent, or otherwise unable to communicate.

An advance directive is a legal document. In Texas it does not have to be drawn up by a lawyer or notarized but does have to be witnessed. An oral statement suffices when done in the presence of two witnesses and the attending physician. Witnesses cannot be physicians, nurses, hospital personnel, fellow patients, or persons who will have claim against a person's estate.[69]

Under Texas law (Consent to Medical Treatment Act), the following people have the option to make medical decisions for an incompetent person: spouse, sole child who has written permission from the other children to act alone, majority of children, parents, a person whom the patient clearly identified before becoming ill, any living relative, or a member of the clergy (surrogate).[70]

Ethics in Business

Lee indicates that all organizations should develop a policy on ethics. Business ethics helps people find the best way to satisfy the demands of competing interests. Ethics is part of corporate culture. Ethical organizations try to satisfy all of their stockholders, are dedicated to high purpose, are committed to learning, and try to be the best at whatever they do. Leaders of ethical organizations have the moral courage to change direction, hire brilliant subordinates, encourage innovation, stick to values, and persist over time. Polaroid established internal conferences on ethics in 1983 and 1984. These included philosophers, ethicists, and business professors who looked at the language and concepts of ethics. The conferences were broadened to include leadership and dilemma workshops to apply the knowledge to company cases.[71]

Nurse managers can explore similar modes of studying ethics. They can do so with clinical nursing staff. This will include looking at how business is done versus how it should be done. It will set the organizational climate for ethical decision-making. Ethics can be built into orientation, management development, participative management, and policies and procedures.

According to Beckstrand, "The aims of practice can be achieved using the knowledge of science and ethics alone."[72] To apply Beckstrand's theory to nursing management, nurse managers would apply their knowledge to change the nursing work environment to realize a greater good where and when needed.

Donley states that a health care system should be built based on values promoting both the individual and the common good.[73] Current dilemmas in nursing are partly due to limitations in nursing management knowledge. Changes are needed that address values and goals. There could be a hierarchy of values in managing practice. Nurse managers need to determine how much decision-making power clinical nurses want and how much managers can delegate. A theory of ethics should be meshed with a theory of nursing management that is congruent with a theory of ethical conduct for clinical nurses.

Both clinical nurses and managers use scientific knowledge to determine whether conditions support change. The intrinsic value of the management actions should be given careful thought and should be debated by nurse managers who consciously attempt to practice management that realizes the highest good. The manager is more apt to be successful if scientific management knowledge is applied.

Ethics in management translated into nursing theory can be summed up as follows:

1. Nurse managers can influence the ethical behavior of nursing personnel by treating them ethically.
2. Nurse managers have a code of ethics that peers have agreed on (see Appendix 11-1). They enter into ethical dilemmas when they go against that code.
3. Nurse managers fall into moral dilemmas when they go against their internal values.
4. Although ethical and moral dilemmas differ, an ethical nurse manager is a moral nurse manager.
5. Ethical functions can be confronted by three questions:
   a. "Is it legal?" This question resolves some dilemmas but not when nonsensical laws and policies are involved.
   b. "Is it balanced?" The nurse manager should aim for a win-win solution.
   c. "How will it make me feel about myself?" The nurse manager should consider the impact of each action on her/his self-respect.
6. Nurse managers with positive self-images usually have the internal strength to make the ethical decision.
7. An ethical leader is an effective leader.
8. Nurse managers should apply six principles of ethical power:
   a. The chief nurse executive promotes and ensures pursuit of the stated mission or purpose of the nursing division, since this statement reflects the vision of practicing nurses. Although the mission statement should be reviewed periodically, goals or objectives are set for yearly achievement.
   b. Nurse managers should build an organization to win, thereby building up employees through pride in their organization.
   c. Nurse managers should work to sustain patience and continuity through a long-term effect on the organization.
   d. Nurse managers should plan for persistence by spending more time following up on education and activities that build commitment of personnel.
   e. Nurse managers should promote perspective by giving their staff time to think. They should practice good management for the long term.
   f. Nursing service managers should consider developing an organization-specific code of ethics expressed in observable and measurable behaviors.[74]

A code of ethics should be ingrained in employees to create a strong sense of professionalism. Such a code should be the basis of a planned approach to all management functions of planning, organizing, leading, and evaluating. Nursing employees can help develop the code of ethics, can help implement it, and can determine its associated rewards and punishments. A code of ethics should be read and signed by employees and regularly reviewed and revised.

Contents of a code of ethics include definition of ethical and unethical practices, expected ethical behavior, enforcement of ethical practices, and rewards and punishments. To be objective, a code of ethics specifies rules of conduct. To be effective, it should be applied to all persons.[75]

Multicultural Aspects of Nursing

While nurses have attended to the multicultural aspects of patient care through the decades, the importance of such aspects has received increasing attention during recent years. The term *multicultural* relates to such characteristics as race, gender, religion, cognitive diversity, sexual orientation, age, and class. It also relates to all of the ideas and habits a social or ethnic group learns, practices, shares, and transmits from generation to generation.

An ethnic group may be both a minority and a majority—for example, the French-Canadians are a majority in Quebec province and a minority in other provinces of Canada. Ethnic groups have cultural needs relating to their beliefs, values, and lifestyles. They have distinct *learned* knowledge and skills that are socially inherited. Ethnic groups have distinct eating habits, ways of raising children, political beliefs, and beliefs related to health and illness.[76] Knowledge of a patient's culture assists the caregiver in preventing stress and morbidity in caring for that patient.[77]

Signals of stress are culturally grounded.[78] As an example, persons from different cultures respond to pain differently. Patients from some cultures are stoic about pain and illness, whereas others are emotional and expressive. Through interview and observation, the professional nurse assesses the cultural needs of the patient as she or he assesses the patient's other needs. Among the needs assessed are the need for an interpreter—sometimes because of language or other communication limitations. Language is sometimes a challenge for political reasons. Some groups want the official U.S. language to be English. The professional nurse transcends the political argument. If a patient cannot speak English, the caregiver obtains a translator from the family or other source to translate for the patient. Communication is enhanced when nurses respect and appreciate diversity of culture. The world's largest over-the-phone interpreting service with over 140 languages is available from AT&T. Some agencies hire bilingual employees if the need is great enough. Other agencies retain interpreters to help explain things to patients and calm their fears.[79] Another aspect of multicultural nursing is the need to communicate with low-literacy patients. Most oral and written communications for these patients should be at a fourth to sixth grade reading level.[80]

Since diet is important in treating most diseases and in maintaining health, nurses and other health care workers should establish which foods and beverages a person from another culture will consume and how these foods should be prepared. National studies on illnesses have used predominantly male subjects. These studies have led to wrong conclusions in treating female patients. Studies have also led to wrong conclusions in treating pain in women, as a result of which, women may have inadequate pain management.[81]

Nurses may need to do self-examination to identify their personal biases and prejudices regarding cultural issues. Such issues may center around religious differences, superstitions, and customs related to space and colors, and questions related to survival, sharing, protecting the environment, and even intelligence. Educators are exploring the concept of people having multiple (seven) intelligences: linguistic, logical-mathematical, spatial, bodily-kinesthetic, musical, interpersonal, and intrapersonal. A dominant intelligence may become the conduit for developing another or others.[82] This knowledge may help in assessing patients' needs.

Cultural goals are defined by nurses to fit the assessed needs of patients, including equity, tolerance, and acceptance. Cultural awareness leads to responsible action and empowerment. Desirable cultural outcomes include being accepted, being valued, being loved, having a sense of belonging, cooperation in reaching decisions, and resolving problems. As caregivers learn the cultural beliefs of other ethnic groups, they become less idealistic and more understanding. Conflict is tempered by conformity and commonality.

Summary

Nurse managers work with staff consisting of clinical practitioners. Educated in nursing management, they can assist these practitioners in their work according to the models of such theorists as Orem, Kinlein, Roy, Newman, Levine, Johnson, Peplau, and Orlando.

Several modalities of nursing have evolved over the past 50 years. Functional nursing, the oldest nursing practice modality, is a method in which each staff member is assigned a particular nursing function, such as administering medications, admitting and discharging patients, and making beds and serving meals. Later, team nursing became the modality of choice for many hospital nursing services. Under the leadership of a professional nurse, a group of nurses work together to provide patient care. Team nursing rests on theoretical knowledge related to philosophy, planning, leadership, interpersonal relationships, and nursing process.

During the past three decades, the modality of total patient care through primary nursing has evolved. With primary nursing, the total care of a patient and a case load is the responsibility of one primary nurse.

Joint or collaborative practice by a physician–nurse team has developed as a modality of nursing in a very few hospitals. The latest development is case management, a method of practicing nursing that incorporates any modality but in which the knowledgeable nurse becomes the case manager, making or facilitating all clinical nursing decisions about a case load of patients during an entire episode of illness.

As new technologies of patient treatment develop and the health care delivery system evolves around managed care, nurses need avenues to pursue the ensuing ethical dilemmas. Nursing practice is further complicated by the need for multicultural assessments as part of the nursing process and its outcomes.

APPLICATION EXERCISES

EXERCISE 11-1

Use your student group or form an ad hoc committee of nurses to plan for needed implementation of nursing theory in a nursing unit. Make a management plan. The following format may be used for all management plans. To help make a decision, access the Internet and locate applications of theories of Orem, Roy, Margaret Newman, Levine, Johnson, Peplau, and Orlando.

MANAGEMENT PLAN

PROBLEM:

OBJECTIVE:

ACTIONS	TARGET DATE	ASSIGNED TO	ACCOMPLISHMENTS

EXERCISE 11-2

Evaluate case management as practiced in the agency in which you are employed or to which you are assigned as a student. Do this by gathering and analyzing data that

1. Describe the model of case management being used.
2. Identify the standards used to trigger the case management process.
3. Trace the continuum of case management from patient's entry through discharge.
4. Measure the achievement of stated outcomes.
5. Relate the nursing modality to case management.

EXERCISE 11-3

Form a group of 6 to 8 peers. Each group member identifies and describes, orally or in writing, an ethical dilemma. Discuss each from the viewpoints of care for the patient and support for the caregiver. What are the implications for interpersonal relationships among caregivers and care recipients?

EXERCISE 11-4   Set up two teams to debate the following:

"Professional nurses should intervene in instances where they observe unethical conduct or illegal or unprofessional activities."

VERSUS

"Professional nurses should *not* intervene in instances where they observe unethical conduct or illegal or unprofessional activities."

Select a moderator. Divide the group into two teams. These may be divided by viewpoints. Decide on rules for selection first and then decide on rules of procedure. For example, each speaker from each side may be allowed to speak to a question for three minutes.

Consider the following questions:

1. What is the individual responsibility of the professional nurse employee in instances where he or she observes unethical conduct or illegal or unprofessional activities by the employer?
2. What is the responsibility of professional nursing organizations when they are made aware of such instances?
3. What is the responsibility of community organizations if they are made aware of such instances?

Consider the following:

- Accreditation action
- Government action (Medicare)
- Publicity (media)
- Prevention

EXERCISE 11-5   Examine organizational policies related to patients' rights as well as statements made by nursing associations and hospital associations and articles in professional journals. What authority or source would lead one to believe that the patient has a right to know his or her nursing diagnosis, the goals of care related to that diagnosis, and the nursing actions prescribed to meet those goals? What authority or source would lead one to believe that the patient has a right to assist in the planning of his or her nursing care? What authority or source would lead one to believe that the patient has a right to know what to expect as a result of his or her nursing care?

EXERCISE 11-6   Read the work of M. L. Leininger (see references). With a group of your peers, discuss application of Leininger's theory of culture care. Outline the steps to follow in assessing, diagnosing, and identifying outcomes for the cultural needs of patients. Describe how you would apply these steps in clinical practice. Outline the characteristics of a culturally competent professional nurse.

NOTES

1. H. A. Bush, "Models for Nursing," *Advances in Nursing Science* (January 1979), 13–21.
2. G. L. Dickson, and H. Lee-Villasenor, "Nursing Theory and Practice: A Self-Care Approach," *Advances in Nursing Science* (October 1982), 29–40.
3. T. Jaarsma, R. Halfens, M. Senten, H. H. Abu Saad, and K. Dracup, "Developing a Supportive-Educative Program for Patients with Advanced Heart Failure within Orem's General Theory of Nursing," *Nursing Science Quarterly*, (summer 1998), 79–85.
4. Sister C. Roy, "Adaptation: A Basis for Nursing Practice," *Nursing Outlook* (April 1971), 254–257; K. Frederickson, "Using a Nursing Model to Manage Symptoms: Anxiety and the Roy Adaptation Model," *Holistic Nursing Practice* (January 1993), 36–43.
5. Ibid.
6. M. F. Mastal, and H. Hammond, "Analysis and Expansion of the Roy Adaptation Model: A Contribution to Holistic Nursing," *Advances in Nursing Science* (July 1980), 71–81.
7. K. Frederickson, op. cit.
8. M. C. Silva, and J. M. Sorrell, "Testing a Nursing Theory: Critique and Philosophical Expansion," *Advances in Nursing Science* (June 1992), 12–23.
9. V. F. Engle, "Newman's Conceptual Framework and the Measurement of Older Adults' Health," *Advances in Nursing Science* (October 1984), 24–36.

10. Ibid.

11. Ibid.

12. M. E. Levine, "Adaptation and Assessment: A Rationale for Nursing Intervention," *American Journal of Nursing* (November 1966), 2450–2453.

13. Ibid.

14. A. C. Rawls, "Evaluation of the Johnson Behavioral System Model in Clinical Practice," *Image* (February 1980), 12–16.

15. A. K. Derdiarian, "The Relationships Among the Subsystems of Johnson's Behavioral System Model," *Image* (winter 1990), 219–225.

16. L. Thompson, "Peplau's Theory: An Application to Short-Term Individual Therapy," *Journal of Psychosocial Nursing* (August 1986), 26–31.

17. H. E. Peplau, "Interpersonal Relations: A Theoretical Framework for Application in Nursing Practice," *Nursing Science Quarterly* (spring 1992), 13–18; P. Schafer, "Working with Dave. Application of Peplau's Interpersonal Nursing Theory in the Correctional Environment," *Journal of Psychosocial Nursing and Mental Health Services* (September 1999), 18–24.

18. N. J. Schmieding, "Putting Orlando's Theory into Practice," *American Journal of Nursing* (June 1984), 759–761; I. J. Orlando, *The Discipline and Teaching of Nursing Process: An Evaluative Study* (New York: G. P. Putnam's Sons, 1972); I. J. Orlando, *The Dynamic Nurse–Patient Relationship: Function, Process, Principles* (New York: G. P. Putnam's Sons, 1961).

19. A. G. Wiens, "Patient Autonomy in Care: A Theoretical Framework for Nursing," *Journal of Professional Nursing* (March–April 1993), 95–103.

20. M. B. Happ, "Sociotechnical Systems Theory," *Journal of Nursing Administration* (June 1993), 47–54.

21. D. P. Newcomb, and R. C. Swansburg, *The Team Plan: A Manual for Nursing Service Administrators*, 2nd ed. (New York: Putnam, 1953, 1971), 56.

22. G. D. Marram, M. W. Schlegel, and E. O. Bevis, *Primary Nursing: A Model for Individualized Care* (Saint Louis: Mosby, 1974), 1.

23. Ibid., 16–17.

24. C. M. Fagin, "The Economic Value of Nursing Research," *American Journal of Nursing* (December 1982), 1844–1849.

25. J. C. Lyon, "Models of Nursing Care Delivery and Case Management: Clarification of Terms," *Nursing Economic$* (June 1993), 163–169.

26. The National Joint Practice Commission, *Guidelines for Establishing Joint or Collaborative Practice in Hospitals* (Chicago, IL: Neely Printing, 1981).

27. Ibid.

28. L. W. Koch, S. H. Puzaki, and J. D. Campbell, "The First 20 Years of Nurse Practitioner Literature: An Evolution of Joint Practice Issues," *Nurse Practitioner* (February 1992), 62–66, 68, 71.

29. J. Herman, and S. Ziel, "Collaborative Practice Agreements for Advanced Practice Nurses: What You Should Know," *AACN Clinical Issues* (August 1999), 337–342.

30. "Toward a Fully-Integrated CareMap™ and Case Management System," *The New Definition* (spring 1993), 1.

31. "Part 1: Rationale for Care-Provider Organizations," *The New Definition* (summer 1994), 1.

32. Ibid.

33. Ibid.

34. Ibid.

35. "Quantifying, Managing, and Improving Quality Part I: How CareMaps® Link CQI to the Patient," *The New Definition* (spring 1992), 1.

36. Ibid.

37. "Quantifying, Managing and Improving Quality Part III: Using Variance Concurrently," *The New Definition* (fall 1992), 1–2.

38. D. Y. Brockopp, M. Porter, S. Kinnaird, and S. Silberman, "Fiscal and Clinical Evaluation of Patient Care," *Journal of Nursing Administration* (September 1992), 23–27.

39. M. Rogers, J. Riordan, and D. Swindle, "Community-Based Nursing Case Management Pays Off," *Nursing Management* (March 1991), 30–34.

40. J. C. Lyon., op. cit.

41. K. Bower, *Case Management by Nurses*, 2nd ed. (Washington, DC: American Nurses Publishing, 1992), 33–34.

42. R. Williams, "Nurse Case Management: Working with the Community," *Nursing Management* (December 1992), 33–34.

43. A. G. Strong, "Case Management and the CNS," *Clinical Nurse Specialist* (summer 1992), 64.

44. J. Thomas, "Package Deals," *Nursing Times* (15 July 1992), 48–49.

45. G. F. Dowling, "Case Management Nursing: Indications for Material Management," *Hospital Material Management Quarterly* (February 1991), 26–32.

46. A. G. Strong, and N. V. Sneed, "Clinical Evaluation of a Critical Path for Coronary Artery Bypass Surgery Patients," *Progress in Cardiovascular Nursing* (January–March 1991), 29–37.

47. S. H. Servais, "Nursing Resource Applications Through Outcome Based Nursing Practice," *Nursing Economic$* (May–June 1991), 171–174, 179.

48. K. Zander, "Case Management Series," (summer 1994), op. cit.

49. K. Bower, op. cit., 7–8.

50. The University of Iowa College of Nursing, *CHAOS* (May 2000).

51. M. G. Titler, and J. M. McCloskey, eds., "On the Scene: University of Iowa Hospitals and Clinics: Outcomes Management," *Nursing Administration Quarterly* (fall 1999), 31–65.

52. Report of the Special Committee on Biomedical Ethics, *Values in Conflict: Resolving Ethical Issues in Hospital Care* (Chicago: American Hospital Association, 1985).

53. Ibid.

54. A. J. Davis, "Helping Your Staff Address Ethical Dilemmas," *Journal of Nursing Administration* (February 1982), 9–13.

55. M. Flaherty, "Search for Answers: Drug Trials Create Ethical Balancing Act," *HealthWeek* (30 August 1999), 1, 10; R. Noble-Adams, "Ethics and Nursing Research. 1: Development, Theories and Principles," *British Journal of Nursing* (July 1999), 888–892; M. L. Dwyer, "Genetic Research and Ethical Challenges: Implication for Nursing Practice," *AACN Clinical Issues* (November 1998), 600–605; C. H. Kawas, C. M. Clark, M. R. Farlow, D. S. Knopman, D. Marson, J. C. Morris, L. J. Thal, and P. T. Whitehorse, "Clinical Trials in Alzheimer Disease: Debate On the Use of Placebo Controls," *Alzheimer Disease Associated Disorders* (July–September 1999), 124–129; M. Brommels, "Sliced Down to the Moral Backbone? Ethical Issues of Structural Reforms in Healthcare Organizations," *Acta Oncology*, 38(1), 1999, 63–69.

56. L. E. Mortenson, "Are Oncology Nurses too Expensive?" *Oncology Nursing Forum* (January–February 1984), 14–15.

57. Committee on Ethics, American Nurses' Association, *Ethics in Nursing: Position Statements and Guidelines* (Kansas City, MO: American Nurses' Association, 1988).

58. J. E. Sauer, "Ethical Problems Facing the Healthcare Industry," *Hospital & Health Services Administration* (September–October 1985), 44–53.

59. M. C. Berger, A. Seversen, and R. Chvatal, "Ethical Issues in Nursing," *Western Journal of Nursing Research* (August 1991), 514–521.

60. C. Scanlon, and C. Fleming, "Confronting Ethical Issues: A Nursing Survey," *Nursing Management* (May 1990), 63–65.

61. S. Pennington, G. Gafner, R. Schilit, and B. Bechtel, "Addressing Ethical Boundaries Among Nurses," *Nursing Management* (June 1993), 36–39.

62. A. Landers, "Pain-Free Death Is a Right Worth Defending," *San Antonio Express-News* (17 June 1994), 5J.

63. L. L. Curtin, "Creating Moral Space for Nurses," *Nursing Management* (March 1993), 18–19.

64. L. L. Curtin, "When the System Fails," *Nursing Management* (August 1992), 21–25.

65. P. Konstam, "Values-Based System Focuses on Ethics," *San Antonio Light* (12 December 1992), D 1.

66. S. Buchanan, and L. Cook, "Nursing Ethics Committees: The Time Is Now," *Nursing Management* (August 1992), 40–41.

67. Sec 4206, "Medicare Provider Agreements Assuring the Implementation of the Patient's Right to Participate in and Direct Health Care Delivery Affecting the Patient," *Congressional Record-House* (26 October 1990), H12456–H12457.

68. C. P. Murphy, M. A. Sweeney, and D. Chiriboga, "An Educational Intervention for Advance Directives," *Journal of Professional Nursing* (January–February 2000), 21–30; D. W. Molloy et al., "Systematic Implementation of an Advance Directive Program in Nursing Homes: A Randomized Controlled Trial," *JAMA* (15 March 2000), 1437–1444; J. L. Geller, "The Use of Advance Directives by Persons with Serious Mental Illness for Psychiatric Treatment," *Psychiatric Quarterly* (spring 2000), 1–13; J. G. Burt, "Compliance with Advance Directives: A Legal View," *Critical Care Nursing Quarterly* (November 1999), 72–74.

69. Bexar County Hospital District, "Understanding Advance Directives: Your Rights as a Patient," (San Antonio, Texas, 1991).

70. P. Premack, "Medical—OK Law Has a Key Change," *San Antonio Express-News* (23 July 1993), 11D.

71. C. Lee, "Ethics Training: Facing the Tough Questions," *Training* (March 1986), 30–33, 38–41.

72. J. Beckstrand, "The Need for a Practice Theory as Indicated by the Knowledge Used in the Conduct of Practice," *Research in Nursing and Health* (December 1978), 175–179.

73. Sr. R. Donley, "Ethics in the Age of Health Care Reform," *Nursing Economic$* (January–February 1993), 19–23.

74. K. C. Fernicola, "Take the High Road . . . to Ethical Management: An Interview with Kenneth Blanchard," *Association Management* (May 1988), 60–66.

75. M. Mizock, "Ethics—The Guiding Light of Professionalism," *Data Management* (August 1986), 16–18, 29.

76. H. A. Robinson, "Weaving the Tapestry of Diversity," *National Forum* (winter 1994), 3–5; S. Dobson, "Bringing Culture into Care," *Nursing Times* (9 February 1983), 53, 56–57.

77. J. Doku, "Approaches to Cultural Awareness," *Nursing Times* (26 September 1990), 69–70.

78. C. F. Diaz, "Dimensions of Multicultural Education," *National Forum* (winter 1994), 9–11.

79. L. Morgan, "Making the Connection," *HealthWeek* (20 July 1998), 13.

80. M. Habel, "Get Your Message Across to Low-Literacy Patients," *HealthWeek* (12 June 2000), 20–21; S. P. Weinrich, "The High Risk of Low Literacy," *Reflections* (Fourth Quarter 1999), 22–24.

81. A. H. Vallerand, "Gender Differences in Pain," *IMAGE: Journal of Nursing Scholarship* (fall 1995), 235–251.

82. J. H. Gray, and J. T. Viens, "The Theory of Multiple Intelligences," *National Forum* (winter 1994), 22–25.

REFERENCES

"Advance Directives . . . Is the Law Clear?" *Healthcare Alabama* (January–February 1991), 3, 5–7, 21.

American Academy of Nursing. *Primary Care by Nurses: Sphere of Responsibility and Accountability* (Kansas City, MO: The Academy, 1977).

American Nurses' Association. *Nursing: A Social Policy Statement* (Washington, DC: American Nurses' Association, 1994).

"Biomedical Ethics and the Bill of Rights." *National Forum* (fall 1989).

Bircher, A. U. "One Development and Classification of Diagnoses." *Nursing Forum* (January 1975), 11–29.

Blanchard, K., and N. V. Peale. *The Power of Ethical Management* (New York: Fawcett Crest, 1988).

Bower, K. A., and J. G. Somerville. "Managed Care and Case Management Outcome Based Practice: Creating the Environment," Program at Sheraton Grand Hotel, Tampa, Florida, February 15–16, 1988.

Bradshaw, M. J. "Clinical Pathways: A Tool to Evaluate Clinical Learning." *Journal of the Society of Pediatric Nurses* (January–March 1999), 37–40.

Burr, J. A., and T. Chapman. "Some Reflections on Cultural and Social Considerations in Mental Health Nursing." *Journal of Psychiatric Mental Health Nursing* (December 1998), 431–437.

Carr, J. M. "Vigilance as a Caring Expression and Leininger's Theory of Cultural Care Diversity and Universality." *Nursing Science Quarterly* (summer 1998), 74–78.

Carse, J. "Diversity in the World's Religions." *National Forum* (winter 1994), 26–27.

Chase, M. "Cancer Doctors Aim to Improve Chemotherapy." *The Wall Street Journal* (21 May 1992), 88.

Chinn, P. L., and Jacobs, M. K. *Theory and Nursing: A Systematic Approach* (St. Louis: Mosby, 1987).

Ciske, K. I. Response to Zander's "Primary Nursing Won't Work . . . Unless the Head Nurse Lets It." *Journal of Nursing Administration* (January 1978), 26, 43, 50.

Cortes, C. E. "Limits to Pluribus, Limits to Unum." *National Forum* (winter 1994), 6–8.

Dickoff, J., James, P., and Wiedenbach, E. "Theory in a Practice Discipline, Part I. Practice Oriented Theory." *Nursing Research* (September–October 1968), 415–435; Dickoff, J., James, P., and Wiedenbach, E. "Theory in a Practice Discipline, Part II. Practice Oriented Research." *Nursing Research* (November–December 1968), 545–554.

Dixon, E. L. "Community Health Nursing Practice and the Roy Adaptation Model." *Public Health Nursing* (August 1999), 290–300.

Donaldson, T. "Individual Rights and Multinational Corporate Responsibilities." *National Forum* (winter 1992), 7–9.

Etzioni, A. "Too Many Rights, Too Few Responsibilities." *National Forum* (winter 1992), 4–6.

Fadden, T. C. and Seiser, G. K. "Nursing Diagnosis: A Matter of Form." *American Journal of Nursing* (April 1984), 470–472.

Felton, G. "Increasing the Quality of Nursing Care by Introducing the Concept of Primary Nursing: A Model Project." *Nursing Research* (January–February. 1975), 27–32.

Flaherty, M. "Letting Go: Facing the Sensitive Subject of DNR Orders." *HealthWeek* (28 September 1998), 20.

Flanagan, J. "Achieving Partnership: The Contribution of Nursing Education to the Production of a Flexible Workforce." *Journal of Nursing Management* (May 1998), 135–136.

Freed, P. E., and V. K. Drake. "Mandatory Reporting of Abuse: Practical, Moral, and Legal Issues for Psychiatric Home Healthcare Nurses." *Issues in Mental Health Nursing* (July–August 1999), 423–436.

Garcia, M. A., D. Bruce, J. Niemeyer, and J. Robbins. "Collaborative Practice: A Shared Success." *Nursing Management* (May 1993), 72–74, 78.

Goodman, D. "Application of the Critical Pathway and Integrated Case Teaching Method to Nursing Orientation." *Journal of Continuing Education in Nursing* (September–October 1997), 205–210.

Goodman, E. "Health System Relies on Lying." *San Antonio Express-News* (21 April 2000).

Goodpaster, K. E., and G. Atkinson. "Stakeholders, Individual Rights, and the Common Good." *National Forum* (winter 1992), 14–17.

Hellinghausen, M. A. "Closing the Gap: Program Aims to Add More Minorities to Healthcare Professions." *HealthWeek* (6 March 2000), 27.

Henry, B., C. Arndt, M. DiVincenti, and A. Mariner-Tomey, eds. *Dimensions of Nursing Administration: Theory, Research, Education, Practice* (Boston: Blackwell, 1989).

Hoffman, W. M., and E. S. Petry, Jr. "Abusing Business Ethics." *National Forum* (winter 1992), 10–13.

Jonsdottir, H. "Outcomes of Implementing Primary Nursing in the Care of People with Chronic Lung Diseases: The Nurses' Experience." *Journal of Nursing Management* (July 1999), 235–242.

Koleszar, A. J. "The Great Debate." *CWRU* (February 1990), 16–20.

Kols, A. J., J. E. Sherman, and P. T. Piotrow. "Ethical Foundations of Client-Centered Care in Family Planning." *Journal of Womens Health* (April 1999), 303–312.

Koziol-McLain, J., and M. K. Maeve. "Nursing Theory in Perspective." *Nursing Outlook* (March–April 1993), 79–81.

Leininger, M. "Leininger's Theory of Nursing: Culture Care Diversity and Universality." *Nursing Science Quarterly*, 1(4) 1988, 152–160.

Leininger, M. "Culture Care Theory: The Comparative Global Theory to Advance Human Care Theory and Practice." In D. A. Gaut, ed. *A Global Agenda for Caring* (New York: National League for Nursing, 1993), 3–18.

Leininger, M. "Quality of Life from a Transcultural Nursing Perspective." *Nursing Science Quarterly*, 7(1) 1994, 22–28.

Leininger, M. *Transcultural Nursing: Concepts, Theories, Research & Practices*, 2nd Ed. (New York: McGraw Hill, 1995).

McLaughlin, C. "Thinking About Diversity." *National Forum* (winter 1994), 16–18.

Moffic, H. S., and J.D. Kinzie, "The History of Cross Cultural Psychiatric Services." *Community Mental Health Journal* (December 1996), 581–592.

Moore, J. "Senator Says Mental Hospital Abuses Not Limited to Texas." *San Antonio Light* (April 29 1992), D 6.

Morgan, L. "Faith Meets Health." *HealthWeek* (30 August 1999), 15.

Murphy, W. J. "Ethical Perspectives in Neuroscience Nursing Practice." *Nursing Clinics of North America* (September 1999), 621–635.

Nelson-Marten, P., K. Hecomovich, and M. Pangle. "Caring Theory: A Framework for Advanced Nursing Practice." *Advanced Practice Nursing Quarterly* (summer 1998), 70–77.

Newman, M. A. "Nursing Diagnosis: Looking at the Whole." *American Journal of Nursing* (December 1984), 1496–1499.

Nightingale, Florence. *Notes on Nursing* (Philadelphia: J. B. Lippincott, 1959).

Norman-Culp, S. "No Mercy for Dying Man, Wife Says." *San Antonio Express-News* (23 May 1993), 3F.

Parker, R. S. "Measuring Nurses' Moral Judgments." *Image* (winter 1990), 213–218.

Parse, R. R. "Nursing Science: The Transformation of Practice." *Journal of Advanced Nursing* (December 1999), 1383–1387.

Paul, N. "For the Record: Information on Individuals." *National Forum* (winter 1992), 34–38.

Redman, B. K., and S. T. Fry. "Ethical Conflicts Reported by Certified Registered Rehabilitation Nurses." *Rehabilitation Nursing* (July–August 1998), 179–184.

Rogers, M. *An Introduction to the Theoretical Basis of Nursing* (Philadelphia: F. A. Davis, 1970).

Rogers, M., J. Riordan, and D. Swindle. "Community-Based Nursing Case Management Pays Off." *Nursing Management* (March 1991), 30–34.

Rothrock, J. C. "Nursing Diagnosis in the Days of Florence Nightingale." *AORN Journal* (August 1984), 189–190.

Roy, S. C. *Introduction to Nursing: An Adaptation Model* (Englewood Cliffs, NJ: Prentice-Hall, 1976).

Saliba, D., R. Kington, J. Buchanan, R. Bell, M. Wang, M. Lee, M. Herbst, D. Lee, D. Sur, and L. Rubenstein. "Appropriateness of the Decision to Transfer Nursing Facility Residents to the Hospital." *Journal of the American Geriatric Society* (February 2000), 154–163.

Shaw-Taylor, Y., and B. Benesch. "Workforce Diversity and Cultural Competence in Healthcare." *Journal of Cultural Diversity* (winter 1998), 147–148.

Shukla, R. K. "Structure vs. People in Primary Nursing: An Inquiry." *Nursing Research* (July–August 1981), 236–241.

Simpson, R. D., and W. W. Anderson. "Science Education and the Common Good." *National Forum* (winter 1992), 30–33.

Smith, H. L. "Genetic Technologies: Can We Do Responsibly Everything We Can Do Technically?" *National Forum* (winter 1992), 26–29.

Smith, L. S. "Concept Analysis: Cultural Competence." *Journal of Cultural Diversity* (spring 1998), 4–10.

Strong, A. G., and N. V. Sneed. "Clinical Evaluation of a Critical Path for Coronary Artery Bypass Surgery Patients." *Progress in Cardiovascular Nursing* (January–March 1991), 29–37.

Swansburg, R. C. *Team Nursing: A Programmed Learning Experience*, 4 Volumes (New York: G. P. Putnam's Sons, 1968).

Swansburg, R. C. *Management of Patient Care Services* (St. Louis: Mosby, 1976), 172–173.

Swansburg, R. C., and P. W. Swansburg. *Strategic Career Planning and Development for Nurses* (Rockville, MD: Aspen Publishers, 1984), 26–27.

Thomas, J. "Package Deals." *Nursing Times* (15 July 1992), 48–49.

Thomas, L. H. "Qualified Nurse and Nursing Auxiliary Perceptions of Their Work Environment in Primary, Team, and Functional Nursing Wards." *Journal of Advanced Nursing* (March 1992), 373–382.

Thomas, N. M., and G. G. Newsome. "Factors Affecting the Use of Nursing Diagnosis." *Nursing Outlook* (July–August 1992), 182–186.

Thorns, A. R., and J. E. Ellershaw. "A Survey of Nursing and Medical Staff Views On the Use of Cardiopulmonary Resuscitation in the Hospice." *Palliative Medicine* (May 1999), 225–232.

Tritsch, J. M. "Application of King's Theory of Goal Attainment and the Carondelet St. Mary's Case Management Model." *Nursing Science Quarterly* (summer 1998), 69–73.

VanLeit, B. "Using the Case Method to Develop Reasoning Skills in Problem-Based Learning." *American Journal of Occupational Therapy* (April 1995), 349–353.

Williams, R. "Nurse Case Management: Working with the Community." *Nursing Management* (December 1992), 33–34.

Williams, R. "Cultural Safety—What Does It Mean for Our Work Practice?" *Australia New Zealand Journal of Public Health* (April 1999), 213–214.

Wong, F. K. "The Nurse Manager as a Professional–Managerial Class: A Case Study." *Journal of Nursing Management* (November 1998), 343–350.

Yamashita, M. "Newman's Theory of Health as Expanding Consciousness: Research on Family Caregiving in Mental Illness in Japan." *Nursing Science Quarterly* (fall 1998), 110–115.

Yoder, M. E. "Nursing Diagnosis: Application During Perioperative Practice." *AORN Journal* (August 1984), 183–188.

Zander, K. S. "Primary Nursing Won't Work . . . Unless the Head Nurse Lets It." *Journal of Nursing Administration* (October 1977), 19–23.

APPENDIX 11-1
ASNSA Code of Ethics

PREAMBLE

This code of ethics is intended to give direction to and facilitate accomplishment of the goals of nursing service administration through the integrity and expertise of practitioners in the field of nursing service administration. Effective executive functioning demands that nursing service administrators affirm and accept the responsibility to practice their profession according to the highest professional nursing and management standards.

Nursing service administrators believe in the worth and dignity of man. Nursing service administrators share responsibility for the multifaceted delivery of health care and are committed to maintain standards of excellence in facilitating an environment for the provision of nursing care. Nursing service administrators are prepared to undertake a valid and consistent approach to the solution of patient care problems.

This code of ethics is applicable to professional individuals having responsibility as nursing service administrators in any health care setting and complies with existing policies of the American Hospital Association.

ACCOUNTABILITY

Nursing service administrators must meet four primary accountabilities: to the consumer; to themselves in accomplishing their responsibilities as nursing service administrators and for and to the staffs for whom they are responsible; to the chief executive officer or chief operating officer of the health care agency; and to the American Society for Nursing Service Administrators.

Nursing service administrators are expected to adhere to the Guidelines of Ethical Conduct and Relationships for Health Care Institutions formulated by the American Hospital Association. They are expected to utilize the standards of nursing practice as determined by professional nursing. Therefore, the nursing service administrator shall:

1. Maintain and support interpersonal relationships within the organization that will assure an environment conducive to humane and appropriate care of those served

2. Continually strive to merit the confidence and respect of patients, staff, and community through quality and scope of nursing services

3. Cooperate with other disciplines engaged in or supportive of health services

4. Develop, implement, and periodically review nursing service organization and management, professional policies, practices, standards of performance, and activities for quality assurance

In matters of professional and personal ethics, the nursing service administrator has a duty to:

1. Observe at all times the existing local, state, and federal laws as a minimum guide for fulfillment of responsibilities

2. Conduct activities on behalf of and within the health care agency in a manner that is honest and ethical

THE GOVERNING BODY AND CHIEF EXECUTIVE/OPERATING OFFICER

Effectiveness in nursing service administrative performance depends on mutual respect and harmonious relationships between the nursing service administrator, the chief executive/operating officer, and the governing authority. Such accord can be maintained best when functions and prerogatives of each are carefully defined, understood, and followed.

In the fulfillment of defined functions the nursing service administrator shall:

1. Exercise authority required to conduct nursing service activities of the organization in accordance with nursing and health care agency policies adopted by the governing body

2. Demonstrate personal integrity and professional competence with capable leadership that merits confidence and respect

3. Consider as a major factor the corporate interest in all matters affecting the nursing service administrator's role and responsibility

(continued)

MEDICAL STAFF

The nursing service administrator shall promote effective channels for exchange of thinking and decision making between the medical staff and nursing service administration.

To effect the above, the nursing service administrator shall:

1. Promote coordination, supportive mechanisms, and understanding; through colleagueship with the medical staff to carry out responsibilities and activities with respect to quality of nursing care provided patients
2. Enhance, through appropriate channels, the policies established for the rights and responsibilities of patients

NURSING STAFF

The nursing service administrator shall strive to enhance the knowledge and expertise of nursing service personnel to assure the highest level of care to the patient.

To effect the above, the nursing service administrator shall:

1. Establish and implement appropriate philosophy, objectives, policies, and standards for nursing care of patients in concert with corporate policies and resources
2. Provide and implement a departmental plan of administrative authority clearly delineating accountability and responsibility for all categories of nursing personnel
3. Establish staffing requirements for nursing services and recommend and implement policies and procedures to assure an appropriate and competent nursing staff
4. Estimate needs for supplies, facilities, and equipment and implement an effective evaluation and control system
5. Initiate, utilize, and participate in studies and research projects designed for the improvement of patient care and health care agency services
6. Provide and implement a program of continuing education for all nursing personnel
7. Facilitate an environment for professional nursing practice that enables staff to continue to learn and students to have clinical experience in nursing
8. Assume responsibility for preparation and management of both operating and capital equipment budgets for nursing services

INTERDEPARTMENTAL RELATIONSHIPS

The nursing service administrator shall foster an effective interdepartmental relationship between nursing service and all other departments existing in the health care setting. The nursing service administrator coordinates the needs of nursing service with those of supporting departments and, together with general administration and department heads, plans solutions to problems related to the welfare of the patient and staff.

AGENCY RELATIONSHIPS

Nursing service administrators shall maintain a spirit of cooperation with representatives of other health care organizations where there is a sharing of common objectives. They assist other nursing service administrators and their organizations through participation in activities and services that will improve the quality of patient care programs. They cooperate with education and planning organizations that contribute to the advancement of health care.

CONFLICT OF INTEREST

Nursing service administrators shall conduct their personal and professional relationships in such a way as to assure themselves, their organizations, and the public that decisions they make are in the best interest of the patient and the organization. Exercise of judgment is required to determine whether a potential conflict of interest exists. A conflict of interest exists when a nursing service administrator is in a position, apart from the remuneration received from employment, to profit directly or indirectly through the application of personal or administrative authority. The nursing service administrator shall endeavor to avoid conflict of interest by providing full disclosure to the chief executive/ operating officer and the governing body of any potential conflict of interest.

SYSTEMS CONFLICT

Because of the need to coordinate and participate in the operation of the larger health care system, nursing service administrators are often elected and appointed to the governing bodies of health-related organizations, such as planning bodies, state and national hospital associations, and other health care organizations. Inherent in such positions is a potential conflict of interest because of the duality of interest of the nursing service administrator. Such duality of interest is acceptable only when there is no conflict of interest.

CONFIDENTIAL INFORMATION

Confidential information belongs to the health care agency. Use of it by nursing service administrators, their business associates, friends, or relatives for their own gain is a violation of the code of ethics.

P332-500-10/1/78

*A committee to administer this code of ethics will provide a clarifying and supportive function to nursing service administrators.

Source: Reprinted with permission of the American Organization of Nurse Executives.

CHAPTER 12

Decision-Making and Problem-Solving

Russell C. Swansburg, PhD, RN

Introduction

Decision-making is essential to problem-solving. It is doubtful that anyone would argue with that statement. Nurses already know how to make decisions, don't they? They have been doing so since they were small children. Certainly these decisions were not always made after careful deliberation and by consciously following specified steps in a process. Nurses may not have known how they did it; they just did it. Thus, a nurse might be thinking, "I wouldn't be where I am professionally if I didn't know how to make decisions, so I'll go to the next chapter."

Wait! How often have nurses made bad decisions? Why were the decisions bad? How do nurses avoid making similar errors in future decisions? How do they deal with indecision?

This chapter explores the answers to these questions. Complex decision-making is a part of any level of nursing. To function successfully, the nurse must consistently demonstrate the ability to solve problems in rapidly changing and uncertain situations in which indecisiveness or poor decisions are costly. The ability to foster organizational decision-making and problem-solving is an essential personal skill for nurses. This chapter deals with models and strategies that nurses can use to successfully strengthen personal skills and further develop the decision-making and problem-solving abilities of staff members.

The theory of decision-making, a required competency for all professionals, is an essential component of the nursing process and the management process. Good decisions require outside information on how other people view the world of nursing and make decisions about their care.

The Decision-Making Process

Definition

Since everyone is involved at some time in making decisions, it may be assumed that innate abilities, past experience, and intuition form the basis for making successful decisions. Decisions are often made by choosing among known alternatives. But what about unknown alternatives? Making a choice is not the only element of decision-making. The process, which usually involves a systematic approach of sequenced steps, should be adaptable to the environment in which it is used. Lancaster and Lancaster define decision-making as a systematic, sequential process of choosing among alternatives and putting the choice into action. This definition acknowledges natural and learned abilities while providing order and continuity to the process of decision-making.[1]

Empirical evidence shows that speedy decision-makers are needed in today's environment. Such decision-makers consider more alternatives, more batches of options at one time. They are themselves, experienced mentors or they rely on older, experienced mentors. Speedy decision-makers thoroughly integrate strategies and tactics. They juggle budgets, schedules, and organizational options simultaneously. They constitute the winning culture in decision-making.[2]

Clinical Decision-Making

In the clinical decision-making arena, clinical nurses manage patients' history and physical data, nursing diagnoses, nursing interventions, and nursing outcomes data to effect therapeutic results.[3] Many decision support systems are available in the medical treatment of patients. Research has shown that a majority of patients prefer to leave decision-making to their physicians. Patients' decision-making activity decreases with age and severe illnesses and increases with education.[4] Information on decision-making related to individual protocols abounds. This literature includes decision-making about cancer treatments, cardiovascular disease, growth hormone (GH) therapy, triage practices, and computer systems related to clinical decision-making models in general.[5] Nurse practitioners use these decision support systems while developing additional ones. Such nurse practitioner support systems are already being reported in relation to general practice.[6]

A review of the literature yields a number of decision-making models. Four models are covered in this chapter.

The Normative Model

This model is at least 200 years old. It is assumed to maximize satisfaction and fulfills the "perfect knowledge assumption" that "in any given situation calling for a decision, all possible choices and the consequences and potential outcome of each are known."[7] Seven steps are identified in this analytically precise model:

1. Define and analyze the problem.
2. Identify all available alternatives.
3. Evaluate the pros and cons of each alternative.
4. Rank the alternatives.
5. Select the alternative that maximizes satisfaction.
6. Implement.
7. Follow up.

The normative model for decision-making is unrealistic because of its assumption that there are clear-cut choices between identified alternatives.

The Decision-Tree Model

Various adaptations of decision-tree analysis are found in the literature; the essential elements described in the 1960s are standard. All factors considered important to a decision can be represented on a decision tree. Vroom arranged answers to seven diagnostic questions in the form of a decision tree to identify types of leadership style used in management decision-making models. The questions focus on protecting the quality and acceptance of the decision and deal with adequacy of information, goal congruence, structure of the problem, acceptance by subordinates, conflict, fairness, and priority for implementation.[8] Magee and Brown depict decision trees as starting with a basic problem and using branches to represent "event forks" and "action forks." The number of branches at each fork corresponds to the number of identified alternatives. Every path through the tree corresponds to a possible sequence of actions and events, each with its own distinct consequences. Probabilities of both positive and negative consequences of each action and event are estimated and recorded on the appropriate branch. Additional options (for example, delaying the decision) and consequences of each action-event sequence can be depicted on the decision tree. Computer simulations of decision trees are now available and can be adapted to a limited number or a highly complex network of branches involved in the decision-making process. Normal analysis of the tree is conducted by computing predicted consequences of all event forks (the right-hand edge of the tree), substituting that value for the actual event fork and its consequences, and selecting the action fork with the best expected consequences. Both the optimal strategy and its expected consequences will be determined. Quantitative analysis in the form of decision trees can be used for any type problem but may be unnecessary in simple problems involving limited consequences.[9]

The Descriptive Model

Simon developed the descriptive model based on the assumption that the decision-maker is a rational person looking for acceptable solutions based on known information. This model allows for the fact that many decisions are made with incomplete information because of time, money, or people limitations; it also allows for the fact that people do not always make the best choices. Simon wrote that few decisions would ever be made if people always sought optimal solutions. Instead, he contended, people identify acceptable alternatives. The following are the steps in the descriptive model[10]:

1. Establish an acceptable goal.
2. Define subjective perceptions of the problem.
3. Identify acceptable alternatives.
4. Evaluate each alternative.
5. Select an alternative.
6. Implement a decision.
7. Follow up.

The descriptive model may lend itself well to nurses faced with daily decisions that must be made rapidly and that will have significant consequences. Steps in the model are not unlike those in the familiar nursing process, although the sequencing is different. Readers may readily identify conditions in their own environments similar to those described by Simon and see immediate application of this model.[11] Lancaster and Lancaster illustrated the use of this model for nursing administrators.[12]

Exhibit 12-1 has been developed by the author after many years of experience using the descriptive model.

The Strategic Model

Strategic decision-making usually relates to long-range planning. As an example, hospitals merge and nursing departments are affected. Among the decisions that are made are the need for one top manager or department head versus two or more, whether to decentralize and eliminate middle managers, and what operational strategies will prevent duplication and maximize the use of scarce resources and provide for their efficient use. Nagelkerk and Henry used a model by Mintzberg, Raisinghani, and Theoret (the MRT model) to design and test the nature of strategic decision-making that entailed substantial risk. They worked with chief nurse executives employed in six acute care hospitals with 400 or more beds each.[13] The model is depicted in Exhibit 12-2.

In applying this model, participants used mixed scanning of general and specific information from subordinates to identify complex problems. To develop potential solutions they gathered facts from hospital documents. They made their selection of the best single solution by "(1) screening solutions using predetermined criteria, (2) identifying the costs and benefits as nearly as possible, and (3) selecting the single best solution."[14]

It was concluded that top managers make these final choices using intuition, formal analysis, and knowledge of organizational politics. In making good choices, top managers do extensive planning, communicating, and politicking.

In this research project, successful strategies for decision-making were reported as follows[15]:

1. Building extensive networks of individuals and groups who would provide them with resources at local, state, and national levels.
2. Searching the nursing, hospital, and business literature.
3. Being knowledgeable and involved in the politics of their organization and professional organizations.
4. Communicating regularly and repeatedly about decision-making activities to organization members, especially those in the hospital's dominant coalition—usually the chief executive officer, finance manager, and chief of the medical staff.
5. Directing most of their time and energy toward the accomplishment of their plans.

Since the model proved promising in strategic decision-making, it needs further testing, particularly in the area of human resource development and investment in human capital. As described in this work, strategic decision-making was the domain of top management. With current changes in health care organizations to flatter, leaner ones, input from self-managed work teams may be profitable.

Steps in the Process

From these and other models of decision-making, seven general steps of the process have been identified. Goals and objectives may be set prior to beginning the general process. They will answer the question, "What do we want the outcome or results of this decision to be?" When new products or services are the outcome, the goals and objectives are established first and problems or decisions are then forecast (step 1 of Exhibit 12-1). (Managers who wish to reverse steps 1 and 2 may do so.)

The problem must be identified (step 2 of Exhibit 12-1). Although this step may seem simple, recognizing and defining the problem is complex because of the diversity of individual perceptions. Because all individuals affected by the problem should be involved in discussing it, authority for decision-making should be delegated to individuals at the level of impact. When this is impossible, representatives of various affected groups may provide input. Each representative may have a different perspective as to what the outcome should be. Nurses should make certain that the identified problem is one that requires their attention and cannot be handled alone by those involved. Collecting

EXHIBIT 12-1

The Decision-Making Process Including Cost–Benefit Analysis

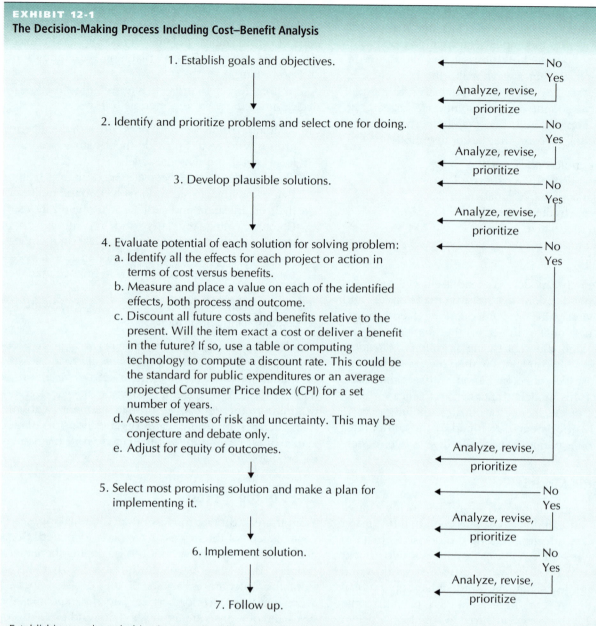

1. Establish goals and objectives.

2. Identify and prioritize problems and select one for doing.

3. Develop plausible solutions.

4. Evaluate potential of each solution for solving problem:
   a. Identify all the effects for each project or action in terms of cost versus benefits.
   b. Measure and place a value on each of the identified effects, both process and outcome.
   c. Discount all future costs and benefits relative to the present. Will the item exact a cost or deliver a benefit in the future? If so, use a table or computing technology to compute a discount rate. This could be the standard for public expenditures or an average projected Consumer Price Index (CPI) for a set number of years.
   d. Assess elements of risk and uncertainty. This may be conjecture and debate only.
   e. Adjust for equity of outcomes.

5. Select most promising solution and make a plan for implementing it.

6. Implement solution.

7. Follow up.

Establishing goals and objectives requires that decisions be made as to how they will be achieved. A first decision may be setting the priority in which they will be carried out. Decisions do not relate only to problems. They relate to development of plans and programs to accomplish nursing goals and objectives. When the best alternative does not work, another decision on whether to start over from step 1 is required, especially if other alternatives have less chance of success. The cost versus the benefit of the solution is introduced at step 4.

factual information in addition to subjective perceptions is essential. Logical and systematic fact-finding includes questioning all sources for divergent opinions and objective data. When the difference between desired and present situations or outcomes is significant, it may signal recognition of the problem.

Once the problem has been identified, the nurse must then evaluate the potential for a solution and determine the priority of the problem. Reitz suggests three approaches to setting priorities for problems[16]:

1. Deal with problems in the order in which they appear.
2. Solve the easiest problems first.
3. Solve crisis problems before all others. A decision will depend on the time and energy that can be devoted at that time. When a high-priority problem

EXHIBIT 12-2
Model of the Strategic Decision Process

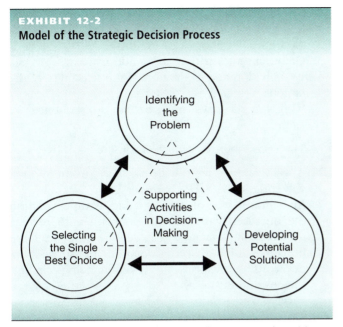

Source: Reprinted from "The Structure of 'Unstructured' Decision Processes" by Henry Mintzberg, Duru Raisinghani, and Andre Theoret, published in *Administrative Science Quarterly*, 21, 2, (July–August 1990), 20, by permission of Administrative Science Quarterly. © 1990 by Administrative Science Quarterly.

with limited potential for resolution is identified, the decision-maker may be forced to give it lower priority until more information is collected and acceptable alternatives can be found. The fact that needed information is missing may help define the real problem underlying the perceived one.

The third step in decision-making is *gathering and analyzing information related to the solution* (step 3 of Exhibit 12-1). This step involves defining, through a series of activities, the specifications to be met by the solution. A thorough information search may be needed to validate that the problem has been correctly identified. This search should include knowledge of organizational policy, prior personal experience or training, or the experience of others. Externally, the nurse begins to identify alternatives, comparing the potential solutions with the desired outcome and the desired outcome with available resources. In organizational settings, data base information systems may provide this information quickly. Establishing goals with measurable objectives helps focus the search for alternatives. Certainly to be considered while comparing potential alternatives is the cost, the time required and available, and the capabilities of those who will be involved in implementing a decision.

Once again, it is essential to involve in these discussions the individuals who will be affected by the choice. Irrelevant, insignificant, and extraneous factors must be eliminated from consideration. Gaining a com-

mitment to implement a decision before the choice is made supports the process. It is possible to reach a point of overload when the searcher has received information too quickly or in too great a quantity to process. Research indicates that the quantity of information sought has a direct, positive correlation with the degree of anticipated risk in the decision to be made. The personal confidence of the decision-maker also affects the amount of information required to support decision-making choices. Less searching is required by the nurse who recognizes patterns or similarities to previously encountered problems and confidently makes a choice of alternatives.

The forth and fifth steps in decision-making are *evaluating all alternatives and selecting one for implementation* (steps 4 and 5 of Exhibit 12-1). In the evaluation of alternatives, possible positive and negative consequences and the estimated probability of each choice are identified. A common approach involves identifying the best and worst possible outcomes to an alternative and then the outcomes that fall between the two extremes. As each alternative is evaluated, additional options may become apparent. Disagreement may stimulate the imagination and produce better solutions.

The effects of making no decision must be weighed against the effects of each proposed solution. Each alternative must be systematically evaluated for its efficiency and effectiveness in accomplishing the desired outcome and for the likelihood of achieving it with available or obtainable resources. The advantages and disadvantages of each alternative are identified during these steps to determine risk factors in possible outcomes. Identifying the solution that best satisfies specifications should receive attention before any compromises, concessions, or revisions are made by involved parties. The alternative that provides the greatest probability of an acceptable desired outcome using available resources is most likely to be selected.

A sixth step in the decision-making process is to *act on or implement the selected alternative* (step 6 of Exhibit 12-1). The knowledge and skills of the decision-maker transform the alternative into action by completing any necessary plans involving sequencing steps and preparing individuals to implement the solution, all the while effectively communicating the process with all involved.

Orton suggests asking seven questions to increase the success of one's decision choice[17]:

1. Does the quality of the decision really make a difference?
2. Do I have all the information I need to make the decision alone?
3. Do I know what I'm missing? Do I know where to find the information? Will I know what to do with the information I'm given?

4. Do I need anybody's commitment to make sure this succeeds?
5. Can I gain commitments without offering participation in the decision?
6. Do those involved in the decision share the organization's goals?
7. Is there likely to be conflict about the available alternatives?

A final step in the process of decision-making is to *monitor the implementation and evaluate outcomes* (step 7 of Exhibit 12-1). The nurse compares actual results with anticipated outcomes and makes modifications as needed to accomplish the desired outcome. Evaluation criteria obtained from measurable objectives provide feedback for testing the validity and effectiveness of the decision against the actual sequence of events in the process. Determination of flaws or gaps in the process may assist the decision-maker to monitor the process more closely in the future and prevent the recurrence of problems. The effective decision-maker consciously follows these seven steps in a logical sequence.

Cost–Benefit Analysis

Cost–benefit analysis has a major role to play as a decision-making tool. Is the expenditure justified in terms of the return or benefit on the investment? Exhibit 12-1 illustrates the addition of cost–benefit analysis to the decision-making process. Additional reference to cost–benefit analysis is found in Chapter 10, on Budgeting.

Cost–benefit analysis should be as objective as possible. Many actions can be quantified and a value placed on them. Others are qualitative and should be evaluated on a rational basis.[18]

Prescriptive Decision Theory

Prescriptive decision theory uses decision-making rules that are more clearly related to the rational modes of thinking—to left-brain thinking. Descriptive decision theory, on the other hand, looks for patterns, regularities, or principles related to the process by which people actually make decisions.

The defining attributes of a decision are[19]:

1. Making a deliberate mental choice.
2. Taking action based on indication or evidence.
3. Choosing between two or more options.
4. Bringing doubt or debate to an end by committing to certain actions or inactions.
5. Expecting to accomplish certain goals.

The antecedents of a decision are:

1. Consideration of a matter that causes doubt, wavering, debate, or controversy.
2. Awareness of choices or options.
3. Gathering information about alternatives.
4. Examination and evaluation of the feasibility of the various alternatives.
5. Weighing the risks and possible consequences of each option.

The consequences of a decision are:

1. A stabilizing effect, with an end to the doubt, wavering, debate, or controversy.
2. An action in one of the following ways: to reaffirm the decision with full implementation, to reverse the decision, to stand by the decision but curtail full implementation, a consideration of subsequent decisions in response to ever-changing circumstances and desires.

Pitfalls of Decision-Making

Although information technology is having an increasing effect on decision-making, pitfalls in the process stem more from individuals than from computers. Individuals are still resistant to change involving risk and new ideas. Such attitudes stifle not only individuals but also groups. When nurses find themselves resisting, they should analyze their behavior toward the goal of becoming more imaginative and creative. It is important to move away from becoming authoritarian and controlling. If the nurse chooses to control decision-making and omit from the process those affected by the decision, less commitment to implementing the decision is a natural result. When feasible, the nurse may use a team approach to decision-making, as in a matrix organization. Group decision-making usually produces greater commitment to putting the selected alternative into action and working for success. Team decision-making is especially effective in patient care.

Other pitfalls of decision-making include inadequate fact-finding, time constraints, and poor communication.

Failing to systematically follow the steps of the decision-making process will likely result in unanticipated results.

Improving Decision-Making

Basic precepts other than those already mentioned include educating people so they know how to make decisions, securing top management support for decision-making at the lowest possible level, establishing decision-making checkpoints with appropriate time limits, keeping informed of progress by ensuring access to first-hand information, using statistical analysis when possible to pinpoint problems for solution,[20] and staying open to use of new ideas and technologies to analyze problems and identify alternatives. Computers can be used to support decision-making through data-based management systems. Numerous strategies and tools are available to improve decision-making abilities.

A successful nurse is one who stays informed about decisions being made at different levels of the organization after appropriately delegating these responsibilities and who deals only with those decisions requiring his or her level of expertise, supports implementation of decisions, and credits the decision-maker. McKenzie states that managers who make all decisions themselves convey a lack of trust in the ability or loyalty of their subordinates. Selective delegation of decision-making gains the support of staff members and raises their self-esteem. They gain a sense of belonging and develop loyalty. Delegation leads to leadership. Leaders share authority and power rather than impose it. This is not to say that leaders do not ever make decisions without input from subordinates. This may be necessary on occasion and is acceptable to subordinates who know they participate in decisions that rely on their level of knowledge and experience.[21] Wrapp wrote that good managers don't make policy decisions. Instead, they concentrate on a limited number of significant issues, identify areas where they can make a difference, judge how hard to force an issue, give a sense of direction to the organization through open-ended objectives, and spot opportunities that permit others to "own" their own ideas and plans for implementation. Wrapp's description of the successful manager portrays a motivator, knowledgeable and skilled in both decision-making and problem-solving, who serves as a role model for others.[22]

Consensus Building

One of the strong points of decision-making by Japanese leaders is consensus building. When a major change is to occur, Japanese leaders may spend months and even years gaining consensus of internal customers and even of some external customers such as suppliers. When the change is initiated, all concerned parties have had input into the decision-making process and so get behind it to make it successful. They are stakeholders with a perception of a shared future. Kanter would probably label this a synergy, since it encourages cooperation of all groups. Partnerships among groups require consultation and cooperation. Such partnerships are egalitarian, with members talking about work and its tasks. These members search for consensus on goals that lead to successful outcomes for the corporation, the employees, and shareholders.[23]

Group-think and consensus building are somewhat of a paradox. To build consensus, one listens to all parties, uses their ideas, and brings them onto the team by involving them in critical thinking and realistically considering their ideas. Group-think aims for fast solutions with minimal critical thinking and participant input.

The Role of Intuition

Intuitive reasoning abilities have a place in the decision-making process for intuitive reasoning abilities. Intuition is a powerful tool for guiding decision-making. So-called left-brain activities, such as analytical and logical thinking, mathematics, and sequential information processing are essential in decision-making and problem-solving. But right-brain functions allow people to simultaneously process information, conceive and use contradictory ideas, fantasize, and perceive intuitively. Intuition is defined as the power to apprehend the possibilities inherent in a situation. It is a subspecies of logical thinking and integrates information from both sides of the brain—facts and feeling cues.[24] Nurses who can think intuitively have a sense of vision—they generate new ideas and ingenious solutions to old problems. Agor reported research involving 2,000 managers using a Myers-Briggs Type Indicator (MBTI) for measuring intuitive ability. The MBTI is widely used to measure intuition. Initial findings showed intuitive ability varying by managerial level, with higher ability in top-level managers than in middle- or lower-level managers.

Factors cited by middle- and lower-level managers that impeded the use of intuition included lack of confidence, time constraints, stress factors, and projection mechanisms such as dishonesty and attachment. Follow up of the 200 top executives who scored in the top 10% of the first study revealed that all but one used intuitive ability as a tool in guiding decisions. These managers stated that their intuitive ability stemmed from years of knowledge and experience. From this research, Agor identified eight conditions in which intuitive ability seems to function best[25]:

1. When a high level of uncertainty exists.
2. When little previous precedent exists.
3. When variables are less scientifically predictable.
4. When "facts" are limited.
5. When facts don't clearly point the way to go.
6. When analytical data are of little use.
7. When several plausible alternative solutions exist to choose from, with good arguments for each.
8. When time is limited and there is pressure to come up with the right decision.

Nurses can certainly identify with each of these decision-making situations. It should be gratifying to know that research has supported the use of intuition in decision-making. Research findings suggest that decision-making in clinical practice is both a rational and intuitive process.[26] Research also indicates "that intuition occurs in response to knowledge, is a trigger for action and/or reflection and thus has a direct bearing on analytical processes in patient/client care."[27] Intuition is based on rational factors of knowledge and experience.[28] However, it is stressed that there are appropriate times for using intuition as an *adjunct* to the logical steps of decision-making—*not* where objective data are complete. Because basic nursing education stresses the need for assessing facts and avoiding personal opinions, it may be difficult for some nurses to activate intuition for decision-making. Agor has identified techniques and exercises used by executives to activate and expand their intuitive decision-making abilities, including relaxation and mental/analytical techniques. A full account of Agor's research is beyond the scope of this chapter; the reader is referred to Agor's extensive writings on the subject of intuitive decision-making.[29]

Intuition is observed in individuals and in groups and is a creative and powerful attribute. Groups use intuition to reach consensus, particularly where information is incomplete. Consensus in a group leads to selection of a solution to a problem or to the making of a decision. Intuition can be developed through group brainstorming sessions, group visualization, and quiet thinking time.[30]

The human brain has a specialized region for making personal and social decisions, which is located in the frontal lobes at the top of the brain and is connected to deeper brain regions that store emotional memories. Injury or stroke damage to this area causes personality changes, and the person can no longer make moral decisions. This knowledge has implications for behavior related to intuitive versus rational decision-making.[31]

Decision-making involves critical thinking. As the nurse becomes more expert, the process becomes more intuitive, and the expert nurse automatically processes the decision-making action as a consequence of a high level of knowledge and experience. The decision-making process is fostered by training, feedback, and the expansion of nursing knowledge. Case studies are good vehicles for teaching critical thinking.[32]

Nurses make critical decisions about resources affecting patient care. Resources include staff, equipment, supplies, bed space, time, and patient assignments to staff. Expert nurses make different decisions than do novice nurses. Nurses make decisions requiring intelligence and judgment, personal and professional

values, ethics, law, political reality, organizational culture, norms of classes, and economics.[33] Intuitive nurses have clinical skills, incorporate a spiritual component in their practice, are interested in the abstract nature of things, are risk takers, are extroverted, and express confidence in their intuitions.[34]

Organizational Versus Personal Decisions

Various models for decision-making have been identified, and specific steps involved in the process, including the role of intuition, have been described. Now the question is raised of when to make an organizational or a personal decision.

Organizational decisions relate to organizational purpose; constant refinement of organizational purpose is required because the organizational environment changes. This process provides opportunities for participative management styles, thereby giving subordinates the prerogative and responsibility of professional decision-making.[35]

When are organizational decisions necessary? It would be easy to say we deal with professionals who are capable of making decisions related to their practice. An effective manager would not make decisions for competent professionals. However, incapacity of subordinates, uncertain instructions, novel conditions, conflicts, or failure of authority to make effective decisions or to make decisions at all may cause decisions to be appealed to a higher authority. Effective organizational decisions require collaboration and consultation with those having specialized knowledge.

From an organizational standpoint, decisions may be analyzed on the basis of futurity, impact, or qualitative or value factors, and whether the decision is recurrent, rare, or unique. *Futurity* is defined as the length of time over which the decision will affect the organization in the future and the time required to reverse its impact. *Impact* refers to the number of individuals or departments affected and is a determinant of the level at which the decision is made. When *qualitative or value factors* of philosophy or ethics are involved, decisions must be made at a higher level. The last characteristic refers to the *uniqueness* of the decision; *recurrent* decisions are made following a rule or principle already established.[36]

But what about institutional policy? Historically, decision-making in nursing has been authoritarian, with minimal input from nursing staff, particularly when it involves institutional policy. Nurses have also been limited in their professional autonomy. Literature on the sociology of professions has indicated that a professional person has an ultimate or independent decision-making authority granted by society on the basis of unique knowledge and skill. This viewpoint gave physicians control over nurses. The traditional definition of autonomy no longer applies: Patients now demand more input in decision-making, and, increasingly, patient care technology requires nurses to make independent life-and-death decisions. McKay redefined professional autonomy as "both independent and interdependent practice-related decision-making based on a complex body of knowledge and skill."[37] Primary nursing promotes nurse accountability, intraprofessional and interprofessional consultation, and an assertive synthesis of nursing and medical care plans. Interdependent decision-making promotes professional autonomy.

Since nurse caregivers are functioning with increasing professional autonomy, nurse managers are moving into more executive positions in health care administration. Nurse managers recognize the advantages of nurses being involved in strategic institutional decisions such as those concerning major programs, policies, promotions, personnel, and budgets. In addition to enhancing professional autonomy, the involvement of nurses in decision-making has resulted in higher job satisfaction, better morale, lower turnover, improved communication, improved professional relationships with peers and colleagues from other disciplines, and higher productivity.[38]

Blegen and others at the University of Iowa studied nurses' preferences for decision-making autonomy in Iowa hospitals. They found that nurses wanted a more independent level of authority and accountability in 12 of 21 patient-care decisions, including those that concern patient teaching, pain management, preventing complications, clarifying and advancing orders, scheduling and discussing the plan of care with the patient, consulting with other providers, and arranging daily assignments and schedules. They also found that nurses wanted to make group decisions about such matters as setting policies, procedures, unit goals, job descriptions and standards, quality improvement, and job performance. Nurse managers desired to increase decision-making by staff nurses. It would appear that nurse managers should provide the impetus for more involvement in decision-making by staff nurses by asking them what they want and actively involving them. The latter would include training and education. Staff nurses may want decision-making autonomy in areas where they are expert and competent.[39]

Many nurses equated decision-making autonomy with nurse professionalism. Most nurses are nonautonomous since they are not self-employed. Research studies do not always support the premise that decision-making autonomy increases job satisfaction or performance or decreases nurse turnover.[40]

The nurse manager can maximize the opportunity for staff nurses to be involved in interdependent decision-making by involving them at all levels of patient-care decision-making, especially on interdisciplinary institutionwide committees. Strategies that have proven successful in involving nurses in accomplishing this include decentralization to the unit level, committee systems, and governance systems.[41]

Nurses who pursue holistic nursing practice encourage clients to make decisions about health and health care issues. Decisions about health care policy are not controlled by health care professionals. They are made by the business sector and according to sociopolitical and economic variables.

Nurses need to become policy analysts, since analysts use communication networks or structures as strategy to action. Communication with decision-makers is crucial to effecting decision-making. Nurses use networking and professional relationships to influence decision-makers. They arrive at positions on health care policy through interest groups. Membership in professional associations, committees, and interest groups, plus communication with or as analysts, leads to participation in policy decision-making and changes in the primary health care system.[42]

Shared governance is an organizational administrative model that has been used as a vehicle for increasing staff-nurse participation in decision-making and problem-solving. It often involves multidisciplinary groups. Shared governance has as its object the provision of a trusting and nonjudgmental environment in which nurses, along with others, use the decision-making and problem-solving processes to make productive changes in organizations. Improved communication is a product of the shared governance process.[43]

> **Research indicates that promotion of decision-making by nurse managers is a factor in retention of critical care nurses.[44] Research also indicates that increased academic education is associated with better decision-making in practice.[45]**

Problem-Solving Process

At this point, one may be wondering about the relationship between decision-making and problem-solving. The first step in decision-making was to identify the problem. But problem-solving can involve the making of several decisions. The best way to define the relationship between the two is to define the steps of problem-solving.

Steps in the Process

The steps of the problem-solving process are the same as the steps of the nursing process and the decision-making process: assess and analyze, plan, implement, and evaluate. Assessment includes systematic collection, organization, and analysis of data related to a specific problem or need. It involves logical fact-finding, questioning all sources, and differentiating between objective facts and subjective feelings, opinions, and assumptions. Knowledge and experience guide the data collection and analysis of data. Before the process goes any further, assessment should also determine whether a commitment exists to implement a decision or an action.[46] Making certain that there is no readily apparent solution also saves the time of all the people who may become involved in problem-solving. Once the problem is identified, it must be determined whether it requires other than routine handling—that is, whether it is a rare or unique situation rather than a recurrent one. This leads to the second step of problem-solving: planning.

Planning involves several phases. In nursing terms, we determine priorities, set goals and measurable objectives, and plan interventions. Management literature essentially says the same thing: break the problem down into components and establish priorities; develop alternative courses of action; determine probable outcomes for each alternative; decide which course is best in relation to resources, goals, risks, and the like; and decide on and make a plan of action with a time table for implementation.[47]

When determining priorities, nurses should relate the problem to the corporate mission. Decisions involve choosing among alternative courses of action. They must have an acceptable effect on those directly involved, other areas affected, and the entire organization. Plans should include when and how to alter a course of action when undesired results occur.

The third step is implementation of the plan. The nurse should keep informed of the status of the process because it is unlikely that she or he will be directly involved. This is the one step in the process most likely to be delegated to subordinates. Implementation requires knowledge and skills appropriate to the specific alternatives selected.

Evaluation, the final step in problem-solving, includes determining how closely goals and objectives were met, the success or failure of actions taken in resolving the problem, and whether the plan should be terminated because the problem has been resolved or whether it should be continued, with or without modification.

Effective problem-solving requires that the practitioner be frequently at a high cognitive level: the level of abstract thinking. The essential difference between problem-solving and decision-making is that in the former, the thinking process works to solve a problem, whereas in the latter, it serves to reach a goal or condition. Students learn to do problem-solving by actually solving client's problems. In doing so, student and client collaborate. Computer simulations are available for problem-solving. Students progress through several levels of cognitive problem-solving and practice: novice, advanced beginner, competent, and proficient. A few interactive video discs are available for practice in solving clinical problems.[48] Many strategies are available through the Internet.

Group Problem-Solving

While each step of the problem-solving process can be approached by an individual, input from all affected individuals or areas promotes more complete data collection, creative planning, successful implementation, and evaluation indicating problem resolution. Managerial problem-solving groups are often formed in organizations, with the expectation that the group's effect will prove to be greater than the sum of its parts. Brightman and Verhoeven state that:

> [a] team of problem-solvers has greater potential resources than an individual, can have a higher motivation to complete the job, can force members to examine their own beliefs more carefully and can develop creative solutions.[49]

Summary

Decision-making and problem-solving occur concurrently with all major functions of nursing. Four models of the cognitive thinking skills involved in decision-making are presented: the normative model, the decision-tree model, the descriptive model, and the strategic model.

Decision-making involves having an objective, gathering data pertaining to the objective, analyzing the data, identifying and evaluating alternative courses of action to achieve the objective, selecting an alternative (the decision), implementing it, and evaluating the results. Nurses make the best decisions through knowledge and use of the theory of decision-making combined with intuitive ability developed over years of experience.

Although problem-solving is not the exact equivalent of decision-making, it employs a similar thinking process. Decision-making is different from problem-solving in that the objective does not have to pertain to a problem. It can be an objective that relates to change, to progress, to research, and to implementation of any operational or management plan.

APPLICATION EXERCISES

EXERCISE 12-1

The following exercises may be done individually or as a group. You may want to work with a group of your peers.

Case Study: You are Ms. Carrie Platt. You have been director of nursing of Mason General Hospital for 1½ years. Mason General is a 500-bed general hospital in a metropolitan area, serving a population of 700,000. The city has four other hospitals and a University Medical Center. A local ADN nursing program is affiliated with your hospital. Today is Monday, March 20. During the past week, on Thursday, March 16, and Friday, March 17, you were away from the hospital to conduct a two-day workshop. It is 8 A.M. and you have just arrived at the hospital. You must leave the hospital at 8:50 A.M. in order to be at the airport at 9:10 A.M. There has been an unexpected death in the family and you will be gone the entire week. You notice that the in-basket contains several items. You should make decisions about these things before leaving.

INSTRUCTIONS: Three decision-making exercises appear on the following pages. Each exercise is composed of a memorandum or other message-carrying device and a decision worksheet format. Use the worksheet format to list ideas for action and arrive at a decision. If the information given lacks essential details, make any assumptions necessary. Possible examples of decisions include the following:

1. Take immediate action and state what the action is.
2. Delegate the action to another person and state who the person is.
3. Postpone the action; state to what time.
4. Other course; please specify.

A. MEMORANDUM

TO: Ms. Platt SUBJECT: Poor charting of I&O
FROM: Kay Campbell, Nurse Manager–5 N Date: March 17

The I&O record on Mrs. East in 517 is incomplete for evening and night shifts for her postoperative period. She went into shock in the recovery room and is in renal failure. Dr. Blake is *extremely* upset about the lack of thorough charting of I&O. One of the evening aides heard Mr. East call his lawyer about the possibility of a lawsuit. We thought you needed to be aware of this situation.

DECISION WORKSHEET

SUBJECT ALTERNATIVES	DECISION ANALYSIS	DECISION SELECTED	DECISION

B. MEMORANDUM

TO: Ms. Platt SUBJECT: Uniform Regulations
FROM: Mrs. Back, In-service Instructor TE: March 17

The meeting with the nursing assistants regarding uniform regulations has been scheduled for March 21 at 10:00 A.M. in In-service Room 406. We appreciate your offer to discuss this matter with the nursing assistants.

DECISION WORKSHEET

SUBJECT ALTERNATIVES	DECISION ANALYSIS	DECISION SELECTED	DECISION

(continued)

EXERCISE 12-1
(continued)

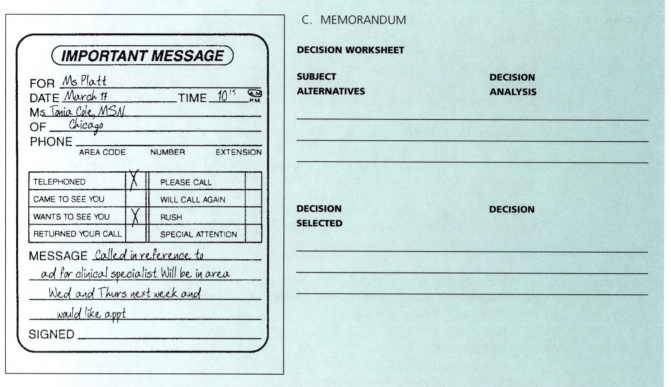

IMPORTANT MESSAGE

FOR _Ms Platt_

DATE _March 17_   TIME _10¹⁵_ A.M. / P.M.

Ms _Tonia Cole, MSN._

OF _Chicago_

PHONE _____

AREA CODE   NUMBER   EXTENSION

TELEPHONED	X	PLEASE CALL	
CAME TO SEE YOU		WILL CALL AGAIN	
WANTS TO SEE YOU	X	RUSH	
RETURNED YOUR CALL		SPECIAL ATTENTION	

MESSAGE _Called in reference to_
ad for clinical specialist. Will be in area
Wed and Thurs next week and
would like appt

SIGNED _____

C. MEMORANDUM

DECISION WORKSHEET

SUBJECT	DECISION
ALTERNATIVES	ANALYSIS

_____

_____

_____

DECISION	DECISION
SELECTED	

_____

_____

_____

NOTES

1. W. Lancaster and J. Lancaster, "Rational Decision Making: Managing Uncertainty," *Journal of Nursing Administration* (September 1982), 23–28.
2. T. Peters, "This Is CNN: Chaos Is the Future of Business," *San Antonio Light* (3 March 1992), B9.
3. P. Nolan, "Competencies Drive Decision Making," *Nursing Management* (March 1998), 27–29.
4. N. K. Arora and C. A. McHorney, "Patient Preferences for Medical Decision Making: Who Really Wants to Participate?" *Medical Care* (March 2000), 335–341; S. H. Babic, P. Kokol, M. Zorman, and V. Podgorelec, "The Influence of Class Discretization to Attribute Hierarchy of Decision Trees," *Student Health Technology Information*, 68, 1999, 676–681.
5. R. D. Shankar and M. A. Musen, "Justification of Automated Decision Making: Medical Explanations as Medical Arguments," *Proceedings AMIA Symposium* (1999), 395–399; P. W. Jamieson, "A New Paradigm for Explaining and Linking Knowledge in Diagnostic Problem Solving," *Journal of Clinical Eng* (September–October 1990), 371–380; M. F. Gerdtz and T. K. Bucknall, "Why We Do the Things We Do: Applying Clinical Decision-Making Frameworks to Triage Practice," *Accident Emergency Nursing* (January 1999), 50–57; J. Dowie, "What Decision Analysis Can Offer the Clinical Decision Maker. Why Outcome Databases Such as KIGS and KIMS Are Vital Sources for Decision Analysis," *Horm Res*, 51 Suppl 1, 1999, 73–82; C. A. Taylor, M. T. Draney, J. P. Ku, D. Parker, B. N. Steele, K. Wang, and C. K. Zarins, "Predictive Medicine: Computational Techniques in Therapeutic Decision Making,"

Computer Aided Surgery, 4(5), 1999, 231–247; L. G. Balneaves and B. Long, "An Embedded Decisional Model of Stress and Coping: Implications for Exploring Treatment Decision Making by Women with Breast Cancer," *Journal of Advanced Nursing* (December 1999), 1321–1331; M. Mazumdar and J. R. Glassman, "Categorizing a Prognostic Variable: Review of Methods, Code for Easy Implementation and Applications to Decision Making About Cancer Treatments," *Statistical Medicine*, (15 January 2000), 113–132.
6. M. Offredy, "The Application of Decision Making Concepts by Nurse Practitioners in General Practice," *Journal of Advanced Nursing* (November 1998), 988–1000; S. D. McGuinness and S. Peters, "The Diagnosis of Multiple Sclerosis: Peplau's Interpersonal Relations Model in Practice," *Rehabilitation Nursing* (January–February 1999), 30–33.
7. W. Lancaster and J. Lancaster, op. cit., 23.
8. V. H. Vroom, "A New Look at Managerial Decision Making, Organizational Decision Making," *Organizational Dynamics* (spring 1973), 66–80.
9. R. V. Brown, "Do Managers Find Decision Theory Useful?" *Harvard Business Review* (May–June 1970), 78–89; J. Magee, "Decision Trees for Decision Making," *Harvard Business Review* (July–August 1964), 126; J. Magee, "How to Use Decision Trees in Capital Investment," *Harvard Business Review* (September–October 1964), 79.
10. H. A. Simon, *Administrative Behavior*, 3rd ed. (New York: The Free Press, 1976).
11. Ibid.
12. W. Lancaster and J. Lancaster, op. cit.

13. J. M. Nagelkerk and B. J. Henry, "Strategic Decision Making," *Journal of Nursing Administration* (July–August 1990), 18–23.
14. Ibid., 21.
15. Ibid.
16. J. H. Reitz, *Behavior in Organizations* (Homewood, IL: Richard D. Irwin, 1977), 154–199.
17. A. Orton, "Leadership: New Thoughts on an Old Problem," *Training* (June 1984), 28, 31–33.
18. K. Harrison, "Cost Benefit Analysis: A Decision-Making Tool for Physiotherapy Managers," *Physiotherapy* (July 1991), 445–448.
19. P. Matteson and J. W. Hawkins, "Concept Analysis of Decision Making," *Nursing Forum*, 25(2), (1990), 4–10.
20. D. Graham and D. Reese, "There's Power in Numbers," *Nursing Management* (September 1984), 48–51.
21. M. E. McKenzie, "Decisions: How You Reach Them Makes a Difference," *Nursing Management* (June 1985), 48–49.
22. H. E. Wrapp, "Good Managers Don't Make Policy Decisions," *Harvard Business Review* (September–October 1967), 91–99.
23. R. M. Kanter, *When Giants Learn to Dance* (New York: Simon & Schuster, 1989), 114, 153–155.
24. W. H. Agor, "The Logic of Intuition: How Top Executives Make Important Decisions," *Organizational Dynamics* (winter 1986), 5–18.
25. Ibid., 9.
26. M. P. Watkins, "Decision-Making Phenomena Described by Expert Nurses Working in Urban Community Health Centers," *Journal of Professional Nursing* (January–February 1998), 22–23.
27. L. King and J. V. Appleton, "Intuition: A Critical Review of the Research and Rhetoric," *Journal of Advanced Nursing* (July 1997), 194–202.
28. P. Easen and J. Wilcockson, "Intuition and Rational Decision Making in Professional Thinking: A False Dichotomy?" *Journal of Advanced Nursing* (October 1996), 667–673.
29. W. H. Agor, op. cit.
30. L. Rew, "Intuition: Concept Analysis of a Group Phenomenon," *Advances in Nursing Science* (January 1986), 21–28.
31. S. Blakeslee, "Seat of Morality Inside the Brain," *San Antonio Express-News* (30 May 1994), 24A.
32. L. Casebeer, "Fostering Decision Making in Nursing," *Journal of Nursing Staff Development* (November–December 1991), 271–274.
33. M. L. Botter and S. B. Dickey, "Allocation of Resources: Nurses the Key Decision Makers," *Holistic Nursing Practice* (November 1989), 44–51.
34. V. G. Miller, "Characteristics of Intuitive Nurses," *Western Journal of Nursing Research* (June 1995), 305–316.
35. C. Barnard and M. Beyers, "The Environment of Decision," *The Journal of Nursing Administration* (March 1982), 25–29.
36. R. C. Swansburg, *Management of Patient Care Services* (Saint Louis: C.V. Mosby, 1976), 149–170.
37. P. S. McKay, "Interdependent Decision Making: Redefining Professional Autonomy," *Nursing Administration Quarterly* (summer 1983), 21–30.
38. American Hospital Association, *Strategies: Nurse Involvement in Decision Making and Policy Development* (1984), 1–10.
39. M. A. Blegen, C. Goode, M. Johnson, M. Maas, L. Chen, and S. Moorhead, "Preferences for Decision-Making Autonomy," *Image* (winter 1993), 339–344.
40. D. J. Dwyer, R. H. Schwartz, and M. L. Fox, "Decision Making Autonomy in Nursing," *Journal of Nursing Administration* (February 1992), 17–23.
41. American Hospital Association, op. cit.
42. N. J. Murphy, "Nursing Leadership in Health Policy Decision Making," *Nursing Outlook* (July–August 1992), 158–161.
43. B. Anderson, "Voyage to Shared Governance," *Nursing Management* (November 1992), 65–67; P. Ide and C. Fleming, "A Successful Model for the OR," *AORN Journal* (November 1999), 805–808, 811–813; H. M. Bell, "Shared Governance and Teamwork—Myth or Reality," *AORN Journal* (March 2000), 631–635.
44. D. K. Boyle, M. J. Bott, H. E. Hansen, C. Q. Woods, and R. L. Taunton, "Managers' Leadership and Critical Care Nurses' Intent to Stay," *American Journal of Critical Care* (November 1999), 361–371.
45. E. A. Girot, "Graduate Nurses: Critical Thinkers or Better Decision Makers?" *Journal of Advanced Nursing* (February 2000), 288–297.
46. A. Scharf, "Secrets of Problem Solving," *Industrial Management* (September–October 1985), 7–11.
47. B. Blai, Jr., "Eight Steps to Successful Problem Solving," *Supervisory Management* (January 1986), 7–9.
48. E. Klaasens, "Strategies to Enhance Problem Solving," *Nurse Educator* (May–June 1992), 28–30.
49. H. J. Brightman and P. Verhoeven, "Why Managerial Problem Solving Groups Fail," *Business* (January–March 1986), 24–29; D. E. Shaddinger, "Digging for Solutions," *Nursing Management* (May 1992), 96f, 96h.

REFERENCES

Argyris, C. "How Tomorrow's Executives Will Make Decisions." Reprint from *THINK Magazine*, IBM, 1967.

Argyris, C. *Reasoning, Learning and Action* (San Francisco: Jossey-Bass, 1982), 87, 102.

Beissner, K. L. "Use of Concept Mapping to Improve Problem Solving." *Journal of Physical Therapy Education* (spring 1992), 22–27.

Denton, D. K. "Problem Solving by Keeping in Touch." *Business* (July–September 1986), 40–42.

Galbraith, J. K. *The New Industrial State* (Boston: Houghton Mifflin, 1967).

Goldstein, M., D. Scholthaver, and B. B. Kleiner. "Management on the Right Side of the Brain." *Personnel Journal* (November 1985), 40–45.

Grandori, A. "Prescriptive Contingency View of Organizational Decision Making." *Administrative Science Quarterly* (June 1984), 192–209.

Greiner, L. E., D. P. Leitch, and D. P. Barnes. "Putting Judgment Back into Decisions." *Harvard Business Review* (March–April 1970), 59–67.

Hansten, R. I., and M. J. Washburn. "Individual and Organizational Accountability for Development of Critical Thinking." *Journal of Nursing Administration* (November 1999), 39–45.

Holland, H. K. "Decision Making and Personality." *Personnel Administration* (May–June 1968), 24–29.

Kersey, J. H. Jr. "Responsibility Accounting: Making Decisions Efficiently." *Nursing Management* (May 1985), 14, 16–17.

Kontryn, V. "Strategic Problem Solving in the New Millennium." *AORN Journal* (December 1999), 1042–1044.

Lachman, V. D. "9 Ways to Make Better Decisions." *Nursing 86* (June 1986), 73–74.

Lauri, S., S. Salantera, F. L. Gilje, and P. Klose. "Decision Making of Psychiatric Nurses in Finland, Northern Ireland, and the United States." *Journal of Professional Nursing* (September–October 1999), 275–280.

Leo, M. "Avoiding the Pitfalls of ManagemenThink." *Business Horizons* (May–June 1984), 44–47.

Locke, E. A., D. M. Schweiger, and G. P. Latham. "Participation in Decision Making: When Should It Be Used?" *Organizational Dynamics* (winter 1986), 65–79.

Matteson, P., and J. W. Hawkins. "Concept Analysis of Decision Making." *Nursing Forum*, 25(2), (1990), 4–10.

McKenzie, M. E. "Decisions: How You Reach Them Makes a Difference." *Nursing Management* (June 1985), 48–49.

Miller, M. "Putting More Power into Management Decisions." *Management Review* (September 1984), 12–16.

Newman, M. G. "Improved Clinical Decision Making Using the Evidence-Based Approach." *Annals of Periodontology* (November 1996), i–ix.

O'Neill, E. S. "Strenghtening Clinical Reasoning in Graduate Nursing Students." *Nurse Educator* (March–April 1999), 11–15.

Peters, T. *Thriving on Chaos* (New York: Harper & Row, 1987), 194–210.

Rakich, J. S., and A. B. Krigline. "Problem Solving in Health Services Organizations." *Hospital Topics* (spring 1996), 21–27.

Smith-Love, J., and C. Carter. "Collaboration, Problem Solving, Reevaluation: Foundation for the Heart Center of Excellence." *Progress in Cardiovascular Nursing* (autumn 1999), 143–149.

Southern Council on Collegiate Education for Nursing. *Preparing Nurses for Decision Making in Clinical Practice: A White Paper* (Atlanta: SCCEN, 1985).

Suding, M. J. "Decision Making Controlling the Computer Input." *Nursing Management* (July 1984), 44, 46, 48–52.

Willemsen, M. C., A. Meijer and M. Jannink. "Applying a Contingency Model of Strategic Decision Making to the Implementation of Smoking Bans: A Case Study." *Health Education Resources* (August 1999), 519–531.

CHAPTER 13

Implementing Planned Change

Russell C. Swansburg, PhD, RN

LEARNING OBJECTIVES AND ACTIVITIES

- Identify reasons or need for change in nursing practice and nursing management.
- Match examples of change to Reddin's seven techniques for accomplishing change.
- Match examples of change to Lewin's three stages of change theory.
- Match examples of change to Lippitt's seven stages of change theory.
- Match descriptions of change theory to the correct theorist.
- Identify the causes of resistance to change.
- Develop plans including strategies for overcoming resistance to change.
- Define creativity.
- Develop plans for recognizing and increasing the creativity and innovation of clinical nurses.
- Describe the need for nursing research in a service setting.
- Make a plan for nursing research activity in the service setting.

CONCEPTS: Change theory, creativity, innovation, nursing research.

MANAGER BEHAVIOR: The manager considers change the domain of executive nursing and initiates all efforts for change accordingly.

LEADER BEHAVIOR: A leader encourages all nursing employees to recommend changes in the practice of nursing and in the environment in which nursing is practiced. He or she involves nurses in implementing change and encourages nurses to be creative and involved in nursing research activities.

Introduction

As a catalyst, the nurse causes or accelerates changes by using knowledge and skills that are *not* permanently affected by the reaction to the changes. In essence, the nurse may be considered a change agent. Let us first consider the philosophy embodied in theories of human resource management, theories based on adequate assumptions about human nature and human motivation. Has the nurse organized money, materials, equipment, and personnel in the interests of providing quality services to patients and thereby giving them their money's worth? Have nursing employees had experiences of supervision that have made them passive and resistant to organizational needs? Or do nursing employees work under conditions that inspire them to develop their potential, assume increased responsibility, and work to achieve their personal goals as well as those of the organization? Are clinical nurses able to direct their own efforts?

Machiavelli said, "There is nothing more difficult to take in hand, more perilous to conduct, or more uncertain in its success, than to take the lead in the introduction of a new order of things."[1] With a few notable exceptions, such as the weather, most of the change that takes place in our society is planned. This means that nurse managers can plan with clinical nurses to implement change. It must first be decided that a new skill or technique using a new apparatus or technology is needed to improve patient care and the ability to deliver that care. Then nurse managers and clinical nurses can plan and carry out the changes they want to make.

Spradley defines planned change as "a purposeful, designed effort to bring about improvements in a system, with the assistance of a change agent."[2] Peters writes that planned change is the exception rather than the rule.[3] Change occurs whether one wants it to or not. New technology is developed, and new treatments result, causing personnel and organizational adjustments. These changes need to be controlled or managed. Hence we refer to the process as *planned change*.

The Need for Change

Four general reasons for designing orderly change have been defined by Williams[4]:
1. To improve the means of satisfying somebody's economic wants.
2. To increase profitability.
3. To promote human work for human beings.
4. To contribute to individual satisfaction and social well-being.

To these reasons one must add the climate of the new millennium: that the structures of health care organizations will continue to change as will the structures of other businesses and industries. These changes encompass higher standards and superior performance, constant innovation in technology and corporate structure, the accomplishment of doing more for less, teamwork, customer preference, employee versus employer loyalties, industry regulations, corporate ownership, increased opportunities, shrinking resources, increased competition, more transactions, more paperwork, and more complexity.[5] The need for organizational change may involve not only the whole system but also each of its units. This change will require management of the political dynamics and transition as well as motivation of constructive behavior.[6]

The basic motivation for change could be that orderly change needs to be designed to improve patient care while lowering costs and increasing nursing's economic status. It could be that the organization would profit by being able to do more for less or at the same cost or by improving its reputation for quality of care. Or, change could improve individual satisfaction and social well-being for both patients and staff members.

Implementing planned change will alter nursing's status quo. New programs of patient care will modify existing relationships among nursing personnel and between them and other members of the health care team.

Change can help achieve organizational objectives as well as individual ones. Individual nurses and the institution of nursing will grow and prosper if they change with improved technology, especially if that technology will cure disease, save infant lives, prolong life without increasing suffering, and in general promote social improvement.

Other changes include personnel and organizational adjustments, such as constant turnover of personnel or changes in organizational structure. Nurses are certainly aware of changing relationships with those who hold authority and power, changes in responsibility and status, and changes in organizational, departmental, and unit objectives. Some employees resist change, but others welcome it as an opportunity to make adjustments in existing work situations, alter their relationships with their associates, and achieve personal goals.

Structural change will greatly reduce central staffers, perhaps by as much as 80% to 90%. This will include those in human resource development as well as nursing staff development. Central staffers will need to become project creators and network builders for the primary business units—the direct patient care units and the product sales units. As consultants to these units, central staffers can help develop the expertise needed there. Otherwise they can develop independent service centers, selling their services to the business units within the organization and to outside markets.[7] All of this change is needed because of increasing competition, technological advancements, and human resource concerns.[8]

During the past three decades there have been significant changes in the nature of health care organizations, the demands placed on nurse managers, and the needs and motivations of nursing personnel. Successful nurse managers have learned to manage change and have publicly related the role of nursing to being an involved and concerned element of society. They recognize the growing complexity of the health care organization, particularly today's division of nursing, and they recognize the changing values of nurses within the profession. Nurses want opportunities for advancement or promotion, recognition for their work, and more help from their peers and supervisors to improve their job skills. One dramatic change for nurses has been the impetus to develop their professional standards to higher levels by raising their credentials, particularly with regard to education. They have also recognized the need for continuing education to deliver up-to-date services. A glance at the plethora of nursing journals shows nurses' awareness of society's current problems and their increasing involvement with them. These include problems of health, environmental pollution, poverty, ethnic equality, education, civil rights, religion, and advances in genetics. Nurse managers see themselves as agents of change functioning within a profession that draws its basic support from society.

Evidence suggests that technological innovation can cause scientists' and engineers' knowledge to become obsolete in 10 years or less if they do not pursue further education. Parallel evidence could be developed to support the same conclusion about nursing. Today's nurses are more committed to task, job, and profession than they are loyal to an organization. They look at the kind of services provided (short term versus critical versus chronic), management's philosophy (participative versus authoritarian), experimental outlook, and physical and geographical location. Nurses want control over their work environment and are dissatisfied if they have no such control. For these reasons, philosophies and assumptions of nursing management are changing. Nurse managers are changing their management styles, policies, procedures, relationships with subordinates, and employment and compensation practices. Hospital managers are looking at the kinds of health services they offer. Nurse managers are seeking knowledge of community, state, and national affairs; government trends; individual needs; and group motivations. They are learning to function in a computerized world of business systems.

No longer is the nursing worker bound down by threat or ritual. Experienced expert nurses are still in great demand in the job market and are highly mobile. Nurses are willing to work hard, but they desire an environment where there is humor and opportunity to use imagination. Nurse managers change their behavior to suit the changing profile of this new breed of worker. Nurse managers are more flexible and individualized in dealing with employees. Nurse managers are candid, confronting conflict by allowing nurses to express their feelings, thoughts, and reactions. The change in nursing management aims to promote ideas of all people, to encourage attentive listening, and to reward people for becoming personally involved and committed to their work.

Adaptation to change has always been a job requirement for nursing. Nursing personnel work for numerous bosses, including individual patients, physicians, the nurse manager, and a different charge nurse on each shift. Nurse practitioners find their roles changed many times in a day, sometimes as a manager, sometimes as a clinical nurse, sometimes as a consultant, and always in multiple roles.

Among the reasons for change is the evidence that something needs changing. The nurse manager needs to recognize the symptoms, which can be glaring or subtle. An example of the latter would be offhand comments by float personnel, such as, "I'd rather work anywhere than unit 3F" or "Could you send me someplace else?"

The health care system is constantly changing. Changes include a labor force that wants wages comparable to those in other professions, hours of work that fit their personal needs, and the power to make their own professional decisions about patient care. The change often focuses on technology, without consideration for human relationships and political sensitivities. A case in point was the American Medical Association's 1988 failed

push to solve the nursing shortage by proposing a new health care technician. Professional nurses later introduced their own assistive nursing personnel proposals.

Nurses require extensive knowledge of community affairs, government trends and constraints, world affairs, international practices and procedures, the changing nature of individual needs, and group motivation. Even the supply and demand for nurses relate to these many areas. Within nursing, needs change with new computer systems, planning, business, accounting, control, and marketing.[9]

Younger nurses, like other younger professionals, are mobile and have salable skills. They want to use all of their skills and to be collaborative and democratic.[10]

Change is the key to progress and to the future. With it nurses develop new nursing systems that improve patient care and give greater satisfaction to nursing workers.

Change Theory

Some widely used change theories are those of Reddin, Lewin, Rogers, Havelock, Lippitt, and Spradley.

Reddin's Theory

Reddin has developed a planned change model that can be used by nurses. He has suggested seven techniques by which change can be accomplished:

1. Diagnosis.
2. Mutual setting of objectives.
3. Group emphasis.
4. Maximum information.
5. Discussion of implementation.
6. Use of ceremony and ritual.
7. Resistance interpretation.

The first three techniques are designed to give those who will be affected by the change an opportunity to influence its direction, nature, rate, and method of introduction. These individuals are then able to have some control over the change, to become involved in it, to express their ideas more directly, and to propose useful modifications.

Diagnosis (the first technique) is scientific problem-solving. Those affected by the change meet and identify problems and the probable outcomes. Mutual objective setting (technique number 2) ensures that the goals of both groups, those instituting the change and those affected by it, are brought into line. It may be necessary for groups to bargain and compromise. Group emphasis (number 3) is sometimes referred to as *team emphasis*. Change is more successful when supported by a team rather than by a single person. "Groups develop powerful standards for conformity and the means of enforcing them."[11]

Maximum information (number 4) is important to the success of change. Management should make at least four announcements with regard to a proposed change[12]:

1. That a change will be made.
2. What the decision is and why it was made.
3. How the decision will be implemented.
4. How implementation is progressing.

Lewin's Theory

One of the most widely used change theories is that of Kurt Lewin. Lewin's theory involves three stages:

1. *The unfreezing stage*: The nurse manager or other change agent is motivated by the need to create change. Affected nurses are made aware of this need. The problem is identified or diagnosed, and the best solution is selected. One of three possible mechanisms provides input to the initial change: (a) individual expectations are not being met (lack of confirmation), (b) the individual feels uncomfortable about some action or lack of action (guilt-anxiety), or (c) a former obstacle to change no longer exists (psychologic safety). The unfreezing stage occurs when disequilibrium is introduced into the system, creating a need for change.[13]
2. *The moving stage*: The nurse manager gathers information. A knowledgeable, respected, or powerful person influences the change agent in solving the problems (identification). A variety of sources give a variety of solutions (scanning), and a detailed plan is made. People examine, accept, and try out the innovation.[14]
3. *The refreezing stage*: Changes are integrated and stabilized as part of the value system. Forces are at work to facilitate the change (driving forces). Other forces are at work to impede change (restraining forces). The change agent identifies and deals with these forces, and change is established with homeostasis and equilibrium.[15]

Rogers' Theory

Everett Rogers modified Lewin's change theory. Antecedents included the background of the change agent and the change environment. Rogers' theory has five phases: Phase 1, *awareness*, corresponds to Lewin's unfreezing phase; phase 2, *interest*, phase 3, *evaluation*, and phase 4, *trial*, correspond to Lewin's moving phase. Phase 5, *adoption*, corresponds to the refreezing phase. In the adoption phase the change is accepted or rejected. If accepted, it requires interest and commitment.[16]

Rogers' theory depends on five factors for success. These factors are as follows[17]:

1. The change must have the relative advantage of being better than existing methods.
2. It must be compatible with existing values.
3. It must have complexity—more complex ideas persist even though simple ones get implemented more easily.
4. It must have divisibility—change is introduced on a small scale.
5. It must have communicability—the easier the change is to describe, the more likely it is to spread.

Havelock's Theory

Havelock's theory is another modification of Lewin's theory, expanded to six elements. The first three correspond to unfreezing, the next two to moving, and the sixth to refreezing. Havelock's phases are as follows[18]:

1. Building a relationship.
2. Diagnosing the problem.
3. Acquiring the relevant resources.
4. Choosing the solution.
5. Gaining acceptance.
6. Stabilization and self-renewal.

Lippitt's Theory

Lippitt added a seventh phase to Lewin's original theory. The seven phases of his theory of the change process are as follows[19]:

Phase 1: Diagnosing the problem. The nurse as change agent looks at all possible ramifications and involves those who will be affected. Group meetings are held to win the commitment of others. To ensure success, key people in top management and policy-making roles are involved.

Phase 2: Assessing the motivation and capacity for change. Possible solutions are determined, and the pros and cons of each are forecast. Consideration is given to implementation methods, roadblocks, factors motivating people, driving forces, and facility forces. Assessment considers financial aspects, organizational aspects, structure, rules and regulations, organizational culture, personalities, power, authority, and the nature of the organization. During this phase the change agent coordinates activities among a number of small groups.

Phase 3: Assessing the change agent's motivation and resources. The change agent can be external or internal to the organization or division. An external change agent may have fewer bases but must have expert credentials. An internal change agent, on the other hand, knows the people. The process could involve both. The change agent must have a genuine desire to improve the situation, knowledge of interpersonal and organizational approaches, experience, dedication, and a personality to suit the situation. The change agent should be objective, flexible, and accepted by all.

Phase 4: Selecting progressive change objectives. The change process is defined, a detailed plan is made, timetables and deadlines are set, and responsibility is assigned. The change is implemented for a trial period and evaluated.

Phase 5: Choosing the appropriate role of the change agent. The change agent will be active in the change process, particularly in handling personnel and facilitating the change. The change agent will deal with conflict and confrontation.

Phase 6: Maintaining the change. During this phase emphasis is on communication, with feedback on progress. The change is extended in time. A large change may require a new power structure.

Phase 7: Terminating the helping relationship. The change agent withdraws at a specified date after setting a written procedure or policy to perpetuate the change. The agent remains available for advice and reinforcement.

Exhibit 13-1 compares these theories.

It should be noted that all five theories are similar to the problem-solving process itself, indicating that the latter could be used to implement planned change. The nurse manager should select the theory she or he feels most comfortable with after identifying the change to

be made. A management plan is then made to cover the phases of making the change. The planning phase requires gathering data to support a decision for change. To set objectives, the nurse manager would work with the nursing staff who will be affected by the change. Thus, the entire group becomes aware of and interested in the need for change. A relationship is built between the nurse manager and nursing employees. The plan can then become an opportunity made cooperatively, implemented by an enthusiastic group, and evaluated and maintained by the group. Decision-making is implemented by planned change.

Spradley's Model

Spradley has developed an eight-step model based on Lewin's theory. She indicates that planned change must be constantly monitored to develop a fruitful relationship between the change agent and the change system. Following are the eight basic steps of the Spradley model[20]:

1. *Recognize the symptoms.* There is evidence that something needs changing.
2. *Diagnose the problem.* Gather and analyze data to discuss the cause. Consult with the staff. Read appropriate materials.
3. *Analyze alternative solutions.* Brainstorm. Assess the risks and the benefits. Set a time, plan resources, and look for obstacles.
4. *Select the change.* Choose the option most likely to succeed that is affordable. Identify the driving and

---

EXHIBIT 13-1
Comparison of Change Theories

REDDIN	LEWIN	ROGERS	HAVELOCK	LIPPITT
1. Diagnosis 2. Mutual objective setting	1. Unfreezing	1. Awareness	1. Building a relationship 2. Diagnosing the problem 3. Acquiring the relevant resources	1. Diagnosing the problem 2. Assessing motivation and capacity for change 3. Assessing change agent's motivation and resources
3. Group emphasis 4. Maximum information 5. Discussion of implementation 6. Use of ceremony and ritual	2. Moving	2. Interest 3. Evaluation 4. Trial	4. Choosing the solution 5. Gaining acceptance	4. Selecting progressive change objective 5. Choosing the appropriate role of the change agent 6. Maintaining change
7. Resistance interpretation	3. Refreezing	5. Adoption	6. Stabilization and self-renewal	7. Terminating the helping relationship

opposing forces, using challenges that include assimilation of the opposition.

5. *Plan the change.* This will include specific, measurable objectives, actions, a timetable, resources, budget, an evaluation method such as the Program Evaluation Review Technique (PERT), and a plan for resistance management and stabilization.

6. *Implement the change.* Plot the strategy. Prepare, involve, train, assist, and support those who will be affected by the change.

7. *Evaluate the change.* Analyze achievement of objectives and audit.

8. *Stabilize the change.* Refreeze; monitor until stable.

Exhibit 13-2 provides an illustration of this model. In a study of a nursing center for the community elderly, results showed that the use of change theory could determine a client's readiness to change health behaviors.[21]

The New Management Theory

Dunphy and Stace describe a differentiated contingency model for organizational change. It includes two contrasting theories of change, incremental and transformational, and two contrasting methods of change, participation and coercion.

Incremental change assumes that the effective manager moves the organization forward in small, logical steps. The long time frame plus the sharing of information increases confidence among employees and reduces the organization's dependence on outsiders to provide the impetus and momentum for change. The incremental model is similar to the systems approach to change and organizational development. It is used when the organization is ready for predicted future environmental conditions, but adjustments are needed in mission, strategy, structure, and/or internal processes.[22]

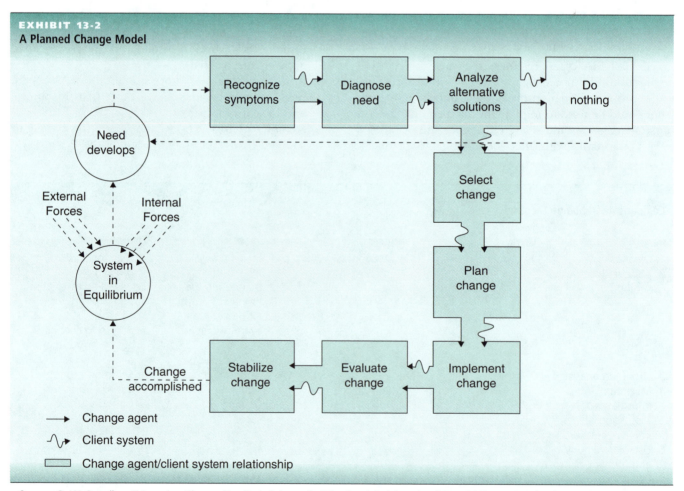

EXHIBIT 13-2
A Planned Change Model

Source: B. W. Spradley. "Managing Change Creatively." *Journal of Nursing Administration* (May 1980). Reprinted with permission of J. B. Lippincott.

An organization may require transformational change on a large scale when there is environmental "creep," organizational "creep," diversification, acquisition, merger, shutdowns, industry reorganization, or major technological breakthroughs. Transformational strategies embody large-scale adjustments in strategy, structure, and process requirements.

Participative methods of change are used to overcome work force resistance. Coercive methods are authoritarian and use force. The contingency model uses a mixture of methods, as dictated by conditions.[23] (See Exhibit 13-3.)

The new theory of management is one of transformation or change. Today the fundamental sources of wealth are knowledge and communication, not natural resources and physical labor. Change means opportunity and danger. Information technology and the computer are the enablers of productivity. Customers have much more power. Computers have replaced middle managers.

Success requires quick responses to changing circumstances. Organizational design should be reconfigurable on an annual, monthly, weekly, daily, or hourly basis. Organizations should be able to develop new products rapidly, have flexible production systems, and use team-based incentives. Big companies are outsourcing many functions. Companies are paying for intellectual labor. Intellectual assets—networks and databases—have replaced physical assets. The most valuable devices will help people cope with change.[24]

Management theory is going through a massive transformation, referred to in management literature as a revolution. The new theory of change process has three steps:

1. **The awakening.** This is when the need for change is realized. During step 1 the leadership articulates why the change is necessary.
2. **Envisioning.** This is a group effort that addresses technical, political, and cultural resistance. During step 2, resistance is dealt with. There will be technical resistance, political resistance related to resource allocation and powerful coalitions, and cultural resistance related to the chain of command, media, and training.
3. **Re-architecting.** This eliminates boundaries and compartments. To get rid of boundaries or ceilings, the hierarchy is de-layered, perks for executives are reduced, and gain-sharing incentive systems are broadened. To get rid of horizontal boundaries or internal walls, cross-functional teams, project teams, and partnership are used. To get rid of external boundaries, alliances are created, customer satisfaction is measured, and teams are built with customers and suppliers.

Leadership skills for the change include[25]:

1. Identify changes in the environment that will affect the business.
2. Lead others to overcome fear and uncertainty in making change.

EXHIBIT 13-3

A Typology of Change Strategies and Conditions for Their Use

	INCREMENTAL CHANGE STRATEGIES	TRANSFORMATIVE CHANGE STRATEGIES
Collaborative Modes	1. Participative Evolution Use when organization is in 'fit' but needs minor adjustment, or is out of fit but time is available and key interest groups favor change.	2. Charismatic Transformation Use when organization is out of 'fit' and there is little time for extensive participation, but there is support for radical change within the organization.
Coercive Modes	3. Forced Evolution Use when organization is in 'fit' but needs minor adjustment, or is out of fit but time is available, but key interest groups oppose change.	4. Dictatorial Transformation Use when organization is out of 'fit' and there is not time for extensive participation and no support within the organization for radical change, but radical change is vital to organizational survival and fulfilment of basic mission.

Source: Reprinted from "Transformational and Coercive Strategies for Planned Organizational Change: Beyond the O.D. Model." by D. C. Dunphy and D. A. Stace. *Organization Studies*, 9(3), (1988), 331. Reprinted with permission of Walter de Gruyter & Co., FB Wiso, Postiach 303421 10728 Berlin, © 1988.

3. Visualize the business in the eyes of the customer.
4. Have a clear vision of the future of the business.
5. Assume responsibility for own mistakes.
6. Build coalition and network across organizational lines to achieve important goals.
7. Lead the change.

Transformation is the process of reinventing an organization. Leaders create an atmosphere of never-ending change. Evaluation is done by peers, superiors, and subordinates. Transformed organizations have no boundaries, employees work up and down the hierarchy, across functions and geography, and with suppliers and customers. Goals center on numbers, total quality, and unity. Celebration is crucial, with emphasis on teamwork and using people's brains, imagination, and dedication. Let the team map the work to do it better and faster. The transformational manager views any process as susceptible to improvement. Reorganization focuses on customer segments and needs.[26]

In this transformation, leadership requires courage, judgment, and visibility. It requires a burning desire to change as health care organizations move to meet a world standard of quality. Managers need to motivate, empower, and educate employees. Managers may practice seven steps to being the best[27]:

1. Determine the world standard in every part of the process of providing care.
2. Use process mapping for the system's parts. Redesign to get rid of inefficiencies. Survey customers.
3. Communicate with your employees as if your life depended on it.
4. Distinguish what needs to be done from how hard it is to do it.
5. Set stretch targets. Let people decide how to reach them. Do not punish.
6. Never stop.
7. Pay attention to your inner self: recreation.

The Change Agent

As one studies change theory, one notes that its application tends to mimic the problem-solving process. The nurse, operating as a change agent, uses change theory to identify and solve problems. This nurse learns to anticipate impending change, including that from interdependent systems, responds to change, and takes direct action to direct its course.

Nurses can compete successfully in the world of health care by doing things a new way. Professional nurses are expected to have the vision to change things, and to be change agents.[28]

Outsiders are resisted as change agents.

> **Nurse managers will learn that leadership is the major characteristic of the change agent. Great leadership is based on the success of others.[29]**

Examples of the Application of Change Theory

Retrenchments involving layoffs do not always use appropriate change theory. As a consequence, considerable unnecessary pressures, including unfavorable publicity, are placed on nurses. The organizational climate becomes tense and disruptive and gives personnel a sense of loss of security. Nurse executives feel tired and drained.

Causes of such problems include policies and plans that are developed after the fact, with few policies developed to deal with employees remaining with the organization. The media can be used to inform the public of changes in the health care system that necessitated the layoff.

The following are among the positive responses that will minimize resistance to the change of retrenchment[30]:

1. Having a strong orientation toward reality, preparedness, knowledge of human behavior, stress management, and openness and honesty in dealing with employees.
2. Developing organization-wide retrenchment plans and policies with the advice of the personnel/human resource management department and legal counsel.
3. Considering the use of consultants.
4. Evaluating the criteria for layoffs: seniority, performance appraisal, and job categories. The principle of last hired, first fired should be weighed against the principle of keeping the best-qualified employees.
5. Having the public relations department (or a consultant) handle publicity.
6. Dealing positively with rumors through newsletters, informal discussions, and open meetings.
7. Reassuring remaining employees by being visible and available. Making frequent rounds.
8. Doing team building with chaplains, psychiatric specialists, and human resource specialists.
9. Forming a nurse manager support group that includes families, friends, colleagues, and nonnursing professional peers.
10. Being fair and honest and handling people with dignity and care.

Transformational change brings radical change to the mission, structure, and organizational culture of an organization. This change may be managed with consultation and employee participation. The nurse manager should keep training personnel abreast of organizational changes. Empowerment is a key factor in managing change, because empowered employees become change agents. Some coping strategies are problem-focused, some emotion-focused.

Exhibit 13-4 lists individual coping strategies and organizational initiatives for coping with change. Change threatens a person's tenure, job role, career path, and status and power within the organization.[31]

Employees need time to adjust to change, sometimes as long as a year or several years. They can use this time to learn new skills and should become well trained. If they are to leave the organization, they need time to prepare résumés and do a job search. All employees should be treated with respect and concern. Whenever possible, change should give employees choices.[32]

Resistance to Change

Resistance to change, or attempting to maintain the status quo when efforts are being made to alter it, is a common response. Change evokes stress that in turn evokes resistance.

Resistance is often based on a threat to the security of the individual, since change upsets an established pattern of behavior. If the problem-solving approach is used, answers should be provided to questions about the impact of the change, including the following: Will the change affect the work standard and subsequent employment, promotion, and raises? Will it mean an increased work load at an accelerated pace? Do employees visualize how they will fit into the picture if this change occurs? In-service education and continuing education may help provide the answers.

Factors that stimulate resistance to change include habits, complacency, fear of disorganization, set patterns of response to change, conservatism, perceived loss of power, ego involvement, insecurity, perceived loss of current or meaningful personal relationships, and perceived lack of rewards.[33]

People are afraid of change because of lack of knowledge, prejudices resulting from a lifetime of personal experience and exposure to others, and fear of the need for greater effort or a higher degree of difficulty.

People have developed fears, biases, and social inhibitions from the cultural environment in which they live. Since they cannot be separated from these cultural factors, it is necessary to find ways of managing them within a system.

Barriers to change include a perception of implied criticism. "You are changing the system because you don't like the way I do it." Employees perceive that machines and systems are replacing them or making their jobs less interesting. As an example, a programmed system could be used by patients to take their own nursing histories.

EXHIBIT 13-4
Strategies for Coping with Organizational Change: Sources of the Strategy

INDIVIDUAL COPING STRATEGIES

Use of coping efforts: problem-focused, emotion-focused

Reliance on internal resources (personality traits, internal locus of control, hardiness, *sense* of mastery)

Use of external resources and social supports (spouse, family, friends, managers, co-workers)

ORGANIZATIONAL INITIATIVES

Communication/Leadership

Empowering individuals to take control of change

Provision of timely and accurate communication

Training in communication

The use of transformational leaders

Unlearning

Promotion of unlearning programs to deal with the removal of old elements of organizational culture; use of pre-merger diagnosis and integration workshops to determine elements of culture incompatibility

Job-Related Tasks

Classification of roles and relationships; establishment of support teams, improving person-job fit; job enrichment

Stress Programs

Provision of stress management interventions, including establishment of fitness and wellness programs

Source: V. J. Callan. "Individual and Organizational Strategies for Coping with Organizational Change." *Work & Stress* (March 1993), 68.

Change may demand the investment of a great deal of time and effort in relearning. If nurses are to be independent practitioners, what happens to those who are not prepared? "Probably the greatest single personal barrier is that individuals do not understand or refuse to accept the reasons for the change or the need for it. Unfortunately, it is not always easy to equate the reasons and the needs and to communicate them in meaningful and compelling language."[34]

People are members of a social system in a community and will resist change if it affects that social system. Social changes that threaten social customs, values, self-esteem, and security are resisted more than technical changes. One member of the social system may influence others even if unaffected by the change.

Other causes of resistance to change include time and pace; different generations of nurses have different rates of change.

Values and Beliefs

Cognitive frameworks are based on values and beliefs about effective means of achieving these values. Nurse managers who value the chain of command, policies, and procedures, and who believe their management experience does not need input from clinical nurses may not look for problems needing change. So long as they are successful, they are strengthened by success that builds their self-respect. This success fosters resistance to any change that threatens the integrity of the framework. People resist discarding their own ideas. Accepting another's idea reduces their self-esteem. They may consider a good idea a unique event to be preserved. Ideas should have life cycles. They shine and then dim and need to be replaced. Ideas need to be put on a depreciable basis.[35]

Change is affected by the crucial differences among geographical regions. Some regions are more open to fast change, whereas others accept slow changes. Cultural changes are affected by religious or political beliefs. People hold fast to meaningful beliefs.[36]

Gillen claims that change stimulates increased levels of energy, which is called *hyper-energy* and is *not* stress. Hyper-energy is the heightened drive a person feels in response to a perceived challenge or threat. If not managed, hyper-energy is used by employees to think of surreptitious ways of preventing change. Hyper-energy can be pooled for collective resistance to change. It distracts employees, causing errors and accidents.[37] Skilled nurse leaders bring employees into the change process so the employees do not view the change as a threat. Employees' hyper-energy is then channeled into involvement in the change process.

One reason for resistance to change is that hierarchical, bureaucratic frameworks with rules achieve stability. It should be kept in mind that both individuals and organizations need such stability through continuity in policies and procedures so that recurring needs can be dealt with routinely and problems do not have to be resolved anew each time they appear.

The major symptoms of resistance to change are refusal; confrontation; covert resistance such as nonpreparation for meetings or misunderstandings of the place or time; incomplete reports; refusal to accept responsibility; uncooperative employees; passive aggressiveness; absenteeism; and tardiness.[38]

Strategies for Overcoming Obstacles to Change

Managed Change

According to Drucker, "One cannot manage change. One can only be ahead of it."[39] Drucker suggests that the manager lead change, viewing it as an opportunity. Change can be led with nurse managers acting as change agents. One of the strategies a nurse manager can use is to hire a consultant to make the diagnosis and recommend programs that will improve the productivity of nurse personnel while giving them job satisfaction. Such measures can include educational programs to improve the areas where problems exist.

Effectively led change leads to improvement of patient care services, raised morale, increased productivity, and meeting of patient and staff needs. Change is an art, the mastery of which can be exhilarating, refreshing, challenging, and exciting, because it represents opportunity. Change is facilitated when nurse employees are assigned to adapt to changing job requirements.

Collection and Development of Data

Nurse managers need to gather data about work so that it can be discussed, analyzed, and used to effect change when indicated. Personnel, particularly managers, can be educated to make and manage change. They will learn about labor power planning and utilization rather than leave this entirely to the human resources department. They will learn about financial management rather than depend on the accounting office personnel to take care of it. These are areas in which effective strategies can be developed to foster external cooperative efforts among chief nurse executives of similar institutions and organizations within a community. Such concepts can be expanded to clinical services. If a division of nursing cannot afford to use such specialists as a full-time mental health nurse practitioner, several organizations can collectively contract for the services of one. Thus, change becomes a cooperative venture.

Integration of computers and automated equipment is essential to the change process, particularly when managers are competing for professional nurses as well as for health care dollars. Within this domain, nurse educators can elicit the advice and skills of nursing management system personnel as impartial third-party critics of the change being effected. These personnel will give nurse educators effective feedback while providing management information support systems.

Preparation for Planning

Preplanning will help overcome many obstacles to change. Planning will keep interpersonal relationships from being disrupted if persons with common frames of reference are brought together. The planner can assist people to meet their goals while minimizing their fear and anxiety. Fear is stimulated by the external threat of change. Anxiety, which is self-induced dread, is internally stimulated. Planning will help people accept the change without fear or anxiety.

In making changes, nurse managers should plan to help people unlearn the old (unfreeze) and use the new (refreeze). Implementation and updating of nursing management information systems can refine much unfreezing and refreezing. Often nurse managers help their staff learn the new without having them unlearn the old. This is a major problem in nursing today because of how the role of nurses is changing.

To prepare a plan carefully, the nurse manager should share information and decision-making, work for common perception and understanding, and support and reinforce the nursing staff's effort to effect change. Clear statements of philosophy, goals, and objectives are needed in preparing for change.

Beyers recommends that nurse executives be involved in the following elements of strategy planning[40]:

1. Product/market planning.
2. Business unit planning.
3. Shared resource planning.
4. Shared concern planning.
5. Corporate-level planning.

Nursing in all areas, both clinical and managerial, must consider competition. The patient will go where there is higher-quality nursing care, which results from effectively planned and managed change. Nurse educators should perform market surveys to determine the nursing products and services that consumers want.[41] This activity itself will constitute change and will result in changes.

Looking at the theory of the business of the health care organization and of nursing, what needs to be abandoned? This may include products, services, markets, distribution channels, and every end-user who does not fit the theory of the business. End-users do not need many present-day organizations to get information; they use the Internet to obtain information on providers and services. Nursing's goal is to improve this information and these services in the interest of survival and progress. The opportunity is with maintaining physical and mental functioning of individuals and populations. Drucker suggests managers look at windows of opportunity[42]:

- The organization's own unexpected successes and unexpected failures, but also the unexpected successes and unexpected failures of the organization's competitors.
- Incongruities, especially incongruities in the process, whether of production or distribution, or incongruities in customer behavior.
- Process needs.
- Changes in industry and market structures.
- Changes in demographics.
- Changes in meaning and perception.
- New knowledge.

Plans will list everyone on whom the change depends and their level of involvement. Who will oppose and who will support the change? The dominant coalition in the organization and the forces that will stimulate change should be identified and their support enlisted. Appropriate current events should be noted through reading and meetings, highlighting those that will enhance the mission of the organization and for which the clinical nurses will claim or share ownership.[43] This activity brings new ideas and new knowledge to stimulate and justify the need for change.

Planning will also require thinking in multiple time frames: changes to be effected in six months, one year, and so on. The nurse manager should identify the trade offs between nursing and other departments, between clinical and management staffs, and within the change process itself, and list ways to enlist support.[44]

Nurse managers need to be careful not to overplan. They should leave some room for the people who will implement the change to exercise intelligent initiative. They need to be sure that the rewards or benefits to individuals and to the group are carefully communicated. If people want a change to work, they will make it happen. Change leads to real innovation and, although it creates uncertainty and discomfort, requires nurse leaders to have the knowledge and skills to manage it.[45]

Training and Education

The frequency of training and education should match the frequency of change. Nursing personnel will require constant staff development programs to keep from depreciating in knowledge and competence. From initial hiring and orientation, change should be portrayed as an integral part of the nurse's job.[46] Nurse managers should inform employees of the pressures that make change necessary.

Rewards

Rewards for old behavior patterns should be removed after the individuals have been helped to see the reasons for the proposed change. Employees need to see the necessity for the new behaviors and should be given real incentives, financial or nonfinancial. Here is where job standards come in. The job standards should incorporate the new methods or skills and phase out the old ones. To provide an incentive, performance appraisal can be based on the new standards. Time must be allowed and opportunity provided for retraining. Nonfinancial rewards include enriching jobs and encouraging self-development. Such activities can satisfy individual needs.

Using Groups as Change Agents

Groups in themselves are often effective change agents. When the group appears to work in harmony and to have well-understood goals, it may be used to institute the change. If the idea can be planned in the group, it will be implemented more successfully. A group is more willing than most individuals to assume risks. Planning should make clear the need for change and provide an environment in which group members identify with such need. Objectives should be stated in clear, concise, and qualitative terms. Administrative policy should contain broad guidelines with understandable procedures for achieving the objectives, and the guidelines and procedures should be communicated to the group. The procedures they contain also need to be understood.

As agents of change, nurse managers need to utilize staff talents by using temporary work teams to solve specific problems and effect change. They need to participate on interdisciplinary task forces and prepare people for job mobility through experiences planned to facilitate it. Third-party critics may help diagnose and solve problems.

The informal group can promote and support change. It can be formed by enlisting the help of a strong leader and by forming a strong group that will communicate its perception of needed change to nurse managers and educators.[47]

Communications

Too often change is announced by rumor when it should be clearly introduced. Since changes split teams and kill friendships, causing productivity to drop, employees should be told about upcoming changes before they become a rumor.[48] Announcements should be factual and comprehensive and should state objectives, nature, methods, benefits, and drawbacks of the change. An announcement made face-to-face will be better received.

Discussion of implementation should give people maximum information. The discussion should cover the rate and method of implementation, including the first steps that will be taken and the sequence and people involved in each element.

Ceremonies may be effective in various aspects of the change. They are useful for retirements; promotion; introduction of a new coworker, superior, or subordinate; a move to a new job; start of a new system; and reorganization. When used well, ceremonies focus on the importance of the ongoing institution and underline the importance of individual loyalty to that institution and its positions. They convey that the organization and the employees are both needed.

As change agent, the nurse manager discusses with people reasons for resisting change. When people understand the real reasons for the change, they are not as resistant to it. They should be encouraged to sound off.

Planned change needs to be successfully communicated to all employees, even those who are not directly or immediately involved. Verbal announcements can be followed up with written ones and progress reports. Change occurs smoothly in direct proportion to the positive and democratic behavior that demonstrates management's philosophy and practice at all levels from the top down. Communication includes body language and tone of voice as well as words.[49]

The Organizational Environment

Nurse managers could be more successful if they paid attention to the organizational environment into which change is introduced and the manner in which it is done. Managers need to be committed to a change and to support it by actions that express their attitudes. When the nurse leader attempts to impose change on people in an authoritarian manner, people often resist it. Concern for employees is as important as concern for patients. Managers can establish an environment for change by doing the following:

1. Emphasizing relationships with and between groups.
2. Bringing out mutual trust and confidence.
3. Emphasizing interdependence and shared responsibility.
4. Containing group membership and responsibility by limiting individuals from belonging to too many

groups and ensuring that the same responsibilities are not given to several groups.

5. Having a wide sharing of control and responsibility.
6. Resolving conflict through bargaining or problem-solving discussions.[50]
7. Permitting job movement to facilitate careers.
8. Anticipating and rewarding change, thus institutionalizing it.[51]
9. Modifying the nursing organizational structure to accommodate changes that provide growth and development.
10. Promoting a can-do attitude.
11. Providing predictability and stability by maintaining job security, sharing bad news early, and shifting concern to teamwork and process improvement.[52]

When the organizational climate changes, employees change behaviors. A desired organizational climate fosters high-quality patient care.[53]

Anticipating Potential Failures

Although preparation is the key to successful change, it should include anticipation of potential failure. Three questions need to be answered before actions for change begin. First, nurse leaders should determine what the risks are and how much they are willing to expend in terms of resources. Second, they should decide who would do the work. Third, they should have a flexible agenda and plan what will be done when it goes wrong.

Mistakes will happen. The importance of the change will determine how much risk the nurse leader is prepared to take. For example, one might risk a great deal and reorganize an entire unit to achieve the goal of having professional nurses perform as case managers. Changes can be introduced in one unit, evaluated, and modified before being extended to other units.

The positive aspect of resistance to change is that it pushes the change agent to plan more carefully, listen with sympathetic understanding, and reexamine goals, functions, priorities, and values. When properly addressed, resistance uses less of peoples' energy. Other effective responses to resistance are showing respect for honest questions and differences of opinion, altering of strategy and tactics, altering of composition of groups, and proceeding in an objective, firm, assertive, and non-judgmental manner.[54]

Creativity and Innovation

Creativity Defined

Creativity is defined in *Webster's New Twentieth Century Dictionary, Unabridged, second edition,* as "artistic or

intellectual inventiveness." *Innovation* is defined as "the introduction of something new." These definitions suggest that the terms are interchangeable. A person could say that creativity is the mental work or action involved in bringing something new into existence, while innovation is the result of that effort.[55] If one wishes to differentiate the two, one might say that a nurse can create or invent a new nursing product, process, or procedure (creativity) or can effect change by putting a new product, process, or procedure into use (innovation). Creativity is a way of using the mind.[56] Research indicates that creativity is *not* intelligence.[57]

Creativity is the fuel of innovation.[58]

Why Creativity?

Business leaders argue that creativity yields profits. With creativity, new products can be developed and a company can compete. New methods are also fruits of creativity. For many years nurses have tended to think that selling their services like a product is mercenary or unethical. This thinking has changed as nurses have acquired more education and become more autonomous. More professional nurses have become entrepreneurs in establishing business enterprises. Sister Reinkemeyer predicted this development when she wrote, "university programs try to produce independent personalities and thinkers capable of facing some of the modern scientific and psychosocial changes in nursing."[59]

A constant flow of new ideas is needed to procure new products, services, processes, procedures, and strategies for dealing with the changes occurring in every sphere of endeavor: technology, social systems, government, and everyday living. Health care is big business.

Drucker advocates a reporting system to call attention both to things that go wrong and to those that go better than expected, forecasted, or budgeted. Following his advice, nurses would be entrepreneurs if the organization did not penalize them for it. He also states that entrepreneurship should neither be mixed with operations and rewards nor put at the bottom of the organization to be killed. Instead, good people should be put to work in the new enterprise, with a full-time person in charge. Even if the organization is middle-sized, it can have some people working in a new service. Although innovation needs order, it does not need excess policy. It requires reception and a market to be successful.[60]

Innovation is the key to survival and growth of health care and nursing. Entrepreneurs create the new and different. They change values. Entrepreneurial nurses create new businesses with new products and services within organizations. It takes up to ten years for a professional nurse to be totally competent. Both nurse and organization benefit from entrepreneurship. The nurse gains personal satisfaction, rewards, and recognition while the organization survives and prospers.[61]

Establishing a Climate for Creativity

For creativity to prosper, the organization should provide a warm intellectual environment that gives employees recognition, prestige, and an opportunity to participate. Employees will gain a sense of ownership and commitment by being involved in planning their work and making decisions. Nurse managers promote creativity through sensitivity that gives people the attention they want and treats them as distinct individuals. Professionally competent managers inspire creativity by taking risks, as well as by showing confidence, giving praise and support, being nourishing, using tact, and having patience.[62]

Metamanagement

Metamanagement describes a cooperative effort of entrepreneurial or creative managers, strategic planners, and top management. It is:

> [a] planning framework that cuts across organizational boundaries and facilitates strategic decision-making about current practices and future directions; a flexible and creative planning process that stimulates in-house entrepreneurial thinking and behavior; and a consistent and accepted value system that reinforces management's commitment to the organization's strategy, and stresses teamwork, organizational flexibility, open communication, innovation, risk taking, high morale and trust.[63]

Nurse managers practicing metamanagement will plan the organizational structure—its dynamics, nature, and position. They will perform as an innovative, committed, enlightened, disciplined, and courageous group willing and able to restructure thinking and organizations, and generate and execute successful plans for a profitable nursing business. They will stimulate the input of the clinical nurses, thereby generating direction for the nursing organization and occupation.

The following task-related actions by nurse managers will help to develop and maintain a creative climate[64]:

1. Providing freedom to experiment without fear of reprimand.
2. Maintaining a moderate amount of work pressure.
3. Providing challenging yet realistic work goals.
4. Emphasizing a low level of supervision in performance tasks.
5. Delegating responsibilities.
6. Encouraging participation in decision-making and goal setting.
7. Encouraging use of a creative problem-solving process to solve unstructured problems.
8. Providing immediate and timely feedback on task performance.
9. Providing the resources and support needed to get the job done.

Creative Problem-Solving

Creative problem-solving starts by using vague or ill-defined problems as challenges. Problems can be attacked intuitively to generate as many ideas as possible. Solutions may create new challenges and new cycles of creative problem-solving. Research indicates that both the right and left cerebral hemispheres contribute to the maintenance of multiple word meanings in highly creative persons.[65]

There are several theories of creative problem-solving. Lattimer and Winitsky suggest the following[66]:

1. *Thinking.* Identify the factors to be used in solving an issue or developing a strategic plan. The choice is between a risk-free alternative and one that involves risk.
2. *Decomposing.* Break down the situation into components—alternatives, uncertainties, outcomes, consequences; work with each and combine the results for a decision.
3. *Simplifying.* Determine the important components and concentrate on them. What are the most crucial factors and most essential relationships? Then make intuitive judgments.
4. *Specifying.* Establish the value of key factors, the probabilities for the uncertainties, and preferences for the outcomes.
5. *Rethinking.* Was the original analysis sensible regarding omissions, inclusions, order, and emphasis?

Godfrey recommends an alternative theory of creativity that has the following five steps[67]:

1. *Perception.* Realizing there is a problem.
2. *Preparation.* Research, data collection, and arrangement of information to define the problem.
3. *Ideation.* Analysis and structure of a variety of formats that stimulate analogies and images; brainstorming.
4. *Incubation.* Withdraw and relax when the flow of ideas ends. The unconscious takes off and forms images of possible solutions.
5. *Validation.* Test a solution.

Drucker indicates that every corporation needs a strategy for innovation. He suggests four strategies for innovation, as follows[68]:

1. *The first with the mostest.* Be first in the market and the first to improve a product or cut its price. This discourages prospective competitors.

2. *The second with the mostest.* Let someone else establish the market. Satisfy markets with narrow needs and specific capabilities. Provide excellent products for big purchasers with narrow needs. Offer new features. This strategy is evident in the competitive health care market, where certain corporations have specialized in psychiatric services, rehabilitation services, or drug-dependency services.

3. *The niche strategy.* Corner a finite market, making it nonprofitable for others. When the niche becomes a mass market, change the strategy to remain profitable.

4. *Making the product your carrier.* One product carries another. This has been done by medical supply companies whose electronic thermometers are the basis for sales of disposable covers and intravenous pumps are the basis for sales of fluid administration sets.

Creativity Training

Training can help people be creative. It can teach them to develop creative thinking skills and logic techniques that can lead to successful results. General Electric established creativity training for its engineers in 1937. Many other companies also provide creativity training. Before developing creativity training, nurse educators should establish some general concepts about the new products, techniques, markets, and so forth they want employees to bring into existence.

Creativity training aims to increase the creative capacity or creative behavior of individuals or groups. The techniques of creativity training can include brainstorming, synectics, morphological analysis, forced fit, forced relationships, brainwriting, visualization, cueing, lateral thinking, and divergent thinking.[69] Refer to the article by Gordon and Zemke for a more detailed explanation of these creativity techniques.

Other Approaches

Nurses will be motivated to be creative when nurse leaders encourage them to express their ideas openly and accept divergent ideas and points of view. Other motivators of creativity by nurses include providing assistance to develop new ideas, encouraging risk-taking while buffering resisting forces, providing time for individual effort, providing opportunities for professional growth and development, encouraging interaction with others outside the group, promoting constructive intragroup and intergroup competition, recognizing the value of worthy ideas, and exhibiting confidence in workers.[70]

Research studies indicate that creative behavior is inherent in human nature and can be developed. Elements or pieces necessary for creating something new exist and must be arranged in new and useful combinations. Excessive motivation, caused by high rewards for performance or anxiety over possible failure, has been proven to inhibit creativity. It causes people to pursue ideas down blind alleys.

The following are actions for producing original, goal-oriented ideas[71]:

1. Assemble the separate elements that will be creatively combined to produce a product or a new procedure. The problem must be identified in terms of usefulness of this product or process. If a known element is missing, what is available to replace it?

2. Use the available and assembled elements in combinations that produce original ideas.

3. Remove inhibitions to creativity such as excess motivation, anxiety, fear of taking risks, dependence on authority, or habitual modes of thinking and talking about things. Creativity is not confined to a small, exclusive set of gifted people. Language contains the potential for creative thought, and everyone has the potential.

4. Study techniques of creativity so that the elements can be used.

Characteristics of a Creative Person

Creative people, including nurses, have a broad background of knowledge. They have the mental skills of curiosity, openness, sensitivity to problems, flexibility, ability to think in images, and capability of analysis and synthesis.[72] Nursing leaders possess the attributes of teamwork, global thinking, multitasking, creativity, and flexibility so important to the health care marketplace. They have integrated clinical and business principles and are a source of knowledge and skills to make their organizations prosper.[73]

In addition, traditional evaluation will need to be upgraded to deal with such socially constructed decision-making processes as evolve from information systems. Evaluation must keep pace with human judgments resulting from complexity, uncertainty, theory, change, and control.[74]

Creative nurses use their knowledge to stimulate their sensory perceptions. In addition to solving problems, they create new problems to solve by formulating questions about the whys and hows of established practices. To foster independence and creative talents, nurse managers will assume that creative nurses are not odd or eccentric. As a consequence, barriers will not be erected among peer groups. Nurse managers will communicate and cooperate with clinical nurses to set new goals or new practices for achieving goals.[75]

Creative people have been considered different from other people. This difference has been described by one writer: "The public would have him nearsighted but farseeing, brilliantly innovative but absentminded, widely acclaimed but impervious to applause, capable of highly involved abstract thinking but naive and eccentric in his everyday reasoning. The truth of the matter is that the creative person *is* different but is *not* a monster strangely mysterious and incomprehensible."[76] An individual may appear to have been gifted with a brilliant intellect. During childhood this individual may have been the curious type who searched for books to read and tasks to do that satisfied his or her curiosity. Searching for the approval and encouragement of parents, friends, or teachers but not receiving it, he or she may have become somewhat of a loner.

Creative individuals value the work and association of other creative individuals. They stimulate each other to think and perhaps even to be competitively creative. Creative people can tolerate ambiguity; they have self-confidence, the ability to toy with ideas, and persistence.[77]

As an example, a clinical nursing coordinator set up her own cancer clinic. She convinced the physicians of her ability to perform the functions and of the clinic's benefit to them and to the patients. Patients now make direct appointments with this clinic, which has expanded to become a health screening clinic for women. In addition to coming for a Pap test and breast examination, clients have a history taken by the nurse practitioner. They are referred to the physician only when there is evidence of pathology. Many patients now come for personal health counseling.

In another instance, an assistant to the director of nursing questioned the time-honored practice of nurses counting narcotics and controlled drugs three times a day. With the advice of legal counsel, it was determined that this was being done only because it had become common practice. As a result, policy has been changed so that the narcotics and controlled drugs are inventoried by the pharmacist when the medications are ordered each morning and by the unit manager before leaving at the end of the shift. Discrepancies are reported to the nurse manager. Thus, nurses have lost another nonnursing function. In the clinical arena a major change is taking place as nurses move to evidence-based practice. To accomplish this requires that nursing education programs teach skills needed to appraise, synthesize, and diffuse the best evidence into practice. Nurse managers and administrators will provide the resources.[78]

Managing Creativity

The nurse manager can encourage creativity through interpersonal relationships that establish trust. This requires acceptance of differing behaviors and ideas and a willingness to listen. It requires friendliness and a spirit of cooperation. It will also require respect for the feelings of others and a lack of defensiveness.[79]

Creative nurses produce a lot. They are unconventional and individualistic. Their critical skills are problem awareness and specification, skills that lead to problem resolution.[80]

Nurse managers can plan to nourish creativity in nursing personnel by doing the following:

1. Noting the creative abilities of those who develop new methods and techniques.
2. Providing time and opportunity for people to do creative work. This can be planned during the performance appraisal process.
3. Recognizing that those who are masters or experts in nursing work in clinical practice, teaching, research, and management.
4. Encouraging nursing personnel to become involved in new nursing endeavors at work, in the community, and in professional organizations, as well as undertaking other activities that increase knowledge and skills.
5. Encouraging risk-taking and acceptance of personal responsibility.

To encourage creativity, hire creative people. Usually they have taken time off to learn. Hire a few genuine off-the-wall sort of people. Weed out the dullards. Support generous sabbaticals. Measure curiosity. Seek out curious work. Model the way. Teach curiosity. Make it fun. Change the pace.[81]

Successful companies hire and keep creative employees who will create and market new products. They keep people by knowing how to manage, motivate, and reward them. Venture teams composed of persons with diverse expertise and experiences usually accomplish more than individuals alone. Human resources planning includes recruitment of employees with this expertise and experience. Venture teams are used by such firms as Motorola and the 3M Company.

Creative venture team members include those with technical skills and people skills. They have members who are practical problem-solvers and team players. They include artists, scientists, and businesspersons. They must be decisive.

Successful companies do extensive interviewing before hiring. They then do extensive training. They seek people who are genuine in their desire to create new products and serve the customer.

Performance appraisal rewards risk-taking and intelligent effort that may result in failure.

Innovation results in profitability. Successful companies reward generation of new ideas from within and adoption from without. Performance evaluation should help marginal performers do better. Six-month evaluations are recommended. Peer evaluation and feedback are effective.

Innovative companies do technical audits of individual units to rate them on technical factors, business factors, and overall viability. Reward systems include freedom for creative individual research; freedom to fail; fellowships; in-house grants; autonomy; choice of own venture team; pay raises based on performance, not on seniority; three-track career systems—scientific, managerial, and research; in-house promotions; peer recognition awards; banquets; plaques; and letters of appreciation. Reward teams to foster cooperation. Research confirms results. Reward individuals when someone has gone "the extra mile," to encourage the newcomer, to thank someone who is leaving, when someone's contribution has been ignored by the team, to stir up the team from group-think, and when members differ greatly in their choice of rewards.

Encourage careers through empowerment to raise self-esteem, through leading by example, continuing education, and sabbaticals. Motorola spent $60 million on training and $60 million on lost work time to re-educate its employees in 1989.[82]

The Relationship of Nursing Research to Change

The Need for Nursing Research

Although there are many predictions of the future directions of health care, the future will probably differ from all of them. Nursing research is essential to preparing for the future and for competition within the health care system. Nurse managers should have good information to keep nursing competitive with other caregivers in providing patient care. They should also have the knowledge to be competitive among employers and in a global economy. This requires the development and employment of nursing scientists who are researchers. Employment of these nursing researchers will commit nurses to developing research in managing human beings to their full potential. It is an investment that keeps people, the future human capital, from depreciating.[83]

Nursing research improves nursing practice. A profession grounds practice in scholarly inquiry. Nurse educators will improve the quality of nursing practice when they promote nursing research and the application of the findings of nursing research. Nursing research will validate the discipline of nursing.[84]

Nurse managers, clinical nurses, instructors, and others are often eager to effect change. They like to try something new, to apply the latest technologies; they

can do so through the nursing research process. There are two kinds of research activities: those in which nurses are the subjects and those in which they develop their own nursing research program. Real research requires preparation and time.

Nursing Research in the Service Setting

It follows, then, that if there is to be research in nursing, and if it is to be part of the organizational goals, there must be planning. Plans incorporate a budget, a staff, and defined problems for research. Staff nurses working in clinical jobs and management personnel usually do not have time for this kind of research. They can use the results of such research and apply them to their situation to build better health care delivery systems.[85]

A nursing position filled by a scholar will enhance the chances that a nursing research program will be successful. A scholar will have the knowledge to increase nursing research of a high intellectual and professional caliber. A nurse researcher can promote the reunification model of nursing education and nursing service through joint appointments and joint nursing research endeavors, supporting cooperation between service and education.

Nursing faculty tend to disengage from practice because of the numerous demands of their teaching roles. One reason that faculty focus on wellness may be their disengagement from practice. Since nursing faculty are often well-prepared scientists, nursing managers should find ways to budget money for released time from faculty duties. Faculty may then do clinical practice and the service agency reimburses the school for the faculty member's work. A coalition will benefit all nurses because faculty will be recognized for research activities that keep them up-to-date, and managers will benefit from improved patient care.[86]

Nursing administration scholars will allow clinicians adequate time to develop their projects. They will provide a resource link to help clinicians find research partners with whom they can pursue relevant nursing research.[87]

A survey of nursing deans indicated increased demand for well-prepared nurse researchers. Researchers were most highly needed in the psychosocial and biophysical domains. Also needed would be those in health care delivery systems and administration, education, and methodology and instrumentation. All areas of research are important to the profession and the development of its theory base.[88] The National Center for Nursing Research has focused on funding for training in biological theory and measurements in nursing research.[89]

Nurse managers and administrators can improve the use of nursing research findings by encouraging replication of nursing studies, having research findings translated into understandable language, and rewarding nurses for implementing research findings. Otherwise, too much new nursing knowledge will continue to be unused.[90]

Nurse managers can facilitate the implementation of nursing research findings through specific continuing education programs and by providing sources of help in developing research activities, identifying available library services, and using computer networks. They should keep clinical nurses informed on institutional review policies. Seed money can often be found by institutional administrators. Research forums may be held once or twice a year. Research awards are excellent forms of recognition. They are even better when supported by funds for presentation when papers are accepted by professional organizations.[91]

Establishing a research program in a clinical institution requires administrative support, including funds for staffing, supplies, and equipment. The program coordinator may be established in the nursing division or the research and development department. Goals and priorities need to be established for the types of research to be done: education, administration, program evaluation, methodological, case study, and clinical nursing. A nursing research program requires a budget, funding, and strategies. One strategy may be to focus on research and not be distracted by other activities. Nursing research should focus on outcomes that will have values for clients and for nurses and nursing (see Exhibit 13-5).[92]

Efforts are being made to use research findings to change nursing practice. Laschinger and others designed a project to use the findings of research in nursing administration. Students chose the area of job satisfaction. They presented themselves as an external consultant team and chose the Conduct and Utilization of Research in Nursing (CURN) model as an approach. One project was to develop a program using research findings for nurse managers in an agency. The exercise represents a method for nurse managers and administrators to use research findings in nursing administration.[93]

To build a nursing research culture, nurse managers should create an environment that fosters it. This can be achieved by using the learning process. Resource individuals are academic nursing faculty and nurses prepared in research methodology at the graduate level. The nurse leaders provide continuing education to promote interest in nursing research. They support this interest with internal and external funding as pay for performance in productive research activities.[94]

The Nursing Research Process

The nursing research process includes both scientific and technical steps. The format for writing up research is a problem-solving one and includes the following sections[95]:

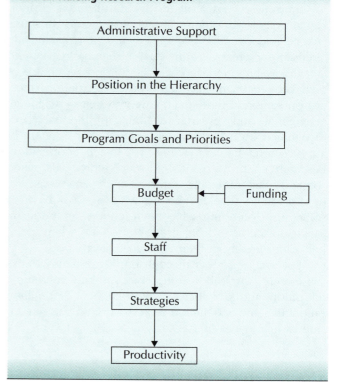

EXHIBIT 13-5
Framework for Establishing a Clinical Nursing Research Program

Source: L. Marchette. "Developing a Productive Nursing Research Program in a Clinical Institution." *Journal of Nursing Administration* (March 1985), 26. Reprinted with permission of J. B. Lippincott, Williams and Wilkins.

1. *Introduction.* Includes an overview of the problem and tells why the research is being done.
2. *Statement of the problem.* An explicit and precise expression of the research question.
3. *Purpose of the study.* Answers the question, What is the long-range goal of the research, the ultimate purpose that will be achieved by the findings? The statement also relates to current nursing concerns and the motivation for the study. If readers of a study cannot determine its purpose, they should read no further.
4. *Review of the literature.* A summary of the studies previously published and their results and a statement indicating what this study will add. The review should present a conceptual framework for the study; concepts and theories documented in previous studies; and evidence to support the approach. It should also indicate how the proposed study goes beyond what has already been achieved. The dependent variables to be measured and the independent variables to be manipulated should be identified.
5. *Hypothesis.* A formal statement of the research question, of what relationships are being tested and

how they are to be measured. The variables are specifically defined.

6. *Methodology, or design.* Describes the setting, the subjects, how the subjects are chosen, procedures, analysis, and data collection. Measurement techniques used will be those appropriate to the hypothesis.

7. *Analysis.* A statistical test that measures the effect of the independent variable.

8. *Results.* Answers the research question objectively. The presentation of results stays within the parameters of the designed study.

9. *Discussion.* Includes any unexpected results as well as the conclusions reached.

This format can be used to evaluate research reports. Steps 1 through 5 indicate how to develop a research proposal; plans for steps 6 through 9 should be included in the proposal.

The Research Question

The research question comes from many intensive hours of thought, literature review, and reflection. It avoids value judgments and opinions. The research question needs more than one variable. It may be a question or a statement. The researcher begins by getting thoughts down on paper and by writing an annotated statement of the question without concern for grammar, which will be refined later. A literature search is undertaken to find out what facts are known about the subject, including relationships and their level of confidence.

Written abstracts are made by the researcher, including types of studies and categories of variables. The researcher also defines the independent and dependent variables and has peers critique them. Questions answered include the following: Are these variables related so that change in one is apt to produce change in the other? What variables other than the one

to be tested could influence the variable(s) to be measured?[96] See Exhibit 13-6 for a sample research question.

According to Lindeman and Schantz, a good research question will meet the following criteria[97]:

1. It can be answered by collecting observable evidence or empirical data.

2. It contains reference to the relationship between two or more variables.

3. It follows logically and consistently from what is already known about the topic.

Lindeman and Schantz state that experimental studies should not be done if no descriptive ones exist.[98]

The Research Design

The research design is the blueprint created to answer the research question. It follows development of the research question, the literature search, and statement of the hypothesis. The following are six elements of a good research design:

1. *Setting.* This is the place where research will be done. There must be enough cases or variables specific to the intent of the research, thereby strengthening internal and external validity and the ability to generalize.

2. *Subjects.* Subjects should be profiled and limited to those most useful in answering the research question. Their human rights will be protected. When there is a lack of consensus among the research community on the relative efficacy of the treatments, the equipoise standard can be used. Equipoise is a standard to be used when treatment interventions confer benefit regardless of the subject's perception.[99]

3. *Sampling.* This is the method for choosing the sample size or number of subjects. Increasing the size of a sample adds strength, power, and meaningfulness

---

EXHIBIT 13-6
Sample Research Question

RESEARCH QUESTION
What is the difference in attendance between continuing education (CE) programs that are based on a needs survey and those that are not? (This question is researchable, while "Should a CE needs survey be done?" is not.)

TEST	**OTHER FACTORS**	**MEASURE**
Independent variable: the variable being tested, examined, or manipulated. Provides measurement of the dependent variable.	Extraneous variables: conditions, behaviors, or characteristics known to exist but not considered of primary importance to the research. The research design may or may not control for these.	Dependent variables: the variables being measured, studied, or investigated to evaluate the impact of the first variable. The outcome or criterion: what will result from the study?
Needs survey	*Cognitive mapping, rewards, threats, personal needs*	*Attendance at CE programs*

Source: Adapted from C. A. Lindeman and D. Schantz. "The Research Question." Journal of Nursing Administration (January 1982), 6–10. Reprinted with permission of J. B. Lippincott, Williams and Wilkins.

4. *Treatment.* Subjects of the sample are assigned to groups—experimental versus control—randomly. They are manipulated to increase the difference between the groups.
5. *Measurement.* Statistical tests are selected to measure the differences between the groups. A reliable instrument produces consistent results. A valid instrument measures what it claims to measure.
6. *Communicating the results.* Data are analyzed and results reported to others. Findings related to the research question are given first, followed by surprise data.[100]

Research Strategies

Nursing Research in a Health Care Agency

Utilization of nursing research findings is poor in all spheres of nursing. This is improving as nurse administrators establish nursing research programs within their organizations. Once the nurse administrator, with input from practicing nurses, defines the objectives of a nursing research program, a decision can be made regarding the organizational design for it. If resources are so scarce that additional budgeted personnel cannot be hired, a standing research committee can be established. A standing committee will promote stability by maintaining effective protocols and standards. The committee chair should have research expertise.

Since program resources are a determinant of the scope of the research program, the nurse administrator will need to establish a budget related to the objectives. This may include reallocation of money, generation of external funding, or revenue-generating activities by the professional nursing staff.

Budget permitting, the nurse administrator may hire a research specialist, full- or part-time. Sometimes a budgeted position is shared by another nurse specialist. It could be a joint appointment with the college of nursing faculty.[101]

A research consortium can be established as a cooperative venture with other organizations within the community. This can include such organizations as hospitals, home health care agencies, and nursing homes.

Given a larger budget, the nurse executive can establish a research department as a separate cost center. Such a department will have direct accountability and clearly structured authority. It can even be self-supporting. Success will reflect strong commitment and will give increased visibility. Exhibit 13-7 shows examples of nursing research studies from one institution.

The ultimate purpose of service-based nursing research is to improve patient care. Nursing management research will answer questions related to the management of resources used in providing patient care. As practicing nurses become aware of the availability of

---

EXHIBIT 13-7

Nursing Research Studies Completed at Northeast Georgia Medical Center, 1986–1988

"A Comparison Study of Three Self-Monitoring Blood Glucose Meters," Shannon Garner, R.N., Debbie Cleland, R.N., and Susan Stone, R.N.

"The Recruitment and Retention of Registered Nurses in a Hospital Setting," Susan Stone, R.N., and Dan Walter, M.B.A.

"A Comparison Study of Heparinized Saline and Normal Saline in Maintaining INT Catheter Patency," Susan Stone, R.N., NGMC IV team.

"The Perceived Personal Needs of Families of Acute Brain-Injured and Spinal Cord–Injured Patients," Tracy Carlisle, R.N., and NGMC neuroscience nursing staff.

"ICU Mortality Prediction Model," Susan Stone, R.N., Ruth Kunkle, R.N., NGMC ICU Nursing Staff.

"Nurses' Attitudes Towards Alcohol-Dependent Clients," Joan Burnham, R.N., North Georgia College.

"The Effects of Music Therapy on Critically Ill Patients in an ICU Setting," Sonja Chaffin, R.N., Angela Chambers, R.N., Fran Rusk, R.N., and Susan Stone, R.N., NGMC ICU Nursing Staff.

"Nurse Retention: Staff Nurse Perspectives," D. Patricia Gray, R.N., Susan Stone, R.N., NGMC neuroscience nursing staff.

"The Effects of Nocturnal Bottle-Feeding Patterns on Infant Weight and Maternal Satisfaction," Gay Mortimer, R.N., and Susan Stone, R.N., NGMC newborn nursery staff.

Source: Reprinted with permission of Northeast Georgia Medical Center, 743 Spring Street, Gainesville, GA 30501-3899. The author visited this hospital and noted that while administration provided seed money, nursing research was expected to pay for itself through improved practice and cost savings.

---

competent nurse researchers, they will refer research questions to them.

Four phases occur in the application of research findings to practice[102]:

1. Evaluation of the strength of the research design.
2. Evaluation of the feasibility and desirability of making the change in practice.
3. Planning the introduction and implementation of the change.
4. Using a pretest and posttest to evaluate the effect of the proposed change on practice.

Milieu

A University of Michigan study of the Conduct and Utilization of Research in Nursing (CURN) model included participating hospitals with milieus that supported research. These milieus were found to include an active clinical faculty for such resources as undergraduate and graduate students, existing research programs, influential nurse administrators, and librarians. Each facility had experienced, degree-prepared nurses with flexible, autonomous roles that facilitated research. These nurses perceived nursing research to have increased the status and visibility of nursing on both the education and practice sides.[103]

Organizational Considerations

Once nurse administrators decide that nursing research will be a component of the nursing organization, they must plan the program design within the organizational structure. The mission, philosophy, and objectives will give direction to a nursing research program design. Input can be obtained from interested professional nurses at the planning stage. This can be done through an ad hoc committee that defines clear objectives for both clinical and administrative research activities. These objectives can include those for research conducted to satisfy departmental, personal, and interdisciplinary needs of the institution, graduate students, staff, faculty, and others. Other ad hoc committees can be formed to conduct research studies or to evaluate and implement research findings. Their composition will be determined by their objectives and by interest and expertise of participating nurses.

Research Strategies

Protocols can be developed to benefit the entire institution. A hospital-wide research department or committee can include nurses. Such a committee can standardize procedures for approval, evaluation, and implementation of all research.

Staff development programs can support interest in the nursing research program. Instructors can communicate to the nursing staff the relevance of nursing research studies and teach nursing staff their roles. The nursing staff can be provided with rewards of nursing research in the form of money, improved care, and prestige. This will be supplemented with consistent communication in memoranda, study abstracts, literature, references, presentations, seminars, and conferences.[104] Exhibit 13-8 presents details of an actual research study.

Pressure is increasing to produce research that is congruent with societal need. This pressure reflects the public's view of costs versus benefits, of societal need

---

EXHIBIT 13-8
ICU Mortality Prediction Model

PURPOSE

As health care resources become limited and the cost of intensive care increases, reliable methods are needed to predict patient outcomes in the critical care setting. Determination of those patients who are most likely to benefit from the intensive care unit (ICU) could be useful to evaluate the need for admission and to estimate resources required for the ICU.

Northeast Georgia Medical Center (NGMC) was invited to participate in a national study funded by the National Center for Health Service Research Grant HS 04833. The purpose of this study was to describe the severity of illness of patients admitted to ICU and to predict the mortality of ICU patients based on clinical variables assessed on admission.

STUDY DESIGN

A sample of 100 consecutive patient admissions was drawn from the ten-bed NGMC ICU. Each ICU nurse was instructed on the use of the ICU mortality prediction model (MPM) admission and discharge forms. Each MPM admission form was completed by an ICU nurse within four hours of the patient's admission to the ICU. Following patient discharge, the MPM discharge forms were completed and each was reviewed by the clinical nursing researcher.

Confidentiality and anonymity were assured. Logistic regression and analysis were used to interpret the data.

RESULTS

One hundred patients participated in the study. The mean patient age was 53 years. Fifty-eight percent were admitted to surgical service; 26 percent to medical service; 16 percent to neurological service. Average patient acuity according to the Medicus Patient Classification System was 3.91. Two of the patients were categorized as "do not resuscitate" by the physician.

The *actual* ICU mortality rate was 7 percent. The *predicted* ICU mortality rate, according to the ICU Mortality Prediction Model, was 16.5 percent. Among the other sixteen hospitals included in the study, the average predicted mortality rate was 17 percent. The predicted mortality range was 10 to 31 percent.

The average probability of dying among the living was 0.138 for NGMC. The average probability of dying among the dead was 0.519 for NGMC. Ninety-one of the 100 patients were correctly classified by the MPM. There were no patients who died who were predicted to live. For the ten highest calculated probabilities, 6.59 patients were expected to die and four actually died.

Source: Reprinted with permission of Northeast Georgia Medical Center, 743 Spring Street, Gainesville, GA 30501-3899.

versus scientific interest. Heads of U.S. corporations indicate that most innovation today is coming from industry rather than from the research community. Americans tend to waste research money. Five major international research priorities are: "human resources, cultural concerns (effect of socioeconomic status and culture on health practices, patterns of illness, and styles of intervention), health of women and children, models for delivery of nursing care, and models for education." Nursing research should result in a significant payoff to the public.[105]

Summary

Ability to manage planned change is a necessary competency of all nurses, since it represents viability of the nursing organization. Since planned change is a necessity, nurse managers create the climate for its receptivity by nursing personnel. Change, the key to innovation and the future, has its basis in change theory.

Lewin's change theory is widely used by nurses and involves three stages: unfreezing, moving, and refreezing. In the unfreezing stage, employees are made aware of needed changes. A plan for change is made and tested in the moving stage. During the refreezing stage, the change becomes a part of the system, establishing homeostasis and equilibrium.

Rogers, Havelock, and Lippett each modified Lewin's original change theory. Reddin's theory has many similarities, and all have common elements of problem-solving and decision-making.

Resistance to change is evoked by stress from threatened security of affected employees. It can be overcome by planning that involves those who will be affected, particularly if they can see a benefit. Established values and beliefs, imprinting, time perspectives, and hyper-energy all stiffen resistance to change.

The nurse as change agent is the manager of change and thus requires knowledge of the theory of change. Education and training are necessary for nursing personnel who will be affected. Intrinsic and extrinsic rewards are another management tool. Using groups to effect change will help absorb the risks of change, since risks are part of the process.

Creativity and innovation are important aspects of nursing that lead to better practice as new knowledge and skills are applied. The result is change that leads to maintenance of a competitive share of the health care market, thus ensuring the position of nursing.

Nursing educators can promote change through nursing research, thus committing nursing to a clinical practice based on scholarly inquiry. Promotion of nursing research effects change through application of research findings. Nursing research can be income-enhancing when it produces more effective and efficient nursing prescriptions.

Change involves nursing managers in many functions of nursing. It requires planning. The organization is adapted to accommodate the changes. The nurse manager uses communication, leadership, and motivation theory to overcome resistance and gain support in making the change work. The implemented change is continually evaluated to keep it working and effective.

APPLICATION EXERCISES

EXERCISE 13-1   Select a change that needs to be made in managing nursing personnel or in nursing care of patients. The needed change may originate from the results of research or from a notable problem. Decide which change theory or theories to use and make a plan for the change.

EXERCISE 13-2   Ascertain whether your unit of employment has a business plan. If not, develop one with your peers. If there is a business plan, note whether it needs updating, and if so, update it. Will this process result in any changes within the unit?

EXERCISE 13-3   Organize a group of professional nurses to:
Explore the theory of the nursing business within an organization (hospital, nursing home, home health care, professional organization).
Identify products and activities to be abandoned.
Identify products or activities to be developed. Select one for a pilot test.

EXERCISE 13-4   You may complete the following exercise as an individual or as a group.
Scenario: It was obvious to the entire nursing staff of a community hospital that the work load was decreasing. There were empty beds on every unit. Deliveries on the obstetrical unit were down to an average of one per day, and the daily census of the postpartum unit and newborn nursery was four to six patients. Work load and patient census on the pediatric unit were likewise low. Rumors were rampant. One was that the pediatric and obstetrical units would be combined. Another was that they would both be closed and their patients would be combined with medical-surgical patients on other units. A third rumor was that the other community hospital was having similar problems and that negotiations were under way to combine several specialty services between the two institutions. It was even rumored that one would become an extended-care facility and that the management of both hospitals would be combined. Worries of nursing staff gave way to gossip among various groups in corridors, at coffee breaks, in the dining room, and everywhere employees chanced to meet, including areas to which patients were transported, such as the x-ray lab, the physical therapy room, and the medical laboratory. Employees were concerned most about job security and institutional stability—whether there would be jobs for all of them and whether the job benefits would be the same if they worked at either hospital. At a clinical nurse managers' meeting, the director of nursing was asked if any of the rumors were true. She stated that the administrator would make an announcement at the appropriate time and that until then the staff should continue with its work. That afternoon the local newspaper announced a merger of the two hospitals, describing in detail the missions and services each would provide to the community. No reference was made to the plans for employees.
Prepare a business plan (management plan) that embodies application of change theory that would be best under the preceding scenario.

EXERCISE 13-5   Scan the previous year's issues of ten different nursing journals and answer the following:
How many articles report *research* in:
Management or administration?_____
Teaching?_____
Practice?_____

EXERCISE 13-6   Identify a published research study from one of the journals you used for Exercise 13-5. What was the research question? How does it meet the criteria of Lindeman and Schantz? Evaluate the study, using the steps of the research process outlined in this chapter.

EXERCISE 13-7   Identify a published research study from one of the journals used for Exercise 13-5 and apply the results. Use change theory to make a business or management plan for doing this.

EXERCISE 13-8

Form a group of your peers and have each member identify something that can be improved in nursing. This may be a policy or a procedure; a change in a form to make its use more effective; an interdepartmental protocol, such as how tests are scheduled or patients transported or handled; or a change in clinical practice. Using change theory, each person makes a plan for improvement and discusses it with the peer group. When the group decides the plan merits implementation, present it to nursing administration where you work or are assigned as a student.

EXERCISE 13-9

Scan several nursing journals for the past year. Select research findings you would like to use in clinical nursing. Select a model for implementation such as the Conduct and Utilization of Research in Nursing (CURN) model. (See J. A. Horsley, J. Crane, and J. Bingle, "Research Utilization as an Organizational Process," *Journal of Nursing Administration*, 8, 7 (1978), 4-6). Prepare a plan and implement the findings.

EXERCISE 13-10

Explore the idea of creating a nursing research council. Consider its mission, philosophy, and objectives. If there is enough interest among the nurses in the organization in which you work, make a management plan to launch the council as an organizational entity.

EXERCISE 13-11

Use the Internet to look at some of the practices of highly profitable companies. What business practices do they use that could be used in the health care industry? Pay particular attention to practices related to creativity, innovation, and research. Is there evidence of the application of change theory?

NOTES

1. W. J. Reddin, "How to Change Things," *Executive* (June 1969), 22–26.
2. B. W. Spradley, "Managing Change Creatively," *The Journal of Nursing Administration* (May 1980), 32–37.
3. T. Peters, "Vote for Change but Follow Through," *San Antonio Light* (7 May 1991), B2.
4. E. G. Williams, "Changing Systems and Behavior," *Business Horizons* (August 1969), 53–58.
5. R. M. Kanter, *When Giants Learn to Dance* (New York: Simon & Schuster, 1989), 9–26.
6. D. A. Nadler and M. L. Tushman, "Organizational Frame Bending: Principles for Managing Reorganization," *Executive* (March 1989), 194–204.
7. T. Peters, "Winds of Change Hit Central Staffs," *San Antonio Light* (19 November 1991), E3.
8. T. J. Covin and R. H. Kilmann, "Participant Perceptions of Positive and Negative Influences on Large-Scale Change," *Group & Organizational Studies* (June 1990), 233–248.
9. R. D. Brynildsen and T. A. Wickes, "Agents of Changes," *Automation* (October 1970).
10. Ibid.
11. W. J. Reddin, op. cit.
12. Ibid.
13. B. W. Spradley, op. cit.; L. B. Welch, "Planned Change in Nursing: The Theory," *Nursing Clinics of North America* (June 1979), 307–321.
14. Ibid.
15. Ibid.
16. L. B. Welch, op. cit.
17. Ibid.
18. Ibid.; K. Oates, "Models of Planned Change and Research Utilization Applied to Product Evaluation," *Clinical Nurse Specialist* (November 1997), 270–273.
19. L. B. Welch, op. cit.
20. B. W. Spradley, op. cit.
21. C. M. Kreidler, J. Campbell, G. Lanik, V. R. Gray, and M. A. Conrad, "Community Elderly. A Nursing Center's Use of Change Theory as a Model," *Journal of Gerontological Nursing* (January 1994), 25–30.
22. D. C. Dunphy and D. A. Stace, "Transformational and Coercive Strategies for Planned Organizational Change: Beyond the O. D. Model," *Organizational Studies*, 9(3), (1988), 317–334.
23. Ibid.
24. T. A. Stewart, "Welcome to the Revolution," *Fortune* (13 December 1993), 66–80.
25. N. M. Tichy, " Revolutionize Your Company," *Fortune* (13 December 1993), 114–118.
26. "A Master Class in Radical Change," *Fortune* (13 December 1993), 82–96.
27. Ibid.
28. J. V. Roach, "U.S. Business: Time to Seize the Day," *Newsweek* (4 April 1988), 10; M. Beyers, "Getting on Top of Organizational Change: Part 1, Process and Development," *Journal of Nursing Administration* (October 1984), 32–39; D. H. Freed, "Please Don't Shoot Me: I'm Only the Change Agent," *Health Care Supervision* (September 1998), 56–61.

29. N. H. Busen and M. E. Jones, "Leadership Development: Educating Nurse Practitioners for the Future," *Journal of the American Academy of Nurse Practitioners* (March 1995), 111–117; A. Kennedy, "Attila the Hun: Leadership as a Change Agent," *Hospital Material Management Quarterly* (February 1996), 29–37.

30. J. Feldman and D. Daly-Gawenda, "Retrenchment: How Nurse Executives Cope," *Journal of Nursing Administration* (June 1985), 31–37.

31. V. J. Callan, "Individual and Organizational Strategies for Coping with Organizational Change," *Work & Stress* (March 1993), 63–75.

32. D. Rosenberg, " Eliminating Resistance to Change," *Security Management* (January 1993), 20–21.

33. E. G. Williams, op. cit.

34. M. J. Ward and S. G. Moran, "Resistance to Change: Recognize, Respond, Overcome," *Nursing Management* (January 1984), 30–33.

35. R. E. Hunt and M. K. Rigby, "Easing the Pain of Change," *Management Review* (September 1984), 41–45.

36. Ibid.

37. D. J. Gillen, "Harvesting the Energy from Change Anxiety," *Supervisory Management* (March 1986), 40–43.

38. M. J. Ward and S. G. Moran, op. cit.

39. P. F. Drucker, *Management Challenges for the 21st Century* (New York: HarperCollins, 1999), 73.

40. M. Beyers, "Getting on Top of Organizational Change: Part 2. Trends in Nursing Service," *Journal of Nursing Administration* (November 1984), 31–37.

41. Ibid.

42. P. F. Drucker, *Management Challenges for the 21st Century*, 81–85.

43. M. Beyers, op. cit.; D. J. Gillen, op. cit.

44. D. J. Gillen, op. cit.

45. G. McPhail, "Management of Change: An Essential Skill for Nursing in the 1990s," *Journal of Nursing Management* (July 1997), 199–205.

46. R. E. Hunt and M. K. Rigby, op. cit.

47. M. J. Ward and S. G. Moran, op. cit.

48. Report on Victor E. Dowling's Change Theory, "How to Wage the War on Change," *Electrical World* (October 1990), 38–39.

49. D. Levick, "How Do You Communicate? Managing the Change Process," *Physician Executive* (July 1996), 26–29.

50. R. E. Endres, "Successful Management of Change," *Notes & Quotes* (November 1972), 3.

51. R. E. Hunt and M. K. Rigby, op. cit.

52. Report on Victor E. Dowling's Change Theory, op. cit.

53. M. Beyers, op. cit.

54. W. J. Ward and S. G. Moran, op. cit.

55. D. P. Newcomb and R. C. Swansburg, *The Team Plan: A Manual for Nursing Service Administrators*, 2nd ed. (New York: Putnam, 1971), 136–172.

56. R. L. Lattimer and M. L. Winitsky, "Unleashing Creativity," *Management World* (April 1984), 22–24.

57. J. Gordon and R. Zemke, "Making Them More Creative," *Training* (May 1986), 30ff.

58. M. J. Gilmartin, "Creativity: The Fuel of Innovation," *Nursing Administration Quarterly* (winter 1999), 1–8.

59. Sr. M. H. Reinkemeyer, "A Nursing Paradox," *Nursing Research* (January–February 1968), 8.

60. A. J. Rutigliano, "An Interview with Peter Drucker: Managing the New," *Management Review* (January 1986), 38–41; "Peter Drucker on Managing the New," *Newsweek* (October 1998), S6–S7.

61. J. Manion, "Nurse Intrapreneurs: The Heroes of Health Care's Future," *Nursing Outlook* (January–February 1991), 18–21.

62. R. R. Godfrey, "Tapping Employees' Creativity," *Supervisory Management* (February 1986), 16–20.

63. R. L. Lattimer and M. L. Winitsky, op. cit.

64. A. G. Van Gundy, "How to Establish a Creative Climate in the Work Group," *Management Review* (August 1984), 24–25, 28, 37–38.

65. R. A. Atchley, M. Keeney, and C. Burgess, "Cerebral Hemispheric Mechanisms Linking Ambiguous Word Meaning Retrieval and Creativity," *Brain Cognition* (August 1999), 479–499.

66. R. L. Lattimer and M. L. Winitsky, op. cit.

67. R. R. Godfrey, op. cit.

68. P. F. Drucker, "Creating Strategies of Innovation," *Planning Review* (November 1985), 8–11, 45.

69. J. Gordon and R. Zemke, op. cit.

70. A. G. Van Gundy, op. cit.

71. S. Glucksberg, "Some Ways to Turn on New Ideas," *Think* (IBM), (March–April 1968), 24–28.

72. R. R. Godfrey, op. cit.

73. C. S. Kleinman, "Nurse Executives: New Roles, New Opportunities," *Journal of Health Administration Education* (winter 1999), 15–26.

74. G. Southon, "IT, Change and Evaluation: An Overview of the Role of Evaluation in Health Services," *International Journal of Medical Information* (December 1999), 125–133.

75. D. P. Newcomb and R. C. Swansburg, op. cit.

76. H. Levinson, "What an Executive Should Know About Scientists," *Notes & Quotes* (Hartford: Connecticut General Life Insurance Company, November 1965), 1.

77. R. R. Godfrey, op. cit.

78. M. A. Rosswurm and J. H. Larrabee, "A Model for Change to Evidence-Based Practice," *Image*, 31(4), 1999, 317–322.

79. A. G. Van Gundy, op. cit.

80. J. Gordon and R. Zemke, op. cit.

81. T. Peters, "Lack of Curiosity May Kill Business," *San Antonio Light* (11 August 1990), B2.

82. A. K. Gupta, and A. Singhal, "Managing Human Resources for Innovation and Creativity," *Resource Technology Management* (May–June 1993), 41–48.

83. T. R. Horton, "Poised for Tomorrow," *Newsweek* (5 October 1987), S–4.

84. M. L. McClure, "Promoting Practice-based Research: A Critical Need," *Journal of Nursing Administration* (November–December 1981), 66–70; American Hospital Association, *Strategies: Integration of Nursing Research into the Practice Setting* (Chicago: AHA Nurse Executive Management Strategies, 1985).

85. R. C. Swansburg, *Management of Patient Care Services* (St. Louis, MO: C. V. Mosby, 1968), 334.

86. M. L. McClure, op. cit.

87. K. P. Krone and M. E. Loomis, "Developing Practice-Relevant Research: A Model That Worked," *Journal of Nursing Administration* (April 1982), 38–41.

88. L. N. Sherwen, C. A. Bevil, D. Adler, and P. G. Watson, "Educating for the Future: A National Survey of Nursing Deans About Need and Demand for Nurse Researchers," *Journal of Professional Nursing* (July–August 1993), 195–203.

89. M. J. Cowan, J. Heinrich, M. Lucas, H. Sigmon, and A. S. Hinshaw, "Integration of Biological and Nursing Sciences: A 10-Year Plan to Enhance Research and Training," *Research in Nursing & Health* (16: 1993), 3–9.

90. L. R. Bock, "From Research to Utilization: Bridging the Gap," *Nursing Management* (March 1990), 50–51.

91. H. J. Krouse and S. D. Holloran, "Nurse Managers and Clinical Nursing Research," *Nursing Management* (July 1992), 62–64; A. Retsas, "Barriers to Using Research Evidence in Nursing Practice," *Journal of Advanced Nursing* (March 2000), 599–606.

92. L. Marchette, "Developing a Productive Nursing Research Program in a Clinical Institution," *Journal of Nursing Administration* (March 1985), 25–30.

93. H. K. S. Laschinger, S. Foran, B. Jones, K. Perkin, and P. Boran, "Research Utilization in Nursing Administration," *Journal of Nursing Administration* (February 1944), 32–35.

94. G. C. Polk, "Building a Nursing Research Culture," *Journal of Psychosocial Nursing*, 27(4), 1989, 24–27.

95. C. A. Lindeman and D. Schantz, "The Research Question," *Journal of Nursing Administration* (January 1982), 6–10; D. Schantz and C. A. Lindeman, "Reading a Research Article," *Journal of Nursing Administration* (March 1982), 30–33.

96. C. A. Lindeman and D. Schantz, op. cit.

97. Ibid.

98. Ibid.

99. D. P. Olsen, "Equipoise: An Appropriate Standard for Ethical Review of Nursing Research?" *Journal of Advanced Nursing* (February 2000), 267–273.

100. D. Schantz and C. A. Lindeman, "The Research Design," *Journal of Nursing Administration* (February 1982), 35–38.

101. American Hospital Association, op. cit.

102. E. A. Hefferin, J. A. Horsley, and M. R. Ventura, "Promoting Research-Based Nursing: The Nurse Administrator's Role," *Journal of Nursing Administration* (May 1982), 34–41.

103. K. P. Krone and M. E. Loomis, op. cit.

104. American Hospital Association, op. cit.

105. E. Larson, "Nursing Research and Societal Needs: Political, Corporate, and International Perspectives," *Journal of Professional Nursing* (March–April 1993), 73–78.

REFERENCES

Ayers, A. F. "Defined Objectives Helping Management to Reach for Stars." *Presidential Issue* (1988–89), 70–72, 74.

Barker, S. B., and R. T. Barker. "Managing Change in an Interdisciplinary Inpatient Unit: An Action Research Approach." *Journal of Mental Health Administration* (winter 1994), 80–91.

Barry-Walker, J. "The Impact of Systems Redesign on Staff, Patient, and Financial Outcomes." *Journal of Nursing Administration* (February 2000), 77–89.

Beasley, P. "Ways to Boost Creativity in the Workplace." *The Knoxville News Sentinel* (7 May 2000), J1.

Blake, L. "Reduce Employees' Resistance to Change." *Personnel Journal* (September 1992), 72–76.

Bolster, C. "Work Redesign: More than Rearranging Furniture on the Titanic." *Aspen Advisor* (6: 1991), 4–7.

Bolton, L. B., C. Aydin, G. Popolow, and J. Ramseyer. "Ten Steps for Managing Organizational Change." *Journal of Nursing Administration* (June 1992), 14–20.

Brink, P. J., and Wood, M. J. *Basic Steps in Planning Nursing Research*, 4th ed. (Sudbury, MA: Jones and Bartlett, 1994).

Brockopp, D. Y., and M. T. Hastings-Tolsma. *Fundamentals of Nursing Research*, 2nd ed. (Sudbury, MA: Jones and Bartlett, 1995).

Brothers, J. "Some Techniques that Can Help You . . . Turn a Drawback into a Strength." *Parade Magazine* (10 April 1994), 4–6.

Buckley, D. S. "A Practitioner's View on Managing Change." *Frontier Health Service Management* (fall 1999), 38–43, 49–50.

Coeling, H. V. E., and J. R. Wilcox. "Using Organizational Culture to Facilitate the Change Process." *ANNA Journal* (June 1990), 231–236.

Drenkard, K. "Executive Journey: From 1,300 FTEs to None." *Nursing Administration Quarterly* (fall 1997), 57–63.

Dumaine, B. "Payoff from the New Management." *Fortune* (13 December 1993), 103–104, 108, 110.

Golembienski, R. T., and Ben-Chu Sun. "Public-Sector Innovation and Predisposing Situational Features: Testing Covariants of Successful QWC Applications." *PAQ* (spring 1991), 106–131.

Helle, P. F. "Creativity: The Key to Breakthrough Changes, How Teaming Can Harness Collective Knowledge." *Hospital Materials Management Quarterly* (August 1999), 7–12.

Ingersoll, G. L., J. C. Kirsch, S. E. Merk, and J. Lightfoot. "Relationship of Organizational Culture and Readiness for Change to Employee Commitment to the Organization." *Journal of Nursing Administration* (January 2000), 11–20.

Lane, A. J. "Using Havelock's Model to Plan Unit-Based Change." *Nursing Management* (September 1992), 58–60.

Lesic, S. A. "Using Instrumental Leadership to Manage Change." *Radiology Management* (May–June 1999), 44–52, 53–56.

Lynn, M. R. "Poster Sessions: A Good Way to Communicate Research." *Journal of Pediatric Nursing* (June 1989), 211–213.

Lyth, G. M. "Clinical Supervision: A Concept Analysis." *Journal of Advanced Nursing* (March 2000), 722–729.

Manz, C. "Preparing for an Organizational Change: The Managerial Transition." *Organizational Dynamics*, 19 (1990), 15–26.

Marshall, Z., and N. Luffingham. "Does the Specialist Nurse Enhance or Deskill the General Nurse." *British Journal of Nursing* (11–24 June 1998), 658–662.

Marszaleck-Goucher, E., and V. D. Eelsenhans. "Intrapreneurship: Tapping Employee Creativity." *Journal of Nursing Administration* (December 1988), 20–22.

McGregor, D. *Leadership and Motivation* (Cambridge, MA: M.I.T. Press, 1966), 15–16.

McGuire, D. B., and M. E. Ropka. "Research and Oncology Nursing Practice." *Seminar in Oncology Nursing* (February 2000), 35–46.

Merchant, J. "Task Allocation: A Case of Resistance to Change?" *Nursing Practice*, 4(2), (1991), 16–18.

Munhall, P. L., and C. O. Boyd. *Nursing Research: A Qualitative Perspective*, 2nd ed. (Sudbury, MA: Jones and Bartlett, 2000).

Murphy, F. A. "Collaborating with Practitioners in Teaching and Research: A Model for Developing the Role of the Nurse Lecturer in Practice Areas." *Journal of Advanced Nursing* (March 2000), 704–714.

Noble-Adams, R. "Ethics and Nursing Research. 2: Examination of the Research Process." *British Journal of Nursing* (22 July–11 August 1999), 956–960.

Peters, T. "Ingersoll-Rand Retools the Way It Makes Tools." *San Antonio Light* (12 February 1991), D1.

Petro-Nustas, W. "Evaluation of the Process of Introducing a Quality Development Program in a Nursing Department at a Teaching Hospital: The Role of a Change Agent." *International Journal of Nursing Studies* (December 1996), 605–618.

Rempusheski, V. F. "Incorporating Research Role and Practice Role." *Applied Nursing Research* (February 1991), 46–48.

Rodger, M. A., and L. King. "Drawing Up and Administering Intramuscular Injections: A Review of the Literature." *Journal of Advanced Nursing* (March 2000), 574–582.

Ryan, M., K. H. Carlton, and N. S. Ali. "Evaluation of Traditional Classroom Teaching Methods Versus Course Delivery Via the World Wide Web." *Journal of Nursing Education* (September 1999), 272–277.

Thurston, N. E., S. C. Tenove, and J. M. Church. "Hospital Nursing Research Is Alive and Flourishing." *Nursing Management* (May 1990), 50–53.

Wilson, H. S., and S. A. Hutchison. *Applying Research in Nursing: A Resource Book* (Menlo Park, CA: Addison Wesley, 1986).

Zeira, Y., and J. Aredisian. "Organizational Planned Change: Assessing the Chances for Success." *Organizational Dynamics* (spring 1989), 31–45.

CHAPTER 14

Organizing Nursing Services

Russell C. Swansburg, PhD, RN

LEARNING OBJECTIVES AND ACTIVITIES

- Define *organizing*.
- Apply or illustrate selected principles of organizing.
- Evaluate selected elements of organizational development.
- Describe a bureaucracy.
- Identify the components of a nursing care delivery system.
- Analyze an organizational structure.
- Use a set of standards to evaluate line and staff relationships of a nursing organization.
- Distinguish among various forms of organizational structures.
- Use a set of standards to evaluate departmentation.
- Describe an informal organization.
- Use a set of standards to evaluate an organizational chart.
- Identify characteristics of organizational effectiveness of a nursing organization, including symptoms of malorganization.

CONCEPTS: Organizing, bureaucracy, role theory, organizational development, autonomy, accountability, organizational culture, organizational climate, team building, organizational structure, adhocracy, nursing care delivery system, differentiated practice, flat organization, tall organization, organization chart, organizational effectiveness, informal organization.

MANAGER BEHAVIOR: The manager maintains the nursing organization to support a bureaucratic structure through adherence to basic principles of organizing.

LEADER BEHAVIOR: The leader works with nursing employees to develop a modified organizational structure that supports autonomy, accountability, and culture and climate conducive to satisfied patients, families, nurses, physicians, and other staff.

Organizational Theory

Once plans are made; the mission, purpose, or business for which the organization exists has been established; the philosophy and vision statements have been developed and adopted; and the objectives have been formulated, resources are organized to sustain the philosophy, achieve the vision, and accomplish the mission and objectives of the organization. Organizations develop as goals become too complex for the individual and have to be divided into units that individuals can manage.[1]

Fayol referred to the organizing element of management as the form of the body corporate and stated that the organization takes on form when the number of workers rises to the level requiring a supervisor. It is necessary to group people, distribute duties, and adapt the organic whole to requirements by putting essential employees where they will be most useful. An intermediate executive is the generator of power and ideas.[2] The body corporate of the nursing organization includes executive management and its staff, departmental managers (middle managers), operational managers (first-line managers), and practicing professional and technical nursing personnel. Reformed organizations eliminate middle management, with operational managers becoming the department heads. Professional nursing personnel manage the performances of technical nursing personnel. In a theory of nursing management, nurse managers have as their object the development of a nursing organization that facilitates the work of clinical nurses.

Definitions of Organizing

Urwick referred to organizing as the process of designing the machine. The process should allow for personal adjustments, but these will be minimal if a design is followed. It should show the part each person will play in the general social pattern, as well as the responsibilities, relationships, and standards of performance. Jobs should be put together along the lines of functional specializations to facilitate the training of replacements. The organizational structure must be based on sound principles, including that of continuity, to provide for the future.[3]

Organizing is the grouping of activities for the purpose of achieving objectives, the assignment of such groupings to a manager with authority for supervising each group, and the defined means of coordinating appropriate activities with other units, horizontally and vertically, that are responsible for accomplishing organizational objectives. Organizing involves the process of deciding which levels of organization are necessary to accomplish the objectives of a nursing division, department or service, or unit. For the unit, it would involve the type of work to be accomplished in terms of direct patient care, the kinds of nursing personnel needed to accomplish this work, and the span of management or supervision needed.

Principles of Organizing

Following is a discussion of the established principles of organizing.

Principle of Chain of Command

The chain of command principle states that organizations are established with hierarchical relationships within which authority flows from top to bottom to be satisfying to members, economically effective, and successful in achieving goals. This principle supports a mechanistic structure with a centralized authority that aligns authority and responsibility. Communication flows through the chain of command and tends to be one-way—downward. In a modern nursing organization, the chain of command is flat, with line managers and technical and clerical staffs that support the clinical nursing staff. Communication flows freely in all directions, with authority and responsibility delegated to the lowest operational level.

Principle of Unity of Command

The unity-of-command principle states that an employee has one supervisor and that there is one leader and one plan for a group of activities with the same objective. This principle is still followed in many nursing organizations but is increasingly being modified by emerging organizational theory. Primary nursing and case management modality support the principle of unity of command, as does joint practice. Professional nurses and others frequently engage in matrix organizations in which they answer to more than one supervisor.

Principle of Span of Control

The span-of-control principle states that a person should be a supervisor of a group that he or she can effectively supervise in terms of numbers, functions, and geography. This original principle has become elastic—the more highly trained the employee, the less supervision is needed. Employees in training need more supervision to prevent blunders. When different levels of nursing employees are used, the nurse manager has more to coordinate. Some management experts recommend up to 75 employees answering to one supervisor.[4]

Principle of Specialization

The principle of specialization is that each person should perform a single leading function. Thus there is a division of labor: a differentiation among kinds of duties. Specialization is thought by many to be the best way to use individuals and groups. The chain of command joins groups by specialty, leading to functional departmentalization. Self-directed teams modify this principle and are discussed in Chapters 15 and 16.

The hierarchy or scalar chain is a natural result of these principles of organizing. It is the order of rank from top to bottom in an organization. These principles of organizing are interdependent and dynamic when used by nurse managers to create a stimulating environment in which to practice clinical nursing.

Bureaucracy

Bureaucracy evolved from the early principles of administration, including those of organizing. Max Weber coined the term bureaucracy. Bureaucracy is highly structured and usually includes no participation by the governed. The principles of chain of command, unity of command, span of control, and specialization support bureaucratic structures. These structures do not work in their pure form and have been greatly adapted in today's organizations.

Among the historical strong points of bureaucratic organizations is their ability to produce competent and responsible employees. They perform by uniform rules and conventions; are accountable to one manager who is an authority; maintain social distance with supervisors and clients, thereby reducing favoritism and promoting impersonality; and receive rewards based on technical qualifications, seniority, and achievement.

The characteristics of bureaucracy include formality, low autonomy, a climate of rules and conventionality, division of labor, specialization, standardized procedures, written specifications, memos and minutes, centralization, controls, and emphasis on a high level of efficiency and production. These characteristics frequently lead to complaints about red tape and to procedural delays and general frustration.[5]

Using the bureaucratic model as a reference, Hall studied ten organizations evaluating the following six dimensions: division of labor, hierarchy of authority, employee rules, work procedures, impersonality, and technical competence. He found varying degrees of each of these dimensions. An organization could be highly bureaucratized in one dimension but not in others. Highly bureaucratic structures would have a high degree of bureaucracy in each of the six dimensions. Bureaucracy is a matter of degree among organizations. Similar organizations may have similar degrees of bureaucracy.[6]

Hall also found that age and size of organization do not relate to its degree of bureaucratization. The "technical qualifications" dimension did not appear to correlate with the other five dimensions. It is the rational aspect of bureaucracy. A high degree of impersonality develops in organizations that deal with large numbers of customers or clients.[7]

This study has significance for nursing administration. The scale can be used for testing in health care organizations and in nursing divisions. It can be used to measure and compare the six dimensions of bureaucracy.

Professionalism and Bureaucracy

Hall studied the relationship between professionalization and bureaucratization. For a study using both structural aspects and attitudinal attributes of a profession, his findings were as follows[8]:

1. Attitudes are strongly associated with behavior: professional organizations, certification.
2. Nurses are high in professionalism in terms of belief in service to the public, belief in self-regulation, and sense of calling to the field, but are low in feeling of autonomy and using the professional organization as reference point.
3. Nurses are high in bureaucratization, except for technical competence.
4. Autonomous organizations have less hierarchy of authority. (Autonomous organizations are those that promote autonomy of professional practitioners.)
5. An organization's size does not affect hierarchy.
6. Autonomous organizations have less division of labor.
7. Autonomous organizations have fewer procedures.
8. Autonomous and heteronymous organizations emphasize technical competence. (These organizations promote differences in practice patterns among autonomous practitioners of nursing.)
9. Professionalism increases with decreased division of labor, decreased procedures, decreased impersonality, and increased autonomy. Hierarchy is accepted if it serves coordination and communication functions.
10. Bureaucracy inhibits professionalism.

The conclusion would be that the less bureaucratic the organization, the more nurses perceive themselves as professionals.

Nurse managers need to move from bureaucratic management to transformational leadership, thereby empowering professional nurses in a world in which technology, communication, and political, economic, demographic, and social forces are constantly reshaping the health care system.[9]

Role Theory

Role theory indicates that when employees receive inconsistent expectations and little information, they will experience role conflict, which leads to stress, dissatisfaction, and ineffective performance. Role theory supports the chain-of-command and unity-of-command principles. Multiple lines of authority are disruptive, divide authority between profession and organization, and create stress. They force employees to make choices between formal authority and professional colleagues. The result is role conflict and dissatisfaction for employees and reduced efficiency and effectiveness for organization. Role conflict reduces trust of and personal liking and esteem for the person in authority; it reduces communication and decreases employee effectiveness. Management that provides for the following can reduce role conflict and ambiguity:

1. Certainty about duties, authority, allocation of time, and relationship with others.
2. Guides, directives, policies, and the ability to predict sanctions as outcomes of behavior.
3. Increased need fulfillment.
4. Structure and standards.
5. Facilitation of teamwork.
6. Toleration of freedom.
7. Upward influence.
8. Consistency.
9. Prompt decisions.
10. Good, prompt communication and information.
11. Using the chain of command.
12. Personal development.
13. Formalization.
14. Planning.
15. Receptiveness to ideas by top management.

16. Coordinating work plans.
17. Adapting to change.
18. Adequacy of authority.

The implications for nurse managers are obvious. Role conflict and role ambiguity are separate dimensions, role conflict being more dysfunctional. Some employees, however, find stress rewarding.[10]

In a changing work environment, nurses are required to perform in new roles and under new circumstances. Managers provide the education and support needed by nurses who are coping with their role changes. Management support addresses the potential and real needs deficits nurses will confront. The goal is to prevent role insufficiency by thoroughly preparing nurses to function in new roles. Managers may opt to do this through role modeling. Clear understanding of role changes and planned programs to support them will reduce role stress and prevent role strain.[11]

Effective use of role theory has a positive impact when making changes in a nursing care delivery system. Role ambiguity, role stress, and role strain are minimized through educational programs aimed at socializing nurses into their new roles. Effective communication improves role changes.[12]

Nurses acquire more personal power and incentives as they move up the managerial hierarchy. Nurse managers are motivated by the content of their work and the tasks and responsibilities assigned to their positions. Upper-level managers and supervisory-level nurses have firm beliefs in their competence and regard their roles as meeting professional goals.[13] With the restructuring of health care organizations, particularly hospitals, a whole new approach to organizing is required. It will include application of the theory related to culture, climate, team building, and role theory, among others.

Organizational Development

Organizational development deals with changing the work environment to make it more conducive to worker satisfaction and productivity. An underlying premise is that "people planning" is as important as technical and financial planning. Organizational development allows managers to attend to the psychological as well as the physical aspects of organizations. Change is the terrain by which organizational development applies.

Organizational development can sustain the favorable or desirable aspects of bureaucracy. Change can be employed to modify the undesirable aspects of bureaucracy. There is room for directive as well as nondirective leadership within organizations. Nurse managers have to be strong and tough in supporting the values of clinical nurses. They have to be proactive in planning, designing, and implementing new organizational structures and work environments. The object is to develop people, not to exploit them. Organizational development emphasizes personal growth and interpersonal competence.[14]

Autonomy and Accountability

Among the psychological and personality attributes of organizational development are autonomy and accountability, crucial elements of nursing professionalism. A professional nurse is obliged to answer for decisions and actions. This would be achieved using a management by results (MBR) approach. This approach defines performance standards incorporating acceptable behavior and results. It includes tracking for progress, performance feedback, making adjustments, and personnel accountability.[15]

Characteristics of professional autonomy include self-definition, self-regulation, and self-governance. Professional nurses respond to demographic changes in society by defining and reshaping the content of nursing practice. They address societal needs, including the needs for increased care for the elderly and the control of resources. Autonomy will be strengthened by unbundling the hospital bill and by direct reimbursement for nursing services by third-party payers.

Self-governance for nursing includes a nursing administrator hired or elected with input from nurses, self-employment of nurses, approval of nursing staff privileges by peer review with privileges revoked by the nursing staff organization, and case management.[16]

Argyris describes people as complex organizations who work for an organization for their own needs or gains. These needs exist in varying degrees or at varying depths that must be understood by organizations. People seek out jobs to meet their needs. They develop and live on a continuum from infancy to adulthood that is reflected throughout life and work and leisure.[17] Exhibit 14-1 shows the developmental continuum.

Ridderheim describes a hospital administrator's action to change a management style that was paternalistic, used downward communication, encouraged dependency, and inhibited management development. In an opinion survey, employees scored high on patient care and personal pride in work but low in decision-making ability. The following are among the changes made by the administrator after organizational assessment and consultation[18]:

1. Decisions were turned back to operating managers, giving them freedom to act within broad policy guidelines.
2. Operating management was restructured in an executive operating committee (EOC) that included the administrator and assistants for medical staff affairs,

EXHIBIT 14-1
Developmental Continuum

INFANT	ADULT
Dependent	Independent
Submissive	Autonomous
Few abilities	Many abilities
Shallow abilities	Deep abilities
Short time perspective	Long time perspective
Frustrated by	Motivated or inspired by
Lack of self-control	Self-control
Being controlled	Self-direction
Directive (authoritarian) leadership	Job involvement
Lack of self-actualization	Participative (democratic) leadership (electing own leaders)
Lack of opportunity to learn	Self-actualization
Lack of opportunity to advance	Opportunity to learn
Repetitive work	Opportunity to advance
Dull work	Variety in work
Lack of equipment	Interesting work
Lack of information	Resources to do job
Low pay	Feedback
Powerlessness	High pay
Fractionalized jobs	Autonomy and responsibility
Lack of education restricting job opportunity to lower levels	Job enlargement
Structured jobs that inhibit individual growth	Education that increases job opportunity at higher levels
Overstaffing	Opportunity for independent thought, action, growth, and feelings of accomplishment
Specialization of tasks	Understaffing (perform multiple roles)
Routine work	Generalization and wholeness of jobs
Responds by	Rewards for learning
Fighting for redesign or control (union)	Self-governance
Leaving (turnover)	Complex work
Psychological apathy or indifference	Responds by
Becoming oriented to payoffs of being market-oriented or instrumentally oriented	Allocating own tasks
Absenteeism	Staying
Daydreaming	Seeking out intrinsic rewards
Aggression toward supervisors	Increasing productivity
Aggression toward coworkers	Focusing on job content
Restricting output	Attendance
Making mistakes or errors	Being industrious and attentive
Postponing difficult tasks or decisions	Being innovative
Focusing on pay, fringe benefits, hours of work	Cooperating
Lack of interest in work	Participation
Alienation	Accepting responsibility
Decreased job rating associated with	Focusing on self-direction, self-expression, individual accomplishment, opportunity to use abilities or help people
Reduced community participation	Increased job rating associated with
Decreased leisure involvement	Increased community participation
Decreased political activity	Increased leisure involvement
Decreased participation in voluntary activities, culture, cerebral skills, group activities	Increased political activity
Being solitary	Increased participation in voluntary activities
Being withdrawn	

Source: Reprinted from "Personality and Organization Theory Revisited" by Chris Argyris, published in *Administrative Science Quarterly*, 18, 2 (June 1973): 141–167 by permission of *Administrative Science Quarterly*. © 1973 by *Administrative Science Quarterly*.

operations, facilities, patient care, personnel, and finance. Each assistant had policy-making status.

3. A core group was established at lower levels of management to focus on the technical interests and objectives of the hospital.

4. Task forces were established for special projects.

5. A team was set up to monitor terminations, retirements, recruitments, advancements, and demotions.

6. Performance standards were developed for each manager.

7. Team-building seminars were held.

8. After nine months, progress was critiqued at a retreat, first by the EOC, then by subordinate managers.

9. Achievement in relation to goals, individual growth, and teamwork was stressed over seniority.

10. Subsequent surveys showed improvement in job satisfaction, supervisory concern for employees, supervisory emphasis on goal achievement, and work group emphasis on teamwork, decision-making practices, and motivational conditions.

Culture

Organizational culture is the sum total of an organization's beliefs, norms, values, philosophies, traditions, and sacred cows. It is a social system that is a subsystem of the total organization. Organizational cultures have artifacts, perspectives, values, assumptions, symbols, language, and behaviors that have been effective.

Organizational cultures include communication networks, both formal and informal. They include a status/role structure that relates to characteristics of employees and customers or clients.

Such structures also relate to management styles—whether authoritative or participatory. Management style impacts on individual behavior. In a health care setting, these structures promote either individuality or teamwork. They relate to classes of people and can be identified through demographic surveys of both employees and patients.

The basic mission of the organization is part of its culture: employment, service, learning, and research. There is a technical or *operational arm* for getting the work done. Also, there is an *administrative arm* of wages and salaries, of hiring, firing, and promoting, of report making and quality control, of fringe benefits, and of budgeting.

The artifacts of an organizational culture may be physical, behavioral (rituals), or verbal (language, stories, myths). Verbal artifacts result from shared values and beliefs. They include traditions, heroes, and the party line and result in ceremonies that embody rituals. They include ceremonies to reward years of service, the annual picnic, the Christmas party, and the wearing of badges and insignia.[19]

Metaphors are used to characterize personalities and work styles[20]:

1. The military—language includes such terms as *battle zone, tight ship, captain, troops, battles, campaigns, enemies,* and *stars.* Award ceremonies also contain military metaphors.

2. Sports—terms such as *teams, stars,* and *quarterback* are used. Award ceremonies may also reflect the sports metaphor.

3. Anthropology—terms include *family, novice, big daddy, big momma, elder,* and *prodigal son.*

4. Television—terms include *sitcom, soap opera, country club, playground, nursery,* and *jungle.*

5. Mechanistic—terms such as *factory, assembly line,* and *well-oiled machine* are used.

6. The "zoo"— terms such as *sly fox, chicken,* and *top dog* appear.

Perspectives are shared ideas and actions. They relate to decision-making methods. For example, the social, technical, and managerial systems or subsystems will either support innovation or demand conformity.[21]

Dress, personal appearance, social decorum, and physical environment are all part of the organizational culture. They will require strict compliance through written or implied rules.

Values are the general principles, ideals, standards, and sins of the organization. Basic assumptions are the core of the culture. They include the beliefs that groups have about themselves, others, and the world.

> **Corporate culture denotes the personality of a business. If pride is valued, the culture may denote pride in how employees dress and how the facilities look. If productivity is thought to be increased by employees seeing themselves as part of a cause, the dress may be casual. Culture is created by necessity.**[22]

Corporate culture is a concept created in people's minds. It originates as a vision of the leader and spreads throughout the company and sets the tone of the organization. Culture is termed *climate* or *feel* by some people. What does the leader do to nurture the feeling desired in his or her department? Culture is created by such rites and rituals as[23]:

- Casual day—workers wear jeans and sport shirts to create an atmosphere of creativity and friendship.
- Birthing rooms and sibling birth participation programs to promote family health.
- Focus on quality, service, and reliability.
- A strong communication network.
- Face-to-face contacts.
- Name tags with only first names.

- Open parking.
- Open dining.

Culture is evident in the way workers relate to time, trust of each other, and authority relationships. It is evident in the dress and personal appearance of workers; promotion policies from within or outside; and where to take meal breaks. Every organization has heroes to model and antiheroes to be avoided. Artifacts of an organization include its written materials such as the organizational chart. A project team could evaluate an organization's culture and recommend changes. A clinical nurse specialist (CNS) could act as team leader.[24] Exhibit 14-2 lists suggested questions for organizational assessment.

Culture and the Manager

When outputs or productivity decreases in amount or kind, managers look at the social, technical, and managerial systems that are part of the organizational culture. They know that people behave in accordance with their understanding of the organization's norms and values. If they want to be successful, they identify these norms and values and apply their efforts in conformity with them. They gather data on needs: market analysis, attitude surveys, management statements, directives, and climate surveys. Then they address the real needs. These will include a marketing campaign to build strong customer relations. They continually do self-criticism, looking at usefulness of projects, plans, programs, and products.[25]

A successful manager identifies and accepts the prevailing culture before making changes. It is more difficult to change a culture at the level of basic beliefs, values, and perspectives. It is easier to change technical and administrative systems.

Changing the culture uncovers the sacred cows and taboos, among which are diploma graduates, collective bargaining, mission, the competition, layoffs, converting positions, education, and clinical ladders. Organizational culture focuses on work life. There is potential for conflict between a collection of differing personal norms of individuals and opposing cultural norms of the organization.[26]

Managers and personnel who survive in a culture learn how to support the values and norms of that culture. Their conformity impedes change and innovation. The social, technical, and managerial systems are changed through organizational development. Organizational culture is far more difficult to change because it operates at the level of basic beliefs, values, and perspectives. Change in the organization often involves revolution and conflict, so it is a tough issue. To change culture may require installing a new leader.[27] See Exhibits 14-3, 14-4, and 14-5.

Research indicates that a strong culture that encourages participation and involvement of employees in shared decision making, emphasizing customers, stockholders, and employees, and of leadership from managers at all levels positively affects an organization's performance. Such organizations outperform competitors 2:1 in return on investments and sales. The organizational culture can be influenced by the CEO.[28] See Exhibit 14-6.

EXHIBIT 14-2
Suggested Questions for Organizational Assessment

- What were your first impressions when you initially came to this unit/institution?
- From this first impression, what factors were most pleasing for you to encounter?
- What factors were most anxiety-provoking?
- What do "they" say about the nurses who work on this unit/at this hospital?
- How can *you* tell that a nurse works on this unit/at this hospital?
- What is the most interesting story you ever heard about this unit/hospital?
- What do you think this story tells you?
- What is most helpful in contributing to excellent nursing care on this unit/at this hospital? Why?
- What is the most significant barrier to the delivery of excellent nursing care at this institution?
- Who, in this environment, is a hero? Why?
- What does it mean to be "the best"?
- What is the most important lesson, good or bad, that you've learned here? How did you learn it?

Source: Reprinted from "Assessment of Organizational Culture: A Tool for Professional Success" by C. Caroselli, with permission of *Orthopedic Nursing*, © May/June 1992:60.

EXHIBIT 14-3
OD Cycle: System Change

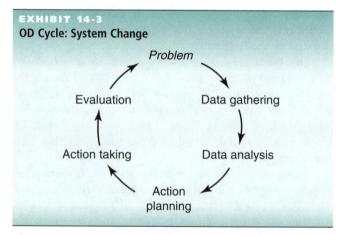

Source: "Organizational Development: System Change or Culture Change?" by William G. Dyer, et al. *Personnel* (February 1986). © 1986 American Management Association, New York. Reprinted by permission. All rights reserved.

EXHIBIT 14-4
Organizational Development Cycle: Culture Change

1. A crisis calls into question the leader's assumptions. → 2. There is a breakdown of symbols, beliefs, and structure.

   ↑   ↓

6. The new leadership establishes new symbols, beliefs, and   3. New leadership emerges with a new set of
   structure to sustain the new culture.   assumptions.

   ↑   ↓

5. If the crisis is solved and new leaders are given credit for ← 4. Conflict occurs between the old and new cultures.
   the improvement, they become the new cultural elite.

Source: "Organizational Development: System Change or Culture Change?" by William G. Dyer, et al. *Personnel* (February 1986). © 1986 American Management Association, New York. Reprinted by permission. All rights reserved.

EXHIBIT 14-5
Differences between System Change and Culture Change

SYSTEM CHANGE	CULTURE CHANGE
1. Problem-oriented	1. Value-oriented
2. More easily controlled	2. Largely uncontrollable
3. Involves making incremental changes in systems	3. Involves transforming basic assumptions
4. Focuses on improving organization output/measurable outcomes	4. Focuses on the quality of life in an organization
5. Diagnosis involves discovering nonalignments between subsystems	5. Diagnosis involves examining dysfunctional effects of core assumptions
6. Leadership change is not essential	6. Leadership change is crucial

Source: "Organizational Development: System Change or Culture Change?" by William G. Dyer, et al. *Personnel* (February 1986). © 1986 American Management Association, New York. Reprinted by permission. All rights reserved.

Organizations all have cultures, and large ones have subcultures. With time and effort nurse managers can change the culture of their organization to improve performance. Culture change is accomplished through strategic planning, the first step being the creation of a vision of desired values and outcomes. Suggestions for culture change include[29]:

1. Emphasize quality.
2. Use available knowledge of processes that have worked in other organizations.
3. Create partnerships for care and an organizational structure and philosophy of shared ownership and participation.
4. This requires collaboration, shared decision-making, and problem-solving work experience. It includes patient and family, physicians, nurses, other caregivers, and support and administrative staff. They use clinical pathways and clinical practice guidelines. Collaboration requires joint rounds, caregiver commitment, and total commitment of top management. Information is shared and communications are free flowing.
5. Redesign the roles and responsibilities of managers as well as caregivers and support staff. Practices that do not work are abandoned. Patient and family become a part of the entire process.

The various subcultures of an organization need to come into line with each other and with the corporate strategy (strategic fit) to achieve a corporate culture for success. Three essential components of value-based management are persuasion, negotiation, and compromise. An effective leader persuades people to have a similar perception of the truth so they will work together. "Negotiation is the art of coordinating different perceptions of the truth so that people can work together efficiently to achieve the common goal. Compromise is the art of identifying and trading off non-essentials so that the integrity of each party is intact as they work together to achieve mutual goals." [30]

Successful organizations have leaders and staff that share clear strategic visions, perform identifiable activities with confidence and within achievable time frames, and attain specific goals by department.

The culture of the workplace determines whether professional nurses stay with or leave an organization.[31]

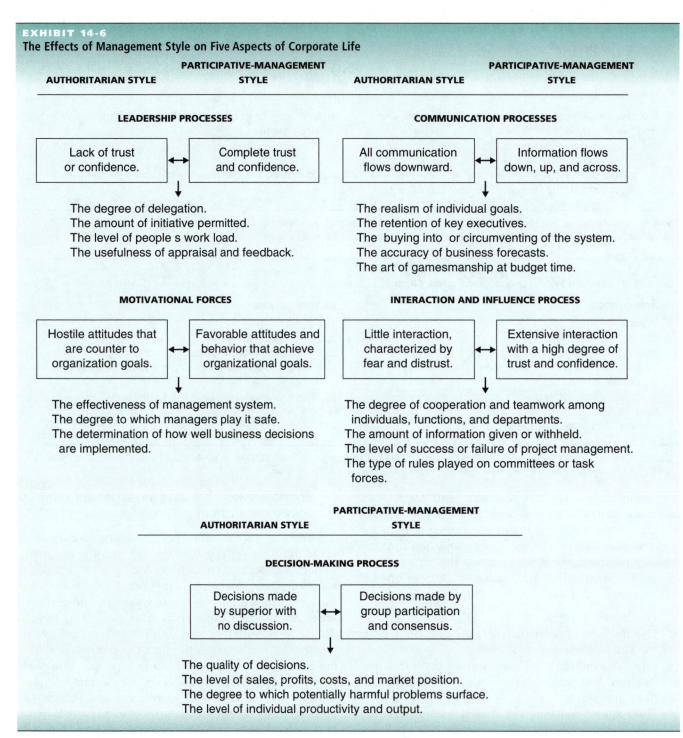

EXHIBIT 14-6
The Effects of Management Style on Five Aspects of Corporate Life

| | PARTICIPATIVE-MANAGEMENT | | PARTICIPATIVE-MANAGEMENT |
| AUTHORITARIAN STYLE | STYLE | AUTHORITARIAN STYLE | STYLE |

LEADERSHIP PROCESSES   **COMMUNICATION PROCESSES**

Lack of trust or confidence. ⟷ Complete trust and confidence.   All communication flows downward. ⟷ Information flows down, up, and across.

The degree of delegation.
The amount of initiative permitted.
The level of people s work load.
The usefulness of appraisal and feedback.

The realism of individual goals.
The retention of key executives.
The buying into or circumventing of the system.
The accuracy of business forecasts.
The art of gamesmanship at budget time.

MOTIVATIONAL FORCES   **INTERACTION AND INFLUENCE PROCESS**

Hostile attitudes that are counter to organization goals. ⟷ Favorable attitudes and behavior that achieve organizational goals.   Little interaction, characterized by fear and distrust. ⟷ Extensive interaction with a high degree of trust and confidence.

The effectiveness of management system.
The degree to which managers play it safe.
The determination of how well business decisions are implemented.

The degree of cooperation and teamwork among individuals, functions, and departments.
The amount of information given or withheld.
The level of success or failure of project management.
The type of rules played on committees or task forces.

| | PARTICIPATIVE-MANAGEMENT |
| AUTHORITARIAN STYLE | STYLE |

DECISION-MAKING PROCESS

Decisions made by superior with no discussion. ⟷ Decisions made by group participation and consensus.

The quality of decisions.
The level of sales, profits, costs, and market position.
The degree to which potentially harmful problems surface.
The level of individual productivity and output.

Research and Organizational Culture

Ideas, values, and symbols relate to and transform attitudes, feelings, and behavior. Bureaucracy has survived and expanded within organizations. Most cultural changes within organizations occur within the bureaucratic structure. Nurse leaders should initiate and support cultural changes that not only keep the enterprise profitable and economically fit but also preserve the caring behavior of nurses.

Through qualitative research Ray developed the theory of differential caring. Differential caring has multiple meanings, including:

- Humanistic—empathy, love, and concern.
- Political–legal—decision-making, liability, and malpractice.
- Ethical–religious—trust, respect, acts of "brotherly" love, and ideals of "doing unto others."
- Economic—budget management and economic well-being.
- Technological/physiological—use of machinery.
- Educational—information, teaching, education programs.
- Social—communication, social interaction and support, interrelationships, involvement, intimacy, knowing clients and families, humanistic potential for compassion and concern, love and empathy.

A formal theory of bureaucratic caring emerged from the substantive theory of differential caring (see Exhibit 14-7). The challenge for nurse managers is to create an organizational culture that supports the theory of bureaucratic caring.[32]

Fleeger studied organizational culture to arrive at the characteristics of consonant and dissonant cultures indicated in Exhibit 14-8. She recommends that managers promote a consonant culture through the following[33]:

- Strategic planning sessions promoting employees' involvement.
- Identifying conflict situations as opportunities for creative change.

EXHIBIT 14-7
Differential Caring in an Organizational Culture: Caring Categories of Administrators

ROLE	DOMINANT CARING DESCRIPTORS	STRUCTURAL CARING CATEGORIES
Nonnurse administrators	Empathy	Social
	Communication	Political
	Economic management	Economic
	Effective competition	Spiritual
	Responsibility/attitude	Ethical
Nurse administrators	Empathy	Social
	Communication	Political
	Time management	Economic
	Rapport	Spiritual
	Budget decisions	
	Spiritual concern	

Source: M. A. Ray. "The Theory of Bureaucratic Caring for Nursing Practice in the Organizational Culture." *Nursing Administration Quarterly*, winter 1989, 37. © 1989 Aspen Publishers. Reprinted with permission.

EXHIBIT 14-8
Characteristics of Consonant and Dissonant Cultures

CONSONANT CULTURES	DISSONANT CULTURES
Collective spirit	Mismatch between professional and organizational goals
Golden rule norm	Stronger union affiliations than organizational
One superordinate goal	Little staff representation on committees
Frequent management/staff interactions	Low staff participation in decision-making
Clinical expertise valued	Do not have primary care models
Professional and organizational goals similar	Competitive spirit
Goals same across work units	Them versus us norm
High cooperation between units	Low staff/management interactions
Primary care model promoting autonomy and independence	Staff feel undervalued
Formal and informal systems to address conflicts	Mismatch between values and outcomes
Match between values and outcomes	Nurse managers seen as outside occupational
All nurses seen as members of same occupational group	Double standards exist for behaviors
All members seen as working toward same goal	Groups feel others not working toward common goal
Behavior norms same for everyone	Myths, stories, symbols not caring or positive

Source: M. E. Fleeger. "Assessing Organizational Culture: A Planning Strategy." *Nursing Management* 24, no. 2 (February 1993): 40.

EXHIBIT 14–9
Ideal Culture Profile (n = 26 registered nurses)

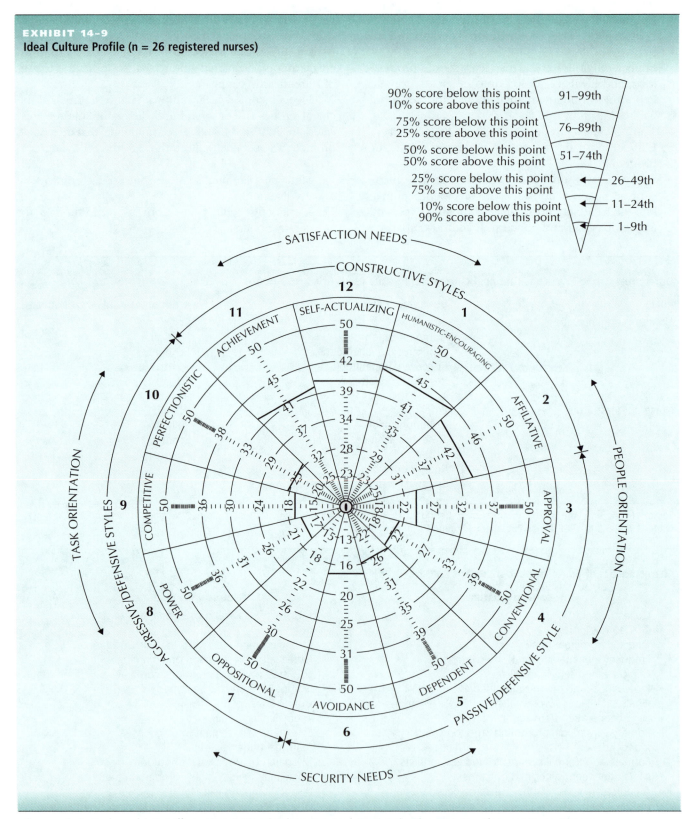

Source: R. A. Cooke and J. C. Lafferty, Organizational Culture Inventory. Reprinted with permission of Human Synergistics. © Copyright 1989.

- Planning job redesign and job-enrichment activities in stagnant departments where personnel demonstrate signs of stagnation.
- Increasing both formal and informal staff interactions.
- Adapting a nursing care model that promotes autonomy and responsibility.

It takes a well-planned and well-executed unit orientation to integrate new employees into the corporate culture and subculture. The object is to achieve a fit between employee and organization. The Organizational Culture Inventory (OCI) is an instrument that can be used to measure culture as perceived by employees. It was used to profile the "ideal" nursing culture as described by a small group of nurses representing several hospitals (see Exhibit 14-9). Such instruments can be used to measure organizational culture to define what needs preservation versus what needs changing.[34]

Leadership styles are determined by the organization's structure and culture.[35]

Climate

The organizational climate is the emotional state and the perceptions and feelings shared by members of the system. It can be formal, relaxed, defensive, cautious, accepting, trusting, and so on. It is the employees' subjective impression or perception of their organization. The employees of major concern to nurse managers are the practicing nurses. Practicing nurses create or, at the very least, contribute to the creation of the climate perceived by patients.

Managers create the climate in which practicing nurses work. If managers trust them, practicing nurses will provide them with good information to keep their managers informed. This climate promotes the concept that most hands-on employees can perform routine management, accounting, engineering, and quality tasks. Well-trained, well-equipped, and self-managed work teams, the members of which are also good salespersons, can perform 90% of expert staff work. The object of expert staff is to spread knowledge fast.[36]

Organizational climate relates to the personality of an organization and can be changed. Following are six sociological dimensions of organizational climate:

1. Clarity in specifying certification of the organization's goals and policies. This is facilitated by smooth flow of information and management support of employees.
2. Commitment to goal achievement through employee involvement.

3. Standards of performance that challenge, promote pride, and improve individual performance.
4. Responsibility for one's own work fostered and supported by managers.
5. Recognition for doing good work.
6. Teamwork—a sense of belonging, mutual trust, and respect.

The environmental dimensions of climate include room attractiveness, illumination, and the shape of the furniture. The foregoing facets of organizational climate can be measured using the supervisory climate survey shown in Exhibit 14-10.[37]

Practicing nurses want a climate that will give them job satisfaction. They achieve job satisfaction when they are challenged and their achievements are recognized and appreciated by managers and patients. They achieve satisfaction from a climate of collegiality with managers and other health care providers, in which they have input into decision-making.

Practicing nurses want a climate that provides good working conditions, high salaries, and opportunities for professional growth through counseling and career development experiences that will enable them to determine and direct their professional futures. They want a climate of administrative support that includes adequate staffing and shift options. It has been known for years that the personnel shortage, frustration, failure, and conflict in nursing required sweeping changes in intrinsic and extrinsic rewards, including career development programs that increase the ability of professional nurses to develop their self-esteem through self-actualization.

Management climate surveys measure clarity and understanding of an organization's goals, effectiveness of decision-making processes, integration, cooperation, vitality, leader effectiveness, openness and trust, job satisfaction, opportunities for growth and development, level of performance, orientation and accountability, effectiveness of teamwork and problem-solving, and overall confidence in management. Surveys may be used to make a diagnosis and to[38]:

- Establish new strategic directions.
- Clarify an organization's mission, objectives, and goals.
- Identify managers and supervisors' training and development needs.
- Reallocate resources.
- Prepare a foundation for cultural change.
- Revise hiring priorities using a patterned interview to "select in" those who share the same values.

Many studies have been done to determine work climate within business, industry, and health care organizations. Climate and philosophy result from the

EXHIBIT 14-10
Supervisory Climate Survey

INSTRUCTIONS

For each of the statements below draw a circle around one of the following: A—Always; F—Frequently; O—Occasionally; S—Seldom; N—Never.

For example, if you feel that you are frequently encouraged to come up with new and original ideas, you would circle the F in the following question:

A   F   O   S   N   1. We are encouraged to come up with new and original ideas.

Use only one evaluative letter code for each answer.

A	F	O	S	N	1. I have the opportunity to review my overall performance and effectiveness with my supervisor.
A	F	O	S	N	2. There is much respect between management and other personnel in this group.
A	F	O	S	N	3. In this organization, the rewards and encouragements you receive for effective performance outweigh the threats and criticisms.
A	F	O	S	N	4. Our people are encouraged to make decisions when the situation demands an immediate decision.
A	F	O	S	N	5. In this group I am given a chance to participate in setting the performance goals for my job.
A	F	O	S	N	6. The rooms in which we hold meetings for decision-making are conducive to good interpersonal communication.
A	F	O	S	N	7. I feel that I am a member of a well-functioning team.
A	F	O	S	N	8. My supervisor is easily accessible to all of his or her employees.
A	F	O	S	N	9. We are encouraged to come up with new and original ideas.
A	F	O	S	N	10. In this group we are rewarded in proportion to how well we do.
A	F	O	S	N	11. As a group we can disagree without becoming disagreeable.
A	F	O	S	N	12. People are proud to belong to this group.
A	F	O	S	N	13. In this group what constitutes good performance has been identified.
A	F	O	S	N	14. Most of our meetings are held in attractive rooms.
A	F	O	S	N	15. The results I am supposed to achieve in my job are realistic.
A	F	O	S	N	16. In meetings we may sit wherever we wish.
A	F	O	S	N	17. In this group people demonstrate strong commitment to achieving group performance.
A	F	O	S	N	18. Things seem to be well organized in my group.
A	F	O	S	N	19. There is good communicative balance in my group.
A	F	O	S	N	20. People in this group help each other in solving job-related problems.
A	F	O	S	N	21. In this group people come to meetings well prepared.
A	F	O	S	N	22. We can disagree with our boss and not fear any form of reprisal.
A	F	O	S	N	23. I am involved in setting my own performance goals and in understanding how they relate to the overall goals of my group.
A	F	O	S	N	24. My supervisor does a good job in recognizing good performance.
A	F	O	S	N	25. Our overall organizational climate is a positive one.

Score the Supervisory Climate Survey in the following manner: Always, 4 points; Frequently, 3 points; Occasionally, 2 points; Seldom, 1 point; Never, 0 points.

Your organizational climate is excellent if you scored 90 to 100 points, good if you scored 80 to 89 points, average if you scored 70 to 79 points, fair if you scored 60 to 69 points, and poor if you scored less than 60 points.

Source: H. E. Munn, Jr. "Organizational Climate in the Health Care Setting." *The Health Care Manager*, October 1984, 27. Reprinted with permission. Copyright © 1984 Aspen Publishers.

corporate culture, and changing the culture leads to climate change. One head nurse designed and implemented a project to motivate the nursing staff of a medical unit to better service and greater self-satisfaction. She designed an "employee of the month" motivational strategy that included measurable performance criteria. While the staff was initially disinterested, they eventually increased their interest and participation. Productivity also increased, as did emergence of talents. The strategy culminated in a recognition ceremony. The employee of the month received a free lunch or dinner, and his or her picture was put on the bulletin board. By the end of six months, 25 of 144 employees had earned the title of employee of the month, their voluntary participation indicating that it met some of their needs.[39]

Other studies indicate the following:

1. Nurse managers are satisfied by an increased variety of clinical and management skills and their ability to see the results of their work. The nurse managers who scored high on autonomy were less constrained and were also satisfied with their pay.[40]

2. Practicing clinical nurses reported obtaining satisfaction from patient and family care; education; a variety of work experiences; interaction with staff members; their paycheck; mental challenges; being needed; friendly staff and physicians; observed patient improvement; patients' compliments; knowledge of a job well done; exciting and unpredictable work; the ability to contribute, learn and achieve; the availability of senior professionals to assist and teach; developing new staff; and having predictable work schedules.[41]

3. The behavior of professional nurses is positively affected by charge nurses who give honest pep talks, keying in on feelings; make fair and equitable assignments; handle orders efficiently; help when the work load is great; listen to complaints and ideas and promote cooperation; treat their staff as resource persons for clinical expertise and value their opinions; and are up to date in knowledge and skills and teach others.

4. Behavior was negatively affected by charge nurses who were two-faced or phony, gossiped and took advantage, favored friends in making assignments, ignored questions and refused advice or help, did not help with patients when the need arose, did not communicate orders, did not follow suggestions they asked for, were disorganized, and did not know policies and procedures.

5. Staff nurses put high value on self-esteem and self-fulfillment, achievement, recognition, tasks assigned, advancement, and responsibility.[42]

6. Senior students indicate that practicing nursing meets their self-esteem needs. Sources of job satisfiers include personal satisfaction (77.5%), collegial relationships (43.75%), security (12.5%), choice of work area (12.5%), and hours (11.25%).[43]

7. Customers' views of the organizational climate of a bank indicated these features important to them: convenience, short waiting time, personal friendly service, full-service banking, safety, and decoration. These features were evident in the caliber of employees who helped each other in serving customers, treated all customers equally, and appeared happy.[44]

8. Medical–surgical and psychiatry practice areas have the greatest potential for problems with job satisfaction and would require the greatest attention to organizational climate by nurse managers.[45]

9. Humor is motivating, stimulates creativity, and improves job performance. A positive work climate is created by steering conversations to the positive; brainstorming negative statements to make them humorous; keeping humorous things around you; encouraging laughter, which boosts the heart rate, blood circulation, and energy exchange; and never using put-down humor.[46]

Satisfied caregivers described organizational climate as being high in responsibility, warmth, support, and identity.[47] A desired climate is one in which there are positive relationships and openness characterized by esprit, intimacy, and humanistic thrust. Group climate can be measured using such instruments as Fiedler's Leader Match Scales and the Organizational Climate Description Questionnaire. Group climate contributes to staff retention and to personal and organizational success.[48]

The nursing climate makes use of the individual practicing nurse's skills and motivational potential. Obsolete nursing organizational structures and communication can be changed. Nursing management practice can be brought in line with technological and environmental changes and the aspirational and value changes of practicing nurses. Rules, habits, and bureaucratic process can be modified to enable nurses to use their potential energy and creativity. New nursing management philosophies, styles, and structures can be developed to relate to nurse providers and consumers of nursing products and services. Communication, trust, and involvement can be established among nurse managers and practicing nurses. The organizational climate for educated nurses can provide for personal enrichment and involvement in decisions—a piece of the action. Practicing nurses who are given problems to solve will solve them. Otherwise nurses are oversupervised and underled!

Nurse managers should emphasize those management tasks or activities that stimulate motivation in nursing employees. They can then establish an organizational climate that supports such activities. This climate will include motivational characteristics or "satisfiers" to keep practicing nurses happy. Productivity will increase with fair compensation plus the intrinsic motivators of task identity or degree of completion of a whole piece of work with the visible outcome of patients who improve in health status, are maintained in comfort, or die peacefully as a consequence of nursing action. In the ideal climate, nurses will be able to use a variety of skills and talents to achieve this impact, acting with autonomy while receiving adequate feedback.

Nurse managers should establish a management strategy to support new nurses and involve them in decision-making. They should not merely plug them into vacant slots but rather should match them to job choices and follow-up to determine that all goes well.

Nurse managers should establish a climate in which discipline is applied fairly and uniformly. Nurses whose work is unsatisfactory should be discharged, following policies and procedures that protect their rights. The entire work climate should clearly promote employee rights. It should indicate that their ideas are being used. Nurse managers should promote competitive wages and fringe benefits by staying informed of the personnel policies of their competitors.

The nurse manager will work to establish an organizational climate that provides incentives for clinical nurses; places them on committees; is creative and equitable in all staffing matters; emphasizes pride; promotes participation; rewards seniority and achievement; and reduces boredom and frustrations. This nurse manager will rate high in labor relations.[49]

Nurse managers should learn to use organizational climate surveys to find out the issues and concerns of practicing clinical nurses. They can then establish strategies that produce the climate that motivates their nurses to increased productivity.

Nurse managers who fail are no different from other managers. They fail when they go about business as usual, do not learn the business, apply their technical skills quickly, ignore organizational problems, ignore strategic business needs, treat all responsibilities equally, take on too many conflicting priorities, promise without delivering, try to do other line managers' jobs, do not respond adequately to higher concerns, represent selective interests, do not evaluate the anticipated impact of their actions on other people and projects, have poor timing, do not criticize themselves, do not market and merchandise their wares, are insensitive to internal client needs, and fail to understand the organization's culture.[50]

If nurse managers believe that trust is a key element of recognition and that recognition and trust are desirable elements of organizational climate, they will eliminate signs of distrust. Physical signs of distrust include time clocks and signs forbidding certain activities. The successful nurse manager hires practicing nurses who can be trusted and then trusts them. She or he supports subordinates without rescuing them or smothering them.

Nurse managers need management education and training. Such training should be given before nurses move into a management role and should continue to be provided by the organization and sought after by the individual. Management training is less expensive than turnover among practicing nurses. Educated nurse managers will evoke an organizational climate of serenity, camaraderie, solidarity, and identification with the organization—a climate of excellence. Such a climate will stir up and excite nurses' energies by providing opportunities. Nurse managers and practicing nurses can work together to manage the work and the work environment so that energy is channeled into accomplishing personal and organizational goals.[51]

The job environment has become a major builder or destroyer of self-esteem and self-actualization. There are many sources of knowledge available for improving organizational climate. It remains for nurse managers to selectively learn and use them.

Job satisfaction is not a right of employees but a joint employer–employee responsibility. There are mutual benefits. Values and expectations should be rational. The employee makes a careful career choice and works to satisfy it. The employer provides an enabling organizational climate. This will include matching employee and job through a realistic pre-employment interview, fostering job satisfaction, and being honest and truthful. There are no substitutes for either the nurse manager or the practicing nurse.

A study of organizational climate and its effect on scientists indicated that scientists perceived structure as related to organizational climate. The research did not support this relationship, as the structural data were poor. Flat organizations and large organizations tended to have scientists with more autonomy. Scientists perceived the climate as more competent, potent, responsible, practical, risk-oriented, and impulsive when performance reviews were tied to compensation programs. Scientists had greater autonomy over projects, assignments were general, and there were more informal research budgets. Risk-orientation decreased with increased performance reviews. These organizational climate factors improved performance and job satisfaction.[52]

Activities to Promote a Positive Organizational Climate

1. Developing the organization's mission, philosophy, vision, goals, and objectives statements with input

from practicing nurses, including their personal goals.

2. Establishing trust and openness through communication that includes prompt and frequent feedback and stimulates motivation.

3. Providing opportunities for growth and development, including career development and continuing education programs.

4. Promoting teamwork.

5. Asking practicing nurses to state their satisfactions and dissatisfactions during meetings and conferences and through surveys.

6. Marketing the nursing organization to the practicing nurses, other employees, and the public.

7. Following through on all activities involving practicing nurses.

8. Analyzing the compensation system for the entire nursing organization and structuring it to reward competence, productivity, and longevity.

9. Promoting self-esteem, autonomy, and self-fulfillment for practicing nurses, including feelings that their work experiences are of high quality.

10. Emphasizing programs to recognize practicing nurses' contributions to the organization.

11. Assessing needed threats and punishments and eliminating them.

12. Providing job security with an environment that enables free expression of ideas and exchange of opinions without threat of recrimination, which may manifest as downscaled performance reports, negative counseling, confrontation, conflict, or job loss.

13. Being inclusive in all relationships with practicing nurses.

14. Helping practicing nurses to overcome their shortcomings and to develop their strengths.

15. Encouraging and supporting loyalty, friendliness, and civic consciousness.

16. Developing strategic plans that include decentralization of decision-making and participation by practicing nurses.

17. Being a role model of performance desired of practicing nurses.

Team Building

The commonly used terms related to the state of "feelings" of an organizational climate are *high morale* or *low morale*. *Morale* is a state of mind that refers to the zeal or enthusiasm with which someone works. A person who works courageously and confidently, with discipline and willingness to endure hardship, would be manifesting high morale. Low morale is evident in the person who is timid, cowardly, devious, fearful, diffident, disorderly, unruly, rebellious, turbulent, or indifferent as a result of job dissatisfaction and organizational

milieu. Morale is a motivation factor related to productivity and product or service quality outcomes. Firms want high morale among employees and use activities to promote it.

A team is a group of two or more workers interdependently striving for a common purpose or mission. The team members depend on one another. The team leader will emerge (if not appointed) as the person sustaining the confidence of the group. The leader will sustain the team's confidence through his or her expertise in the team's purpose or mission and by the enthusiasm expressed by his or her verbal and nonverbal behavior. High enthusiasm by the leader will spark high enthusiasm within the group, thereby boosting group morale and stimulating the group's *esprit de corps*, a spirit and sense of pride and honor.

Among the leader roles are those of guide, marketer, teacher, visionary, team builder and player, intrapreneur, and idea broker.[53] The conditions for team building are collaboration, commitment, motivation, willingness, and timely feedback. Team building has as a goal the raising of performance by combining results. It permits risk taking, encourages trust, and builds confidence. A strong team will have knowledge, be receptive and flexible, and promote freedom and openness. Team building is not needed when communications are working well for group and organizational needs.[54]

One continually hears such remarks as "This organization does not care about the employees!" or "This organization really cares about its employees!" It goes without saying that nurse managers want to hear the positive statement. People who have low morale are not satisfied with their work. Dissatisfied workers will not contribute positively to *esprit de corps*.

Today's nurse managers will be effective if they are informed about nursing personnel's values. These include the following:

1. Work conflicts with family responsibilities and leisure activities, so some people want fewer hours or more flexible hours. The nurse manager determines how many hours each worker wants of work per day, per week, per month, and per year. The result is matched with the givens.

   a. What are the legal givens?

   b. What are the organizational givens? Are they flexible? Can a person contract to work shorter than 8-hour shifts? Shifts of 10 and 12 hours and even 16 hours are commonplace. Under what conditions can a person work 4-hour shifts, 6-hour shifts, or some variation such as three 10-hour shifts and two 5-hour shifts? Can the beginning and ending times of shifts be set at other than 7:00 A.M., 3:00 P.M., 7:00 P.M., and

11:00 P.M.? Why not 12:00 P.M. and 12:00 A.M. or other times?

c. When child care services are provided, are they available only during an employee's shift or can an employee use them when off duty? Can use fees be waived, reduced, or purchased with vouchers given as awards for service? Is sick child care available?

2. The fast pace of the information age creates impatience. Everyone wants the rewards of being at the top. They want to live the lifestyle of the rich and famous depicted in television soap operas. This drive overrides any sense of loyalty. People know they cannot all reach the top so they want to be involved in decisions about their work. What can be done to involve them at the unit level, department level, division level, and organization level?

3. People want inside knowledge about their organization. Some view this as a right. This desire can be accommodated by a solid communication plan that can be made to work by building quality assurance into the plan. This need should be addressed regularly, without fail, and actions under the plan should be made to meet their stated purpose of providing employees with information.

These values are consistent with those of people in other occupations in today's society.[55]

Nurse managers should create a humanistic environment for nursing employees, one that fosters trust and cooperation. Such an environment treats employees, rather than technology and buildings, as the most important asset. It is one in which minor rules are sometimes bent, complaints and ideas are heard, and self-worth and self-esteem are highlighted.

Nurses who have high self-esteem or self-worth are energetic and confident, take pride in their work, and have genuine respect and concern for patients, visitors, colleagues, and others. Their self-worth is evident in their behavior, including in their language. They are committed to excellence in patient care. These nurses have high morale. They work with *esprit de corps*.

The objective of team building is to establish an environment of cohesiveness among shift personnel and among different shifts of a unit. This is extended to other units, the department, and the division. The first step in team building is to find out why nursing employees are unhappy or dissatisfied. This can be accomplished through a questionnaire, although an open meeting is probably better. The meeting will be more productive if it is held away from the unit to eliminate interruptions and the shadow of the organization.

The head nurse or other manager can assume the leadership or allow the group to select a leader. In any event, the nurse manager will have to explain what the effort is all about and what the group is supposed to accomplish. To set a positive note, the nurse manager should, if possible, begin identifying group satisfactions.

Next, the leader focuses on identifying problems and setting their priorities for action. If the nurse manager can assume the role of facilitator rather than leader, the group will probably proceed at a faster pace. The meeting style is a participatory management one, with group ownership of activities and outcomes. The leader guides the members in defining each member's role on the team.

Problems or dissatisfactions are identified, and a calendar is established for addressing them. It is important to make a schedule of meetings and keep a list of attendees for all phases of team-building activities. Meetings should be held at times when most of the staff can be there. They should be short, focused on the problems, and followed in priority sequence. It is best for the team to make a brief management plan that includes the problem, objectives, actions the team can accomplish on its own authority, actions needing management support, persons assigned specific responsibilities, target dates, and a list of accomplishments.

As the plan is put into effect it should be communicated to the entire staff of the unit, department, or division. Evaluation should occur on a continuous basis to keep the momentum going. Each person can be encouraged to fulfill commitments, and everyone's accomplishments should be recognized. Although members of each shift can work on their own plans, an occasional open forum of personnel on all three shifts is essential for intershift problems.

Once the team is functioning, team building focuses on work production. Some meeting time should always be dedicated to morale, motivation, team skills, and discussion of team direction.[56]

Jacobsen-Webb reported the use of the SELF Profile (Personal Dynamics, Inc., Minneapolis, MN) in a team-building exercise. Team members were given the SELF Profile to diagnose their behavioral patterns as *self*-reliant, *e*nthusiastic, *l*oyal, or *f*actual. Teams were formed based on the four behavioral types. The leadership position changed with the problem-solving task and the type of expert needed. The team leader, who tapped skills of team members and built commitment through effective group process, maintained a democratic and participatory climate. Progress was tracked through use of Program Evaluation Review Technique (PERT) charts. When conflicts surfaced, they were discussed and resolved through the team with input from each behavior style. This process increased self-esteem and subsequent successful collaboration. It also increased skills of assertion, aggression, deference, interpersonal comfort, empathy, decision-making, and effective communication.[57]

Recognition of the individual worth of each nurse is an important morale builder. It gives the individual self-esteem. Managers can stimulate self-esteem with praise that promotes a sense of competence, success, and worth. Nurse managers have to feel worthy before they can nurture that feeling in subordinates. Each nurtures the other. Managers who have self-esteem are not afraid to explore their personal feelings with colleagues or subordinates.

Professional nurses can think very highly of themselves while believing that others do not think highly of them. This tends to cause them to dominate others and so to become feared and rejected. Ultimately these nurses band together and punish others as well as themselves.

Those professional nurses who think highly of themselves and believe that others do too, take risks in their personal relationships. They give and seek praise, love, support, and participation. All grow stronger and feel more worthy.

Many professionals depend on their jobs as a large source of self-esteem. For this reason, nurse managers should aspire to building a milieu that develops and enhances the self-esteem of all nurses. Such a milieu promotes outstanding performance.

Praise is even more important when the environment is beset with shortages and stresses. Managers gain self-esteem from the success of their employees. They must supplement it with outside activities such as sports, hobbies, recreation, volunteer work, and work in service and professional organizations.[58]

Recognition can be made with a special plaque, commendation in a local paper or other medium, group social activities, gifts, and group service activities. Consider the benefits of scheduled versus surprise recognition activities. Nave and Thomas suggest 50 specific techniques to boost employee morale.[59] (See Exhibit 14-11.)

Many simple things can be done to improve the working environment. Involving the best workers in the decision-making process rewards the best performers and alerts others. One group had a monthly "warm fluffy day" when they complimented each employee and gave them a cotton ball on a pin. It produced spirit![60]

Team building is a part of the self-directed work team organizational concept. Developing teams to their top potential is a tough job. The team leader identifies training needs of the team and of individual members. He or she also runs interference for the team, acts as liaison in negotiation for scarce resources, arranges publicity for accomplishments, and keeps abreast of information on outside events affecting the team. When conflicts arise from perceptions that some team members are doing more than their share of work or that the wrong members are getting promoted, the team leader manages them. The dream team collaborates with enthusiasm to get a job done well. Self-directed work teams and team building would continue to increase.[61]

Although people will participate in team building, they still want to retain their individuality. Nurse managers provide leadership that is flexible, fair, and mindful of tasks and people; that inspires; and that models the role of professional nurse.[62] Team building and self-managed work teams require continuous efforts by team leaders to maintain effective functioning.

Developing an Organizational Structure

An organizational structure for a division of nursing must meet the needs of that division as written in the statements of mission, philosophy, vision, values, and objectives. Most existing institutions already have an organizational structure. Before the structure is changed, the nurse managers should engage in a systematic analysis as well as do some sound thinking about altering the organization's design and structure, starting with objectives and strategy.

Objectives have already been discussed. Strategy covers the key activities of nursing that determine the purpose of the organizational structure. Nursing strategy will indicate the present business of nursing, its future business, and what its business should ideally be. The organizational structure allows, supports, and promotes nursing functions consistent with organizational mission, philosophy, vision, values, and objectives.

A newer concept in the theory of organizations is that the organizational structure affects the strategic decision-making process. Historically, changes in organizational structure have followed changes in strategy such as unit volume, geographic dispersion, and vertical and horizontal integration. The organizational form determines the decision-making environment: it delimits responsibilities and communication channels, controls the decision-making environment, and facilitates information processing.[63]

Strategic decision-making requires wide expertise from numerous levels. In nursing, managers should seek broad input from clinical nurses. This can be done through task forces, committees, project teams, or ad hoc groups. Nurse executives should make conscious decisions to delimit centralization, formalization, and complexity, particularly in large organizations. The object is conscious integration. Decentralization and participation are discussed in Chapter 16.

EXHIBIT 14-11

Fifty Specific Techniques to Boost Employee Morale

The following are 50 of the techniques identified to boost employee morale. In reviewing them, keep in mind that there is no best answer for anyone. The best techniques are those that best suit your organization.

1. Supervisors greet employees with a handshake as the employees begin their shifts.
2. Supervisors write personal notes such as Thank You or Happy Birthday on payroll checks.
3. Members of employee groups meet regularly with management representatives to promote understanding and carry out activities of mutual interest.
4. Employees and management work side by side once a year on a community help project.
5. Employers are personally congratulated by supervisors when they exceed their goals.
6. Supervisors personally introduce new hires to each employee.
7. An employee's years of service are noted each year on the anniversary date of employment on a plaque or poster in the lobby.
8. When department supervisors enter the employee lounge, they treat all employees who happen to be there to a cup of coffee.
9. Supervisors personally hand employees in their department a silver dollar at Christmas as a "little something extra."
10. Relations with retired employees are maintained by means of an annual breakfast and personal delivery by the supervisors of a box of Christmas candy each year.
11. A cash reward is given each month to the employee with the "best idea" for the firm.
12. Part-time employees are invited to all social events.
13. The chief executive officer periodically has "brown bag" luncheon discussions with employees at which their concerns are addressed.
14. Employees are allowed to accept telephone calls at any time.
15. Letters of commendation are sent to employees for performance above and beyond normal expectations. Copies of the letter are included in the employees' personnel files.
16. The plant manager cooks at the supervisors' picnic. At another firm, supervisors serve the food at a company picnic.
17. Birthday cards are signed by the president of the firm or immediate supervisor and are sent to the employees' homes.
18. Free popcorn is always available for employees and customers.
19. Employee birthdays are celebrated with cake and by singing "Happy Birthday."
20. The safety department issues a monthly "safety for the family" newsletter that is mailed directly to the employees' homes.
21. Free meals are provided in the company cafeteria for employees working on special days such as Christmas and Thanksgiving.
22. At irregular intervals managers provide food for employees to munch in the break area.
23. Soft drinks, coffee, and/or snacks are provided for staff at departmental meetings.
24. Flexible working hours are permitted during slow work times.
25. Morale-building meetings are held at which management informs employees of the firm's successes.
26. Brief meetings are scheduled for all new employees with staff from the business office, security, facilities management, and the like to familiarize new hires with policies and procedures.
27. A worker is recognized by being named Employee of the Week or Employee of the Month. The recognition takes many forms, including presentation of a plaque, lunch with the president or supervisor, gifts, and mention in the company newsletter.
28. An activities committee has been established to plan social events, and new employees are introduced to a member of this committee so they become aware of company activities.
29. Snacks are available during employees' first break each day.
30. Employees missing one day or less due to illness or injury during the year receive a gift.
31. Factory eating areas are decorated on special occasions.
32. Free coffee is provided on special days.
33. Once a quarter, 10 to 12 employees selected by random drawing are taken on a guided tour of all plant facilities and have lunch on the house in the plant cafeteria.
34. A Halloween costume contest is held each year, employees wear their costumes the work day, and the winner receives one day off with pay.
35. Receptions are given for every employee who retires.
36. In each month that new accounts exceed an established figure, all employees are taken out for dinner.
37. An annual awards banquet is held for employees on the last working day before a holiday.
38. Annual parties for occasions such as Christmas are given by the company.
39. An appropriate gift is distributed to all employees daily, weekly, or monthly, when a production record is established.
40. A cash drawing is held each month that there is no employee time lost due to accident. Variation: A drawing is held each month for employees who have not missed time due to injury or illness.
41. An annual employee appreciation dinner is given by the company.
42. Lunch and entertainment are provided "on the grounds" for all employees two or three times each year.

(continued)

EXHIBIT 14-11 (continued)

43. Some food for snacking is supplied by the company on a daily basis.
44. Positive comments on an employee by a customer result in the employee receiving a silver pin. Three such compliments during the year earn a gold pin.
45. Special food items are given to all employees on occasions such as Thanksgiving or Christmas.
46. Occasional boat rides on a cruiser are made available to all employees.
47. Company-wide potluck luncheons are held.

48. One firm sponsors a daily 15-minute radio program on which one of the employees is recognized/spotlighted.
49. When a new safety record is reached, employees receive a small memento and attend a cook-out hosted by management.
50. Lunch is provided for all employees on the last working day before a holiday.

Source: J. L. Nave and B. Thomas. "How Companies Boost Morale." *Supervisory Management*, October 1983, 29–33 © 1983, American Management Association, New York. Reprinted by permission. All rights reserved.

Work Activities and Functions

Work activities and functions to be analyzed and encompassed in identifying the building blocks of organization include the following:

1. The operating work at the unit level includes primary nursing care (the basic mission, not the method or modality of nursing); operational nursing management, commonly referred to as nurse manager activities; and support activities essential to the application of primary nursing care, such as training and clerical work. Management at the unit level includes management of the clinical component of direct nursing care and management of nonnursing or indirect activities.
2. In any health care institution, top management functions will need to be performed. In a small division, the nurse manager will be top manager of the department and a member of top management of the institution. Within a large division with multiple missions and objectives, there will likely be enough functions and activities for a top management team in the division of nursing. The chair will still be a member of top management of the institution, functioning at the strategic planning level in both instances.
3. A technostructure of staff of varying size, depending on the size of the institution, will support the management and clinical components of the nursing organization. These will include experts in such areas as infection control, staff development, oncology nursing, and quality improvement. In some organizations, they are labeled *consultants*.

Context

There are certain contextual variables that relate to an organization's structure, such as size, technology, organizational charter or social function, environment, interdependence with other organizations, structuring of activities, concentration of authority, and line of control of work flow.[64]

Organizational Charter or Social Function

Nursing organizations exist within institutions that are either government-owned, private not-for-profit, or private for-profit. Government-owned organizations are impersonally founded and highly centralized, with concentrated authority. Impersonality of origin increases the level of control of work flow. Since many health care organizations are impersonal in origin, they are highly centralized with increased line control of work flow of professional nurses.

A study of a random sample of 46 organizations stratified by size and product or purpose concluded that[65]:

1. Public accountability did not affect structuring of activities, including line of control of work flow.
2. Public accountability increased concentration of authority by standardization of personnel policies but relied on professional line subordinates for work flow control.
3. Increased accountability decreased or dispersed concentration of ownership with control.
4. Impersonally founded organizations are more dependent on the founding organization. Publicly accountable organizations are more dependent on external power.
5. High dependence is associated with impersonally founded, publicly accountable, or vertically integrated organizations; contracted specialties; smallness of units; low status; and little representation in policy-making.
6. Low dependence is associated with personal foundation, low public accountability, little vertical integration, few contract specialties, and the unit being the parent organization.

Since professional nurses want autonomy of decision-making in their clinical practice, these findings need to be substantiated by nursing research. There is empirical evidence to substantiate them in the initiation of nursing administration strategies. Nursing is an occupation with a history of public accountability, a desirable characteristic. Nurse managers, knowledgeable of the impersonality aspects of public accountability, will initiate strategies to increase and allow the desired autonomy and accountability of clinical nurses in order to increase their independence, their status, and their representation on policy-making entities. This is especially true in an environment in which health care organizations are pursuing vertical integration and mergers that decrease independence.

Size

Larger organizations tend to have more specialization and more formalization than small ones. The larger the size, the more decentralized the organization and the more standardized the procedures for selection and advancement of personnel. Bureaucracy increases with increased size and decreased personal integration.[66]

Increased size of an organization requires that managers differentiate employees into work groups, functions, departments, or work centers with described tasks. They are also differentiated into hierarchical levels. These differentiations are done to exercise management control, coordination, or integration. They are also done to buffer the core technology of an organization and to prepare it to respond to variety in the external environment.[67]

Contingency theory was used to study the technology, size, environment, and structure in 157 nursing subunits located in 24 hospitals in the Canadian province of Alberta. The theory postulated that the wide range of differences in organizational structure vary systematically with such factors as technology, size, and environment. It was found that increased subunit beds decreased the registered nurse (RN) ratio and increased the measure of bureaucratization of professionals. There was no relationship between decentralization of the subunit and size and little relationship between size and role specificity.[68] These findings would support those of Pugh and others who found no relationship between size and concentration of authority, between size and line control of work flow, or between size and autonomy.[69]

Technology

Technology is defined as "the sequence of physical techniques used on the work flow of the organization, even if the physical techniques involve only pen, ink, and paper." The more rigid and highly integrated the technology, the greater is the structuring of activities and procedures and the more impersonal the control. Complex technology emphasizes administration.[70]

Within nursing subunits, uncertainty in the technology *decreased* role specificity and decentralization and *increased* decentralization from the head nurse. A lack

of an adequate knowledge base by nurses was related to their perceptions of the uncertainty in the technology. This led to intuitive care for complex social–psychological problems. Increased instability and uncertainty of technology increased the RN ratio. Uncertainty in the technology decreased specificity and decentralization from physicians while increasing decentralization from the head nurse. Bureaucracy increased with a decreased ratio of RNs to other types of nursing personnel.[71]

Sophisticated technology increases perceptions of complexity and of increased use and development of skills, thereby creating higher job satisfaction. This finding can be generalized across services with similar technology levels and across organizations. Higher technology leads to higher job satisfaction, a possible reason for nurses aspiring to work in areas of critical care.[72]

Such findings give credibility to nursing management education. Nurse managers can use them to justify differentiated practice, since complex technology requires more advanced education and by inference staff development that sustains more advanced knowledge and skills. Education can thus be related to performance and pay.

Other Contextual Variables

Age did not relate to structuring of activities or line of control of work flow. Older organizations tended to be more decentralized and to have more autonomy.[73]

Product is related to control of work flow. If the product is nonstandard goods, there is impersonal control of work flow. If the product is a standard consumer service, there is decreased supervisor line control of work flow.[74] Health care organizations produce both standard and nonstandard consumer services.

Technology, size, and environment do not operate totally independently in their interaction with structure. More research is needed to discover the combination of contextual variables that interact with specific political processes to produce structure. Nurse managers need to be experienced and competent and to exert powerful leadership that will establish the context within which nurses' values can be implemented. Such a context will include more highly educated RNs, less bureaucratization, more clerks, increased documentation using information technology, and increased decentralization.

Forms of Organizational Structure

A mixture of two common forms of organizational structures—hierarchical and free-form—is needed in nursing.

Hierarchical Structure

A hierarchical structure is commonly called a *line structure* (see Exhibit 14-12). It is the oldest and simplest

EXHIBIT 14-12
A Hierarchical Organizational Structure

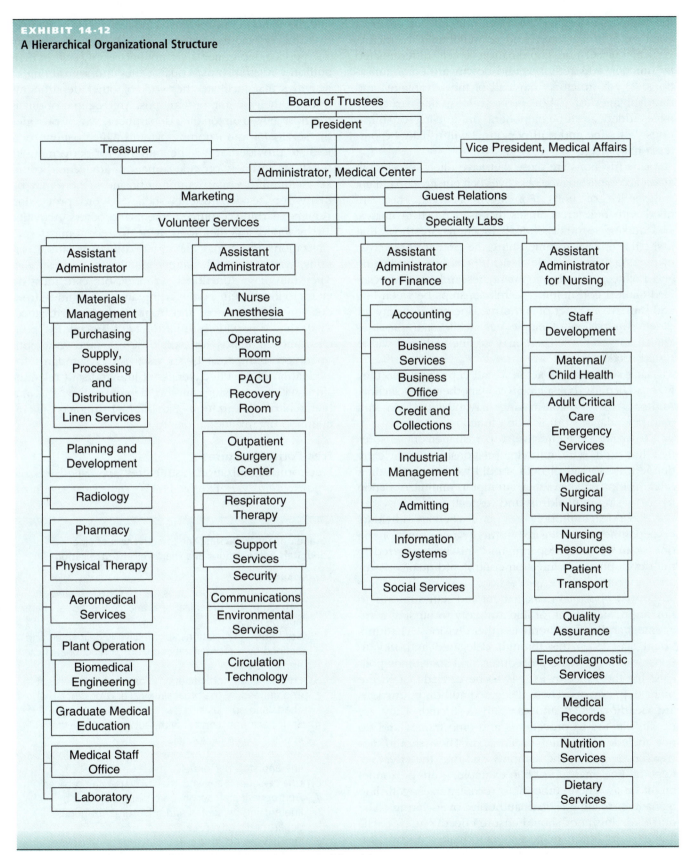

Source: Courtesy University of South Alabama Medical Center, Mobile, Alabama.

form and is associated with the principle of chain of command, bureaucracy and a multitiered hierarchy, vertical control and coordination, levels differentiated by function and authority, and downward communications. These structures have all of the advantages and disadvantages of a bureaucracy. Most line structures have added a staff component. In nursing organizations, both line and staff personnel will usually be professional nurses.

Line functions are those that have direct responsibility for accomplishing the objectives of a nursing department (or service or unit). For the most part, they are filled with registered nurses, licensed practical nurses, and nursing technicians. Staff functions are those that assist the line in accomplishing the primary objectives of nursing. They include clerical, personnel, budgeting and finance, staff development, research, and specialized clinical consulting. The relationships between line and staff are a matter of authority. Line has authority for direct supervision of employees, while staff provides advice and counsel. There may be line authority within a staff section.

Line sections may act in a staff capacity when they give advice or consultation to another line section. Authority for decision-making may be based on staff recommendations but is a line function.

To make staff effective, top management ensures that line and staff authority relationships are clearly defined. Personnel of both should work to make their relationships effective; they attempt to minimize friction by increasing mutual trust and respect.

Functional authority takes place when an individual or department is delegated authority over functions in one or more other departments. This has occurred in the development of infection control and quality-assurance systems where professional nurses have line authority to hospital management and staff authority to nursing management, or line authority to nursing management and staff authority to other divisions. The functional staff does this through delegated authority to consult and prescribe procedures, and sometimes policies, for the function as it is to be carried out in the other departments. These delegated authority functions are clearly defined and carefully restricted. They are usually limited to procedures and time frames and do not include personnel or context. They should not weaken or destroy the authority and thus the effectiveness of line managers. For example, staff personnel might be assigned authority to recruit nurses, with line managers retaining final authority over hiring. The nurse administrator should ensure effective use of staff functions by line managers so as to make effective use of the advice of experts and reduce duplication of effort of line managers. Staff gives information that will facili-

tate the solution of problems. Line managers in an effective and cooperative relationship seek such information.

Service departments are not necessarily staff in their authority relationships. Usually, they are a grouping of activities that facilitate the work of other departments through their operating functions. An example of this is the hospital's maintenance department, which provides the service of a functioning plant in which patient services are provided. It has the authority for performing its functions and may provide some staff advice and counsel. Within a hospital, as in any business, there may be many service departments such as word processing centers, learning resource centers, and others. Activities are grouped together to provide for economical specialization. There may be service units for labor relations, contracts, legal matters, purchasing, and others. They may have functional authority, but care must be taken to keep them from causing divided loyalties, from delaying performance, and from displaying arrogance. They should provide for uniformity of procedures, policies, and standards for skilled service and a smooth operation. Exhibit 14-13 shows a set of standards for evaluation of the effectiveness of line and staff relationships within a nursing division, department, or unit in a hierarchical organization. Exhibit 14-14 depicts several common organizational patterns.

Free-Form Structures

Free-form organizational structures are called *matrix organizations* (see Exhibit 14-15). The matrix organiza-

---

EXHIBIT 14-13

Standards for Evaluating the Effectiveness of Line and Staff Relationships in a Hierarchical Organization

STANDARDS

1. Line authority relationships are clearly delineated and defined by the organizational and/or functional charts and policies.
2. Staff authority relationships are clearly delineated and defined by the organizational and/or functional charts and policies.
3. Functional authority relationships are clearly delineated and defined by the organizational and/or functional charts and policies.
4. Staff personnel consult with, advise, and provide counsel to line personnel.
5. Service personnel functions are clearly understood by line and staff personnel.
6. Line personnel seek and effectively use staff services.
7. Appropriate staff services are being provided by line nursing personnel and other organizational departments or services.
8. Services are not being duplicated because of line and staff authority relationships.

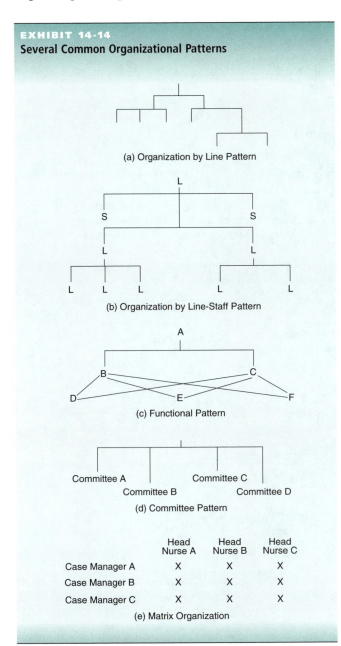

EXHIBIT 14-14
Several Common Organizational Patterns

(a) Organization by Line Pattern

(b) Organization by Line-Staff Pattern

(c) Functional Pattern

(d) Committee Pattern

	Head Nurse A	Head Nurse B	Head Nurse C
Case Manager A	X	X	X
Case Manager B	X	X	X
Case Manager C	X	X	X

(e) Matrix Organization

Source: B. S. Barnum and R. M. Kerfoot. *The Nurse As Executive*, 4th ed. (Gaithersburg, MD: Aspen, 1994), 66. Reprinted with permission. Copyright © Aspen Publishers.

tion design enables timely response to external competition and facilitates efficiency and effectiveness internally through cooperation among disciplines.

A matrix organization has the following characteristics[75]:

1. Maintenance of old-line authority structures.
2. Specialist resources obtained from functional areas.
3. Promotion of formation of new organizational units.
4. Decision-making done at the organizational level of group consensus, the first-line management level.
5. The exercising of authority by the matrix manager over the functional manager.

6. Cooperative planning program development and allocation of resources to accomplish program objectives.
7. Assignment of functional managers to teams that respond to the chief of the functional discipline and matrix manager.

Matrix nursing organizational structures have the following advantages[76]:

1. Improved communication through vertical and horizontal control and coordination of interdisciplinary patient care teams.
2. Increased organizational adaptability and fluidity to respond to environmental changes.
3. Increased efficiency of resource use with fewer organizational levels and decision-making closer to primary care operations.
4. Improved human resource management because of increased job satisfaction with achievement and fulfillment, improved communication, improved interpersonal skills, and improved collegial relationships.

Matrix nursing organizational structures have the following disadvantages[77]:

1. Potential conflict because of dual or multiple lines of authority, responsibility, and accountability relationships.
2. Role ambiguity.
3. Loss of control over functional discipline as a result of a multidisciplinary team approach.

A matrix management structure superimposes a horizontal program management over the traditional vertical hierarchy. Personnel from various functional departments are assigned to a specific program or project and become responsible to two bosses—a program manager and their functional department head. Thus, an interdisciplinary team is created with core and extended team members. A longitudinal study of a geriatrics matrix team program showed initial increased costs offset after a year by decreased acute care readmission rates, emergency room use, and nursing home placement. Mortality was significantly decreased and function ability of patients increased.[78]

Adhocracy

"Adhocracy" models of organization are like matrix models. There are simple teams or task forces that exist on an ad hoc basis. They are formed, complete their goals, and are disbanded; and new groups are then formed to meet changing and dynamic mission and objectives.[79]

Matrix and adhocracy models employ participatory management. Xerox is an example of a company that has successfully used self-managing work teams. They once exceeded cost-reduction targets of $3.7 million by $1 million.

EXHIBIT 14-15
Fully Evolved Matrix Organization

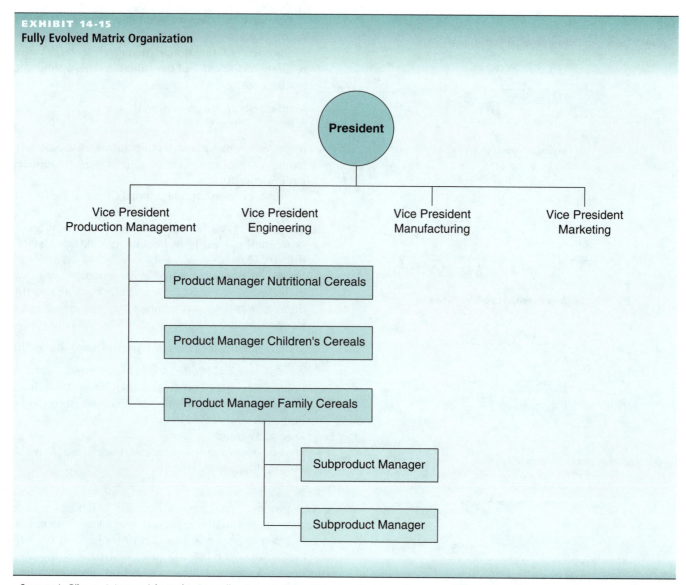

Source: J. Gibson, J. Ivancevich, and J. Donnelly. *Organizations: Behavior, Structure, Processes*, 9th ed. (Burr Ridge, IL: Irwin, 1997), 340.

The expert is the authority who leads the team. Companies that use work teams are consultative organizations that delegate rather than tell. They encourage maverick behavior and reward results. Of 360 manufacturing companies studied, the 41 that were most successful had fewer employees per sales dollar; encouraged risk taking; had fewer headquarters staff; had decentralized decision-making; and had self-contained units or cost centers.[80]

Restructuring Nursing Organizations

The survival of many hospitals is threatened as they compete for growth and a competitive edge in the marketplace. For this reason, Flarey indicates that the gov-erning boards may need to be reconstituted. Members of governing bodies should focus on patient care. Many hospitals include the chief nurse executives in governing board meetings as active participants.[81]

Kanter defines synergies as "interactions of businesses that would provide benefits above and beyond what the units could do separately."[82] Synergies are both a good and a consequence of restructuring in which organizations are downsized (employees cut), demassed (middle management cut), and decentralized. The aim of restructuring is to achieve synergies from the value of adding up the parts to create a whole.[83] One of the elements of restructuring would be to build a synergistic model of a governing body. A synergistic model for the governing body as suggested by Flarey is depicted in Exhibit 14-16.

EXHIBIT 14-16
A Synergistic Model for a Governing Body

GOVERNING BODY FUNCTION	CONTRIBUTION OF NURSE EXECUTIVE
1. Defining mission	• Patient and community advocate: provides focus of consumer needs and views. • Incorporates nursing philosophy and mission. • Educates nursing staff on agency's mission.
2. Quality of care	• Quality-of-care expert. • Presents evaluations and quality issues to the board. • Influences hospital-wide decision making regarding quality and health services.
3. Strategic planning	• Shares in responsibility of executive management in developing and implementing the strategic plan. • Meshes goals of the nursing department with organization's plan. • Presents nursing strategic plan.
4. Financial viability	• Participates on finance committee. • Oversees largest department operating budget. • Obtains resources for patient care. • Introduces productivity measures to create synergies.
5. Reduce risk and liability	• Acts as a guardian of the institution's welfare. • Presents policy and procedures focusing on potential liability. • Presents nursing risk-management plan and program. • Interprets standards and legislation affecting nursing service delivery.
6. Community relations	• Represents the agency in community-service programs and relations. • Presents community perspectives and needs regarding the agency's role in health-services delivery.
7. Organizational growth	• Interprets and communicates needs and visions of the nursing department and community in planning for growth. • Supports and assists the chief executive officer in implementing strategic vision and plan.
8. Policy development	• Educates trustees in issues regarding the delivery of care. • Represents nursing in overall policy development.
9. Service development	• Presents proposals for the enhancement of care services. • Provides a clinical focus to planning. • Acts as consultant to planning needs and operational needs.
10. Decision-making	• Represents the voice of nursing in overall governance and decision making. • Provides insights from a nurse- and client-centered focus.

Source: D. L. Flarey. "The Nurse Executive and the Governing Body: Synergy for a New Era." *Journal of Nursing Administration* 21, no. 12 (December 1991): 13. Reprinted with permission of J. B. Lippincott.

Old organizational forms do not work in today's health care environment. Sovie recommends development of special project teams to design the required structure and system change. She gives the following as the first five steps of restructuring:

1. Create an organizational culture marked by commitment to high-quality care and superior, responsive service to all users including patients, families, physicians, nurses, and other staff.

2. Redesign the organizational structure to flatten it and eliminate or reduce barriers among departments, disciplines, and services.

3. Empower the staff; invest in employee education and training; and create mechanisms to ensure information flow.

4. Develop special project teams to design the required system changes; nurture and promote innovation and pilots of new approaches.
5. Celebrate accomplishments, innovators, and champion care for the caregivers; support, recognize, and reward.

The goals are improvement of patient care, organizational success, and staff satisfaction.[84]

Restructuring of organizations includes downsizing and elimination of middle managers (see Exhibit 14-17). As a consequence of this, the hands-on workers are empowered to provide clients (customers, patients) what they need and want. Before they can be empowered, hands-on nursing workers need to have management training for their new roles. The span of control is greater when hands-on workers are educated, trained, motivated, stable, and empowered. Such workers neither want nor need micromanagement. The manager with a widened or expanded span of control now becomes mentor, guide, facilitator, and coach.

Small departments can be consolidated under one department head through empowerment. One example would be physical therapy, occupational therapy, endoscopy, neurodiagnostics, sleep disorders, social services, and respiratory therapy. Issues of loss of power and authority arise and must be resolved so that job shrinking and empowerment can occur. Managers who spend time protecting their turf decrease productivity of their workers.

Nurse managers of their units can do all hiring; resolve patient complaints; budget authority associated with staffing and patient losses; and provide orientation to new managers. Middle managers can be incorporated into the structure as nurse managers of units or in staff functions, such as case managers. Clearly, the span of control for top managers can increase as first-line managers are empowered.

Empowerment increases responsiveness. It is better to eliminate jobs through attrition than to fire personnel. Excess managers should be turned back into service performers.[85]

Downsizing is a common organizing activity in today's corporate world, including in health care organizations and institutions. The goals of downsizing are to decrease costs and increase profits. While decentralization and participatory management are identified with downsizing, the goals are not always the same. The latter have increasing job satisfaction and increased productivity as primary goals.

Companies are now reporting that the hoped-for results of downsizing have not occurred. There have been huge emotional and financial costs to employees and significant costs to American corporations. Between 1983 and 1993, Fortune 500 companies eliminated 4.7 million people from their payrolls. Job cuts do not necessarily lead to improved productivity. Gains in production are frequently traced to firms with growing employment. Mass layoffs do not inspire worker loyalty. Workers should be well prepared for restructuring.[86]

Business is adapting organizational structures because of marketplace demands related to greater rates of change and a higher competitive intensity and because of information technology. Health care organizations should do the same. What services should a business offer and what should it divest? Hospitals are high cost producers. The excessive vertical integration since diagnosis-related groups (DRGs) may be to blame. The emerging organizational structure is messy: some resources need to be centralized to improve productivity by responding to customers' needs. A good organization will have key aspects of both consistency and inconsistency.[87]

When reengineering organizations, leaders should use key strategies such as emotional management, professional empowerment, and empowerment by values. Staff members are given room to grow and to learn from their mistakes.[88]

Excessive organizational structures are inhibitors to quick responses to change. Get staff out into the field. This includes accounting, purchasing, personnel, and others. There should be only three to five layers of management in the total organization. Every CEO should look at the corporate structure from the perspective of increasing the span of control through reduction of layers of management. Matrix organization brought about de facto centralization as groups were wired to groups by dotted lines on organization charts. The most effective present-day management structure is supervisor, department head, and boss. In health care organizations, this would be nurse manager, nurse executive, and hospital administrator.

Winning companies have three to nine fewer levels of management. Winning companies have workers doing their own maintenance, self-inspection, direct costing, and just-in-time inventory management. Winning companies have few people at headquarters level. They decentralize database management, eliminate approval signatures, retrain middle managers, and increase spending authority at unit level.[89]

Mergers and acquisitions result in unified management teams with single executive managers. As examples, one CEO replaces two to several, one assistant administrator for nursing replaces two to several, and one department head replaces two to several. Desirable characteristics include a highly visible chief nurse executive, a professional practice model of patient care, nursing diagnosis as the basis for nursing care delivery, and collaborative practice among professions.

EXHIBIT 14-17
Restructured Nursing Department

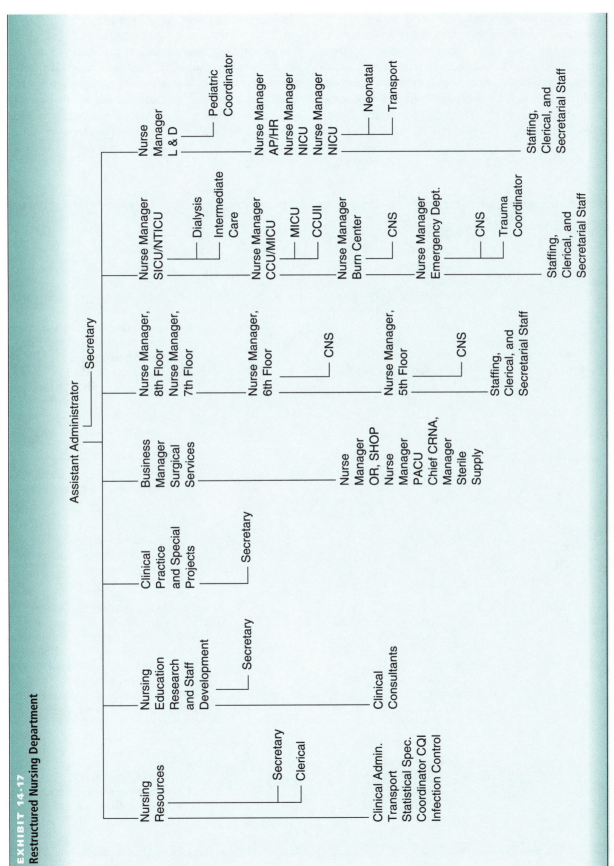

Source: Courtesy University of South Alabama Medical Center, Mobile, Alabama.

An organizational analysis should be done to gain the theory and skills needed to intervene in complex organizational systems. Areas analyzed include formal organizational structure, power bases, leadership, communication system, and organizational climate (see Exhibit 14-18). Used to prepare clinical nurse specialists, it could be used by nurse managers and practicing CNSs.[90]

The Organization of Work

Work is organized according to the stages in the process. In some areas, the work moves to the skills and tools, good examples being coronary care nursing and operating room nursing. Sometimes a team moves different skills and different tools to the work, for example, when an operating room team moves to a delivery

---

EXHIBIT 14-18
Organizational Analysis

AREAS TO BE ASSESSED	DATA COLLECTION STRATEGIES		ANALYSIS CRITERIA

A. Formal organizational structure	A. Obtain a copy of the following:
	Philosophy and objectives—hospital and nursing
	Organization charts (table of organization (TO))
	Hospital, nursing, job descriptions—nursing
		(5%)	A. 1. Provides philosophies and objectives of hospital and nursing
			  a. Discusses compatibility of the two re formal mission
			  b. Discusses congruence between own philosophy of nursing and nursing department's philosophy
			2. Includes nursing job descriptions
			  a. Relates how CNS job description compares to New York State Nurses Association's position statement
			  b. Comments on appropriateness of other relevant nursing job descriptions
			3. Provides organizational charts

B. Power bases	B. Refer to TO Documents Observations Interviews	(2%)	B. 1. States where power bases lie—formal and informal 2. Names and describes sources of power identified
C. Decision-making and policy-making bases	C. Refer to TO—Superimpose informal decision-making network on TO Documents Observations Interviews	(5%)	C. 1. States where formal bases lie 2. Identifies informal networks 3. Describes extent to which nursing is represented on major decision-making bodies in hospital and influences major decisions 4. Discusses extent of nursing staff's participation at unit level; in what issues? 5. Describes methods used in decision and policy making
D. Leadership	D. Documents Observations Interviews	(2%)	D. 1. Relates predominant leadership styles of unit head nurse and CNS 2. Describes nursing staff's response to styles used

(continued)

EXHIBIT 14-18 *(continued)*

AREAS TO BE ASSESSED	DATA COLLECTION STRATEGIES		ANALYSIS CRITERIA
E. Communication system	E. Refer to TO Staff communication books and all other communication methods Documents Observations Interviews	(4%)	E. 1. Discusses a. Direction of flow b. Openness of communication; clarity; distortions; omissions; overload c. Primary sources of and participants in communication re task accomplishment (sociogram may be used) 2. Identifies formal and informal methods of communication
F. Organizational climate	F. Refer to Clark and Shea, pp. 29–30, for Walton's guidelines for analyzing the organizational climate Census and patient reports Analysis of staffing and assignments Professional development Activities Interviews Documents Observations	(3%)	F. 1. Discusses degree of individual autonomy 2. Describes compensation, working conditions, assignments 3. Relates opportunities for continued professional and personal growth
G. See criteria		(8%)	G. For each area A–E, based upon your clinical work as a CNS and the analysis, identifies and discusses the organizational-environmental factors that facilitate and inhibit nursing management and the functioning of the CNS
H. See criteria		(3%)	H. Based on G, identifies at least one potential, realistic project for planned change to be implemented in the spring semester

Source: M. Reddecliff, E. C. Smith, and M. Ryan-Merritt. "Organizational Analysis: Tool for the Clinical Nurse Specialist." *Clinical Nurse Specialist*, fall 1989, 135. With permission of Williams & Wilkins.

room to perform a cesarean section. We certainly find combinations in nursing.

Much of the work in nursing is accomplished by a functionally structured organization. Clarity is an advantage of the functional structure, since the individuals know where they stand and they understand their tasks. Functional structures are usually stable. A disadvantage is that sometimes the task neither relates to the whole structure nor contributes to the common purpose. Functional structures are rigid, and frequently they neither prepare nurses for the future nor train nor test them.

Functional organizations become costly when friction builds up and requires coordinators, committees,

meetings, troubleshooters, and special dispatchers. Functional organizations make low psychological demands on people; people in such organizations tend to focus on their efforts only. Small functional organizations are economical and foster good communications. These organizations are good when one kind of work is done. Usually they require that decisions be made at the top. Nurses within them have narrow visions, skills, and loyalties. Employees of such organizations focus on function rather than on results and performance. The functional process does not usually apply to top management positions or to performance of innovative work by employees.

The team organization has been tried in nursing for the past half century. It has been used mainly at the operating or primary-care level rather than at top or middle management levels. "A team is a number of people—usually fairly small—with different backgrounds, skills, and knowledge, and drawn from various areas of the organization (their home) who work together on a specific and defined task. There is usually a team leader or team captain."[91]

In health care institutions, patients see the physician as team leader. However, the team leader uses the resources of the entire organization; in many cases it is the nurse who identifies, recommends, and coordinates these resources.

A team must have a continuing mission, which nursing has. The team should be highly flexible without a rigid chain of command. Like all organizational structures, in business, industry, or health care institution, the team organization needs clear and sharply defined objectives. Leadership decides on decision and command authority, and the team is responsible for accomplishing the tasks or mission. Team members know each other's function, but leadership must first establish clarity of objectives and in everybody's role. Everyone on the team should know the whole work and be adaptable and receptive to innovation. The team leader gives continuing attention to clear communications and clear decision-making. A team should be kept small for top management work and for innovative work. Otherwise, the team design complements the functional design. A combination may consist of employees who work in teams but produce work organized on the functional principle. This approach seems to work best in nursing and is probably better than either organizational structure in its pure form.

Knowledge work is best for team design. Use of a functional axis manages people and their knowledge, whereas use of a team axis manages work and task. The team may be the key to making functional design effective. Team organization is a difficult structure requiring great self-discipline.

Nursing Care Delivery Systems

Managed care and case management appear to be leading innovations in health care delivery. Benefits are controlled costs, improved outcome monitoring, reduced bureaucracy, less travel time for patients, and fewer people to sort out or confront. Patient care needs and outcomes should be assessed and evaluated by nurses. Priority of patient care tasks should be determined by nurses who refer needs to others. This is the essence of work redesign that will retain nursing autonomy and influence.[92]

Some health care institutions integrate standards of practice into their nursing care delivery systems. Structure and process standards are stated as outcome standards and are used to measure the overall effectiveness of the nursing division. The integration is accomplished throughout the core committees of the nursing division, including quality assessment, policy and procedure, job description, and other committees. This is done through nursing care plans and the computer system. The nursing care plans may be generic or individual and include nursing diagnosis/problems, intervention/discharge plans, and goals. [93]

Example # 1—Nursing Practice Model
Valley Baptist Medical Center (VBMC) in Harlingen, Texas, built a nursing practice model that included unit action committees on each nursing unit, a comprehensive integrated tool called the restorative care path, variance analysis, permanent care teams with clinical managers, assistant clinical managers, licensed vocational nurses, nursing assistants, and collaborative nurse physician practice with a physician–nurse liaison committee. Since credentialing and recredentialing of physicians is considered the ultimate form of peer review, it should be considered for peer review of nurses.[94]

Example # 2—Group Practice
Nursing group practice at Catherine McAuley Health System "is a formal membership of professional nurses who contract to provide nursing care for a specific patient population." Nurses may contract privately or as employees of an organization. They provide 24-hour coverage 365 days a year. The group's staffing for cardiothoracic surgery includes 16 nurses, two certified surgical technologists, and one clinical nurse manager who reports to the clinical director of operating room services. The group eliminated the first-line manager, making the clinical nurse manager a resource facilitator, liaison, and mentor. A supportive climate emphasizes trust, accountability, and responsibility. The criteria for group practice membership include clinical competence and leadership ability. Evaluating peers use a clinical ladder with described behaviors. The practice model is shared governance: practice, education, and quality assurance councils.

The following are suggested activities to implement a group practice:

- Define roles and organization structure.
- Determine program costs.
- Decide on membership criteria and staffing mix.
- Set salary guidelines (e.g., hourly or salaried status).
- Work with the hospital administration in writing policies and planning for implementation.

- Plan to evaluate the success of the program using specific, predetermined instruments.

Staff satisfaction, cost, and quality assurance all improved. Turnover rate decreased. Problems such as surgical complications and poor communications were prevented. Products and techniques were changed to reduce costs. Turnaround times were faster. Financial recognition was made quarterly. Incorrect sponge and instrument counts were reduced 25%.[95]

Example # 3—Helper Model

The helper model of health care delivery is widespread. It matches RNs with nurse aides. To work efficiently, the helper model requires the following[96]:

1. Experienced RNs at the competent or proficient levels of practice.
2. Permanent RN/nurse aide pairs.
3. Enhanced primary nursing.
4. Support for agency and float nurses.
5. Policy for attendance that targets incentive and reward programs.
6. Thoroughly prepared RNs/nurse aides.
7. Support systems.
8. Follow-up inservices.

Example # 4—Differentiated Practice

Role theory underlies the concept of differentiated practice, which defines the levels of competence within which two categories of RNs will practice: nurses with bachelor's degrees and those with associate degrees.

The BSN (bachelor of science in nursing) level is the professional practice level; the ADN (associate degree in nursing) is the associate or technical practice level. These practice levels can function within a variety of different delivery systems, including team and primary systems. The premise for differentiated practice is that professional practice exercises the nurse's autonomous decisions, including personal acceptance of risks and responsibilities in making professional judgments. Extended education at a BSN level or higher is required preparation for this role at the professional practice level.[97]

The differentiated group professional practice (DGPP) model has three major components of which differentiated care delivery is one[98]:

1. Group governance.
2. Differentiated care delivery.
3. Shared values.

A differentiated practice system or delivery model has the following components:

1. Differentiated registered nurse (RN) practice.
2. Use of nurse extenders.
3. Primary case management.

Differentiated care delivery is designed so that nurses with varying educational preparation and work experience can most efficiently use their knowledge and skills, while delegating nonnursing tasks to assistive personnel. Nurse extenders are delegated tasks rather than patient assignments.[99]

The differentiated practice role has three basic components:

1. Provision of direct care.
2. Communication with and on behalf of patients.
3. Management of patient care.

A differentiated practice maximizes available registered nurse resources for efficiency and effectiveness. "Differentiated practice is a strategy that calls for licensed and practicing nurses to be used in accord with their respective experience, ability, and formal and continuing education. Further, differentiated practice is defined as both a human resource deployment model and an alternative to primary nursing and case management." It is role differentiation. More education and experience are needed for cognitive skills.[100]

In an ethnographic study of differentiated practice in an operating room it was found that introduction of a new role requires insight into setting and an emphasis on staging and orientation of employees to the new role.[101] Otherwise, introduction of a new role can create turmoil and job insecurity.

To use the differentiated practice mode, the nurse's knowledge and skills are assessed (see Exhibit 14-19).

EXHIBIT 14-19
Differentiated Practice Assessment

RN PROFESSIONAL
BSN prepared
Makes complex decisions and interactions
Cost management of supplies, clinical alternatives, flexible scheduling of personnel, and case loads
Structures the unstructured
Cognitive role and highly skilled tasks
Care manager
Independent judgments, initiative, problem solving
Coaches self-managed work team
Manages all resources, fiscal and material
Consults with other disciplines
Discharges patients

RN ASSOCIATE OR TECHNICIAN
Non-BSN RN
Assists the professional nurse
Performs high-skill tasks such as chemotherapy
Special tests and procedures
May lead self-managed work team coached by professional nurse
Direct care provider
Uses common, well-defined diagnoses
Works in structured settings and situations

Styles and others advocate differentiated credentialing. What are the goals and what would differentiated credentialing accomplish? In the practice environment, cost effectiveness often calls for varied nursing personnel. It is essential that the professional level be designated. To gain public respect and rights of self-determination, nursing must adhere to the professional norm. Role-delineated relationships with other health professionals and incentives for improvement are dependent on identification of professional status. In brief, higher standards of care, clear public recognition and specificity in authority, accountability, roles and responsibilities, and rewards for the professional nurse are the goals of the entry effort.

The proposed solution might work like this: BSN education, RN licensure, followed with national generalist certification with the title CPN (certified professional nurse), and then a differentiated practice with recognition/reimbursement.[102]

Tall (Vertical) Versus Flat (Horizontal) Organizations

Line organizations are considered to be tall or vertical organizations, whereas matrix and adhocracy models are considered to be flat or horizontal organizations. In a study of the effects of tall versus flat organizational structures on job satisfaction of managers, flat organizations were found to decrease need deficiencies in selected indicators of self-esteem and self-actualization. Tall organizations decrease need deficiencies for selected indicators of security, social needs, and self-esteem. Overall, there was "no difference between tall and flat organizations in terms of perceived need deficiencies." Flat organizations are not superior to tall organizations for managers.[103] Research is needed along these lines for practicing nurses.

Future organizations will be unstructured, flat, flexible, and decentralized; that authority will come from competence; leaders will change with goals. There will be no formal job descriptions. Employees will be salaried collegial groups of equals who will respond quickly to change. Vertical integration will diminish with microprocessor technology in communication through artificial intelligence and robotization. People will go from manufacturing to service, transportation, communication, and recreation industries. Employees will telecommute from home. Telecommuting programs already exist in over 450 companies. The mother and/or father will be able to stay at home and have an improved quality of work life.[104]

Vertical integration "offers, either directly or through others, a broad range of patient care and support services operated in a functionally unified manner."[105] Vertical integration allows control and coordination of ambulatory care, long-term care, home care, medical products supply, and even wellness and health-promotion activities to pro-

mote referral to the core business of inpatient acute care. This vertical integration helps a hospital gain market share.

Product or service lines are gained or integrated through such means as:

- Internal development of new services.
- Acquisition of another service or organization.
- Formal merger.
- Lease or sale/lease back arrangement.
- Franchise.
- Joint venture.
- Contractual agreement.
- Loan guarantee.
- Informal agreement or affiliation.

Vertical (pyramid) structures frighten employees and threaten their security. Employees are deprived of association and ability for commitment. Vertical structures do not work because of more hierarchy, more supervision, more manuals, executive suites, privileged policy, special titles, more divisions, departments, sections or groups, and executive trimmings.

The following do work: horizontal structures; temperance; leaders who treat key managers and employees alike; elevating human resources; clear tasks and goals, and agreed-on tasks, goals, and objectives; few reports; and no rank, no boss, no seniority. The result is committed employees participating in decisions and accepting responsibility.[106]

Mechanistic Versus Organic Structures

Organic structures maximize satisfaction, flexibility, and development. They emphasize greater use of human potential and greater human worth and importance. Within organic structures, job design stresses personal growth and responsibility. There is decentralization of decision-making, control, and goal-setting processes. Communication flows in all directions. Generalization is emphasized in a climate that is informal.[107]

Mechanistic (bureaucratic) organizations support many of the opposite characteristics: group formality, external pressures, structuring of activities, and centralization of authority with high control. Structural variables do not necessarily relate to work satisfaction. Mechanistic organizations can produce high satisfaction among co-workers in formal groups. The classic dysfunctions of bureaucracy do not necessarily exist at lower levels of organizational structure. Organic structures probably lead to more flexible and innovative managerial behavior.[108]

Analyzing Organizational Structures in a Division of Nursing

Analyzing the organizational structure of a division of nursing entails six main steps, which should be used when major organizational problems occur, such as friction among department heads over authority, staffing problems, and the like. These steps also apply to organizing a new corporation, division, or unit and to reorganizing. They are as follows:

Step 1.

Compile a list of the key activities determined by the mission and objectives of patient care. The written philosophy and vision statements will help by indicating important values to be considered. Once this list is completed, it must be analyzed. Group similar activities together. What are the central load-carrying elements? Most will be related to primary care, and philosophy will usually dictate that excellence of patient care is a requirement for the accomplishment of objectives.

Whenever the strategy changes, the organizational structure should be reviewed and analyzed. This includes changes in mission, philosophy, vision, objectives, and the operational plan for accomplishing the objectives. The analysis of key activities can be done according to the kinds of contributions made. These will include the following:

1. Results-producing activities related to direct patient care, such as training, recruiting, and employment.
2. Support activities, which may include those related to vision or future, values and standards, audit, advice, and teaching.
3. Hygiene and housekeeping activities.
4. Top management activities to include "conscience" activities such as vision, values, standards, and audit as well as managing people, marketing, and innovation.

Service staffs such as those performing advisory and training support should be limited. They should be required to abandon an old activity before starting a new one. Prevent them from building empires as a career. Informational activities are the responsibility of top management though they stem from support activities such as controller and treasurer. There must be a system for disseminating information. Hygiene and housekeeping need the attention of nurses if they are to be done well and cheaply. This does not mean that nurses will do these tasks, but that nurses will recognize their importance and support and facilitate their being done by the appropriate departments. Contract services are the answer in some instances.

Consider whether the groups of key activities should be rank-ordered in the sequence in which they will occur.

Step 2.

Based on the work functions to be performed, decide on the units of the organization. Decision analysis will be important here, since it must be decided which kinds of decisions will be required and who will make them.

Decisions involving functions of future commitments may have to be a top management function, depending on the degree of futurity of a decision and the speed with which it can be reversed. It will be necessary to analyze the impact of decisions on other functions, the number of functions involved being an important factor. Qualitative factors such as decisions involving ethical values, principles of conduct, and social and political beliefs will have to be analyzed. The frequency of the decision will influence its placement: Is it recurrent or is it rare? In principle, all decisions should be placed at the lowest level and as close to the operational scene as possible.

Step 3.

Decide which units or components will be joined and which separated. Join activities that make the same kind of contribution. This will require relations analysis and will be related to the sequence of key activities or functions.

Step 4.

Decide on the size and shape of the units or components.

Step 5.

Decide on appropriate placement and relationships of different units or components. This will result from the relations analysis (Step 3). There should be the smallest possible number of relationships, with each being made to count.

Step 6.

Draw or diagram the design and put it into operation. This will result in an organizational chart or schema.

Departmentation

These steps should be used when major organizational problems occur, such as friction among department heads over authority and staffing problems. They also apply to organizing a new corporation, division, or unit and to reorganizing an established entity.

Steps 3, 4, and 5 involve *departmentation*, the grouping of personnel according to some characteristic. Departmentation is an organizing process.

For departmentation purposes, functional specialties are formed from clusters of units with similar goals. In most of our health care institutions, the functions of nursing are grouped into a division or department. Within that division or department are further groupings of nursing personnel by specialization, such as medical, surgical, pediatric, and obstetric. Sometimes the grouping is further broken down into areas of subspecialization. This process is termed *functional departmentation*. Clients may also be grouped according to degree of illness, such as minimal, intermediate, or intensive care.

There are advantages and disadvantages of functional departmentation. Among the advantages are focus on the basic activities of the enterprise through a logical and time-proven method of organizing, efficient use of specialized personnel, simplified training, and tight control by top administration. A big disadvantage for nursing is that people tend to develop tunnel vision about their specialty and the service or unit within which they work.

Time departmentation is common within health care organizations. Personnel are grouped by shift. This has important implications for administration as the activities of shifts have to be grouped according to qualifications and numbers of personnel on any shift.

Territorial departmentation involves grouping of activities according to geography or physical plant. This is more common in merged organizations with geographically separated units. Some activities, such as staff development, may be assigned by territory and specialization as well as being grouped by function.

Territorial departmentation should encourage participation in decision-making in provision of health services to a wider population base and be of a nature that will prevent illnesses and injuries. There may be justification for the exploration and formation of consortiums using the principle of territorial departmentation. For example, several small hospitals in an area could contract for consultant services in research, clinical nurse specialist services, or nursing education services.

In addition to functional, time, and territorial departmentation, there is the fourth option, product departmentation. This approach has implications for health care, although its ultimate achievement may not always be immediately practical. Increasingly, the products of nursing care are focused on the health needs of populations—those who need not only the illness care but also the care that keeps aging populations healthy; that maintains health and prevents injury and disease in the large group who take voluntary risks such as smoking, reckless driving, poor eating, poor exercising, or using artificial mood changers; that provide health care by promoting a clean environment; that modify the health risks associated with human reproduction; and that decrease the need for illness care. In the vertically integrated organization, product line departmentation is common in today's health care institutions.

Departmentation could be done on the basis of consumer needs or demands. There is a distinct possibility that health care institutions will offer people a choice of services in the future, thereby giving them the opportunity to select those services that will be covered by third-party payers and those that will be paid for out-of-pocket. Also, the times the services will be given and who will be giving them may well be part of the choice.

There may be no pure form of departmentation that will work in the health care institution. It may be more important to look at all the variables in order to group

people to facilitate successful production of health care services. In the matrix organization, product and functional forms of departmentation are combined. Projects have managers who move products through production stages in coordination with managers of each production stage. We will see more use of matrix organizations in nursing as health care takes on new dimensions.

At the present, nursing services are usually organized using a mix of departmentations. So long as the system is based on logic, it will provide a viable and efficient organization. Use Exhibit 14-20 to evaluate departmentation of nursing service activities and personnel.

EXHIBIT 14-20
Standards for Evaluation of Departmentation

1. Nursing activities have been grouped to attain goals and sustain the enterprise.
2. Nursing activities have been grouped for intradepartmental and interdepartmental coordination.
3. Personnel roles have been designed to fit the capabilities and motivation of persons available to fill them.
4. Personnel roles have been designed to help employees contribute to departmental or unit objectives.
5. Personnel roles provide optimum and economic job enlargement.
6. Nursing activities have been grouped for full use of resources, people, and material.
7. Nursing activities have been grouped for optimum cost benefits.
8. Nursing activities have been grouped to match special skills to special needs.
9. Nursing activities have been grouped to achieve an optimum management span.
10. Nursing activities and personnel have been grouped for optimum correlation for decision making and problem solving.
11. Nursing activities have been grouped to achieve minimal levels of management by providing for delegation of responsibility and authority to the lowest competent operational level.
12. Nursing activities and personnel have been grouped to eliminate duplication of staff services and centralized services of specialists.
13. Nursing activities and personnel have been grouped to facilitate production of products and services that will promote health of individuals and groups.
14. Nursing activities and personnel have been grouped to promote soundness of industrial relations programs and fiscal policies and procedures.
15. Nursing activities have been grouped to fulfill time demands of shifts.
16. Nursing activities have been grouped to achieve priorities and allow for change and flexibility in achievement of objectives.
17. Nursing activities have been grouped to facilitate training of employees.
18. Nursing activities have been grouped to facilitate communication.

Organization Charts

Most nursing organizations have made graphic representations of the organizing process in the form of organization charts. These charts usually show reporting relationships and communication channels. Line charts show supervisor and supervisee relationships from top to bottom of the nursing organization. Hierarchical relationships exist on which communication channels follow the line of authority to and through the chief nurse executive. (Refer to Exhibits 14-12, 14-14, 14-15, and 14-17.)

Staff charts show the advisory relationship of specialists or experts who are extensions of the nurse administrators. These types of charts usually depict the title or rank of each line and staff officer position in the authority relationship structure. They denote the delegation of authority and responsibility as well as the direction of accountability for the goals of the nursing division.

Organization charts distribute the nursing responsibilities. These responsibilities may be divided according to one function or a combination of functions: contiguous geography, similar techniques, similar objectives, or like clientele.

Organization charts are sometimes referred to as schemas. Decentralized schemas are flatter because there are fewer levels of control or management. Managers have more freedom to act, and the emphasis is on results.

There are advantages to having a current organization chart. Such charts should show clear relationships. They show employees who their supervisor is and supervisors who they supervise. They could facilitate coordination and communication. They can prevent intrigue, frustration, and duplication of effort, and promote decision-making, efficiency, and adherence to policy. They can tie the structure together and show inconsistencies and complexities. One must remember that organization charts have limitations. They will show formal authority structure only; they will show what was rather than what is if they are outdated and obsolete. Organization charts may confuse authority with status.

The success of nursing and of health care organizations depends on service to the customer. The focus then is on job function, and the organization chart should reflect this rather than show titles or names. Look at the traditional organization chart. It tells the employee who the boss is, and it often becomes a plan for empire building and for abdication of responsibility.

A circular organizational chart was developed at Our Lady of the Way Hospital, Martin, Kentucky. This chart reflected the hospital's increased reliance on team processes throughout the organization and significantly reduced the number of reporting assignments.[109]

Exhibit 14-21a depicts the organizational detail of the circular organization chart at Our Lady of the Way Hospital. Exhibit 14-21b depicts the relationships of the board, councils, and committees of such an organization.[110]

A new way of drawing organizational charts is the organigraph, which is a map offering an overview of a company's functions and the way people organize themselves at work. The organigraph is said to help managers see untapped opportunities by showing where ideas flow, what parts are connected to one another, and how processes and people should come together.[111]

Exhibit 14-22 shows how to evaluate an organization chart of a nursing division or department or unit.

The Informal Organization

Every formal organization has an informal one. The informal organization meets the needs of individuals with similar backgrounds, values, hobbies, interests, and physical proximity. It meets their needs for sharing experiences and feelings. Some administrators try to hinder the effects of informal organizations because they facilitate the passing of information. The information may be rumor, but the best way to combat rumor is by free flow of truthful information. Only that information which might violate individual privacy or the survival and health of the enterprise should be kept

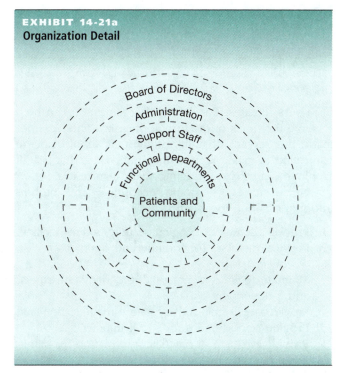

EXHIBIT 14-21a
Organization Detail

Board of Directors
Administration
Support Staff
Functional Departments
Patients and Community

Source: Used with permission from *Hospital and Health Services Administration*, 42, 2 (summer 1997): 243–254 (Chicago: *Health Administration Press*, 1997).

EXHIBIT 14-21b
Board, Councils, and Committees

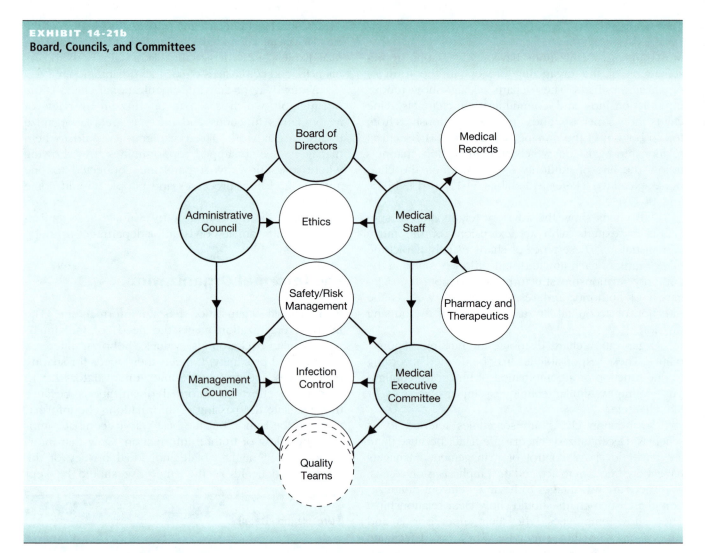

Source: Used with permission from *Hospital and Health Services Administration*, 42, 2 (summer 1997): 243–254 (Chicago: *Health Administration Press*, 1997).

from subordinates. The informal organization can help to serve the goals of the formal organization if it is not made the servant of administration. It should not be controlled. A major shortcoming in its use is that not all employees are part of the informal organization.

Nurse managers should encourage and nurture informal organizations that:

1. Provide a sense of belonging, security, and recognition.
2. Provide methods for friendly and open discussion of concern.
3. Maintain feelings of personal integrity, self-respect, and independent choice.
4. Provide an informal and accurate communication link.
5. Provide opportunities for social interaction.
6. Provide a source of practical information for managerial decision-making.
7. Are sources of future leaders.

Problems can include creation of conflicting loyalties, restricted productivity, and resistance to change and management's plans.[112]

Minimum Requirements of an Organizational Structure

1. *Clarity*—Nurses need to know where they belong, where they stand in relation to the quality and quantity of their performances, and where to go for assistance.
2. *Economy*—Nurses need as much self-control of their work as they can possibly be given. They need to be self-motivating. There should be the smallest possible number of overhead personnel

EXHIBIT 14-22
Evaluating Organizational Function

Answer the following questions as a final evaluation of your organizing function within a department or unit. For those checked No, plan changes so that they will result in effective organizing. Then implement the management plan.

	YES	NO
1. Is there evidence that organizing is an intentional and ongoing function of the division, department, service, or unit?	_____	_____
2. Is there evidence that organizing changes as plans, goals, or objectives change?	_____	_____
3. Is there evidence that managers are developed or replaced to fit organizational changes emerging from changed plans and objectives?	_____	_____
4. Are organizational managerial relationships clearly structured to give security to individual managers?	_____	_____
5. Has authority been delegated to appropriate levels of managers?	_____	_____
6. Is there evidence that delegation of authority has been balanced to retain control of appropriate administrative functions by the chief nurse executive?	_____	_____
7. Is information dissemination clearly separated from decision making?	_____	_____
8. Is the authority delegated commensurate with the responsibility?	_____	_____
9. Is there evidence of acceptance of responsibility and authority by subordinate managers?	_____	_____
10. Is there evidence that subordinate managers have the power to accomplish the results expected of them?	_____	_____
11. Is there evidence that authority and responsibility have been confined within divisional, departmental, service, or unit boundaries?	_____	_____
12. Is there evidence of balance in support and use of staff functions?	_____	_____
13. Is there evidence of balance in support and use of functional authority?	_____	_____
14. Is there evidence of maintenance of the principle of unity of command?	_____	_____
15. Is there evidence of efficient and effective use of service departments?	_____	_____
16. Is there evidence of too many levels of managers (overorganization)?	_____	_____
17. Is there evidence of unneeded line assistants to managers (overorganization)?	_____	_____
18. Is there evidence that the nursing division, department, service, or unit is organized to facilitate accomplishment of its specified objectives by its personnel?	_____	_____
19. Is there evidence that the nursing division, department, service, or unit structure has been modified to fit human factors after being organized to accomplish its specified objectives?	_____	_____
20. Is there evidence that the nursing division, department, service, or unit is organized to accomplish planning for recruiting and training to meet present and future personnel needs?	_____	_____
21. Is there evidence that the organizational process is flexible enough to adapt to changes in its external and internal environment?	_____	_____
22. Are changes in organization justified, based on deficiencies, experience, objectives, purpose, and plans?	_____	_____
23. Is there evidence that the organizing process is balanced between inertia and continual change?	_____	_____
24. Is there evidence that all nursing personnel know the organizational structure and understand their assignments and those of their co-workers?	_____	_____
25. Is there evidence that the nursing organizational charts are widely used?	_____	_____
26. Is there evidence that nursing organizational charts provide comprehensive information to all workers?	_____	_____
27. Is there evidence that there are job descriptions and job standards for every job and that they are widely used by nursing managers?	_____	_____
28. Is there evidence that nursing employees are all oriented to the nature of the nursing organizing process?	_____	_____
29. Is there evidence that the organizing process within the nursing division, department, service, or unit prevents waste or unplanned costs?	_____	_____
30. Is there evidence that the nursing organization has an effective span of control by managers?	_____	_____
31. Are the lines of authority within the nursing organization clear?	_____	_____
32. Is there evidence that the management information system is effective?	_____	_____
33. Is there evidence that each employee has only one supervisor?	_____	_____
34. Is there evidence that the CNE has absolute responsibility for subordinate nursing managers?	_____	_____
35. Is there evidence that all nursing managers are able to effect their leadership abilities?	_____	_____

necessary to keep the division and units operating and well maintained.

3. *Direction of vision*—Nurse managers must direct their vision and that of their employees toward performance, toward the future, and toward strength. Nurses must understand their own tasks and the common tasks, the common ones being those of the organization. They should see that their tasks fit the common tasks of the organization so that the structure helps communication.

4. *Decision-making*—Nurses should be organized to make decisions on the right issues and at the right levels. They should be organized to convert their decisions into work and accomplishments. The chair of the department of nursing and the staff make all nursing decisions and see that nursing work is done.

5. *Stability and accountability*—Nurses should be organized to feel community belongingness. They can adapt to show objectives requiring changes in their functions and productivity.

6. *Perception and self-renewal*—Nursing services should be organized to produce future leaders. The organizational structure should produce continuous learning for the job each nurse holds and for promotion.

To apply design principles that are appropriate, the nurse manager uses a mixture of all that are productive.

Principle: Organizational needs derive from the statements of mission and objectives and from observation of work performed.

Principle: Organizational design and structure develop to fit organizational needs, so that people perform and contribute to achieving the work of the division of nursing.

Principle: A formal organization should be flexible and based on policy that promotes individual contributions to the achievement of organizational objectives.

Principle: A formal organization is efficient when it promotes achievement of objectives with a minimum of unplanned costs or outcomes. Most results should be planned for, should give satisfaction to supervisors and employees, and should not occasion waste and carelessness. When grouping activities for organizing purposes, the supervisor or administrator should examine the benefits and disadvantages of alternative groupings.

Principle: A formal organization should build the least possible number of management levels and forge the shortest possible chain of command. This eliminates stresses and levels of friction, slack, and inertia.

Organizational Effectiveness

The product or output of an organization is termed *organizational effectiveness* (OE). There should be a relationship between organizational effectiveness and organizational performance (OP). Nurse managers define the goals and provide the resources for both organizational effectiveness and organizational performance. They have many dimensions, which can include:

1. Patient satisfaction with care.
2. Family satisfaction with care.
3. Staff satisfaction with work.
4. Staff satisfaction with rewards, intrinsic and extrinsic.
5. Staff satisfaction with professional development: career, personal, and educational.
6. Staff satisfaction with organization.
7. Management satisfaction with staff.
8. Community relationships.
9. Organizational health.

Nurse administrators control these dimensions of organizational effectiveness. Proactivity is more successful in developing them than is reactivity.[113]

The organizational effectiveness of hospitals could be improved if administrators would enter into general or limited partnerships with nurses. Hospitals have moved to vertical integration to capture the lost revenues of retrospective reimbursement. General hospitals have entered into services such as home care, long-term care, psychiatric care, rehabilitation, hospice care, rental and sale of durable medical supplies, and many other profit-making services. Although they call for general or limited partnerships with physicians, they ignore nurses as a potential source of partnerships for profit. Instead, the not-for-profit status of hospital inpatient beds is reputed to be maintained by policies that tie nursing to charity and idealism rather than to viability and profitability. Such statements as the following validate this tie: "Keeping nursing care in the not-for-profit hospital corporation preserves the oldest tradition of hospitals—their role in serving the needy."[114]

Nurses can overcome this attitude by themselves becoming proactive. As an example, nurses could plan a limited partnership that would provide contract nurses through a staffing agency owned by them. They could offer a hospital a contract to provide needed personnel on a first priority basis, surplus personnel being provided for other institutions. The contract could provide for up-to-date continuing education of the agency nurses through cooperative arrangements with the contracting hospital. Profits would be shared and nurses would perceive that the hospital supported nursing entrepreneurship, thus contributing to their morale and professional esteem. Other ventures could be added to improve OP as well as OE and to give nurses a sense of ownership.

Vertical integration, mergers, linkages, and multi-hospital systems have created more and new corporate nurse roles. The corporate nurse is physically and organizationally removed from daily nursing service operations. As such, the corporate nurse reviews data from a number of hospitals and organizations, comparing outcomes. Having access to much data and many specialties, and serving on corporate committees, the corporate nurse creates a personal power base. She or he can develop systems for member organizations in such areas as management education, nursing division policy, search and selection of nurse executives, research, quality assurance, risk management, and others.[115]

Symptoms of Malorganization

A symptom of malorganization is recurring problems. They indicate the focus is on the wrong elements of the business when it should emphasize key activities, major business decisions, performance, and results rather than secondary problems. Another symptom of malorganization is too many meetings attended by too many people. Such meetings are poor tools for accomplishing work. An alternative is to give individual assignments and only meet to report and avoid duplication. Committees are instruments of participation and communication and must be made productive. Too many management levels are another symptom of malorganization.

Principle: Build the least possible number of management levels and forge the shortest possible chain of command. This eliminates stresses and levels of friction, slack, and inertia.

If people always have to worry about other people's feelings, there is overstaffing. If the organization is put together to get the job done, layers of coordinators are not needed. Fit the chart to the organization and its needs rather than drawing a chart and building the organization to support it.

Summary

There is no best design for a nursing organization, nor are there universal design principles. Nurse managers need to work for an ideal organizational structure, and they need to be pragmatic. They should build, test, concede, compromise, and accept. They should design the simplest organization for getting the job done. They should focus on key activities to produce key results. The organization is productive when the people are performing care that meets clients' needs and for which employees have a sense of accomplishment.

An organization can be shaped through:

1. Job enlargement that is qualitative—meaningful, interesting, and intellectually rewarding.
2. Making the structure more manageable. Increasing clinical nurses' autonomy reduces the organization's size.
3. Increasing the span of control of the manager.
4. Shortening the hierarchy.
5. Involving the employees in participation.
6. Decentralization.
7. Increasing the employee's stake in his or her own performance.
8. Increasing creativity while maintaining fiscal responsibility.
9. Replacing direction and control with advice.
10. Meeting employees' needs.

The nursing management function of organizing is an evolving one. It evolves as nurse managers learn and apply the knowledge gained from research and experience in business and industry. They further develop the organizing function through nursing research and experience in nursing management.

APPLICATION EXERCISES

EXERCISE 14-1   Use the list entitled "activities that promote a positive organizational climate" in this chapter as a point of discussion for a group of your peers. Assess the organizational climate in the organization in which you are a student or an employee.

EXERCISE 14-2   Read the following articles:

Bruhn, J. G., "Creating an Organizational Climate for Multiculturalism," *Health Care Supervision* (June 1996), 11–18.

Butcher, A. H., "Supervisors Matter More Than You Think: Components of a Mission-Centered Organizational Climate," *Hospital Health Services Administration* (winter 1994), 505–520.

Counte, M. A., G. L. Glandon, D. M. Oleske, and J. P. Hill, "Total Quality Management in a Health Care Organization: How Are Employees Affected?" *Hospital Health Services Administration* (winter 1992), 503–518.

DeLellis, A. J., "Creating a Climate of Mutual Respect Among Employees: A Workshop Design," *Health Care Supervision* (June 1997), 48–56.

Gibson, J. M., "Using the Delphi Technique to Identify the Content and Context of Nurses' Continuing Professional Development Needs," *Journal of Clinical Nursing* (September 1998), 451–459.

Jones, L. C., T. D. Guberski, and K. L. Soeken, "Nurse Practitioners: Leadership Behaviors and Organizational Climate," *Journal of Professional Nursing* (November–December 1990), 327–333.

Keuter, K., E. Byrne, J. Voell, and E. Larson, "Nurses' Job Satisfaction and Organizational Climate in a Dynamic Work Environment," *Applied Nursing Research* (February 2000), 46–49.

Mattiasson, A. C. and L. Andersson, "Organizational Environment and the Support of Patient Autonomy in Nursing Home Care," *Journal of Advanced Nursing* (December 1995), 1149–1157.

Piscopo, B., "Organizational Climate, Communication, and Role Strain In Clinical Nursing Faculty," *Journal of Professional Nursing* (March–April 1995), 113–119.

Answer the following questions:

What characteristics of organizational climate were evident in these articles?
How did these characteristics impact negatively or positively on professional nurses?
What actions could be taken to improve any negative impacts on professional nurses' performance?
Compare them with the list of activities that promote a positive organizational climate. Add activities missing from this list.

EXERCISE 14-3   Refer to Exhibit 14-11, "Fifty Specific Techniques to Boost Employee Morale." Make a list of similar activities found in the organization in which you work as a student or employee.

EXERCISE 14-4   Use Exhibit 14-13, "Standards for Evaluating the Effectiveness of Line and Staff Relationships in a Hierarchical Organization," to evaluate the nursing division, department, service, or unit in which you work as a student or an employee. Involve your colleagues.

EXERCISE 14-5   Explore the concept of the high-tech home care nurse operationalizing the trend to bring critical care nursing and medical services directly into the home care environment. Make a business plan to develop high tech home care as a new product.

Carruth, A. K., S. Steele, B. Moffett, T. Rehmeyer, C. Cooper, and R. Burroughs, "The Impact of Primary and Modular Nursing Delivery Systems on Perceptions of Caring Behavior," *Oncology Nursing Forum* (January–February 1999), 95–100.

McNeal, G. J., "Care of the Critically Ill Client at Home," *Nursing Clinics of North America* (September 1998), 267–278.

McNeal, G. J., "Telecommunication Technologies in High-Tech Homecare," *Nursing Clinics of North America* (September 1998), 279–286.

EXERCISE 14-6 Organize a team to study the concepts of circular organizational charts and organigraphs. Draft a circular organizational chart for a department or unit of the organization in which you work or are a student. Outline a process for doing an organigraph of a nursing unit and implement it.

EXERCISE 14-7 Describe the form of the organizational structure of the nursing division and unit on which you work as a student or employee. Discuss the changes that could be made to make it more functional.

EXERCISE 14-8 Use Exhibit 14-22, "Evaluating Organizational Function," to evaluate the nursing organization chart of the organization in which you work as a student or employee.

NOTES

1. C. Argyris, "Personality and Organization Theory Revisited," *Administrative Science Quarterly*, 18, 1973, 141–167.
2. H. Fayol, *General and Industrial Management*. Trans. by C. Storrs (London: Sir Isaac Pittman & Sons, 1949), 53–61.
3. L. Urwick, *The Elements of Administration* (New York: Harper & Row, 1944), 37–39.
4. T. Peters, *Thriving on Chaos* (New York: Harper & Row, 1987).
5. J. L. Gibson, J. M. Ivancevich, and J. H. Donnelly, Jr., *Organizations: Behavior, Structures, Processes*, 8th ed. (Burr Ridge, IL: Richard D. Irwin, Inc., 1994), 539–541.
6. R. H. Hall, "The Concept of Bureaucracy: An Empirical Assessment," *The American Journal of Sociology* (July 1963), 32–40.
7. Ibid.
8. R. H. Hall, "Professionalization and Bureaucratization," *American Sociological Review* (February 1968), 92–104.
9. D. Sofarelli and D. Brown, "The Need for Nursing Leadership in Uncertain Times," *Journal of Nursing Management* (July 1998) 201–207.
10. J. R. Rizzo, R. J. House, and S. I. Lirtzman, "Role Conflict and Ambiguity in Complex Organizations," *Administrative Science Quarterly*, 15, (1970), 150–162.
11. M. Warda, "The Family and Chronic Sorrow: Role Theory Approach," *Journal of Pediatric Nursing* (June 1992), 205–210; D. A. Revicki and H. J. May, "Organizational Characteristics, Occupational Stress, and Mental Health in Nurses," *Behavioral Medicine* (spring 1989), 30–36.
12. J. A. MacLeod and S. Sella, "One Year Later: Using Role Theory to Evaluate a New Delivery System," *Nursing Forum* (April–June 1992), 20–28.
13. J. O. Miller and S. J. Carey, "Work Role Inventory: A Guide to Job Satisfaction," *Nursing Management* (January 1993), 54–62.
14. D. Dunphy, "Personal and Organizational Change—Status and Future Direction," *Work and People* (February 1983), 3–6.
15. J. Johnson and K. Luciano, "Managing by Behavior and Results—Linking Supervisory Accountability to Effective Organizational Control," *The Journal of Nursing Administration* (December 1983), 19–26.
16. E. C. Dayani, "Professional and Economic Self-Governance in Nursing," *Nursing Economic$* (July–August 1983), 20–23.
17. C. Argyris, op. cit.
18. D. S. Ridderheim, "The Anatomy of Change," *Hospital & Health Services Administration* (May–June 1986), 7–21.
19. D. J. del Bueno and P. M. Vincent, "Organizational Culture: How Important Is It?" *Journal of Nursing Administration* (October 1986), 15–20.
20. Ibid.
21. W. G. Dyer and W. G. Dyer, Jr., "Organizational Development: System Change or Culture Change?" *Personnel* (February 1986), 14–22.
22. B. Pfister, "Philosophy, Attitudes in Workplace Define the Personality of a Business," *San Antonio Express-News* (17 January 1999), 1K, 3K.
23. W. W. Moore, "Corporate Culture: Modern Day Rites & Rituals," *Healthcare Trends and Transitions* (March 1991), 8–13, 32–33.
24. C. Caroselli, "Assessment of Organization Culture: A Tool for Professional Success," *Orthopedic Nursing* (May–June 1992), 57–63.
25. R. L. Desatnick, "Management Climate Surveys: A Way to Uncover an Organization's Culture," *Personnel* (May 1986), 49–54, 14–22.
26. D. J. del Bueno and P. M. Vincent, op. cit.
27. W. G. Dyer and W. G. Dyer, Jr. op. cit.
28. R. L. Desatnick, op. cit.
29. M. D. Sovie, "Hospital Culture—Why Create One?" *Nursing Economic$* (March–April 1993), 69–75.
30. L. L. Curtin, "Creating a Culture of Competence," *Nursing Management* (September 1990), 7–8.
31. J. Donald, "What Makes Your Day? A Study of the Quality of Worklife of OR Nurses," *Canadian Operating Room Nursing Journal* (December 1999), 17–27.
32. M. A. Ray, "The Theory of Bureaucratic Caring for Nursing Practice in the Organizational Culture," *Nursing Administration Quarterly* (winter 1989), 31–42.
33. M. E. Fleeger, "Assessing Organizational Culture: A Planning Strategy," *Nursing Management* (February 1993), 39–41.
34. C. Thomas, M. Ward, C. Chorba, and A. Kumiega, "Measuring and Interpreting Organizational Culture," *Journal of Nursing Administration* (June 1990), 17–24.
35. S. Stordeur, C. Vandenberghe, and W. D'hoore, "Leadership Styles Across Hierarchical Levels in Nursing Departments," *Nursing Research* (January–February 2000), 37–43.
36. T. Peters, "Experts' Strengths Can Be a Weakness," *San Antonio Light* (24 September 1991), B3.
37. H. E. Munn, Jr., "Organizational Climate in the Health Care Setting," *The Health Care Supervisor* (October 1984), 19–29.

38. R. L. Desatnick, op. cit.

39. M. Holt Ashley, "Motivation: Getting the Medical Units Going Again," *Nursing Management* (June 1985), 28–30.

40. M. B. Guthrie, G. Mauer, R. A. Zawacki, and J. D. Conger, "Productivity: How Much Does This Job Mean?" *Nursing Management* (February 1985), 16–20.

41. L. R. Campbell, "What Satisfies . . . and Doesn't?" *Nursing Management* (August 1986), 78.

42. R. L. Jenkins and R. L. Henderson, "Motivating the Staff: What Nurses Expect from Their Supervisors," *Nursing Management* (February 1984), 13–14.

43. T. K. Crout and J. C. Crout, "Care Plan for Retaining the New Nurse," *Nursing Management* (December 1984), 30–33.

44. B. Schneider, "The Preceptor of Organizational Climate: The Customer's View," *Journal of Applied Psychology* (March 1973), 248–256.

45. C. Joiner, V. Johnson, J. B. Chapman, and M. Corkrean, "The Motivating Potential in Nursing Specialties," *The Journal of Nursing Administration* (February 1982), 26–30.

46. S. Felgelson, "Mixing Mirth and Management," *Supervision* (November 1989), 6–8.

47. D. A. Gillies, M. Franklin, and D. A. Child, "Relationship Between Organizational Climate and Job Satisfaction of Nursing Personnel," *Nursing Administration Quarterly* (summer 1990), 15–22.

48. M. J. Hern-Underwood and L. L. Workman, "Group Climate: A Significant Retention Factor for Pediatric Nurse Managers," *Journal of Professional Nursing* (July–August 1993), 233–238.

49. B. Conway-Rutkowski, "Labor Relations: How Do You Rate?" *Nursing Management* (February 1984), 13–16.

50. R. L. Desatnick, op. cit.

51. G. K. Gordon, "Developing a Motivating Environment," *The Journal of Nursing Administration* (December 1982), 11–16.

52. E. E. Lawler, III, D. T. Hall, and G. R. Oldham, "Organizational Climate: Relationship to Organizational Structure, Process and Performance," *Organizational Behavior and Human Performance* (November 1974), 139–155.

53. K. Russell-Babin, "Team Building for the Staff Development Department," *Journal of Nursing Staff Development* (September–October 1992), 231–234; S. P. San Juan, "Team Building: A Leadership Strategy," *Journal of the Phillippine Dental Association* (June–August 1998), 49–55.

54. D. Heming, "The Titanic Triumvirate: Teams, Teamwork and Team Building," *CJOT* (February 1988), 15–20.

55. D. L. Niehouse, "Job Satisfaction: How to Motivate Today's Workers," *Supervisory Management* (February 1986), 8–11.

56. K. Russell-Babin, op. cit.

57. M. Jacobsen-Webb, "Team Building: Key to Executive Success," *The Journal of Nursing Administration* (January–February 1985), 16–20.

58. C. Logan, "Praise: The Powerhouse of Self-Esteem," *Nursing Management* (June 1985), 36, 38.

59. J. L. Nave and B. Thomas, "How Companies Boost Morale," *Supervisory Management* (October 1983), 29–33.

60. P. Cornett-Cooke and K. Dias, "Teambuilding: Getting It All Together," *Nursing Management* (May 1984), 16–17.

61. "Managing a Dream Team," *Modern Materials Handling* (January 1993), 23.

62. J. W. Frederickson, "The Strategic Decision Process and Organizational Structure," *Academy of Management Review* (April 1986), 280–297.

63. D. S. Pugh, D. J. Hickson, C. R. Hinings, and C. Turner, "The Context of Organization Structures," *Administrative Science Quarterly* (March 1969), 91–114; P. Leatt and R. Schneck,

"Technology, Size, Environment, and Structure in Nursing Subunits," *Organizational Studies*, 3(3), (1982), 221–242.

64. D. S. Pugh, D. J. Hickson, C. R. Hinings, and C. Turner, op. cit.

65. Ibid.

66. M. Roznowski and C. L. Hulin, "Influences of Functional Specialty and Job Technology on Employees' Perceptual and Affective Responses to Their Jobs," *Organizational Behavior and Human Decision Processes* (October 1985), 186–208.

67. P. Leatt and R. Schneck, op. cit.

68. D. S. Pugh, D. J. Hickson, C. R. Hinings, and C. Turner, op. cit.

69. Ibid.

70. P. Leatt and R. Schneck, op. cit.

71. Ibid.

72. M. Roznowski and C. L. Hulin, op. cit.

73. D. S. Pugh, D. J. Hickson, C. R. Hinings, and C. Turner, op. cit.

74. Ibid.

75. M. L. McClure, "Managing the Professional Nurse: Part I. The Organizational Theories," *The Journal of Nursing Administration* (February 1984), 15–21; M. M. Timm and M. G. Wavetik, "Matrix Organization: Design and Development for a Hospital Organization," *Hospital & Health Services Administration* (November–December 1983), 46–58; American Organization of Nurse Executives, *Organizational Models for Nursing Practice* (Chicago: American Hospital Association, 1984).

76. Ibid.

77. Ibid.

78. J. G. Newman and R. Boissoneau, "Team Care and Matrix Organization in Geriatrics," *Hospital Topics* (November–December 1987), 10–15.

79. B. Fuszard, "'Adhocracy' in Health Care Institutions," *Journal of Nursing Administration* (January 1983), 14–19; R. H. Waterman, Jr., *Adhocracy—the Power to Change* (New York: W. W. Norton, 1990).

80. R. H. Guest, "Management Imperatives for the Year 2000," *California Management Review* (summer 1986), 62–70.

81. D. L. Flarey, "The Nurse Executive and the Governing Body," *Journal of Nursing Administration* (December 1991), 11–17.

82. R. Kanter, *When Giants Learn to Dance* (New York: Simon & Schuster, 1989), 36.

83. Ibid., 57–67.

84. M. D. Sovie, "Redesigning Our Future: Whose Responsibility Is It?" *Nursing Economic$* (January–February 1990), 21–26.

85. A. Lewis, "Too Many Managers: Major Threat to CQI in Hospitals," *Quality Review Bulletin* (March 1993), 95–101.

86. L. Genasci, "Downsizing Not Always Effective, Experts Say," *San Antonio Express-News* (24 July 1994), 3H.

87. P. Kaestle, "A New Rationale for Organizational Structure," *Planning Review* (July–August 1990), 20–22, 27.

88. S. Staring and C. Taylor, "A Guide to Managing Workforce Transitions," *Nursing Management* (December 1997), 31–32.

89. T. Peters, *Thriving on Chaos* (New York: Harper & Row, 1987), 424–438.

90. M. Reddecliff, E. L. Smith, and M. Ryan-Merritt, "Organizational Analysis: Tool for the Clinical Nurse Specialist," *Clinical Nurse Specialist* (fall 1989), 133–136.

91. P. F. Drucker, *Management: Tasks, Responsibilities, Practice* (New York: Harper & Row, 1973), 564.

92. D. L. del Bueno, "Paradigm Shifts—What's Good and Not So Good for Health Care," *Nursing & Health Care* (February 1993), 100–101.

93. M. McAllister, "A Nursing Integration Framework Based on Standards of Practice," *Nursing Management* (April 1990), 28–31.

94. R. A. Adams and A. R. Rentfro, "Strengthening Hospital Nursing: An Approach to Restructuring Care Delivery," *Journal of Nursing Administration* (June 1988), 12–19.

95. C. E. Schmekel, "Nursing/Group Practice," *AORN Journal* (May 1991), 1223–1226, 1228.

96. K. M. Metcalf, "The Helper Model: Nine Ways to Make It Work," *Nursing Management* (December 1992), 40–43.

97. M. Manthey, "Delivery Systems and Practice Models: A Dynamic Balance," *Nursing Management* (January 1991), 28–30.

98. D. Milton, J. Verren, C. Murdaugh, and R. Gerber, "Differentiated Group Professional Practice in Nursing: A Demonstration Model," *Nursing Clinics of North America* (March 1992), 23–29.

99. Ibid.

100. K. S. Ehrat, "The Value of Differentiated Practice," *JONA* (April 1991), 9–10.

101. C. Graph, K. Roberts, and K. Thornton, "An Ethnographic Study of Differentiated Practice in an Operating Room," *Journal of Professional Nursing* (November–December 1999), 364–371; N. Smith-Blair, B. L. Smith, K. J. Bradley and C. Gaskamp, "Making Sense of a New Nursing Role: A Phenomenological Study of an Organizational Change," *Journal of Professional Nursing* (November–December 1999), 340–348.

102. M. Styles, S. Allen, S. Armstrong, M. Matsurra, D. Stannard, and J. S. Ordway, "Entry: A New Approach," *Nursing Outlook* (September–October 1991), 200–203.

103. L. W. Porter and E. E. Lawler, III, "The Effects of 'Tall' Versus 'Flat' Organization Structure on Managerial Job Satisfaction," *Personnel Psychology* (summer 1964), 135–148.

104. R. H. Guest, op. cit.

105. D. A. Conrad and W. L Dowling, "Vertical Integration in Health Services: Theory and Managerial Implications," *Health Care Management Review* (fall 1990), 9–22.

106. G. Klaus, "Horizontal Organization," *Executive Excellence* (November 1989), 3–5.

107. J. L. Gibson, J. M. Ivancevich, and J. H. Donnelly, Jr., op. cit., 540–543.

108. D. C. Pheysey, R. L. Payne, and D. S. Pugh, "Influence of Structure at Organizational and Group Levels," *Administration Science Quarterly*, 16, (1971), 61–73.

109. M. M. Fanning, op. cit.

110. M. M. Fanning, "A Circular Organization Chart Promotes a Hospital-Wide Focus On Teams," *Hospital Health Services Administration* (summer 1997), 243–254.

111. H. Mintzberg and L. Van der Heyden, "Organigraphs: Drawing How Companies Really Work," *Harvard Business Review* (September–October 1999), 87–94, 184.

112. P. E. Han, "The Informal Organization You've Got to Live With," *Supervisory Management* (October 1983), 25–28.

113. K. Cameron, "A Study of Organizational Effectiveness and Its Predictors," *Management Science* (January 1986), 87–112.

114. Ibid.

115. M. Beyers, "Getting On Top of Organizational Change: Part 3. The Corporate Nurse Executive," *The Journal of Nursing Administration* (December 1984), 32–37.

REFERENCES

American Nurses' Association. *Standards of Clinical Nursing Practice* (Washington, DC: American Nurses' Publishing, 1991).

American Nurses' Association. *Scope and Standards for Nurse Administrators* (Washington, DC, American Nurses' Publishing, 1995).

Antrobus, S., and A. Kitson. "Nursing Leadership: Influencing and Shaping Health Policy and Nursing Practice." *Journal of Advanced Nursing* (March 1999), 746–753.

Badovanic, C. C., S. Wilson, and D. Woodhouse. "The Use of Unlicensed Assistive Personnel and Selected Outcome Indications." *Nursing Economic$* (July–August 1999), 194–200.

Bailey, K. L. "Establishing Private Duty in a Medicare World." *Caring* (September 1998), 29–31.

Bichan, M. S., M. J. Hegge, and T. E. Stenvig. "A Tiger by the Tail: Tackling Barriers to Differentiated Practice." *The Journal of Continuing Education in Nursing*, 22(3), 109–112.

Bigelow, B., and M. Arndt. "The More Things Change, the More They Stay the Same." *Health Care Management Review* (winter 2000), 65–72.

Bowen, M., K. J. Lyons, and B. E. Young. "Nursing and Health Care Reform: Implications for Curriculum Development." *Journal of Nursing Education* (January 2000), 27–33.

Call, A. "Building Bridges." *Nursing Times* (2 December 1992), 44–45.

Clark, D. A., P. F. Clark, D. Day, and D. Shea. "The Relationship Between Health Care Reform and Nurses' Interest in Union Representation: The Role of Workplace Climate." *Journal of Professional Nursing* (March–April 2000), 92–96.

Cody, M. "Vertical Integration Strategies: Revenue Effects in Hospital and Medicare Markets." *Hospital Health Services Administration* (fall 1996), 343–357.

Collins, C., and A. Green. "Public Sector Hospitals and Organizational Change: An Agenda for Policy Analysis." *International Journal of Health Planning Management* (April–June 1999), 107–128.

Coluccio, M. and K. Havlick. "Shared Leadership in a Newly Merged Medical Center." *Nursing Administration Quarterly* (winter 1998), 36–39.

Dawkins, C., D. Oakley, J. Davis, and N. Erwin. "Collaboration as an Organizational Process." *Journal of Nursing Education* (April 1991), 189–191

Dennis, K. E. "Nursing's Power in the Organization: What Research Has Shown." *Nursing Administration Quarterly* (fall 1983), 47–60.

Dienemann, J., and T. Glazner. "Restructuring Nursing Care Delivery Systems." *Nursing Economic$* (July–August 1992), 253–258, 310.

Galvin, K., C. Andrewes, D. Jackson, S. Cheesman, T. Fudge, R. Ferris, and I. Graham. "Investigating and Implementing Change Within the Primary Health Care Nursing Team." *Journal of Advanced Nursing* (July 1999), 238–247.

Gardner, D. L. "Assessing Career Commitment: The Role of Staff Development." (November–December 1991), 263–266.

George, J. R., and L. K. Bishop. "Relationship of Organizational Structure and Teacher Personality Characteristics to Organizational Climate." *Administrative Science Quarterly* (1971), 467–475.

Glazner, L. "Understanding Corporate Cultures: Use of Systems Theory and Situational Analysis." *AAOHN Journal* (August 1992), 383–387.

Glover, D. "Everett Hospitals to Unify Management." *Seattle Post-Intelligencer* (21 July 1993), B2.

Hansten, R. I., and M. J. Washburn. "Individual and Organizational Accountability for Development of Critical Thinking." *Journal of Nursing Administration* (November 1999), 39–45.

Hart, S. K., and M. N. Moore. "The Relationship Among Organizational Climate Variables and Nurse Stability in Critical Care Units." *Journal of Professional Nursing* (May–June 1989), 124–131.

Haynie, L., and B. Garrett. "Developing a Customer-Service and Cost-Effectiveness Team." *Journal of Healthcare Quality* (November–December 1999), 28–29, 32–34.

Heilriegel, D., and J. W. Slocum. "Organizational Climate: Measures Research and Contingencies." *Academy of Management Journal* (June 1972), 255–280.

Hirsch, J. "Organizational Structure and Philosophy." *Nursing Administration Quarterly* (summer 1987), 47–51.

Hodgetts, R. M. *Management: Theory, Process, and Practice*, 5th ed. (Orlando, FL: Harcourt, Brace 1990), 138–231.

Ingersoll, G. L., J. C. Kirsch, S. E. Merk, and J. Lightfoot. "Relationship of Organizational Culture and Readiness for Change to Employee Commitment to the Organization." *Journal of Nursing Administration* (January 2000), 11–20.

Jablin, F. M. "Formal Structural Characteristics of Organizations and Superior-Subordinate Communication." *Human Communication Research* (summer 1982), 338–347.

Jones, L. C., T. D. Guberski, and K. L. Soeken. "Nurse Practitioners: Leadership Behaviors and Organizational Climate." *Journal of Professional Nursing* (November–December 1990), 327–333.

Joyce, W. F., and J. Slocum. "Climate Discrepancy: Refining the Concepts of Psychological and Organizational Climate." *Human Relations*, 11, (1982), 951–972.

Kerfoot, K. "The Culture of Courage." *Nursing Economic$* (July–August 1999), 238–239.

King, C., and A. Koliner. "Understanding the Impact of Power in Organizations." *Seminars in Nursing Management* (March 1999), 39–46.

Koloroutis, M., and J. K. Moe. "Assessment: The First Step in Creating a more System-Wide Approach to Nursing Practice." *Journal of Nursing Administration* (February 2000), 97–103.

Krampitz, S. D., and M. Williams. "Organizational Climates: A Measure of Faculty and Nurse Administrator Perception." *Journal of Nursing Education* (May 1983), 200–206.

Laschinger, H. K., C. Wong, L. McMahon, and C. Kaufmann. "Leader Behavior Impact On Staff Nurse Empowerment, Job Tension, and Work Effectiveness." *Journal of Nursing Administration* (May 1999), 28–39.

Lehrman, S., and K. K. Shore. "Hospitals' Vertical Integration into Skilled Nursing: A Rational Approach to Controlling Transaction Costs." *Inquiry* (fall 1998), 303–314.

Miller, E. "Reengineering the Role of the Nurse Manager in a Patient-Centered Care Organization." *Journal of Nursing Care Quality* (August 1999), 47–56.

Mills, P. K., and B. Z. Posner. "The Relationships Among Self-Supervision, Structure, and Technology in Professional Service Organizations." *Academy of Management Journal* (June 1982), 437–443.

Payne, R. L., and R. Mansfield. "Relationships of Perceptions of Organizational Climate to Organizational Structure, Context, and Hierarchical Position." *Administrative Science Quarterly*, 18, (1973), 515–526.

Perryman-Starkey, M., P. A. Rivers, and G. Munchus. "The Effects of Organizational Structure On Hospital Performance." *Health Services Management Research* (November 1999), 232–245.

Peters. T. "McKenzie Exemplifies Structureless Corporation of Future." *San Antonio Light* (12 November 1992), B1, B8.

Pillar, B., and D. Jarjoura. "Assessing the Impact of Reengineering on Nursing." *Journal of Nursing Administration* (May 1999), 57–64.

Poulton, B. C. "User Involvement in Identifying Health Needs and Shaping and Evaluating Services: Is It Being Realized?" *Journal of Advanced Nursing* (December 1999), 1289–1296.

Pritchard, R. D., and B. W. Karasick. "The Effects of Organizational Climate on Managerial Job Performance and Job Satisfaction." *Organizational Behavior and Human Performance*, 9, (1973), 126–143.

Schaffner, J. W., S. Alleman, P. Ludwig-Beymer, J. Muzynski, D. J. King, and L. J. Pacura. "Developing a Patient Care Model for an Integrated Delivery System." *Journal of Nursing Administration* (September 1999), 43–50.

Seago, J. A. "Evaluation of a Hospital Work Redesign: Patient-Focused Care." *Journal of Nursing Administration* (November 1999), 31–38.

Shortell, S. M., R. H. Jones, A. W. Rademaker, R. R. Gillies, D. S. Dranove, E. F. Hughes, P. P. Budetti, K. S. Reynolds, and C. F. Huang. "Assessing the Impact of Total Quality Management and Organizational Culture on Multiple Outcomes of Care for Coronary Artery Bypass Graft Surgery Patients." *Medical Care* (February 2000), 207–217.

Spitzer-Lehman, R., K. J. Yahn. "Patient Needs Drive an Integrated Approach to Care." *Nursing Management* (August 1992), 30–32.

Swansburg, R. C. Self-Study Module-27-77: *The Organizing Function of Nursing Service Administration* (Hattiesburg, MS: School of Nursing, University of Southern Mississippi, 1977).

Swansburg, R. C. *Nurses & Patients: An Introduction to Nursing Management* (Hattiesburg, MS: Impact III, 1978).

Swansburg, R. C. *Management of Patient Care Services* (St. Louis: Mosby, 1976).

Theile, J. R. "The Anatomy of an Organization." *Nursing Administration Quarterly* (winter 1983), 42–45.

Tushman, M., and D. Nadler. "Organizing for Innovation." *California Management Review* (spring 1986), 74–92.

Valanis, B. "Professional Nursing Practice in an HMO: The Future Is Now." *Journal of Nursing Education* (January 2000), 13–20.

Van Mullem, C., L. J. Burke, K. Dohmeyer, M. Farrell, S. Harvey, L. John, C. Kraly, F. Rowley, M. Sebern, K. Twite, and R. Zapp. "Strategic Planning for Research Use in Nursing Practice." *Journal of Nursing Administration* (December 1999), 38–45.

Walston, S. L., and R. J. Bogue. "The Effects of Reengineering: Fad or Competitive Factor." *Journal of Healthcare Management* (November–December 1999), 456–476.

Wong, F. K. "The Nurse Manager as a Professional-Managerial Class: A Case Study." *Journal of Nursing Management* (November 1998), 343–350.

CHAPTER 15

Committees and Other Groups

Russell C. Swansburg, PhD, RN

- Define *committee*.
- Distinguish between standing and ad hoc committees.
- Use a set of standards to evaluate nursing committees.
- Discuss group dynamics and the roles played by group members.
- Analyze the phases of groups.
- Analyze committee effectiveness.
- Define *groupthink* and give examples.
- Describe the characteristics of various group techniques.
- Describe the characteristics of self-directed work teams.

CONCEPTS: Committee, ad hoc committee, standing committee, group dynamics, focus group, groupthink, quality circles, self-managed work team.

MANAGER BEHAVIOR: The manager supports committees as part of the organizational structure..

LEADER BEHAVIOR: The leader promotes shared governance through the committee structure and wide use of group dynamics.

Committees Defined

A committee is a group form that evolves out of a formal organization structure. Committees are formed to make collective use of knowledge, skills, and ideas. They blend the good characteristics of several to many individuals—a reason for making careful appointments or selections. The principle of synergy underlies committee activity; it puts the thinking power of a selected group together for the most effective outcome. What is the optimal number of people to produce the desired outcome of synergy? The answer is difficult because it depends on the goals to be addressed, the characteristics of the committee members, and the environment within which these members function. The goal is to aim for the best combination of skills and energies.[1]

Committees as Groups

Because the work of organizations is accomplished by groups, many persons have studied the dynamics of group function. Although all groups are not committees, the management of a group of employees whose goal is to accomplish the objectives of the enterprise is similar to the leadership and management of a committee whose goal is to accomplish selective objectives. In the 1920s, researchers at Harvard Business School found that worker morale and productivity were positively influenced by small, informal work groups.[2]

In the world of the nurse manager, work is performed by individuals and by groups. Primary nursing has become a much used modality, or method, of practicing nursing because it gives professional nurses more autonomy than do other modalities. It adds accountability, as nurses are continuously responsible for patients from admission through discharge. Case management adds group dynamics to the autonomy, since the case manager is responsible for functioning in a collaborative practice with other professional nurses and with physicians. Case management also uses managed care as a medium to keep the patient on the critical path from admission through discharge. Case management can extend through the illness episode to include home care even at the critical care level.

Committees are formal groups that can serve useful functions in the organizational process of nursing and administration. In addition to being organizational entities, committees are a part of managerial planning, and, in turn, they make plans. They are directed by leaders who are appointed by management or elected by constituents determined by management. Since professional nurses want autonomy but are mostly employed by organizations, formal groups, including committees, are a medium for promoting autonomy by giving them a voice in managing the organization. A committee's effectiveness can be controlled internally and externally. A committee that does not serve a useful function should be evaluated and restructured. When no longer needed, it should be selectively abandoned.

There are two common types of committees: *standing* and *ad hoc*, or *special*. Standing committees are advisory in authority, although some may have collective authority to make and implement decisions. They have continuity as organizational entities. Ad hoc committees are formed to fulfill a specific purpose and are disbanded on achievement of their purpose.

Stevens advocated the use of groups for management and stated that they can greatly increase productivity when used effectively. Nurse managers need to be able to function in groups to promote problem-solving and acceptance of responsibility. The group can function within an administrative council and demonstrate its ability to manage itself by preparing agendas, reviewing status of agenda topics, obtaining and using learning aids, and handling meetings. In short, it is possible to structure the business of groups and to direct and control the behavior of group members.[3]

Fuszard and Bishop use the term *adhocracy* to refer to the use of ad hoc committees in nursing organizations. They credit Toffler with originating the term. Applying adhocracy to nursing, a group would be formed to accomplish a specified mission, after which it would be dissolved. It could be called a *task force*, a *project team*, or an *ad hoc committee*. Team members would be those nurses with the special qualifications needed to accomplish the task.[4]

> In nursing, a project team would form around each patient, each member chosen for special expertise relevant to the patient's unique needs. The team would exist as a group only for a single patient. Its members would solve problems, share expertise, make decisions, implement these decisions, and evaluate their effectiveness, using open-systems feedback to monitor and modify the treatment plan. Once the project is completed and the patient discharged, the group of experts would disband to assume roles in other projects needing such expertise.[5]

Benefits of Committees

Committees can transmit useful information in two directions—toward administrators or managers and toward employees. They encourage and involve participation of interested or affected employees in the management of the nursing enterprise. Their advice can be helpful, and they can promote understanding of objectives and programs by other employees. They can promote loyalty. Some of the new ideas that keep nursing an open sociotechnical system come from committees. Committees provide face-to-face meeting of individuals for the purposes of gathering information, seeking advice, making decisions, negotiating, coordinating, and thinking creatively to resolve operational problems and improve the quality of services rendered by the organization.

Committees provide a pool of people with specific skills and knowledge that can be assimilated into plans of action. They can bridge gaps between departments or units. They can use the pooled expertise of specialists and people with special talents and leadership abilities. They give people an opportunity to participate in the social process of group dynamics. They can help reduce resistance to change. Supervision, control, and discipline can be reduced through committee activities. Care quality can be improved, personnel turnover reduced, and harmony promoted through committee work.

All of the positive or beneficial outcomes of committees can be achieved if the committees are appropriately organized and led. Otherwise, committees become liabilities to the organizing process by wasting time and money, deferring decisions or providing wrong information for the making of decisions, promoting too many compromises and stagnation, or using administrators to avoid decision-making.

Organization of Committees

Every committee should have a purpose and short-range objectives, and every standing committee should have long-range objectives. Objectives need to be translated into plans of action with time frames and precise responsibility. Assignments should be given well in advance of the meeting so that presentations are ready at the time of the meeting. Committee chairs are accountable to a specific administrator, who provides guidance to them through consultation. Committee members should be chosen according to their expertise and their capacity to represent the larger group. Committees should be of manageable size for discussion and disagreement. They should have prepared agendas and effective chairs. Exhibit 15-1 contains standards for evaluating nursing committees.

Nursing should be represented on most health care institution committees and always on those whose activities will affect nursing. It should have representation that will be effective in determining the outcomes of a health team approach to patient care services. In effect, nurses should determine how they will practice nursing. The organizational standards presented in Appendix 15-1 meet the goals of shared governance.

Group Dynamics

Each member of a group plays a role in achieving the work of the group. Since each member has a unique personality and individual abilities, the group leader needs to know how groups function to facilitate effectiveness. Original studies of group dynamics were done through observations of informal groups. The Hawthorne studies of 1924–1932 were conducted in four phases designed to discover what would make workers increase their output. The results of the studies indicate that employees respond to identification with their groups and to the interpersonal relationships with members of their small groups by increasing their output.

Through interpersonal relationships, group members perform task roles, group-building and maintenance roles, and individual roles. In the performance of these roles, the group members share the power of the organization and its management.

EXHIBIT 15-1
Standards for Evaluating Nursing Committees

1. The committee has been established by appropriate authority: by laws, executive appointment, or other.
2. Each committee has a stated purpose, objectives, and operational procedures.
3. There is a mechanism for consultation between chairs and persons to whom they report.
4. Each committee meeting has a published agenda.
5. Committee members are surveyed beforehand to obtain agenda items, including problems, plans, and sharing of news.
6. Each committee has an effective chair.
7. Recorded minutes of each committee's meetings are used to evaluate the committee's effectiveness in meeting stated objectives.
8. Committee membership is manageable and representative of the expertise needed and the people affected.
9. Nurses are adequately represented on all appropriate institutional committees.

Group Task Roles

Each member of a group performs a role related to the task of the group or committee to arrive cooperatively with the other group members at a definition of and solution to a common problem. Benne and Sheats identify twelve group task roles, each of which may be performed by a group member or by the leader; one person may perform several roles. These roles are as follows[6]:

1. Initiator–contributor, a group member who proposes or suggests new group goals or redefines the problem. (This may take the form of new procedures or group restructuring. There may be more than one initiator–contributor functioning at different times within the group's lifetime.)
2. Information seeker, a group member who seeks a factual basis for the group's work.
3. Opinion seeker, a group member who seeks opinions that reflect or clarify the values of other members' suggestions.
4. Information giver, a group member who gives an opinion indicating what the group's view of pertinent values should be.
5. Elaborator, a group member who suggests by example or extended meanings the reason for suggestions and how they could work.
6. Opinion giver, a group member who states personal beliefs pertinent to the group discussion.
7. Coordinator, a group member who clarifies and coordinates ideas, suggestions, and activities of the group members or subgroups.
8. Orienter, a group member who summarizes decisions or actions and identifies and questions differences from agreed-on goals.
9. Evaluator critic, a group member who compares and questions group accomplishments and compares them to a standard.
10. Energizer, a group member who stimulates and prods the group to act and to raise the level of their actions.
11. Procedural technician, a group member who facilitates the group's action by arranging the environment.
12. Recorder, a group member who records the group's activities and accomplishments.

Group-Building and Maintenance Roles

Individual members of the group work to build and maintain group functioning. Again, each role may be performed by a group member or by the leader, and one person may perform several roles. The following are the seven group-building roles[7]:

1. Encourager, a group member who accepts and praises the contributions, viewpoints, ideas, and suggestions of all group members with warmth and solidarity.
2. Harmonizer, a group member who mediates, harmonizes, and resolves conflicts.
3. Compromiser, a group member who yields his or her position within a conflict.
4. Gatekeeper and expediter, a group member who promotes open communication and facilitates participation to involve all group members.
5. Standard setter or ego ideal, a group member who expresses or applies standards to evaluate group processes.
6. Group-observer and commentator, a group member who records the group process and uses it to provide feedback to the group.
7. Follower, a group member who accepts the group members' ideas and listens to their discussion and decisions.

Individual Roles

Group members also play roles to serve their individual needs. To keep individual roles from disrupting the group's activities in meeting its objectives, selected group members are frequently trained in group dynamics. This training is particularly important for the group leader. These individual roles are not suppressed but are managed by the leader and the other trained leaders. The following are the eight individual roles[8]:

1. Aggressor, a group member who expresses disapproval or vetoes the values or feelings of other members through attacks, jokes, or envy.
2. Blocker, a group member who persists in expressing negative points of view and resurrects dead issues.
3. Recognition-seeker, a group member who works to focus positive attention on himself or herself.
4. Self-confessor, a group member who uses the group setting as a forum for personal expression.
5. Playboy, a group member who remains uninvolved and demonstrates cynicism, nonchalance, or horseplay.
6. Dominator, a group member who attempts to dominate and manipulate the group.
7. Help-seeker, a group member who manipulates members to sympathize with expressions of personal insecurity, confusion, or self-depreciation.
8. Special interest pleader, a group member who cloaks personal prejudices or biases by ostensibly speaking for others.

All group roles were developed at the First National Training Laboratory in Group Development in 1947. Nurse managers with a working knowledge of group dynamics can use their knowledge to assemble groups.

Such knowledge is important in the selection of chairs of committees, task forces, and other groups of clinical nurses. It is equally important when selecting nurses for organization committees if nursing is to gain power and recognition for its contributions to the mission and objectives of the corporate entity.

Group training will give members awareness of the roles they play and opportunity to manage themselves so that they become more productive. Group training has evolved into a science that contributes to a theory of nursing practice and nursing management. Self-analysis or self-evaluation and development of sensitivity to others to make oneself productive within group settings is a part of these theories. Nurse managers benefit from training in group dynamics and may include it in a continuing staff development program for professional nurses. This can be done through actual role-playing of group missions.

Phases of Groups

Groups have a natural history of development. The following are five generally accepted phases of a group.

1. *Forming or orientation phase.* This is the phase during which group members are discovering themselves. They want uniqueness; they want to belong while maintaining personal identity. They test each other for appropriate and acceptable behavior. This is the time to exchange information, discover ground rules, size up each other, and determine fit.

When forming these groups the nurse manager will include experts, affected constituencies, people who will implement the solution, persons with different problem-solving styles, and equal numbers of sensing/thinking and intuitive/feeling individuals. The group leader will develop the *explicit* norm of constructive conflict: disagreement, multiple definitions, minority opinions, devil's advocate, professional management, and a "group wins" psychology. *Implicit* norms are avoided because they bring bias to the group process by imposing individual values and beliefs. The leader helps members fit into the group, providing structure, guidelines, and norms, and making them comfortable.

2. *Conflict or storming phase.* During this phase, group members jockey for position, control, and influence. Leadership struggle and increased competition take place. The leader helps members through this phase, assisting with roles and assignments.

3. *Cohesion or norming phase.* Roles and norms are established, with a move toward consensus and objectives. Members reach a common understanding of the true nature of the opportunity to reach the group's goals. They will diagnose the root cause of the problem, the deviation from expected performance. They

will be open to alternative definitions with multiple views. Morale and trust improve, and the negative is suppressed. The leader guides and directs as needed.

4. *Working or performing phase.* Members work with deeper involvement, greater disclosure, and unity. They complete the work. The leader may intervene as needed.

5. *Termination phase.* Once goals are fulfilled, the group terminates. The leader guides the members to summarize discussions, express feelings, and make closing statements. The group is reluctant to break up. A celebration can help.[9]

Group Cohesiveness

Group cohesiveness includes the forces (bundle of properties) acting on the members of a group to preserve group integrity. These forces deal with and overcome disruption and conflict. Among the forces are such beliefs as the power of influence of the group, the personality of individual members of the group, and the mission or goals of the group. Cohesiveness is demonstrated by mutual understanding and support, improvements in self-esteem, and successful completion of the mission and goals of the group. Cohesive groups have a positive valence, the combination of members' inputs leading to a strengthening of group processes and outcomes.[10]

Knowledge of group dynamics is needed by nurse managers to improve leadership competencies and facilitate group discussion and communication. Groups are a common feature of a majority of experiences of all nurses in such roles as outcome management, team coordination, and teaching of students and patients and families.[11]

Selected Group Techniques

A number of group techniques have been developed to make groups effective and productive. Among these are the Delphi technique, brainstorming, the nominal group technique, and focus groups.

Delphi Technique

Originally developed by the Rand Corporation as a technological forecasting technique, the Delphi technique pools the opinion of experts. This technique can be used in nursing management to pool the opinions of a group of leaders in the field. Each round of questioning has three phases. For example, the group is polled for input, which is analyzed, clarified, and codified by the investigator and given as feedback to the experts; the experts are polled for further commentary on the composite of the first round. This process can continue for three to five rounds. See Exhibit 15-2 for an example of a format for round one of a Delphi technique.[12]

Members of the group using the Delphi technique may never have the opportunity to meet personally, since most of the activities are done through correspondence or electronically.

Brainstorming

As a group technique, brainstorming seeks to develop creativity by free initiation of ideas. The object is to elicit as many ideas as possible. The following are the steps in the brainstorming technique:

1. The leader instructs the group, giving the leader the topic or problem and telling him or her to respond

---

EXHIBIT 15–2
Delphi Technique, Round One

	Desirability			Feasibility			Timing probability (year by which probable event will have occurred)		
	High	Average	Low	High	Likely	Unlikely	10%	50%	90%
1. Case management will become dominant in nursing in a majority of hospitals.									
2. A majority of hospitals will have unbundled the hospital bill to cost and charge nursing services.									

Source: Adapted from R. M. Hodgetts. *Management: Theory, Process and Practice*, 5th ed. (Orlando, FL: Harcourt Brace, 1990), 286. Reprinted with permission.

positively with any ideas or suggestions relative to it. No critical responses are allowed.

2. The leader lists on a poster or chalkboard all ideas and suggestions as they are given and encourages their generation.

3. Ideas and suggestions are evaluated only after each group member has contributed all possible ideas and suggestions.

One variation on brainstorming, the Gordon technique, keeps the subject area general to elicit more ideas. Success depends on the skills of the group leader. A second variation of brainstorming is the Phillips 66 buzz session, used for large groups. The large group is broken down into smaller groups of six members each. Each conducts a brainstorming session for 6 minutes and then reports to the large group.[13]

The Nominal Group Technique

In this technique, the problem or task is defined. Members independently write down ideas about it, trying to make the ideas more problem-centered and of higher quality. Each member presents ideas to the group without discussion. The ideas are summarized and listed. Next, the members discuss each recorded idea to clarify, evaluate, and assign a priority to each decision. The results are averaged and the final group decision is taken from the pool. The process takes about 1.5 to 2 hours and results in a sense of accomplishment and closure.[14] Nominal group technique is a reliable evaluation tool as well as an efficient group teaching technique.[15]

Focus Groups

Focus group methods stem from consumer market research. They do not provide quantitative research but a phenomenologic approach to qualitative research. Focus groups offer descriptions of the vicarious experiences of the participants. Groups of 8 to 12 participants meet as a group with a moderator who facilitates focused discussion on a topic.

Focus groups have been used to develop nurse retention programs. Some of the objectives of focus groups are to[17]:

1. Provide an intellectual forum for innovative solutions to chronic problems.

2. Encourage a specific communication process whereby a different breadth and depth of interaction, spontaneity, and cross-fertilization can occur, allowing participants to pick up ideas from one another. Ultimately, group ownership of ideas occurs.

3. Allow for necessary ventilation of workplace irritants.

4. Provide an excellent opportunity for management to hear and translate constructive criticism in a neutral, nonemotional environment.

5. Provide an environmental process whereby groups can visualize, define, and appreciate the size and complexity of the problem as well as the solution.[16]

6. Focus groups are used within qualitative research studies as a methodology. Perceptions of members of groups are frequently analyzed using focus group techniques. These perceptions include those about client-centered care, expanded roles of professional nurses, experiential learning, cultural diversity, workplace stress, community population characteristics, substance-abuse prevention, resident abuse in long-term care, and relationships between lifestyles and disease prevention.

The three phases of the focus process are:

Phase 1: Gathering data of internal and external conditions related to the group's objectives.

Phase 2: Designing the study—type and size of sample, group discussion method, and focus group format. Identify three to four groups of 8 to 12 participants. During this phase, the role of moderator is defined and the script is developed.

Phase 3: Implementing the plan and providing participant confidentiality.[18]

Group Leaders

Group leaders may be formal, informal, or specialized. Formal leaders are appointed by management or elected by management directive; they carry line authority and the power to discipline and control group members. Informal leaders emerge from the group process. Their influence inspires cooperation and mediation, and group members reach consensus about their contributions to the effective functioning of the group in their quest of goals. Specialized leaders are often temporary leaders who have a special skill or ability that is needed by the group at a particular point in time.

Participative management requires commitment of individuals to work toward shared goals as well as profitability. A dynamic leader inspires people to put spirit into working for a shared goal. The leader can use symbols, posters, slogans, T-shirts, and memorable events. The leader must believe in people and support a theory of leadership that espouses self-direction, self-control, commitment, responsibility, imagination, ingenuity, creativity, and effort. How the leader behaves toward peer group members will demonstrate these beliefs.[19] Leaders can make committees and meetings effective by having an extensive knowledge of group dynamics. They will keep the group on course by convincing each member of the genuine need for input and by personal sensitivity to group processes. They will draw in the shy and the quiet. They will politely cut off the garrulous and protect the weak. While controlling the squashing reflex in themselves, they will encourage a clash of ideas by mitigating domination by cliques. They will refrain from being judgmental. Being a group leader requires a thinking, skilled performance based on knowledge and ability acquired through management education and training.[20]

To influence people you must be viewed as having power. Power to influence groups includes[21]:

1. Preparing prior to the meeting.
2. Dressing to influence, to be included, and to the next level position.
3. Being aware of body language such as posture, facial expression, arm position, and eye contact. Noting attention, messages being received, and agreement.
4. Touching people on the forearm or the back of the hand to transmit confidence, reassurance, praise, and security. Saying the person's name.
5. Using space expansion—greater height, raised head, standing position.
6. Planning meetings for your own office, or seating yourself at the 1 o'clock position in relation to the leader.
7. Being attentive. Listening for information, concerns, and emotional overtones. Clarifying and repeating to verify.
8. Overcoming resistance to new ideas by giving others ownership, proposing new ideas in a What-would-happen-if? framework; developing a Yes pattern; being an initiator.
9. Speaking clearly and with enthusiasm. Using declarative sentences. Tape recording and evaluating your speech within a group.
10. Learning how to negotiate. Going for win–win results, giving deadlines for completing tasks, and getting concession even after the final negotiation.

Williams lists ten commandments for group leaders[22]:

1. Thou shalt consider the type of group best suited to tackle thy task: advisory, small project team of experts, larger brainstorming group.
2. Thou shalt know thy communication style and its strengths and weaknesses.
3. Thou shalt choose thy members wisely: knowledge, intelligence, motivation, and personality style.
4. Thou shalt be the champion for the group's task.
5. Thou shalt get a few things straight among participants before proceeding: regular meetings, mission, authority.
6. Thou art empowered to demand things of thy participants (without being dictatorial!).

7. Thou shalt have thy logistical house in order before any meeting: necessity for meeting, next activity, agenda with differentiation among presentation, discussion, and decision items, out two days in advance, set start and finish times, guests to be invited, and recorder. Stick to the agenda and summarize all actions and decisions before adjourning.
8. Thou shalt keep thy members and interested parties thoroughly apprised of the progress of thy group toward completion of the tasks: minutes within two days.
9. Thou shalt act as consensus-builder, not lord-high executioner: reach a decision that all members fully support.
10. Thou shalt promote mutual respect and discourage personal attacks among thy members: encourage all members and never belittle anyone.

In one example, a unit manager decided to use group problem-solving techniques to solve the problem of "lack of documented teaching." Group members indicated they felt unprepared to teach, lacked a uniform method of documentation, were uncomfortable with patients' responses, and were bothered by many interruptions. As a result of brainstorming this problem, the assistant unit managers developed, directed, and did inservice teaching on a one-on-one basis. Documentation was done in the nurses' notes. Compliance for documented teaching increased from 89% to 97% as measured the month before and the month after the inservice education.[23]

Making Committees Effective

Purposes of Committees

Organizations, through meetings, promote communication. In one year the cost of meetings in U.S. companies is several billion dollars and executives spend as much as 60% of their time in meetings. For this reason, nurse managers should evaluate the purposes and functions of committees, particularly of standing committees. Evaluation should be both normative and summative and should determine whether committees are accomplishing their purpose or are wasting the time and talents of many people who are required to attend the meetings. Are unnecessary meetings being held?

Meetings fulfill deep personal and individual needs. Their effective use by groups improves productivity. Types of committees are determined by organizational objectives and functions. Committees can be effectively used to implement major policy changes, to accomplish a job, and to plan strategically. Problems requiring research and planning are better assigned to individuals. Day-to-day decisions should be handled by line managers.[24]

A major purpose of using groups or committees is to involve personnel in participatory management that gives representation of employees at all levels a share in the decision-making process. According to Dixon, this goal can be accomplished by having[25]:

1. Enough groups to ensure representation at all levels.
2. Standing committees, ad hoc committees, town hall meetings, and small meetings so that all levels feel represented.
3. Representation by visible managers to ensure support.
4. Control of employees.
5. Planned absence of managers at selective meetings to encourage discussion.
6. Stimuli to employee participation with tangible results.
7. Members solicited as volunteers, appointed by managers, or selected by employees.
8. Technical assistance to identify problems, promote communication, and solve problems.
9. A focus on the power of the group to act on its own recommendations, have its own budget, or access company resources.

American health care organizations are confronted with a hostile and turbulent environment of expanded demands, inflation, competition, shortages of professional nurses at times, and intrusion by other groups. Professional nurses are more highly educated and have higher expectations for extrinsic reward and intrinsic satisfiers such as autonomy and challenge. They want to participate and to impact organizational performance and employee satisfaction positively.

Mohrman and Ledford's recommendation for successful employee participation can be used by nurse managers. Success depends on design and implementation of the participation group process. Participation groups are designed to[26]:

1. Be effective in group problem-solving.
2. Be effective within the larger organization as well as within the division or unit of nursing. This can be expanded to include appropriate professional and service organizations.
3. Achieve legitimacy.
4. Acquire resources and approval for their ideas.
5. Motivate others in the organization to accept, implement, and support their group solution.

Advantages of Committees

In addition to allowing for participation in decision-making, committees allow for group deliberations and coordination. Research comparing two groups of interviewees in a public employment agency has shown that the more competitive the group, the less productive it is.

On the other hand, in the more competitive group, the more competitive the individuals, the more productive they are. A cohesive group reduces anxiety, curbs competitive tendencies, fosters friendly personal relationships, and makes the group more productive. Personnel ratings that focus on production records increase anxiety and decrease cohesiveness and productivity. Supervisors who decrease employee anxiety and increase employee cohesiveness will increase efficiency and productivity. This model could be used in nursing management research on group effect on productivity.[27]

Another advantage of committees is their use as a medium of communication. Committees should not, however, supplant such communication techniques as personal executive action, written communications, individual and conference telephone calls, audio tapes, and closed-circuit television.

Meetings also provide an opportunity for managers to relate to employees. They provide a variety of input and a collective depth of knowledge on which to make quality decisions. Meetings bring together people who advance more approaches to a problem. They blend concrete experiences, reflective observations, active experiments, and abstract conceptualization. Through group dynamics, committees increase acceptance of solutions and commitment to implementation of their decisions. Also, groups take risks.[28]

Disadvantages of Committees

Committees can waste time. Attendees become cynical, often benefiting more from the recreational than the educational aspects of a meeting. Committees do not always use the organization's own experience in a meaningful way. This can be remedied by using organizational personnel and events as part of the program.[29]

Participants complain that committee meetings and conferences do not allow enough individual input, lead to compromise, are expensive, sometimes have weak leaders who are dominated by other members, and act as substitutes for weak executives who cannot make decisions. If not trained, committee participants may arrive at premature decisions, especially those that are popular with a majority of members, and they may not change decisions when better approaches are found. Without trained leadership, committees can be dominated by one person, suffer disruptive conflicts, and be tormented by individuals who must win at all costs.[30]

Improving Committee Effectiveness

Nurse managers can improve the effectiveness of standing and ad hoc committees by establishing minimal ground rules, including the following[31]:

1. Establish clearly stated objectives. For ad hoc or specialized meetings, discuss the goals before planning the meetings. Base the goals on advancing the clinical and business goals of nursing. See Appendix 15-1.
2. Establish a committee structure to support the clearly stated objectives (see Exhibit 15-3).
3. Plan all meetings and events to meet the goals and objectives.
   a. Keep the committee or event at a manageable size. Define membership. *Assemblies* begin at 100 and increase in size. They observe and listen but may have little participation. *Councils* comprise 40 to 50 persons who listen or comment. *Committees* should include approximately 10 to 12 persons who all participate on an equal footing.
   b. Draw up a point-by-point agenda and send it to the attendees. Include the purpose of the meeting. Since the sequence of the agenda is important, the following points are helpful:
      (i) Put dull items early and "star" items last.
      (ii) Decide whether to place divisive items early or late.
      (iii) Plan a time for starting important items.
      (iv) Limit committee meetings to 2 hours or less.
      (v) Schedule meetings to begin 1 hour before lunch or 1 hour before the end of the workday.
      (vi) Avoid extraneous business on the agenda.
      (vii) Read the agenda and write in comments before the meeting.
   c. Tailor the meeting room to the group and prepare it beforehand.
   d. Prepare for the meeting by learning the subject matter and by preparing audiovisual materials to support it. Bring input via videotaped interviews from people who do not attend. Make events memorable.
   e. Time the agenda items. New or controversial subjects usually take more time. Attention spans diminish after the first hour. Use time efficiently, including mealtimes.
   f. Referee and set the pace of the meeting. Summarize and clarify as needed.
   g. Promote lively participation by involving attendees in the program with a warm-up getting-acquainted phase, a conflict phase, and a total collaboration phase. Bring out the personal goals of the individuals.
   h. Listen to what others say so there will be a sharing of knowledge, experience, judgments, and folklore.
   i. Bring the meeting to a definite conclusion by obtaining decisions and commitments.

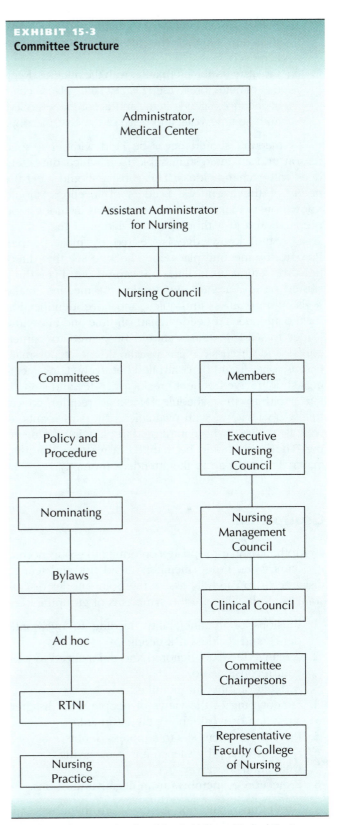

EXHIBIT 15-3
Committee Structure

Source: Courtesy University of South Alabama Medical Center, Mobile, Alabama.

j. Follow up as necessary to eliminate loose ends. Evaluate whether the meeting's purpose was achieved.

k. Circulate useful information with the minutes. Keep the minutes brief, listing time, date, place, chair, attendance, agenda items and action, time ended, and the time, date, and place of the next meeting.

A meeting should never be held without a solid reason and an interesting subject on which the attendees will exchange ideas. This subject should meet the needs of the attendees. Leaders of meetings should know how to make them successful. This includes good preparation and a thorough knowledge of the subject area. Useful knowledge is desired by most people. Prepare the meeting place and check to see that directions for setting up facilities are carried out. Everything should be in readiness. In running the meeting, make registration painless and quick, and have identification for the attendees if needed. Start on time and allow the leader to lead. Meetings should be geared to participants, and discussion groups should be kept small. Discussions should be controlled but lively. Long meetings should have frequent breaks for coffee and stretching. Hold to the schedule. Meetings require critical follow-up reviews, with evaluations by participants as well as by those who contributed to planning the meeting. The latter should be thanked in writing. Promised materials should go to the attendees promptly.

Groupthink

Groupthink is inappropriate conformity to group norms. It occurs when group members avoid risk and fear to disagree or to carefully assess the points under discussion. The following are the symptoms of groupthink[32]:

1. Illusions of invulnerability, leading to overconfidence and reckless risk-taking.
2. Negative feedback ignored and rationalized to prevent reconsideration.
3. A belief of inherent morality.
4. Stereotyping of the views of people who disagree as wrong or weak and badly informed.
5. Pressure on members to suppress doubts.
6. Self-censorship by silence about misgivings.
7. Unanimous decisions.
8. Protection of members from negative reactions.

Groupthink will not occur when members are aware of the potential for it. Groups are considered effective when their resources are well used; their time is well used; their decisions are appropriate, reasonable, and error-free; their decisions are implemented

and supported by group members; problem-solving ability is enhanced; and group cohesion is built by promoting group norms and structuring cooperative relationships. The group's leader should teach group members cures for groupthink that include the following[33]:

1. Acting as devil's advocate.
2. Considering unlimited alternatives.
3. Thinking critically.
4. Providing increased time for discussion.
5. Changing directions.
6. Surveying people affected by the problem under discussion.
7. Seeking other opinions.
8. Constructing challenging group measures.
9. Including input from people in the group who do not agree with you.

Quality Circles

Quality circles are a participatory management technique that uses statistical analyses of activities to maintain quality products. The technique was introduced in Japan through the teaching of Dr. W. Edwards Deming after World War II. The concept is to use statistical analysis to make quality improvements. Workers are taught the statistical concepts and use them through trained, organized, structured groups of 4 to 15 employees, called *quality circles*. Group members share common interests and problems and meet on a regular basis, usually an hour a week. They represent other employees from whom they gather information that they then bring to the meetings.[34]

The quality circle process has become widespread in Japan, raising the quality of Japanese manufacturing to worldwide eminence. It involves workers in the decision-making process. Quality circles have spread to major manufacturing companies and to some health care institutions in the United States.

Quality circles are similar to other elements of participatory management. Employees are trained to identify, analyze, and solve problems. Because they are involved in the process, they make solutions work because they identify with ownership. As a result of being recognized, they develop goodwill toward their employers.

Quality circles are effective when facilitators, leaders, and members are trained in group dynamics and quality circle techniques. Leaders act as peers to generate ideas for operational improvements and problem elimination. In the process, all quality circle members reach consensus before decisions are recommended or implemented. Training occurs during regular quality circle meetings and continues during subsequent meetings.[35]

The premise of quality circles is that problems can best be resolved by the people affected and who are usually members of a peer group.

Because quality circles contribute to the knowledge base of human behavior and motivation, the process is important to the development of nursing management theory. This theory will be learned and used by nurse managers concerned with developing job satisfaction for professional nurses who deliver quality nursing care. The objects of quality circles are participation, involvement, recognition, and self-actualization among clinical nurses caring for patients.

Quality circles should meet successful group design guidelines, including the following[36]:

1. Participation groups must include or have access to the necessary skills and knowledge to address problems systematically. All actors in the process need training. Support people participate only as needed.
2. Formalized procedures enhance the effectiveness of the group. Systematic records should be kept and the formal schedules of meetings adhered to.
3. Participation groups are integrated horizontally and vertically with the rest of the organization to promote communication. Accomplishments are publicized through award dinners and publicity in in-house newspapers. Organized higher-level support groups hear the ideas of lower-level groups. All are limited by usual formal and informal communication mechanisms and routes.
4. Groups are a regular part of the organization and not a special or extra activity. They are composed of members of natural work groups. Results are measured in terms of ongoing organizational objectives and goals.
5. Normal accountability processes operate, using the same skills, habits, and expectations as general organizations.
6. Groups manage themselves and are assisted by leaders and facilitators who are peer group members.
7. Participation occurs in such areas as decisions about job enrichment, hiring, training in problem-solving and other management skills, and business conditions, pay based on skill mastery, gain sharing, and union-management relationships based on mutual interests.
8. They require administrative support.

Research indicates that productivity and morale are strongly improved when employees participate in decision-making and in planning for change. It is important that participation include goal setting because it will lead to higher goals and higher levels of acceptance and performance. This research has been supported by meta-analysis. Research also shows that highly nonparticipatory jobs cause psychological and physical harm. *It is an ethical imperative to prevent harm by enabling employees to participate in work decisions.* Mental health is positively influenced by feelings of interest, a sense of accomplishment, personal growth, and self-respect.[37] Nurse managers will use this knowledge in managing clinical professional nurses.

Participation in manager selection by nursing staff increases their support, management knowledge and skills, and ability to write resumes and prepare for interviews. It increases management's knowledge of the nursing staff. It reduces conflict and favoritism and increases the new manager's power. Such participation by nursing staff can be stressful to managing candidates, and it is time consuming.[38]

Among the disadvantages of quality circles are the potential for disagreements between management and labor and resistance from unions. When the group is led by a member of management, it runs the risk of violating the National Labor Relations Act, "if it is shown that the employer has attempted to manipulate or administrate a labor organization." Flarey recommends that quality circles stay away from such topics as wages, grievances, labor disputes, or conditions of work. They may focus on issues such as productivity enhancement, patient satisfaction, nurse–patient relationships, quality care outcomes, charting methods, and delivery systems. Participation should be voluntary. The circle group should not act as an agent or representative for a larger group of employees. Employees should be paid for time spent in quality circles, so as not to violate the provisions of the Fair Labor Standards Act that requires compensation of one and one-half times for hours worked over 80 in a 14-day period.[39]

Quality circles sometimes evolve into self-directed work teams, which may be evaluated by focus groups. Self-directed work teams involve employees in decisions of organizations.[40]

Self-Managed (Self-Directed) Work Teams

Self-managed teams tend to give workers a high degree of autonomy and control over their immediate behavior. Workers are organized into teams on the basis of relatively complete task functions. Workers make such decisions as who will work on what machine or work operation, how to address interpersonal difficulties within the group, and how to resolve quality problems.

The change to self-managed work teams requires training of management personnel who are uncomfortable with the process and find their status and power threatened. Managers have to unlearn traditional autocratic approaches with punitive emphasis and tight controls on the work force. Managers are trained to overcome feelings of threat and resentment to change; to perceive workers as mature and responsible; to believe that workers can train each other; to believe that peer pressure can overcome absenteeism and that a self-managed team gives them time to develop key people; and to believe they can be a resource to team members and a support group among themselves. They will be facilitators who work with the group. Managers can make the transition to new roles with modified behavior and attitudes.[41]

One of the activities that self-managed work teams can do effectively is problem-solving, a powerful service strategy that gets everyone working toward top performance. Employees feel that their ideas and efforts are valued. Once the self-managed work teams are formed, problem-solving may be introduced in five steps as follows[42]:

1. Brainstorming to identify problems. Team members are asked to describe problems they have observed or experienced.
2. Once all problems are listed, team members are asked to vote on paper for the three problems they believe are most significant. The votes are tallied and the most important problem is presented.
3. Brainstorming for possible solutions to the problem. The most promising solution is selected. Team members are assigned to investigate the solution and gather further information to report on later. The meeting is then closed.
4. At the next meeting, the team reports their findings, which are discussed, including positive and negative aspects.
5. The team chooses the solution through discussion and general agreement. Team members share the responsibility for putting the solution to work.

Self-directed work teams and work groups are successfully used to reduce cost per unit-of-service, improve service and customer satisfaction, determine optimal staffing levels, and reduce the number of layers of organization. These teams do tasks that require both technical and management skills, thereby increasing productivity.[43]

Summary

Synergy—putting the thinking power of a selected group together for the most effective outcome—defines a committee's primary function. Committees provide employees with a representative voice in the management of organizations.

A standing committee has continuity as an organizational entity, whereas an ad hoc committee is formed for a purpose and disbanded when that purpose is fulfilled.

Adhocracy represents a system in which a project team exists for a single patient and disbands when the patient is discharged.

Committees can facilitate communication, promote loyalty, pool special human resources, reduce resistance to change, and give people opportunities to work together. They should have purposes, objectives, and operational procedures.

Chairs of committees need knowledge and skills of group dynamics, which can be provided through staff-development programs for all nurses desiring it.

Groups work in five phases:

1. Forming or orientation phase.
2. Conflict or storming phase.
3. Cohesion or norming phase.
4. Working or performing phase.
5. Termination phase.

Group techniques include the Delphi technique, brainstorming, the nominal group technique, and focus groups, among others. Group leaders either are appointed (formal leaders) or emerge from the group (informal leaders).

Committees can waste time if they make a premature decision or do not accomplish their objectives. They can be made effective by application of the management functions of planning, organizing, directing (leading), and controlling (evaluating).

Quality circles have emerged as a participatory management technique that uses statistical analysis of activities to maintain quality products. Quality circles have the characteristics of groups and use group dynamics but are a regular part of the organization whose members are established work groups.

Groupthink, in which the entire committee conforms to group norms, should be prevented by training in group processes.

Self-managed work teams increase participatory management by broadening jobs and increasing employee cohesiveness.

Committees can lead to improved productivity.

APPLICATION EXERCISES

EXERCISE 15-1	Attend meetings of several committees for the purpose of identifying behavior of members in group task roles. Identify the role each member is playing. Write a brief summary of your observations. Do the same for members in group-building and maintenance roles and members in individual roles.

EXERCISE 15-2	Examine the collective minutes of an ad hoc committee. Identify the phases of the committee and link each phase with recorded behaviors. Summarize your findings.

EXERCISE 15-3	1. Use Exhibit 15-4, "Checklist for Evaluating Meeting Effectiveness," and Exhibit 15-1, "Standards for Evaluating Nursing Committees," to evaluate a nursing meeting in the organization in which you work as a student or as an employee.
	2. When the minutes of the same meeting have been distributed, use Exhibit 15-4 to evaluate them. Is there a difference between the actual meeting and the minutes? What is it? How can the process be improved? Make a management plan (using the following format) to improve the committee's meetings and/or the minutes. Be tactful and use a positive approach in your planning.

MANAGEMENT PLAN

OBJECTIVE:

ACTIONS	TARGET DATES	ASSIGNED TO	ACCOMPLISHMENTS

EXHIBIT 15-4

Checklist for Evaluating Meeting Effectiveness

STANDARDS	YES	NO
1. The meeting started on time.	_____	_____
2. A quorum existed.	_____	_____
3. The meeting agenda is on a schedule.	_____	_____
4. The agenda for the meeting reflects the purpose of the committee.	_____	_____
5. The chair acts as an equal member of the group, taking no special considerations.	_____	_____
6. The chair follows the agenda.	_____	_____
a. Dull items are scheduled early, star items last.	_____	_____
b. Divisive items are strategically placed.	_____	_____
c. Important items have a starting time.	_____	_____
d. The agenda avoids "any other business."	_____	_____
e. Meetings are scheduled for one hour before lunch or one hour before end of work day.	_____	_____
f. The chair is well prepared for the meeting.	_____	_____
g. The chair referees, paces, summarizes, and clarifies discussion.	_____	_____
h. The meeting concludes with definite decisions and a commitment to them.	_____	_____
i. The chair follows up on necessary items.	_____	_____
j. Useful information is circulated with the minutes.	_____	_____
7. The chair allows adequate time for discussion.	_____	_____
8. The chair facilitates participation by all members.	_____	_____
9. Items requiring further study are referred to smaller groups as projects. Timetables for results are established.	_____	_____
10. Managers attend meetings when needed to ensure support.	_____	_____
11. Managers plan absences from selected meetings to encourage discussion.	_____	_____
12. Technical assistance is provided to facilitate meeting success.	_____	_____

NOTES

1. D. C. Mosley, P. H. Pietri, Jr., and L. C. Megginson, *Management: Leadership in Action*, 5th ed. (New York: HarperCollins, 1996), 456.

2. E. Mayo, *The Human Problems of Industrial Civilization* (Boston: Harvard Business School, 1946).

3. B. J. Stevens, "Use of Groups for Management," *Journal of Nursing Administration* (January 1975), 14–22.

4. B. Fuszard and J. K. Bishop, "'Adhocracy' in Health Care Institutions," in *Self-Actualization for Nurses*, ed. B. Fuszard (Rockville, MD: Aspen, 1984), 90–99.

5. Ibid.

6. K. D. Benne and P. Sheats, "Functional Roles of Group Members," *Journal of Social Studies* (winter 1948), 41–49.

7. Ibid.

8. Ibid.

9. L. L. Northouse and P. G. Northouse, *Health Communication: A Handbook for Health Professionals* (Englewood Cliffs, NJ: Prentice-Hall, 1985); H. J. Brightman and P. Verhowen, "Running Successful Problem Solving Groups," *Business* (April–June 1986), 15–23.

10. L. S. Beeber and M. H. Schmitt, "Cohesiveness in Groups: A Concept in Search of a Definition," *Advances in Nursing Science* (January 1986), 1–11.

11. J. Tipping, R. F. Freeman, and A. R. Rachlis, "Using Faculty and Student Perceptions of Group Dynamics to Develop Recommendations for PBL Training," *Academic Medicine* (November 1995), 1050–1052; S. H. Cook and H. Matheson, "Teaching group Dynamics: A Critical Evaluation of an Experiential Programme," *Nursing Education Today* (February 1997), 31–38; J. W. Krejci and S. Malin, "Impact of Leadership Development on Competencies," *Nursing Economic$* (September–October 1997), 235–241; R. Abusabha, J. Peacock, and C. Achterberg, "How to Make Nutrition Education More Meaningful Through Facilitated Group Discussions," *Journal of the American Dietetic Association* (January 1999), 72–76.

12. R. M. Hodgetts, *Management: Theory, Process and Practice*, 5th ed. (Orlando, FL: Harcourt Brace 1990), 286.

13. D. C. Moseley et al., op. cit., 197.

14. L. L. Northouse and P. G. Northouse, op. cit., 240–241.

15. G. Lloyd-Jones, S. Fowell, and J. G. Bligh, "The Use of the Nominal Group Technique as an Evaluative Tool in Medical Undergraduate Education," *Medical Education* (January 1999), 8–13; R. C. Swansburg, "Nominal Group Technique," in *Innovative Teaching Strategies in Nursing*, 2nd ed., ed. B. Fuszard (Gaithersburg, MD: Aspen 1995), 93–100.

16. M. B. DesRosier and K. C. Zellers, "Focus Groups: A Program Planning Technique," *Journal of Nursing Administration* (March 1989), 20–25.

17. S. Ekblad, A. Marttila, and M. Emilsson, "Cultural Challenges in End-of-Life Care: Reflections from Focus Groups' Interviews with Hospital Staff in Stockholm," *Journal of Advanced Nursing* (March 2000), 623–630; D. J. Corring and J. V. Cook, "Client-Centered Care Means That I Am a Valued Human Being," *Canadian Journal of Occupational Therapy* (April 1999), 71–82; M. Hind, D. Jacjson, C. Andrewes, P. Fulbrook, K. Galvin, and S. Frost, "Exploring the Expanded Role of Nurses in Critical Care," *Intensive Critical Care Nursing* (June 1999), 147–153; B. J. Dewar and E. Walker, "Experiential Learning: Issues in Supervision," *Journal of Advanced Nursing* (December 1999), 1459–1467; J. L. Dreachslin, "Conducting Effective Focus Groups in the Context of Diversity: Theoretical Underpinnings and Practical Implications," *Qualitative Health Research* (November 1998), 813–820; A. M. Jinks and R. Daniels, "Workplace Health Concerns: A Focus Group Study," *Journal of Management in Medicine*, 13(2–3), (1999), 95–104; E. Hildebrandt, "Focus Groups and Vulnerable Populations. Insight into Client Strengths and Needs in Complex Community Health Care Environments," *Nursing Health Care Perspectives* (September–October 1999), 256–259; H. Reiskin, S. Gendrop, A. Bowen, P. Wright, and E. Walsh, "Collaboration Between Community Nurses and Nursing Faculty Using Substance Abuse Prevention Focus Groups," *Nursing Connections* (summer 1999), 31–36; S. P. Hirst, "Resident Abuse: An Insider's Perspective," *Geriatric Nursing* (January 2000), 38–42; R. J. Lowry and M. A. Craven, "Smokers' and Drinkers' Awareness of Oral Cancer: A Qualitative Study Using Focus Groups," *British Dental Journal* (December 1999), 668–670.

18. M. B. DesRosier and K. C. Zellers, op. cit.

19. N. Dixon, "Participative Management: It's Not as Simple as It Seems," *Supervisory Management* (December 1984), 2–8.

20. L. Caramanica, "What? Another Committee?" *Nursing Management* (September 1984), 12–14; A. Jay, "How to Run a Meeting," *Journal of Nursing Administration* (January 1982), 22–28.

21. T. A. Kippenbrock, "Power at Meetings: Strategies to Move People," *Nursing Economic$* (July–August 1992), 282–286.

22. B. Williams, "Ten Commandments for Group Leaders," *Supervisory Management* (September 1992), 1–2.

23. J. N. Shultz, "Group Dynamics Can Change Attitudes," *Nursing Management* (November 1992), 95–97.

24. B. J. Stevens, op. cit.

25. N. Dixon, op. cit.

26. S. A. Mohrman and G. E. Ledford, Jr., "The Design and Use of Effective Employee Participation Groups: Implication for Human Resource Management," *Human Resource Management* (winter 1985), 413–428.

27. P. M. Blau, "Cooperation and Competition in a Bureaucracy," *The American Journal of Sociology* (May 1984), 530–535.

28. R. L. Veninga, "Benefits and Costs of Group Meetings," *Journal of Nursing Administration* (June 1984), 42–46.

29. R. M. Kanter, "Toward the World's Best Corporate Conference," *Management Review* (May 1986), 7–9.

30. R. L. Veninga, op. cit.

31. A. Jay, op. cit; B. Y. Auger, "How to Run an Effective Meeting," *Commerce* (October 1967); R. C. Swansburg, *Management of Patient Care Services* (St. Louis: Mosby, 1976); R. M. Kanter, op. cit.; B. J. Stevens, op. cit.; B. J. Stevens, *The Nurse as Executive*, 4th ed. (Gaithersburg, MD: Aspen, 1995); H. S. Rowland and B. L. Rowland, eds., *Nursing Administration Handbook*, 4th ed. (Gaithersburg, MD: Aspen, 1997).

32. E. H. Rosenblum, "Groupthink: The Peril of Group Cohesiveness," *Journal of Nursing Administration* (April 1982), 27–31; H. S. Rowland and B. L. Rowland, op. cit.; M. Leo, "Avoiding the Pitfalls of Management Think," *Business Horizons* (May–June 1984), 44–47.

33. Ibid.

34. The theory for quality circles was actually developed by Frederick Hertzberg and W. Edwards Deming of the United States approximately 50 years ago. S. Johnson, "Quality Control Circles: Negotiating an Efficient Work Environment," *Nursing Management* (July 1985), 35A–34B, 34D–34G; A. M. Goldberg and C. C. Pegels, *Quality Circles in Health Care Facilities* (Rockville, MD: Aspen, 1984).

35. Ibid.

36. S. A. Mohrman and G. E. Ledford, Jr., op. cit.

37. M. Sashkin, "Participative Management Remains an Ethical Imperative," *Organizational Dynamics* (spring 1986), 62–75.

38. N. Ertl, "Choosing Successful Managers: Participative Selection Can Help," *Journal of Nursing Administration* (April 1984), 27–33.

39. D. L. Flarey, "Quality Circles and Labor Relations Issues," *Nursing Economics* (September–October 1989), 266–269, 280.

40. T. F. Gilbertson, "Self-Directed Work Teams in Marketing Organizations," *Journal of Hospital Marketing*, 13(1), (1999), 87–95; J. L. Dreachslin, P. L. Hunt, and E. Sprainer, "Key Indicators of Nursing Care Team Performance: Insights from the Front Line," *Health Care Supervisor* (June 1999), 70–76.

41. C. C. Manz, D. E. Keating, and A. Donellon, "Preparing for an Organizational Change to Employee Self-Management: The Managerial Transition," *Organizational Dynamics* (autumn 1990), 15–26.

42. K. L. Seelhoff, "Six Steps to Team Problem Solving," *Hotels* (August 1992), 26.

43. G. M. Brandon, "Flattening the Organization: Implementing Self-Directed Work Groups," *Radiology Management* (March–April 1996), 35–42; D. E. Yeatts and E. Schultz, "Self-Managed Work Teams: What Works?" *Clinical Laboratory Management Review* (January–February 1998), 16–26.

REFERENCES

Baker, K. G. "Application of a Group Theory in Nursing Practice." *Supervisor Nurse* (March 1980), 22–24.

Basford, P., and C. Downie. "How to . . . Organize Brainstorming." *Nursing Times* (4 April 1990), 63.

Blanchard, M. A., L. E. Rose, J. Taylor, M. A. McEntee, and L. L. Latchaw. "Using a Focus Group to Design a Diabetes Education Program for an African American Population." *Diabetes Education* (November–December 1999), 917–924.

Blejwas, L., and W. Marshall. "A Supervisory Level Self-Directed Work Team In Health Care." *Health Care Supervisor* (June 1999), 14–21.

Butterfield, P. G. "Nominal Group Process as an Instructional Method with Novice Community Health Nursing Students." *Public Health Nursing* (March 1988), 12–15.

Challinor, P. "Meetings: The Challenge." *Nursing Standards* (September 1999), 40–46.

Chow, J. D. "Wanna Know a Secret?" *ANS Advanced Nursing Science* (December 1999), 49–61.

Coenen, A., D. M. Weis, M. J. Schank, and R. Matheus. "Describing Parish Nurse Practice Using the Nursing Minimum Data Set." *Public Health Nursing* (December 1999), 412–416.

Damron, D., P. Langenberg, J. Anliker, M. Ballesteros, R. Feldman, and S. Havas. "Factors Associated with Attendance in a Voluntary Nutrition Education Program." *American Journal of Health Promotion* (May–June 1999), 268–275.

Donald, J. "What Makes Your Day? A Study of the Quality of Worklife of OR Nurses." *Canadian Operating Room Nursing Journal* (December 1999), 17–27.

Dreachslin, J. L., P. L. Hunt, and E. Sprainer. "Key Indicators of Nursing Care Team Performance: Insights from the Front Line," *Health Care Supervisor* (June 1999), 70–76.

Eason, F. R. "Quality Circles—A Summation for Inservice Educators: Using Circles to Increase Staff Nurse Participation in Problem Solving." *Journal of Nursing Staff Development* 4(3), (1988), 131–132.

Galavotti, C., and D. L Richter. "Talking About Hysterectomy: The Experiences of Women from Four Cultural Groups." *Journal of Women's Health Gender Based Medicine* 9 (suppl 2), (2000), S63–67.

Gans, J. S., and E. F. Counselman. "Silence In Group Psychotherapy: A Powerful Communication." *International Journal of Group Psychotherapy* (January 2000), 71–86.

Helmer, F. T., and S. Gunatilake. "Quality Control Circles: A Supervisor's Tool for Solving Operational Problems in Nursing." *Health Care Supervisor* (July 1988), 63–71.

Hughes, J. A., and R. A. Pakieser. "Factors That Impact Nurses' Use of Electronic Mail (E-mail)." *Computers in Nursing* (November–December 1999), 251–258.

Hyett, K. "A Meeting of Minds." *Nursing Times* (18 February 1987), 53–54.

Jackson, S., and C. Stevenson. "What Do People Need Psychiatric and Mental Health Nurses For?" *Journal of Advanced Nursing* (February 2000), 378–388.

Kirchhoff, K. T., V. Spuhler, L. Walker, A. Hutton, B. V. Cole, and T. Clemmer. "Intensive Care Nurses' Experience With End-of-Life Care." *American Journal of Critical Care* (January 2000), 36–42.

Leebov, W. "Problems, Plans, and Sharing: A Format for Productive Meetings." *Supervisory Management* (June 1984), 35–37.

Llewelyn, S., and G. Fielding. "Forming, Storming, Norming and Performing." *Nursing Mirror* (21 July 1982), 14–16.

Pitt, S. E., J. D. Brandt, C. Tellefsen, J. S. Janofsky, M. E. Cohen, E. D. Bettis, and J. R. Rappeport. "Group Dynamics in Forensic Pretrial Decision-Making." *Journal of the American Academy of Psychiatry and Law* 25(1), (1997), 95–104.

Roberts, V. "The Head Nurse Meeting: Who, What, When and Where." *Nursing Management* (August 1985), 10, 12.

Sarvela, P. D., D. R. Holcomb, and J. A. Odulana. "Designing a Safety Program for a College Health Service." *JACH* (March 1992), 231–233.

Schirm, V., T. Albanese, and T. N. Garland. "Understanding Nursing Home Quality of Care: Incorporating Caregivers' Perceptions Through Structure, Process, and Outcome." *Quality Management Health Care* (fall 1999), 55–63.

Schmele, J. A., M. E. Allen, S. Butler, and D. Gresham. "Quality Circles in the Public Health Sector: Implementation and Effect." *Public Health Nursing* (September 1999), 190–195.

Smeltzer, C. H. "Brainstorming: A Process for Cost Reduction." *Nursing Economic$* (January–February 1992), 74–75.

Thomas, B. "Using Nominal Group Technique to Identify Researchable Problems." *Journal of Nursing Education* (October 1983), 335–337.

APPENDIX 15-1
Nursing Council By-Laws

ARTICLE I
NAME

1.1 The name of this Committee shall be the Nursing Council.

ARTICLE II

The purpose of this Council shall be:

2.1 To ensure excellence in nursing care which will return patients to their best possible state of health or will enable them to die with dignity.

2.2 To provide a climate which will promote and support the practice of professional nursing.

2.3 To provide a forum for the discussion of management and patient care concerns.

The function of the Council shall be:

2.4 To ensure excellence in nursing care.
   a. Through the development and support of ad hoc committees.
   b. Through the support of USA Standards of Care.

2.5 To develop nursing service employees to their fullest potential.
   a. Through the development and support of ad hoc committees.
   b. Through the support of USA Standards of Care.

ARTICLE III
MEMBER

The members of this Council shall be:

3.1 All members of Nurse Manager Council Group, Clinical Council, Executive Council, committee chairs, and representatives from the USA College of Nursing.

ARTICLE IV
OFFICERS

The officers shall consist of:

4.1 Chair, Vice-Chair, and Parliamentarian
   a. All officers shall be elected by secret ballot.
   b. A majority of votes cast will be required to be elected.
   c. In the event a majority of votes is not achieved by the first ballot, a run-off between two candidates having the most votes shall be required.
   d. Ballots shall be counted by the Administrative Secretary and RTN I.
   e. Officers shall serve for one year and are eligible for reelection for one consecutive term.

4.2 Officers, together with the Assistant Administrator of Nursing, shall constitute a governing board.

4.3 In the event of a vacancy:
   a. The Vice-Chair replaces the Chair.
   b. The Parliamentarian shall replace Vice-Chair.

   c. The new Parliamentarian will be appointed by the governing body.

4.4 Duties of the officers:
   a. The Chair shall work closely with the other officers of the Council. The Chair and other officers shall meet one week prior to each regular meeting for the purpose of developing and distributing the agenda and establishing time limits for discussion. The Chair is responsible to the Council for the smooth and effective functioning of its committees. The Chair is a voting member of the Executive Council and is responsible to the Council for communicating recommendations to the Executive Council. The Chair shall function according to the guidelines established in *Robert's Rules of Order.*
   b. The Vice-Chair shall assume the duties of the Chair in his or her absence and shall serve as Chair of the nominating committee.
   c. The Parliamentarian shall oversee that the Business of Nursing Council is conducted according to *Robert's Rules of Order.*

4.5 Qualifications for office—Must be members of Nursing Council.

ARTICLE V
MEETINGS

5.1 Regular meetings shall be held quarterly.

5.2 The annual meeting shall be held in November, at which time annual reports of officers and Chair shall be read and officers elected.

5.3 Special meetings shall be called by the Chair. The purpose of the meeting shall be stated in the call and at least two days notice will be given.

ARTICLE VI
QUORUM

A quorum of the Council shall be one-third of the membership. The presence of a quorum shall be documented in the minutes.

ARTICLE VII
COMMITTEES

7.1 Policy and Procedures Committee
   a. Purpose
      1. To establish guidelines, policies, and instructions for performance of procedures in accordance with the current standards of nursing practice for personnel of the Department of Nursing. The guidelines are specific and prescribe the precise action to be taken under a set of circumstances.
      2. To annually appraise policies and procedures followed by nurses, and to develop new policies to meet present and future needs.

(continued)

3. To assure compliance between nursing policy and hospital policy.

b. Membership

1. Members shall be appointed from each of the divisions within the Department of Nursing and from the USA College of Nursing. One member shall be appointed from each of the following: Executive Council, Staff Development, and Nursing Resources. Two members shall be appointed from the USA College of Nursing. Three members (one Nurse Manager or Clinical Specialist, one staff RN, and one LPN) shall be appointed from each of the following divisions: Medical Surgical, Maternal Child, Critical Care, and Special Services.

2. Each member shall have an alternate appointed to attend in the member's absence.

3. Members are to be appointed to serve a two-year term, beginning January 1 of each year.

4. Each representative may be reappointed for one consecutive term. Only one-half of the membership shall turn over annually.

c. Meetings

1. The policy and procedures committee shall meet at least six times annually.

2. The time, date, and place of meetings shall be determined by the Chair.

3. Minutes of the meeting shall be recorded and kept on file in Nursing Service.

4. The Chair of this committee shall be elected by its membership.

d. Duties

1. To accept written recommendations from an individual or committee regarding the need for a policy or procedure.

2. Identify independently the need for a policy or procedure.

3. To research the literature and other resources to determine common, accepted nursing practice.

4. To develop policy and procedures statements.

5. To annually review and revise as necessary all current policies and procedures.

6. To report to Nursing Council at each regular meeting.

7. To prepare a written annual report outlining the accomplishments of the committee. The report shall be prepared by the Chair of the committee and submitted to the Chair of the Nursing Council.

7.2 Nominating Committee will meet during the last quarter prior to the annual meeting as called by the Chair. The slate of nominees shall be presented to Council for consideration one month prior to the annual meeting.

7.3 By-Laws

a. Purpose—To review the by-laws of the Nursing Council and make recommendations to the Council for by-laws revision.

b. Membership

1. A Chair shall be elected from Nursing Council following the annual meeting.

2. Members shall be volunteers from Nursing Council.

c. Meetings

1. The Chair shall determine the frequency, time, date, and place of meetings.

2. Minutes of the meeting shall be recorded and kept on file in Nursing Service.

7.4 Ad Hoc Committees

a. Purpose—To provide a vehicle by which specific tasks or programs can be assumed by a committee.

b. Membership

1. Membership shall follow the same format as for standing committees, unless the council decides that a smaller, more specific group, will be more appropriate.

2. Members can be appointed by Nursing Council or the committee may elect its Chair during its first meeting.

c. Meetings

1. During the first meeting, the committee shall:
   a. Define its purpose.
   b. Outline the necessary steps to achieve the purpose.
   c. Establish a tentative timetable.

2. Minutes of the meetings shall be recorded and kept on file in Nursing Service.

d. Duties

1. The committee Chair shall report to Nursing Council during regular meetings.

2. When the committee has completed its task, a final recommendation is made to Nursing Council for approval. Upon acceptance of this final recommendation, the Ad Hoc Committee is dissolved.

7.5 RTN-I

a. Purpose—To provide a forum for the discussion of topics relating to the practice of professional nursing at USAMC.

b. Membership

1. RTN from each unit or area and float pool for term of one year.

2. Any RTN may attend as an observer.

(continued)

3. Adviser chosen by the committee and approved by administration. The adviser is a non-voting member.
4. Officers are chosen by the committee.

c. Duties

1. To identify problems related to professional nursing and recommend solutions to Nursing Council.
2. To disseminate information to coworkers.
3. To review at monthly meetings all approved new and/or revised policies and procedures.
4. To accept and assume responsibility for projects delegated by Nursing Council.
5. To report to Nursing Council at each regular meeting. The report shall include:
   a. Problems identified concerning professional nursing.
   b. Recommendations for the solution of the identified problems.
   c. Progress on delegated projects.
   d. Summary of monthly committee activities.
6. To prepare an annual written report outlining the accomplishments of the committee. This report shall be prepared by the committee Chair and submitted to the Chair of Nursing Council.

7.6 Nurse Practice Committee

a. Purpose

1. To assist in identifying potential or actual problems related to quality of care, recommend corrective action, develop and plan for corrective action, and review effectiveness of corrective actions until an acceptable level of compliance is obtained. An additional charge of the committee is to develop and/or revise Nursing Standards of Care and Practice.

b. Membership

1. The Clinical Administrator for Nursing Practice shall assume position of Chair.

2. The Nurse Practice Committee is comprised of a Registered Nurse from each nursing unit within the hospital.

c. Duties

1. To review and evaluate Quality Assurance monitoring.
2. To evaluate the effectiveness of previous actions taken to improve care based on follow-up and tracking.
3. To plan appropriate actions that will improve the delivery of nursing care and affect patient outcomes.
4. To communicate and implement the planned action and follow-up at the unit level.
5. To identify trends for potential monitoring and evaluation.
6. To report Quality Assurance analysis to Nursing Council at each regular meeting.

d. Meetings

1. The committee will meet at least monthly or as called by the Chair.
2. Each committee member will receive written notice prior to meetings for attendance.
3. An annual written report summarizing the accomplishments of the committee shall be prepared by the Chair and shall be presented to Nursing and Executive Council.

ARTICLE VIII
PARLIAMENTARY AUTHORITY

The business of this group shall be conducted according to the *Robert's Rules of Order.*

ARTICLE IX
AMENDMENTS

The by-laws may be amended at any regular meeting by a majority vote. Any member of Council may present an amendment for vote.

The proposed amendment must be presented to the Committee in writing one month prior to voting.

Source: Courtesy of the University of South Alabama Medical Center, Mobile, Alabama.

CHAPTER 16

Decentralization and Participatory Management

Russell C. Swansburg, PhD, RN

LEARNING OBJECTIVES AND ACTIVITIES

- Describe decentralization.
- Give examples of the reasons for decentralization.
- Define *participatory management*.
- Give examples of the reasons for participatory management.
- Describe activities that promote participatory management.
- Illustrate the advantages and disadvantages of decentralization and participatory management.
- Illustrate the characteristics of Theory Z.
- Illustrate the structure of decentralization and participatory organizations.

CONCEPTS: Decentralization, participatory management, autonomy, vertical integration, horizontal integration, job enrichment, personalization, self-directed work teams, shared governance, entrepreneurship, gain-sharing, pay equity.

MANAGER BEHAVIOR: Appoints nursing personnel to all organization committees.

LEADER BEHAVIOR: Involves nursing personnel in strategic planning to develop and implement appropriate processes for decentralization and participatory management. Measures staff satisfaction before and after.

The U. S. health care system is a $1 trillion industry without a definition of its product. Until population outcome measures are developed and rewarded for, we will not solve the twenty-first century challenge of maximizing health outcome improvement for the resources available.

D. A. Kindig[1]

Decentralization

Description

Decentralization refers to the degree to which authority is shifted downward within an organization to its divisions, branches, services, and units. Decentralization involves the management components of planning, organizing, leading, and controlling or evaluating. It includes the delegation of decision-making power, authority, responsibility, and accountability. Decentralization of these functions represents a management philosophy and reflects the management style of the chief executive officer and the chief nurse executive. Decentralization within organizations varies in degree but is never total. Decentralization also includes changes in organizational structures and delegation of tasks. Decentralization has been driven by changes in reimbursement and quality pressures that have resulted in the redesign of the nursing practice environment, evolvement of the nurse administrator role into the role of chief of nursing practice, and decentralization of acute care to home care settings. Making decentralization successful is a team effort that requires continuous evaluation to achieve and maintain its goals and objectives. Top management bears ultimate responsibility for the success of an organization and the achievement of goals, objectives, outcomes, and profit or loss.[2]

The United States Compared with Japan and Europe

In Japan, when workers are asked who is in charge, they respond, I am! The Japanese style of management is a fad of the present era. Japan has an entirely different culture from that of the United States. The Japanese studied U.S. management and modified it to fit their culture. They have learned to manage complex organizations by using the concepts of Theory Z, which William Ouchi developed after studying Japanese systems and similar management approaches in the United States. The following are the basic management principles of Theory Z[3]:

- Long-term employment.
- Relatively slow process of evaluation and promotion.
- Broad career paths.
- Consensus decision-making.
- Implicit controls with explicit measurements.
- High levels of trust and egalitarianism.
- Holistic concern for people.

Although long-term employment is fast disappearing in the United States, at least one nursing organization has reversed this process. Theory Z has been combined with the Marker professional model. This model is an outgrowth of primary nursing but expands its concepts to encompass the entire professional environment. It is the easiest model to implement on a new unit. There is no nurse manager, just a resource nurse whose function is to remind the nurses they are empowered to act. Committees are established on nursing practice, patient and family education, nursing education, and fiscal accountability. The four basic premises of the Marker model are that nurses have the following[4]:

1. A decentralized hierarchy
2. The ability to function collectively
3. Twenty-four-hour accountability
4. Direct access to clients

Decentralization is a U.S. business strategy that was instituted in the 1960s to aid in the penetration of European markets. Decentralization is considered necessary for the successful management of large firms. Both Europe and Japan have more family-held firms. Japanese firms retain collective, centralized, and strongly hierarchical organizational structures. Managerial reward systems in the United States usually emphasize individual rather than group performance, although this is changing with implementation of self-managed work teams.[5]

The United States has more formal business education schools than do Europe and Japan. European firms tend to provide management education and training in-house. Annually, U.S. colleges and universities produce over 78,000 graduates with master's degrees in business; whereas Great Britain produces approximately 1,500 annually, and Japan and Germany fewer.

The United States produces professional managers who move from firm to firm. Japan has strong patterns of corporate loyalty and long-term employment. The United States has professional associations for man-

agers; management is more tolerant of mergers, organizational development; and new ideas, such as strategic planning matrices, entrepreneurship, and the concept of corporate culture. U.S. firms hire more outside consultants and adopt external management ideas, such as worker representation on corporate boards of directors, flextime work schedules, and worker participation in job design. Organized labor is weaker in the United States than in either Japan or Europe.[6]

When Theory Z was implemented at Chrysler, activities included[7]:

1. Building a cohesive top management team. Members trust each other.
2. Creating a strategic vision, and communicating it effectively. The vision of the future includes a strategy to gain a competitive edge and is exciting and inspiring.
3. Building strong personnel support systems within the organization. Such systems should reinforce the company's belief in its people and permit employees to build broad careers. This will give workers security by committing them to lifelong careers, and thus will provide a work force that is stable and trained. Primary personnel systems will provide for regular organizational effectiveness surveys to monitor the health of the system. Employees will be rewarded by fair and competitive compensation programs, including bonus or profit-sharing plans. Employees will be involved in a broad, formal job selection and placement process. Effective, regular performance reviews will reflect development of employees. Specific educational opportunities will be reimbursed. Every personnel transaction will be viewed as a significant opportunity to encourage, motivate, and establish trust.
4. Creating a participative organizational structure to facilitate problem-solving and consensus building. All employees are motivated to become committed to goals. An outside facilitator may be used. The participatory organization structure can be created by eliminating meddling managers and staff, reducing reporting levels, widening the span of control, and cutting the number of managers and staff. Employees will be given jobs and trusted to do them. Participatory organizational structures are rigid, with agreed-on forms, operational plans, and timetables for action. The managers manage by "wandering around." Proper forums for participation include committees, policy boards, and task teams.
5. Providing leadership. Change requires good commonsense leaders who have strong beliefs in people and are committed to excellence. They will practice group leadership skills, including decision

by consensus. When the leadership team is prepared, it tells the employees where the organization is headed. The leadership will put human, personal, informal, and measured effort into making the system work and keeping it alive.

Reasons for Decentralization

Health care organizations are among the most complex in the world. Because their complexity increases with size, decisions are better managed at the specific site from which they originate. Communication does not have to travel up and down an organizational hierarchy. Sound decisions can be made and action taken more promptly when decision-making is decentralized.

The variety and depth of nursing management problems have increased. Patient care must keep moving; delay in a diagnostic procedure or treatment can delay progress toward recovery and discharge, thereby increasing expense. Staffing is a complicated process that must account for many variables, a few of which are physician absences due to education, vacation, or illness; seasonal fluctuations resulting from factors such as school vacations; the random nature of tertiary care for conditions such as heart attacks, strokes, trauma, and cancer; third-party payer requirements; government rules and regulations related to patients and employees; coordination of multiple activities; increased technology with increased specialization; environmental and human stress; the complexity of managing human beings, including those with dual careers as nurses and homemakers; complaints; quality improvement; and staff development.

The object of decentralizing nursing is to manage decisions in their specific area of origin, thereby facilitating communication and effectiveness. Decentralization also supports role clarification to prevent overlapping and duplication of individual work.[8]

Studies have shown that decentralized decision-making increases productivity, improves morale, increases favorable attitudes, and decreases absenteeism. One could conclude that decentralized decision-making is good for health care institutions because it is good for nursing personnel. Research on the decentralization of decision-making confirms the hypothesis that it enhances job enrichment and job enlargement, and decentralization affects employees' organizational commitment positively through job satisfaction and professional autonomy.[9]

Managers have difficulty believing that complex systems will work better without central controllers. In the decentralized firm the front-line workers seek out information and solve problems, thereby processing much more information. Larger numbers of people use less-distorted information from customers, distributors, vendors, and fellow front-line employees. There is more parallel processing of information, with no-holds-barred communication across, up, down, inside, and beyond official borders. Work teams communicate directly with whom they need to, resulting in cumulative learning and increased readiness. Feedback loops are faster with instant responses. More time is spent problem-solving and more problems are solved. There is higher accountability and less control. Decentralization can be overdone, usually because it is only half done.[10]

Change in the patient care delivery system is made at the unit level in a decentralized organization. Nurse managers as department heads have 24-hour-a-day responsibility. To meet unit needs, staff development is also decentralized, creating the need for better communication. Decentralization among units may be done with a calendar of events or computer bulletin boards announcing staff development activities on a daily, weekly, or monthly basis. The screens can be printed at user units. Communication can also be improved with planning days done on a 6-month basis. Centralized strategies include a master schedule to coordinate equipment, software, books, and subscription purchases and to coordinate forms. Clinical nurses responsible for unit staff development need to have master's degrees including education in teaching techniques and principles of adult education.[11]

Bowling Green State University decentralized library databases and other information services by putting computers in dormitory rooms, an action that has become widespread. Every health care organization will benefit from making all possible electronic information available to all workers on the job.[12] Professional nurses need access to the Internet at their workstations.

Magna International, a large auto parts company, has 75 stand-alone operating plants of 150 to 200 workers each. Magna sets pay by averaging the labor costs of its closest regional competitors. Every Magna worker has a major role in the day-to-day company operations, and every Magna worker receives a guaranteed share of the company's pretax profits. Motivation comes from having a piece of the action. Workers are needed who use empowerment well.[13]

Decentralization will not solve all of the ills of managing health care institutions. To reform the health care system requires collaboration of all stakeholders. Collaboration includes compromise and accommodation. The empirical evidence for decentralization includes benefits of increased job satisfaction and organizational commitment, reduced turnover, reduced role conflict, a clarified relationship between performance and reward, increased productivity, and improved staff performance.

Research indicates "that nurses are twice as likely to be sanctioned for poor performance than rewarded for good performance." Nurses are penalized for participation—it is added to their work load without a time-added factor. Research also indicates that shared governance has sometimes failed because old values of supervision have prevailed. To succeed, end users need to have and control the budget. They decide which decisions they want to input and then give input that is used. Decision makers need training to become proficient in these activities. Managers are trained in group process. Reducing staff turnover costs that can amount to $50,000 to $100,0000 per single registered nurse position will soon pay for real participation.[14]

Unit managers are being included on collective bargaining teams in some organizations, which is especially effective in geographically dispersed business units. Gains include empowerment of unit managers, linking pay with productivity, closer contact between employees, and easier introduction of technical and organizational change.[15]

To decentralize is to empower. Tom Peters suggests the following activities to empower employees[16]:

1. Give production people wide latitude to act when confronting a problem.
2. Take all employees seriously—listen to them and talk and act as if you hear them.
3. Delegate, that is, give ownership.
4. Give high spending authority.
5. Require relatively infrequent formal reporting.
6. Have high standards, live them, transmit them to employees, demand them.
7. Have a crystal-clear vision.
8. Believe in people wholeheartedly.
9. Let employees bite off more than they can chew.
10. Really let go. Do not take back. Give psychological ownership.
11. Love and respect your people.
12. Provide effective leadership and horizontal management to all employees.
13. Act to destroy bureaucracy.

The judgments of experts are no more reliable than those of the people doing the job. More judgments equal more chances of unreliability.[17]

Decentralization embodies the concept of participatory management, including shared governance.

Participatory Management

Implementation of a philosophy of decentralized decision-making by top management sets the stage for involving more people—perhaps even the entire staff—in making decisions at the level at which an action occurs. Both decentralized management and participatory management delegate authority from top managers downward to the people who report to them. In doing so, objectives or duties are assigned, authority is granted, and an obligation or responsibility is created by acceptance. The employee is accountable for results.[18]

In nursing, as in other organizations, delegation fosters participation. A first-line manager with delegated authority will contact another department to solve a problem in providing a service. The first-line manager does not need to go to his or her department head, who in turn would contact the department head of the other service, creating a communication bottleneck. The people closest to the problem solve it, resulting in efficient and cost-effective management. The following sections detail some of the characteristics of participatory management.

Trust

Participatory management is based on a philosophy of trust. The employee is trusted to complete the task, with periodic progress reports and a final review with management. The time and rate of participation should be managed to control stress. The entire task or decision should be delegated as much as possible. Increasingly, professional nurses want to control their nursing practice. The manager can facilitate control by teaching them to make complete operational plans, including structuring priorities and setting deadlines. Such plans provide a documented standard for joint review. Managers who empower and facilitate employee performance communicate trust. This process will demonstrate the employee's capabilities and reveal shortcomings.

Motorola has had a participatory management program in effect since 1968, with almost all of its thousands of U.S. employees involved in it at some stage. These three basic ideas of their program embody trust[19]:

1. Every worker knows his or her job better than anybody else.
2. People can and will accept responsibility for managing their own work if that responsibility is given to them in the proper way.
3. Intelligence, perspective, and creativity exist among people at all levels of the organization.

Commitment

Personal involvement in managing a nursing service requires commitment from the chief nurse and other nurse managers. Managers should be highly visible to the staff, supporting and nurturing them in the process. In turn, the staff should also be committed, a characteristic they will develop from association with the committed managers. They gain this commitment from seeing their bosses out at the production level where patients are being treated, from cooperating with their colleagues and managers in a spirit of teamwork, and from acquiring feelings of accomplishment.

Nursing commitment comes from knowing that the purpose of the organization is patient care and that the managers are working with the nurses to produce that care. Staff share in making decisions and in coming to consensus with the bosses. This experience in participation "turns them on and tunes them in" so that they do not want to be lazy or mediocre or to featherbed. Commitment inspires staff to be industrious, outstanding, and productive. Under participatory management, commitment is elicited, not imposed.

Professional nurses are motivated to develop their human skills, resulting in increased self-esteem. They have a sense of accomplishment and feel that their accomplishments have been supported by management. They feel they are expanding their worth through their work.

Professional nurses demand professional courtesies. When they are not extended, nurses resort to deviant behavior. Additionally, they tend to align themselves with colleagues and professional associations for recognition and evaluation. They also frequently recommend each other for awards.[20]

Goals and Objectives

Conflict resolution is a major requirement or goal of participatory management. Conflict is inevitable when human beings work together, but it is not productive during process or to outcomes. In nursing, as in other occupations, conflict produces stress and results in turnover and absenteeism. Employees can be sensitized to deal with potential and real conflict and to take action to reduce its destructive consequences: fear, anger, distrust, jealousy, and resentment. Reducing the destructiveness of conflict can be accomplished by establishing a climate of openness with procedures for problem-solving, persuasion, bargaining, and dealing with organizational politics. The goal is to reduce adversarial relations, which is accomplished through joint planning and problem-solving and facilitating employee consultation.[21]

A key goal for a nursing organization is to keep itself healthy. Participatory management encourages a healthy work environment. Participation will make maximum use of employees' abilities without relinquishing the ultimate authority and responsibility of management. Professional nurses want to have input into decisions but do not want to do the job of managers. They want the support of managers, to be able to talk with them and to be informed. Without this support, nurses develop anger and hostility, which results in absenteeism and lower productivity.

Goal-setting activities can occur with reasonably frequent performance review and feedback. Nursing personnel bring their goals and objectives to conferences with managers. The process is reciprocal, with the manager and employee together developing goals and objectives that are challenging, clear, consistent, and specific. Nurses and managers will both be motivated, healthy stress will be increased, and undesirable stress will be reduced.

Career development programs for professional nurses help to reduce conflict and inspire loyalty to an organization. Provided with job information, nurses can set goals for themselves that relate to promotion, tenure, and job security. Differences in work attitudes and personal aspirations are recognized. There is less professional role conflict. New employees, who are young and fresh out of college, should be given information about the nature of the organization, current and future availability of jobs, career opportunities and career ladders, and management goals and responsibilities. Managers learn about the professional nurse employees' aspirations and expectations and should help them set a course and monitor it.[22] (Conflict resolution is a major goal of participatory management and is discussed in Chapter 23, Conflict Management.)

The motivation of professional nurses should be stimulated by incentives, which should include financial rewards and recognition for effective involvement. Participation can result in promotion or changes in work assignments. Incentives keep nurses working to achieve their goals and objectives.

Autonomy

Autonomy is the state of being independent, of having responsibility, authority, and accountability for one's work and personal time. Professional employees indicate they want autonomy for practicing their profession and in making decisions about their work. They do not want their decisions made for them by hospital administrators, physicians, or others. They want to be treated as equal partners and colleagues in the health care delivery system. This desire for autonomy has increased as nurses have developed increasingly sophisticated knowledge and skills and have used them with effective results.

Professional nurses want autonomous control over conditions under which they work, including pace and content. Such decisions are often in conflict with management's coordination role, a conflict that can be mitigated by involving professional nurses in delegating coordination of activities.[23]

Professional nurses are willing to assume and accept responsibility and to be held accountable for a charge.

They want the authority, the rightful and legitimate power to fulfill the charge. This authority comes from their expert knowledge and skill, their license, their position, and their peers.[24]

The autonomy of professional nurses is evident in an organization in which management trusts nurses by giving them freedom to make decisions and take actions within the scope of their knowledge. Nurses are thus free to exercise their authority. This freedom is legitimized in the bylaws of their departments and in job descriptions, performance appraisals, and management support of their decisions. Nurses' independent behavior includes acknowledging mistakes, taking action to correct them, and preventing them from happening again.

The professional nurse is accountable for the consequences of his or her actions.

Accountability is the "fulfillment of the formal obligation to disclose to referent others the purposes, principles, procedures, relationships, results, income, and expenditures for which one has authority."[25]

The relationship between responsibility, authority, autonomy, and accountability is depicted in Exhibit 16-1.

To have autonomy, nursing employees should be involved in setting their own goals and be allowed to determine how to accomplish their goals. This principle applies to all nursing employees. When professional nurses work with other nursing employees, they should facilitate participation and input from these groups. This approach promotes interest, trust, and commitment.[26]

A study of nurse autonomy found variations in perceptions of whether the nurses were expected to exhibit autonomy and of whether they were supported in exhibiting it. The typical nurse exhibiting the highest level of autonomy was a female with a master's degree practicing in a clinical administrative role in the emergency room who perceived an expectation to function autonomously to a high degree. The typical nurse exhibit-

ing the lowest level of autonomy was a male staff nurse in the operating room or post-anesthesia with less than a master's degree who perceived an expectation to practice autonomously to a low extent or was unsure of the expectation for autonomy. No change was found in the perceived levels of autonomy from studies done 15 years before. Highest scores were found among nurses practicing in the emergency room, psychiatry, and critical care, areas where institutions and physicians grant the greatest autonomy. Nurses at the master's level exhibited the highest scores in autonomy. Below that level, poor role definition, role confusion, and poor role modeling contribute to a socialization process that encourages all nurses to act the same. Conversely, nurses in administrative roles have clearer role expectations and correspondingly higher scores on autonomy. Apparently, they are not empowering their practice staff to have the same level of autonomy. The authors state that their findings may indicate that "hospitals do not expect or support autonomy in registered nurses."

To foster greater autonomy, nurses need to be included in decision-making, policy setting and financial decisions. They need role clarity and to be educated at a higher level for autonomous practice. Greater attention needs to be paid to role modeling to facilitate understanding of nursing's independent, dependent, and interdependent aspects. When elements are identified within one area of practice that promote autonomy, they need to be incorporated into other areas as well.[27]

A study of graduating students at one university indicated that the students ranked high on individual autonomy. It would appear that lack of professional status is not due to lack of autonomy in individual nurses. Therefore, consideration must be given to the denial of autonomy by employing institutions as the root cause. Nurses probably arrive at their first job with more autonomous attitudes than do women in other industries. Serious consideration should be given to the role that institutions play in blocking nurses' efforts at achieving professional autonomy. Nursing education should address this issue by looking critically at existing programs and working to educate nurses who will be able to claim their rightful professional status.[28]

Other Characteristics

Participation in management should be inclusive rather than exclusive, but it should be voluntary. The climate of the organization, as set by the philosophy of managers, will motivate (or fail to) professional nurses to participate at a level consistent with their goals and desires. Participation is increased by facilitators who are enthusiastic and expert.

The participatory management environment promotes change and growth, fostering originality and creativity.

EXHIBIT 16-1
Interlocking Major Concepts

CONCEPT	KEY ASPECTS
Responsibility	The charge
Authority	The rightful power to act on the charge
Autonomy	Freedom to decide and to act
Accountability	Disclosure regarding the charge

Source: F. M. Lewis and M. V. Batey. "Clarifying Autonomy and Accountability in Nursing Service: Part 2." *Journal of Nursing Administration*, October 1982. Reprinted with permission of J. B. Lippincott.

The professional nurse employee recognizes that conditions can be changed; changes are real; managers listen and are supportive; and suggestions are evaluated and used or are discussed when rejected. In the Motorola participative management program, employees submit "I recommend" suggestions that require posted answers within 72 hours. The answers can be discussed with management, a process that promotes employees' trust of management.[29]

All of these characteristics exact a large investment from professional clinical nurses and their leaders. They are required to put great effort into learning new skills and relationships. Until it is established and working, they face increased ambiguity and uncertainty about the process. They also cope with the psychological pain and discomfort related to changing beliefs and attitudes.

Participation may be temporary when it is specific to a task. It takes time. Because participation involves risk, many people will not voluntarily choose it, therefore it has to be managed for success. Participatory management will not work automatically and will not work in every situation.

Structure of Decentralized and Participatory Organizations

Flat organizational structures are characteristic of decentralized management. Traditional hierarchical structures with increasingly authoritative levels of management frighten employees, threaten their need for security, and make them uncomfortable. Economic events of the past decade favor horizontal organizational structures with no rank, no boss, and no seniority. Flat organizational structures are flourishing. They are increasing management–employee association and commitment and reducing the number of managers and manuals, titles, and executive suites.[30] In nursing, there are reports of the elimination of nurse manager positions, with committees of professional nurses elected by unit staff to manage unit activities. These nurses' efforts are facilitated by the new breed of leaders, who are democratic, participative, and laissez-faire (or free rein), and who involve their followers in making decisions, setting objectives, establishing strategies, and determining job assignments. These nurse leaders place emphasis on people, employees, and followers and their participation in the management process. They are employee centered and relationship centered.

Decentralized organizational structures are compatible with primary nursing. Decisions are made, goals are set, peer review and evaluation take place, schedules are made, and conflicts are resolved by primary nurses. Levels of practice are built into staffing.[31]

Each nursing unit in a hospital is usually as big as other departments, such as the medical laboratory or pharmacy, and should be considered a department on the same level. This organizational structure increases accountability and teamwork. Care, staffing, budget, equipment, education, and environment should be planned to more accurately reflect the needs of the individual unit. Staffing for each unit becomes the responsibility of each department head; floating is eliminated because each unit has its own part-time (float) staff. However, there can still be a central staffing coordinator.

Decentralized organizations call for increased involvement by the staff development department, which can also be decentralized. Each department (unit/specialty) is autonomous, with its own specific goals. Cooperation and sharing of ideas are increased, and goals and output are evaluated. Continuity of care is improved with a single department head and elimination of float personnel from other units. The department head is responsible for the hiring, training, performance, evaluation, and termination of personnel.

Top Management

What is the role of top management under a decentralized system with participatory management? Its role is directed toward results. Top management shares in planning and implementing the program. Because effective controls are needed to monitor performance of lower-level units, top managers use computers to assist in making decisions and developing controlling techniques for decentralization.

In one research study, 18 of 20 hospitals had some decentralization; 77% had some decentralization down to the unit level. The overriding purpose was to increase worker satisfaction. Decentralization resulted in increased morale and job satisfaction and greater motivation among managers and workers. Personnel development, flexibility, and effective decision-making all increased; conflict decreased, along with operational costs, negative attitudes, and underutilization of managers. The work force stabilized and became more effective and efficient.

The study indicated that most managers do not understand the concept of delegation, are not effective communicators, do not concentrate on goals, and do not delegate according to the abilities and interests of their employees.[32]

With the dynamics of decentralization, each unit works with its own budget; job descriptions are clear, concise, flexible, and current; in-service training is effective; performance standards are clear; employee recognition occurs; and accountability is enforced at all times.

Vertical Versus Horizontal Integration

Vertical integration combines decentralization with integration. When businesses and industries decentralize operations into product lines and subsidiaries, each unit maintains its partnership and identity within the corporate structure. Before the advent of the prospective payment system and competition among hospitals, the industry was largely characterized by horizontal integration of departments within divisions. Some examples are nursing; operations related to patient care services, such as pharmacy, physical therapy, and occupational therapy; operations related to plant management, including housekeeping; and finance.

As competition increased, hospitals began the quest to diversify into new markets. New corporate structures that included umbrella corporate management with subsidiary companies were formed. As hospitals struggle for survival they have chosen vertical integration as a means of capturing lost revenues through control of inputs and outputs. Whether all efforts at vertical integration will be successful depends on the market share of products and services captured. Recent studies indicate moderate effects on operating costs as a result of hospital mergers.

Among the objectives of vertical integration are[33]:

1. Conversion of internal cost centers into revenue producers. An example is medical supply and durable medical equipment. Heretofore, hospitals would refer discharged patients to hospital or medical equipment companies to purchase dressings, wheelchairs, and the like. Some hospitals have formed their own companies to sell and rent medical supplies and equipment to ambulatory patients and to other subsidiaries within the corporate structure. Profits go to the hospital subsidiary instead of to the medical supply company.
2. Development of new and expanding markets for hospitals. These include home health care, which was formerly referred to a public health agency or private home health care agency. Referrals have increased dramatically with early discharge of patients. Hospital corporations have also formed health insurance companies such as preferred provider and health maintenance organizations.

From another viewpoint, that of functions rather than structure, organizations have focused on the vertical dimensions of decentralized decision-making. This vertical dimension aims for representation by levels of employees, thereby restricting decentralization to a single function or issue considered to be of primary importance to the organization. Recently, health care has focused on issues of marketing and quality control, in which decisions are made up or down the hierarchy.

Horizontal integration is also important to the success of participatory management. Integration of the decentralized decision-making process horizontally or laterally links traditionally separate functional hierarchies. The objective is to improve communication across functions, with mutually influential inputs from different interest groups whose individual values, objectives, and loyalties have previously been compartmentalized into obstructions to lateral integration. The organizational structure and functions require adaptation to models that will support participatory processes.[34] Organizational integration requires a merger of information technology that reports results for all organizational entities.[35] Health care systems are sometimes horizontally and vertically integrated for maximum service integration, service delivery, patient capture, and medical education.[36]

Process of Participatory Management

In the process of participatory management, professional nurses are involved in making decisions that affect them and in setting their own work standards. This process involves training, changed roles for supervisors, changed roles for unions, and communication. It also involves preparing managers for changed organizational structures. Participation requires the understanding and support of many levels of people in the organization.

As organizations grow, they are frequently geographically dispersed. In hospitals, this dispersion can occur as new services or products are added. Home health care is an example. When the mission is established, it is frequently housed in another building and sometimes in another part of the community. Geographic dispersion tends to result from vertical integration and to increase decentralization.

Health care organizations grow as they establish new missions for wellness, sports medicine, outpatient surgery, freestanding emergency and surgical centers, birthing centers, and auxiliary services and clinics of many kinds. Both diversity of specialization and geographic distribution encourage decentralization and delegation of decision-making authority, responsibility, and accountability.

> **Decentralization tends to increase when organizational growth is internal rather than external.**

As these products and services grow, it is more difficult to manage them effectively from a central office. It is important to have well-qualified product managers and unit managers, particularly when there is a great diversity of products and services.

Hospitals are highly differentiated entities, as are many functions within them. Political differences emerge as each department or function recruits its own experts. Separate functions produce uncertainty; output for one is input for another. Examples of this dynamic are pharmacy and nursing, or the operating room vis-à-vis other nursing departments. Matrix management and project management are systems that aim to improve lateral coordination and cooperation.

Within a hierarchy, participation based on interaction and influence will succeed to the extent that it can operate independently of other parts of the organization. Product management will be done across organizational functions, so managers must attend to the quality of lateral arrangements, including integration of line and staff functions, such as production and marketing or production and education.

Uncertainty is associated with information processing. One function must know how its inputs affect another's outputs and vice versa. The greater the uncertainty, the greater is the need for information. Uncertainty leads to a heavy information-processing load, which leads to differentiation with its subsequent problems and the need for lateral integration. Problems of lateral integration constrain and inhibit participation. In contrast, specialists and experts dominate participatory structures because of their ability to make highly complex technical decisions. Structurally, the optimum conditions for participation include uncertainty plus facilitation of the integration of differentiated interest groups. The participants are approached systematically, and the organization is restructured laterally.[37]

Even small companies are enlisting front-line workers as active participants in rethinking the business, organizing the work, and hiring new employees. Front-line workers are given information such as monthly sales figures and quarterly financial reports. Decentralization and employee participation and empowerment create turmoil. Managers respond with training and coaching.

Some companies hire new employees only after worker interview and approval (along with prospective manager and personnel professional). When teams hire members, the teams need training to ensure that hiring laws are not violated.[38]

Training

Managers at all levels of nursing should subscribe to the philosophy of participatory management if it is to be successful. All managers and employees must unfreeze the present system of attitudes and values. This unfreezing process will require a comprehensive, well-planned training program. Training will promote a sense of job security by preparing everyone for changed roles. Staff members at every level learn the reasons for participatory management, the advantages and disadvantages, and the roles they will play.

Managers might be threatened by the concept of participatory management if they perceive that their authority is being diminished. Their training program will require that their competencies be assessed. This training will include developing managers' abilities to be frank with employees, to be willing to admit to past failures, and to encourage contributions from their workers and be influenced by them. Managers need to learn to deal with justifying the existence of their jobs.[39]

More than one thousand businesses in the United States are involved in some form of participatory management. Many nursing organizations subscribe to the notion of participatory management to some degree. Centralized management and authority are becoming history in the development of the science of human behavior.[40]

Because they have been subjected to centralized, authoritarian management for so long, nursing personnel will need to be schooled in the process of participatory management. This will include training to make input into collaborative decision-making.

In participatory management a complementary relationship exists between managers and practitioners, rather than a hierarchical one. Training is done to prepare staff and prevent insecurity. Availability of managers qualified to function in participatory management increases decentralization. Training of supervisors will focus on changes in their needs as well as their functions. Supervisors will learn to gain self-fulfillment from delegating and team building.[41]

Management training of supervisors will include group dynamics, problem-solving, planning, and decision-making. Such training can occur through conferences, workshops, and seminars. It should be rewarding and continuous to be successful. It will relieve the threats supervisors feel from challenges by employees, from exposure of their weaknesses, from perceived loss of prestige and power, and from "digging in" to keep control.[42]

Changed Roles of Supervisors

Decentralization with participative management means that roles must be redefined and coordinated to prevent conflict. Nurse managers and primary nurses have increased management responsibility. For some, this will mean decreased hands-on clinical responsibility. Supervisors of nurse managers have decreased responsibility for unit management and become mentors, role models, and facilitators. With a flattened organizational structure, some may lose jobs while others have the overall scope of their responsibility increased.[43]

In one experiment in decentralized patient education, all clinical nurses caring for patients became the teachers. The assistant head nurse became the facilitator, that is, the person responsible for planning and developing objectives for patient education programs and for promoting staff interest and participation in all phases. The education department became the resource available to coordinate teaching programs in support of the primary nurse. The advantages of decentralized versus centralized patient education are summarized in Exhibit 16-2.[44]

As supervisors learn to delegate authority, they modify the climate that promotes deviant behavior by giving professional nurses what they want: the authority to manage themselves. Because authority gives the supervisors initiative in performing their jobs and freedom to question managers, managers should expect loyalty in return. The profession of nursing does not employ nurses; organizations do. Participatory management is a process in which there must be an ongoing dialogue with constraints: nurses will control their profession; management uses its input to set objectives and priorities and to review output. Nurse employees cannot control the enterprise, and management cannot compromise the professional or ethical standards of professional nurses.[45]

In participatory management, the supervisor facilitates rather than directs the work force. Traditional supervising functions are delegated downward. There must be clear delineation of managers' basic responsibilities, distinct from their behavioral or management style. Managers can gain satisfaction from their ability to make clinical nurses successful and satisfied. The interpersonal skills and conceptual abilities demanded of supervisors will increase. Supervisors should be chal-lenged and should have a future. Supervisors promote implementation of committee decisions, listen, and offer assistance.[46]

Because fewer supervisors will be needed, career development programs for college-educated nurses must provide them promotional opportunities as clinical practitioners, managers, teachers, or researchers.

Supervisors are important to the success of decentralized decision-making and employee involvement in the management of nursing and the health care system. They should be taught to manage under employee involvement programs. They need to learn that they will have more time to plan and organize work and to be creative. Their jobs can be expanded upward, but they should keep in contact with employees and encourage participation by everyone.

Changed Roles of Unions

Decentralized decision-making and participatory management are not processes that give comfort to unions. Unions may view these processes as threats to their survival and to membership and as a prelude to efforts to decertify. Decentralization plans should include participation by union membership that emphasizes the common interests of union and management. Both entities want mutual trust, quality of work life, and employee involvement. Both want job security for their employees and members; successful participatory management programs give security a high priority.

Some employers will promote decertification of unions while working to bond employees to them through involvement. Others will cooperate with their unions and promote their active support; in this instance, traditional prerogatives of management are sometimes subjected to union influence. The risk-benefit ratio of mutual union-management involvement will have to be weighed by both sides.

EXHIBIT 16-2
Decentralized Versus Centralized Teaching

DECENTRALIZED

1. Utilizes all nursing and health personnel for education
2. Each nurse assumes professional responsibility for patient education.
3. Provides education to maximum number of patients and families.
4. Educator(s) currently practicing in the clinical area. Possess up-to-date clinical skills and knowledge. Usually less formal training in education.

CENTRALIZED

1. Specified individuals responsible for teaching patients and/or coordinating patient teaching activities.
2. Concentrates responsibilities and accountability on individuals whose specific function is patient education.
3. Number of patients reached may be limited.
4. Educator(s) have more formal training in educational approaches. Clinical skills may or may not be in current use.

Source: S. Malkin and P. Luteri. "A Community Hospital's Approach: Decentralized Patient Education." *Nursing Administration Quarterly* 4, 2, (1980), 103–104. Reprinted with permission of Aspen Publishers. © 1980.

The union's role will have to be defined. The goal is good labor-management relations. If they are to play a role, union shop stewards will be trained with company supervisors. There will need to be a memorandum of understanding for keeping grievance and contractual issues outside of the employee involvement program.[47]

Because market-based reforms have paid little attention to changes for nurses, some nurses have turned to union representation.[48]

Communication

Good communication within the nursing organization is essential to an effective employee participation program. Good communication is effective communication; it is evident in employees who are informed about the business of nursing. Such employees know what management is saying and what management's intentions are. Management knows what employees are saying and how it squares with the perceptions management is working to develop. Broken communication contributes to stress and leads to direct economic losses through low productivity, grievances, absenteeism, turnover, and work slowdowns or strikes.

Flat organizational structures promote effective communication. Managers plan the vehicles, content, and intent of effective communication, and they monitor the process. Supervisors are important to effective communication and, as another aspect of their changed roles, work to ensure its openness. Management attitudes should promote truth, frankness, and openness.

Participation enhances commitment and interdepartmental and intradepartmental communication. In medium-sized and large organizations, a communication center will operate 24 hours a day. Message delivery will be facilitated. Computers will be used to communicate instantly, nurse to nurse, nurse to manager, manager to nurse, and nurse to others. Messages will be hand-delivered when necessary.

Decentralization requires a movement away from mainframe information processing toward distributed systems of smaller computers. Doing so increases flexibility and control at lower organizational levels, giving users heightened feelings of ownership of the system. Packaged software then offers fast relief for specific application needs. End user involvement with computer application increases.[49]

With direct communication the middle person is eliminated and time is saved. The problem of missing medical laboratory or radiology reports is taken up between the primary nurse or the nurse manager and the manager of the department immediately responsible.[50]

Increased representation of clinical nurses on hospital and departmental committees improves communication. The goal is to facilitate the flow of information, not embody it in the authority of a management position. Management by objectives, group brainstorming, and quality circles are vehicles of effective communication used in participatory management.

Advantages of Participatory Management

The following is a list of advantages of participatory management as cited by writers in business, industry, and health care, including nursing[51]:

1. High trust and mutual support
2. Eliminated full-time-equivalent positions; fewer levels of management; fewer specialized departments
3. Increased accountability of managers and employees
4. Reduced ambiguity in work requirements for practitioners and employees as a result of improved communication
5. Enhanced role for the clinical nurse; self-supervision; active involvement of employees in identifying and solving problems; encouragement of employee contributions; career development
6. Increased independence of the nursing division
7. Legal clarity
8. Increased efficiency resulting from higher nurse-to-patient ratios
9. Teamwork

In teamwork, people become cooperative and independent as a result of increased motivation and initiative.

10. Improved organizational communication, with nurses being briefed on all phases of the nursing business, including revenues, costs, and strategic plans, thereby increasing employees' understanding of the organization
11. Decreased absenteeism
12. Increased effectiveness and productivity; improved quality of work; higher level of mastery
13. Uplifted morale and motivation at work; increased excitement from fluctuating participation (participation makes work and values visible)
14. Fresh ideas for management decision-making and problem-solving
15. Identification of potential leaders
16. Fostering within professionals a strong sense of identification with employer's goals and objectives
17. Decreased turnover and increased stability of work force

18. Increased commitment as attitudes become positive
19. Less overtime
20. Lower cost
21. Better utilization of professional nurses as participants' skills and talents are discovered and enhanced
22. Increased job satisfaction
23. Recognition of contributions because participation increases individual and organizational capacities to learn, adapt, and develop toward higher levels of excellence
24. Improved quality of care. Also, positive outcomes result from inclusion of family careers in community dementia management
25. Establishment of worker-management ergonomics teams that design and implement changes in training and work practices result in fewer musculoskeletal symptoms as well as improvements in job satisfaction
26. Participation in design and implementation of shift systems results in resolution of shift staffing problems and improved ergonomics

27. Instruments exist for measuring the outcomes of participatory strategies

Exhibit 16-3 is a model of how participatory management works.

Practice and Research

In the Motorola participatory management program, factory-level employees in Plan I belong to groups of 50 to 250 people who set targets and valid standards that measure current cost, in-process quality, product deliveries, inventory levels, and housekeeping and safety. Representatives belong to working committees that review ideas, recommendations, and issues of waste and quality. The committees solve problems and send recommendations to a representative steering committee for review. Committee involvement of workers improves communication. Improved product quality or customer satisfaction is evident in increased sales and profits and results in financial bonuses to employees. In this process, each employee can see the effect of his or

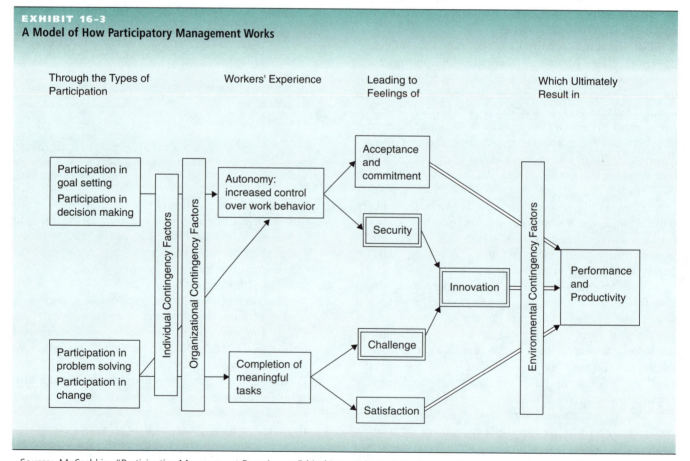

EXHIBIT 16–3
A Model of How Participatory Management Works

Source: M. Sashkin. "Participative Management Remains an Ethical Imperative." *Organizational Dynamics*, Spring, 1986, 64. Reprinted by permission of American Management Association, New York. All rights reserved.

her contributions on the group and feel a sense of accomplishment. In one instance, as a result of the participatory management process at Motorola, a 4% loss of gold went to zero in 2 months. Production volume at one plant went up 33% with fewer employees. Team spirit and a sense of cooperation existed between management and employees, who worked with less supervision.[52]

Research studies have reported greater motivation and satisfaction when subordinates participate in performance appraisal. Research also indicates that mutual goal setting improves performance, increases productivity, satisfies employees' need for fulfillment and self-actualization, and thus contributes to the well-being of the organization. Participatory management develops mature, healthy, self-directed personalities among employees.[53]

Disadvantages of Participatory Management

Some of the disadvantages of participatory management are as follows[54]:

1. Occasional failures will occur.
2. Initiation of programs takes time and money.
3. Policies and procedures must be changed.
4. It is sometimes difficult to determine which responsibilities are whose, even though other ambiguities are reduced.
5. The budget office and other offices or departments have to deal with several units in nursing service rather than a single department.
6. Lacking knowledge of the process, employers do not want it imposed on them. They give excuses such as: employees have too little attachment to the organization, are not interested in work, and have a weak commitment to the work ethic; employees and managers do not get along; employees have a poor assessment of their supervisors; and employees have low regard for organization-wide openness.
7. It is difficult to change management style to true participation.
8. Employees who view management as being autocratic perceive participatory performance appraisal as being insincere, patronizing, and manipulative. The person who initiates it has gone "soft."
9. Self-evaluation is threatening because the employee feels exposed to the views of others.

All of these disadvantages will be overcome by a committed chief nurse executive who prepares and implements a plan with supervisors and educators who are prepared psychologically, politically, and technically. The chief nurse executive selects and develops key people (the human beings developing human beings), works at a long-range future, and is accessible.

Activities Involving Nurses in Participatory Management

Some of the activities that can be used to involve nurses in participatory management are job enrichment, personalization, primary nursing, self-directed work teams, shared governance, entrepreneurship, gain-sharing, and pay equity.

Job Enrichment

Job enrichment satisfies the motivation to fulfill higher-order needs, including variety within and among jobs and a strategy that challenges by emphasizing performance output over job processes. Job enrichment creates jobs with greater responsibility and more flexibility and promotes personal development.

Enrichment requires preparation and careful implementation. By focusing on the whole job, it makes maximum use of and expands employee skills. It includes decision-making authority. Growth from job enrichment prevents apathy, burnout, and alienation. Employees can choose to assume more responsibility for particular assignments. Lateral transfers are supported with job postings and project assignments. Output, not the process used to produce it, is evaluated. Professionals respond to orders from other professionals, an indication that professional nurses will respond best to enrichment programs developed by competent professional nurse managers whose management styles promote participation and involvement. Enrichment works best with hard workers who like to work best with friendly people.[55]

Job enrichment and redesign are related to the employee's needs for learning, challenge, variety, increased responsibility, and achievement.

Herzberg's two-factor theory (hygiene factors vs. motivation factors) is one approach to job enrichment: growth and motivation factors are achievement, recognition, work, responsibility, and advancement. Reducing hygiene factors such as salary, job security, and working conditions, reduces dissatisfaction among employees but does not motivate them.

A job characteristics model structures work for effective performance, personal rewards, and job satisfaction. Job characteristics are variety, task entity, task significance, autonomy, and job-based feedback.

The Japanese style of management practices teamwork, group consciousness, harmony, training, and lateral transfers.

Quality of work life approaches consider tasks, physical work environment, social environment within the organization, the administrative system, and the relationship between life on and off the job.

Job enrichment is affected by the workers' expressed interest. (See Exhibit 16-4.)

How should the organizational structure be changed to accommodate job enrichment? The job clarification plan relates to the new organizational structure. In addition to the job characteristics model described in Exhibit 16-4, suggested procedures for a job design or redesign program include[56]:

- Define the system's goals.
- Define the relevant tasks and activities.
- Interview.
- Define unique characteristics and restraints.
- Cluster tasks.
- List intervention techniques.
- Relate techniques to requirements and assumptions.
- Define the level of implementation.
- Pull into a picture.
- Screen generalities.
- Develop an implementation process.
- Adapt job design and the process of design.

Research indicates that increased job enrichment and increased quality of communication predict the development of greater self-efficacy of employees.[57]

Personalization

Personalization is a strategy that focuses on people and knowledge, not numbers and politics. Those who use personalization stress empathy and involve professionals in making critical decisions that affect them. Career development opportunities are facilitated by advertising jobs, allowing transfers, giving feedback to job applicants, allowing and providing liberal training and development, and promoting based on objective measures.[58]

Primary Nursing

Primary nursing as a modality of nursing care delivery makes nursing worthwhile work, enhances nurses' self-esteem through performing a complete function, produces results of a personal endeavor, and realizes collegial and collaborative relationships.[59] In a hospital setting where primary nursing is practiced, decentralization of patient care delivery systems provides the most efficient nursing care. Primary nurses are accountable. The ideal environment for self-governance is primary nursing with a stable, mature, self-directed, skilled, and committed staff trained in leadership skills.[60]

> A comparative study of highly enriched jobs (primary nursing) and jobs with a low level of enrichment indicated that "personnel occupying highly enriched jobs reported significantly higher work motivation and satisfaction with the management than the personnel occupying jobs with a low level of enrichment."[6]

Other nursing modalities that are compatible with participatory management are modular nursing, team nursing, case management, and collaborative practice models.

Self-Directed Work Teams

A self-directed work team is a functional group of typically 8 to 15 employees. The team shares responsibility for a particular unit of production, including units of service or information. Members are cross-trained in all the technical skills necessary to complete the tasks assigned. Members have the authority to plan, implement, and control all work processes. Members are responsible for scheduling, quality, and costs—responsibilities have been clearly defined in advance. Exhibit 16-5 compares a self-directed team management model with a traditional management model. The nine characteristics of a self-directed work team are compared with those of a traditional work group in Exhibit 16-6. Employers indicate that self-directed work teams improve quality, increase productivity, decrease operating costs, and foster greater commitment from workers. Employees state that they feel "in on things," involved in decisions, challenged, and empowered, and employees also have increased job satisfaction.

Self-directed work teams have leaders. During early phases, the leader is appointed by upper management. As the team grows and changes, it selects its leader. Eventually, the role rotates. The team leader is an internal facilitator. Middle managers are trained to become external facilitators.[62]

Self-managed work teams are empowered to make all decisions about the work they do. For example, Federal Express and IDS claim productivity up 40% with self-managed work teams. A survey of Fortune 1,000 companies indicates that 68% use self-managed work teams, although only 10% of workers are in them.

Quality circles are on the decline because of lack of empowerment. They satisfy the egos of managers who want to retain control. They work parallel to producers of work, not within them.

To make self-managed teams successful employers should do the following[63]:

EXHIBIT 16-4

Job Characteristics Model for Job Redesign

	JOB ENRICHMENT	JOB CHARACTERISTICS	JAPANESE-STYLE MANAGEMENT	QUALITY OF WORK-LIFE APPROACHES (SOCIOTECHNICAL MODEL)
Description	Based on motivation-hygiene theory. Focuses on changes in job content.	Based on job characteristics research. Focuses on job content.	Based on Japanese experience. Deals with organizational, job, and managerial factors.	Based on a variety of experiences in many countries and many types of organizations.
Motivational Assumptions	Two different needs are involved: increasing motivation and reducing dissatisfaction. Factors involved in increasing motivation relate to human characteristics; factors involved in reducing dissatisfaction relate to pain avoidance.	Work motivation is based on three psychological states: the knowledge of results, experienced responsibility, and experienced meaningfulness. These are achieved through five core job characteristics: task significance, skill variety, autonomy, task identity, and job feedback.	Motivation is based on "wa" (teamwork) or family-like norms and the organizational culture.	Motivation is based on jobs designed according to sociotechnical criteria and the capacity of individuals to make choices in designing their work.
Critical Techniques	• Direct feedback. • A client relationship. • A learning function. • The opportunity for each person to schedule his or her own work. • Unique expertise. • Control over resources. • Direct communications. • Personal accountability.	• Combining tasks. • Forming natural unity of work. • Establishing client relationships. • Using vertical loading. • Opening feedback channels.	• Intensive socialization. • Lifetime employment. • Competitive education. • Rotation and slow promotion. • Behavior evaluation. • Work-group task assignments. • Nonspecialized career paths. • Open communication. • Consultational decision making.	• Technical systems changes. • Job changes. • Participation/consultation. • Structural changes. • Pay/reward systems. • Compressed shift schedules. • Training and recruitment. • The operating philosophy statement. • Collective agreement modifications. • Group management.
Implementation Procedures	• Interview to identify critical changes in the person's feelings. • Group results into general motivation/hygiene categories.	• Diagnose the need for change. • Assess motivation and satisfaction. • Assess the motivational potential of the job.	• Concern for employees. • Compensation. • Audit the organizational philosophy. • Define the desired philosophy. • Implement the change. • Develop interpersonal skills.	• Define the need for change. • Obtain agreement. • Hold search conference. • Form action group. • Analyze the technical system.

(continued)

EXHIBIT 16-4 (continued)

	JOB ENRICHMENT	JOB CHARACTERISTICS	JAPANESE-STYLE MANAGEMENT	QUALITY OF WORK-LIFE APPROACHES (SOCIOTECHNICAL MODEL)
Implementation Procedures	• Brainstorm changes. • Screen for generalities, vagueness, and horizontal and vertical suggestions. • Avoid participation. • Set up a controlled experiment.	• Assess particular job problems. • Assess readiness for change. • Implement changes, conduct training, and assess the impact.	• Test. • Involve the union. • Stabilize employment. • Install systems for slow promotion and career development. • Implement.	• Analyze the social system. • Develop design hypotheses. • Implement and evaluate. • Adjust to normal operations. • Implement in other settings.
Implementation Requirements	Worker participation or consultation is appropriate.	Worker participation or consultation is appropriate.	Emphasis on diagnosis or consultation is appropriate. Quality circles require involvement.	Broad-based participation. Emphasis is on "philosophy" of organization with corresponding job involvement.
Job Classification Changes	Many supervisory tasks should become workers' responsibilities. Emphasis is on doing tasks at higher classification levels.	Emphasis is on enlarging the job and doing tasks at the same classification level. Some higher-level tasks may be appropriate.	Requires major changes in job-classification structure, although quality circles may not affect the classification plan.	Emphasis is on the development of a "philosophy" of organization with corresponding changes in the job-classification plan emphasizing teamwork.
Types of Settings or Occupations	Probably more successful with operational/production jobs in which tasks can be defined and broken down.	Probably more successful with operational/production jobs in which tasks can be defined and broken down.	Focus is on changing the management approach based on concepts of Japanese management.	Focus is on changing the management approach based on sociotechnical needs.
Issues	• Criteria of motivation may be questioned. • No role for union. • Relatively easy to implement because of limited scope, although it suggests workers should perform higher-level tasks.	• Criteria of motivation may be questioned. • Undefined union role. • Relatively easy to implement because of limited scope. • Consultational in nature.	• Criteria of motivation may be cultural. • Undefined union role. • May be culturally bound and require value changes. • Attempts to shift decisions to workers.	• Criteria of motivation are based on the situation. • Requires union role. • Implementation requires value changes.
Key Employee Questions	Do workers need more responsibility, variety, growth?	Do workers need more responsibility, variety, growth?	Do workers need more responsibility, variety, growth? Do workers desire to work in teams in making decisions? Do workers see the organization as part of their identity?	
Key Classification Questions	What job design ideas can be implemented without changing the job-classification plan? What job-classification plan adjustments should be made, and when would they be appropriate?		What job design ideas can be implemented without changing the job classification plan? What structural adjustments should be made? How should the job-classification plan be altered to respond to structural changes?	

Source: J. B. Cunningham and T. Eberle. "A Guide to Job Enrichment and Redesign." *Personnel*, February 1990, 59. Reprinted by permission of American Management Association, New York. All rights reserved.

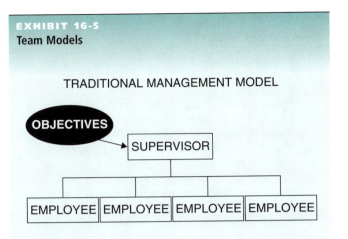

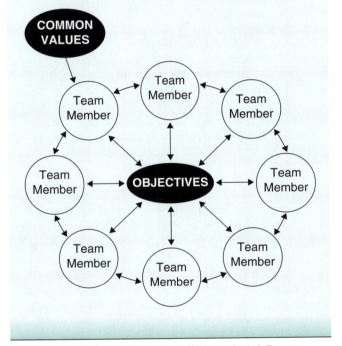

Source: L. Ankarlo. *Implementing Self-Directed Work Teams* (Boulder, Colo.: Career Track Publications, 1992), 5. Reprinted with permission.

1. Empower the teams with decision-making.
2. Provide teams with electronic mail communication systems so teams can talk with each other.
3. Create teams only for work that can be done by teams.
4. Make teamwork the centerpiece of a pay-for-performance system.
5. Inspire teams to increase morale, productivity, and innovation.
6. Use the right team for the right job. Form a problem-solving team to solve a problem; then disband it. Use work teams to do the day-to-day work. Work teams should be self-managed, have power to change the order of things, and have budgets.

TRADITIONAL	SELF-DIRECTED
Top-down	Bottom-up
Unilateral	Consensus
Narrow focus	Big picture
Narrow training	Ongoing diverse training
Move up	Move around
Helplessness	Empowerment
Stuck/complacent	Challenged/innovative
Internal competition	External competition
Work together	Work and celebrate

Source: L. Ankarlo. *Implementing Self-Directed Work Teams* (Boulder, Colo.: Career Track Publications, 1992). Reprinted with permission.

7. Create a hierarchy of teams that make decisions on the spot. To build the 777, Boeing used three layers of teams: A top management team to see that the plane was built correctly and on time; leader teams from engineering and operations to oversee the work teams; and cross-functional work teams. A fourth layer of airplane integration teams with access to everyone in the organization was added later. Problems were identified and solved early.
8. Maintain trust and morale. When restructuring, bring employees into the process. Plan for job loss by retraining, reassigning, retiring, and attrition.
9. Tackle people problems head on by spending time to get people to work together.

Virtual teams are work teams whose members talk by computer, fly in and out of the organization and team participation as needed, and take turns as leader.[64]

Shared Governance

Shared governance is defined as the allocation of control, power, or authority among mutually interested parties. Data supporting reduction in turnover and increases in levels of nursing satisfaction are evidence of successful outcomes of shared governance processes. The principles of shared governance are more consistent with the principles of professionalism than are the principles of participatory management. The following are the main principles of shared governance[65]:

1. Shared governance is not a form of participatory management. Participatory management means allowing others to participate in decisions over which a line manager has control.

2. Shared governance is not management driven. All activities that are neither direct caregiving nor related to that process are in support of it.

3. Shared management has no locus of control. Accountabilities of a role are attributed to the role from within the role; they can never be assigned, nor can they be given away.

4. Models should be based on a clinical rather than an administrative organization.

5. Governance should be representative in nature, not democratic.

6. Representatives should be elected, not selected.

7. Bylaws should provide a system of checks and balances, and they should be passed by a majority vote of the entire nursing staff.

Three models of shared governance are the congressional model, the unit-based model, and the councilor model. All three models delineate four broad areas of accountability: practice, quality, education, and management. Accountabilities of practice include practice standards, job descriptions, care delivery systems, and nursing representation in hospital-wide committees. Accountabilities for quality include practice standards, job descriptions, the care delivery system, and nursing representation in hospital-wide committees. Accountabilities for quality include delineation of data sources, evaluation criteria, evaluation processes, mechanisms for quality improvement, credentialing, peer review, and research. Education accountabilities include needs assessment, incorporation of new standards of research, and evaluation of educational endeavors. Accountabilities of management include provision of resources, including human and financial resources, implementation of council or committee decisions, interdepartmental problem-solving, and facilitation of staff problem-solving, decision-making, and leadership.[66]

Under collaborative governance, managers become integrators, facilitators, and coordinators. Clinical managers are educated in decision-making, team building, group dynamics, goals and objectives development, interviewing skills, budgeting, disciplining, and rewarding. Unit personnel develop policy. Structure is kept informal except for areas governed by law, regulations, and efficiency, in which representative central committees operate. Unit personnel decide whether their unit will be "open" in which case personnel float in and out, or "closed." For the system to work, all unit employees must buy into the system. It takes years to build successful collaborative governance. A successful system is in a constant state of flux and chaos. This system is based on 12 shared beliefs (see Exhibit 16-7).[67]

To prepare for self-management, there must be a committed administration, a prepared staff, time, a will-

EXHIBIT 16-7
Twelve Shared Beliefs

1. Knowledge is power.
2. Given adequate information, people will make appropriate decisions.
3. Individuals are unique in their contributions.
4. A sense of purpose results when organizational and personal values are congruent.
5. Maximum productivity results when organizational and personal values are congruent.
6. Risk-taking, with or without success, is growth.
7. People are honest and trustworthy and will work hard to achieve their full potential.
8. Individuals are accountable and responsible for their practice.
9. All problems identified are mutually owned and responsibility for resolution begins with problem identification.
10. Weaknesses and strengths are the same characteristics used differently. (Weaknesses are strengths in excess.)
11. Our decisions will acknowledge federal and state regulations and reasonable economic restraints.
12. Full cooperation with other divisions must be maintained to fulfill the hospital's mission.

Source: J. Jacoby and M. Terpstra. "Collaborative Governance: Model for Professional Autonomy." *Nursing Management*, February 1990, 42. Reprinted with permission.

ingness to make mistakes and move on, and managers who are able to relinquish decision-making power over daily operations. Those responsible for fostering self-management must prepare for a fundamental change in the perception of "self as manager" and "subordinate" roles and responsibilities. In self-management, it is more important than ever for management to set and communicate clear expectations. Without a safe environment, self-management will fail because people will avoid changing or taking risks. Ongoing training and information sessions, with feedback and practice, are fundamental to the success of the new model. Gaining trust of staff and first-line supervisors and managers is made possible through modeling self-management principles and practices in the administrative structure of the organization.[68]

Although it appears that shared governance is expanding, a persistent question relates to whether its benefits are being objectively evaluated. Research studies show that nurses gain job satisfaction and growth satisfaction from working in a nurse-managed special care unit with a shared governance management model.[69] Surveys of nurses involved in horizontal integration through hospital acquisition indicate that nurses value shared governance and professional nursing autonomy.[70] Descriptive reports of shared governance organizations report the following:

- Shared governance decentralizes decision-making, disperses power, increases participatory management, and enlarges the span of control. It can be unit based, department based, or organization based.[71]
- Shared government involves staff in management, education, quality, and practice issues that support changes in skill-mix and patient-focused care systems.[72]
- Shared governance as an organizational structure supports vertical integration, product line development, and an organizational culture with strong relationships.[73]

Entrepreneurship

As decentralization and vertical integration strategies are implemented in health care organizations, a great opportunity exists for professional nurses to be involved in entrepreneurship. Nurses can form small companies with the support of government agencies and private businesses. Such companies require venture capital, which can, with sufficient preparation, be obtained from government and the private health care industry. As an example, in the face of greater professional nurse shortages, health care agencies could find it advantageous to contract with corporate nurse personnel agencies or vertical integration spin-offs that become, for example, nurse staffing subsidiaries, durable medical goods subsidiaries, and clinical nursing care subsidiaries.

The following five strategies promote entrepreneurship[74]:

1. Decentralize.
2. Give actual responsibility and authority to key executives.
3. Let executives express their managerial skills and give them a chance to make their own business mistakes on the road to excellence.
4. Monitor these executives and encourage them to make business decisions on their own, so that they can measure the results of these decisions not only in dollars and cents, but in terms of the effects on the people involved.
5. Establish a basic corporate policy that people are the biggest asset of the company, and make it clear that the development of these people will contribute greatly to the company's strength.

Entrepreneurship in nursing will be good for professional nurses and the health care industry because it will create independent thinkers who are motivated to be productive, creative, and more competitive in the marketplace. They will become like other business people who have a strong desire to control their own careers.

Gain-Sharing

Gain-sharing is a group incentive program in which employees share in the financial benefits of improved performance. It has many of the same advantages and disadvantages as other methods of participatory management. Top management is sensitive to the employees' goals, and employees identify with the organization through greater involvement.

Initiation of gain-sharing takes a long-term plan that includes application of these three phases of the change process[75]:

1. Unfreezing: Do an organizational diagnosis, a management questionnaire on gain-sharing, a bonus calculation, and an employee attitude survey.
2. Moving: Establish employee ownership with a task force of employees, meetings, and training of employees and managers. Involve everyone at once.
3. Refreezing: Institutionalize the plan, continued training, improved motivation and communication, goals, periodic reviews, periodic elections to task forces or committees, and annual reviews.

The results of gain-sharing are measurable: savings, improved labor-management relations, fewer grievances, less absenteeism, and reduced turnover. Gain-sharing adds money to intrinsic rewards. Stock ownership and profit sharing are economic rewards similar to gain-sharing. Gain-sharing, stock ownership, and profit sharing may not be legally possible in not-for-profit organizations. However, increased financial benefits can be made available through legal means such as merit pay, certification pay, and clinical promotions. Also, vertically integrated corporations have profit-making ventures under their corporate umbrellas.

All gain-sharing programs must be appropriately installed by employers to achieve maximum employee motivation, participation, and trust in management.

Pay Equity

Pay equity between management and employees is an issue of participatory management. Employees resent announcements of huge salary increases, fringe benefits, and perquisites for top management. Incentive programs for employees are a part of participatory management programs. Employees receive intrinsic satisfaction from public recognition and praise, but they also obtain extrinsic rewards from financial bonuses, stock options, and profit sharing.[76]

Professional nurses, like other professional workers, frequently respond negatively to the strategy of linking financial benefits to promotion into management. They want financial reward for accomplishing personal and organizational objectives that increase productivity and reduce turnover and absenteeism. These rewards can be in the form of nonmanagerial advancement of salary, status, recognition, autonomy, and responsibility. It is accomplished through *dual ladders*, that is, clinical promotions that match management promotions. It preserves their professional career opportunities with financial rewards based on graduated pay scales that can be objectively measured through levels of achievement culminating in mastery.

Pay equity has progressed in nursing, although civil rights legislation, collective bargaining, and job evaluation systems have not resulted in hoped-for outcomes. The educational system in nursing may be counterproductive to pay equity.[77]

Summary

Decentralization disburses authority and power downward to the operational units of an organization. Japanese organizations practice decentralization by eliciting consensus decision-making in management. Decentralization in nursing organizations facilitates communication and effective decisions, and clarifies roles.

Increased productivity, improved morale, increased favorable attitudes, and decreased absenteeism are the products of decentralized decision-making. Decentralization supports participatory management, the characteristics of which are trust, commitment, involvement of employees in setting goals and objectives, autonomy, inclusion of employees in decision-making, change and growth, originality, and creativity.

Decentralized and participatory organizations are usually flat or horizontal, employee and relationship centered. They are vertically integrated to enhance revenue production by developing new markets for health care organizations.

Training is essential to the success of participatory management because managers are often threatened by loss of authority. They have to be prepared for their new roles. Practicing nurses need to be able to perform as collaborators in the management of the nursing organization and the health care institution. With their new roles comes increased accountability for practicing nurses. Managers become facilitators.

Decentralization and participatory management are consistent with union participation. A memorandum of agreement is needed to keep grievance and contractual issues outside the employee involvement program. Some employers will opt to promote union decertification while bonding employees to the organization through participatory management.

Increased participation of nurses on organizational boards and committees will improve communication. Communication among units and departments becomes direct and, hence, faster and more accurate.

Although participatory management has numerous benefits or advantages, it also has some disadvantages. Among these disadvantages are occasional failures, occasional difficulty in fixing responsibilities, and difficulty in changing employee perceptions of previously authoritarian management.

Nurses can be involved in participatory management through activities such as job enrichment, personalization, primary nursing, case management, entrepreneurship, gain-sharing, and pay equity.

APPLICATION EXERCISES

EXERCISE 16-1   This is a group exercise.

1. Form groups of six to eight persons each.
2. Select group leaders and recorders.
3. List characteristics of decentralization and participatory management evident in your organization. (15 minutes)
4. List characteristics of centralized management evident in your organization. (15 minutes)
5. List changes you would like to see implemented to increase decentralization of decision-making in your organization. (20 minutes)
6. Report. (20 minutes)

EXERCISE 16-2   Delegation from nurse managers to clinical nurses is a part of the participatory management process. Mature nurse managers accept the principle of delegation, which leads to a more productive and enjoyable relationship with clinical nurses. Use Exhibit 16-8 to audit your ability to delegate duties to licensed practical nurses, nursing assistants, and other professional registered nurses when appropriate.

1. Review your own delegation audit. Choose three areas you intend to refine, assign them priorities, and outline three steps to improve performance in each area.
2. Narrate an experience in delegating that convinced you of the importance of exercising this basic responsibility and strengthened your confidence in your ability to delegate effectively.
3. Use the standards listed in Exhibit 16-9 to evaluate decentralization of authority in the division, department, service, or unit in which you work.

EXHIBIT 16-8
Delegation Audit

How effective are you in

	LOW					HIGH
1. Establishing work priorities for your subordinates?	1	2	3	4	5	6
2. Giving subordinates the necessary freedom and authority to work effectively?	1	2	3	4	5	6
3. Building confidence through guidance and direction?	1	2	3	4	5	6
4. Defining requirements clearly but not rigidly when you delegate work?	1	2	3	4	5	6
5. Relinquishing work you would like to do to others who can do it as well?	1	2	3	4	5	6
6. Spelling out the purpose and importance of a task, as well as other related duties?	1	2	3	4	5	6
7. Assigning someone to coordinate your activities when you are away?	1	2	3	4	5	6
8. Taking advantage of others' specialized skills when delegating?	1	2	3	4	5	6
9. Injecting challenge and motivation into tasks that you delegate?	1	2	3	4	5	6

TOTAL = _____
AVERAGE (total divided by 9) = _____
INTERPRETATION: Average Score of: 5–6—Terrific; 3–4—So-So; 1–2—You're "Doing," not "Delegating"

Source: E. C. Murphy. "Delegation—From Denial to Acceptance." *Nursing Management*, January 1984, 56. Permission requested and granted.

EXHIBIT 16-9
Standards for Evaluating Decentralization of Authority in a Nursing Division, Department, Service, or Unit

STANDARDS
1. Authority for decision making is delegated to the lowest operating level consistent with:
   a. Competence of subordinate managers
   b. Responsibility and accountability
   c. Economic management of enterprise
   d. Costs involved
   e. Need for uniformity and innovation of policy
   f. Management philosophy
   g. Subordinate managers' desires for independence
   h. Development of subordinate managers
   i. Need for evaluation and control
   j. Physical location of subordinate managers
   k. Organizational dynamics
2. Delegated authority is clear, specific, certain, and written. It is known by each subordinate manager.
3. Delegated authority supports the organizational, departmental, service, and unit goals, policies, standards, and plans.
4. Delegated authority is consistent with requirements of regulatory agencies, private and governmental.

NOTES

1. D. A. Kindig, "Purchasing Population Health: Aligning Financial Incentives to Improve Health Outcomes," *Nursing Outlook*, (January–February 1999), 15–22.

2. D. C. Moseley, P. H. Pietri, Jr., and L. C. Megginson, *Management: Leadership in Action*, 5th ed. (New York: Harper & Row, 1996), 274–277; H. Shoemaker and A. El-Ahraf, "Decentralization of Nursing Service Management and Its Impact on Job Satisfaction," *Nursing Administration Quarterly* (winter 1983), 69–76; I. H. Aas, "Organizational Change: Decentralization in Hospitals," *International Journal of Health Planning Management* (April–June 1997), 103–114; M. K. Anthony, "The Relationship of Authority to Decision-Making Behavior: Implications for Redesign," *Research in Nursing and Health* (October 1999), 388–398; R. Gross and B. Rosen, "Decentralization in a Sick Fund: Lessons from an Evaluation," *Journal of Management in Medicine*, 10(1), 67–80; J. Wasem, "A Study on Decentralizing from Acute Care to Home Care Settings in Germany," *Health Policy* (September 1997), 41, s109–129; E. Ross, C. MacDonald, K. McDermott, and G. Veldhorst, "The Chief of Nursing Practice: A Model for Nursing Leadership," *Canadian Journal of Nursing Administration* (January–February 1996), 7–22.

3. C. W. Joiner, Jr., "SMR Forum: Making the 'Z' Concept Work," *Sloan Management Review* (spring 1985), 57–63.

4. M. Boyd, L. Collins, J. Pepitone, E. Balk, and P. Kapustay, "Theory Z as a Framework for the Application of a Professional Practice Model in Increasing Nursing Staff Retention on Oncology Units," *Journal of Advanced Nursing* 15 (1990), 1226–1229.

5. R. Edfelt, "A Look at American Management Styles," *Business* (January–March 1986), 51–54; B. O'Reilly, "Reengineering the MBA," Fortune (24 January 1994), 38–40, 42.

6. Ibid.

7. C. W. Joiner, Jr., op. cit.

8. B. J. A. Simons, "Decentralizing Nursing Service: Six Months Later," *Supervisor Nurse* (October 1980), 59–64; R. B. Fine, "Decentralization and Staffing," *Nursing Administration Quarterly* (summer 1977), 59–67.

9. H. Shoemaker and A. El-Ahraf, op. cit.; S Acorn, P. A. Ratner, and M. Crawford, "Decentralization as a Determinant of Autonomy, Job Satisfaction, and Organizational Commitment Among Nurse Managers," *Nursing Research* (January–February 1997), 52–58.

10. T. Peters, "Letting Go of Controls," *Across the Board*, (June 1991), 14–15, 18.

11. A. Haggard, "Decentralized Staff Development," *The Journal of Continuing Education in Nursing* 15(3), (1984), 90–92.

12. R. Pastore, "PCs Take Command on Campus," *Computer World* (4 March 1991), 40.

13. L. Montgomery, "Subassemblies and Parts: Magna International," *F. W.* (14 April 1992), 57.

14. D. Allen, "Decentralization: Problems and Approaches," *Aspen's Advisor for Nurse Executives* (November 1990), 1,3–5.

15. J. Purcell, "How to Manage Decentralized Bargaining," *Personnel Management* (May 1989), 53–55.

16. T. Peters, *Thriving on Chaos* (New York: Harper & Row, 1987), 2, 9, 230, 525, 545–550.

17. T. Peters, "Human Judgment Is Simply Unreliable," *San Antonio Light* (23 April 1991), C2.

18. D. C. Moseley, P. H. Pietri, and L. C. Megginson, op. cit., 274–277, 349, 582.

19. W. J. Weisz, "Employee Involvement: How It Works at Motorola," *Personnel* (February 1985), 29–33; G. W. Poteet, "Delegation Strategies: A Must for the Nurse Executive," *Journal of Nursing Administration* (September 1984), 18–27.

20. J. A. Raelin, C. Sholl, and D. Leonard, "Why Professionals Turn Sour and What to Do," *Personnel* (October 1985), 28–41.

21. R. B. Fine, op. cit.; R. E. Walton, "From Control to Commitment in the Workplace," *Harvard Business Review* (March–April 1985), 77–84.

22. J. A. Raelin, C. Sholl, and D. Leonard, op. cit.

23. Ibid.

24. M. V. Batey and F. M. Lewis, "Clarifying Autonomy and Accountability in Nursing Services: Part I," *Journal of Nursing Administration* (September 1982), 13–17.

25. F. M. Lewis and M. V. Batey, "Clarifying Autonomy and Accountability in Nursing Services: Part II," *Journal of Nursing Administration* (October 1982), 10.

26. J. E. Bragg and I. R. Andrews, "Participative Decision Making: An Experimental Study in a Hospital," in B. Fuszard, *Self-Actualization for Nurses* (Rockville, MD: Aspen, 1984), 102–110.

27. S. S. Collins and M. C. Henderson, "Autonomy: Part of the Nursing Role?" *Nursing Forum* 26(2), (1991), 23–29.

28. S. Boughn, "Nursing Students Rank High in Autonomy at the Exit Level," *Journal of Nursing Education* (February 1992), 58–64.

29. W. J. Weisz, op. cit.

30. G. Klaus, "Corporate Pyramids Will Tumble When Horizontal Organizations Become the New Global Standard," *Personnel Administrator* (December 1983), 56–59.

31. E. A. Elpern, P. M. White, and A. F. Donahue, "Staff Governance: The Experience of the Nursing Unit," *The Journal of Nursing Administration* (June 1984), 9–15.

32. H. Shoemaker and A. El-Ahraf, op. cit.

33. T. S. Snail, "Organizational Diversification in the American Hospital," *Annual Review of Public Health* 19 (1998), 417–453.

34. C. W. Clegg and T. D. Wall, "The Lateral Dimension to Employee Participation," *Journal of Management Studies* (October 1984), 429–442.

35. B. A. Friedman, "Orchestrating a Unified Approach to Information Management," *Radiology Management* (November–December 1997), 30–36.

36. D. M. James, "An Integrated Model for Inner-City Health-Care Delivery: The Deaconess Center," *Journal of the National Medical Association* (January 1998), 35–39.

37. C. W. Gregg and T. D. Wall, op. cit.

38. M. Levinson, "Playing with Fire," *Newsweek* (21 June 1993), 46–48; M. Levinson, "When Workers Do the Hiring," *Newsweek* (21 June 1993), 48.

39. W. J. Weisz, op. cit.

40. R. E. Walton, op. cit.

41. B. J. Simons, op. cit.

42. M. H. Schuster and C. S. Miller, "Employee Involvement: Making Supervisors Believers," *Personnel* (February 1985), 24–28.

43. B. J. Simons, op. cit.

44. S. Malkin and P. Lauteri, "A Community Hospital's Approach: Decentralized Patient Education," *Nursing Administration Quarterly* (winter 1980), 101–106.

45. J. A. Raelin, C. Sholl and D. Leonard, op. cit.

46. R. E. Walton, op. cit.

47. M. H. Schuster and C. S. Miller, op. cit.

48. D. A. Clark, P. F. Clark, D. Day, and D. Shea, "The Relationship Between Health Care Reform and Nurses' Interest in Union Representation: The Role of Workplace Climate," *Journal of Professional Nursing* (March–April) 2000, 92–96.

49. M. A. Robinson, "Decentralize and Outsource: Dial's Approach to MIS Improvement," *Management Accounting* (September 1991), 27–31.

50. C. L. Cox, "Decentralization: Uniting Authority and Responsibility," *Supervisor Nurse* (March 1980), 28, 32.

51. H. Shoemaker and A. El-Ahraf, op. cit.;" M. P. Lovrich, "The Dangers of Participative Management: A Test of Unexamined Assumptions Concerning Employee Involvement," *Review of Public Personnel Administration* (summer 1985), 9–25; W. J. Bopp and W. P. Rosenthal, "Participatory Management," *American Journal of Nursing* (April 1979), 671–672; J. A. Fanning and R. B. Lovett, "Decentralization Reduces Nursing Administration Budget," *The Journal of Nursing Administration* (May 1985), 19–24; G. W. Poteet, op. cit.; C. L. Cox, op. cit.; R. E. Walton, op. cit.; S.R. Hinkley, Jr., "A Closer Look at Participation," *Organizational Dynamics* (winter 1985), 57–67; B. B. Arnetz, "Staff Perception of the Impact of Health Care Transformation On Quality of Care," *International Journal of Quality Health Care* (August 1999), 345–351; L. Chenoweth and K. Kilstoff, "Facilitating Positive Changes in Community Dementia Management Through Participatory Action Research," *International Journal of Nurse Practitioners* (September 1998), 175–188; B. A. Evanoff, P. C. Bohr, and L. D. Wolf, "Effects of a Participatory Ergonomics Team Among Hospital Orderlies," *American Journal of Internal Medicine* (April 1999), 358–365; A. Gissel and P. Knauth, "Knowledge-Based Support for the Participatory Design and Implementation of Shift Systems," *Scandinavian Journal of Work Environmental Health* 24 (Suppl. 3) (1998), 88–95; L. A. Linnan, J. L. Fava, B. Thompson, K. Emmons, K. Basen-Engquist, C. Probart, M. K. Hunt, and J. Heimendinger, "Measuring Participatory Strategies: Instrument Development for Worksite Populations," *Health Education Research* (June 1999), 371–386.

52. W. J. Weisz, op. cit.

53. M. P. Lovrich, op. cit.; M. H. Schuster and C. H. Miller, op. cit.

54. H. Shoemaker and A. El-Ahraf, op. cit.; M. P. Lovrich, op. cit.; W. J. Weisz, op. cit.; C. L. Cox, op. cit.

55. J. A. Raelin, C. Sholl, and D. Leonard, op. cit.; H. Shoemaker and A. El-Ahraf, op. cit.; R. E. Walton, op. cit.

56. J. B. Cunningham and T. Eberle, "A Guide to Job Enrichment and Redesign," *Personnel* (February 1990), 56–61.

57. S. K. Parker, "Enhancing Role Breadth Self-Efficacy: The Roles of Job Enrichment and Other Organizational Interventions," *Journal of Applied Psychology* (December 1998), 835–852.

58. J. A. Raelin, C. Sholl, and D. Leonard, op. cit.

59. J. E. Bragg and I. R. Andrews, op. cit.

60. M. R. Probst and J. M. Noga, "A Decentralized Nursing Care Delivery System," *Supervisor Nurse* (January 1980), 57–60; E. A. Elpern, P. M. White, and A. F. Donahue, op. cit.

61. M. Kivimaki, P. Voutilainen and P. Koskinen, "Job Enrichment, Work Motivation, and Job Satisfaction in Hospital Wards: Testing the Job Characteristics Model," *Journal of Nursing Management* (March 1995), 87–91.

62. L. Ankarlo, *Implementing Self-Directed Work Teams* (Boulder, CO: Career Track, 1992); workshop: Implementing Self-Directed Work Teams, San Antonio, TX 1993.

63. B. Dumaine, "The Trouble with Teams," *Fortune* (5 September 1994), 86–88, 90, 92.

64. Ibid.

65. T. Porter-O'Grady, *Implementing Shared Governance* (St. Louis, MO: Mosby 1992).

66. Ibid.

67. J. Jacoby and M. Terpstra, "Collaborative Governance: Model of Professional Autonomy," *Nursing Management* (6 February 1990), 42–44.

68. Presentation by T. Maldonado (San Antonio, TX: Incarnate Word College, 1992).

69. H. M. Bell, "Shared Governance and Teamwork—Myth or Reality," *AORN Journal* (March 2000), 631–635; R. Song, B. J. Daly, E. B. Rudy, S. Douglas and M. A. Dyer, "Nurses' Job Satisfaction, Absenteeism, and Turnover After Implementing a Special Care Unit Practice Model," *Research in Nursing and Health* (October 1997), 443–452; M. Gavin, D. Ash, S. Wakefield and C. Wroe, "Shared Governance: Time to Consider the Cons as Well as the Pros," *Journal of Nursing Management* (July 1999), 193–200.

70. V. M. George, L. J. Burke and B. L. Rodgers, "Research-Based Planning for Change: Assessing Nurses' Attitudes Toward Governance and Professional Practice Autonomy After Hospital Acquisition," *Journal of Nursing Administration* (May 1997), 53–61.

71. S. B. Prince, "Shared Governance. Sharing Power and Opportunity," *Journal of Nursing Administration* (March 1997), 28–35.

72. G. Joiner and J. Wessman, "Expanding Shared Governance Beyond Practice Issues," *Recruitment, Retention, Restructuring Research* (November–December) 1997, 4–7.

73. P. Aikman, I. Andress, C. Goodfellow, N. LaBelle and T. Porter-O'Grady, "System Integration: A Necessity," *Journal of Nursing Administration* (February 1998), 28–34.

74. R. E. Levinson, "Why Decentralize?" *Management Review* (October 1985), 50–53.

75. L. L. Hatcher and T. L. Ross, "Organizational Development Through Productivity Gainsharing," *Personnel* (October 1985), 42, 44–50; R. E. Walton, op. cit.

76. R. E. Walton, op. cit.

77. C. Tiffany and L. R. Lutjens, "Pay Equity: It's Still with Us." *Journal of Professional Nursing* (January–February 1993), 50–55.

REFERENCES

Afo, G. V., J. A. Thomason, and S. E. Karel. "Better Management for Better Health Services." *World Health Forum* 12(1991), 161–167.

Boissoneau, R. and B. Schwada. "Participatory Management: Its Evaluation, Current Usage." *AORN Journal* (November 1989), 1079–1086.

Brider, P. "The Move to Patient-Focused Care." *American Journal of Nursing* (September 1992), 26–33.

Clifford, M. "Can Do, Make Do." *Far Eastern Economic Review* (5 March 1992), 53–54.

Cummings, C. and R. McCaskey. "A Model Combining Centralized and Decentralized Staff Development." *Journal of Nursing Staff Development* (January–February 1992), 22–25.

Dixon, I. L. "Continuous Quality Improvement in Shared Leadership." *Nursing Management* (January 1993), 40–41, 44–45.

Dixon, N. "Participative Management: It's Not as Simple as It Seems." *Supervisory Management* (December 1984), 2–8.

Doering, L. "Recruitment and Retention: Successful Strategies in Critical Care." *Heart and Lung* (May 1990), 220–224.

Ertl, N. "Choosing Successful Managers: Participative Selection Can Help." *The Journal of Nursing Administration* (April 1984), 27–33.

Gentile, G. "Fun Becoming Part of Corporate Culture." *The Augusta Chronicle* (30 July 1989), 7.

Goliembiewski, R. T. and B. Sun. "Positive-Findings Bias in Quality of Work Life Research: Public-Private Comparisons." *Public Productivity & Management Review* (winter 1989), 145–154.

Hillebrand, P. L. "12 Commandments to Communication in a Decentralized System." *Nursing Management* (August 1992), 56–57.

Johnson, L. M., J. R. Happel, J. Edelman, and S. J. Brown. "A Model of Participatory Management with Decentralized Authority." *Nursing Administration Quarterly* (fall 1983), 30–36.

Kabb, M. "Participatory Management in Nursing as an Alternative to Traditional Management." *Health Matrix* (April 1989), 39–44.

Manthey, M. "Empowering Staff Nurse: Decision on the Action Level." *Nursing Management* (February 1991), 16–17.

Muczyk, J. P. and B. C. Reimanu. "Has Participative Management Been Oversold?" *Personnel* (May 1987), 52–56.

Ondrack, D. A. and M. G. Evans. "Job Enrichment and Job Satisfaction in Quality of Working Life and Nonquality of Working Life Work Sites." *Human Relations* (September 1986), 871–889.

O'Toole, J. "Employee Practices at the Best Managed Companies." *California Management Review* (fall 1985), 35–65.

Pesut, D. J. "Self-Regulation, Self-Management and Self-Care." *South Carolina Nurse* (summer 1992), 22–23.

Rauer, R. "Practicing Participative Management." *Nursing Management* (June 1990), 48A–48B, 48F, 48H.

Sashkin, M. "Participative Management Remains an Ethical Imperative." *Organizational Dynamics* (spring 1986), 62–75.

Schaffner, R. J. and C. C. Bowman. "Increasing the Impact of the Clinical Nurse Specialist through Activity in a Shared Governance Organization." *Clinical Nurse Specialist* 6(4), (1992), 211–216.

Solomon, J. "The Fall of the Dinosaurs." *Newsweek* (8 February 1993), 42–44.

Van Gorder, B. "Moving Back to Centralization." *Credit Magazine* (May–June 1990), 12–13, 15–16.

Vian, J. J. "Theory Z: 'Magic Potion' for Decentralized Management." *Nursing Management* (December 1990), 34–36.

Vlcek, D. J., Jr. "Decentralization: What Works and What Doesn't." *The Journal of Business Strategy* (fall 1987), 71–74.

Wagel, W. H. "Working (and Managing) Without Supervisors." *Personnel* (September 1987), 8–11.

Zelman, W. N. and D. L. Parham. "Strategic, Operational, and Marketing Concerns of Product-Line Management in Health Care." *Health Care Management Review* (winter 1990), 29–35.

CHAPTER 17

The Directing (Leading) Process

Russell C. Swansburg, PhD, RN

Directing or leading is best done with maximum attention to employee participation and employee self-management.

LEARNING OBJECTIVES AND ACTIVITIES

- Define *directing*.
- Identify the nature of the directing function of nursing management relative to the physical acts of directing.
- Make a plan for delegating duties, tasks, and responsibilities.
- Make a plan for using management by objectives (MBO).
- Use a set of standards for evaluation of the directing function.

CONCEPTS: Directing (leading), delegating, management by objectives, organizational development.

MANAGER BEHAVIOR: Implements management plans through the process of supervision.

LEADER BEHAVIOR: Develops and implements management plans through the process of delegating decision-making to the lowest organizational entity. Encourages management by objectives and other directing (leading) activities that develop the conditions for human effectiveness and thence organizational effectiveness.

Introduction

In describing the functions of management, Fayol stated that the manager must know how to handle people and must be able to defend his or her point of view with confidence and enthusiasm. The manager learns continuously and educates people at all levels for success in their assigned tasks.[1]

Fayol stated that command occurs when the manager gets "the optimum return from all employees of his (sic) unit in the interest of the whole concern."[2] To do this, the manager must know the personnel, eliminate the incompetent, be well-versed in binding agreements with employees, set a good example, conduct periodic audits, confer with chief assistants to focus on unity of direction, not become mired in detail; and have as a goal unity, energy, initiative, and loyalty among employees.[3] Fayol defined *coordination* as creating harmony among all activities to facilitate the working and success of the unit.[4] In modern management, command and coordination are labeled directing or leading.

According to Urwick, it is the purpose of command and the function of directing to see that individual interests do not interfere with the general interest.[5] Command (directing) protects the general interest and should ensure that each unit has a competent and energetic head. Command functions to promote esprit de corps and to carefully select a staff that can be of most service.[6] It was Urwick's premise that bringing in new blood rather than promoting from within may excite resentment. Urwick indicated the need for a grievance procedure, for common rules to be observed by all, and for regulations that allow for self-discipline. Managers should explain regulations and cut red tape. They should "decarbonize," that is, clean out rules and regulations as needed.[7]

Rowland and Rowland stated that directing "initiates and maintains action toward desired objectives" and is "closely interrelated with leadership."[8] These authors suggested that a manager's choice of leadership style will be the major factor in exercising the directing function. Among the activities of directing are delegation, communication, training, and motivation.[9]

Leading has become a more acceptable term for the directing function. All of the effective principles of nursing management are to be applied by nurse leaders. They begin with accomplishing the mission, goals, and objectives of a division, department, or unit. Because statements of mission, goals, objectives, philosophy, and vision direct the work of all nursing personnel, it is important that they be functional. All leading or directing activities will be guided by these statements. The actions of nurse leaders should inspire nursing personnel to produce services and products that please customers and maintain the vitality of the organization. The following are activities related to the leading or directing function[10]:

1. Implementing the theory (knowledge) base of nursing.
2. Making and using strategic and tactical plans with input from nursing personnel. Facilitating operational planning.
3. Facilitating the achievement of the organizational mission, vision, goals, and objectives.
4. Providing and maintaining resources: people, supplies, and equipment.
5. Maintaining morale.
6. Providing education and training programs to maintain competency.
7. Providing, interpreting, and maintaining standards in the form of policies, procedures, rules, and regulations.
8. Facilitating maximum communication
9. Coordinating among disciplines.
10. Providing leadership.
11. Facilitating and maintaining intrapersonal relationships.
12. Counseling and coaching.
13. Acting to inspire trust, teamwork, and cooperation.
14. Resolving conflict.
15. Using controlling (evaluating) processes that increase and maintain quality and productivity.
16. Facilitating group dynamics.
17. Organizing human resources.
18. Maintaining the physical plant.
19. Assisting personnel with directing their own careers.
20. Promoting the implementation of new nursing roles involving nurse practitioners and case managers who direct all activities related to process and outcomes.
21. Facilitating nursing research and implementing research evidence in practice.

Although the developing theory of human relations management supports new approaches to directing, it should be remembered that the nurse manager oversees the work of nursing personnel. It is incumbent on nurse managers to have up-to-date knowledge and skills so they can develop satisfied nursing workers. This requires that nurse managers facilitate and coach nursing workers in becoming self-managers who produce quality outcomes; that they work cooperatively

within nursing and among other disciplines; do peer review; maintain their knowledge and abilities; and hold themselves accountable for their performances.

In the 9,9-oriented Grid® style developed by Blake and Mouton, the directing function of management is described by the following statement: "I keep informed of progress and influence subordinates by identifying problems and revising goals or action steps with them. I assist when needed by helping to remove barriers."[11]

> What separates good leaders from great leaders is the understanding and development of their facilitation skills.[12]

Directing and Nursing Management

Directing is a physical act of nursing management, the interpersonal process by which nursing personnel accomplish the objectives of nursing. To understand fully what directing entails, the nurse manager examines the conceptual functions of nursing management, that is, planning and organizing.[13] From the statement of mission or purpose, the statement of beliefs or philosophy, the vision statement, and the written objectives of the organization, the nurse manager develops management plans, the process by which methods and techniques are selected and used to accomplish the work of the nursing unit. Directing is the process of applying the management plans to accomplish nursing objectives. It is the process by which nursing personnel are inspired or motivated to accomplish work. Three of the major elements of directing are embodied in supervision of nursing personnel: motivation, leadership, and communication[14] (discussed in Chapters 18, 19, and 20, respectively).

Nurse managers know something of the nature of human beings. Subordinates are hired as total human beings and have to be managed as total human beings who respond to many institutions within society: church, school, government, family, service organizations, professional societies, and all of the other social groupings. Similarities and differences exist between supervisors and subordinates, who are complex human beings with known and conscious needs for physiological well-being, safety, achievement, and human associations. People react to the stresses and strains of a fast-paced society and may need some time for solitude if they are to function effectively and survive. Most individuals place their own concerns before those of others. They enjoy work when the benefits exceed the costs, and they take a job that meets their established priorities for income and, perhaps, social life.

People can be led and will accept leadership for various reasons, among them admiration, power, income, and safety. The zest with which they pursue achievement of the objectives of the nursing division, department, service, or unit will correspond with the leader's ability to create an internal environment that inspires them to work at the levels of their capabilities. It is inherent in the acceptance of an administrative position that the person develop and use leadership abilities. These include:

- Identification of training and education needs of individuals and establishment of programs to meet such needs.
- Establishment of a system of performance appraisal to identify personal competencies; assignments and promotions based on competency, including performance.
- Development of trust and subsequent delegation of responsibility and authority for decision-making.

A good leader will contribute to creating a work environment that has the following properties:

1. Jobs that offer a living wage as well as adequate work.
2. Group identity and group purpose, that is, the opportunity to work with others.
3. Pleasant surroundings and coworkers.
4. Interesting work.
5. Recognition that employees' work is valued and well done.
6. Opportunity for accomplishment and challenge.
7. Harmony between organizational and individual goals: equality of opportunity to be safe and secure, to achieve differently, and to have choices about shifts; to have job enlargement, and to be recognized as an individual.

Like other human beings, a nurse leader who is also a nurse manager is in many ways different from subordinates. He or she is the one who persuades the group to work to achieve organizational objectives. The nurse leader knows more about organizational policies, goals, new programs, and plans for change. He or she is believed to have good judgment based on a breadth of experience. He or she controls the careers of subordinates. The nurse leader is expected to behave in a socially acceptable manner, to exhibit personal qualities acceptable to subordinates, and to demonstrate skill in leadership, communication, and motivation techniques.

Effective directing increases subordinates' contributions to achievement of nursing management goals and creates harmony between nursing management goals and nursing workers' goals. Effective directing is the management function wherein the nurse manager acts as facilitator and coach. The effective facilitator and coach provides the education needed for primary nurses and case managers to become leaders and man-

agers. Nurse managers teach nursing personnel to manage themselves in self-managed teams. Personnel learn to do planning, self-scheduling, personnel management, and budgeting; effect change; make decisions and solve problems; and build teams for doing research.[15]

> **Nurse managers encourage and inspire their workers every step of the way.**

Delegating

Delegating, a technique of time management, is a major element of the directing function of nursing management.[16] It is an effective management competency by which nurse managers get the work done through their employees. One of the criticisms of new nurse managers is that they emerge from clinical nurse roles and fail to identify with their management roles. These nurses have been rewarded for their nursing, not for their skill in leading other nurses. Delegation is a part of management; it requires professional management training and development to accept the hierarchical responsibilities of delegation.

> **Nurse managers need to be able to delegate some of their own duties, tasks, and responsibilities as a solution to overwork, which leads to stress, anger, and aggression.**

As nurse managers learn to accept the principle of delegation, they become more productive and come to enjoy relationships with the staff. They learn to delegate by purposefully thinking about the delegation process, by carefully planning for it, by gaining knowledge of clinical nurses' capabilities, by planning and implementing effective interpersonal communications, and by being willing to take risks. As they learn to delegate, they are freed of daily pressures and time-consuming chores and have time to manage.

The following list suggests ways for nurse managers to successfully delegate[17]:

1. Train and develop subordinates. It is an investment. Give them reasons for the task, authority, details, opportunity for growth, and written instructions, if needed.
2. Plan ahead. It prevents problems.
3. Control and coordinate the work of subordinates but do not peer over their shoulders. To prevent errors, develop ways of measuring the accomplishment of objectives with communication, standards, measurements, feedback, and credit. Nursing employees want to know the nurse manager's expectations of them. They understand expectations when clear,

consistent messages and behavior exist that prevent confusion. They understand expectations from clearly defined jobs, work relationships, and expected results.

4. Follow up by visiting subordinates frequently. Spot potential problems of morale, disagreement, and grievance. Expect employees to make suggestions to improve work and use the feasible ones.
5. Coordinate to prevent duplication of effort.
6. Solve problems, and think about new ideas. Encourage employees to solve their own problems, and then give them the autonomy and freedom to do so.
7. Accept delegation as desirable.
8. Specify goals and objectives.
9. Know subordinates' capabilities, and match the task or duty to the employee. Be sure the employee considers the task or duty important.
10. Agree on performance standards. Relate managerial references to employee performance.
11. Take an interest.
12. Assess results. Expect what is clearly and directly asked for as the deadline for completing and reporting arrives. The nurse manager should accept the fact that employees will perform delegated tasks in their own style.
13. Give appropriate rewards.
14. Do not take back delegated tasks.

Build professional nurses' self-esteem by delegating as much of the authority for nursing practice as possible. Professional nurses want authority over their practice and can be educated to perform management tasks related to it. Nurse managers will determine what authority to delegate through communication with clinical nurses. Authority should be commensurate with assigned responsibility. As professional nurses gain individual self-esteem, organizational self-esteem follows. Employees respond to participation in decision-making and gain satisfaction with their jobs and the organization.

Organizational self-esteem will be built by[18]:

- Managerial interest in employees' well-being, status, and contributions, and concern and support for their personal problems, personal development, and comfort.
- Job variety from delegation that provides job enlargement, autonomy, significant work, and use of skills and abilities the employees value. Delegating that enlarges an employee's job develops his or her sense of responsibility, general understanding, and job satisfaction. As part of a successful knowledge base, professional nurses learn effective strategies for managing tasks, including increased work loads, establishing priorities, and delegating responsibility.

- A climate or work environment that bolsters cohesiveness and trust.
- Management's faith in and recognition of the rewards of self-direction.

Reasons for Delegating

Five reasons for delegating include[19]:

1. Assigning routine tasks.
2. Assigning tasks for which the nurse manager does not have time.
3. Problem-solving.
4. Changes in the nurse manager's own job emphasis.
5. Capability building.

The nurse manager should be careful not to misuse the clinical nurse by delegating tasks that can be done by nonnurses or nonlicensed personnel. This error can be avoided by consulting with clinical nurses to determine what authority they want.

Techniques for Delegating

Nurse managers at all levels, from nurse executive to department or unit head and from unit head to clinical nurse, can prepare lists of duties that can be delegated. Delegation includes authority to approve, recommend, or implement. The list of duties should be ranked by time required to perform them and their importance to the institution. One duty should be delegated at a time.

What Not to Delegate

Do not delegate the power to discipline, responsibility for maintaining morale, overall control, a "hot potato," jobs that are too technical, or duties involving a trust or confidence.[20] These complicated areas of nursing management require specialized knowledge and skills. Nurse managers who handle these responsibilities should be well-educated in the sciences of management and behavioral technology. Delegating these duties and responsibilities will cause clinical nurses to assume that managers are incompetent to handle these areas of nursing leadership and management.

Barriers to Delegating

Barriers to delegating can exist in the delegator, delegatee, or situation. Exhibit 17-1 lists a number of barriers to delegating.

EXHIBIT 17-1
Barriers to Delegating

BARRIERS IN THE DELEGATOR

1. Preference for operating by oneself.
2. Demand that everyone "know all the details."
3. "I can do it better myself" fallacy.
4. Lack of experience in the job or in delegating.
5. Insecurity.
6. Fear of being disliked.
7. Refusal to allow mistakes.
8. Lack of confidence in subordinates.
9. Perfectionism, leading to excessive control.
10. Lack of organizational skill in balancing workloads.
11. Failure to delegate authority commensurate with responsibility.
12. Uncertainty over tasks and inability to explain.
13. Disinclination to develop subordinates.
14. Failure to establish effective controls and to follow up.

BARRIERS IN THE DELEGATEE

1. Lack of experience.
2. Lack of competence.
3. Avoidance of responsibility.
4. Overdependence on the boss.
5. Disorganization.
6. Overload of work.
7. Immersion in trivia.

BARRIERS IN THE SITUATION

1. One-person-show policy.
2. No toleration of mistakes.
3. Criticality of decisions.
4. Urgency, leaving no time to explain (crisis management).
5. Confusion in responsibilities and authority.
6. Understaffing.

Source: Reprinted, with permission of the publisher, from *The Time Trap* by Alec Mackenzie, © 1972 AMACOM, a division of American Management Association. All rights reserved.

Management by Objectives

Management by objectives (MBO) as a directing element was first advocated by Peter Drucker and made famous by George Odiorne who defined it as[21]:

> . . . a process whereby the superior and subordinate managers of an organization jointly identify its common goals, define each individual's major areas of responsibility in terms of the results expected of him [sic], and use these measures as guides for operating the unit and assessing the contribution of each of its members.

Odiorne further defines MBO as a system for making organizational structures work, of bringing about vitality and personal involvement in the hierarchy by means of statements of what is expected from everyone involved and measurement of what is actually achieved. It stresses ability and achievement rather than personality.[22]

Management by objectives allows the individual nurse to contribute to the common goal of the enterprise while nurse managers focus on the business goals. MBO promotes high standards, focusing on the job and not on the manager or the worker. Applying Drucker's MBO theory accomplishes this; nurse managers are the persons who know what to expect of employees. Just like their nurse managers, nursing staff should know for what they will be held accountable.[23]

Management by objectives spells out the results expected of the clinical nursing unit and of the unit in relation to other units. It emphasizes teamwork and team results and includes short- and long-range objectives, as well as tangible and intangible objectives. Intangible objectives include development of the individual, performance and attitude of workers, and public responsibilities. Objectives should include those that indicate the contributions to higher levels of the enterprise.

Management by objectives allows people to control their own performance, measure themselves, and exercise self-control. Through MBO, clinical nurses make demands of themselves. Nurse managers will assume that clinical nurses want to be responsible, want to contribute, want to achieve, and have the strength and desire to do so. According to Drucker[24]:

> What the business enterprise needs is a principle of management that will give full scope to individual strength and responsibility, as well as common direction to vision and effort, establish team work, and harmonize the goals of the individual with the commonweal. Management by objectives and self-control make[s] the commonweal the aim of every manager. It substitutes for control from outside the stricter, more exacting, and more effective control from inside. It motivates the manager to action, not because somebody tells him (sic) to do something or talks him into doing it, but because the objective task demands it. He acts not because somebody wants him to but because he himself decides that he has to—he acts, in other words, as a free man.
>
> I do not use the word "philosophy" lightly; indeed I prefer not to use it at all; it's much too big a word. But management by objectives and self-control may properly be called a philosophy of management. It rests on a concept of the job of management. It rests on an analysis of the specific needs of the management group and the obstacles it faces. It rests on a concept of human action, behavior, and motivation. Finally it applies to every manager, whatever his level and function, and to any organization whether large or small. It ensures performance by converting objective needs into personal goals. And this is genuine freedom.

Procedure and Process

Training

The training for the MBO process should begin with the nurse managers of the enterprise. Managers will learn the characteristics of the process, the objectives of initiating an MBO program, the procedures to be used, and the methods for evaluating the program's effectiveness. During this training program, nurse managers can simulate the procedures to be used.

Once nurse managers are trained, all nursing employees are given similar training. Employees will be made aware of the necessity for writing and working toward their personal objectives as they seek to achieve those of the organization. They will be taught the value of synergism of personal and organizational objectives and will be asked to bring their written lists of objectives to the first meeting with their superior.

First Meeting

The first MBO meeting should be held in quiet surroundings, with sufficient time for discussion. The nurse manager should put the employee at ease. Most survival and safety needs of nurses are reasonably satisfied. Nurses' social, ego, and self-fulfillment needs are predominant at this time. As the nurse presents each personal objective, the nurse manager relates it to an objective of the enterprise. Thus, the manager creates the conditions for fulfilling the nurse's needs, including the removal of obstacles, encouragement of growth, and provision of guidance.

During this first meeting, the nurse manager and clinical nurse set goals that are specific, promote teamwork, are measurable (in the sense that they can be quantified or described qualitatively), and are attainable. Goals should involve enough risk to challenge but not defeat. They should include objectives that are routine, solve problems, are creative or innovative, and result in personal development.[25]

At the end of the first meeting, both the nurse manager and clinical nurse should be satisfied with the written objectives. Each will have a copy of these objectives. The nurse manager and the clinical nurse will part with an understanding of mutual expectations how future meetings will progress and will have set a time for the next meeting.

Actions

Between meetings, employees perform work that meets their agreed-on objectives. They should periodically review these objectives and summarize their accomplishments.

Second Meeting

Conditions for the second MBO meeting will be the same as for the first meeting. The meeting will provide a time for evaluation of results, review, appraisal, and the setting of further goals.

The employee should be encouraged to spell out gratifying and exhilarating experiences, do self-examination, and relate his or her thoughts about work. The nurse manager should listen and make the employee feel safe while helping them to have a person-to-organization fit.

The manager examines his or her own reactions without criticizing the employee, which helps build trust and confidence as well as an ethical relationship. In doing so, the manager and employee establish an organizational climate for personal and organizational achievement.[26]

Management by objectives should include appraisal of managers by subordinates. Subordinates will appraise how well the manager helps employees do their jobs, supports them, assists with problems, and demonstrates proficiency and visibility.[27]

Both nurse manager and employee should exit the second meeting with a sense of accomplishment. This does not mean the employee will not be made aware of deficiencies or shortcomings. Deficiencies and shortcomings will be recognized in the form of needed additions or changes, increased progress, and even deletions. All will be tied to patient care and organizational development. The feedback process tells the employee what is expected and when an error has been made.

The process will be repeated at intervals, with dates and times agreed on at each meeting. At the end of an appraisal period, a performance results contract will be signed by both the employee and the supervisor and sent to the personnel department to be included in the employee's record. The performance appraisal can be used to identify promotion potential and to determine merit pay increases.

Problems with Management by Objectives

Management by objectives must be viewed as genuine and fair by all employees. It must allow for errors and for adjustments that result from work constraints and individual capabilities. The following are some specific problems of MBO:

1. Top management is not supportive. To be effective MBO must be supported and carried out at all levels, and it must be monitored closely.
2. Inconsistency exists among managers. This can be fixed or avoided by awareness of both parties. Periodic summative evaluation conferences can help uncover these inconsistencies.
3. Goals are too easy or are unattainable. Employees sometimes fear that they will be subjected to goals of increasing difficulty. Frank discussion will help

resolve this problem. Employees have to be able to meet increasing personal needs as they climb the career ladder. These can be recognized and satisfied through MBO.

4. Conflicts between goals and policies exist. When this occurs, policies should give way to goals unless they would violate a safety or legal standard.

5. Accountability is beyond the control of employees. When this occurs, the nurse manager helps modify the goal and makes allowance for the difference, which can be done by decreasing accountability or increasing authority. Factors beyond the employee's control should not be evaluated.

6. Employees have a lack of commitment. Determine the cause if possible and produce interactions that will increase commitment. Discuss the problem frankly, and encourage the employee to be specific in a plan to cope with it. Do not threaten.

Management by objectives is a superb tool if the objectives are "(1) simple, (2) focused on what's important, (3) genuinely created from the bottom up (the objectives are drafted by the person who must live up to them, with no constraining guides), and (4) a 'living' contract, not a form driven exercise." MBO should promote flexibility.[28]

Some management writers recommend management by results (MBR) rather than MBO. When using MBR, managers should be sure the key results include quantity, quality, and the cost of outcomes. Subjectivity and favoritism should be avoided because they sow resentment and distrust. Objectives should be set high and pushed even higher using the new level as the expected base, with quality being the fundamental objective. Workers should be rewarded with bonuses or in any other form possible. It is best to reward groups so that people share information and work together.[29]

When using MBR, follow these principles[30]:

1. Employees are capable of crafting solutions to problems because they know the system and what the problems are.

2. Use budget systems that fund outcomes rather than inputs.

3. Outcomes are measures of the volume of something produced and of quality.

4. Two-thirds of workers today work with their minds.

5. The work force comes from a mosaic society with great cultural diversity.

MBO is a total management process that includes planning, organizing, directing (leading), and controlling (evaluating). Exhibit 17-2 lists the standards for evaluating the directing function of nursing management.

Organizational Development

Management by objectives is needed for organizational development (OD) and vice versa. Organizational development allows the organization to be managed against goals and for results. OD occurs as management skills and organizational processes are applied to shape and develop the conditions for human effectiveness. These are[31]:

- Interpersonal competence. The individual has high expectations, respect for others, honest relationships, freedom to act, and a team orientation.

- Meaningful goals. The goals are understandable, desirable, attainable, and synergistic. The individual influences the goals.

- Helpful systems. Users understand and control systems because systems are goal-oriented and provide feedback. Users adapt to and adopt systems.

- Achievement and self-actualization. As the organization grows, the individual grows. People are committed to goals, are highly motivated, and have high trust and minimal dissatisfaction.

The management philosophy should permit these conditions for human effectiveness to occur. In addition, it should emphasize meaningful work in which the doers are involved in all aspects of the job. Managers should delegate decisions and ensure that the decisions are made, limits are known, support is provided, and accountability is met by evaluating results.

A theory of nursing management explores the cause-effect relationship between clinical nurses and their performances. It has as its objectives the removal of controls that create distrust, fear, and resentment and the promotion of conditions (climate) that provide opportunities for clinical nurses to achieve their goals.

Summary

Effective directing will result in greater harmony in the actions of supervisors and employees and in the achievement of the objectives of personnel as well as of the enterprise. Directing will be most effective when employees have leaders who provide direct personal contacts. Directing that encourages leadership, motivation, and communication techniques and emphasizes the human aspects of managing individuals is most desirable. Effective leadership can be fostered by nursing administrators who desire to improve their directing or leading activities.

EXHIBIT 17-2
Standards for Evaluating the Directing Function

1. Managers have established a medium by which nursing workers feel free to ask for advice, counsel, and consultation.
2. Needed written directions are available in the form of policies, procedures, standards of care, job analyses, job descriptions, job standards, and nursing care plans. They are clearly stated and current and are kept to a minimal number.
3. A training program is in effect that meets nursing employees' needs as they perceive them. They participate.
4. Supervisors are competent in needed knowledge and skills of administration and clinical specialization.
5. Nurse managers periodically work evening, night, weekend, and holiday shifts to keep abreast of clinical and administrative behaviors peculiar to these shifts.
6. The nurse administrator has operationalized the American Nurses Association (ANA) Scope and Standards for Nurse Administrators.
7. The nurse managers have operationalized the ANA Standards of Clinical Nursing Practice.
8. Nurse managers are knowledgeable about and apply the appropriate standards of the Joint Commission on Accreditation of Healthcare Organizations, National League for Nursing, Medicare, and Medicaid.
9. The nurse administrator uses techniques of operations analysis. (This service is available at no charge to member hospitals of the American Hospital Association and its state affiliates.)
10. Nurse managers use a system of management by objectives or results.
11. The nurse administrator works with the consent and knowledge of patients and solicits input from consumers regarding nursing services desired.
12. Nursing unit personnel are organized into and working as direct care personnel and clerical personnel.
13. Nurse managers use the physical plant to the best advantage for patients and personnel.

APPLICATION EXERCISES

EXERCISE 17-1   Look at the statements of mission, philosophy, vision, and objectives of a division of nursing in which you work as a student or an employee.

1. What is the work of the unit or division?
2. What is the inference for the directing function of the unit or division?

EXERCISE 17-2   *Scenario:* Jennie Lynd, RN, has been working in the newborn nursery for one year. Her performance in caring for babies, teaching parents, and supporting other unit personnel has been exemplary. She has been told this. Jennie Lynd tells her nurse manager she is interested in transferring to the pediatric intensive care unit. With a group of your peers, decide how the nurse manager should handle this request.

EXERCISE 17-3   *Scenario:* As a nurse manager, Ms. Pressley, RN, has studied career development theory because she believes that clinical nurses do not really have careers. This is particularly true when a clinical ladder is nonexistent. Ms. Pressley plans to counsel her clinical nurses regularly and to push for a clinical promotion ladder that recognizes advanced competence, education, and certification. This activity falls within the directing category of management. Compare Ms. Pressley's actions with those of several other nurse managers you know or have known. Summarize your findings.

EXERCISE 17-4 Select one or more goals you would like to accomplish in the unit in which you work as a student or employee. Make a management plan to accomplish them. The process should:

1. Cover *your* individual objectives.
2. Be discussed and adjusted with your boss.
3. Have a plan for achieving each objective.
4. Set a time to evaluate accomplishments with your boss.

EXERCISE 17-5 Use Exhibit 17-3 "Standards for Evaluation of the Directing Function," to evaluate one of the entities in the organization where you work as a student or employee. Identify one concrete example for each standard. Summarize your results. If the directing function does not meet the standards, use a problem-solving approach and implement a plan of improvement.

NOTES

1. H. Fayol, *General and Industrial Management*, Trans. by C. Storrs (London: Sir Isaac Pitman & Sons, 1949), 82–96.
2. Ibid., 97.
3. Ibid., 97–98.
4. Ibid., 103.
5. L. Urwick, *The Elements of Administration* (New York: Harper & Row, 1944), 77.
6. Ibid., 81–82.
7. Ibid., 90–96.
8. H. S. Rowland and B. L. Rowland, eds., *Nursing Administration Handbook*, 3rd ed. (Gaithersburg, MD: Aspen, 1992), 10.
9. Ibid., 11.
10. T. Kron and E. Durbin, *The Management of Patient Care: Putting Leadership Skills to Work*, 10th. ed. (Philadelphia: W. B. Saunders, 1987), 155–176; L. M. Douglass, *The Effective Nurse: Leader and Manager*, 3d ed.(St. Louis: C. V. Mosby, 1988), 115; D. Strickland and O. C. O'Connell, "Saving Your Career in the 21st Century," *Journal of Case Management*, (summer 1998), 47–51; A. Retsas, "Barriers to Using Research Evidence in Nursing Practice," *Journal of Advanced Nursing*, (March 2000), 599–606; J. Neal, T. Brown and W. Rojjanasrirat, "Implementation of a Case Coordinator Role: A Focused Ethnographic Study," *Journal of Professional Nursing*, (November–December 1999), 349–355; J. A. Beal, "A Nurse Practitioner Model of Practice in the Neonatal Intensive Care Unit," *MCN American Journal of Maternal Child Nursing*, (January–February 2000), 18–24.
11. R. R. Blake and J. S. Mouton, *The Managerial Grid III*, 3rd ed. (Houston: Gulf Publishing, 1985), 94.
12. T. Schulte, "Facilitating Skills: The Art of Helping Teams Succeed," *Hospital Materials Management Quarterly*, (August 1999), 13–26.
13. C. Arndt and L. M. D. Huckabay, *Nursing Administration: Theory for Practice with a Systems Approach*, 2nd ed. (St. Louis: C. V. Mosby, 1980), 92–106.
14. H. Koontz, C. O'Donnell, and H. Weihrich, *Essentials of Management*, 5th ed. (New York: McGraw-Hill, 1990), 300.
15. R. C. Swansburg, *The Directing Function of Nursing Service Administration* (Hattiesburg, MS: The University of Southern Mississippi School of Nursing, 1977), 3–5.
16. R. E. Schroeder, "Using Time Management to Achieve Balance," *Medical Group Management Journal* (November–December 1998), 20–26, 28.
17. B. B. Beegle. "Don't Do It—Delegate It!" *Supervisory Management* (April 1970), 2–6; J. K. Matejka and R. J. Dunsing, "Great Expectations," *Management World* (January 1987), 16–17.
18. J. K. Matejka and R. J. Dunsing, op. cit.
19. H. S. Rowland and B. L. Rowland, op. cit., 69–70.
20. Ibid.
21. G. S. Odiorne, *Management by Objectives* (New York: Pitman, 1965), 55–56.
22. Ibid.
23. P. F. Drucker, *Management: Tasks, Responsibilities, Practices* (New York: Harper & Row, 1973, 1974), 430–442.
24. Ibid., 441–442.
25. M. L. Bell, "Management by Objectives," *Journal of Nursing Administration* (May 1980), 19–26.
26. H. Levinson, "Management by Whose Objectives?" *Harvard Business Review* (July–August 1970), 125–134.
27. Ibid.
28. T. Peters, *Thriving on Chaos* (New York: Harper & Row, 1987), 603–604.
29. D. Osborne and T. Gaebler, *Reinventing Government* (New York: Plume, 1992), 156–158.
30. Ibid., 160–168.
31. A. C. Beck, Jr., and E. D. Hillman, "OD to MBO or MBO to OD: Does It Make a Difference?" In A. T. Hollingsworth and R. M. Hodgetts, eds., *Readings in Basic Management* (Philadelphia: W.B. Saunders, 1975), 190–196.

REFERENCES

Alexander, E. L. *Nursing Administration in the Hospital Health Care System*, 2nd. ed., (St. Louis: C.V. Mosby, 1978), 198–246.

Barrett, J. *The Head Nurse: Her Changing Role* (New York: Appleton Century-Crofts, 1968), 310–332.

Cain, C., and V. Laschinger. "Management by Objectives: Applications to Nursing." *Journal of Nursing Administration* (January 1978), 35–38.

Campbell, J. M., and E. S. Kinion. "Teaching Leadership/Followership to RN-to-MSN Students." *Journal of Nursing Education* (March 1993), 138–140.

Donovan, H. M. *Nursing Service Administration: Managing the Enterprise* (St. Louis: C.V. Mosby, 1975), 128–154.

Fulmer, R. M. *Supervision: Principles of Professional Management* (Beverly Hills: Glenco Press, 1976), 4.

Gibson, J. L., J. W. Ivancevich, and J. H. Donnelly, Jr. *Organizations: Behavior, Structure, Processes*, 9th ed. (Burr Ridge, IL: Richard D. Irwin, 1997).

Holley, W. H., and K. M. Jennings. *Personnel Management: Functions and Issues* (New York: The Dryden Press, 1983), 237–240.

Jones, C., T. D. Gubereski, and K. L. Soeken. "Nurse Practitioners: Leadership Behaviors and Organizational Climate." *Journal of Professional Nursing* (November–December 1990), 327–333.

McDaniel, C., and G. A. Wolf. "Transformational Leadership in Nursing Service." *Journal of Nursing Administration* (February 1992), 60–65.

McGregor, D. *Leadership and Motivation* (Cambridge, MA: The MIT Press, 1966).

Robin, I. M., R. E. Fry, and M. S. Plovnick, eds. *Managing Human Resources in Health Care Organizations* (Reston, VA: Reston Publishing, 1978), 128–129, 154–161, 182–189, 198, 236–243.

Leadership

Sharon Farley, PhD, RN
PROFESSOR AND EXECUTIVE ASSOCIATE DEAN
INDIANA UNIVERSITY SCHOOL OF NURSING
INDIANAPOLIS, INDIANA

Leadership
Fail to honor people
They fail to honor you
But of a good leader, who talks little
When his work is done, his aim fulfilled
They will all say
"We did this ourselves."

Lao Tsu

LEARNING OBJECTIVES AND ACTIVITIES

- Define *leadership*.
- Explain trait theories of leadership.
- Match examples to Gardner's nine tasks to be performed by leaders.
- Match examples to individual leadership behavioral theorists.
- Match examples to the theory of transformational leadership.
- Discuss similarities between leadership and management.
- Match examples to interpersonal bases of power.

CONCEPTS: Leadership, trait theories of leadership, behavioral theories of leadership, leadership styles, transformational leadership, gender issues of leadership, buffering.

MANAGER BEHAVIOR: Emphasizes problem-solving, results, analysis of failure, tasks, control, decision-making, and decision analysis.

LEADER BEHAVIOR: Focuses on creating spirit and commitment, seeking advice and feedback, empowering constituents, and modeling appropriate behavior as symbols of values and norms.

Introduction

"Florence Nightingale, after leaving the Crimea, exercised extraordinary leadership in health care for decades with no organization under her command."[1]

One of the purest examples of the leader as agenda-setter was Florence Nightingale. Her public image was and is that of the lady of mercy, but under her gentle, soft-spoken manner, she was a rugged spirit, a fighter, a tough-minded system changer. In mid-nineteenth century England a woman had no place in public life, least of all in the fiercely masculine world of the Military establishment. But she took on the establishment and revolutionized health care in the British military services. Yet she never made public appearances or speeches, and except for her two years in the Crimea, held no public position. She was a formidable authority on the evils to be remedied, she knew exactly what to do about them, and she used public opinion to goad top officials to adopt her agenda.

Florence Nightingale was both leader and manager[2].

Leadership Defined

Researchers have studied leadership for decades, but experts still do not agree on exactly what it is. Many persons use the term *leadership* as if it were a magic quality, something one is born with or simply has a talent for. However, like talent for music and art, talent for leadership involves much knowledge and disciplined practice. Many definitions of leadership have been written, among them that of Stogdill, who defines it as "the process of influencing the activities of an organized group in its efforts toward goal-setting and goal achievement."[3] A difference in responsibilities exists among group members, and each member influences the groups' activities. A leader is one others follow willingly and voluntarily.[4]

Stogdill's definition of leadership can be applied to nursing. In nursing practice, goals of patient care are set. Each patient has a nursing care plan that lists the problems that interfere with achieving physical, emotional, and social needs. For each problem, a goal is set and an approach or nursing prescription is written. An interdisciplinary team may identify problems, set goals, and write prescriptions. The team is influenced by the most highly skilled nurse available, the registered nurse who coordinates the care. Each interdisciplinary team member assumes different responsibilities in performing the total team functions.

The same principles may be applied to the entire division of nursing. Usually, the title of the head of the division is assistant administrator, vice president, chair, or director of nursing services. The division head is responsible for influencing all nursing employees toward achieving the stated purpose and objectives of the division of nursing. The nurse administrator is influenced by a stated philosophy or statement of beliefs about the kinds of services to be rendered by the personnel of the division of nursing. The total staff includes personnel in different job categories, including nurse managers, nursing case managers of shifts and clinical nursing personnel, each with different responsibilities.

Gardner defines leadership as "the process of persuasion and example by which an individual (or leadership team) induces a group to take action that is in accord with the leader's purposes or the shared purposes of all."[5] Numerous other definitions of leadership exist. Embodied in these definitions are the terms *leader, follower* or *constituent, group, process,* and *goals.* One would conclude that leadership is a process in which a person inspires a group of constituents to work together using appropriate means to achieve a common mission and common goals. Constituents are influenced to work together willingly and cooperatively, with zeal and confidence and to their greatest potential.[6]

Leadership is a social transaction in which one person influences others. People in authority do not necessarily exert leadership. Rather, effective people in authoritative positions combine authority and leadership to assist an organization to achieve its goals. Effective leadership satisfies four primary conditions[7]: (1) a person receiving a communication understands it, (2) this person has the resources to do what is being asked of him or her, (3) the person believes the behavior being asked of her or him is consistent with personal interests and values, and (4) the person believes the request is consistent with the purposes and values of the organization.

According to McGregor[8],

There are at least four major variables now known to be involved in leadership: (1) the characteristics of the leader; (2) the attitudes, needs, and other personal characteristics of the followers; (3) the characteristics of the organization, such as its purpose, its structure, the nature of the task to be performed; and (4) the social, economic, and political milieu.

Leadership is a highly complex relationship that changes with the times. Such changes are brought about by management, unions, or outside forces. In nursing, changes in leadership are wrought by nursing management, nursing educators, nursing organizations, unions, and the expectations of the clientele—patients and their families.

Talbott said, "Leadership is the vital ingredient that transforms a crowd into a functioning, useful organization."[9] The theme seems always to be the same: "Leadership is the process of sustaining an initiated action. It is certainly not a matter of pointing in a direction and just letting things happen. Leadership is the conception of a goal and a method of achieving it; the mobilization of the means necessary for attainment; and the adjustment of values and environmental factors in the light of the desired end."[10]

In all of the definitions, leadership is viewed as a dynamic, interactive process that involves three dimensions: the leader, the followers, and the situation. Each dimension influences the others. For instance, the accomplishment of goals depends not only on the personal attributes of the leader but also on the follower's needs and the type of situation.[11]

Leadership Theories

Trait Theory

Much of the early work on leadership focused on the leader. This research was directed toward identifying intellectual, emotional, physical, and other personal traits of effective leaders. The underlying assumption was that leaders are born, not made.

After many years of research, no particular set of traits has been found that predict leadership potential. There are several possible reasons for this failure. According to McGregor, "Research findings to date suggest that it is more fruitful to consider leadership as a relationship between the leader and the situation than as a universal pattern of characteristics possessed by certain people."[12] This statement implies that leadership is a human relations function and that different situations may require quite different characteristics from a leader. Is it not to a large degree universally accepted in nursing that authoritarian power is effective in times of crisis but that otherwise it promotes instability?

Despite the shortcomings of the trait theory, some traits have been identified that are common to all good leaders. Exhibit 18-1 lists some of the 20 most important qualities (traits) of a leader as cited by 3,032 Latinos in a recent nationwide study.

Gardner's Leadership Studies

Two major treatices of Gardner's writings that relate to the traits of leadership are *The Tasks of Leadership* and *Leader-Constituent Interaction.* A brief summary of

EXHIBIT 18-1
What Makes a Leader?

The 20 most important qualities of a leader, as cited by 3,032 Latinos in a recent nationwide survey. Some traits appear similar because they were named in response to an open-ended question, not chosen from a prepared list.

1	Honest/Trustworthy/Integrity	50.4%	11	Just/Impartial/Fair	2.3%
2	Intelligent/Educated/Experienced	7.5%	12	Strong Leader/Assertive	1.7%
3	Respectful/Respects the People	4.6%	13	Skilled Communicator	1.2%
4	Serve/Help the Community	4.3%	14	Patriot/Loves Country	1.2%
5	Loving/Compassionate/Kind	4.1%	15	Hard Working/Strong Work Ethic	0.8%
6	Strong Moral Values/Ethical Person	2.9%	16	Good Listener/Accessible	0.6%
7	Good Person/Responsible	2.8%	17	Dedicated/Committed	0.6%
8	Religious/Spiritual/Persona de Fe (Person of Faith)	2.8%	18	Charismatic/Visionary	0.5%
			19	Goal Oriented/Efficient	0.3%
9	Courageous/Tenacious	2.7%	20	Common Sense/Wise/Good Judgment	0.3%
10	Humble/Sincere	2.6%			

Source: J. Castillo. "Latinos List Top Qualities." *San Antonio Express-News* (22 January 2001), 1.

Gardner's ideas on these topics follows.[13] Gardner identifies nine tasks to be performed by leaders[14]:

1. Envisioning goals. These include a vision of the best a group can be, solving problems, and unifying constituencies. Goals may involve extensive research. They may be shared, and they come from many sources. Long-term goals lend greater stability than do short-term goals.

2. Affirming values. Communities have "shared assumptions, beliefs, customs, ideas that give meaning, ideas that motivate." These include norms or values. Values embody religious beliefs and secular philosophy. Society celebrates its values in art, song, ritual, historic documents, and textbooks. People will strive to meet standards that affirm their values and motivate them. Values must be continually rebuilt or regenerated, with leaders assisting to rediscover and adapt traditions to the present. Leaders reaffirm values verbally, through policy decisions, and through their conduct.

3. Motivating. Leaders stimulate people to serve society and solve its problems. They balance positive attitudes and acts with reality. They look toward the future with confidence, hope, and energy. Loss of confidence breeds rigidity, fatalism, and passivity. Poverty affects morale, learning, and performance negatively. Leaders correct the circumstances of negative attitudes and defeat. Involving employees in decisions gives them a sense of power and ownership. Leaders bring resolve to failure, frustration, and doubt and use intuition and empathy to solve problems.

4. Managing. Leadership and management overlap. Leaders set goals, plan, fix priorities, choose means, and formulate policy. They also build organizations and institutions that outlast them. Leaders keep the system functioning by setting agendas and making decisions. Leaders mold public opinion and exercise political judgments.

5. Achieving workable unity. Leaders function in a pluralistic society in which conflict is necessary if there are grievances to be settled. Conflict is also necessary in commercial competition, settling civil suits, and bringing justice to the oppressed. Conflict must be resolved to achieve cohesion and mutual tolerance, internally and externally. Society is fragmented and must not be polarized. Conflict resolution requires political skills: brokering, coalition formation, mediating conflicting views, de-escalation of rhetoric and posturing, saving face, and seeking common ground. People must trust each other most of the time to prevent or resolve conflict. Leaders raise the level of trust.

6. Explaining. Leaders must communicate effectively. They teach.

7. Serving as a symbol. Leaders speak for others. They represent unity, collective identity, and continuity.

8. Representing the group. All human systems are interdependent. Leaders view events affecting them broadly.

9. Renewing. Leaders blend continuity with change. They are innovators who awaken the potential of others. They visit the front lines and keep in touch. Leaders sustain diversity and dissent, and they change the social order.

Leader-Constituent Interaction

Charismatic Leaders

Gardner defines "charisma" as the quality that sets one person apart from others: supernatural, superhuman, endowed with exceptional qualities or powers. Charismatic leadership can be good or evil. Charismatic leaders emerge in troubled times and in relation to the state of mind of constituents. They eventually run out of miracles and "white horses," even though the leaders are magnetic, persuasive, and spellbinding.

Masses of people will often follow the charismatic leader. Such masses have historically been labeled unstable. The worry about mob rule and instability still exists. Social disorder is embodied in the Constitution of the United States.

Influence of Constituents on Leaders

Constituents and leaders have an equal influence on each other. Constituents confer the leadership role. Good constituents select good leaders and make them better. In politics, constituents may follow any leader unless they are bureaucratic constituents (such as government employees) who feel constrained to mute their support. Loyal constituents support leaders who help them meet their needs and solve problems.

Influence of Leaders on Constituents

Leaders choose to be leaders. They must adapt their leadership style to the situation and their constituents. In doing so, they weigh the following considerations: the degree of structure they want in relationships with constituents; the degree or hierarchy of authority, formality, discipline, constraint, and control; and the amount of focus on task versus people.

Leaders influence their superiors and their subordinates and have the courage to defy their constituents. Sam Houston was a leader of this type. He opposed the secession of Texas from the United States, going contrary to his constituents. A leader may show different faces to pluralistic groups of constituents, including special interest groups.

Transforming Leaders

Transforming leaders respond to people's basic needs, wants, hopes, and expectations. They may transcend the political system or even attempt to construct it in order to operate within it. Transforming leadership is innovative and evolutionary.

The best leadership may be that which focuses on self-development and self-actualization. Leaders should develop the strengths of constituents and make them independent.[15]

Many of Gardner's leadership qualities embody concepts of management.

Behavioral Theories

Among the behavioral research and theories are those of Douglas McGregor's Theory X and Theory Y, Rensis

Likert's Michigan studies, Blake and Mouton's managerial Grid® and Kurt Lewin's studies. Each of these is described here in more detail.

McGregor's Theory X and Theory Y

McGregor related his theories to the motivation theories of Maslow. McGregor stated that each person is a whole individual living and interacting within a world of other individuals. What happens to this person happens as a result of the behavior of other people. The attitudes and emotions of others affect this person. The constituent is dependent on the leader and desires to be treated fairly. A successful relationship is desired by both and depends on the action taken by the leader.

Security is a condition of leadership. Constituents need security and will fight to protect themselves against real or imagined threats to these needs in the work situation. Leaders must act to give constituents this security through avenues such as fair pay and fringe benefits. Unions act to solidify job security.

A leader provides a further condition for effective leadership by creating an atmosphere of approval for constituents. Such an atmosphere is created through the leader's manner and attitude. Given the genuine approval of their leader, constituents will be secure. Otherwise, they will feel threatened, fearful, and insecure.

Knowledge is another condition of effective leadership espoused by McGregor. Employees have security when they know what is expected of them, including[16]:

- Knowledge of overall company policy and management philosophy.
- Knowledge of procedures, rules, and regulations.
- Knowledge of the requirements of the subordinate's job duties, responsibilities, and place in the organization.
- Knowledge of the personal peculiarities of the constituent's immediate leader.
- Knowledge by the constituent of the leader's opinion of his or her performance.
- Advance knowledge of changes that may affect the constituent.

Consistent discipline is another condition for effective leadership. People are met with approval when they do their jobs according to the rules. They should know what to expect in terms of disapproval when they break these rules. Leaders should be consistent in setting standards and expecting constituents to meet them. Even discipline must occur in an atmosphere of approval.

Security encourages independence, another condition for effective leadership. Insecurity causes a reactive fight for freedom. Security that stimulates independence is desired. Constituents need to be actively independent by becoming involved in contributing ideas and suggestions concerning activities that affect them. When

EXHIBIT 18-2
Likert's Leadership Systems

AUTHORITATIVE		DEMOCRATIC	
SYSTEM I **EXPLOITATIVE-AUTHORITATIVE**	**SYSTEM II** **BENEVOLENT-AUTHORITATIVE**	**SYSTEM III** **CONSULTATIVE-DEMOCRATIC**	**SYSTEM IV** **PARTICIPATIVE-DEMOCRATIC**
Top management makes all decisions	Top management makes most decisions	Some delegated decisions made at lower levels	Decision making dispersed throughout organization
Motivation by coercion	Motivation by economic and ego motives	Motivation by economic, ego, and other motives such as desire for new experiences	Motivation by economic rewards established by group participation
Communication downward	Communication mostly downward	Communication down and up	Communication down, up, and with peers
Review and control functions concentrated in top management	Review and control functions primarily at top	Review and control functions primarily at the top but ideas are solicited from lower levels	Review and control functions shared by superiors and subordinates

Source: Adapted from R. Likert. *The Human Organization* (New York: McGraw-Hill, 1967), 4–10. © 1967. Reproduced with permission of McGraw-Hill Book Co.

workers are secure and encouraged to participate in solving the problems of work, they provide new approaches to solutions. They work to achieve the goals of the organization and feel they are a part of it.

With security and independence, constituents develop a desire to accept responsibility. The level of responsibility can be increased at a pace commensurate with preservation of constituents' security. Having security gives constituents pleasure and pride. Leaders need security before they can delegate responsibility to constituents.

All constituents need a provision for appeal, that is, an adequate grievance procedure by which they can take their differences with their superiors to a higher level in the organization. Leaders who do the jobs expected of them, and who treat constituents in ways that meet their needs and give them security achieve self-realization and self-development.[17]

McGregor's Theory X and Theory Y are further discussed in Chapter 19, Motivation.

Likert's Michigan Studies

Likert and his associates at the Institute for Social Research at the University of Michigan did extensive leadership research. They identified four basic styles or systems of leadership: System I, exploitative-authoritative; System II, benevolent-authoritative; System III, consultative-democratic; and System IV, participative-democratic. These systems are summarized in Exhibit 18-2.

A measuring instrument for evaluating an organization's leadership style was developed by Likert's group. It contains 51 items and encompasses variables of the concepts of "leadership, motivation, communication, interaction-influence, decision-making, goal setting, control, and performance goals."[18]

It is generally conceded that leadership behavior improves in effectiveness as it approaches System IV.

Blake and Mouton's Managerial Grid®

The Managerial Grid® is a two-dimensional leadership model. Dimensions of this model are tasks or production and the employee or people orientations of managers. Grid synopsis describes the model[19]:

Grid® Synopsis. Two key dimensions of managerial thinking are depicted on the Grid®: *concern for production* on the horizontal axis, and *concern for people* on the vertical axis. They are shown as nine-point scales, where 1 represents low concern, 5 represents an average amount of concern, and 9 is high concern.

These two concerns are interdependent; that is, although concern for one or the other may be high or low, they are integrated in the manager's thinking. Thus, both concerns are present to some degree in any management style. Study of the Grid® enables one to sort out various possibilities and the attitudes, values, beliefs and assumptions that underlie each approach. When one is able to objectively see one's own behavior compared to the soundest approach, it provides motivation to change in order to more closely approximate the soundest management style. When group members come to share 9, 9 values, beliefs, attitudes, and assumptions, they develop personal commitment to achieving group goals as well as their individual goals. In doing so they develop standards of mutual trust and respect that cause them to elevate cooperation and communication.

Blake and Mouton contend that the 9, 9 style is the one most likely to achieve highest quality results over an extended period of time. The 9, 9 style, unlike the others, is based on the assumption that there is no inherent conflict between the needs of the organization for performance and the needs of people for job satisfaction.

Finally, as an orienting framework, the Grid® serves as a road map toward more effective ways of working with and through others. When group members have this common frame of reference for what constitutes effective and ineffective approaches to issues of mutual concern, they are enabled to take corrective action based on common understanding and agreement about the soundest approach and objectivity when actions taken are less than fully sound.

Exhibits 18-3A–C illustrate general management application of the Grid®, whereas Exhibit 18-3D illustrates its application to the job of the nurse administrator.

Kurt Lewin's Studies

Lewin's leadership studies were done in the 1930s. Lewin examined three leadership styles related to forces within the leader, within the group members, and within the situation. These three leadership styles are summarized in Exhibit 18-4.

Other behavioral studies include the Ohio State studies, which use a quadrant structure that relates leadership effectiveness to initiating structure, with emphasis on the task or production, and consideration, with emphasis on the employee. These studies identified four primary leadership styles, as illustrated in Exhibit 18-5.

The Ohio State Researchers used the Leader Behavior Description Questionnaire. Items related to "initiating structure" and "consideration" describe how leaders carry out their activities. Both factors are considered simultaneously rather than on a continuum. As to which combination works best, the situation determines the style.[20]

Problems with Leadership Questionnaires

According to Phillips and Lord, the accuracy of leadership questionnaires is debatable. Yet they are often the only feasible way to measure leadership in real-world settings. Some researchers consider reliable questionnaires accurate. However, these authors contend that any systematic sources of variance, such as leniency error, halo, or implicit theories, can produce high internal consistency. Factor structures produced solely on the basis of implicit leadership theories do not tell users of these questionnaires anything about accuracy.

The Leader Behavior Description Questionnaire was flawed by having subjects form an overall leadership impression before completing it. Questionnaires can be improved by requiring "observers to distinguish between the presence and absence of specific, conceptually equivalent behaviors in videotaped stimulus materials."[21]

Most questionnaire-based leadership research has been conducted in laboratory settings. The results are biased by the fact that some conditions do not exist in typical field settings. Research participants do not know or have contact with the target leader; thus the behavioral-level accuracy of their responses is limited. Phillips and Lord make the following suggestions to improve research techniques of existing behavioral description questionnaires[22]:

1. Assess whether the level of accuracy required for the purpose is classification or behavioral.
2. Assess whether the level of accuracy produced by the chosen measurement technique is classification or behavioral.
3. Evaluate the research setting for potential biases "such as rote knowledge of performance, leniency in describing superiors, or other relevant rater characteristics."
4. If biases exist, judge whether they are likely to be confounded with substantive variables of interest to the user.
5. Collect global measures of leadership and leniency during the measurement process.

Leadership questionnaires are useful when used and interpreted appropriately.

Leadership Style

Other studies of leadership focus on style, including contingency-situational leadership models that focus on a combination of factors, such as the people, the task, the situation, the organization, and a number of environmental factors. These models combine theories of Fred F. Fiedler; Paul Hersey, Kenneth H. Blanchard, and D. E. Johnson; and William J. Reddin, whose contributions are discussed in the following section.

Fiedler's Contingency Model of Leadership Effectiveness

There must be a group before there can be a leader. Fiedler indicates three classifications that measure the kind of power and influence the group gives its leader. The first and most important of these is the relationship between the leader and the group members. Personality is a factor, but its influence depends on the group's perception of the leader. Second is the task structure, the degree to which details of the group's assignment are programmed. If the assignment is highly structured, the leader will have less power. If the assignment requires planning and thinking, the leader will be in a position to exert greater power. Third is the positional power of the leader: It should be noted that great power does not yield better group performance. The best leader has

EXHIBIT 18-3A–C
The Leadership Grid Figure

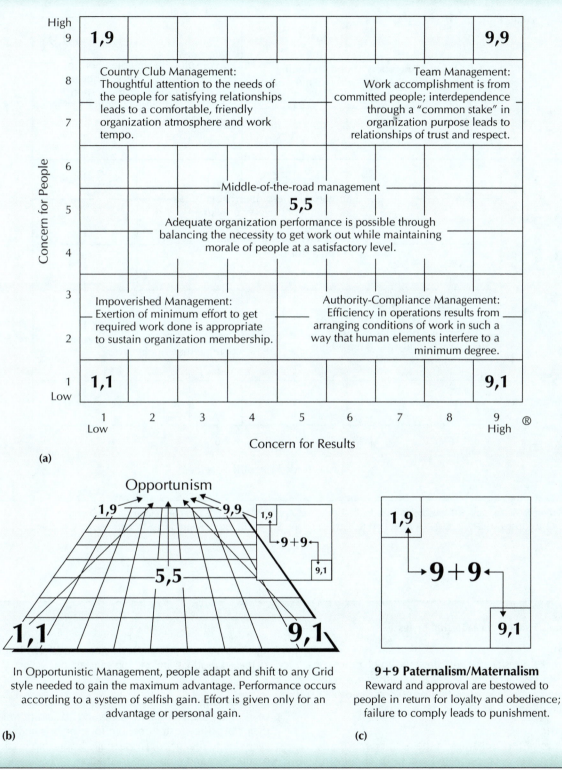

(a)

Opportunism

In Opportunistic Management, people adapt and shift to any Grid style needed to gain the maximum advantage. Performance occurs according to a system of selfish gain. Effort is given only for an advantage or personal gain.

(b)

9+9 Paternalism/Maternalism
Reward and approval are bestowed to people in return for loyalty and obedience; failure to comply leads to punishment.

(c)

Source: The Leadership Grid® figure, Paternalism figure, and Opportunism Figure from *Leadership Dilemmas*—Grid Solutions, by Robert R. Blake and Anne Adams McCanse (Houston: Gulf Publishing Company). (Grid figure: p. 29, Paternalism figure: p. 30, Opportunism figure: p. 31). Copyright 1991 by Scientific Methods, Inc. Reproduced by permission of the owners.

EXHIBIT 18-3D
The Nurse Administrator Grid®

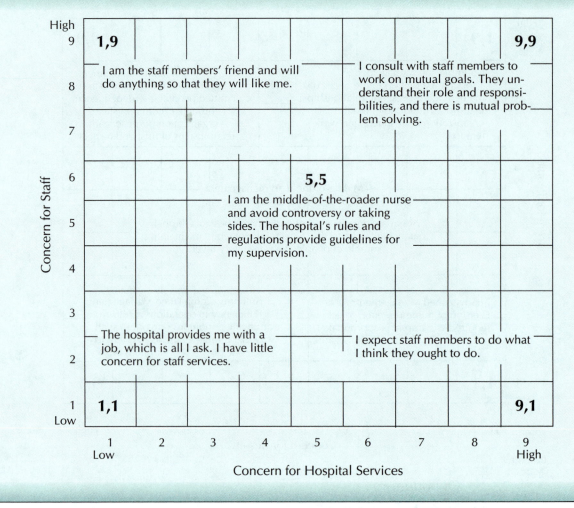

Source: Robert R. Blake, Jane S. Mouton, and Mildred Tapper. *Grid Approaches for Managerial Leadership in Nursing* (St. Louis: C. V. Mosby, 1981), 2. © 1984 by Robert R. Blake and Jane Srygley Mouton. Reproduced by permission of owners.

EXHIBIT 18-4
Kurt Lewin's Studies of Leadership Styles

AUTOCRATIC
Leaders make decisions alone. They tend to be more concerned with task accomplishment than with concern for people. Autocratic leadership tends to promote hostility and aggression or apathy and to decrease initiative.

DEMOCRATIC
Leaders involve their followers in the decision-making process. They are people-oriented and focus on human relations and teamwork. Democratic leadership leads to increased productivity and job satisfaction.

LAISSEZ-FAIRE
Leaders are loose and permissive and abstain from leading their staff. They foster freedom for everyone and want everyone to feel good. Laissez-faire leadership results in low productivity and employee frustration.

Source: From *Management: Concepts and Applications*, 2d ed., by Leon Megginson et al. Copyright © 1986 by Harper & Row. Reprinted by permission of HarperCollins Publishers.

EXHIBIT 18-5
Scores of Five Leaders: Initiating Structure and Consideration

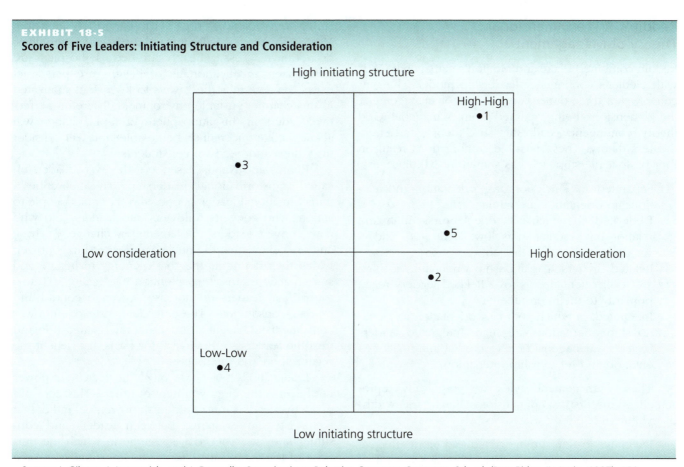

Source: J. Gibson, J. Ivancevich, and J. Donnelly. *Organizations: Behavior, Structure, Processes*, 9th ed. (Burr Ridge, IL: Irwin, 1997), 150.

Note: The Ohio State researchers measured leaders' tendencies to practice these two leadership behaviors and were able to depict them graphically. Exhibit 18-5 shows behaviors of five different leaders. Individual 1 is high on both initiating structure and consideration; individual 4 is low on both dimensions.

Research indicates there are more complicated interactions of the two dimensions. Effective leaders may have equal amounts of initiating structure and consideration.

been found to be one who has a task-oriented leadership style. This style works best when the leader has great influence and power over group members. When the leader has moderate influence over group members, a relationship-oriented style works best.

The organization shares responsibility for a leader's success or failure. Leaders can be trained to learn in which situation they do well and in which they fail. The job can be fitted to the leader. The appointee can be given a higher rank or can be assigned constituents who are nearly equal in rank and status. Most appointees can be given sole authority or can be required to consult with the group. The appointee can be given detailed instructions or independence. A highly successful and effective leader avoids situations in which failure is likely. That leader seeks out situations that fit his or her leadership style. Knowledge of strengths and weaknesses helps in choosing this style.[23]

Fiedler's theory is one of situations. Leadership style will be effective or ineffective depending on the situation.

Life Cycle Theory of Hersey and Blanchard

Hersey, Blanchard, and Johnson follow a situational approach to leadership. A person's leadership style focuses on a combination of task behaviors and relationship behaviors. Focus on task behaviors is "characterized by endeavoring to establish well-defined patterns of organization, channels of communication, and ways of getting jobs accomplished." Focus on relationship behavior relates to "opening up channels of communication, providing socio-emotional support, actively listening, 'psychological strokes,' and facilitating behaviors."[24] These definitions evolve from the Ohio State Leadership Quadrant as shown in Exhibit 18-5.

Reddin's Three-Dimensional Theory of Management

Reddin combined Blake and Mouton's managerial Grid® with Fiedler's contingency leadership model. The outcome was a three-dimensional theory of management, the dimensions being adapted from Managerial Grid theory, contingency leadership style theory, and effectiveness theory. These possible combinations result in four basic leadership styles as shown in Exhibit 18-6.

1. Separated, in which both task orientation and relationship orientation are minimal.
2. Dedicated, in which task orientation is high and relationship orientation is low. Dedicated leaders are dedicated only to the job.
3. Related, in which relationship orientation is high and task orientation is low. Related leaders relate primarily to their constituents.
4. Integrated, in which both task orientation and relationship orientations are high. Integrated leaders focus on managerial behavior, combining task orientation and relationship orientation.

These management styles are graphically represented by the first two dimensions (height and width) of Exhibit 18-6.

- Executive leaders are integrated and more effective than are compromiser leaders, who are less effective integrated leaders.
- Developer leaders are related and more effective than missionary leaders, who are less effective related leaders.
- Bureaucrat leaders are separated and more effective than deserter leaders, who are less effective separated leaders.
- Benevolent autocrat leaders are dedicated and more effective than autocrat leaders, who are less effective dedicated leaders.

The range of effectiveness is a continuum. As in other theories of leadership, the effective behavior of the leader is relative to the situation. Effective leaders apply leadership styles after assessing situations.[25]

Transformational Leadership

The health care system is experiencing tremendous change and chaos, and the problems of the organization are increasingly complex. Health care organizations are restructuring and redesigning the way patient care is delivered to meet the challenges of these changes. In addition, health care is becoming prohibitively expensive for many Americans. Hospitals and emergency rooms are financially burdened by the uninsured who

suffer from violence, drug overdose, and HIV infection. Many people, especially in rural areas and inner cities, do not have access to health care because hospitals are downsizing and a shortage of health care personnel exists. Leaders must find ways to keep staff motivated in this chaotic, unstable environment. Therefore, effective leaders in this atmosphere of rapid change will acknowledge uncertainty, be flexible, and will consider the values and needs of constituents.[26]

Bennis and Nanus describe a theory of leadership called transformational leadership. They describe a transformational leader as one who "commits people to action, who converts followers into leaders, and who may convert leaders into agents of change."[27] These authors believe that the nucleus of leadership is power, which they define as the "basic energy to initiate and sustain action translating intention into reality."[28] Transformational leaders do not use power to control and repress constituents. These leaders instead empower constituents to have a vision about the organization and trust the leaders so they work for goals that benefit the organization and themselves.

Leadership is thus not so much the exercise of power itself as it is the empowerment of others. This does not mean that leaders must relinquish power, but rather that reciprocity, an exchange between leaders and constituents, exists. The goal is change in which the purpose of the leader and that of the constituent become enmeshed, creating a collective purpose. Empowered staff become critical thinkers and are active in their roles within the organization. A creative and committed staff is the most important asset that an administrator can develop.[29]

Transformational leaders will mobilize their staff by focusing on the welfare of the individual and humanizing the high-tech work environment. For the future, experts favor a leadership style that empowers others and values collaboration instead of competition.[30] People are empowered when they share in decision-making and when they are rewarded for quality and excellence rather than punished and manipulated. When the environment is humanized and people are empowered, they feel part of the team and believe they are contributing to the success of the organization. Leaders who share power motivate people to excel by inspiring them to be part of a vision rather than punishing them for mistakes.[31] In nursing, empowerment can result in improved patient care, fewer staff sick days, and decreased attrition. Nurses who are transformational leaders have staff with higher job satisfaction and who stay in the organization for longer periods.[32]

Nurse executives who like to feel in charge may feel threatened by the concept of sharing power with staff. So they need to be personally empowered to assist in the empowerment of others. They will have a

EXHIBIT 18-6
Reddin's Three-Dimensional Management Styles

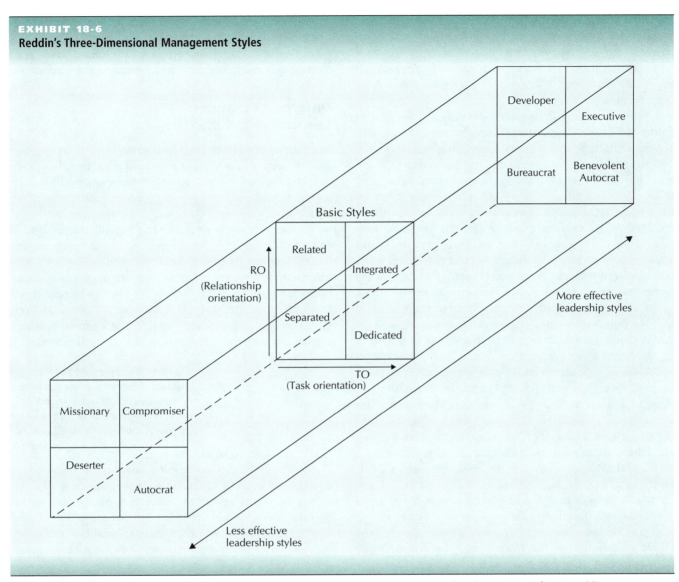

Source: W. J. Reddin. *Managerial Effectiveness* (New York: McGraw-Hill, 1970), 230. Reprinted with permission of W. J. Reddin.

sense of self-worth and self-respect and confidence in their own abilities. Bennis and Nanus believe the most important, essential trait of successful leaders is having positive self-regard.[33] Self-regard is not, however, self-centeredness or self-importance; rather, leaders with positive self-esteem recognize their strengths and do not emphasize their weaknesses. Interestingly, a leader who has positive self-regard seems to create in others a sense of confidence and high expectations. Techniques used to increase self-worth include the use of visualization, affirmations, and letting go of the need to be perfect.[34]

Through research and observations, Bennis defined four competencies for dynamic and effective transformational leadership: (1) management of attention, (2) management of meaning, (3) management of trust, and (4) management of self.[35] The first competency is the management of attention, achieved by having a vision

or sense of outcomes or goals. Vision is the image of a realistic, attainable, credible, and attractive future state for an organization.[36] Vision statements are written to define where the health care organization is headed and how it will serve society. They differ from mission and philosophy statements in that they are more futuristic and describe where energies are to be focused.[37]

People are committed to visions that are mutually developed, are based on a sense of quality, appeal to their values and emotions, and are feasible yet challenging.

The second leadership competency is management of meaning. To inspire commitment, leaders must communicate their vision and create a culture that sustains the vision. Creating a culture or social architecture as described by Bennis and Nanus is "intangible, but it governs the way people act, the values and norms that are subtly transmitted to groups and individuals, and the construct of binding and bonding within a company."[38] Barker believes that "social architecture provides meaning and shared experience of organizational events so that people know the expectations of how they are to act."[39]

Nursing leaders transform the social architecture or culture of health care organizations by using group discussion, agreement, and consensus building, and they will support individual creativity and innovation. To do this, Barker believes that the nurse transformational leader will pay attention to the internal consistency of the vision, goals, and objectives; selection and placement of personnel; feedback; appraisal; rewards; support; and development.[40] For example, rewards and appraisals must relate to the goals, and the vision must be consistent with the goals and objectives. Most importantly, all the elements must enhance the self-worth of individuals, allow creativity, and appeal to the values of nurses. For many nurse leaders, these are new skills that will take time and support from mentors to develop.

Because vision statements are a new concept to many, nursing leaders should provide opportunities for staff to openly explore feelings, criticize, and articulate negative reactions. Face-to-face meetings between nursing leaders and staff are desirable because in reactions involving trust and clarity, memorandums and suggestion boxes are not substitutes for direct communication.[41]

The third competency is the management of trust, which is associated with reliability. Nurses respect leaders whose judgment is sound and consistent and whose decisions are based on fairness, equity, and honesty. Staff can be heard to comment about leaders they trust with a statement such as "I don't always agree with her decision, but I know she wants the best for the patients." Bennis believes that "people would much rather follow individuals they can count on, even when they disagree with their viewpoint, than people they agree with but who shift positions frequently."[42]

The fourth competency is management of self, which is knowing one's skills and using them effectively. It is critical that nurses in leadership positions recognize when they lack management skills and then take responsibility for their own continuing education. Incompetent leaders can demoralize a nursing unit and contribute to poor patient care. When leadership skills are mastered by nurse leaders, stress and burnout are reduced. Nurse leaders thus need to master the skills of leadership.[43]

Although effective leaders are supportive of shared power and decision-making, they continue to accept responsibility for making decisions even when their decisions are not popular. Constituents like to have their wishes considered, but there are times when they want prompt and clear decisions from a leader, especially in times of crisis.[44] Transformational leaders are flexible and able to adapt leadership styles to the chaos and rapid change occurring in the current health care environment.

Differences Between Leadership and Management

Managers come from the "headship" (power from position) category. They hold appointive or directive posts in formal organizations. They can be appointed for both technical and leadership competencies, usually needing both to be accepted. Managers are delegated authority, including the power to reward or punish. A manager is expected to perform functions such as planning, organizing, directing (leading), and controlling (evaluating). Informal leaders, by contrast, are not always managers performing those functions required by the organization. Leaders often are not even part of the organization. Florence Nightingale, after leaving the Crimea, was not connected with an organization but was still a leader.

> Zaleznik indicates that the manager is a problem solver who succeeds because of "persistence, tough-mindedness, hard work, intelligence, analytical ability, and, perhaps most important, tolerance and good will."[45]

Managers focus on results, analysis of failure, and tasks, management characteristics that are desirable for nurse managers. Effective managers also need to be good leaders. Managers who are leaders choose and limit goals. They focus on creating spirit and in doing so, they develop committed constituents. Manager-leaders do this by seeking advice and solutions to problems. They ask for information and provide positive feedback. Leaders understand the power of groups. They empower their constituents, making their subordinates strong—the chosen ones, a team infused with purpose. Mistakes are tolerated by manager-leaders who challenge constituents to realize their potential.

Managers emphasize control, decision-making, and decision analysis. As manager-leaders, they are concerned with modeling appropriate behavior as symbols of values and norms. Effective manager-leaders are technically capable and provide assurance in crises.

Managers focus inward but add the leadership dimension of connecting their group to the outside world, focusing intense attention on important issues. They escalate issues and complaints up the organization to be handled quickly and appropriately, rather than try to control them.[46]

Although managers are sometimes described in less glowing terms than leaders, successful managers are usually successful leaders. Leadership is a desirable and prominent feature of the directing function of nursing management.

Similarities Between Leadership and Management

Gardner asserts that first-class managers are usually first-class leaders. Leaders and leader-managers distinguish themselves beyond general run-of-the-mill managers in six respects[47]:

1. They think longer term—beyond the day's crises, beyond the quarterly report, beyond the horizon.
2. They look beyond the unit they are heading and grasp its relationship to larger realities—the larger organization of which they are a part, conditions external to the organization, global trends.
3. They reach and influence constituents beyond their jurisdiction, beyond boundaries. Thomas Jefferson influenced people all over Europe. Gandhi influenced people all over the world. In an organization, leaders overflow bureaucratic boundaries—often a distinct advantage in a world too complex and tumultuous to be handled "through channels." Their capacity to rise above jurisdictions may enable them to bind together the fragmented constituencies that must work together to solve a problem.
4. They put heavy emphasis on the intangibles of vision, values, and motivation and understand intuitively the nonrational and unconscious elements in the leader-constituent interaction.
5. They have the political skill to cope with the conflicting requirements of multiple constituencies.
6. They think in terms of renewal. The routine manager tends to accept the structure and processes as they exist. The leader or leader/manager seeks the revisions of process and structure required by ever-changing reality.

Good leaders, like good managers, provide visionary inspiration, motivation, and direction. Good managers, like good leaders, attract and inspire. People want to be led rather than managed. They want to pursue goals and values they consider worthwhile. Therefore, they want leaders who respect the dignity, autonomy, and self-esteem of constituents.[48]

Effective nurse executives combine leadership and management.

Mitchell describes five major requirements for every executive, implying that being an executive requires the attributes of a leader[49]:

1. Adjustment to a complex social environment of several or many units
2. Ability to influence and guide subordinates
3. Emotional and intellectual maturity as a preparation for leadership
4. Ability to think through and make decisions, and to translate decisions into effective action
5. Capacity to see beyond the immediate or surface indications and, with experience, to acquire perspective.

Effective nurse leader-managers will work to achieve these same requisites.

That a relationship between leadership and management exists seems scarcely arguable. Leadership is a subsystem within the management system. It is included as an element of management science in management textbooks and other publications. In some, the term *leading* has replaced the term *directing* as a major function of management. In such a context communication and motivation would be elements of leadership, a concept that could be debated according to management theorists' philosophical bent.

Management includes written plans, clear organizational charts, well-documented annual objectives, frequent reports, detailed and precise job descriptions, regular evaluations of performance against objectives, and the administrative ordering of theory.[50] Nurse managers who are leaders can use these tools of management without making them a bureaucratic roadblock to autonomy, participatory management, maximum performance, and productivity by employees.

Leadership Versus Headship

A job title does not make a person a leader, nor does it cause a person to exercise leadership behavior over subordinates. This is as true of nurses as it is of personnel in industry or the military services. It is a mistake to refer to the dean of a college, a professor of nursing, a nurse administrator, a supervisor, a nurse manager, or any nurse as a leader by virtue of position. That person is in a headship position rather than a leadership one, because "leadership is more a function of the group or situation than a quality which adheres to a person appointed to a formal position of headship."[51] A person's behavior will indicate whether that person also occupies a functional leadership position.

Gardner writes that not all people in positions of high status are leaders. Some are chief bureaucrats or custodians. Their high status does have "symbolic values and traditions that enhance the possibility of leadership" since people have higher expectations of people in headship positions.[52] Authority embodied in a title or position of headship is legitimized power; it is not leadership.[53]

Leadership is an attempt to influence groups or individuals without the coercive form of power.

Appointed heads are not selected by persons they will direct. Appointed heads frequently work toward organizational goals while ignoring the personal goals of employees. Their authority comes from higher in the organization and not from their influence within the group.

In cases in which heads are elected by the group, they keep their positions only as long as they satisfy the members' needs for affiliating with the organization. They are responsible only to the group, whereas the appointed head is usually responsible to both the appointive authority and the group. Nurses who are elected to chair committees or preside over professional organizations will not be reelected unless they satisfy the members' needs.

Appointed heads may lack the freedom to choose relationships with subordinates because their supervisors do not allow it. They will have authority and power without being accepted by the group. If appointed nurse managers are allowed to and can exercise their leadership abilities, they can be accorded leadership status by the group. The nurse managers will understand and motivate employees in order to be trusted by them.[54]

Preparation of Nursing Leaders

Gardner believes that 90% of leadership can be taught.[55] Education begins in basic nursing education programs. To develop risk-taking behaviors and self-confidence, students should be encouraged to create new solutions and to disagree and debate and should be allowed to make mistakes without fear of reprisal. Faculty should encourage and support students who exercise their leadership abilities in projects and organizations on campus and in the community.

When nurses graduate and enter the work force, most are not ready to assume a leadership role. They require opportunities for self-discovery to understand their strengths and for skill building. This skill building occurs through on-the-job training, along with support from peers and mentorship from effective leaders. These mentors must be dynamic, not status-quo-seeking, role models who teach nurses how to preserve sameness. Tack writes that to prepare leaders for the future, they must be mentored by "those who see the world differently and project a dramatically different future, those who tend to shake things up rather than follow established precedents."[56]

Organizational managers, including nurse executives, will teach managers the nature of leadership. They will train nurse managers in leadership skills, and will put managers in the proper environment to learn leadership. This will include "starting up an operation, turning around a troubled division, moving from staff to line, working under a wise mentor, serving on a high-level task force and getting promoted to a more senior level of the organization."[57]

Nurse executives and managers should be trained to coach their constituents on leadership skills. Constituents can be trained to help managers in leadership. Leaders can listen and articulate, persuade and be persuaded, use collective wisdom to make decisions, and teach constituents to relate or communicate upward.

Gender Issues

Because the majority of nurses are women, it is essential to understand the gender issues. Research indicates that gender differences do exist in leadership styles and competencies.[58] Masculinity has been associated with being task oriented and using the direct approach for solving problems. Femininity has been characterized as being people-oriented and supportive, sharing feelings and caring for others. Desjardins and Brown conducted two-hour interviews of 72 college presidents that included questions concerning, for example, power, conflict resolution, and learning style. The findings indicated that the majority of women practiced leadership in a care-connected style.[59] This orientation, first described by Gilligan, values intimacy and nurturing in interactions with others.[60] The majority of menmade decisions is in the justice and rights mode, as was first described by Kohlberg in his work on moral reasoning.[61] This style of decision-making values autonomy, objectivity, and fairness.

Rosener's research seems to support the thesis that leadership style is connected to gender issues. Rosener describes four major areas of difference in the women leaders whom she studied. First, these women tend to encourage participation; second, they share power and information more readily; third, they attempt to enhance the self-worth of others; and fourth, they energize others.[62]

It is important to remember that the modes and traits described by both researchers are gender-related but not gender specific. Women and men fall into both modes, but more men are found in the justice and rights mode.[63] Also Rosener's work seems to indicate that men operate more often out of what Rosener sees as management transactions, exchanging rewards for services rendered or punishments for poor performance. Men, she found, also work more out of the power of their positions.[64]

Gender issues as they relate to leadership in health care organizations have not been well studied. Dunham and Klahefn found that male and female nurse executives are not more likely to exhibit transformational leadership rather than transactional leadership, which focuses more on day-to-day operations.[65] Borman's research on executives in health care organizations indicates that women, more than men, identify connections to others and flexibility as important characteristics of leaders.[66] The literature points out that flexibility may be a desirable attribute in a rapidly changing or restructured organization; therefore, women may have an advantage over men.[67]

Gender differences in leadership style and competencies do not translate into one style being better than the other. However, if nurses are sensitized to gender differences, they will accept and utilize individuals for their unique leadership strengths instead of resisting them. This accepting atmosphere will encourage nurses (both men and women) to develop self-confidence and become strong leaders.

Research is needed on gender issues related to nursing leadership.

Nursing and Leadership Health Care Policy

Nursing is usually conspicuous by its absence from lists of national leaders. National consumers do not perceive nurse leaders as having power. The health care system has failed to recognize nurses as professionals with knowledge useful in creating solutions to complex problems. Cutler's perspective of nursing educators and nursing service personnel is that they have been the product of directive and authoritarian leadership.[68]

Historically, nurses have avoided opportunities to obtain power and political muscle. The profession now understands that power and political savvy will assist in achieving its goals to improve health care and to increase nurses' autonomy. Also, if the health care system is to be reformed, nurses must participate individually and collectively. Nurses need to find ways to influence health care policy-making so their holistic voice is heard.[69] Milio believes that nurses have the capacity for power to influence public policy and recommends the following steps to prepare[70]:

1. Organize.
2. Do homework: Learn to understand the political process, interest groups, specific people, and events.
3. Frame arguments to suit the target audience by appealing to cost containment, political support, fairness and justice, and other data relevant to particular concerns.
4. Support and strengthen the position of converted policymakers.
5. Concentrate energies.
6. Stimulate public debate.
7. Make the position of nurses visible in the mass media.
8. Choose as the main strategy the most effective one.
9. Act in a timely fashion.
10. Maintain activity.
11. Keep the organizational format decentralized.
12. Obtain and develop the best research data to support each position.
13. Learn from experience.
14. Never give up without trying.

Nurses in leadership positions are most influential.[71]

Buffering

Nursing leaders can act as buffers or advocates for nurses. In doing so, they protect constituents from internal and external pressures of work. Nurse managers can reduce barriers to clinical nurses completing their clinical work.

Buffering protects practicing clinical nurses from external health system factors, from the health care organization, from other supervisors and employees, from top administrators, from the medical staff, and from themselves when their behavior jeopardizes their careers. Buffering is another facet of the theory of leadership related to management and requires leadership training.

The nurse practitioner, the extended-role nurse, staff nurses, and ancillary personnel can be protected by buffering action by nurse managers. Professional nurses do not want to have additional responsibilities delegated if they are already under severe pressure and stress. Delegation of decision-making is power; delegation of work is drudgery. Professional nurses are there to motivate not dissatisfy.

Smith and Mitry suggest three methods of buffering, the benefits of which will be improved performance, better morale, increased loyalty, a healthier organization, and respect for leaders[72]:

1. Coordinating work, that is, support services and standardized records
2. Insulating by intervening with pressure groups and creating unity of command
3. Evaluating the impingement

Management writers say there is a difference between leadership and managers, but their textbooks and writings on the subject all include leadership content. It can be stated unequivocally that professional nurses want to be led, not directed or controlled. Also, nurse managers can learn the concepts, principles, and laws that will assist them in becoming effective leader-managers.

Different situations require different leadership styles. The leader-manager assesses each situation and exercises the appropriate leadership style. Some employees want to be involved; others do not. There must be a fit between the leader and constituents. The leader demonstrates this by changing style and training others until a transition is made. A flexible leadership style is necessary and vital.

Summary

The theory of nursing leadership is a part of the theory of nursing management. Leadership is a process of influencing a group to set and achieve goals. There are several major theories of leadership. One of the earliest is the trait theory, which suggests that leaders have many intellectual, personality, and ability traits. Trait theory has been succeeded by other leadership theories indicating that managers, including nurse managers, can learn the knowledge and skills requisite to leadership competencies.

Behavioral theories of leadership include McGregor's Theory X and Theory Y, Likert's Michigan studies, Blake and Mouton's Managerial Grid, and Lewin's studies.

Other studies of leadership focus on contingency-situational leadership styles and factors such as people, tasks, situations, organizations, and environment. Theorists include Fiedler; Hersey, Blanchard, and Johnson; Reddin, and Gardner.

John W. Gardner's study of leadership includes the nature of leadership, identification of leadership tasks, leader-constituent interaction, and the relationship between leadership and power.

Bennis and Nanus define a theory of leadership they call transformational. This leadership method involves change in which the purposes of the leader and follower become intertwined. The effective leader creates a vision for the organization and then develops a commitment to the vision. Bennis and Nanus believe that the wise use of power is the energy needed to develop commitment and to sustain action.

Nurse managers should learn to practice leadership behaviors that stimulate motivation within their constituents, practicing professional nurses, and other nursing personnel. These behaviors include promotion of autonomy, decision-making, and participatory management by professional nurses. It should be noted that these behaviors are facilitated by effective nurse manager-leaders.

APPLICATION EXERCISES

EXERCISE 18-1   Name a nurse you consider to be an outstanding leader and state why you consider her or him to be outstanding.

EXERCISE 18-2   Brower describes the leader in politics as a person of stature who can rally the people, a person with outstanding ability and character. He says there is an emotional bond between the leader and the led, a "bond which must exist between a leader and his people if either is to confront greatness."[73] He thinks that the abrasive strains of television may have irreparably damaged the bond between leader and led. Television shows leaders in their weaknesses because it constantly focuses on them. Formerly it had been thought that such talent as Jefferson pictured in a natural aristocracy would freely rise to the top. American leaders would be people of ability and morality; they would be wise and virtuous. According to Brower, "Leadership, a relationship, depends very much on the basis of current enthusiasm or negation. Indeed it cannot exist at all in this country without the consent of the governed. We may very well be short on leadership because we are short on ourselves."[74]

Assuming that the characteristics of leadership are universally applicable to occupations, to government, to business, to industry, and certainly to service institutions and professions, list three characteristics described by Brower and apply them to nursing.

EXERCISE 18-3   Kurt Lewin suggests that there are three leadership styles: autocratic, democratic, and laissez-faire.

1. Which leadership style does your supervisor exhibit?
2. List three of his or her activities or decisions that illustrate the style.
3. How does your supervisor's leadership style affect your work and attitude?

EXERCISE 18-4   Gardner asserts that first-class managers are usually first-class leaders. He believes that leaders and leader-managers distinguish themselves beyond the general run of managers in six respects. Give brief examples of how nurses you know fit all or some of the six characteristics.

EXERCISE 18-5   From the theory of leadership described in this chapter, describe and discuss actual examples of leadership demonstrated by persons in your organization. Consider:

1. Gardner's nine tasks performed by leaders
2. A charismatic leader
3. A transforming leader
4. McGregor's Theory X and Theory Y
5. Likert's authoritative and democratic systems
6. Leadership style
7. The implications for staff development

NOTES

1. J. W. Gardner, *The Nature of Leadership: Introductory Considerations* (Washington, DC: Independent Sector, January 1986), 8.
2. J. W. Gardner, *The Tasks of Leadership* (Washington, DC: Independent Sector, March 1986), 15; E. Huxley, *Florence Nightingale* (New York: G. P. Putnam's Sons, 1975).
3. C. R. Holloman, "Leadership or Headship: There Is a Difference," *Notes & Quotes* (January 1969), 4; C. R. Holloman, "'Headship' vs. Leadership," *Business and Economic Review* (January–March 1986), 35–37.
4. L. B. Lundborg, "What Is Leadership?" *The Journal of Nursing Administration* (May 1982), 32–33.
5. J. W. Gardner, *The Nature of Leadership*, 6.
6. C. R. Holloman, op. cit., A. Levenstein, "So You Want to be a Leader?" *Nursing Management* (March 1985), 74–75; G. R. Jones, "Forms of Control and Leader Behavior," *Journal of Management* (fall 1983), 159–172; D. McGregor, *Leadership and Motivation* (Cambridge, MA: MIT Press, 1966), 70–80.
7. R. K. Merton, "The Social Nature of Leadership," *American Journal of Nursing* (December 1969), 2614–2618.
8. D. McGregor, op. cit., 73.
9. C. M. Talbott, "Leadership at the Man-to-Man Level," *Supplement to the Air Force Policy Letter for Commanders* (August 1971), 13.
10. D. G. Mitton, "Leadership: One More Time," *Industrial Management Review* (fall 1969), 77–83.
11. J. Kilpatrick, "Conservative View," *Sun-Herald* (Biloxi, MS), (February 1974), 4.
12. D. McGregor, op. cit., 75.

13. J. W. Gardner, The Tasks of Leadership, op. cit; *The Heart of the Matter: Leader-Constituent Interaction; and Leadership and Power* (Washington, DC: Independent Sector, October 1986).
14. J. W. Gardner, *The Tasks of Leadership*, 7.
15. J. W. Gardner, *The Heart of the Matter: Leader-Constituent Interaction*.
16. D. McGregor, op. cit., 55–57.
17. Ibid., 49–65.
18. R. Likert, *The Human Organization* (New York: McGraw-Hill, 1967), 4–10.
19. The Grid® synopsis was furnished courtesy of Scientific Methods, Inc., Box 195, Austin, TX, 78747.
20. L. Megginson, D. Mosley, and P. Pietri, Jr., *Management: Concepts and Applications*, 3rd ed. (New York: Harper & Row, 1989), 346–347, 352–353.
21. J. S. Phillips and R. G. Lord, "Notes on the Practical and Theoretical Consequences of Implicit Leadership Theories for the Future of Leadership Measurement," *Journal of Management* (spring 1986), 33.
22. Ibid.
23. F. E. Fiedler, "Style or Circumstance: The Leadership Enigma," *Notes & Quotes* (March 1969), 3; L. Megginson, D. Mosley, and P. Pietri, Jr. op. cit.
24. P. Hersey, K. H. Blanchard, and D. E. Johnson, *Management of Organizational Behavior: Utilizing Human Resources*, 7th ed. (Englewood Cliffs, NJ: Prentice-Hall, 1996), 134–135.
25. W. J. Reddin, *Managerial Effectiveness* (New York: McGraw-Hill, 1970), 230; R. M. Hodgetts, *Management: Theory, Process and Practice*, 4th ed. (Orlando, FL: Academic Press, 1986), 319–320.

26. A. M. Barker, "An Emerging Leadership Paradigm," *Nursing and Health Care* (April 1991), 204–207.

27. W. Bennis and B. Nanus, *Leaders: The Strategies for Taking Charge* (New York: Harper & Row, 1985), 3.

28. Ibid., 15.

29. S. P. Lundeen, "Leadership Strategies for Organizational Change: Applications in Community Nursing Centers," *Nursing Administration Quarterly* (fall 1992), 60–68.

30. M. W. Tack, "Future Leaders in Higher Education: New Demands and New Responses," *Phi Kappa Phi Journal* (winter 1991), 29–31; C. Desjardins and C. O. Brown, "A New Look at Leadership Styles," *Phi Kappa Phi Journal* (winter 1991), 18–20.

31. W. Bennis and B. Nanus, op. cit.

32. F. Medley and D. R. Larochelle, "Transformational Leadership and Job Satisfaction," *Nursing Management* (September 1995), 64JJ–64NN.

33. W. Bennis and B. Nanus, 57.

34. A. M. Barker, op. cit.

35. W. Bennis, "Learning Some Basic Truisms About Leadership," *Phi Kappa Phi Journal* (winter 1991).

36. W. Bennis and B. Nanus, op. cit.

37. A. M. Barker, *Transformational Nursing Leadership: A Vision for the Future* (Baltimore: Williams and Wilkins, 1990).

38. W. Bennis and B. Nanus, op. cit.

39. A. M. Barker, "An Emerging Leadership Paradigm," op. cit., 207.

40. Ibid.

41. J. W. Gardner, *The Heart of the Matter: Leader-Constituent Interaction*, op. cit.

42. W. Bennis, "Learning Some Basic Truisms About Leadership," op. cit., 24.

43. R. P. Campbell, "Does Management Style Affect Burnout?" *Nursing Management* (March 1986), 38A–38B, 38D, 38F, 38H.

44. J. W. Gardner, *The Heart of the Matter: Leader-Constituent Interaction*, op. cit.

45. A. Zaleznik, "Managers and Leaders: Are They Different?" *Harvard Business Review* (May–June 1977), 68.

46. J. H. Zenger, "Leadership: Management's Better Half," *Training* (December 1985), 44–53.

47. J. W. Gardner, *The Nature of Leadership*, 12.

48. J. H. Zenger, op. cit.

49. W. N. Mitchell, "What Makes a Business Leader?" *Notes & Quotes* (July 1968), 2.

50. J. H. Zenger, op. cit.

51. C. R. Holloman, "Leadership or Headship: There Is a Difference," op. cit.

52. J. W. Gardner, *The Nature of Leadership*, op. cit., 6.

53. Ibid.

54. C. R. Holloman, "'Headship' vs. Leadership," op. cit.

55. J. W. Gardner, *The Nature of Leadership: Introductory Considerations*, op. cit.

56. M. W. Tack, op. cit., 30.

57. J. H. Zenger, op. cit.

58. C. Desjardins and C. O. Brown, op. cit.

59. Ibid.

60. C. Gilligan, *In a Different Voice: Psychological Theory and Women's Development* (Cambridge, MA: Harvard University Press, 1982).

61. L. Kohlberg, *The Philosophy of Moral Development, Moral Stages and the Idea of Justice* (San Francisco, CA: Harper and Row, 1981).

62. J. Rosener, "Ways Women Lead," *Harvard Business Review* (November–December 1990), 19–24.

63. C. Desjardins and C. O. Brown, op. cit.

64. J. Rosener, op. cit.

65. J. Dunham and K. A. Klahefn, "Transformational Leadership and the Nurse Executive," *The Journal of Nursing Administration* (April 1990), 28–34.

66. J. S. Borman, "Women and Nurse Executives: Finally, Some Advantages," *The Journal of Nursing Administration* (October 1993), 34–40.

67. S. Helgesen, *The Female Advantage* (New York: Doubleday, 1990).

68. M. J. Cutler, "Nursing Leadership and Management: An Historical Perspective," *Nursing Administration Quarterly* (fall 1976), 7–19.

69. N. J. Murphy, "Nursing Leadership in Health Policy Decision Making," *Nursing Outlook* (July–August 1992), 158–161.

70. N. Milio, "The Realities of Policy Making: Can Nurses Have an Impact?" *The Journal of Nursing Administration* (March 1984), 18–23.

71. Ibid.

72. H. L. Smith and N. W. Mitry, "Nursing Leadership: A Buffering Perspective," *Nursing Administration Quarterly* (spring 1984), 45–52.

73. B. Brower, "Where Have All the Leaders Gone?" *Life* (8 October 1971), 70B.

74. Ibid.

REFERENCES

Aroskar, M. "The Challenge of Ethical Leadership in Nursing." *Journal of Professional Nursing* (May 1994), 270.

Bennis, W. *On Becoming a Leader* (Reading, MA: Addison Wesley, 1994).

Blanchard, K. H., and A. B. Sargent "The One Minute Manager is an Androgynous Manager." *Nursing Management* (May 1986), 43–45.

Buhler, P. "Managing in the 90s." *Supervision* (March 1993), 17–19.

Catton, J. J. "Applying Leadership to People Problems." *Supplement to the Air Force Policy Letter for Commanders* (September 1971), 30.

Davis, C. K., D. Oakley, and J. A. Sochalsk. "Leadership for Expanding Nursing Influence on Health Policy." *The Journal of Nursing Administration* (January 1982), 15–21.

Dixon, D. L. "Achieving Results Through Transformational Leadership." *The Journal of Nursing Administration* (December 1999), 17–21.

Dunham-Taylor, J. "Identifying the Best in Nurse Executive Leadership: Part 2, Interview Results." *The Journal of Nursing Administration* (July–August 1995), 24–31.

Dunning, H. F. "Nobody Can Give You Leadership." *Notes & Quotes* (September 1963), 3.

Feinberg, M. R. *Effective Psychology for Management* (Englewood Cliffs, NJ: Prentice-Hall, 1965), 133–141.

French J., and B. Raven. "The Basis of Social Power," In D. Cartwright, ed. *Studies in Power* (Ann Arbor: Institute for Social Research, University of Michigan, 1959).

Gevedon, S. "Leadership Behaviors of Deans of Top-Ranked Schools of Nursing." *Nursing Education* (May 1992), 221–224.

Glucksberg, S. "Some Ways to Turn on New Ideas." *Think (IBM)* (March–April 1968).

Goldberg, D. "What Makes a Leader?" *Mississippi Press* (23 November 1978), 6D.

Gunden, E., and S. Crissman. "Leadership Skills for Empowerment." *Nursing Administration Quarterly* (spring 1992), 6–10.

Hodgetts, R. M. *Management: Theory, Process and Practice*, 5th ed. (Orlando, FL: Harcourt, Brace, Jovanovich, 1990).

Jennings, E. E. "The Anatomy of Leadership." *Notes & Quotes*, 274 (March 1962), 1, 4.

Jones, G. R. "Forms of Control and Leader Behavior." *Journal of Management* (fall 1983), 159–172.

Kaprowski, E. J. "Toward Innovative Leadership." *Notes & Quotes*, 351 (August 1968), 2.

Keenan, M. J., P. S. Hoover, and R. Hoover. "Leadership Theory Lets Clinical Instructors Guide Students Toward Autonomy." *Nursing and Health Care* (February 1985), 83–86.

Koontz, H. "Challenges for Intellectual Leadership or Management." *Notes & Quotes*, 315 (August 1965), 1, 4.

Levenstein, A. "Where Nurses Differ." *Nursing Management* (March 1984), 64–65.

Levenstein, A. "Leadership Under the Microscope." *Nursing Management* (November 1984), 68–69.

Lorentzon, M. "Authority, Leadership, and Management in Nursing." *Journal of Advanced Nursing* (April 1992), 525–527.

Manthey, M. "Leadership: A Shifting Paradigm." *Nurse Educator* (September–October 1992), 5–14.

McDaniel, C., and G. A. Wolfe. "Transformational Leadership in Nursing Service: A Test of Theory." *Journal of Nursing Administration* (February 1992), 60–65.

Pike, O. "Rutan, Yeager Showed What Leadership is About." *Mobile Press Register* (January 1987), 4A.

Podsakoff, P. M., W. D. Todor, and R. S. Schuler. "Leader Expertise as a Moderator of the Effects of Instrumental and Supportive Leader Behaviors." *Journal of Management* (fall 1983), 173–185.

Smith, H. L., F. D. Reinow, and R. A. Reid. "Japanese Management: Implications for Nursing Administration." *The Journal of Nursing Administration* (September 1984), 33–39.

Yanker, M. "Flexible Leadership Styles: One Supervisor's Story." *Supervisory Management* (January 1986), 2–6.

CHAPTER 19

Motivation

Russell C. Swansburg, PhD, RN

CONCEPTS: Motivation, content theories of motivation, process theories of motivation, self-esteem, self-actualization, self-concept.

MANAGER BEHAVIOR: Provides extrinsic conditions of work in quality and quantity that maintain minimal job satisfaction.

LEADER BEHAVIOR: Directs human resource personnel to develop working conditions to satisfy and retain the best workers at high levels of productivity.

Theories of Motivation

Motivation is a concept used to describe both the extrinsic conditions that stimulate certain behavior and the intrinsic responses that demonstrate that behavior in human beings. The intrinsic response is sustained by sources of energy, termed *motives*, often described as needs, wants, or drives. All people have motives. Motivation is measured by observable and recorded behaviors. Deficiencies in needs stimulate people to seek and achieve goals to satisfy these needs.

- Why do some registered nurses pursue an area of nursing specialization to the extent of continuously acquiring new knowledge and skills that enable them to make rapid and accurate nursing diagnoses and prescriptions?
- Why does a pediatric nurse pursue development of a role that extends professional practice into areas such as teaching parents to enjoy their children, providing follow-up health observations of high-risk newborns, and teaching health practices to the parents of newborns after they have been discharged to their homes?
- Why does that nurse go a step further and teach others to extend his- or herself and then write articles to provide the information for everyone?
- Why does a mental health nurse pursue a role in off-duty time as a cotherapist of a group in addition to rotating shifts as a staff nurse?
- Why does another nurse work to sell the concept and then conduct a psychodrama therapy program and ask for the privilege of answering mental health consultations for medical and surgical patients?
- Why does a professional nurse work many hours as a committee member for a district nurses' association?
- Why do some nurses perform in a positive manner and others negatively?
- Why do some people always act with truthfulness and integrity to support principles they believe in, whereas others remain silent and passive?
- Why are some nurses goal-oriented and others not? Why are some nurses actively dedicated to improving

the quality of people's lives, whereas others merely exert minimal effort to maintain it?

- What makes some nurses come on duty on time, work hard and without error, maintain a pleasant demeanor, and meet all standards of performance, appearance, and behavior, whereas others do just the opposite? Some persons do not do well in an organization. This does not mean that these persons are not useful; the organization may be lacking the means of making them productive, useful, satisfied employees.

The answer to the preceding questions is motivation. Some nurses are motivated to excel and be creative; others put forth just enough effort to do the job. To get goods and services to the customer, managers care about people and their motivation. Managers' beliefs about motivation are reflected in their personal management styles.

Theories of motivation have been classified into content theories and process theories.[1] Work motivation theories have also been classified as dealing either with exogenous causes or with endogenous causes.[2] *Exogenous theories* focus on motivationally relevant independent variables that can be changed by external agents, such as organizational incentive and rewards, and social factors, such as leader and group behavior. There are seven exogenous theories: motive–need theory, incentive–reward theory, reinforcement theory, goal theory, personal and material resource theory, group and norm theory, and sociotechnical system theory. Exhibit 19-1 summarizes some approaches to improving work motivation using these theories. Exogenous theories are content theories, of which four are presented here.[3]

Content Theories

Content theories of motivation focus on factors or needs within a person that energize, direct, sustain, and stop behavior. The most widely recognized work in motivation theory is that of Maslow. Although not universally accepted, because of its lack of scientific evidence or research base, Maslow's work is universally known.

Many managers attempt to use Maslow's work as they turn to a human behavior approach to management.

Much has been said in support of Maslow's theories of motivation relative to human needs and goals. Like every science, nursing is a human creation stemming from human motives, having human goals, and being created, renewed, and maintained by human beings called nurses.

As are other scientists, nurses are motivated by physiological needs, including that for food; needs for safety, protection, and care; social needs for gregariousness, affection, and love; ego needs for respect, standing, and status, leading to self-respect or self-esteem; and a need for self-fulfillment or self-actualization characterized by integrity, responsibility, magnanimity, simplicity, and naturalness. Many nurses, but not all, are also motivated by cognitive needs for knowledge and understanding. They voraciously question others, read textbooks, journals, and patients' charts; and regularly pursue courses in their specialties and in the liberal arts, particularly the humanities. Other nurses are motivated by aesthetic needs for beauty, symmetry, simplicity, completion, and order and by their need to express themselves. How many of these needs are related to a nurse's desire to keep learning and applying new knowledge and skills? What can the nurse manager do to spark in a nurse the motive of curiosity that sets in motion a desire to understand, explain, and systematize? These and many other human needs may serve as the primary motivations for a person pursuing a career in nursing who wants to update and expand knowledge and skills. The motivation may be a feeling of identification and belonging with people in general, love for human beings, a desire to help people, the need to earn a living or express oneself, or a combination of all these needs working together. Certainly an individual's needs are diverse and unique.[4]

Alderfer, who reduced Maslow's hierarchy of needs from five to three, developed a second content theory of motivation: existence (E), relatedness (R), and growth (G), thus the term *ERG theory*. In comparing Alderfer's scheme with Maslow's, existence needs are equivalent to physiological and safety needs; relatedness needs to belongingness, social, and love needs; and growth needs to self-esteem and self-actualization.

Whereas Maslow's theory proposes that the next level of needs emerges when the predominant (satisfaction–progression) ones have been fulfilled, Alderfer's theory adds a frustration–regression process. When higher-level needs are frustrated, people will regress to the satisfaction of lower-level needs.[5]

Limited research is available to support or sustain the ERG theory. As with other theories of motivation, nurse leaders should become familiar with it and use its implications as appropriately as possible.

Herzberg did research on a third content theory, which he labeled a two-factor theory of motivation. One set of factors—dissatisfiers—is extrinsic conditions or hygiene factors. They include salary, job security, working conditions, status, company policy, quality of technical supervision, and quality of interpersonal relations among peers, with supervisors, and with subordinates. They must be maintained in quantity and quality to prevent

EXHIBIT 19-1
Approaches to Improving Work Motivation

EXOGENOUS VARIABLES

IMPERATIVE AND PROGRAMS	1. PERSONAL MOTIVES AND VALUES	2. INCENTIVES AND REWARDS	3. REINFORCEMENT	4. GOAL-SETTING TECHNIQUES	5. PERSONAL AND MATERIAL RESOURCES	6. SOCIAL AND GROUP FACTORS	7. SOCIOTECHNICAL SYSTEMS
Motivational imperative	Workers' motives and values must be appropriate for their jobs	Make jobs attractive, interesting, and satisfying	Effective performance must be positively reinforced but not ineffective performance	Work goals must be clear, challenging, attainable, attractive	Provide needed resources and eliminate constraints to performance	Interpersonal and group processes must support goal attainment	Personal, social, and technological parameters must be harmonious
Illustrative programs	Personnel selection Job previews Motive training Socialization	Financial compensation Promotion Participation Job security Career development Considerate supervision Job enrichment Benefits Flexible hours Recognition "Cafeteria" plans	Financial incentive plans Behavioral analysis Praise and criticism Self-management	Goal setting Management by objectives Modeling Quality circles Appraisal and feedback	Training and development Coaching and counseling Equipment Technology Supervision Methods improvement Problem-solving groups	Division of labor Group composition Team development Sensitivity training Leadership Norm building	Quality of worklife programs Sociotechnical systems designs Organizational development Scanlon plan

Source: R. A. Katzeil and D. E. Thompson. "Work Motivation." *American Psychologist* (February 1990), 147. Copyright 1990 by the American Psychological Association. Reprinted by permission.

dissatisfaction. These conditions become dissatisfiers when not equitably administered, causing low performance and negative attitudes. The other set of factors—satisfiers—are intrinsic conditions or motivators, which include achievement, recognition, responsibility, advancement, the work itself, and the possibility of growth. They create opportunities for high satisfaction, high motivation, and high performance. The individual must be free to attain intrinsic conditions. Both factors, hygiene and motivation, must be done simultaneously. Herzberg's research has been criticized for its limited sample of 200 accountants and engineers and for being simplistic.[6]

McClelland proposed and researched a fourth content theory of motivation closely associated with learning concepts, the learned needs theory. The three primary groups of learned needs acquired from the culture are the need for achievement, the need for affiliation, and the need for power.

McClelland used the Thematic Apperception Test (TAT) to measure the need for achievement. He contended that needs can be learned through organizational and nonorganizational meetings. Persons high in the need for achievement want to set their own performance goals, which they prefer to be moderate and achievable. They want immediate feedback, and they like responsibility for solving problems.[7]

Many nursing personnel enjoy working together and are motivated by these affiliations. In some situations, such as in nursing homes, nurses do not get the recognition they need from clients, so they look for it from colleagues. Many nursing personnel want to talk and socialize with each other on the job. They enjoy and prefer group-centered work activities, teamwork, interdependence, dependability, and predictability. The nurse educator works with these nurses to maintain this affiliation need at a mutually acceptable level.[8]

Process Theories

Endogenous theories deal with process or mediating variables such as expectancies and attitudes "that are amenable to modification only indirectly in response to variation in one or more exogenous variables." Four endogenous theories are[9]:

1. Arousal–activation theory, which focuses on internal processes that mediate the effects of conditions of work on performance.
2. Expectancy–valence theory, which focuses on people's expectations that their efforts will result in good performance and thence on valued outcomes.
3. Equity theory, which focuses on fair treatment; inputs from the employee will result in equal inputs from the employer.

4. Intention–goal theory, which focuses on performance being determined by commitment to goals.

Most behavior within organizations is learned behavior: perceptions, attitudes, goals, emotional reactions, and skills. Practice that occurs during the learning process results in a relatively enduring change in behavior.

Skinner advanced a process theory of motivation called *operant conditioning*, also called *behavior modification*. Learning occurs as a consequence of behavior. Behaviors are the operants; they are controlled by altering the consequences with reinforcers or punishments, as illustrated in Exhibit 19-2.

Positive or desired behaviors should be rewarded or reinforced. Reinforcement motivates, increasing the strength of a response or inducing its repetition. Continuous reinforcement speeds up early performance. Intermittent reinforcement at fixed or variable ratios sustains performance. Research indicates higher rates of response, with ratio rather than interval schedules. Reinforcers tend to weaken over time, and new ones have to be developed.

Undesirable organizational behavior should not be rewarded. Negative reinforcement occurs when desired behavior occurs to avoid negative consequences of punishment. Although frequently used, punishment creates negative attitudes and can increase costs. Behaviorists believe that people will repeat behavior when consequences are positive.

Behavior modification research uses a scientific approach. Application of behavior modification is occurring in large companies. Benefits or results claimed include improved attendance, productivity, and efficiency and cost savings. Reinforcers center on praise, recognition, and feedback. The problem-solving method is used to apply behavior modification[10]:

1. Identify and define (observe and measure) the specific behavior.
2. Measure or count the occurrences.
3. Analyze the antecedents, behaviors, and consequences (ABCs) of the behavior.
4. Perform positive reinforcement, negative reinforcement, punishment, or extinguish the behavior. Positive reinforcement is best because people repeat behavior that is rewarded and avoid behavior that is punished.
5. Evaluate changes. Provide feedback for reinforcement or correction. Give positive reinforcement while discussing areas that need improvement. Give feedback at all steps of performance, not just at outcomes. Follow-up reinforcement motivates people to put plans into effect because of the attention generated: somebody cares and is paying attention. Structured follow-up can include review

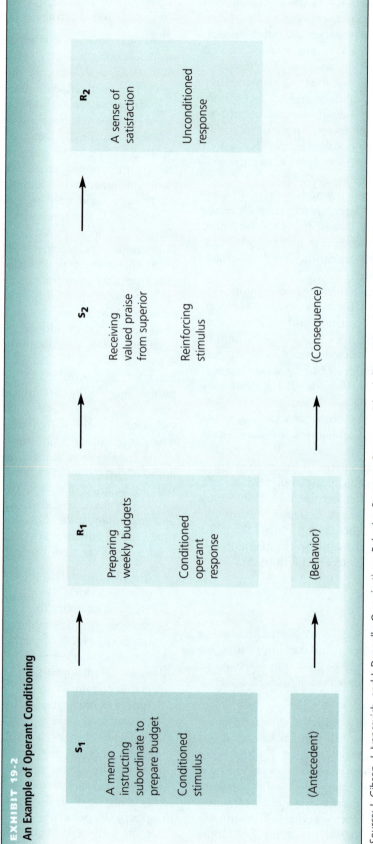

EXHIBIT 19-2
An Example of Operant Conditioning

S₁		**R₁**		**S₂**		**R₂**
A memo instructing subordinate to prepare budget	→	Preparing weekly budgets	→	Receiving valued praise from superior	→	A sense of satisfaction
Conditioned stimulus		Conditioned operant response		Reinforcing stimulus		Unconditioned response
(Antecedent)	→	(Behavior)	→	(Consequence)		

Source: J. Gibson, J. Ivancevich, and J. Donnelly. *Organizations: Behavior, Structure, Processes*, 9th ed. (Burr Ridge, IL: Irwin, 1997), 150.

sessions between clinical nurse and nurse leader, interdisciplinary or intradisciplinary team review of outcomes, review of collected data, or direct consultation.

Critics of the behavior modification theory consider rewards to be bribes.

A second process theory of motivation is Vroom's expectancy theory, which postulates that a person voluntarily controls most behaviors and therefore is motivated. There is an effort-performance expectancy, or a person's belief that a chance exists for a certain effort to lead to a particular level of performance. The performance–outcome expectancy or belief of this person will have certain outcomes. Given choices, the individual selects the one with the best expected outcome. Research on expectancy theory is increasing although not systematic or refined. This process is a complicated one in which unconscious motivation is avoided.[11]

Equity theory is a third process theory. Persons believe they are being treated with equity when the ratio of their efforts to rewards equals those of others. Equity can be achieved or restored by changing outputs, attitudes, the reference person, inputs or outputs of the reference person, or the situation. Research on equity theory has focused on pay.[12]

A fourth process theory of motivation is the goal-setting theory of Locke. This theory is based on goals as determinants of behavior. The more specific the goals, the better the results produced. Research indicates that goals are a powerful force. Goals must be achievable; their difficulty level should be increased only to the ceiling to which the person will commit. Goal clarity and accurate feedback increase security.[13]

Maslow

Maslow's theory of motivation is a positive one and is based on a holistic–dynamic theory. At the base of a needs system are the physiologic needs, based on homeostasis, a condition of constancy of body fluids, functions, and states. The constancy is maintained automatically by uniform interaction of counteracting processes. It should be noted that human beings do not just eat; they eat selectively to maintain homeostasis. The same is probably true of other physiological needs, although not all physiological needs are homeostatic. Some are relatively independent of each other while at the same time interdependent. For example, smoking may satisfy the hunger need in some persons. Some needs are in opposition to each other, such as the tendency to be lazy and the desire to be industrious.

Maslow proposed that human needs are organized in a hierarchy of prepotency: Higher needs emerge as lower ones are satisfied. When the physiological needs are satisfied, they no longer motivate the human being. However, a person tolerates deprivation of a long-satisfied need better than one that has been long or previously deprived.

When unsatisfied, physiological needs are the most prepotent, the strongest, of human needs. A starving person will steal food and perform other acts that threaten the person's safety. The dominance of a physiological need changes the individual's philosophy for the future.

Safety needs are the second group in the hierarchy. Among these are security, protection, dependency, and stability; freedom from anxiety, chaos, and fear; need for order, limits, structure, and law; and strength in the protector. Satisfaction of these needs influences a person's values and philosophy of life. What threatens the safety of nursing? Are nurses threatened by increased consumer interest in their shortcomings, which may lead to consumer control of practice? What motivates people? Is it a fear of the high cost of extended illnesses and results of poor care? The average person likes law, order, predictability, and organization, which may be one reason that people resist change. Insurance programs, job tenure, and savings accounts are expressions of safety needs. People prefer familiar to unknown things. Today's managers are often threatened by the new generation of personnel who question regulations and use the law to achieve their goals.

Once the physiological and safety needs have been satisfied, the needs for love, affection, and belongingness emerge. Most nurses in practice today have had their physiological and safety needs satisfied. Now they want to be part of a group or family with love, acceptance, friendliness, and a feeling of belonging. Are these needs thwarted by frequent moves? How are the needs of the individual, as well as those of the organization, satisfied? A society that wants to survive and be healthy will work to satisfy these needs. Otherwise, people will be maladjusted and exhibit severe emotional and behavioral pathology.

Two categories emerge under the fourth set of needs, the esteem needs. All people share these needs. First, they desire strength, achievement, adequacy, mastery and competence, confidence before the world, independence, and freedom. Second, they desire reputation or prestige, status, fame and glory, dominance, recognition, attention, importance, dignity, or appreciation. A person whose self-esteem is satisfied has feelings of self-confidence, worth, strength, capability, adequacy, usefulness, and being needed in society. For self-esteem to be stable and healthy, it must be based on known or deserved respect. The reason for self-esteem must be known and recognized by its recipient.

Finally, at the pinnacle of the hierarchy of needs is the emotional gold, that is, the need for self-actualization, the effort of people to be what they can be. Nurses want to become everything that they are capable of becoming, achieve their potential, be effective nurses, be creative, and meet personal standards of performance.

Certain conditions are prerequisites to satisfying basic needs. When basic needs are thwarted, the individual feels threatened. These conditions include:

- Freedom to speak—communication
- Freedom to do what one wishes to do without harming others—choice of jobs, friends, and entertainment
- Freedom to express oneself—creativity
- Freedom to investigate and seek for information
- Freedom to defend oneself—justice, fairness, honesty, and orderliness in the group

Human beings want to gain new knowledge, to solve problems, to bring order, and to explore, and they will voluntarily face dangers to do so.

The hierarchy of needs is not a simple classification. Individuals order their needs differently, some placing self-esteem before love. Others place creativity before all else. Certain people have low levels of aspiration. Permanent loss of love needs results in a psychopathic personality.

A long-satisfied need may become undervalued. A person who has never been deprived of a particular need does not regard the need as important. If two needs emerge, a person will probably want the more basic one satisfied first. People who have loved and been well loved and who have had many deep friendships can hold out against hatred, rejection, or persecution.

Most normal persons in our society have partially satisfied and partially dissatisfied basic needs at the same time. They may have more satisfied physiological needs and correspondingly fewer satisfied self-actualization needs. New needs emerge gradually and are more often unconscious than conscious. Basic needs are common throughout different cultures. Most behavior is multidetermined: all of the basic needs are involved. A single act of an individual could be analyzed to show how it addresses physiological needs, safety needs, love needs, esteem needs, and self-actualization needs. Not all behavior is internally motivated; some is stimulated externally. Some is highly motivated, some weakly, and some not at all. Some is expressive and some rote. A gratified or satisfied need is not a motivator of behavior. Healthy persons are primarily motivated by the need to develop and actualize their fullest potential and capabilities.

Usefulness to Nurse Managers

Motivational theory has been used in a number of studies of behavior modification for smoking cessation, weight control, exercising, and general reduction of cardiovascular risk factors. To date, modifying risk-taking behavior has had limited positive results. For example, because nicotine has been touted as a highly addictive substance, motivational theory may have to be combined with other treatment regimens to sustain cessation of smoking. The same may be true of other risk-taking behaviors. This area presents an opportunity for nurses to expand motivational research to include identifying factors that contribute to sustaining risk-taking behavior including psychological profiles.[14] Results of such research are important in managing patients and personnel.

Although many theories exist and much has been written about motivation, there is no easy way to motivate employees. Human motivation is diverse, subtle, and complex. To use the available information on motivation effectively, the nurse manager will study it and select and use those elements that appear to be practical and workable.

Some theories of motivation are contradictory. They provide useful knowledge when used selectively and carefully. Theories of motivation are really constructs because they cannot be directly observed and measured.[15]

Knowledge of motivation theories is essential to improving the job performance of employees. Individual employees have different needs and goals. Nurse managers will learn and use motivation theories selectively.

Dissatisfactions

Nurse managers who apply learned approaches to change within nursing organizations could alleviate dissatisfactions of nurses.

Productivity

Nurses respond negatively and become dissatisfied when managers use force, control, threats, and repeated applications of institutional power. Productivity decreases or stagnates. The new breed of nurses questions authority and gives loyalty to those who earn it. An attitude of mutual respect between clinical nurses and managers is essential to productivity.

To promote mutual respect, free interaction and communication must take place in which expectations are clarified and feedback on performance is given through role modeling of expected and desired performance. In addition, promises that cannot be fulfilled must be avoided. In more than seven of ten working relationships, the employee does not know what is expected of her or him. Expectations must be clear. In a productivity attitude test developed and administered to production workers by Pryor and Mondy over a 2-year period, 75% of respondents said that their supervisors did not keep promises they made. Broken promises anger employees and decrease productivity.[16]

Nurse managers are powerful models for staff. They are emulated, whether their example is good or bad. The obvious implication is that nurse managers will do self-assessment and modify their behavior to assume roles beneficial to both staff and organization.

Like other workers, nurses work to survive and meet their needs and aspirations. The complexity of the technological environment of patient care can lead to specialization and the depersonalization of jobs and work. This alienates nursing employees, and the quality of their work declines.

Nurse as Knowledge Worker

Drucker indicates that knowledge workers are productive only with self-motivation, self-direction, and achievement. No one dominant dimension to working exists. People are motivated to work based on Maslow's hierarchy of needs. Even when satisfied, a human need remains important. Economic rewards that are not properly dispensed create dissatisfaction with work and become deterrents to job satisfaction and productivity.[17]

Nurses are knowledge workers. Their basic economic needs are related to other human needs or human values. Performing work of equal difficulty, they want economic rewards of equal value to those of other knowledge workers. Pay is part of the social or psychological dimension of nurses. They also want increased rank, power, and status, commensurate with other knowledge workers.

More formal education and skills translate into higher real incomes and increased living standards. Boosts in investments in education, research and development, and updated equipment result in increased productivity. Ideas rather than physical resources result in added economic value. Highly skilled workers can switch jobs more easily and therefore spend less time unemployed. Money invested in education is an investment in the economic health and future of the United States.[18] Education makes fear a demotivator. Educated people are mobile. Nurses can move laterally to jobs in other organizations.

The nurse as knowledge worker is self-directed and takes responsibility. Rewarding and reaffirming self-direction and responsibility produce learning; fear produces resistance. Psychological manipulation is only a replacement for the carrot-and-stick approach to management. It does not work.

The role of discipline is to eliminate marginal friction. If used to drive nurses, discipline causes resentment and resistance; it demotivates. Direction and control are useless in meeting ego needs. Needs thwarted or otherwise not satisfied lead to sick or negative behavior. To focus on needs already satisfied is ineffective; however, employees will demand more of what they already have unless attention is given to self-esteem and self-actualization. In such a situation money becomes the only means available to satisfy needs. Nurses want it to purchase material goods and services. Inflation increases the demand because it takes more money to satisfy other desires. This increased demand, however, destroys the usefulness of money and material rewards as incentives and managerial tools.

Nurses are independent adults who want to be treated with dignity and respect—as adults and partners. The organizational perspective should be that it is practicing clinical nurses who achieve health care productivity gains, and not capital spending and automation.

Nursing personnel retreat from association and identification with organizations in which they cannot meet their perceived care requirements. Nurses may believe they are competent and able to do good work; however, they are dissatisfied because organizational resources are not allowing them to live up to the standard of care they consider appropriate. Nurses care; and because they care, they are dissatisfied.

Satisfactions

Science of Human Behavior

How do we apply the knowledge of the social sciences so that our human organizations will be truly effective? We have the knowledge, just as we have the knowledge of physical sciences to develop alternative sources of energy such as solar, tidal, atomic, and geothermal energy. Application of vast knowledge in both physical and social sciences is expensive and time-consuming.

Theory X and Theory Y

Although Douglas McGregor died in 1964, his theories of leadership and motivation live on. Unfortunately, his Theory X (ascribed to Sigmund Freud) has not been replaced by his Theory Y. Theory X, as he described it for the world of business, is summarized in the following points[19]:

1. Management is responsible for organizing the elements of productive enterprise—money, materials, equipment, people—in the interest of economic ends.
2. With respect to people, this is a process of directing their efforts, motivating them, controlling their actions, modifying their behavior to fit the needs of the organization.

3. Without this active intervention by management, people would be passive—even resistant—to organizational needs. They must therefore be persuaded, rewarded, punished, controlled—their activities must be directed. This is management's task—in managing subordinate managers or workers. We often sum it up by saying that management consists of getting things done through other people.

Behind this conventional theory there are several additional beliefs—less explicit, but widespread:
4. The average man is by nature indolent—he works as little as possible.
5. He lacks ambition, dislikes responsibility, and prefers to be led.
6. He is inherently self-centered, indifferent to organizational needs.
7. He is by nature resistant to change.
8. He is gullible, not very bright, the ready dupe of the charlatan and the demagogue.

How many nurse managers demotivate practicing nurses by falling into the trap of voicing the very statements embodied in Theory X? How may nurse managers motivate practicing nurses by applying the following precepts of Theory Y?[20]

1. Management is responsible for organizing the elements of productive enterprise—money, materials, equipment, people—in the interest of economic ends.
2. People are not by nature passive or resistant to organizational needs. They have become so as a result of experience in organizations.
3. The motivation, the potential for development, the capacity for assuming responsibility, the readiness to direct behavior toward organizational goals are all present in people. Management does not put them there. It is the responsibility of management to make it possible for people to recognize and develop these human characteristics for themselves.
4. The essential task of management is to arrange organizational conditions and methods of operation so that people can achieve their own goals *best* by directing *their own* efforts toward organizational objectives.

McGregor's Theory Y was used to change personnel behavior in a skilled nursing facility. An "audit process created unit expectations which provided a sense of accomplishment, personal growth and motivation to seek more responsibility." The staff was provided with extensive in-service education. "Noting," the leaving of notes for the responsible staff person to correct noncompliance, was accepted as peer review to foster responsibility and accountability. The goal was to manage personnel to meet their needs for self-respect and improvement.[21]

Nurse Managers and Motivation

The first manager to tackle the problem of productivity was Robert Owen (1771–1858) in his textile mill in Lanark, Scotland, in the 1820s. Owen is pictured as a manager who related to the work, the worker, the enterprise, and the manager.[22]

Nurse managers should apply techniques, skills, and knowledge, including knowledge of motivational theory, to help people obtain what they want out of nursing work. At the same time these efforts should be directed so as to achieve the objectives of the institution and the division of nursing.

To persuade people to apply their skills to achieve nursing and organizational goals requires many things on the part of the nurse manager: brilliance and sensitivity to people; energy and negotiating skills; gaining people's attention so that their aspirations and emotions are melded with those of a leader, the profession, and the organization for which they work; integrity so that people will be controlled only to the extent necessary.

To successfully lead today's nurses toward accomplishing the goals of nursing, nurse leaders should do motivational research or at least be aware of the findings of motivational research and apply them to personnel management. Through intuition, observation, and knowledge, the nurse's objectives are mixed with those of leaders (and thus those of nursing management and the nursing profession). The objectives will be restated so that when approved by the group they are seen as desirable ones to attain. This process requires intellectual skills that open nurses' hearts and minds, analysis of their perceptions, and synthesis of their perceptions with those of leadership. To achieve results will require mental agility, emotional intensity, and communication and negotiation skills.

Several authors make a good case for saying that one person cannot motivate another and that motivation lies within the individual. Everyone has motivation. If the theories of motivational psychology can be studied, accepted, and applied, such an approach is compatible with the knowledge that human beings have needs that motivate them.

Motivational research is a prime subject for continuing education for nurse leaders.

The choice of action lies with the individual. Incentives should be meaningful to the individual, and motivation should be stimulating on an individual basis. The organization has a set of standards it wants met in providing care that is satisfactory to patients. Nurses want remuneration for providing that care, which they provide best as part of an organized group. Interaction between employee and employer is essential to a contract. For interaction to be successful, rapport and involvement must exist. A successful contract depends on the employer's authority to give or withhold rewards and the employee's level of aspiration. Does the nurse want to advance if risks increase? To find out nurses' needs and aspirations, ask them. Note their individual responses to a variety of work assignments and incentives. A person will seldom respond to being a number. Personnel policies must provide support to supervisors. Communication that identifies needs is not an invasion of privacy but rather a realistic approach that leads to mutual trust and frankness among people.[23]

Motivation is an emotional process; it is psychological rather than logical. The nurse leader should first learn how a nurse wants to feel and then help that nurse use the tools that will encourage attainment of those feelings. These tools may derive from associations with people on the job that make the nurse feel accepted, performance of those acts for which he or she is highly skilled, and recognition for a satisfactory performance.

As previously stated, motivation is basically an unconscious process. When asked why she or he did a certain thing, a nurse may not be able to give an answer. Even though people's basic motives are hidden and intangible, their actions or behavior makes sense to them.

Motivational patterns are learned early and followed for years. There is no conscious selection, judgment, or decision-making involved in 95% of what people do.

Each person is unique, with the key to one's behavior lying within the self. A leader uses judgment to figure out why each person reacts in a given way to a certain situation. Within each individual, motivating needs differ from time to time. The key is to figure out which need is currently predominant.

Human beings, including nurses, motivate themselves. The nurse leader will provide or deprive practicing nurses of the opportunity to satisfy their needs[24]:

The motivational theory under discussion asserts that man if he is freed to some extent, by his presence in an affluent society, from the necessity to use most of his energy to obtain the necessities of life and a degree of security from the major vicissitudes—will by nature begin to pursue goals associated with his higher-level needs. These include needs for a degree of control over his own fate, for self-respect, for using and increasing his talents, for responsibility, for achievement both in the sense of status and recognition and in the sense of personal development and effective problem solving. Thus freed, he will also seek in many ways to satisfy more fully his physical needs for recreation, relaxation, and play. Management has been well aware of the latter tendency; it has not often recognized the former, or at least it has not taken into account its implication for managerial strategy.

Hard Approach Versus Soft Approach to Nursing Management

What are the effects of a hard approach to personnel management such as coercion and disguised threats, close supervision, and tight controls over behavior? Experience has shown that such an approach causes counterforces, including the restriction of output, militant unionism, and subtle but effective sabotage of the objectives of management.

Nurses turn to labor organizations when they fail to achieve results from their supervisors and when authoritarian managers manage from the top down. These managers use job descriptions, performance standards and evaluations, rules, pay incentives, promotions, management objectives, and dismissal threats. Nurses are not consulted on any of these management tools and activities.

The soft approach to personnel management, such as permissiveness, satisfying people's demands, and achievement of harmony, has been proved to cause indifferent performance, with expectations of receiving more and giving less. As a consequence, many managers try to take a middle-of-the-road approach.

Observation and the evidence of the social sciences indicate that employees' behavior shapes itself to management perceptions. This behavior does not result from inherent nature but from the nature of organizations, management philosophy, policy, and practice. The nurse leader looks for simple, practical, immediate ideas to solve personnel problems. There are no magic wands, but that does not mean there are no solutions.

Solutions

Career Planning

Career planning is a continuous process of self-assessment and goal setting. It is a cooperative venture between the organization and the employee, the career counselor (who could be a mentor or sponsor) and the individual nurse. Career planning is an organized system with short- and long-term career goals fitted to those of the organization.

To build a career development program requires major effort. An advisory committee can be formed. Staff development personnel can be career counselors. The real goal is the self-development of a career plan for every nurse, a plan fostered by the nursing organization. For this reason the individual nurse is best involved in the entire career development program from its inception. Most nurses will benefit from participation in a career development program, even if it improves only the quality of their working lives. The following outline stresses the major activities of a career development program[25]:

1. Assess the future goals and labor power needs of the nursing organization relative to recruitment, promotion, hiring, placement, retention, and turnover.
2. Develop job structures with career paths and qualifications, including career opportunities within the nursing organization.
3. Recruit qualified applicants, including those already employed within the nursing organization.
4. Assess each applicant for personal expectations. Why are they making this career choice? What are their needs, motivators, and job satisfiers? What stresses make them frustrated and dissatisfied? What stresses excite them? What are their career goals? How does their present performance relate to their career goals? What are their competencies and interests? What potential performance will be needed to achieve their career goals?
5. Develop an individual career development plan for the individual nurse.
6. Provide developmental opportunities for the individual nurse to achieve career goals.

Communication

Producing quality nursing products and services requires highly motivated practicing nurses. Nurse leaders can motivate nurses by sharing information about the organization. Consultative leaders consult with nurses on problems, solutions, and decisions and share information about results.

Teamwork

Nurse leaders can motivate practicing nurses by encouraging teamwork. Teams can be built from work groups to discuss and resolve work-related issues. Teams should have identifiable output; inclusive membership; leaders with carefully circumscribed authority; agreement on purpose; rules of procedure; and measurable goals, resources, and feedback. Teams are successful because they pool interpersonal skills, knowledge, and the expertise needed to accomplish goals effectively and efficiently.

By using teams Hewlett-Packard has cut labor costs, reduced defects, solved vendor problems, eliminated jobs, decreased inspections, cut scrap production, and reached targets ahead of schedule. Teamwork helps workers achieve personal recognition, raise self-esteem, and increase motivation and commitment. It is stimulated by trust, support, completion, acknowledgment, communication, and agreement.[26]

Teamwork raises the spirits of nurses during a time of economic recession, cutbacks, and curtailment of capital expenditures.

Teamwork is used to clarify the purpose or mission of a department or unit, to define a vision of the process and product of team effort, to identify blocks and barriers to team members' vision, to look at ways the work group members support each other, to make requests and agreements about how each can work better with others on the team, and to plan the team's work goals and activities and commit each member to accomplishing them. The result would be an effective team in which each member feels personally satisfied.[27]

Team processes are developmental. A summary of the developmental stages of teams as described by Farley includes four stages: orientation, adaptation, emergence, and production. Farley describes the characteristics, team leader tasks, member tasks, and ideal outcomes for each of these four stages.[28]

Self-Esteem

Having self-esteem means having a stable, firmly based, usually high evaluation of oneself. Self-esteem involves having self-respect and self-confidence. Being held in esteem by others because of one's personal accomplishments and reputation provides status and recognition; makes one feel appreciated and respected; and increases one's self-esteem. It satisfies one's desire to have strength among family, friends, colleagues, supervisors, patients, visitors, and others.[29]

Self-esteem is gained through strength, achievement of goals, adequacy, mastery, confidence, and independence. Exhibit 19-3 shows examples of self-esteem based on strength. Self-esteem entails satisfying the desire for achievement of personal, professional, and organizational goals, as illustrated in Exhibit 19-4. Self-esteem comes from satisfaction of the desire for adequacy, that is, feeling worthwhile as a person in society and as a worker. (See Exhibit 19-5.) Self-esteem involves satisfying the desire for mastery of and competence in the knowl-

---

EXHIBIT 19-3
Examples of Self-Esteem Through Strength

1. Educators have strength when they know that other employees want to hire them because of their demonstrated influence with nurses, physicians, and others. They have self-esteem when this gives them satisfaction.
2. Nurse administrators have strength when chosen by top management to expand their spheres of responsibility to direct other departments and when recognized by other administrators for skills and knowledge—being consulted by legislators or leaders in nursing and health care. They have self-esteem when this gives them satisfaction.

> **EXHIBIT 19-4**
> **Examples of Self-Esteem Through Achievement of Goals**
>
> 1. A professional nurse satisfies the desire for self-esteem by running for and winning a government office or an office in some service or professional organization.
> 2. A professional nurse satisfies the desire for self-esteem by achieving credentials such as certification, an advanced degree, or computer skills.
> 3. A professional nurse manager satisfies a desire for self-esteem by lowering the absenteeism and turnover rates of personnel in the nursing division.

> **EXHIBIT 19-5**
> **Examples of Self-Esteem Through Adequacy**
>
> 1. A professional nurse feels that she is a good wife and mother because she can work a schedule compatible with her husband's, be involved in the activities of her family, and save money for her children's college education.
> 2. A staff nurse in the recovery room feels she has the time to assess, plan, and give good care and attend to good documentation of care. She even has an opportunity to obtain reading references needed to keep professional knowledge and skills updated.

> **EXHIBIT 19-7**
> **Examples of Self-Esteem Through Confidence**
>
> 1. A professional nurse goes to work confident of being able to perform as well as any other nurse, and better than some; confident of being able to learn whatever is needed to do a job well; confident that her or his abilities will be recognized and credit given; that full merit pay will be earned; that the employers' standards as well as those of the ANA, the JCAHO, and other internal and external agencies can be met.
> 2. A professional nurse decides to win support and run as a candidate for president of the district nurses' association and wages a successful campaign.

> **EXHIBIT 19-8**
> **Examples of Self-Esteem Through Independence**
>
> 1. A supervisor decides to learn something about joint practice as a modality of nursing and obtains information and writes a position paper on it. The administrator suggests making a plan to practice it. The supervisor sets a specific schedule to orient and gain approval of, first, the clinical nurses and then the physicians who use the unit.
> 2. Clinical nurses are given complete freedom to manage the care of their patients, including coordination with personnel of x-ray, medical laboratory, nutrition and food service, and with physicians and others.

edge and skills needed to perform a role as a member of a family, and as a citizen and in clinical practice, management, education, or research. (See Exhibit 19-6.) Self-esteem comes from acquiring a feeling of confidence in the face of the world. (See Exhibit 19-7.) Self-esteem involves satisfying the desire for independence and freedom. A person must be free to speak, to act without hurting others, to express herself or himself, to investigate and seek information, and to defend herself or himself. Each person must be treated with justice, fairness, honesty, and orderliness in the group (see Exhibit 19-8).

Other terms can be used to describe self-esteem. These include valuing oneself or estimating one's worth. Our goal is to value ourselves highly, to consider ourselves favorably, to appreciate and think well of ourselves. We also want others to have a high regard for us, to honor and admire us.

> **EXHIBIT 19-6**
> **Examples of Self-Esteem Through Mastery**
>
> 1. A nurse educator involves clinical nurses in preparing strategic objectives for a unit. The plan is approved by the organization's administrators.
> 2. A clinical nurse is selected to implement a theory of nursing about which the nurse is considered an authority.

In terms of Maslow's hierarchy of needs, self-esteem is a higher-level need in the ego category. It emerges after physiological, safety, belongingness, and love needs are fairly well gratified. Although self-actualization needs are higher in the hierarchy, this hierarchy does not follow the same order in everyone. Rarely are self-esteem needs fully satisfied.

> **People want a good reputation and to have prestige; they want respect or esteem from others. They want to be recognized, to have attention, to be important, and to be appreciated.**

People meet their esteem needs in different ways. They are influenced by culture, including the culture of the organization in which they work. The ends or results of achieving self-esteem are more important than the roads taken to achieve those ends or results. All human beings want to be esteemed, unless they are pathological. Persons lacking self-esteem feel inferior, weak, helpless, and discouraged. They become indolent, passive, resistant to change, irresponsible, and unwilling to follow a dialogue. In the workplace, persons lacking self-esteem focus on salary and fringe benefits, making unreasonable demands for economic benefits. They can become neurotic or emotionally sick when they lack self-esteem.[30]

Meeting the self-esteem needs of employees is of great significance to managers in nursing, as everywhere. Most nurses work in bureaucratic organizations such as hospitals, home health care agencies, nursing homes, and clinics. In such places, work is organized to meet many concerns such as those of the organization, physicians, and the routines and personnel of other departments. The lower levels of the hierarchy have few opportunities to meet nurses' ego needs. Nurses schedule care of their patients around everyone else. They are the servants of the organization.

Direction and control are useless in motivating professional nurses whose social, ego, and self-fulfillment needs are predominant. Intellectual creativity is a characteristic of professional nurses who do not get ego satisfaction from wages, pensions, vacations, or other benefits of work. The job itself must be satisfying and fun if professional nurses are to satisfy their self-esteem needs. Professional nurses get their ego needs met by having a voice in decision-making. They will commit to organizational objectives when they are allowed to determine the steps to take to achieve them. Nurses want to collaborate with other professionals, both internal and external to the environment in which they work.

Full use of their talents and training is another desire of professional nurses. They want critical attention paid to the nature of nursing as a clinical practice discipline, to the organization of nursing functions, and to job challenges. They *do not* want close and detailed supervision. One reason for the success of primary nursing has been the control professional nurses have over the nursing of patients who are their primary responsibility. This success will continue if management gives attention to a career development plan. Such a plan's logical evolution is a joint practice in which physicians and nurses collaborate to give total care to patients. Professional nurses want opportunities to develop within their professional careers as clinical nurses. Career ladder progression must relate to clinical practice.[31]

What can management do to meet nurses' needs for self-esteem? Management can set the conditions under which professional nurses become committed to organizational goals and exercise self-control and self-direction, which leads to creativity.

Strategic planning by top management can involve professional clinical nurse participation. Is not the end result accomplished through professional nursing? The strategic plan can then be submitted to the department level for input by clinical nurses and other professionals. They will critique the plan, strengthen it, and make it one to which nurses can commit. This management process will be a difficult task, the accomplishment of which gives professional nurses new knowledge and skills, opportunity for creativity, and recognition and prestige in the eyes of others, thus meeting nurses' ego needs for self-esteem.

In the area of performance evaluation, nurse managers can again set the stage for meeting the self-esteem needs of professional nurses who want to be evaluated, promoted, rotated, and transferred in terms of their clinical or other personal career motivations. Self-evaluation in which individuals plan and appraise their contributions to organizational objectives promotes self-esteem. Conventional performance appraisal attacks it.[32]

It is obvious that management can create the conditions under which professional nurses can meet their esteem needs. Management can make nurses feel good about themselves by providing adequate staffing to give good nursing care, by correct placement and orientation to achieve mastery, independence, and freedom, by respecting them for a job well done, and by encouraging deserved respect from coworkers and employees.[33]

> **What do managers get from their jobs? Freedom? Social satisfaction? Opportunities for achievement? Knowledge? The ability to create? Who gets the reward and for what? Who must provide the opportunities for increased dignity, achievement, prestige, and social satisfaction?**

Self-esteem involves the personhood of all professional nurses, be they managers, clinical nurses, researchers, or teachers. Each person should enrich the esteem of the other person and should be the peer pal, mentor, sponsor, and guardian of the person within the profession. Esteem results in leading and influencing. One can listen to other people, treat them as individuals, show earnest exhilaration in responding to their creativity, offer ideas for improvement, and share the excitement of their successes and victories. Success provides a good positive self-image and builds self-esteem. It avoids the pain of failure.[34]

Self-Actualization

Self-actualization was defined by Maslow as an ego need at the top of the needs hierarchy. Self-actualization does not exist in isolation. In some persons, it may be no stronger than is the love and belonging need or the self-esteem need.

Self-actualized persons are:

- Able to distinguish the real world, seeing reality more clearly than do others.
- Comfortable with and attracted to the unknown.
- Creative in whatever they do and perceive.
- Less defensive and less artificial than are others, accepting and adjusting to their own shortcomings.
- Uncomfortable not doing something to improve their shortcomings, prejudices, jealousies, envy, and other faults of humanity.

Self-actualized persons have many other qualities; they:

- Have autonomous codes of ethics yet are the most ethical of persons.
- Are able to conform easily when no great issues are involved.
- Accept their own nature, human nature, the realities of social life, and the constraints of physical reality.
- Are problem-centered, not ego-centered.
- Have broad and universal values.
- Are deeply democratic, as opposed to authoritarian, by nature and thus respect others.
- Have a strong sense of right and wrong, of good and evil.
- Are not interested in hostile humor. Their humor is of a philosophical bent, stated only to produce a laugh.
- Are self-movers.
- Are detached and objective in conditions of turmoil.

Self-actualized people like solitude and privacy. Although they generally want to help the human race and can sometimes feel like strangers in a strange land, their relationships with others are profound and their circle of friends is small. They love children and humanity but can be briefly hostile when deserved or for the good of others. In social terms, self-actualized people are godly but not religious. They are not conventional, but they conform to social graces with toleration. They can be radical.

Maslow indicates that living at the higher need level is good for growth and health, both physically and psychologically. Self-actualized persons live longer, have less disease, sleep and eat better, and enjoy their sexual lives without unnecessary inhibitions. For them, life continues to be fresh, thrilling, exciting, and ecstatic. They count their blessings.

Self-actualized people have mystic or peak experiences. These are natural experiences. Happiness can cause tears. It comes from transcendence of appreciation for poetry, music, philosophy, religion, interpersonal relationships, beauty, or politics. They can have the peak experience from doing or sensing.

Self-actualized people merge or unify dichotomies, such as selfishness, considering every act to be both selfish and unselfish. They perceive work as play and duty as pleasure. The purpose of higher needs is a "healthward" trend—when people experience them, they place a higher value on them.

Self-actualized people are "metamotivated." Their motivations are for character growth, character expression, maturation, and development. They place more dependence on self-development and inner growth than they do on the prestige and status of others' honor.

Self-actualizing people are not perfect. They can be (or can be perceived to be) joyless; mundane; silly, wasteful, or thoughtless in habits; boring, stubborn, or irritating; superficially vain or proud; partial to their own productions, family, friends, or children; temperamental; ruthless; strong and independent of others' opinions; shocking in language and behavior; concentrated to the point of absent-mindedness or humorlessness; mistaken; or needing improvement. They can feel guilt, anxiety, sadness, self-castigation, internal strife, and conflict.

> **Self-actualized people develop detachment from the culture. They become autonomous and accepting.**

The satisfaction of higher needs requires more preconditions, such as more people, larger scenes, longer runs, more means and partial goals, and more subordinate or preliminary steps. To achieve the higher needs requires better environmental conditions.

Pursuit and gratification of higher needs have desirable civic and social consequences: loyalty, friendliness, and civic consciousness. People who are living at this level make better parents, spouses, teachers, and public servants. They also create greater, stronger, and truer individualism. They are synergistic.

One possible conclusion is that the self-actualized person achieves a highly satisfactory quality of life and that this quality of life extends from the gratified self-actualized person into society. The social environment of work, family, community, government, and the like can positively influence gratification or satisfaction of the higher-level needs.

Applying these insights to nursing, the nurse leader would selectively apply knowledge and skills of the social and behavioral sciences to creating an environment or climate in which practicing nurses could become self-actualized. In doing so, nurse managers themselves become self-actualized, and the products and services of nursing increase in quantity and quality.

Although critics of Maslow's work say it is based on too narrow a population, the theory is widely accepted and used. Maslow analyzed the profiles of 60 subjects, including Lincoln, Jefferson, Einstein, and Frederick Douglas. He suggested that the self-determined population might be limited to being from 5% to 30% of the total, another forecast criticized by other scientists.[35]

Self-Concept

Self-concept has been analyzed as a nursing diagnosis. Its components are in body image, self-esteem, and personal identity. The nursing diagnoses under Human Responses Pattern, Perceiving, include body image disturbance, personal identity disturbance, and chronic low or situational self-esteem disturbance. Self-concept results from experience and is a determinant of behavior. LeMone adapted Roy's definition of self-concept as follows[36]:

> Self-concept is a composite of thoughts, values, and feelings that one has for one's physical and personal self at any given time formed from interactions with the environment and with other people, and directing one's behavior.

Maslow emphasized self-actualization as the motivating force in developing one's unique self-concept.

Other Activities to Stimulate Motivation

Motivation is stimulated by activities such as job enrichment; praise; empowerment; employee stock ownership plans; lateral promotions; inclusion in organizational actions; and focus on vision, values, and strategy. (Some of these activities or strategies have been discussed in other chapters.)

All employees should be able to describe the values of their employer (see Exhibit 19-9). These values are identified, defined, prioritized, and communicated through means such as booklets and orientation programs. Values are critical in empowerment. Managers should emphasize the value of people by trusting, respecting, and encouraging them. They should tie rewards to values of teamwork, innovation, safety, growth, and profitability and provide employees with financial and nonfinancial rewards.

Taking the following actions capitalizes on the power of a value-driven management system[37]:

- Identify, define, and prioritize critical values through communication and involvement at all organizational levels, including board support.
- Measure the organization's perceptions of the defined values and possible areas of conflict.
- Assess customer-client perceptions of the degree to which they feel company actions conform to these values.
- Audit current management practices to evaluate the extent to which they direct, support, and reinforce desired outcomes.
- Modify leadership styles, management systems, and action programs to close the gap between desired and perceived behaviors.
- Develop a reward system that reinforces selected values and confronts and acts on the lack of performance.

Managers should motivate employees by including them in the group's mission. Employees are motivated by detailed explanations, praise, tangible rewards, and constructive criticism. They need time to improve unsatisfactory performance, and when they cannot do so, they should be encouraged to seek another post within the organization.[38]

Firms are using flexible work plans (see Exhibit 19-10) to cut costs and keep the best people. These plans, which reduce forced layoffs, include the following (the companies surveyed included DuPont, Philadelphia Newspapers, IBM, and Avon Products)[39]:

- Paternity leave or work-at-home policies. Of firms surveyed in 1987 by Hay/Haggins Company, none had such policies. By 1991, nearly half offered paternity leave, and 14% offered telecommuting options.

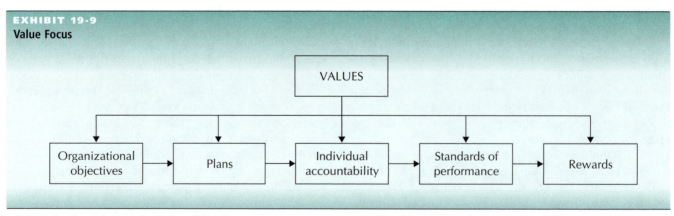

EXHIBIT 19-9
Value Focus

VALUES

Organizational objectives → Plans → Individual accountability → Standards of performance → Rewards

Source: Reprinted from L. Ginsburg and N. Miller. "Value-Driven Management." *Business Horizons* (May–June 1992), 24. Copyright 1992 by the Foundation for the School of Business at Indiana University. Used with permission.

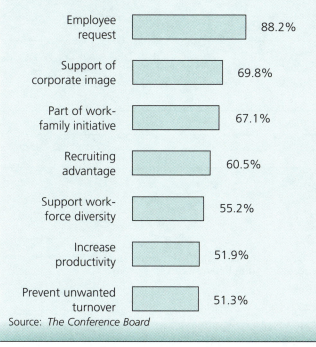

EXHIBIT 19-10
Flexible Work Plans

FAVORITE ARRANGEMENTS
Percentage of companies on the Conference Board's Work-Family Research and Advisory Panel with these flexible work arrangements:

REASON	PERCENTAGE
Personal leave	97.0
Part-time work	94.7
Flextime	92.4
Family/medical leave	89.4
Telecommuting	75.8
Compressed work week	68.7
Job sharing	67.4
Sabbaticals	39.5
Phased retirement	30.8

REASONS FOR FLEXIBLE PLANS
Top seven reasons companies initiate flexible work plans:

Employee request	88.2%
Support of corporate image	69.8%
Part of work-family initiative	67.1%
Recruiting advantage	60.5%
Support work-force diversity	55.2%
Increase productivity	51.9%
Prevent unwanted turnover	51.3%

Source: *The Conference Board*

Flexible hours policies increased from 35% in 1987 to 40% in 1991. These numbers have expanded greatly. Website http://search.yahoo.com lists dozens of new work-at-home jobs. There is even a work-at-home online magazine. Website http://sprint.snap.com has hundreds of thousands of pages on flexible hours and on paternity leave policies.

- Reduced workweek schedules, job sharing, unpaid leaves of absence, and early retirement.
- Rearranged workdays to allow parents to attend children's school functions or meet other personal and family needs.
- Childcare assistance.

Setting personal goals is a way of planning ahead. Doing so provides momentum to employees because it means that they have decided to pursue what they want and obtain the necessary qualifications. It is important that they recognize their personal limitations and abilities and use that awareness to initiate the changes needed to achieve their goals. Social and leadership goals gained from aspects of living, such as family, community, and church, are often overlooked credentials for achieving self-improvement and self-fulfillment.

Summary

To summarize:

1. A person is motivated.
2. A person has goals.
3. Management has goals.
4. A condition or environment needs to be established whereby a person can achieve personal goals and vice versa.
5. The person is rewarded by work achievements that are successful. Management practice provides the setting for success, perhaps by removing constraints or giving other intrinsic rewards. High-level ego needs are met on the job.
6. A cooperative interaction is fostered between manager and employees, because employees participate in decisions affecting them.
7. Motivation occurs.
8. Personal and motivational goals are met as the nurse is motivated to be ambitious and responsible, to show initiative, to be proud of fellow nurses and the employing institution, to welcome change, and to demonstrate individual abilities.

The following law will apply to successful leadership in nursing: Find out where nurse persons want to go and what they want to accomplish, and bring these goals into line with those of the organization. Then nurses will accomplish organizational goals as they achieve their own.

APPLICATION EXERCISES

Use Exhibit 19-11, Future Goals Worksheet, to develop a list of goals. Once you have them written down, you can evaluate them using Exhibit 19-12, Goal Evaluation Checklist.

EXHIBIT 19-11
Future Goals Worksheet

You will want to set goals in at least three areas:

1. **Personal Goals.** What would you really like to do with your life? Write down the personal goals you want to accomplish. Examples are "Become a role model for the profession," "Achieve as a writer in the field of staff development," or "Serve people who need but lack the means to buy health care."

   _____

   _____

2. **Family Goals.** Do you want to save money to travel? To put yourself and your family through school? To supplement a primary income? To buy something special? You may want to discuss these goals with your spouse and children, but write down your family goals.

   _____

   _____

3. **Professional Goals.** Do you want to become a professor, a director of nursing, a consultant in nursing care of cancer patients, a clinical researcher, something outside of nursing altogether? Write down your professional goals.

   _____

   _____

EXHIBIT 19-12
Goal Evaluation Checklist

STANDARDS FOR EVALUATING GOALS	YES	NO
1. I have reviewed my short-range goals within the past 3 months.	_____	
2. I have reviewed my long-range goals within the past year.	_____	
3. My goals reflect my personal philosophy or beliefs and the purpose or reason I want to achieve them.	_____	
4. My goals can be measured or verified as being achieved.	_____	
5. I have set my goals in the priority or sequence in which I want to accomplish them.	_____	
6. My goals are clear to me. They are specific and indicate actions to take to achieve them.	_____	
7. My goals are flexible and realistic so that I will have as many opportunities as possible.	_____	
8. I have the resources to accomplish my goals.	_____	
9. My goals are stated for a specific job.	_____	

Small Group Session

1. Write a statement that provides a vision of what you want to accomplish in stimulating the motivation of your peers or employees. (20 minutes)
2. Outline a process for accomplishing this vision. (20 minutes)
3. Report.

EXERCISE 19-3 Complete Exhibit 19-13, Checklist for Assessing Job Satisfaction, and use it to develop goals that you can achieve. Don't forget that all responsibility for personal satisfaction in life is ultimately your own. We have to take action to help ourselves, to be informed, to become better educated, to improve our interpersonal relationships, and to make our lives meaningful.

EXHIBIT 19-13
Checklist for Assessing Job Satisfaction

IN MY CURRENT JOB I AM	YES	NO OR INSUFFICIENT
Happy with being able to help others.		
Intellectually stimulated and challenged.		
Given opportunity to progress educationally.		
Learning new skills.		
Sharpening old skills.		
Learning a new discipline.		
Qualifying for more responsibility.		
Qualifying for more respect.		
Given opportunities to attend staff meetings, patient care conferences, and staff-development programs.		
Rewarded for doing my job well.		
Adequately paid.		
Given opportunity for advancement.		
Given opportunity to innovate and be creative.		
Given opportunity to choose shifts and hours of work.		
Given opportunity to be a leader.		
Given opportunity to grow as a bedside nurse.		
Able to trust my supervisors and peers.		
Supported by administration.		
Communicated with by administration.		
Being paid for my total knowledge and experience.		
Confident of job security.		
Working with adequate staffing.		
Feeling satisfied with my accomplishments.		
Supported by nursing management in resolving physician-nurse conflict.		
Able to resolve peer conflict.		
Adequately paid for overtime.		
Given opportunity to schedule extra time off above and beyond holidays and vacation.		
Given opportunity to schedule my working hours.		
Prepared to function as a team leader or charge nurse.		
Supported by competent professional nurses who assist and teach me.		

(continued)

EXHIBIT 19-13 *(continued)*

My job satisfaction could be increased by:

_____

_____

Identify specific steps to gather the information or make the changes that will help you reach your goal.

_____

_____

One of my job satisfaction goals is:

_____

_____

As a step toward reaching this goal I will talk to: _____

about: _____

and I will undertake the following activities myself:

_____

_____

EXERCISE 19-4

Scenario: Ms. Sanchez has been director of nursing of a 250-bed hospital for 8 years. Although her management operation has followed traditional patterns, she has read extensively on the subject and has been taking business administration courses in the evenings at the state university. Ms. Sanchez has decided to make some management changes in her department.

Although meetings with members of the nursing staff had been held on a scheduled basis, they were never productive and served mainly as a medium for information to flow from management downward. Ms. Sanchez carefully planned an agenda for her next staff development faculty meeting and distributed it a week in advance. An item of new business on the agenda was to write specific objectives for these meetings that would benefit the members and ultimately the nursing employees throughout the institution. At the same time, Ms. Sanchez would present a working draft of an operational plan for accomplishing the objectives of the department of nursing. The staff development nurse group would be asked to discuss the departmental mission, philosophy, objectives, and operational plan to determine whether the the statements express a vision that would motivate nursing personnel.

At the meeting, Ms. Sanchez was pleased with the active participation by the members. They had many suggestions for changes and for additional activities that would be helpful in achieving the mission, philosophy, objectives, and operational plan. During the discussion Ms. Sanchez learned about many major dissatisfactions of these personnel. For example, they did not understand the personnel rating system and wanted to know how she arrived at decisions for promotions. One of the suggested activities for accomplishment of objectives was that job standards be written and that they use the ANA standards for nursing practice as a basis for them. They appointed an ad hoc committee to do this, without the prodding of Ms. Sanchez, and they set a target date for completion. It was their intent to help Ms. Sanchez strengthen the objectivity of the rating system, thereby giving them input into the promotion process. The members also made plans to expand the project through inclusion of representatives of the entire nursing staff.

Next, Ms. Sanchez asked if the statements of the department's mission, philosophy, objectives, and operational plan should be presented to all the nursing staff, and a large majority of members

(continued)

EXERCISE 19-4
(continued)

agreed that they should. They also recommended that Ms. Sanchez do this, because the staff would be impressed with being able to discuss these important statements with the boss. A suggestion was made that Ms. Sanchez meet with the staff of each unit; the ad hoc committee members wrote a schedule that was acceptable to her. The committee then decided to assist unit personnel with developing or revising statements of mission, philosophy, and objectives, and operational plans for each of the units and to have them done by a specific date.

Ms. Sanchez discussed means of encouraging the nursing staff to be more productive and better satisfied with their working conditions. Several suggestions were made by the staff development nurse group. These included modifications in policies related to wearing the uniform, staffing, and time schedules. The nurses also stated that many nursing personnel had expressed the desire to become more involved in unit in-service education and other nursing activities but had not been encouraged to do so. Ms. Sanchez said she would welcome all suggestions for change but that she could not guarantee that all would take place immediately, because some would have to be approved by the hospital administrator. If Ms. Sanchez did not agree with any of the recommendations she would tell the people involved the reasons why. They agreed that this was acceptable to them, and the meeting was adjourned. From this scenario:

1. List a fact that encourages or discourages freedom to speak, that is, communication.
2. List a fact that encourages or discourages freedom to do what one wishes to do without harming others, that is, choice of jobs, friends, or entertainment.
3. List a fact that encourages or discourages freedom to express oneself, that is, creativity.
4. List a fact that encourages or discourages freedom to defend oneself, justice, fairness, honesty, or orderliness in the group.
5. List a fact that encourages or discourages freedom to investigate and seek information.

EXERCISE 19-5

Scenario: Ms. Rather is in charge of pediatric unit in-service education and encourages employees to discuss their families and their off-duty activities. They tell her of their hopes and dreams and even of confidential personal happenings. Mr. Pottinger is in charge of in-service education on an intensive care unit. He gives personnel needed supervision and training and supports them well while on duty. He lets it be known that he does not want to know anything about employees' personal lives unless it relates to their work.

1. Which nurse exhibits the best understanding of motivational theory?
2. What knowledge of motivational theory has been exhibited by the nurse you selected?

EXERCISE 19-6

Using Herzberg's two-factor theory of motivation and the items in Exhibit 19-13, Checklist for Assessing Job Satisfaction, do the following:

1. Summarize the results of the extrinsic conditions, hygiene factors, or dissatisfiers related to yourself and your job.
2. Summarize the results of the intrinsic conditions, motivators, or satisfiers related to yourself and your job.

EXERCISE 19-7

Self-Esteem Exercises

1. List the strengths or abilities to influence others that you have and that give you self-esteem. How can you improve them?

(continued)

EXERCISE 19-7
(continued)

2. List the personal, professional, and organizational goals of achievement that will make you think well of yourself. How can you improve them?
3. List the things that make you feel adequate in your personal life and your job. How can you improve them?
4. List two or more major areas in which you have achieved mastery and competence. List one or more in which you desire to achieve mastery and competence.
5. List those qualities that give you confidence in the face of the world. How can they be enlarged or improved?
6. List those areas in which your desire for independence and freedom are limited. How can your independence and freedom be expanded?
7. List those activities telling you that you have a good reputation and the respect of others. Indicate whether your reputation and the respect come from patients, visitors, supervisors, physicians, personnel, or others.
8. List those activities that give you feelings of self-confidence, value, strength, or being useful and needed in the world.
9. List those activities that make you feel inferior, weak, helpless, and discouraged.

EXERCISE 19-8

The following is a list of matched pairs of personal characteristics. Complete the list by circling a characteristic for each pair and write a statement summarizing your personal characteristics. Make a plan to change any personal characteristics you believe should be changed to improve your self-esteem.

Personal Characteristics

A	B	A	B
Vivacious	Languid	Honest	Dishonest
Intelligent	Stupid	Truthful	False
Bright	Dull	Accurate	Deceptive
Clever	Clumsy	Confident	Pessimistic
Funny	Solemn	Respectful	Rude
Courteous	Rude	Pleasant	Obnoxious
Prompt	Late	Candid	Deceitful
Tolerant	Prejudiced	Courageous	Fearful
Gracious	Surly	Decent	Gross
Unpretentious	Complacent	Unselfish	Egotistic
Sincere	Devious	Having integrity	Fraudulent
Friendly	Antagonistic	Sincere	Sly
Humble	Arrogant		

Source: Russell C. Swansburg and Philip W. Swansburg. *Strategic Career Planning and Development for Nurses* (Rockville, MD: Aspen, 1984), 76.

EXERCISE 19-9   The following is one approach to developing standards for the motivation aspects of nursing leadership.

Standards for the Evaluation of the Motivational Aspects of Nursing Leadership

STANDARDS

There is evidence to show that the nurse administrator demonstrates knowledge of:

1. Maslow's hierarchy of needs: The manager demonstrates ability to identify employees' physiological, safety, social, esteem, and self-actualization needs, and to create work situations that help meet their needs.
2. Modern motivational theory that relates needs to behavior.
   2.1 Argyris's immaturity–maturity theory: The manager attempts to make jobs challenging and subordinates as independent as they are capable of being.
   2.2 Herzberg's two-factor theory of motivation: The manager attempts to prevent dissatisfaction through providing hygiene factors and prompt satisfaction through motivators.
   2.3 Expectancy theory and learned behavior: The manager promotes an environment in which subordinates see a high probability of achieving objectives that are desirable, and the manager reinforces satisfactory performance with recognition.
      2.3.1 Vroom's expectancy theory: The manager recognizes the productivity of subordinates and recommends promotions accordingly, causing them to expect such outcomes.
      2.3.2 Porter and Lawler's theory: The manager acts so that subordinates expect rewards based on performance.
   2.4 Equity or social comparison theory: The manager recognizes that subordinates adapt and weigh what they give to the enterprise against rewards or benefits.

Apply the standards for evaluation of the motivational aspects of directing nursing personnel, and determine whether there is adequate evidence to show that nurse managers are using modern motivational theory at division, department, service, or unit levels. Summarize your findings.

If the nurse managers are not meeting the standards, discuss with them how they can devise and implement programs to identify and meet the needs of personnel. Summarize your results.

NOTES

1. R. M. Hodgetts, *Management: Theory, Process, and Practice*, 5th ed. (Orlando, FL: Harcourt Brace Jovanovich, 1990), 460.
2. R. A. Katzell and D. E. Thompson, "Work Motivation," *American Psychologist* (February 1990), 144–153.
3. Ibid.
4. A. H. Maslow, *Motivation and Personality*, 2nd ed. (New York: Harper & Row, 1970); www.accel-team.com/motivation/theory.
5. J. L. Gibson, J. M. Ivancevich, and J. M. Donnelly, Jr., *Organizations: Behavior, Structure, Processes*, 8th ed. (Burr Ridge, IL: Richard D. Irwin, 1994), 151–193.
6. R. M. Hodgetts, op. cit., 478–479; D. McGregor, *Leadership and Motivation* (Cambridge, MA: MIT Press, 1966); http://www.accel-team.com/human_relations.
7. J. L. Gibson, J. M. Ivancevich, and J. M. Donnelly, Jr., op. cit., 176–177.
8. E. C. Murphy, "What Motivates People to Work?" *Nursing Management* (February 1984), 61–62; G. K. Gordon, "Developing a Motivating Environment," *Journal of Nursing Administration* (December 1982), 11–16; http://www.accel-team.com/human_relations.
9. R. A. Katzell and D. E. Thompson, op. cit.
10. J. L. Gibson, J. M. Ivancevich, and J. M. Donnelly, Jr., op. cit., 168–193; K. L. Roach, "Production Builds on Mutual Respect," *Nursing Management* (February 1984), 54–56; R. B. Youker, "Ten Benefits of Participant Action Planning," *Training* (June 1985), 52, 54–56.
11. J. L. Gibson, J. M. Ivancevich, and J. M. Donnelly, Jr., op. cit; www.accel-team.com/motivation/theory.
12. Ibid.
13. Ibid.

14. J. Fleury, "The Application of Motivational Theory to Cardiovascular Risk Reduction," *Image* (fall 1992), 229–239; www.accel-team.com/human_relations.

15. G. K. Gordon, op. cit.

16. K. L. Roach, op. cit.; M. G. Pryor and W. Mondy, "Mutual Respect Key to Productivity," *Supervisory Management* (July 1978), 10–17.

17. P. F. Drucker, *Management: Tasks, Responsibilities, Practices* (New York: Harper & Row, 1973–74), 176, 195–196.

18. P. Konstam, "Greenspan Joins Cry for Better Education," (12 February 1992), G1.

19. D. McGregor, op. cit., 5–6.

20. Ibid., 15.

21. M. Griffin, "Assumptions for Success," *Nursing Management* (January 1988), 32U–32X.

22. P. F. Drucker, op. cit., 23.

23. J. Lancaster, "Creating a Climate for Excellence," *Journal of Nursing Administration* (January 1985), 16–19; L. Ackerman, "Let's Put Motivation Where It Belongs: Within the Individual," *Personnel Journal* (July 1970), 559–562.

24. M. Miller, "Understanding Human Behavior and Employee Motivation," *Notes & Quotes* (1968); D. McGregor, op. cit., 211–212.

25. M. K. Kleinknecht and E. A. Hefferin, "Assisting Nurses Toward Professional Growth: A Career Development Model," *The Journal of Nursing Administration* (July–August 1982), 30–36; J. C. Crout, "Care Plan for Retaining the New Nurse," *Nursing Management* (December 1984), 30–33; R. C. Swansburg and P. W. Swansburg, *Strategic Career Planning and Development for Nurses* (Rockville, MD: Aspen, 1984).

26. M. C. Allender, "Productivity Enhancement: A New Teamwork Approach," *National Productivity Review* (spring 1984), 181–189.

27. P. Cornett-Cooke and K. Dias, "Teambuilding: Getting It All Together," *Nursing Management* (May 1984) 16–17.

28. M. J. Farley, "Teamwork in Perioperative Nursing: Understanding Team Development, Effectiveness, Evaluation," *AORN Journal* (March 1991), 732–733.

29. A. H. Maslow, op. cit.

30. B. Fuszard, ed., *Self-Actualization for Nurses: Issues, Trends, and Strategies for Job Enrichment* (Rockville, MD: Aspen, 1984), 140.

31. D. McGregor, op. cit.

32. B. Fuszard, op. cit.

33. Ibid., 40.

34. Ibid., 207.

35. A. H. Maslow, op. cit.

36. P. LeMone, "Analysis of a Human Phenomenon: Self-Concept," *Nursing Diagnosis* (July–September 1991), 126–130.

37. L. Ginsburg, and N. Miller, "Value-Driven Management," *Business Horizons* (May–June 1992), 23–27.

38. L. Hicks, "Motivation Key to Successful Employment," *San Antonio Express-News*, (17 March 1994), 1E–2E.

39. C. Trost, "To Cut Costs and Keep the Best People, More Concerns Offer Flexible Work Plans," *The Wall Street Journal* (18 February 1992), B1.

REFERENCES

Al-Shehri, A. "The Market and Educational Principle in Continuing Medical Education for General Practice." *Medical Education* (26), (1992) 384–387.

Ash, S. "A Big Job: How to Psych Yourself Up." *Supervisory Management* (April 1992), 9.

Astra, R. L. and S. Singg. "The Role of Self-Esteem in Affiliation." *Journal of Psychology* (January 2000), 15–22.

Barber, A. E., R. B. Dunham, and R. A. Formisano. "The Impact of Flexible Benefits on Employee Satisfaction: A Field Study." *Personal Psychology* (spring 1992), 55–75.

Blanchard, K., and S. Johnson. 1982. *The One Minute Manager* (New York: William Morrow, 1982).

Dearhammer, W. G. "Con: Promotion Calls for Proper Preparation." *Business Credit* (April 1991), 27–28.

Donadio, P. J. "Capturing the Principles of Motivation." *Business Credit* (March 1992), 40.

Dowless, R. "Motivating Salespeople: One Order of Empowerment, Hold the Carrots." *Training* (February 1992), 16, 73–74.

Emblen, J. D., and G. T. Gray. 1990. "Comparison of Nurses' Self-Directed Learning Activities." *The Journal of Continuing Education in Nursing*, 21(2), (1990) 56–61.

Erdman, A. "What's Wrong with Workers?" *Fortune* (10 August 1992), 18.

Farley, M. J. "Teamwork in Perioperative Nursing: Understanding Team Development, Effectiveness, Evaluation." *AORN Journal* (March 1991), 730–738.

Fong, C. M. "A Longitudinal Study of the Relationship Between Overload, Social Support and Burnout Among Nursing Educators." *Journal of Nursing Education* (January 1993), 24–29.

Franklin, A. J. "Invisibility Syndrome: A Clinical Model of the Effects of Racism on African-American Males." *American Journal of Orthopsychiatry* (January 2000), 33–41.

Ginnodo, W. L. "Consultative Management: A Fresh Look at Employee Motivation." *National Productivity Review* (winter 1985–86), 78–80.

Hanks, J. H. "Empowerment in Nursing Education: Concept Analysis and Application to Philosophy, Learning and Instruction." *Journal of Advanced Nursing*, 17 (1992), 607–618.

Hayes, E. "Managing Job Satisfaction for the Long Run." *Nursing Management* (January 1993), 65–67.

Hotter, A. N. "The Clinical Nurse Specialist and Empowerment: Say Good-bye to the Fairy Godmother." *Nursing Administration Quarterly* (spring 1992), 11–15.

"Elton Mayo's Hawthorne Experiments," "Motivation Theory," "Financial Motivation." (2000) http://www.accel-team.com/motivation/hawthorne.

Kipnis, D. "Psychology and Behavioral Technology." *American Psychologist* (January 1987), 30–36.

Leclerc, G., R. Lefrancois, M. Dube, R. Hebert, and P. Gaulin. "Criterion Validity of a New Measure of Self-Actualization." *Psychology Report* (December 1999), 1167–1176.

Lublin, J. S. "Trying to Increase Worker Productivity, More Employers Alter Management Style." *The Wall Street Journal* (13 February 1992), B1, B7.

MacDicken, R. A. "Managing the Plateaued Employee." *Assocation Management* (July 1991), 37–39, 57.

Margotta, M. H., Jr. "Pro: Continuing Education Leads to Promotion." *Business Credit* (April 1991), 26–28.

Maslow, A. H. *Religion, Values and Peak Experiences* (Columbus, OH: Ohio State University Press, 1964).

Maslow, A. H. *Toward a Psychology of Being*, 2nd ed. (New York: Van Nostrand Reinhold, 1968).

Meyers, M. E. "Motivating High-Tech Workers." *Best's Review-Life-Health Insurance Edition* (June 1992), 86–88.

Nikolajski, P. Y. "Investigating the Effectiveness of Self-Learning Packages in Staff Development." *Journal of Nursing Staff Development* (July–August 1992), 179–182.

Pell, A. R. "Motivation: Praise." *Manager's Magazine* 67(8), (1992), 30–31.

Peters, T. "'Gee Whiz' 'Wow' Factors Significant." *San Antonio Light* (21 July 1992), B3.

Peters, T. "'Must Do' Ideas Help Keep Business Afloat." *San Antonio Light* (11 February 1992), B8.

Rigdon, J. E. "Using Lateral Moves to Spur Employees." *The Wall Street Journal* (26 May 1992), B1, B5.

Rondeau, K. V. "Morale Boosters for Off-Shift Staff." *Medical Laboratory Observer* (August 1992), 40–41.

Ross, H. T., and M. M. Oumsby. "Teamwork Breeds Quality at Hearing Technology." *National Productivity Review* (summer 1990), 321–327.

Sayers, W. K. "ESOPs are No Fable." *Small Business Reports* (June 1990), 57–60.

Slotterback, Carla. "Carla Slotterback's Portfolio." (2000) carlaslotter @hotmail.com

White, J. A.. "When Employees Own Big Stake, It's a Buy Signal for Investors." *The Wall Street Journal* (13 February 1992), C1.

Wing, D. M., and J. R. Oertle. "The Process of Transforming Self in Women Veterans with Post-Traumatic Stress Disorder Resulting from Sexual Abuse." *International Journal of Psychiatric Nursing Research* (October 1999), 579–588.

CHAPTER 20

Communication

Russell C. Swansburg, PhD, RN

Between two beings there is always the barrier of words. Man has so many ears and speaks so many languages. Should it nevertheless be possible to understand one another? Is real communication possible if word and language betray us every time? Shall, in the end, only the language of guns and tanks prevail and not human reason and understanding?

Joost A.M. Meerloo[1]

LEARNING OBJECTIVES AND ACTIVITIES

- Illustrate the components of communication.
- Interpret the elements of communication.
- Evaluate the climate for effective communication.
- Distinguish between communication as perception and communication as information.
- Compare communication with feedback to communication without feedback.
- Distinguish among causes of listening habits.
- Explain techniques that will improve listening.
- Distinguish among media of communication.
- Apply the Gunning Mueller Fog Index to an assigned reading.
- Contrast future impacts on communication.

CONCEPTS: Communication, elements of communication, communication climate, perception, feedback, information, listening, media of communication, questions, oral communication, written communication, interviews, human capital.

MANAGER BEHAVIOR: Supports the notion that all communication takes place within the principle of the chain of command.

LEADER BEHAVIOR: Evaluates the communication system within the organization to provide a climate for maximum communication, including provision for feedback to and from employees.

Components

In answering the question of who is involved in communication, one could simply answer, everyone. However, several aspects are to be considered. The first of these is that the person who wants to be heard is involved in communication. For example, the Bantam fried chicken facility wants to sell chicken and wants people to know that it has chicken to sell. Its manager will therefore advertise in an effort to communicate this desire to sell an appetizing product. The manager will advertise through media such as newspapers, billboards, radio, television, and the Internet. All kinds of tempting pictures will be portrayed in these advertisements. If the manager is successful and people buy lots of Bantam fried chicken as a result of the advertisements, then the people have received the message and the manager has communicated to them.

A second aspect of communication occurs when a person seeks out desired information. Suppose a working person is just plain tired of cooking and wants Bantam fried chicken to serve the family for Sunday dinner. That person knows where the nearest location is, having heard or seen it advertised. She or he may have driven past the facility and seen the sign and markings that identify the product. That person may have been reminded of the product in the Sunday paper that morning. Even if the person cannot remember the address, she or he can always refer to the Yellow Pages for an address and phone number or call directory assistance. When a person wants information, there are many sources from which to obtain it. All these sources are media of communication.

Elements of Communication

At least two people are involved in communication: a sender, or provider, and a receiver. A sender usually has something he or she wants to communicate, even if the information is distasteful. A receiver usually has need of some information, whether good or bad. Regardless of the medium, information is transmitted from sender to receiver and a communication occurs.

Whether or not money is exchanged, communication always involves a buyer or a seller. The buying or selling is based on a need. Sometimes the receiver's need to hear is not as acute as the sender wants it to be. An example of this is the communication between a parent and a child. A parent can tell the child to be in by midnight on Saturday. The parent has said the same thing before, however, and when the child did not return by midnight, there were no consequences. As a result, now the child does not even hear the parent, because he or she has no reason to listen. When the child returns after midnight and is then told the hour to be home in the coming 4 weeks will be 8:00 P.M., however, the child does have a reason to listen. Communication now takes place, because the child finds sufficient reason for listening.

Communication is a human process involving interpersonal relationships, and therein lies the problem. In the workplace, some managers view their knowledge of events as power; sharing knowledge through communication is sharing power, and the manager does not want to share. Other managers do not realize the importance of communication in an information age because they are not up-to-date on the advantages of decentralization and participatory management. These managers frequently fall into crisis management, treating the symptoms of poor communication and never identifying the root causes. A third group of managers recognizes that communication is like the central nervous system in that it directs and controls the management process.

More than 80% of a higher-level manager's time is spent on communication: 16% of that time is spent reading; 9% writing, 30% speaking, and 45% listening. Is there any question that communication skills are absolutely essential to career advancement in nursing?[2] Effective communication has three basic principles:

1. Successful communication involves a sender, a receiver, and a medium.
2. Successful communication occurs when the message sent is received.
3. Successful nurse managers achieve successful communication.

Climate for Communication

Organizational climate and culture are discussed in Chapter 14, Organizing Nursing Services. The communication climate should be in harmony with the corporate culture and should be used to encourage positive values, such as quality, independence, objectivity, and client service, among nursing employees. Communication is used to support the mission (purpose or business) and vision of the nursing organization and to tell the consumers or clients that nursing is of high quality. The media used will include performance, nursing records, and marketing. Communication will be objective when it is accurately portrayed with descriptions of factual outcomes judged on the basis of objective outcome criteria.

Nursing literature abounds with evidence of nurses' desire for autonomy and knowledge they may use to communicate their support of autonomy. Nurses also may provide a climate in which the nursing business remains as free as possible of political constraints. When political considerations are imperative, the imperative will be communicated to employees, who make decisions based on the institution's values and beliefs.

Organizational culture is more difficult to change than organizational climate, but both can be modified with managerial effort and skill. The first step for nurse managers is to sample employees' attitudes or ideas of how they receive information and effect communication. Managers and employees know the formal structure, including roles and modes of operation used to inform and communicate. What is the informal structure? It involves people who are heroes or role models who can be involved in communication if they are positive and enthusiastic. Otherwise, they may have to be replaced, particularly if they are destructive.

Cultural Agendas

Cultural agendas publicize the mission or business of the organization. They tell what the organization stands for and on what the nursing division, department, or individual unit places value.

Cultural agendas are used to communicate promotions, new hires, marriages, deaths, and other personal news about personnel. Heroes are highlighted with features that illustrate support of desired values and beliefs: the nurse who presents a paper, authors a book, achieves prominence in the profession or the community; the nurse who is a champion bowler, an elected officer in an organization, an appointed official in the health care system; and the nurse who is a volunteer in community activities. The cultural agendas also are used to publicize nursing units and special achievements such as ongoing research in burn care or rehabilitation.

Cultural agendas are publicized using various media, including newsletters, memorandums, awards ceremonies, and external communications—publications, radio, television, and organizational meetings. Such communications are most effective when they depict the people who are directly involved in the publicized events.

Cultural agendas can be effectively used to change the organizational climate and culture.[3] The nurse leader must establish the climate for effective communication. Wlody recommends the following[4]:

Step I: Review your own communication technique.

Step II: Concentrate the staff's attention on communication as a needed skill that everyone can develop.

Step III: Lead the staff into more positive interaction within the unit.

Step IV: Make daily rounds with the whole team.

Step V: Form a group to reduce stress.

To be an effective communicator, a manager should develop close professional relationships with customers on their turf. Nurse managers can do this by identifying their customers and visiting them. Their customers include their employees, other professionals, patients, families, suppliers, and others. Being a role model shows that the manager cares. Behavior kindles the flames of hope. Success is ensured through partnerships between managers and front-line employees.[5]

Nature of Communication Climate

Important communication occurs between supervisor and employees at the work level where climate is set. A supportive climate encourages employees to ask questions and offer solutions to problems. Exhibit 20-1 compares the characteristics of supportive and defensive communication climates. Nurse leaders would strive for a supportive climate.

A strong relationship exists between good communication skills and good leadership.

Although research in the area of organizational attributes has been limited and the results inconclusive, some evidence shows that organizational size (number of employees) influences communication among subordinates but not between superiors and subordinates. The climate is more open at the top, where higher-level supervisors are more likely to involve subordinates in decision-making. Openness decreases as organizations increase in size, particularly in those with more than one thousand employees. With increased organizational size, communication increases but is perceived by employees to be increasingly closed. That is, more communication occurs but with less openness. Although a narrow span of control increases communication between supervisor and subordinate, an increased span of control is not perceived to decrease openness, thus indicating that the quality of interaction may be more important than is quantity.[6]

A supportive climate will produce clear communication to support productive nursing workers and effective teamwork. It will provide for identification of communication problems by designing instruments to collect data during specified periods of time. Real communication patterns and problems will be diagnosed from analysis of the data and can be related to the communication climate and solved by using problem-solving techniques.

Communication problems have been listed as the source of job dissatisfaction. Organizational communication systems are powerful determinants of an organization's effectiveness. Communication rules are organization-specific and are either explicit or implicit. Explicit rules are codified. They govern formal activities such as access to superiors. Violation of explicit rules may result in sanctions. Implicit rules mimic norms of behavioral expectations and are not codified but mutually shared. Conformation to rules reduces dissonance and maintains stability. A questionnaire may be used to assess communication in six areas: "(1) accessibility of information, (2) communication channels, (3) clarity of messages, (4) span of control, (5) flow control/communication load, and (6) the individual communicators"[7] (see Exhibit 20-2).

Negotiation

When disagreements about the intent of a communication occur, negotiation is indicated to prevent conflict, resignation, or avoidance between supervisor and employee. When there is lack of confidence between supervisor and employee or among employees, nurse managers can solve the communication problem through a climate of openness that restores confidence through agreement and promotes individual autonomy as well as esprit de corps.[8]

Communication and change require negotiation. Two basic types of negotiation are cooperative and competitive. Agreement is the objective in both types. Cooperative or win–win negotiation is best. Negotiation requires knowledge of human behavior and is based on human needs. Nurse managers and employees negotiate cooperatively for win–win outcomes for employees and the institution.

The principles of negotiation are:

- Maintaining self-identity and insight into your own motives, values, perceptions, and skills.
- Understanding others' values without judging them to be better or worse but only different from your own.
- Viewing issues in negotiation from the practical orientation as being potentially solvable.
- Using personal flexibility in terms of analyzing and reacting to issues and behaviors.
- Using skills to repair damaged relationships, including the ability to retreat and regroup in a manner that allows for perceptual openness.

EXHIBIT 20-1
Supportive Versus Defensive Communication Climate

SUPPORTIVE CLIMATE

1. The individual is free to talk to managers at any level of the organization without fear of retribution of any kind. Opportunities for this are planned and made known to the entire staff.
2. Equality: management by objectives supports equality by encouraging two-way communication in which both supervisor and employee evaluate progress and make future plans.
3. Descriptive evaluation with management analysis and employee input. The employee gets information at specific intervals and when indicated.
4. Spontaneity.
5. Problem orientation emphasizes joint view, bringing the employee into the process.
6. Provisionalism encourages adaptation and experimentation.
7. Empathy indicates concern and respect. Managers should use it to counteract neutrality by using nontraditional management techniques.

DEFENSIVE CLIMATE

1. The individual works within traditional management principles of chain of command, line of authority, and span of control.
2. Superiority: pyramids, hierarchies, and chains of command support superiority.
3. Traditional evaluation with one-way communication done on an annual basis.
4. Strategy is kept at the managerial planning level.
5. Control emphasizes the supervisor's view.
6. Certainty is dogmatic; it squelches.
7. Neutrality indicates nonconcern. It is fostered by orientation to numbers as in outcomes, profits, and even standardization of orientation procedures.

Source: Adapted from C. E. Beck and E. A. Beck. "The Manager's Open Door and the Communication Climate." *Business Horizons* (January–February 1986), 15–19. Copyright 1986 by the Foundation for the School of Business at Indiana University. Used with permission.

EXHIBIT 20-2
Communication Assessment Questionnaire

Circle the number representing the extent to which you believe the statement is true for you in your work environment.
1 = the statement is not at all accurate
5 = the statement is completely accurate

1. I have the information I need in order to do my job in the most effective and efficient manner.	1	2	3	4	5
2. I know where I can get the information I need in order to do my job well.	1	2	3	4	5
3. I receive information about my job from					
a. my immediate supervisor	1	2	3	4	5
b. my co-workers	1	2	3	4	5
c. notices posted on bulletin boards	1	2	3	4	5
d. personnel from departments other than nursing	1	2	3	4	5
4. I receive the information about any changes that might affect my job in a timely manner.	1	2	3	4	5
5. The communications I receive are clear and understandable.	1	2	3	4	5
6. I am satisfied with the frequency of communications I have with my immediate superior.	1	2	3	4	5
7. I receive too little information about things that are happening in this organization.	1	2	3	4	5
8. I believe that nursing administration shares critical and pertinent information with nursing personnel.	1	2	3	4	5
9. People in administration effectively communicate with employees.	1	2	3	4	5

Source: M. J. Farley. "Assessing Communication in Organizations." *Journal of Nursing Administration*, 19, 12 (December 1989), 28. Reprinted with permission of J. B. Lippincott.

In the win–win negotiation process the nurse manager will state these principles so that both manager and employee are on equal footing. The following are the steps of the negotiation process[9]:

1. Preparing for negotiation (e.g., introducing a topic at a meeting);
2. Communicating a general overview of what is to be accomplished during the process.
3. Relating the history of why negotiation is required;
4. Redefining the issue to be addressed;
5. Selecting when issues will be worked on;
6. Encouraging discussion during the conflict stage of the issue;
7. Addressing the fall-back or compromise for both parties on the issue;
8. Agreeing in principle during the settlement stage;
9. Recapping and summarizing the agreement; and
10. Monitoring subsequent compliance of the agreement (after settlement).

During the negotiation process, the nurse manager is always positive in explaining ideas, suggestions, and benefits. The nurse manager actively listens to employee responses, gaining perceptions, identifying concerns, and explaining obstacles to these ideas. The manager encourages explanations and suggests ways of overcoming obstacles. Questions are phrased to obtain doubtful discussion and answers.

During negotiation, a supportive environment includes a favorable location.

Successful negotiations have win-win outcomes that indicate progress, maintain self-respect, leave positive feelings, are sensitive to each other's needs, achieve a majority of each other's objectives, and facilitate future negotiation.

Change theory is involved in negotiation.[10]

Open-Door Policy

Communication climate influences the success of an open-door policy. An open-door policy of a nurse manager implies that an employee can walk into the manager's office at any time. Because nurse managers follow schedules, however, it usually is more convenient for both parties when the employee makes an appointment.

The communication climate associated with some organizations has made employees wary of the open-door policy. Line managers are threatened when they see their employees in the boss's office. They find out the reason for the visit by any means possible. Some managers punish the employee by telling them to use the chain of command. Some managers adjust performance evaluations, ostracize the employee, adjust pay increases, or work to fire the employee. This climate quickly teaches the employee not to use the open-door policy.

A nurse manager who believes in the open-door policy will clearly state the rules, including whether the employee needs someone else's permission to make an appointment with the manager. A democratic manager who believes in setting a climate for open communication will encourage visits. Such a manager knows how to deal with confidential communication to protect employees and their supervisors.

Communication as Perception

In nursing, as in other disciplines, communication is perception. Sound is created by the sensory perceptions people have associated with it. The sound aspect of communication is voice. Communication takes place only if the receiver hears and the person hears or perceives only that which he or she is capable of hearing. It is important that the communication be uttered in the receiver's language, and the sender must have knowledge of the receiver's experience or perception capacity.

Conceptualization conditions perception; a person must be able to conceive to perceive. In writing a communication, the writer must work out his or her own concepts first and ask whether the recipient can receive them. The range of perception is physiological, because perception is a product of the senses. However, the limitations to perception are cultural and emotional. Fanatics cannot receive a communication beyond their range of emotions.

Different people seldom see the same thing in a communication, because they have different perceptual dimensions. Drucker has said that to communicate, the sender must know what the recipient, *the true communicator*, is able to see and hear, and why. Perhaps if we focus on the recipient as the true communicator, we will improve communications. The unexpected is not usually received at all or is ignored or misunderstood. The human mind perceives what it expects to perceive. To communicate, the sender must also know what the recipient expects to see and hear. Otherwise, the recipient has to be shocked to receive the intended message.[11]

People selectively retain messages because of emotional associations and receive or reject messages based on good or bad experiences or associations. Communications make demands on people. It is often propaganda and so creates cynics. It demands that the recipient become somebody, do something, or believe something. It is powerful when it fits aspirations, values, and goals. Communication is most powerful when it converts, because conversion demands surrender.

Communication as perception indicates the value of a stated mission, philosophy, and goals. If statistical quality control (SQC) is practiced, it should be applied to organizational communication as part of the total system and to prevent misconceptions.

Communication is the process by which time management, skills, prioritization, planning, and personal involvement are transmitted by managers to establish an SQC program that implements change effectively. As managers effectively implement SQC, they inspire conviction, commitment, and conversion of their workers. The workers are first motivated with conviction of the desirability for change; they are inspired by the leader's attitudes. This leads to commitment to the change and internal conversion to a personal attitude and results in high productivity.

Statistical quality control succeeds in a climate fostering open communication among all managers and workers, commitment to employee involvement, and recognition of individuals and the unit or organization. The climate should be nonthreatening and positive.[12]

There is a major difference in perceptions between patients and clinic managers of patients' accessibility to health care clinics.[13] Patients with less education, a history of chronic heart disease, and a diagnosis of stable angina need special follow-up.[14]

Leveling with Employees

Leveling is being honest with employees. It makes all information, both the good and the bad, known to them. Being honest gives employees a chance to improve. Managers can control the content of negative information, not by concealing it but by sharing ideas, feelings, and information with employees. Nurse managers address issues as they arise. They focus on employee needs, offering help as indicated. Communication is a major factor in a performance evaluation.[15]

Conflict Management

Conflict is often a result of poor communication. Supervisors might react to employee outbursts by:

- Overriding their better judgments.
- Becoming defensive.
- Reprimanding the individual.
- Cutting off further expression of feelings.
- Monopolizing the conversation.

The result is increased frustration for both the employee and the manager.

Baker and Morgan suggest the following techniques for dealing with employee outbursts[16]:

1. Tune into the real message the employee is trying to communicate. Interpret it correctly, and direct a response at the feeling level of the employee.
2. Determine the nature of the feelings being expressed. Be sensitive to them because they are subjective and express the employee's values, needs, and emotions. Feelings are neither right nor wrong, but they represent absolute truth to the individual and usually are disguised as factual statements. Determine if they disguise anger, frustration, hurt, or disappointment.
3. Let the feelings subside by encouraging ventilation. Listen and give emotional support and then summarize what you have heard and interpreted from the outburst.
4. Clarify issues with questions that can be answered yes or no.
5. When impasses occur try "linking" the ideas or feelings the employee has expressed.
6. Allow face saving.
7. Be sure perceptions are accurate by summarizing them and checking them with the employee.
8. Verbalize your feelings as a supervisor by using positive "I" statements.

Communication Direction

For effective communication, the place to start is with the perceptions of the recipients. Listeners do not receive the communication if they do not understand the message. Nurse managers need to know what listeners are able to perceive before they formulate their message. Many nurse managers focus on what they want to say and then cannot understand why the recipient does not understand the message.

The information load should be kept to a minimum to help increase communication. Management by objectives focuses on perceptions of both recipients and senders. Recipients have access to the experience of the manager. The communicative process focuses on aspirations, values, and motivations: the needs of the subordinates. Performance evaluation or appraisal should focus on the recipient's concerns, perceptions, and expectations. Communication then becomes a tool of the recipient and a mode of organization because the employee uses it.

Feedback

Feedback completes or continues communication, making it two-way. Today's workers are better managed in a climate that promotes Theory Y and participation or involvement. Most workers are more affluent and better educated than in the past, have increased leisure time, and retire earlier, all indications of their changed values.

Feedback is one of the most important factors influencing behavior. People want to know what they have accomplished and where they stand. Feedback works best when specific goals are set to note the improvements sought, measurable targets, deadlines, and specific methods of attaining goals.

Effective communication includes giving and receiving suggestions, opinions, and information. If this two-way interaction does not occur, little or no communication takes place.

Communication requires mutual respect and confidence.

One-way communication prevents input or feedback and interaction. It causes nurses to depersonalize their relationships with patients and families. It serves as a barrier between nurses and physicians. It causes distorted communications that result in distorted and inaccurate feedback; scapegoating of peers, patients, and families; emotional blowups, skepticism of all messages; frustration and stress; delay of therapeutic interventions; and negative socioeconomic consequences.[17]

Research on Feedback

Research shows that feedback increases productivity. One study showed an 83% increase in productivity as measured by staff treatment programs and client hours, using the technique of private group feedback. Using the technique of public group feedback, productivity increased 163% in 38 weeks.

When suggestions were answered promptly in a mental health organization of 80 employees, the number of suggestions increased by 222.7% over a 32-week period. In other studies, feedback plus training have been found to be even more effective. A review of 27 empirical studies indicated that objective feedback worked in virtually every case.[18]

A study was done to test the effect of feedback on process versus outcomes of reality orientation in a psychiatric hospital serving elderly patients. Subjects were psychiatric nurses and were divided into three groups: Two groups were given appropriate feedback, whereas the third group did not receive any feedback. The nurses in the process feedback group showed "substantial increases" in process behavior over the control group that did not receive feedback. The nurses in the feedback group had increased patient contacts, but it was not determined whether their patients had increased reality orientation.[19]

Innovation and experimentation may be reduced by feedback that causes people to concentrate on process, methods, and procedures. Nurse managers should focus on outcomes or accomplishments that show that clinical nurses have been creative. New ideas as well as application of results of nursing research should be encouraged, and clinical nurses should be supported to develop proposals and conduct new nursing research. Levenstein recommends[20]:

1. Be clear in your own mind about the criteria you are using to assess staff performance.
2. Clarify ends, and the means are more likely to fall into place.
3. Emphasize flexibility in getting results rather than ritualistic observance of rules and procedures.

Successful synergies require leadership, cooperative management plans, joint incentives, information sharing, computer networks, face-to-face relationships, shared experiences, mutual need, and a shared future.[21] Communication is involved in almost every one of these activities. Kanter goes on to say that the communication imperative is that "More challenging, more innovation, more partnership-oriented positions carry with them the requirement for more communication and interaction."[22]

Information

Although they are interdependent, communication and information are different. Communication is perception; information is logic. Information is formal and has no meaning. It is impersonal and not altered by emotions, values, expectations, and perceptions.

Computers allow us to handle information devoid of communication content, an example being personnel information. Information is specific and economical, based on need by a person and for a purpose. Information in large amounts beyond that which meets a person's needs is an overload.

Communication may not be dependent on information; it may be shared experience. Information should be passed to the person who needs to know it, and that person must be able to receive it and act on it. Perception and communication are primary to information, and as information increases, the communicator or receiver must be able to perceive its meaning.[23] In the interest of time management, nurse managers need skills that sort information according to its import. These skills require clear communication and acute perception.

Listening

Communication takes place between employer and employee; herein lies the crux of the matter. To have satisfied, productive employees, an employer must hear what employees are saying as well as what they are *not* saying. Additionally, to really hear someone requires concentration. Consider, for example, what happens in church on Sunday: The preacher speaks, but the congregation hears only by concentrating on what the preacher is saying. Otherwise, the people supposedly listening to the preacher are planning next week's work or the rest of the day's events. Many managers do not listen effectively to what employees are saying to them and thus discourage the person who perhaps wants to point out a problem but knows that either he or she will not be heard or that the suggestion will have no effect.

One reason nursing personnel find it difficult to listen to a change-of-shift report is that a person can listen four times faster than the 125 to 150 words per minute that are being spoken. The listener who is tuned out may not hear a message about an appointment or a directive regarding a patient. As a result, it is usually more efficient for the person to read a change-of-shift report or listen to it on a tape recorder.

Most working persons are engaged in some form of verbal communication 70% of the waking day, or approximately 11 hours and 20 minutes out of 16 hours. Of that time, 45% is spent listening to what will be 50% forgotten within 24 hours. Another 25% is forgotten in the next two weeks.[24] If this is true of nursing personnel, they will forget 75% of what they hear today within the next two weeks. Some claim that immediately after a ten-minute speech we remember only 50% of what we hear; 25% is considered a good retention level.[25]

By learning the art of listening and observing, managers better understand what employees mean by what they say. They receive cues from employees' words and actions. Managers learn that men and women communicate differently. Learning the art of listening creates a better organization with better relationships and better outcomes.[26]

Causes of Poor Listening Habits

Remember that it is a bad habit to call a subject uninteresting or boring. Listen for useful information from what is considered a dull subject. Sift and screen, separate wheat from chaff, and look for something useful. Be an interested person, and make the subject interesting. Good listeners attempt to hear what is said.

It is a bad habit to criticize the delivery. Concentrate on finding out what the speaker has to say that is interesting or useful. Keep from being overstimulated by the subject.

Otherwise, you mentally prepare an argument or rebuttal and miss what the speaker says. Hear the speaker out before making judgments. Listen for the main idea rather than the facts; identify principles, concepts, and generalizations. Facts merely support the generalizations. Accept the face value of the message rather than evaluate it.

Avoiding eye contact with the speaker is a bad habit that decreases trust. Remember that 60% of a message is nonverbal.

Defensive listening occurs when the speaker's message threatens the listener with blame or punishment for something. It is a bad habit because it prevents accurate listening and perceptions. Defensive listening is stimulated when a person's speech implies a listener's behavior is being evaluated. Defensive response is reduced when the speaker describes behavior objectively.

Speech that indicates the sender is trying to control the receiver evokes defense. People don't want their values and viewpoints controlled and will shut out such messages. They want to have freedom to choose. When the sender solicits the collaboration of the receiver in solving mutual problems, the receiver responds positively.

Receivers defend themselves against perceived strategies to change their behaviors or control them, which they regard as deceitful. They respond to spontaneity and honesty, which they perceive as free of deceit.

Speech perceived as being unconcerned about the group's welfare evokes defense. Speech perceived as being empathetic evokes acceptance. People want to hear speech that indicates they are valued. Gestures can communicate neutrality or empathy.

Speech, verbal or nonverbal, that indicates superiority evokes defense, while speech indicating equality is accepted and supported. Certainty indicates dogmatism and evokes defense. A defensive reaction is reduced by professionalism; such speech indicates the sender wants help, information, data, or input from the listener.[27]

Other reasons supervisors give for not listening include[28]:

- Employees do not expect them to listen.
- Employees have nothing of value to say.
- Listening is not part of their jobs.
- Employees should listen to them.

Active listening is a skill for recognizing and exploring patients' clues, thereby giving health care providers a deeper understanding of the true reasons for the visit, which should result in increased patient satisfaction and improved outcomes.[29]

The speech-comprehension difficulties of aging persons primarily reflect declines in hearing rather than in cognitive ability.[30]

Techniques to Improve Listening

Improving listening ability can be accomplished in many ways. One method is to summarize what is being said for better understanding and retention. The listener should give empathetic attention to the speaker and try to understand the substance of what is being said; seek to be objective and to apply creativity; go beyond the speaker's dialect, stance, gestures, and attire to understand the meaning of the speaker's words; and try to counter his or her own emotionality or prejudice even though the speaker may have opposite convictions.

It is important to discriminate among those to whom one listens. Listen to people who keep you informed and lighten your workload or save time. Listen to those who argue constructively and use those judgments to sharpen your judgment. Know the kind of people who want to listen to you and the situation in which they will try to make you hear. Learn to recognize when you are prone to listen and when not.

Some people give good information, and people should listen to them. These people are trusted troubleshooters, line managers in charge of the bread-and-butter functions of primary patient care, staff specialists who have been delegated special tasks, reliable decision makers. Graciously avoid exaggerators, opportunists, office politicians, gossips, and chronic complainers.[31]

Things said by the speaker's appearance, facial expression, posture, accent, skin color, or mannerisms can turn off the listener. A person who wants to hear must thus put aside all preconceived ideas or prejudices and give the speaker full attention so that the speaker will be motivated to do a better job of communicating. While the person is talking, the listener analyzes what is being said for ideas and facts. The receiver must also listen for feelings—which are the background to the performance—tone of voice, gestures, and facial expressions.

Mnemonics

A *mnemonic* is a device used to help one remember. The following are two examples of mnemonics:

1. AIDA: Capture attention, sustain interest, incite desire, and get action.
2. PREP: Point, reason, example, *and point.*[32]

Such formulas are useful for preparing impromptu comments. The AIDA formula causes the speaker to focus on the listener's needs, interests, and problems. The PREP formula is ideal for spur-of-the-moment speaking. The first point reminds the speaker to clearly express a point of view on the subject. In giving the *reason*, the speaker explains why this is his or her point of view. These reasons should be illustrated with specific *examples* to clarify and substantiate the point: sta-

tistics, personal experiences, authoritative quotes, examples, analogies, anecdotes, and concrete illustrations. In the final point, the speaker brings the speech to a close with a restatement of the initial point of view. These formulas are intended to gain the attention of the listener and to elicit a positive response.

The following are some practical suggestions for encouraging people to listen:

1. Be prepared by answering the questions "Who?" and "What?"
2. Identify and evaluate the purpose of your remarks.
3. Organize and outline the report or speech to convey the facts.
4. Make efficient notes, and use them.
5. Remember that you are part of the package.
6. Make your voice work for you with proper breathing and pitch.
7. Communicate with your eyes.

Because critical thinking skills require interpretation of events based on present experience and factual data collection, they are also communication skills. Conceptualizing, which is a part of both the communication and the critical thinking processes, supports this conclusion. Also, the set of information and belief-generating and processing skills and abilities and the habit (based on intellectual commitment) of using these skills and abilities to guide behavior support the integration of critical thinking ability and communication skills. Managers use their critical thinking ability to identify feelings and become aware of beliefs, values, and attitudes of employees to communicate and respond to their needs. Active listening through use of all the senses is required of managers who need to recognize and respond to verbal and nonverbal messages from employees.[33]

Peters says that managers should become obsessed with listening.[34]

To become a good listener requires practice. Listening to the patient can prevent errors. For example, during a patient's temporary stay in a skilled nursing facility, a medication error was made because the nurse refused to listen to the patients, a husband and wife admitted to the same room. The nurse communicated with a physician who did not know either patient. Unneeded laboratory tests were done and reported late. A further irony was the wife was an RN, the husband was a medical doctor, and both were mentally alert. Every nurse manager and practicing nurse should work at improving his or her listening skills.

Good listeners get out from behind the desk and circulate with their customers. Good listening turns people on. Good listeners provide quick feedback and act on what they hear. Good listeners listen naively and intensely. They give people they want to listen to their phone numbers.

Managers who are good listeners may want to reward acts of meritorious listening.

Listening provides information that facilitates work, notes changes in patients' conditions more quickly and speeds up responses to changes. It brings closure to action and problems. It involves everyone.[35]

People tend to change the focus from listening to talking and telling. They perceive education as a solution to communication problems, whereas listening and adapting are the real solutions.

Listen informally at meals and coffee breaks. Listen formally to feedback about informative newsletters. Listen at no-holds-barred meetings. Listen rather than preach. Train people to listen. Provide employees with opportunities and places to talk and solve problems.

Listening to employees empowers them. A good listener is an engaged listener and takes notes. It is okay to ask so-called dumb questions when one needs information. Knowledge will always be power and should never be hoarded. Because information is frequently leaked before it happens, managers should provide it to the first-line people who need it. Providing information does many things; it[36]:

- Motivates employees by making them potent partners.
- Facilitates continuous improvement.
- Discourages unneeded controls and delays.
- Speeds up problem-solving and decision-making.
- Stirs the juices of competition by stimulating ideas.
- Begets more of the same.
- Abets the flattened organizational pyramid.

To get information flowing requires an extensive training program in basic management skills.[37]

Techniques to improve communication and prevent malpractice claims include: documenting telephone advice to patients, determining when and how to terminate patients, improving communication and listening styles, knowing how to effectively obtain the patient's consent, and implementing careful oversight mechanisms with the receipt of outside diagnostic test results.[38]

Some providers are being taught active listening techniques because malpractice suits are considered to be an expression of anger about some aspect of patient-provider relationships and communications.[39]

Results of Effective Listening

The results of effective listening are that two people hear each other, beneficial information is furnished on which to base right decisions, a better relationship between people is established, and it is easier to find solutions to problems.[40]

Communication across settings is needed to understand nurses' contribution to the care of elderly patients making the transition from hospital to home.[41] Knowledge of the communication dynamics of caring for patients may help providers to design strategies to attain the basic goals of continuity of care.[42]

Communication Media

Meetings

Meetings of all kinds are a medium for communication, often for purposes of information dissemination as well as true communication.

To make his company successful, Robert Davies, founder and president of SBT Corporation, changed his management style. To keep his employees motivated, he decided to include two employees in all management meetings to provide ideas from the production level of the organization. Davies encourages employees to risk telling what they really think through an e-mail suggestion system. This computer suggestion box is connected to all employees via more than 100 stations. It assures anonymity and in six months it has spawned more than 100 suggestions, which must be read and answered. For example, employees kept requesting relaxation of the dress code, which was done and is successful. Even Robert Davies dresses casually, and employees are more comfortable talking with him. Technology combined with listening results in consensus, support for decisions, and a company in which employees do their best.[43]

Supervisors

Supervisors or managers at all levels are also a medium for communication. To be successful in today's complicated environment, the nurse manager should be out and about. Communication includes gathering information for decision-making, spreading the management vision, and letting employees know that leaders care for them. Communication is visibility. By walking around among employees and other customers, the nurse manager can prevent information distortion. This requires visiting and chatting with these knowledgeable people.

The vision stamp is applied on the front line. By walking around, managers facilitate and coach; they do not give orders and conduct inspections. That is the work of the hands-on team.

Some corporate executives have dismantled their offices. They maintain work areas at unit levels, with a system to correspond on the phone or computer and handle mail. They are visible.

Peters recommends the following actions for increasing visible management[44]:

1. Put a note card in your pocket that says, "Remember, I'm out here to listen."
2. Take notes, promise feedback—and deliver. Fix things.
3. Cycle your actions through the chain of command and give managers the credit for fixing things.
4. Protect informants.
5. Be patient.
6. Listen, but preach a little, too, by killing unneeded red tape.
7. Give some, but not much, advance notice and travel alone. Take your own notes.
8. Work some night shifts; take a basic training course.
9. Watch out for the subtle demands you put on others that cut down on their practice of visible management.
10. Use rituals to help force yourself and your colleagues to get out and about.

We live in an information society; communication is the necessary ingredient for accomplishing missions and objectives. An effective communicator is an effective leader. Some managers use models or drawings to get their meanings across. Use *synthesia*, the technique of transforming one sense to another, to communicate. Learn to express ideas graphically to engender employees' understanding, trust, and support. Use symbols of success, not symbols of defeat.

Effective communication creates meaning. It should be an act of persuasion. The right metaphor connects with the listener. The effective manager as leader acts and personifies the message transmitted via the metaphor. This leader transmits the message over and over.[45]

Effective nurse leaders share all the information possible. Employees cannot have too much information about the company. The only information a manager does not share is that protected by law, ethics, and decency.

A nurse manager who holds information as a source of power is not an effective manager or leader.

Recognition programs promote communication. Nurse managers recognize fairly mundane actions, send written notes for work well done, and offer special recognition, such as serving a box of doughnuts or a cake to celebrate an individual or a group achievement. Nurse managers should be sure that all acts of special effort are heartfelt, that is, they should not be phonies. Nurse managers should do a few big rewards and many small ones, be systematic, and celebrate events they would like repeated.[46]

Questions

Asking questions is an important method of communicating. Questions are asked to obtain information; the goal is mutual understanding. The tone of voice must encourage confidence and trust from the person questioned. Facial expression is important as is the physical conduct of the questioner. The nurse manager should always go beyond the answer to a primary question and not flatly agree or disagree with the question.

The following types of questions should be used:

1. Open questions that give the other person the opportunity to freely express thoughts and feelings, rather than closed-end questions that force the receiver to become the sender of information. Questions that can be answered "yes" or "no" do not give information or explanation. In the courtroom, attorneys use them to trap people or clarify a point.
2. Leading questions that give direction to the reply, rather than loaded ones that restrict by putting the respondent on the spot.
3. Cool questions that appeal to reason, rather than heated ones reflecting the emotional state of asker and answerer.
4. Planned questions that are reflective and asked in logical sequence, rather than impulsive ones that just happen to occur to the asker.
5. Complimentary or "treat" questions that tell the respondent that he or she can make an important contribution to the asker's views, rather than trick ones that place the respondent on the spot.
6. Window questions that elicit the respondent's true thoughts and feelings, rather than mirror ones that reflect the point of view of the questioner.

Successful questioning consists of creating and maintaining a climate for communication, asking the right questions in the right way, and listening to the responses.

Questions can be used to improve listening, with their use serving to clarify unclear statements. The questioner should take care not to overawe or threaten the speaker. Questions should be worded and spoken in a nonthreatening way, for example:

"I am sorry I did not hear your comment clearly. Would you mind repeating it, please?" or

"I do not quite understand what you mean by 'capital resource.' Would you explain further, please?"

A listener should never be embarrassed to ask questions that improve his or her understanding of a person's communication. Serious questions that result in clarification of or additional information increase comprehension and clear up misperceptions, thus helping senders and receivers. If the medium is an oral presentation, questions can be written down for use at appropriate times, such as during question periods and breaks, after meetings, and even later at an interview. Thus, the listener can construct thoughtful questions.

When questions are used to clarify a point made by the sender, they can be the closed yes-or-no questions. An example might be, "Do you support the position on nurse autonomy you have just described?"[47]

Oral Communication

Oral communication is the most common form of communication used by executives, who spend 50% to 80% of their time communicating. Because oral communication takes so much time, a nurse manager should use the most effective words. Verbal messages are said to be 7% verbal (word choice), 38% vocal (oral presentation), and 55% facial expression.[48]

An advantage of face-to-face communication is that a person can respond directly to another or others. The larger the group, the less effective is face-to-face communication. An effective message requires knowledge of words and their various meanings as well as of the contexts within which the words can be used. Thus, effective communication may depend on use of the dictionary for correct vocabulary.

When giving a speech, one needs to keep in mind that the members of the audience are usually informed and sophisticated and have access to information. The members of the audience want the speaker to talk things over with them, not to talk to them. The speaker must be sincere and respect the listeners.

To present an effective speech, the speaker needs to:

- Develop an outline and hold to four or five main ideas.
- Put other ideas under the main topic as subordinate ones.
- Open with an introduction.
- Close with a brief summary.
- Type the speech for easy reading.
- Practice by reading the speech.
- Maintain eye contact during the speech.
- Keep the voice and manner informal and conversational.

A speaker should know the audience and its members' knowledge of the subject, intellectual level, attitudes,

and beliefs. Former Vice President Hubert Humphrey said, "The necessary components to build a speech are full understanding of the facts of the subject, thorough understanding of the particular audience, and a deep and thorough belief in what you are saying."[49]

Exhibit 20-3 lists other techniques to use in preparing and giving an effective oral presentation.

Written Communication

Writing is a common medium of communication not only in nursing but in society in general. It comes in massive quantities: memos to be read and passed on, even if they go into someone else's wastebasket; letters that need to be answered; newspapers and magazines that collect in stacks; junk mail; posters and flyers; and notices and newsletters. How should one go about handling all this material? First, make a mental decision to deal with each piece of paper. Establish a system for assigning priorities to the mass of written communications; skim through everything, and then answer or delegate that which can be handled immediately. Put aside whatever can be taken care of at a future date, but do not put things where they will be forgotten. Papers can be placed in a folder according to priority.

When writing, remember that you are writing for the receiver: a reader, viewer, listener, observer, or member of an audience. The receiver is not interested in you as a writer, but only in the message being conveyed. Therefore direct your message to the reader or listener, that is, the receiver; use good marketing techniques; and sell your product.[50]

Exhibit 20-4 lists nine rules to follow when writing.

Words are obviously important to written communication. The writer should put the reader's interest first, begin with a provocative question or striking statement to jar the receiver, and get right to the point: the purpose of the written communication, and the request for action. When writing a letter, a personal letter is always better than a form letter. One should use a friendly tone, with first names and personal pronouns, which express an interest in the reader.

The following are some simple suggestions for communicating effectively through the written word[51]:

- Use active voice verbs to give strength to written communication. About 10% of total words should be verbs.
- Use strong nouns.
- Use the subject and main verb early in the sentence.
- Avoid overuse of adjectives and adverbs, and be specific when using adjectives. State the specific amount such as 100 instead of "much," "any," or "a lot."
- Be as brief as possible.

EXHIBIT 20-3

Techniques for Effective Public Speaking

1. Prepare carefully. What is the goal of your presentation? Is it to inform? Persuade? Entertain? It can be a combination of these and, to be effective, should probably combine at least two, such as entertainment with information or persuasion.

2. Prepare the presentation carefully. Make an outline and develop the content to fit the outline. Start well in advance so that you can read and adjust the material for a smooth flow of ideas.
   a. What is the purpose of the presentation? Did you select the topic, or was it given to you? In either instance, clarify the purpose with the organizers of the event or whoever engaged you to do the presentation.
   b. Prepare an introduction that will gain the attention of the audience. Spark their interest. Humor often helps, but be careful of using cynicism or making derogatory remarks. References to religion, sex, and other controversial subjects should be carefully selected, if used at all. They are better avoided if you wish to persuade or inform, unless they are a part of your topic. Remember, words convey feelings, attitudes, opinions, and facts. Use them to turn the audience on, not off.
   c. Make the main points in the body of the presentation. Support them with appropriate and specific examples.
   d. Prepare or select visual aids to support the key points of the presentation. They are an extension of your presentation designed to appeal to the senses and increase reception.
   e. Know who the audience will be and tailor the message to it. Provide useful material.
   f. Plan for audience participation with questions or appropriate exercises to involve listeners.
   g. Tie the message together with interval summaries and an effective conclusion. How do you want to leave the audience?
   h. If you plan to speak extemporaneously, make notes on cards or put outlines on a visual aid such as a poster, a chalkboard, an overhead transparency, or a slide projection screen.

3. Prepare the environment beforehand. Surroundings are important and should be as attractive as possible. Bear this in mind when you have input into selection.
   a. If you want to speak from a podium, make sure it is in place. If you want to sit, have a table and chair in place.
   b. Check lighting and sound equipment.
   c. Check audiovisual equipment.
   d. Remove unneeded barriers such as screens, furniture, and other movable objects. If pillars are in the way, rearrange your position or the audience seating, if this is possible. Arrange your proximity to the group to facilitate a feeling of closeness.
   e. Prepare your person for the presentation. Wear clothes that present you best. Conventional clothes are best because the audience should focus on your words and not your appearance. Be well-groomed.
   f. Good preparation will help you to be relaxed. Get a good night's sleep the night before the presentation. Plan your schedule so as not to be excited beforehand. Eat and drink moderately. Sit and do deep-breathing exercises immediately before.

4. Be on time and use time effectively.

5. Speak to be heard.
   a. Use your voice, varying pitch, volume, rate, and tone for planned effect.
   b. Practice pronouncing words with which you have trouble.
   c. Pause to enhance your delivery. Short silences emphasize points and allow the audience to think about them.
   d. Make your presentation sound natural even if you read it.

6. Use body language effectively.
   a. Slowly develop the audience's awareness of your nonverbal behavior. Be aware of it yourself.
   b. Maintain eye contact.
   c. Plan your movements: walking, standing. Your posture should convey energy, interest, approval, confidence, warmth, and openness.
   d. Keep the space between you and the audience open.
   e. Use positive gestures.
   f. Use head movements for effect.
   g. Use facial expression for effect.
   h. Know where your hands and feet are at all times.
   i. Be genuine! An audience can quickly identify a fake.

7. Adapt to audience feedback, being sensitive to listeners' interests and moods.
   a. Listen for unrest, shifting in seats, whispering, muttering.
   b. Watch for nonverbal responses. Pay attention to body language, facial expressions, gestures, body movements. Leaning backward or away is perceived as a negative response.
   c. Be prepared to answer questions if there are breaks in the presentation. You may want to plan for them. Repeat them before answering, regardless of whether they are oral or written. You are giving additional information.
   d. Treat your audience with respect in every way, and they will view you as genuine.

EXHIBIT 20-4
Nine Rules to Follow When Writing

1. Empathize. Be sensitive to the needs and desires of those who will read what you are writing. Arouse and maintain the reader's interest by appealing to the mind and emotions. For example, compose a message that will transmit respect for the nurse while offering a credible and unique inspiration to taking nursing histories or preparing nursing care plans. When giving orders, explain why you are asking for the task to be done. You-centered rather than I-centered communications are interesting to the reader or listener. Give people honest and deserved praise, the kind of flattery that makes them feel they are worth flattering. If you are addressing a particular person, a unique human personality, put that person's name in the salutation as well as in the body of the letter or memo. Make an effort to please the receiver by using tact, respect, good manners, and courtesy.

2. Attempt to avoid the COIK ("clear only if known" to the reader or listener already) fallacy. Think of the misunderstandings that could occur in a written message using abstract terms. Your aim should be to create mental pictures using language that is suitable to the experience and knowledge level of the receiver.

3. Do not repeat anecdotes frequently, or the reader will be insulted. Avoid overcommunication, overdetailing, and redundancy. Necessary repetition can be achieved by using pleasant and meaningful examples, illustrations, paraphrasing, and summaries. Repetition is essential to the mastery of a skill.

4. Express yourself in clear, simple language. Lincoln's Gettysburg Address contains 265 words, three-fourths of them of one syllable. Abstract, technical-sounding jargon, cliches, and trite platitudes may cover up insecurity in a writer afraid of committing herself or himself in writing. Avoid archaic commercial expressions, specialized in-house jargon, and fading journalese by writing clearly and concisely.

5. Make yourself accessible to the reader by positively and courteously requesting a response. You can ask a direct question and expect a reply by a certain date. You can also encourage response by giving a special return address, a private box or phone number, writing instructions, a postcard, or a return envelope. Make it easy, desirable, and pleasant for the reader to reply.

6. Use the format of the newspaper story: accuracy, brevity, clarity, digestibility, and empathy. Arouse the reader with a headline opener. Follow it with a summary that tells significant highlights in the opening paragraph. Then tell the details. Here is an example of a memo form that has worked for others.

Date_____   Time_____

To:_____ Subject:_____

From: _____

Objective:_____

1. _____

_____

2. _____

_____

3. _____

_____

7. Break up a solid page of print with a variety of forms: underline, space, italicize, capitalize, enumerate, indent, box, summarize, and illustrate. Make your reading attractive and digestible.

8. Back up what you write by what you do; build a reputation for integrity.

9. Organize your material.
   a. Outline key points.
   b. Compile data into groups according to commonality.
   c. Arrange materials in a logical sequential order:
      (i) Chronological.
      (ii) Cause-effect relationship.
      (iii) Increasing complexity.
   d. Tie the groups together using transitional devices:
      (i) Time-order words (first, later, finally).
      (ii) Guide words (as a result, therefore, on the other hand).
   e. Link the communication with the previous message by referring to:
      (i) Date.
      (ii) Subject.
      (iii) Sender of correspondence.
   f. Furnish appropriate excerpts from past correspondence.

- Use short rather than long words.
- Use sentences that contain one idea and are no longer than 16 to 20 words. Vary the sentence length.
- Write naturally, using friendly conversational language (however, use contractions such as "didn't" and "aren't" with discretion).
- Reread and revise your written communication. Look at the nouns and verbs. Evaluate your sentences; they should be simple, not complex. Determine that you have said what you mean. Eliminate unneeded words.
- You may want to add a personal handwritten note at the bottom.

Written Reports

Written reports should indicate how the nursing objectives are being met. If a 24-hour nursing report is made from the patient units to the director of nursing, the information provided should show progress in relation to the achievement of unit and department objectives. The information should be provided in a simple, functional or practical, and qualitative rather than complex and quantitative manner. In providing the information, the reporter should consider its relative value and purpose, eliminate overlap and duplication, and put the report in perspective. The report should indicate the work load and state pertinent facts describing patients' status, why the patients are hospitalized, and the nursing diagnosis and prescription. The following are other factors to consider in writing useful reports:

1. Size and cost should not exceed their need or strength.
2. A strong report will not be contaminated with individual bias. For that reason, a computer printout has value over a hand-prepared report.
3. A strong report will be useful to many people, providing them with vital information to run the operation.
4. A strong report will have authentic and reliable sources of information, that is, people with knowledge and the skills required to judge what information needs to be transmitted. Some information can be given by clerks, some by technicians, and some, of necessity, by the nurse manager.
5. If the report is going to a group of people with limited time, such as a board of directors, the writer should add an executive summary at the beginning of the report and highlight what he or she wants the readers to act on. This may speed up the response.

Sometimes managers have a tendency to eliminate reports. Although the busy nurse manager may hope that all reports would be eliminated, doing so without consensus sometimes drives reports underground. Because reports and forms tend to proliferate, each should have an elimination date, at which time it will be eliminated unless it is rejustified.

Time is an element common to all reports. The *perpetual report* shows up-to-date events for a full year. As the latest month or quarter is added, the oldest is dropped. This time base deals with the realities of the present and provides consistency, completeness, and effectiveness in reporting.

If top management cannot extract the information it wants from reports, then either the information is unnecessary or the procedures need to be improved. Persons who design reports and reporting procedures should do the following:

1. Gain access to all documents listing the short- and long-range objectives of the unit, department, division, and institution. Objectives should be in agreement and clearly stated in writing. Progress is reported.
2. Establish priorities for reports.
3. Categorize reports, indicating which objectives are supported by each.
4. Determine what top management needs and wants to know, and then screen reports.
5. Test reports for logical patterns that avoid complexity and unwieldy clumsiness.
6. Classify reports according to frequency.
7. Determine the levels through which reports will pass.
8. Determine the point of origin.
9. Coordinate reports with the organizational structure.
10. Check for accuracy and consistency.
11. Account for the total cost of reporting.
12. Obtain the concurrence of all levels of management.

Reports form the nucleus of all management communications, and successful communications are dependent on an intelligently conceived report structure. The reader should be able to read from top to bottom and laterally as well as from bottom to top.

Interviews

Interviewing is a basic tool of communication. A prospective employee is interviewed. When good counseling and guidance techniques are practiced, interviews also are used to apprise employees of their performance. An interview is essential to practicing management by objectives. In disciplining an employee, it is necessary to interview the individual. When an employee leaves, an exit interview is desirable to learn why the person is leaving and to gain ideas for strengthening the personnel management program. Interview questions should be worded to obtain the most beneficial information. The following are suggestions for conducting effective interviews:

1. Use plain and direct language rather than technical, professional, or slang terms.
2. Keep questions short.
3. Use familiar illustrations.
4. Do not assume the person being interviewed knows what you mean or are saying. Check the extent of the interviewee's knowledge beforehand.
5. Avoid improper emphasis so as not to indicate the answer you hope to elicit.
6. Be sure the interviewee attaches the same meaning to words that you do.
7. Be precise in choosing words. Use accurate synonyms and words with one pronunciation.

Organizational Publications

Barnard stated that the first function of an executive is to develop and maintain a system of communication.[52] The bigger the organization, the more difficult it is for the director of nursing to communicate with the employees who give direct care to patients. This problem is further complicated by the requirement that services are provided 24 hours a day, seven days a week. The medium for communication between nurse executives and employees is an organizational publication such as a newsletter or in-house magazine. This procedure does not have to be confined to nursing but can be supported and used by nursing staff. Certainly, the nurse executive will have input into the development and evaluation of such an organizational publication.

According to Tingey a successful organizational publication will fulfill six requirements[53]:

1. It will meet clearly stated objectives related to the process of communications. These objectives will state what the executives of the institution or organization, including nursing, want to accomplish through the publication.
2. The publication will need a competent editor who can provide professional editing and who will ensure that the objectives are met.
3. The editor will need access to the ideas of top management. Thus, the nurse executive must provide the editor with the information needed to inform nursing personnel of changes in policy and procedures.
4. Like management of any area, the objectives of the publication will be developed into a master management plan. This plan will indicate articles and story themes to be used to accomplish each objective.
5. Information about future events will provide personnel with articles that give an anticipatory viewpoint. In nursing this could include the organization's role in supporting continuing education, expected problems involved in collective bargaining, changes in organizational structure, and changes that will affect practice, such as new equipment, new supply products, and new support activities.
6. The editor should know the audience, including their educational level, interests, problems, and attitudes. The publication should be interesting to family members and contacts. An unread publication is useless.

Specific objectives of the publication will be related to the internal technologic environment, the internal social environment, the external environment, company social responsibilities, and organizational dynamics.

Electronic Media

Electronic links are a key to a successful management strategy. To increase productivity in the workplace, nurse managers need to be aware of development within the telecommunications industry. For example, fax machines provide quick and accurate transmission of orders from physicians to nurses. Nurse managers can ask the following questions:

- Will fax machines improve the output of clinical nurses if they can use faxes to get drugs from the pharmacy more quickly and accurately?
- Will fax machines improve response times and the accuracy of diagnostic testing by providing an electronic link to the medical laboratory, radiology, and other departments?
- Will fax machines increase therapeutic response times among clinical nurses, physicians, physical therapists, respiratory therapists, and others?

Numerous other electronic links are available, including use of computer bulletin boards for fast memos and software programs that can be used to control supply inventories and provide just-in-time supplies. Electronic networks provide sources of fast up-to-date information about diagnoses and treatments. Cellular phones, electronic memo pads, and all the latest in telecommunications technology should be evaluated by nurse managers for use within and among patient care units. Evaluation should be a part of the strategic planning process. Their adoption should be evaluated on the basis of value added to individual and corporate performances and cost-benefit analysis.

Even though sophisticated communications technology is in place, managers and employees often fail to communicate. Good communication is the key to achieving personal and organizational effectiveness and a fit of the two. To be effective, information must be transferred in a timely fashion. Information technology is available to do this. Managers are responsible for using available information technology and therefore need to have related competencies. To communicate effectively, managers and employees need training in the skills of information technology.[54] The management information system or nursing information system should be transformed into a customer information system. Lack of electronic memos or faxes or other communications may indicate to personnel and patients that a nurse manager is not listening.

Obtaining Information

Receivers have a responsibility for obtaining information. Professional employees feel some conflict between their personal needs and the demands of the organization. Communication, the giving and receiving of information, helps an employee to control or tolerate this conflict. Assume that management controls information that will be given to employees. A conservative manager will give employees as little information as possible, because this manager believes that too much information will be distorted or misunderstood.

A director of nursing stated that although the registered nurse in the recovery room was totally competent, she would not give her the title of nurse manager and bring her to nurse manager meetings because she would misinterpret the statements made there. The enlightened manager will be direct and honest, believing that employees need all the information they can have to do their jobs. Bad news usually leaks, and trying to keep it covered up only creates distrust and anxiety.

Poor communication is caused by caution and preoccupation with running the department. Some managers tend to treat information as private property. Geography and size effect communication. People tend to protect their egos and prejudices, and employees must seek out information.

Communication of information is a joint responsibility of employer and employee. So if you need to know something, ask. Find out how your organization is developing and what its future prospects are. Learn whether its requirements continue to be compatible with your personal goals.

The Future

People as Capital

Specialization, division of labor, and economics of scale do not work in a service organization. People are the capital resource and return on people is the measurable outcome, not capital in building and machines. The cost basis of service organizations will continue to be in people:

- Good employees want ownership. They want to own stock in the company. They also want psychic ownership in the company. They believe they are entrepreneurs. Within the corporation, "intrapreneurship" is already creating new products and new markets, revitalizing companies from the inside out.
- The service economy produces to meet unique human needs. Ideas come from employees having a rich mix of cultures. Customer demands and needs spur intuition and creativity, leading to new products and services. Medical problems, including nursing problems, are not neatly packaged. They are organic and interdependent, requiring workers who will integrate the specialists to meet the needs of the people.

- Capital must be compounded through education and software. Training and education will reduce general and administrative costs to maintain and increase competition. Information should be bought as a direct cost because a productive employee must be up-to-date and have information to be competent and productive.

Organizations

Organizations that foster personal growth will attract the best and brightest people. Work enlargement yields greater productivity from such people. They want health and fitness and education programs from their employers. They want work integrated into their lives. They want to work in environments that are democratic and allow them to network and to work in small teams. They want work to be fun.

To grow and profit, organizations will have to eliminate their hierarchical orientation and become team-oriented. They will have to emulate the positive and productive qualities of small business. The infrastructure of the organization will give way to networking and people orientation.

Many businesses are striving for monopoly through mergers, acquisitions, and coalitions to control their environments. While success evolves from market feedback, market forces demand change from people and are brutally destructive when people fail. The market will become the arbiter of power, obliterating layers of bureaucracy unless seized by political means.

A successful organization has effective communication at all levels, including the managerial level. Managers are skilled in managing human resources to effect communication. Communication makes employees valuable, contributing members of the corporate team, an important perception. Successful communication reduces conflict by reducing litigation and external intervention by labor unions and regulatory governmental agencies.

A good communication system does the following:

- Aids in cost savings, improves efficiency, and enhances productivity. People who know the system uncover and fix any problems.
- Keeps management better informed as it supports trust.
- Keeps employees informed of the company's plans, policies, goals, philosophies, and requirements. Informed employees act positively.
- Improves morale. Information means a happy employee not swayed by outside influences.
- Makes employees feel they are part of a team. Again, spirit and trust support common goals.
- Maintains a work environment free of outside adversaries and unwanted third-party influences.

- Provides some confidentiality for mutual trust and respect.
- Responds promptly and completely.
- Provides a means for employees to ventilate.
- Provides sufficient information.
- Recognizes employees as individuals.

Employee attitude surveys may be a means of evaluating the effectiveness of company communication. These surveys cover employees' feelings about job duties, working conditions, supervisory and managerial skills, communications, pay, benefits, training, promotional opportunities, personnel policies and procedures, morale, and job security. Analyze results and make and implement a plan to resolve problems. Resurvey after a sufficient period.[55]

Managers

Managers should be retrained to be coaches and facilitators. Some organizations are already doing this. W. L. Gore & Associates have 38 plants, 5,000 employees, and no plant managers. Plant size is limited to 150 employees. As employees develop a following, they become the chosen leaders. Employees have sponsors when they are employed. If a job is not learned within 90 days, the employee is no longer paid. Advocate sponsors are consulted by a compensation sponsor to determine salary based on accomplishment.

Thirty-five percent of American corporations pay managers more than they deliver as value added, that is, the increased production and profit they add as a result of their performance. The manager's new role is that of coach, teacher, and mentor.[56]

Technology

Technology will be linked to the service orientation of surviving, adaptive, customer-oriented organizations. It will shift the cost curve, with labor continuing to have high income because of increased productivity.

Quality will be paramount, requiring that the organizational design and the technology be brought together as enablers for human resources. Computers can supplement, not replace, human capital.

Technology will become overhead. Information technology will be used to solve problems where there is little intelligence and very little collective knowledge. When available, information should be bought and not generated directly to decrease overhead costs and hierarchy. Otherwise, managers must establish entire teams of experts to develop and implement a system that may already be available. It will be cheaper to pay the experts by the minute, because many will be available electron-ically. Thus, contract or consultative labor will replace hired labor, especially in the technological sphere.

Artificial intelligence will be a key enabler that will create generalists. It replaces experts and encapsulates and capitalizes knowledge. Knowledge will be added to machines to become an extension of the user. A symbiotic relationship will exist between the manager and the expert machine.

Survival in the information age will depend on a combination of technology and strategic insights. Service organizations will have to find people who need services and deliver these services to them. During the past 6,000 years, information has belonged to the power structure, which did not trade it, market it, or give it away. The service industries of the information age will market services that are heavily information based.

Technology is always in arrears; people and systems can quickly become obsolete. Managers should go after strategic, not technical, gains. They should not computerize what does not work or maintain obsolete technology in hiring people. Employers must be developed and updated, adjusted to the system, or they will career hop within and outside of the organization. Turnover is expensive, because it throws away assets. Human resource assets generate more value added when they are managed, enriched, and involved in the enterprise.[57]

Summary

Communication occurs between government and governed, between governments, between buyers and sellers, between manufacturers and consumers, between pupils and teachers, between parents and children, and between neighbors, but most important, communication occurs between people *only if they want it to*. The products of lack of communication are too costly to accept: misinformation, misunderstanding, waste, fear, suspicion, insecurity, and low morale.

People have difficulty accepting the fact that communication is not the answer to all problems of human relations and personnel management. A gap exists between senders and receivers that must be recognized before it can be bridged—a gap in background, experience, and motivation.

Good communication is frequently an illusion. It is not achieved with open doors, geniality, or jokes. Communication is aided by listening to what people are really saying and perceiving what they are projecting through their words, facial expressions, tone of voice, and actions. To induce greater numbers of people to accept direction, and not undermine it, these people must be encouraged to participate. They will listen for genuineness in the word of the boss as demonstrated by actions.

APPLICATION EXERCISES

EXERCISE 20-1   Check your in box. If you are not receiving communications from your customers (clinical nursing personnel, patients, and others), start a personal listening ritual. Call three customers a day and ask how they are doing and what their problems are. Listen to their responses.

EXERCISE 20-2   From your communications (calls, memos, etc.), follow-up on complaints or problems. Help resolve them.

EXERCISE 20-3   Have a group of internal and external customers meet with you to discuss communication and information problems. Listen to them. Guide them to good solutions. Facilitate action.

EXERCISE 20-4   Use a group of coworkers to evaluate your current recognition program. Discard those activities that are not working if they cannot be fixed. Give an infusion of excitement to the others. Consider having an "attaboy" and "attagirl" award where customers can pick up a short form and fill it out when they feel especially good about something an employee has done. Recognize the employee immediately at change-of-shift report, breakfast, lunch, dinner, or wherever. Send out ten thank-you notes a month to employees and ten more to customers.

EXERCISE 20-5   Make notes of calendar events and take a box of doughnuts or a cake to them.

EXERCISE 20-6   Be the first to make a contribution to the United Way or other community agency. Lead the charge when supporting a voluntary effort for a community activity. Recognize those who put forth community effort.

EXERCISE 20-7   Walk around your area of responsibility. Note at least one hassle that can be fixed each day (or week or month). Fix it!

EXERCISE 20-8   Identify and analyze your worst failure each month. How can it be fixed? Fix it!

EXERCISE 20-9   Visit customers who call you on the phone. These include employees, patients, suppliers, peers, and others.

EXERCISE 20-10   Make a list of all the information you want employees to have. Schedule meetings with all of them. Give them the information, and leave them with a printed version.

EXERCISE 20-11 Evaluate a sample of your writing using the Gunning Mueller Fog Index in Exhibit 20-5. Evaluate this chapter using the same instrument.

EXHIBIT 20-5
How to Use the Fog Index℠ Scale

In the 1920s, educators began developing readability yardsticks to measure writing complexity. They showed how tabulations of sentence length and specific word use could predict whether readers would understand a written passage. Early readability formulas, however, were too complicated and tedious for practical use.

In 1944, Robert Gunning developed a simple, quick, and reliable way to measure writing complexity, called the Fog Index℠ scale.

The Fog Index℠ score represents the approximate years of schooling needed to comprehend a piece of writing. The higher the Fog Index℠ score, the harder the writing is to read.

FINDING YOUR FOG INDEX℠ SCORE:
Pick a writing sample of a least 100 words, ending with a period. Then, follow these steps:

1. Figure the average number of words per sentence. Treat independent clauses (word groupings within a sentence that could stand alone) as separate sentences. Example: "We studied; we learned; we improved." Such statements should be counted as three sentences, even when commas, semicolons, or dashes are used instead of periods to separate the clauses. Hyphenated words ("twenty-five"), numbers ("25"), and dates ("1994") count as one word. (December 25, 1994 = three words.)

2. Count the words of three syllables or more. Don't count capitalized words, including the first word of each sentence; combinations of short, easy words, like "bookkeeper," "butterfly," or "pawnbroker"; or verbs made into three syllables by adding -ed or -es (such as "created" or "trespasses"). Divide the count by the word length of your writing sample to determine the percentage of long (polysyllabic) words. Example: Sixteen long words in a 130-word sample =12.3%.

3. Add #1 (average sentence length = 14) to #2 (percentage of long words = 12.3). **Total** = 26.3. The Fog Index℠ score equals 26.3 x 0.4 equals 10.52, or 10. (Drop the digits after the decimal point.)

Note: Few readers have more than 17 years of schooling, so any passage above 17 gets a Fog Index℠ score of 17+.

Beware: Don't try to write by this or any formula. Test the complexity of your writing occasionally, using the Fog Index℠ scale on a variety of samples. If your score consistently exceeds 12, you're handicapping your copy—and your readers.

Source: Robert Gunning and Richard A. Kallan. *How to Take the Fog Out of Business Writing*, published by Darnell, 1994. The Fog Index℠ scale is a service mark licensed exclusively to RK Communication Consultants by D. and M. Mueller.

NOTES

1. J. Anderson, "What's Blocking Upward Communication?" *Personnel Administration* (January–February 1968), 5.
2. P. Morgan and H. K. Baker, "Building a Professional Image: Improving Listening Behavior," *Supervisory Management* (November 1985), 34–36; J. A. Griver, "Communication Skills for Getting Ahead," *AORN Journal* (August 1979), 242–249.
3. W. J. Corbett, "The Communication Tools Inherent In Corporate Culture," *Personnel Journal* (April 1986), 71–72, 74.
4. G. S. Wlody, "Communicating In the ICU: Do you Read Me Loud and Clear?" *Nursing Management* (September 1984), 24–27.
5. M. Bice, "Behavior Is the Most Effective Communicator," *Hospitals* (20 October 1990), 78.
6. F. M. Joblin, "Formal Structural Characteristics of Organizations and Superior-Subordinate Communication," *Human Communication Research* (summer 1982), 338–347.
7. M. J. Farley, "Assessing Communication in Organizations," *Journal of Nursing Administration* (December 1989), 27–31.
8. P. S. O'Sullivan, "Detecting Communication Problems," *Nursing Management* (November 1985), 27–30.
9. C. H. Smeltzer, "The Art of Negotiation: An Everyday Experience," *Journal of Nursing Administration* (July–August 1991), 26–30; M. H. Bazerman, J. R. Curhan, D. A. Moore, and K. L. Valley, "Negotiation," *Annual Review of Psychology*, 51, (2000), 279–314.
10. Ibid.
11. P. F. Drucker, *Management: Tasks, Responsibilities Practices* (New York: Harper & Row, 1973), 483.
12. P. Crosby, *Running Things: The Art of Making Things Happen* (New York: NAL-Dutton, 1987).
13. J. Sanchez, G. Byfield, T. T. Brown, K. LaFavor, D. Murphy, and P. Laud, "Perceived Accessibility Versus Actual Physical Accessibility of Healthcare Facilities," *Rehabilitation Nursing* (January–February 2000), 6–9.
14. E. Missik, "Personal Perceptions and Women's Participation in Cardiac Rehabilitation," *Rehabilitation Nursing* (July–August 1999), 158–165.
15. W. D. St. John, "Leveling With Employees," *Personnel Journal* (August 1984), 52–57.
16. H. K. Baker and P. Morgan, "Building a Professional Image: Using 'Feeling-Level' Communication," *Supervisory Management* (January 1986), 20–25
17. G. S. Wlody, op. cit.
18. A. Levenstein, "Feedback Improves Performance," *Nursing Management* (February 1984), 64, 66.
19. A. Levenstein, "Back to Feedback," *Nursing Management* (October 1984), 60–61.

20. Ibid.

21. R. M. Kanter, *When Giants Learn to Dance* (New York: Simon & Schuster, 1989), 108–114.

22. Ibid., 275.

23. P. F. Drucker, op. cit., 487–489.

24. R. Haakenson, "How to Be a Better Listener," *Notes & Quotes* (February 1964), 3.

25. P. Morgan and H. K. Baker, op. cit.

26. L. Sousa, "We Need to Teach Life 101," *San Antonio Express-News* (1 May 1993), 6B; N. J. Foster, "Good Communication Starts with Listening," ncmc@ncmc-mediate.org.

27. J. R. Gibb, "Defensive Communication," *The Journal of Nursing Administration* (April 1982), 14–17.

28. D. E. Shields, "Listening: A Small Investment, A Big Payoff," *Supervisory Management* (July 1984), 18–22.

29. F. Lang, M. R. Floyd, and K. L. Beine, "Clues to Patients' Explanations and Concerns About Their Illnesses: A Call for Active Listening," *Archives of Family Medicine* (March 2000), 222–227.

30. B. A. Schneider, M. Daneman, D. R. Murphy, and S. K. See, "Listening to Discourse in Distracting Settings: The Effects of Aging," *Psychology of Aging* (March 2000), 110–125.

31. N. Stewart, "Listen to the Right People," *Nation's Business* (January 1963), 60–63.

32. J. Guncheon, "To Make People Listen," *Nation's Business* (October 1967), 96–102.

33. J. H. Woods, "Affective Learning: The Door to Critical Thinking," *Holistic Nursing Practitioner* (April 1993), 64–70.

34. T. Peters, *Thriving on Chaos* (New York: Harper & Row, 1981).

35. Ibid.

36. Ibid., 524–532.

37. Ibid.

38. A. V. Irving, "Twenty Strategies to Reduce the Risk of a Malpractice Claim," *Journal of Medical Practice Management* (November–December 1998), 130–133.

39. B. B. Virshup, A. A. Oppenberg, and M. M. Coleman, "Strategic Risk Management: Reducing Malpractice Claims Through More Effective Patient-Doctor Communication," *American Journal of Medical Quality* (July–August 1999), 153–159.

40. N. B. Sigband, "Listen to What You Can't Hear?" *Nation's Business* (June 1969), 70–72.

41. K. H. Bowles, "Patient Problems and Nurse Interventions During Acute Care and Discharge Planning," *Journal of Cardiovascular Nursing* (April 2000), 29–41.

42. M. A. Anderson and L. B. Helms, "Talking about Patients: Communication and Continuity of Care," *Journal of Cardiovascular Nursing* (April 2000), 15–28.

43. R. Davies, "Managing by Listening," *Nation's Business* (September 1992), 1:6.

44. T. Peters, op. cit., 608–613.

45. W. Bennis and B. Nanus, *Leaders: The Strategies for Taking Charge* (New York: Harper & Row, 1985), 14, 33–43, 106–108.

46. Ibid., 366–367.

47. E. D. Nathan, "The Art of Asking Questions," Personnel (July–August 1966), 63–71; M. A. Pulick, "How Well Do You Hear?" *Supervisory Management* (November 1983), 27–31; P. Morgan and H. K. Baker, op. cit.

48. W. D. St. John, "You Are What You Communicate," *Personnel Journal* (October 1985), 40–43; D. Caruth, "Words: A Supervisor's Guide to Communication," *Management Solutions* (June 1986), 34–35.

49. H. P. Zelko, "How to Be a Better Speaker," *Notes & Quotes* (April 1965), 3.

50. R. Wilkinson, "Communication: Listening from the Market," *Nursing Management* (April 1986), 42J, 42L.

51. R. Dulik, "Making Personal Letters Personal," *Supervisory Management* (May 1984), 37–40.

52. C. I. Barnard, *The Functions of the Executive* (Cambridge, MA: Harvard University Press, 1938), 226.

53. S. Tingey, "Six Requirements for a Successful Company Publication," *Personnel Journal* (November 1967), 638–642.

54. E. A. Nalley and J. E. Braithwaite, Jr., "Communication: Key to a Vital Future," *Phi Kappa Phi Newsletter* (June 1992), 1–3.

55. K. L. Gilberg, "Open Communication Provides Key to Good Employee Relations," *Supervision* (April 1993), 8–9.

56. P. A. Strassman and S. Zuboff, "Conversation with Paul A. Strassman," *Organizational Dynamics* (fall 1985), 19–34; A. J. Rutigliano, "Naisbitt & Aburdene On 'Re-Inventing' the Workplace," *Management Review* (October 1985), 33–35.

57. Ibid.

REFERENCES

Auger, B.Y. "How to Run an Effective Meeting." *Commerce* (October 1967).

Collette, C. L. "Understanding Patients' Needs Is the Foundation of Perioperative Nursing." *AORN Journal* (March 2000), 629–630.

Crawford, M. J., and A. S. Kessel. "Not Listening to Patients—the Use and Misuse of Patient Satisfaction Studies." *International Journal of Social Psychiatry* (spring 1999), 1–6.

Davidhizar, R. E., and K. Brownson. "Literacy, Cultural Diversity, and Client Education." *Health Care Management* (September 1999), 39–47.

Finsher, S. "Rework, Revise, Rewrite." *Business* (July–September 1985), 54–55.

Foster, N. J. "Barriers to Everyday Communication." (2000) ncmc@ncmc-mediate.org.

Gelfand, L. I. "Communicate Through Your Supervisors." *Harvard Business Review* (November–December 1970), 101–104.

"Is Anybody Listening?" *Fortune* (September 1950), 77.

Iyengar, S., and A. F. Simon. "New Perspectives and Evidence on Political Communication and Campaign Effects." *Annual Review of Psychology*, 51 (2000), 149–169.

Kennedy, M. M. "Understanding the Demographics of the Evolving Workforce." *Clinical Laboratory Management Review* (September–October 1999), 310–313.

Lynch, E. M. "So You're Going to Run a Meeting." *Personnel Journal* (January 1966), 22+.

Macrae, C. N., and G. V. Bodenhausen. "Social Cognition: Thinking Categorically About Others." *Annual Review of Psychology,* 51 (2000), 93–120.

Patterson, F., E. Ferguson, P. Lane, K. Farrell, J. Martlew, and A. Wells. "A Competency Model for General Practice: Implications for Selection, Training, and Development." *British Journal of General Practice* (March 2000), 188–193.

Peters, T. "Listening to What's Wrong and Right." *San Antonio Light* (20 October 1992), D2.

Severson, M. A., S. J. Leinonen, N. N. Matt-Hensrud, and J. A. Ruegg. "Transcultural Patient Care Committee: Actualizing Concepts and Developing Skills." *Journal of Nursing Staff Development* (July–August 1999), 141–147.

Stevens, R. D., and B. S. Katsekas. "Nursing the Terminally Ill. Being with People in Difficult Times." *Home Healthcare Nursing* (August 1999), 504–510.

CHAPTER 21

eNursing

Richard J. Swansburg, RN, BSN, MSCIS

LEARNING OBJECTIVES AND ACTIVITIES

- Record a synopsis of what your electronic information environment is like today, and try to envision what you believe it will be like in 5 years.
- Differentiate between the various types of networks.
- Illustrate uses for applications software.
- Identify and discuss the purposes of various information systems.
- Develop a confidentiality and security plan.

CONCEPTS: Confidentiality, data, database, information, Internet, intranet, multimedia, network, security, spreadsheet, technology, word processing.

MANAGER BEHAVIOR: Advocates and supports the computer technology that impacts nursing operations.

LEADER BEHAVIOR: Plans, develops, and evaluates information technology that improves nursing operations, including management, education, research, and clinical practice. Does so with input from representative nurses.

Introduction

The changes that have occurred in computers and information technology since 1982 are amazing. In fact, the changes over the past 5 years seem almost unbelievable. We are now beyond the year 2000, and computers are a common part of life. Computers are in automobiles, home appliances, and home electronics. Personal computers are in the home, with access to the Internet. Automatic teller machines, debit cards, and electronic banking are now the norm for dealing with money. Retail services are driven by electronic inventory and point-of-sale systems. Computers and information systems in the workplace are a fact of life.

In 1999, Rutsky wrote[1]:

Today, we are often told, we live not simply in an age of information, but in an age of excessive information. The amount and availability of information seem to be increasing at an exponential rate. We feel that our entire world is moving, changing, mutating, at an accelerated pace. Our interactions with this world of information seem plagued by an increasing sense that we cannot keep up, can't take it all in, that we are being overwhelmed by information, deluged by data: the sense of an "information overload."

This fear of information and other computer phobias are barriers that we cannot accept. The challenge of advocating and using new technology will be critical for the management of health care in constant transition.

> "As the business world changes at an ever-increasing rate, many of us are finding that our jobs require us to constantly enhance our skills and develop new ones—possibly some we never thought we'd need. Today, staying in place means falling behind, and no one can afford to do that in our technology-driven world."[2]

Nurses will have to assimilate the knowledge and expertise required to understand and interact with this constantly changing technology, and then they must be capable of teaching this new knowledge and expertise to others.

Future computer communication will focus on a more simplistic user interface. This user interface will be built around the use of multimedia that interacts with the user through sight, sound and voice; that evolves based on patterns of use; and that seamlessly integrates all the tools, technologies, and information that may be located in geographically distributed and often highly differentiated hardware and software environments. The issue of location has already become somewhat irrelevant with the advent of a global network we call the Internet.

Ethical and legal issues will need to be advanced in scope to address new and changing technology. Concepts of privacy, confidentiality, and security should be instilled in nursing personnel not only in terms of operational guidelines (data and physical security, policies, and procedures) but also in terms of professionalism and responsibility. Control of information needs to be taught as a management issue, not a technical one.

Historical Perspective

The history of the computer began in 1642. Blaise Pascal created a calculating device that could add or subtract with the turning of little wheels. In 1834, Charles Babbage theorized a new machine he called the analytical engine, which was to be programmable and have the ability to calculate and store results. Even though this machine was never built, Lady Augusta Ada Loveless created a set of instructions for it in 1842. She is credited with being the first computer programmer.

Herman Hollerith developed the first electronic computing device in the 1880s. This machine was used to calculate the U.S. census in 1890. The results of the census were completed in 6 weeks, compared with 7 weeks for the census of 1880. In 1909, the electronics world was changed with the development of the vacuum tube by Lee deForest. The term *computer bug* was coined in 1945 when a moth flew into a computer at the Naval Weapons Center. The first electronic computer was developed at the University of Pennsylvania in 1946. It was called the ENIAC (Electronic Numerical Integrator and Computer).

In 1947, John Bardeen, Walter Brattain, and William Shockley achieved a second electronic milestone with the discovery of the transistor. The next monumental change in electronics occurred in 1959, with the creation of the integrated circuit by Jack Kilby and Robert Noyce. The transistor and integrated circuit have reduced the size of computing hardware exponentially. The integrated circuit is the building block of today's computers.

In 1962, John Licklider introduced the idea of a global network. He thought of accessing data from anywhere on a set of globally connected computers. In 1968, the precursor to the Internet appears in the form of ARPANET (Advanced Research Projects Agency Network). In 1971, Ray Tomlinson sent the first electronic message. In 1973, Vinton Cerf and Bob Kahn developed the Transmission Control Protocol (TCP). The debut of the first personal computer (PC) occurred in 1974 in the form of the Altair 8800. In 1980, Tim Berners-Lee created HyperText Markup Language (HTML). In 1981, Xerox pioneered the use of the mouse and graphical user interface (GUI). In 1983, the Department of Defense coined the term Internet; TCP is adopted as the standard protocol, changing it in effect to TCP/IP (Internet Protocol). In 1991, the University of Minnesota develops Gopher, the first browser for surfing the Internet. Finally, in 1993, Dave Thompson and Marc Andreesen introduce the graphical Web browser of today.

Current Information Technology

Today's information technology environment puts us into a period of major transition. The advancement of new technology can be overwhelming. A critical challenge is to prove that this technology will provide for the efficient delivery of quality health care while reducing its cost. A whole new generation of manpower views information technology as a normal part of their lives. They have a different sense of reality that works to the advantage of acquiring, implementing, and using newer technology. Overall, there is a new view that health care does not lag that far behind other industries in the use of emerging technology.

> Looking at the use of technology today, we begin to realize that we are on a boundary between the efficient use of today's knowledge and the desire to implement tomorrow's technology.

There is an incredible amount of new technology in the world today that many of us are not using yet. Instead, we are concentrating on finding solutions to some of the older challenges[3]:

- Moving information between multiple locations and entities
- Sharing this information in real time
- Developing real, effective automated scheduling systems
- Building a totally electronic medical record
- Using Internet-based technologies for professional enhancement and patient care improvement
- Integrating disparate systems
- Working toward a paperless delivery system.

Implementing these solutions is considered a long-range project. The organization must develop and put into practice a business plan for tying the technology together. Doing so often requires re-engineering of the organization, with huge changes needing to be made to its infrastructure and work flow processes. Many organizations are looking for a single vendor to deliver and support turnkey enterprise information technology systems. Unfortunately, mature solutions are not widely implemented, and choice of a vendor results from less than a handful of viable candidates.

Today's technology starts with what is termed *legacy* systems, which are text-based information systems that reside on mini and mainframe computers. These systems continue to be integral due to the inheritance of their historical information and because they provide for the most rapid delivery of information to thousands of concurrent users. Quite often the one true legacy system is the corporate or organizational information system that is used by everyone. There are also secondary information systems, which are specialized departmental information systems relevant to the area in which we work. Then there is applications software that is available for personal and group productivity, including communications, database management, word processing, spread sheets, and personal information management. Finally, we have to include access to the Internet.

All these dissimilar systems usually reside at different locations on different hardware and software platforms. Local area networks (LANs) and wide area networks (WANs) provide connections to access these systems. The standard for a LAN connection is 10- or 100-megabit ethernet running over copper wiring, and the standard for a WAN connection is a T1 data line leased from the local telephone provider. Some organizations have implemented mobile computing. In this environment, health care professionals are issued notebook computers that use wireless radio technology to access the network, allowing end users to take their computers and move about the facility while staying connected to the systems they need.

The newest technology is moving toward the use of interactive multimedia. The user interacts with text, voice, music, images, animation, and video. Two areas of importance budding with this technology include education and telemedicine. Multimedia education material is being developed for patients and health care practitioners alike. Virtual reality is being implemented to simulate medical environments for illustration and training purposes. Telemedicine brings the patient and health care practitioner face to face, regardless of their geographical locations.

Future Information Technology Trends

The future of information technology begins with the resolution of two of today's most pressing problems,

communications bandwidth and the integration of systems. *Bandwidth* refers to the amount of data or information that can be moved across a particular communications media over a given period of time.[4] Optical fiber is currently the material of choice to solve our immediate needs for increased bandwidth. The seamless integration of systems is coming about with the incorporation of the Internet into all of today's emerging technologies.

What we can imagine though, is a wireless world where everything and everyone is connected to a network that is "always on, always there." Objects are alive with intelligence and technologies evolve to change the form of everyday things.[5] Real streaming audio and video will be the norm for the integration of the health care environment. All parties will be connected: patients, doctors, nurses, health care organizations, and so on. Even intelligent equipment will be involved to monitor, make recommendations, and possibly take action. Everything will become part of the electronic medical record.

Simulation, virtual reality, and robotics will become common tools to assist us in performing beyond our current limitations. A wearable computer will be the means for managing all interaction, most likely incorporated into protective eyewear. A video screen will become part of the lens, or a projector will generate holographic images. A microphone will capture speech as well as all other audio input. Speakers will play for us whatever sound requested. An alternative to a wearable computer would be the merging of computer technology directly into our biological processes.

The next big technological revolution is predicted to occur between 2010 and 2020. Assertions from Gordon Moore and Ray Kurzweil support this. Moore declared that integrated circuits were doubling their capacity every 18 to 24 months. This predicts that transistors will be so small around 2010 that they will be incapable of functioning reliably. New advances in technologies will have to be achieved. Kurzweil believes that as evolution proceeds, the period between advances becomes shorter, and the benefits from prior developments interact, causing the rate of progress to accelerate further.[6] New technologies that could exponentially increase the power of computing are now on the foreseeable horizon.

The progress of information technology will improve the quality of life for most of us. Work will become more enjoyable as machines perform some of the manual labor and assist us in the decision support process as well. There will be a price, though, as low-skilled and middle management positions are lost. Personnel will have to constantly upgrade their skills in what will become a lifelong process. Organizations will compete for the more effective, higher skilled workers. These workers will also be in a more favorable position to demand higher salaries and better working conditions.

Computer Networking

Computers alone are potent tools, but they are even more influential when joined as a network. A network can be a mini or mainframe computer with dumb terminals attached to it, or two personal computers connected in your home, or all the computing devices in the world attached to the Internet. Networks are the infrastructure of today's world of electronic technology. They are the conduits by which we use computers to transfer information from one location to another. Networks include a number of components such as client and server computers, client and server network software, network protocols, network adapters, physical transport media, hubs, switches, bridges, routers, and other analog and digital data transmission equipment.

Two standards form the basis for today's networking. They are the establishment of the 802 project by the Institute of Electrical and Electronics Engineers (IEEE) and the adoption of the Open Systems Interconnect (OSI) model by the International Organization for Standardization (ISO). The IEEE 802 project provides standards for the implementation of various network topologies. The OSI model provides a common point of reference for describing the communications process across these networks. Exhibit 21-1 presents the IEEE 802 standards, and Exhibit 21-2 presents the OSI model.

In any discussion of computer networking, two issues need to be explored and understood: the physical representation and implementation of the network, and the logical use of the physical network. Here is an example to help us comprehend the gist of this. Let us say that you work in a hospital where the operating room and labor and delivery are on the same floor. These departments have separate client-server information systems, with a departmental server for each. All of the computers are attached using copper wiring to a hub in a centralized wiring closet. Refer to Exhibit 21-3 as this example is discussed further.

Physically, there could be one network, and logically there could also be one network. However, we are going to divide these computers into two work groups or domains. We can associate the client computers LD1 and LD2 along with the server computer LDSRV as being in the domain LD. Likewise we can associate the client computers OR1 and OR2 along with the server computer ORSRV as being in the domain OR. Clients in either of the domains can be totally unaware that the other domain exists, even though they are both passing

EXHIBIT 21-1

The Institute of Electrical and Electronics Engineers 802 Standards

STANDARD	DESCRIPTION
802.1	Higher-level interface
802.2	Logical link control
802.3	Ethernet
802.4	Token-bus
802.5	Token-ring
802.6	Metropolitan area network
802.7	Broadband
802.8	Fiberoptic
802.9	Integrated services local area network
802.10	Interoperable local area network security
802.11	Wireless local area network
802.12	Demand priority
802.14	Cable-TV-based broadband communication network
802.15	Wireless personal area network
802.16	Broadband wireless access

EXHIBIT 21-2

The Open System Interconnect Model

NO.	LAYER	USAGE
7	Application	Provide application services
6	Presentation	Adapt the data to suit the receiver
5	Session	Set up and maintain a communication session
4	Transport	Transport data between two programs
3	Network	Transport data across a network
2	Link	Transport data across a link
1	Physical	Convert data to elecricity, light, radio

their information on the same physical network. These issues will be expanded on as other topics are discussed in this section.

Local and Wide Area Networks

For all practical purposes, computer network technology can be broken down into two main types, LANs and WANs. A LAN is a network of computers considered to be local to each other, with local meaning that all of the computers are within the same room or building. A WAN is a network of two or more groups of computers

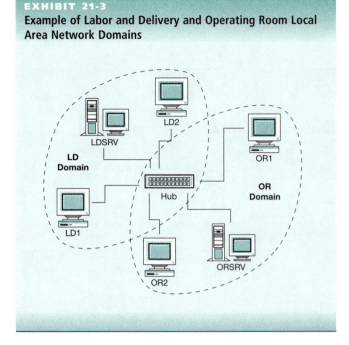

EXHIBIT 21-3

Example of Labor and Delivery and Operating Room Local Area Network Domains

or computing devices that are remote from each other and connected by telecommunications equipment.

When dealing with networks a number of issues need to be addressed, including design, implementation, and management. Depending on the size and needs of the organization, these tasks can range from very simple to extremely complex. Another variable that affects these issues is the willingness of the organization to spend money. Quite often an organization will make a conscience choice to use inferior products and a lower speed network, only to find out that the installed network fails in its purpose.

Planning for the future is necessary when designing a LAN. The possibilities of technologic changes and expansion of the network must be considered. Probably the most important area to concentrate on in the design process is the cabling strategy. A wireless network could be implemented. This would provide for the ultimate in end-user convenience and mobility. Unfortunately, at present, wireless networks have limited bandwidth. Wireless networks appear to be the direction of the future, and thus, wireless bandwidth should improve. Otherwise, a cabling strategy should be promoted that provides for maximum bandwidth, up to currently available gigabit ethernet.

The wiring closet that contains the hubs and switches should be centrally located within the LAN area. Cable lengths between the attached computers and the wiring closet should be minimized. In larger organizations, there should be separate wiring closets for departments with a large number of users, or build-

ings with more than one floor. These wiring closets would all be connected by what is called a backbone LAN. This backbone LAN would also support connections for server computers, routers, and telecommunications equipment. The routers and telecommunications equipment provide WAN access to other organizational sites and the Internet. An example of what a university WAN with a campus and two remote hospital sites might look like is shown in Exhibit 21-4.

Implementation of our network builds on our design. The infrastructure is put in place, and client PCs and servers are attached using network interface cards (NIC). All computers that participate on the network, clients, and servers, must have network software installed to manage the communication between them. For the servers, such network operating systems (NOS) include Microsoft Windows NT, Novell Intranetware, and UNIX. This communication process starts with some type of authentication procedure in which the client is required to login. Once the client has been authenticated, LAN resources are made available based on security policies. These resources typically include shared disk space, software, and printers.

Network management begins before the first client is attached to the network and becomes an ongoing process. Numerous personnel are involved in the practice of network management. Network staff are involved in the installation, configuration, and support of computers, cables, hubs, switches, routers, and telecommunications equipment. Troubleshooting a network problem may require expensive equipment and can be tedious and time-consuming. Routine monitoring should also be done to evaluate capacity and performance and if necessary tune the network. Finally, continuing network administration related to server and user management must be done. Server administration includes the maintenance of shared resources and the daily backup of data. User administration includes the maintenance of client identifications (IDs) and the security relationships between them and shared resources.

Intranets, Extranets, and Virtual Private Networks

Intranets, extranets, and virtual private networks (VPNs) are considered to be private organizational networks that use Internet–World Wide Web technologies for the distribution of information. An organization designs an intranet for internal use by its employees. An organization extends its intranet out onto the Internet as an extranet. This provides for external use of the organization's information and applications by authorized customers, suppliers, and off-site personnel. An organization implements a VPN to provide remote employees secure

EXHIBIT 21-4
Example of a University Wide Area Network

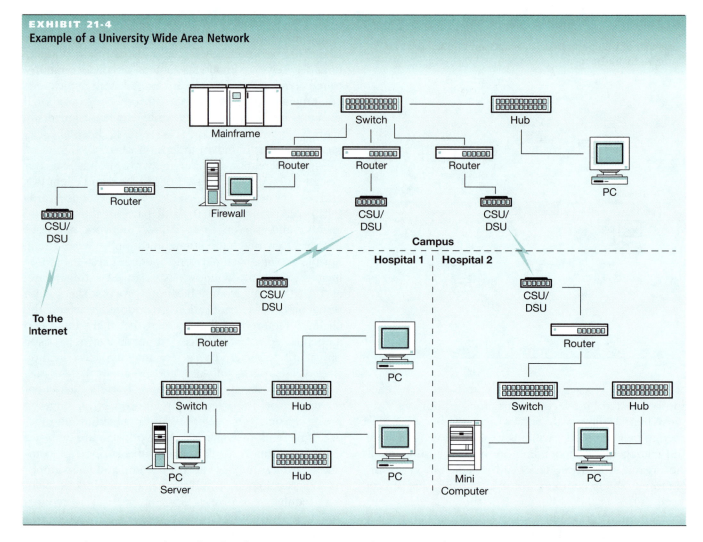

access to their intranet through a local Internet service provider (ISP).

An intranet is fast becoming the standard for integrating organizational data contained in multiple systems. An intranet provides for a simple, consistent interface to information and applications that are easily accessible using any of a number of inexpensive or free Web browsers. A single site or portal can be developed and maintained that provides for centralized access by all parties, in health care, this means doctors, nurses, patients, vendors, and so on. This strategy has the potential to reduce errors and improve the quality of care because information can be kept more current and accurate. Patients and health care providers will be looking at the same information, allowing for direct patient input into care.

An extranet will extend an organization's information beyond its solid boundaries and provide for access from the furthest reaches of the globe. Clinical caregivers will have access to information from patient homes, their own homes, while at off-site education

classes or conferences, and—yes—even while on vacation. Vendors, insurers, and regulating agencies will have a common gateway for obtaining information from and providing information to the health care organization.

A VPN provides the organization with economic and flexible remote access, with the inclusion of a stronger degree of security. Special software can be required on the PC of the client who needs to connect to the intranet of the organization. This software interacts with software on the intranet of the organization to manage authentication and encryption. There are questions to ask before buying or creating a VPN[7]:

- How many people need remote access, and who are they?
- Which hardware, software, and administration costs are involved in a dedicated remote access server?
- Which other long-distance and telecommunications costs are in the mix?
- Which types of additional security does the organization need when using the Internet?

The Internet

What is the Internet? Basically, the Internet is a globally implemented WAN. The Internet is a network of tens of millions of computers connected by the same TCP/IP protocol. Using routers and domain name servers (DNS), the Internet provides us with the capability to communicate with any one of these computers. Add to this the integration of Web browsing technology, open database connectivity and real-time multimedia, and a simple point-and-click environment is created that provides for more interactive and enhanced communications.

Coile wrote[8]:

The arrival of the Internet offers the opportunity to fundamentally reinvent medicine and health care delivery. The "e-health" era is nothing less than the digital transformation of the practice of medicine, as well as the business side of the health industry. The Internet is the next frontier of health care. Internet technology may rank with antibiotics, genetics, and computers as among the most important changes for medical care delivery. Utilizing e-health strategies will expand exponentially in the next five years, as America's health care executives shift to applying IS/IT to the fundamental business and clinical processes of the health care enterprise.

The Internet is already changing the practice of health care and the way professionals interact with patients and other providers. Patient care is being redefined as patients flock to the Internet seeking more information with which to provide greater input into their care. Many websites have been and are being created to supply information and services to patients and their providers. Nurses and physicians are becoming involved by creating their own websites, or they are going to work as advisors to online health care companies. They are assisting in the design of website content and providing information and consultation by answering questions. Health care providers are starting to provide medical treatment over the Internet, which is leading to legal, regulatory, and privacy issues in this new setting.

Certainly, the first step toward this new health care venue is the implementation of electronic medical records. Data and information that can be captured and maintained electronically provide for easier access and faster communication. The logical extension of this information onto the Internet via a private extranet has the potential to improve quality of care and patient and provider satisfaction. Patients can access the Internet from home and complete electronic forms for medical and social histories, lists of allergies and medications, and insurance and payment options. This can be done before a doctor's visit or admission to the hospital. Even after an encounter, patients would be able to review information for accuracy and changes. Doctors and nurses also would have access to this information anytime, anywhere.

The next step in virtual health care proposes to use the Internet to provide all the services of a doctor's visit except that of the physical examination. This lack of touch does bother some patients' rights advocates and the American Medical Association (AMA).[9] The question that begs to be asked, though, is whether this a step in the right direction? Obviously, this change is more significant in the delivery of health care to rural or remote populations where providers are not available. Through the use of computers and multimedia, patients can be evaluated and treated for minor illnesses and injuries. With the addition of emergency medical technicians or advanced practice nurses and diagnostic medical equipment, the treatment of major medical problems becomes more of a reality.

Today, nurses and physicians are already using the Internet for consultation, research, and decision support. Consultation is a normal part of health care delivery. In the past, consultation was done in person or over the telephone, but now with the Internet, it can be done from anywhere. Today, nurses are searching online literature to obtain the most current nursing research about disease processes that are rare or misinterpreted. They are visiting chat rooms and newsgroups to ask questions and seek reassurance and support in their delivery of nursing care. Physicians are using "evidence-based medicine" to access the most recent medical research and practice guidelines. They are using video conferencing at the point of care to consult with peers concerning their evaluation of diagnoses and treatments. Together, nurses and physicians are using all available resources to improve their decision support process. Hopefully, the end result will be that the Internet provides for more timely, accurate information that will reduce errors, improve the quality of care, and decrease costs.

The Internet also is opening up the area of education. The Internet is the ideal vehicle for the delivery of full multimedia instruction on demand. Not only can the patient education process be dealt with, but health care providers also can work toward their continuing or higher education. Internet sites exist that deal specifically with AIDS, diabetes, gerontology, hepatitis, nutrition, oncology, renal disease, wellness, and other health-related topics. These websites provide various degrees of information and education based on ownership and purpose. The primary issue surrounding the use of public websites relates to the quality of information that is provided. Currently, no standards exist for the publication of information unless the site is controlled by a governing organization, for example the

AMA or the Center for Disease Control and Prevention. Private provider extranets can be customized to meet the specific needs of patient populations.

The Internet has made a major impact on continuing education for nurses. Do a search on the Internet and see what results you get. For example, use the search phrase "Alabama continuing education." Literally thousands of courses are being offered by schools, organizations, publications, vendors, and independent educators. The process is as simple as can be. You should start by visiting your state board of nursing website and obtain a list of approved continuing education providers. The board's site may even provide you with a list of providers that have websites. Next, visit the educational provider's website and register with it. This may be as simple as providing your name, address, and telephone number. At this point the process is: register for a course, pay the fee, complete the course requirements, and print your certificate.

Higher education for nursing is also available over the Internet; however, the process does not appear to be as simple as is obtaining continuing education. The reasons being that the admission process does not guarantee acceptance and there may be requirements that cannot be met over the Internet.

Online learning provides up-to-date knowledge in a convenient environment.

At this point, we hope that health care businesses are starting to reengineer their information technology and that strategy is focusing on Internet/extranet/intranet development. There are far too many business aspects of the health care industry that involve information communication between two or more parties. Patient care and education currently are being addressed, what about billing, marketing and human resources, and purchasing, to name a few. The electronic transfer of bills and payments between providers and payers has been taking place for a number of years. Extranets are just now starting to be created that allow providers to check on the status of claims and payers to audit patient care records. What about the consumer? When patients receive bills, it would be convenient for them to be able to connect to the provider and payer's extranets, determine if there is a problem, determine where the problem lies, and communicate on the issues right then.

Marketing is a part of the health care business environment. Organizations market their facilities, products, and services to patients and health care providers. Wouldn't making the organization visible on the Internet seem to make good sense? Organizations can actively recruit patients who are seeking particular services and an openness of information communication.

Organizations can post openings and needs for professional caregivers. Professionals can submit online résumés and communicate with HR personnel directly. What about organizational employees? Shouldn't they be able to access their personnel records to obtain information about education and credentialing, vacation and sick time, and even insurance and retirement benefits?

How about the sale of health care supplies and appliances? Providers should be able to connect to vendors online and order supplies. There could actually be a dynamic inventory system that tracks usage and performs reordering using the Internet. Providers could request bids for products, and vendors could submit responses. Patients could connect to the providers or possibly the vendors directly and purchase their needed supplies and appliances. It is all about cost, convenience, efficiency, and service.

Finally, through all of this, the primary issues of privacy and security must not be overlooked. Today, loss of personal privacy ranks as one of the top concerns of most people. The federal government in 1996 passed the Health Insurance Portability and Accountability Act (HIPAA). This act provided for an initial three-year period to pass legislation that would regulate the health care industry's management of patient records. "The goal is not to inappropriately restrict access, but to restrict inappropriate access."[10] The best ways to deal with the issues of privacy and security will be discussed in greater detail subsequently.

General-Purpose Applications Software

Today's nursing management should be prepared to support the increasing use of information technology in all areas of nursing. Part of this support includes a fundamental degree of computer literacy and the acceptance of the microcomputer as a professional work tool. Many nurses use microcomputers in the performance of their daily duties in areas such as patient care documentation, budgeting, policy and procedure documentation, personnel records, patient and staff education, scheduling, and research and inventory management. Some of the general-purpose applications available for nurses include communications, database management, spread sheets, word processing and publication, personal information management, graphic editing and presentation, and Internet browsers.

A number of office suites exist that integrate these applications into a single bundle. Integrated suites provide the easy ability to share information between applications. For example, spread sheets, database information, and graphics can be inserted directly into word-processed documents such as memos, letters, and reports. When the numbers in a spread sheet are changed or the information in a database is changed, the corresponding information in the memo or report is automatically updated. In addition, all the applications can provide a shared look and feel, with similar menus, toolbars, and keyboard shortcuts. These applications also can incorporate a common macro, scripting, or programming language that allows repetitive and complex tasks to be automated.

Communications

Communications software provides the foundation for accessing other computers. Such access may be in a dedicated manner (the link is maintained even when not in use) or a nondedicated manner (the link is maintained only while being used). Dedicated links tend to be business related, with direct access to the organization's information resources through a LAN connection. Nondedicated links tend to be related to the home or small business, with the need for intermittent access to remote information resources. With the coming of the Internet and digital communications services (such as integrated services digital network [ISDN], digital subscriber line [DSL], and cable modem), dedicated links are becoming the standard, even in homes.

The communications software to support LAN attachments (local and remote) is generally taken for granted. This is because, quite often, the software is provided as part of the operating system installed on microcomputers. In fact, most of the time when a new microcomputer is purchased, the required communications hardware (LAN adapter or modem) is supplied with it. The only outstanding issue revolves around the need for assistance in its setup and configuration. At work there is a dedicated LAN connection; a microcomputer, modem, and remote access software at home can be used to dial into a remote access server and perform computer-related functions as if actually at work.

There still tends to be a need for additional communications software. Quite often there is need for the capability to access IBM mainframes and minicomputers, UNIX systems, and the Internet for information display and print purposes. Internet communications are usually accomplished through the use of free Web browsers such as Microsoft's Internet Explorer and Netscape's Communicator. To access IBM mainframes, 3270 emulation is required; to access IBM AS400s, 5250 emulation is required. To access UNIX systems as well as other ASCII-based mini- and microcomputers, some form of Digital Equipment Corporation (DEC) video terminal emulation is required. All of these terminal emulators are provided by a number of vendors as integrated packages. The particular package usually is standardized by the organization.

Other communications needs may include support of the end user and to move information in the form of a file transfer. When a nurse manager is contacted about a problem by a staff nurse, the nurse manager can access the system and mirror what the staff member is doing. This is also the way a vendor could provide assistance when called about a systems problem. File transfers are becoming a common part of everyday computer usage. Files are transferred over the Internet, over a LAN, to and from host systems (mainframe and minicomputer), and even to computers at home.

Database Management

A computer database is the electronic counterpart to the standard file cabinet and its contents. The database is used to store data and can be manipulated for information much as are paper files. A microcomputer and database management system (DBMS) can be used in place of a manual filing system to handle many information and record-keeping needs. Examples would include personnel records, education records, budget management, and equipment inventory.

A DBMS allows for databases to be constructed by the creation of tables. A *table* is a collection of records composed of data fields that have a common layout. When a data field is defined, its length is set and the type of data that can be stored in it established. Data types can be character or text (allowing letters, numbers, and special symbols), numeric (allowing only numbers), logical (allowing only yes or no, true or false), or date–time (allowing only numbers in a date and time format). (Exhibit 21-5 is an example of an employee table definition.)

Once a table is created, forms or screens can be established to add, modify, or delete information (see Exhibit 21-6 for a sample of a database screen). Queries can be established to display the information in various formats or order. Reports can be established to display the information on paper, transparencies, and labels. (See Exhibit 21-7 for an example of a database report.) Menus with procedures can be created to allow easy access to and execution of these forms, queries, and reports (see Exhibit 21-8 for a sample of a database menu). Advantages to database management are ease in maintaining information, timely retrieval of information, and concurrent access of this information by individuals from different locations.

Spread Sheet

A spread sheet is a tool used to record and manipulate numbers. The original model for the spread sheet was the paper ledger used for business accounting such as

EXHIBIT 21-5
Example of an Employee Table Definition

Database: Nursing.MDB
Table: Employee
Date: Thursday, June 22, 2000

PROPERTIES

Date Created:	6/22/2000 10:25:20	GUID:	Long binary data
Last Updated:	6/22/2000 10:50:08	Name Map:	Long binary data
Order By On:	False	Orientation:	0
Record Count:	0	Updateable:	True

COLUMNS

NAME	TYPE	SIZE	DESCRIPTION
Emp name	Text	30	Employee name. Required, indexed (duplicates OK).
Emp SSN	Text	9	Employee SSN. Required, indexed (no duplicates), primary key. Input mask 000\-00\-0000;;_.
Emp job code	Text	1	Employee job code.
Emp assignment number	Text	3	Employee assignment number.
Emp position number	Text	6	Employee position number. Required.
Emp class code	Text	4	Employee class code.
Emp class title	Text	50	Employee class title.
Emp job status	Text	2	Employee job status.
Emp hire date	Date/Time	8	Employee hire date. Input mask 99/99/0000;0;_.
Emp termination date	Date/Time	8	Employee termination date. Input mask 99/99/0000;0;_.
Emp pay ID	Text	1	Employee pay ID.
Emp license number	Text	20	Employee license number.
Emp license renewal number	Text	20	Employee license renewal number.
Emp license date	Date/Time	8	Employee license date. Input mask 99/99/0000;0;_.
Emp license expiration	Date/Time	8	Employee license expiration date. Input mask 99/99/0000;0;_.
Emp liability insurance	Yes/No	1	Employee liability insurance.
Emp unit	Text	20	Employee unit.
Emp shift	Text	20	Employee shift.
Emp address 1	Text	30	Employee address 1.
Emp address 2	Text	30	Employee address 2.
Emp city	Text	20	Employee city.
Emp state	Text	2	Employee state.
Emp zip	Text	9	Employee zip. Input mask 00000\-9999;;_.
Emp phone	Text	10	Employee phone. Input mask !\(999") "000\-0000;;_.

TABLE INDEXES

NAME	NUMBER OF FIELDS	ORDER
Emp Name	1	Ascending
Emp SSN	1	Ascending
Primary Key	1	Ascending

UNDER PERMISSIONS

Admin   Delete, Read Permissions, Set Permissions, Change Owner, Read Definition, Write Definition, Read Data, Insert Data, Update Data, Delete Data

GROUP PERMISSIONS

Admins   Delete, Read Permissions, Set Permissions, Change Owner, Read Definition, Write Definition, Read Data, Insert Data, Update Data, Delete Data

Users   Delete, Read Permissions, Set Permissions, Change Owner, Read Definition, Write Definition, Read Data, Insert Data, Update Data, Delete Data

EXHIBIT 21-6
Example of a Database Screen

Employee			
Name:	Swansburg, Richard J.	License number:	1-123456
SSN:	123-45-6789	License renewal number:	
Job code:	1	License date:	1/1/1999
Assignment number:	321	License expiration:	12/31/2000
Position number:	98765	Liability insurance:	✓
Class code:	234	Address:	102 Sandy Ridge Road
Class title:	Registered Nurse		
Job status:	E	City:	Mobile
Hire date:	6/4/1979	State:	AL
Termination date:		Zip:	36608-9012
Pay ID:	P	Phone:	(334) 649-1234
Unit:	MICU		
Shift:	Nights		

Record: |◄ ◄ 1 ► ►| ►* of 1

EXHIBIT 21-7
Example of a Database Report

EMPLOYEE LISTING MICU

EMPLOYEE NAME	POSITION	TITLE	HIRE DATE	LICENSE	INSURANCE	PHONE
Adams, Judy M.	97531	RN	7/1/1994	1-468248	Yes	334-434-3557
Armstrong, Sabrina T.	85477	US	3/23/1988		No	601-631-3357
Conner, Rebecca A.	85547	US	6/1/1992		No	334-343-1656
Dawson, John B.	96656	RN	6/15/1998	1-575112	Yes	334-457-9888
Gooden, Amanda W.	84544	US	10/21/1991		No	334-434-5129
Grimes, Sharon N.	91154	RN	6/3/1986	1-223556	Yes	601-631-5451
Hodges, Charles S.	97551	RN	7/10/1982	1-155454	No	334-633-6117
Hooker, Mary Beth	81144	US	8/7/1976		No	334-457-5721
Inge, Janice M.	84198	US	7/10/1982		No	334-434-5199
Johnson, Mary B.	97751	RN	6/6/1972	1-011959	Yes	334-633-7413
Jones, Sandra P.	97494	RN	9/12/1988	1-299114	Yes	334-457-8745
Morris, Barbara R.	97691	RN	6/9/1999	1-591344	Yes	334-633-2424
Nearly, Susan O.	95775	RN	1/15/1997	1-529911	No	334-457-8711
Parker, Frank C.	98511	RN	11/11/1991	1-300551	Yes	601-632-4685
Reynolds, Sara C.	94417	RN	5/27/1991	1-299911	Yes	334-457-9577
Swansburg, Richard J.	98765	RN	6/4/1979	1-123456	Yes	334-649-1234
Williams, Gesina S.	91554	RN	6/8/1995	1-449521	Yes	334-633-7124

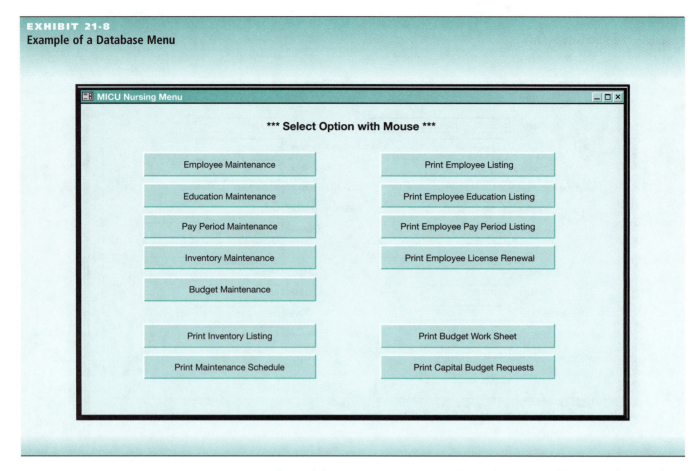

the recording of debits and credits. With the coming of the microcomputer, electronic spread sheets were developed. An electronic spread sheet is a piece of software that turns a microcomputer into a highly sophisticated calculator. Huge quantities of numbers can be recorded, manipulated, and stored quite simply and easily. Nurses can use the information from spread sheets to maintain statistics, create graphics, and plan budgets. (See Exhibits 21-9, 21-10, and 21-11.)

A spread sheet is made up of columns and rows of memory cells. These cells can be varied in size to allow for small or very large numbers. In addition to storing numbers, cells can store text and formulas. Text is used for titles, column and row headers, comments, and instructions. Formulas are used to perform the actual mathematical manipulation (addition, subtraction, multiplication, and division) of memory cells and their numbers. Formulas even provide for special financial, math, and statistical functions such as averages and standard deviations. Formulas are what really make a spread sheet a powerful number-crunching tool. Another important spread sheet capability is graphing, which allows numbers to be displayed in a visually illustrative form. (Exhibits 21-12 and 21-13 are examples of bar and line graphs, respectively.)

Spread sheets are the best tool to use in situations that require the management of a lot of numbers. For this reason, they lend themselves particularly well to financial management, where they speed up processes such as budgeting, forecasting, and developing tables and schedules.

Word Processing and Desktop Publishing

Word processing is the manipulation of words and special characters to produce a printed document. *Desktop publishing* is the manipulation of text and graphics to produce documents of publication quality. Five years ago, the difference between the two was vast. Today, each has incorporated aspects of the other. Among the documents that each can produce are memorandums and letters, policies and procedures, resumes, forms, envelopes and labels, instruction sheets, manuals, posters and signs, books, and newsletters. (Exhibits 21-14 to 21-16 show a few examples.)

Word processing and desktop publishing applications have facilities for the management of multiple document styles. Styles contain formatting codes that are grouped under a single structure. When applied to a section of text or an entire document, they can save

EXHIBIT 21-9
Statistics for New Hires and Terminations

NURSING ORIENTATION STATISTICS

	JAN	FEB	MAR	APR	MAY	JUN	JUL	AUG	SEP	OCT	NOV	DEC	TOTAL
HIRES													
RNs	10	6	8	5	7	27	11	8	13	3	3	5	106
LPNs	3	3	6	1	2	11	5	2	7	4	2	1	47
USs	0	0	0	0	2	1	0	0	2	0	1	0	6
NAs	1	0	0	3	0	2	0	1	1	1	1	0	10
TERMINATIONS													
RNs	11	4	10	6	3	17	8	11	9	5	1	5	86
LPNs	2	5	4	1	3	8	3	5	3	5	1	1	41
USs	0	0	0	1	1	1	0	0	2	0	1	0	6
NAs	1	0	0	2	0	2	0	1	1	1	1	0	10

EXHIBIT 21-10
Pie Graph of New Hires

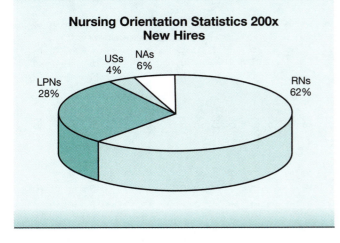

Nursing Orientation Statistics 200x New Hires

- USs 4%
- NAs 6%
- LPNs 28%
- RNs 62%

time and ensure consistency. A library of styles can be created and used among different documents. Styles can establish the following[11]:

- Font type, size, and style, such as **Arial 10-point normal**, *Times New Roman 12-point italic*, and `Letter Gothic 14-point bold`.
- Spacing between lines and paragraphs.
- Margins, tabs, and text alignment.
- Page headers and footers.
- Numbering and outline formats.
- Form size, type, and orientation.

Other tools that are often included in these programs are a spellchecker, a thesaurus, and a grammar checker. The speller contains a dictionary to which the text can be compared. Words not in the program's dictionary can be added to a supplement. When the dictionary is invoked, words that it does not recognize are highlighted. A list of alternative words is generated, along with options to replace, edit, or add a word to the supplement. The thesaurus generates a list of synonyms and antonyms that can be used in place of selected words. The grammar checker is used to check the document for grammar and style errors. It will interpret the presentation of the subject and make recommendations for improvement.

Other utilities are available for performing block functions that operate on words, sentences, paragraphs, or pages within a document. These functions include copying, moving, deleting, formatting, centering, and case conversion. Searching for and replacing particular words or phrases can be done by a simple request. Margins can be justified and words automatically hyphenated within set margins. Pages can be automatically defined and numbered.

Shell documents or templates can be created in which the common content of a document never changes but some areas are reserved for text that will change each time a new document is created from the template. A good example of this is a memorandum or letter that goes out to many different persons. The document and a list of variable information can be created separately and merged for printing.

Personal Information Manager (PIM)

A *personal information manager* (PIM) application is an electronic version of the daily appointment book or day planner. It incorporates an address book, a calendar,

EXHIBIT 21-11

Example of a Departmental Budget

Hospital Information Systems Budget
October 200x–September 200x

Pg 1: Oct 200x–Jan 200x

SUB CODE DESCRIPTION	ORIGINAL BUDGET	BALANCE AVAILABLE	PERCENT USED	OCT 200X CURRENT	OCT 200X YEAR	NOV CURRENT	NOV YEAR	DEC CURRENT	DEC YEAR	JAN 200X CURRENT	JAN 200X YEAR
1600 Student wages	$15,000	$4,084	73	$746	$746	$786	$1,532	$1,145	$2,677	$738	$3,415
1660 Accrued salaries	$0	$0	100		$0		$0		$0	$0	$0
Salaries	$15,000	$4,084	73	$746	$746	$786	$1,532	$1,145	$2,677	$738	$3,415
2110 Medical–surgical supplies	$250	$75	70	$21	$21		$21	$23	$44	$18	$62
2130 Drugs	$0	$0	100		$0		$0		$0	$0	$0
Medical–Surgical Supplies	$250	$75	70	$21	$21		$21	$23	$44	$18	$62
2320 Office supplies	$250	$89	64	$37	$37	$7	$44		$44	$15	$59
2330 Copying and binding	$400	($25)	106	$28	$28	$31	$59	$33	$92	$37	$129
2340 Printing	$0	$0	100		$0		$0		$0		$0
2400 Housekeeping supplies	$100	$25	75	$11	$11	$7	$18		$18		$18
2500 Maintenance supplies	$100	$22	78		$0	$25	$25		$25	$21	$46
2700 Food expense	$0	$0	100		$0		$0		$0		$0
General Supplies	$850	$111	87	$76	$76	$70	$146	$33	$179	$73	$252
3110 Travel	$4,000	$618	85	$76	$0	$1,398	$1,398		$1,398		$1,398
3140 Local travel	$500	$13	97	$46	$46	$42	$88	$38	$126	$41	$167
3160 Workshop and training	$1,500	$522	65		$0		$0		$0	$750	$750
Travel–Entertainment	$6,000	$1,153	81	$46	$46	$1,440	$1,486	$38	$1,524	$791	$2,315
3230 Contract labor	$0	$0	100		$0		$0		$0		$0
3290 Computer software	$2,500	($204)	108	$286	$286		$286	$368	$654		$654
3360 Equipment maintenance/repair	$1,500	$244	84		$0	$128	$128		$128	$227	$355
3370 Maintenance contracts	$3,500	$200	94	$1,500	$1,500		$1,500		$1,500	$1,800	$3,300
3410 Equipment rental	$0	$0	100		$0		$0		$0		$0
3650 Telephone base	$252	$0	100	$21	$21	$21	$42	$21	$63	$21	$84
3660 Telephone, long distance	$0	$0	100		$0		$0		$0		$0
3720 Books and subscriptions	$250	$86	66	$121	$121		$121		$121		$121
Other Expenses	$8,002	$326	96	$1,928	$1,928	$149	$2,077	$389	$2,466	$2,048	$4,514
5050 Minor equipment (<$500)	$3,500	$774	78	$0	$0	$0	$0	$771	$771	$257	$1,028
Minor Equipment Expenses	$3,500	$774	78	$0	$0	$0	$0	$771	$771	$257	$1,028
Total Expenses	$33,602	$6,523	81	$2,817	$2,817	$2,445	$5,262	$2,399	$7,661	$3,925	$11,586

EXHIBIT 21-12
Example of a Bar Graph

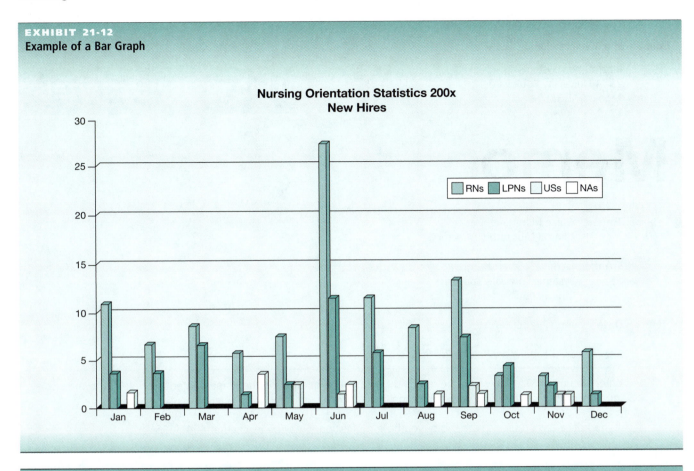

Nursing Orientation Statistics 200x
New Hires

EXHIBIT 21-13
Example of a Line Graph

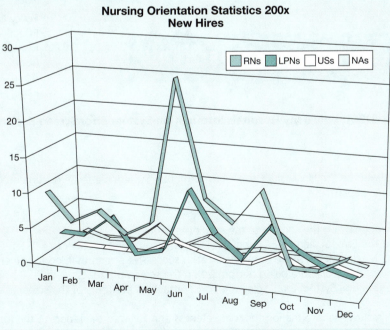

Nursing Orientation Statistics 200x
New Hires

EXHIBIT 21-14
Example of a Memorandum

Information Systems
2534 University Boulevard
Mobile, AL 36608

University Hospitals

Memo

To: Nurse Managers
        Clinical Laboratory Directors

From: Richard J. Swansburg
        Systems Software Specialist
        Information Systems

Date: June 27, 2000

Re: STAT Laboratory Results Printing

When you order STAT lab work, the results should now be printing on the home printer associated with the display terminal or PC that the order was entered on.

If you notice any problems with this or you have a question, I may be reached at 454-3656.

rjs

EXHIBIT 21-15
Example of a Policy

University Hospitals

Policy Number:	5.11
Effective:	April 1998
Revised:	February 2000
Reviewed:	January 2000
Approved:	
Page:	1 of 1

SUBJECT: University Hospitals Information System Error Screen Report

I. POLICY STATEMENT:
All errors screens displayed on the University Hospitals Information System are to be documented and the report sent to the Information Systems department.

II. PROCEDURE:
When an error screen appears on the computer, the employee should:
1. Make a printout of the Error Screen by pressing "PA1" on the computer keyboard.
2. Beginning with the Master Menu, make printouts of each successive screen that led to the error screen.
3. Highlight each step of the procedure being performed on the screen printouts.
4. Complete the "Information System Error Screen Report," attach all printouts of the screens, and forward to the supervisor.
5. The supervisor will review the information for completeness and forward the report to the Information Systems department.

EXHIBIT 21-16

Example of a Form

REQUISITION

Requisition No. _____

Departmental Request No. _____

Date _____ *June 27, 2000* _____

UNIVERSITY HOSPITALS
Mobile, Alabama 36608

To: PURCHASING OFFICE
The following order is requested by:

DIVISION _____ *Information Technology Services* _____ DEPARTMENT _____ *Information Systems* _____ ACCOUNT NO. _____ *75150 - 323* _____

DELIVER TO _____ *Information Systems* _____ ROOM & LOCATION _____ *Room 212, 2nd Floor* _____

QUANTITY	ITEM	UNIT	COST
5	Academic Windows 2000 Professional	$78.95	$394.75
PRICES ARE REQUIRED ON ALL REQUISITIONS		TOTAL	$394.75

CHECK HERE IF YOU ESTIMATED PRICE _____ PRICE QUOTED BY _____

NAMES AND ADDRESSES OF VENDORS IN ORDER OF PREFERENCE (ATTACH ALL QUOTATIONS)

1. GE Capital ITS 3250 Downs Street Mobile, AL 36606 (334) 471-2471	2.	3.
	Quoted Price _____	Quoted Price _____

The authority to issue purchase orders rests solely with the University Hospitals purchasing department. The University Hospitals assumes no obligation except on a previously issued and duly authorized purchase order. Direct orders by departments must show evidence of definite and particular permission.

FOR ACCOUNTING USE		
USE	FUND	AMOUNT

SIGNED _____ REQUESTOR

APPROVED _____ DEPARTMENT HEAD

APPROVED _____ DEAN

APPROVED _____ CONTROLLER

e-mail, a journal, notes, and tasks. It can also include groupware capability that allows direct collaboration with others that share the same PIM software. Today's PIMs reside on two platforms of personal computing that consist of a desktop or notebook computer and a *personal digital assistant* (PDA), which is a computing device small enough to be carried in a pocket. A PDA offers much the same personal information management capabilities as a PIM does on a desktop computer. Quite often, the PDA includes a tool for synchronizing information between the PDA and the desktop system. This allows calendar or contact information to be entered into one system and then be transferred to the other system.

The *address book* component provides a database for storing information about personal and professional contacts. This information includes names, titles, addresses, telephone numbers, e-mail and website addresses, and various other personal and professional information. The address book is a fundamental part of other PIM components and even other applications such as word processing and spread sheets. The *calendar* is a component used to create and schedule appointments and tasks as one-time or recurring events over a given period of time. When a meeting is scheduled, attendees can be invited directly (via e-mail or the groupware feature) from the address book. When invitees acknowledge their availability, their schedules automatically get updated to show the meeting, and the meeting organizer receives an accepted response. Reminders can be assigned to these events to provide notifications of their approaching occurrence.

Tasks can be created, scheduled, and assigned much the same as appointments. A *task* indicates a duty or job that is to be performed. It often includes information related to its priority, start date, due date, percent complete, and status. *Notes* are brief pieces of recorded information that can be assigned to defined categories and associated with events and tasks. A *journal* can be equated with a diary. It provides a recorded account of daily events, experiences, and reflections. These may include conversations, meetings, telephone calls, letters, and work performed. A journal and notes can be quite useful in remembering critical information at a later date. Usually a search tool is provided to find specific words or phrases in the subject or contents.

"E-mail is just the latest chapter in the evolving history of human communication."[12]

E-mail has become a convenient method of corresponding with others instead of using the telephone, fax, or U.S. Post Office. E-mail has become a common part of our personal and professional lives. Quite often,

employees have more than one e-mail account, and the management of e-mail communications has become critical. With this in mind, the e-mail component has become the cornerstone of today's PIM software. It provides us with services that allow us to send and receive our e-mail within the organizational setting and on the Internet. It provides us with rules and folders for separating and storing e-mail based on sender or content. It provides us with tools for archiving and retrieving old e-mail. It provides us with a favorable way to transfer pictures and files with our daily contacts. Can we really imagine life again without e-mail?

Graphics

Another valuable tool is a graphics program that can produce graphics that can be used for presentations, illustrations, and teaching. Graphics can be printed, displayed to a monitor, or projected onto a screen for viewing by large numbers of people. They can also be converted to presentation aids such as overhead transparencies, videotapes, and slides.

In the past, graphics programs focused on the visual display of numerical data in the form of bar, line, and pie graphs. This focus relates to the early use of graphics by business and management. Today, graphics systems can be used in a multitude of ways to visually illustrate almost anything. Features have been incorporated to display graphics such as slide shows and animation. Such presentation capability can be very helpful to the nurse trying to present information related to various business and clinical subjects. See Exhibits 21-17 and 21-18 for examples.

EXHIBIT 21-17

Example of Presentation Graphics to Discuss Coronary Disease

Coronary Disease Risk Factors

- Diabetes
- Family history
- High blood pressure
- High blood cholesterol
- Overweight
- Sedentary lifestyle
- Smoking
- Stress

EXHIBIT 21-18

Example of Presentation Graphic to Discuss the Anatomy of the Eye

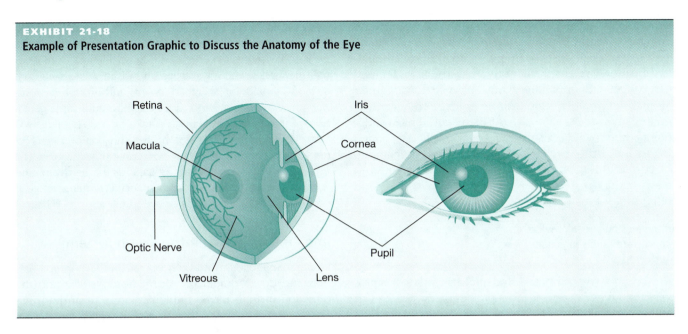

Graphics can be created in a number of ways. They can be created as part of the program in association with some numerical data; they can be scanned; the user can create them freehand; or they can be purchased as an add-on to the graphics program.

Information Systems

Nurses are beginning to find that the demands of working with automation in nursing can be great. Nurses may be asked to interact with specialized and generalized nursing information systems as well as with hospital information systems.

Nursing Information Systems

Nursing information systems are software packages developed specifically for nursing usage. These programs may be explicit to a particular area of nursing application, or they may be general to the support of the nursing services division. Examples of nursing areas that can benefit from unique information systems support include mental health, neonatology, acute care, urology, enterostomal therapy, oncology, maternity, operating room, and infection control.

General nursing information systems have multiple programs, or modules, that are used to perform various clinical, educational, and management functions. Most nursing information systems have modules for classification, staffing, scheduling, personnel management, and report generation. Other modules may be included, such as budget development, resource allocation and cost control, case mix and diagnosis-related groups

(DRGs) analysis, quality management, staff development, modeling and simulation for decision-making, strategic planning, short-term demands for forecasting and work planning, and program evaluation.

Modules for patient classification, staffing, scheduling, personnel management, and report generation are often closely interrelated. Patients are classified according to established acuity criteria. The patient classification information is input into the staffing module, and staffing levels are calculated according to various work load formulas. Also, actual staffing is input and a comparison of census, patient acuity, needed staffing, and actual staffing can be made. Schedules are then prepared using the information from the staffing and personnel records modules.

Analysis and quality management of DRGs are performed to associate patient acuity, quality of care, and DRGs, which is helpful for establishing future guidelines and care needs for patients according to their DRGs. The budget is also supported by the census, patient acuity, and needed staffing patterns. This information is invaluable to support requests for additional full-time and part-time employees. The report generation module allows all of the stored information to be retrieved and output in a timely and presentable manner.

Nursing information systems can be used to improve the effectiveness of patient care while making it more economical. Clinical components include patient history and assessment, nursing care plans, nursing progress notes and charting, patient monitoring, order entry and results reporting, patient education, and discharge planning. These can all be available from virtually any location—from the patient's bedside to the nurses' and doctors' homes.

Clinical nurses can use their nursing information systems to replace manual systems of data recording. This may reduce costs while permitting improved quality of care as well as quality of work life. Clinical nurses can collect and input clinical data and use the computer to analyze it to formulate treatment plans. They can use quantitative decision analysis to support clinical judgments. Automated consultation can be applied to screen for adverse drug reactions, interactions, and preparation of correct dosages. Computers can be programmed to reject orders that could cause problems in these and other areas, thus preventing errors.[13]

Curtin reminds nurses to provide high-touch care in this inhuman high-tech world.[14]

Technology, computers, and information systems provide the knowledge to save or prolong lives. Nurses can return to patients and families control over their lives when families have lost their freedom of action or understanding of events. Nurses can keep control of cybernetics through the exercise of human compassion.[15] High-tech includes the new scientific knowledge of microelectronics, computers, information, sensors, processors, displays, and education. Its objective is the solution of society's total problems, not just those related to health care, including nursing.[16] Helping nurses provide high-touch while using high-tech should be a primary goal of nurse managers.

Hospital Information Systems

Hospital information systems are large, complex computer systems designed to help communicate and manage the information needs of a hospital. They are tools for interdepartmental and intradepartmental use. A typical hospital information system will have components for admissions, medical records, patient accounting, nursing, order entry, and results reporting. Other components can exist for virtually any department and for almost any purpose. Divisions such as nursing (the nursing information system), laboratory, radiology, pharmacy, personnel, and payroll may be so large and complex that they have their own information systems. These systems may stand alone and run independently of the hospital information system but are usually interfaced for information transfer.

Admissions procedures include patient scheduling, admissions, discharges, transfers, and census functions. Medical records procedures include master patient index functions, abstracting (diagnosis/procedure/DRG coding), transcription and correspondence, and medical record locator functions. Business and accounting procedures include patient insurance verification, billing, billing follow-up, billing inquiry, accounts payable, accounts receivable, cash processing, and service master and third-party maintenance.

Hospital information systems tend to be developed with mainframe and minicomputers in mind, although the trend today seems to be toward downsizing and distributed data networks. The advantages and disadvantages of each strategy should be weighed before information systems implementation. Selection, development, and implementation of information systems can take years. This time will vary, depending on the system and the complexity of its applications, and may actually be a continuous process. The initial cost can be millions of dollars for the hardware and software. Continued yearly maintenance is required and can cost hundreds of thousands or even millions of dollars.

Implementation of Information Systems

Nurse managers should be involved in the implementation and development of information systems and the direction of their users. Implementation of an information system requires preparation of a management plan. The first step is to form an implementation committee to assess the current system and what is wanted out of the proposed system. This assessment should lead to a strategic plan, because acquiring an information system requires expenditure of a large amount of human, material, and financial resources.

The procurement process begins by asking vendors to respond to a request for information (RFI). The response will provide the implementation committee with valuable information related to system purpose and capability. From this a request for proposal (RFP) is created and sent to selected vendors. The RFP must be accurate and clearly worded to prevent misinterpretation of system requirements. This formal process is important because the only way of being sure that a vendor understands and promises to meet an information system's expectations is to get it on paper.[17]

Once the available systems have been reviewed and priced, a selection must be made based on which system fits the organization's needs and budget. From here the process proceeds to contract development. A properly designed and negotiated contract is crucial for the protection of the purchaser. A good contract does three things[18]:

1. It ensures that the vendor clearly understands your expectations of the system's capabilities and costs.
2. It provides a means for recovery in the event that the system fails or does not perform properly.
3. It provides a guarantee for continuous maintenance, support, and system updates needed to protect the investment and stay current with ongoing advances in computing.

Once the contract has been signed, the real project implementation begins. A project manager is assigned, a project implementation plan is developed (see Exhibit

21-19), and resources are allocated. Commitment to this process is essential from the bottom level users to executive management.

It has been reported that in 1998, only 26% of organizational information technology projects were successful, which means completed on time, on budget, and with all the features as specified.[19]

Finally, after the information system is live, it must be evaluated to determine if it meets the organization's needs as proposed. If it does, payments must be made to the vendor as per the contract. If it does not, the contract must be reevaluated and a new course of action planned.

Data Warehousing and Knowledge Management

Information and knowledge are valuable commodities in today's complex and competitive health care environment.

EXHIBIT 21-19
Example of a Project Implementation Plan

ID	ACTIVITY	DURATION	START	FINISH
1	UNIVERSITY HOSPITALS RESULTS REPOSITORY PROJECT STARTUP	2.5d	9/11/00	9/13/00
4	ADMINISTRATIVE	120d	9/13/00	2/28/01
5	Project Status Meetings	115.25d	9/15/00	2/23/01
13	Project Steering Committee Meetings	95.25d	9/20/00	1/31/01
19	Quality Assurance Review Visit	2d	9/13/00	9/15/00
20	Project Supervision	120d	9/13/00	2/28/01
21	PROJECT INITIATION	10d	9/14/00	9/27/00
22	Pre-Implementation Planning	1d	9/14/00	9/14/00
24	Project Planning	2d	9/15/00	9/18/00
28	Adapt Network	5d	9/18/00	9/22/00
30	Project Kickoff	7d	9/19/00	9/27/00
35	HARDWARE AND SOFTWARE	12.5d	9/13/00	9/29/00
36	Hardware/Software Installation	12.5d	9/13/00	9/29/00
39	Software Delivery Validation	9d	9/13/00	9/26/00
43	ANALYSIS	58d	9/28/00	12/18/00
44	Results Repository Surveys/Process Flow/Tables	15d	9/28/00	10/18/00
48	Results Repository Interfaces	20d	10/19/00	11/15/00
51	Results Repository Profiles/Procedures	11d	11/16/00	11/30/00
59	Nursing Assessment Surveys/Process Flow/Procedures	11d	11/27/00	12/11/00
63	Nursing Assessment Master Files	3d	12/12/00	12/14/00
65	Nursing Assessment Reports/Project Scope	2d	12/15/00	12/18/00
68	TRAINING	42d	12/18/00	2/13/01
69	Training Preparation	12d	12/18/00	1/2/01
73	Educate Users	30d	1/3/01	2/13/01
77	LIVE EVENT	28d	1/22/01	2/28/01
78	Live Event Preparation	22d	1/22/01	2/20/01
83	Results Repository Live Event	4d	2/23/01	2/28/01
86	Nursing Assessment Live Event	5d	2/22/01	2/28/01
88	Live Event Support	5d	2/22/01	2/28/01
90	POST-LIVE	10d	3/1/01	3/14/01
91	Evaluation and Feedback to Management	10d	3/1/01	3/14/01
92	Monitor Production System	6d	3/1/01	3/8/01
95				

Vast amounts of data are stored in various legacy information systems within health care organizations. These systems were developed to promote throughput and limit redundancy, and not to encourage data analysis and decision support. Data warehousing has become the new means for collecting, structuring, and storing data into repositories that provide for quick retrieval and intuitive analysis. "When designed and used properly, data warehouses lead to more effective business decisions in less time, which can increase a company's competitive advantage."[20]

In a complementary fashion, vast amounts of knowledge are stored in various hypermedia systems (documents, e-mail, and Web pages) within health care organizations. These systems require tools to cull, retrieve, and present these knowledge assets buried within. Knowledge management incorporates *data mining* (discovering hidden information in data) and ad hoc query and reporting services that attempt to tie together the knowledge on a common platform.

> **"Knowledge management encompasses an overarching business strategy aimed at exposing and taking advantage of a company's information, experience, and expertise to serve customers better and respond quickly to changing market conditions."[21]**

Decision Support Systems, Expert Systems, and Predictive Technology

A *decision support system* (DSS) is software that provides personnel with essential information to substantiate the making of decisions. An *expert system* is software that uses a knowledge base, rules, and inference to aid in solving problems. An expert system is associated with a particular discipline, and experts in that field develop the knowledge base, rules, and conclusions. *Predictive technology* refers to the process of using the information content in large, complex databases to understand and predict the actions of various entities in health care, that is, patients, providers, and payers. The purpose is to improve business decisions.[22]

"Organizations that create a strategy and implement DSS tools to provide decision-makers with the critical information they need to face the competition and maintain quality and costs will have the advantage."[23] Additionally, a clinical DSS can be implemented to drive the appropriate process improvement activities required to achieve successful care outcomes.[24] Good DSSs should blend analytical tools with intuitive heuristics to provide insight about complex factors that cannot be built into models. These systems must assist in the modification of analytical results when they contradict what intuition tells us.

Four types of decision-makers exist: analytical, intuitive, accommodating, and integrated. Analytical decision-makers seek to use quantitative, rational, and logical reasoning. They seek a single, predictable cause to a problem, ignoring the unpredictable and simplifying the complex. Intuitive decision-makers consider the whole problem using an unstructured and spontaneous approach to its resolution. Accommodating decision-makers are either analytical or intuitive, but experience has taught them to adopt the other style when appropriate. Finally, integrated decision-makers do not have a dominant style. They reason, analyze, and gather facts that trigger their use of intuition.

Decision support systems should provide for quick and convenient access to data extraction and analysis tools. They should provide a wide range of models for investigation and summarization. They should track experience to factor in past decisions and results. They should allow for the input of values, ethics, morals, and goals. They should help to understand what is known, and to recognize what has been overlooked. They should provide alternatives and their interpretations. In the end, they must be capable of presenting understandable results to the decision-makers.[25]

Expert systems encode the relevant knowledge and experience of experts to make them available to less knowledgeable and less experienced persons. An example would be to take the accumulated knowledge and experience of clinical nurse specialists in neuroscience nursing, encode them in a computer system, and make the system available to clinical nurses working in the neuroscience area. A nurse would identify a situation requiring a decision, the criteria defining the problem, and objectives for handling the situation. The expert system would evaluate the information and provide a listing of alternative ways to manage the situation. The nurse would then evaluate the alternatives and make the decision.

Predictive technology provides organizations with a method to identify and exploit behavioral patterns hidden within their data. It is capable of learning from experience and improving its predictive capabilities over time. In health care, patient interactions that may occur through ambulatory care centers, physicians' offices, business offices, and hospitals can be analyzed to allow health care providers to determine the preferences, usage patterns, and future needs of the patient. Opportunities to apply predictive technology in health care may include[26]:

- The detection of fraud and abuse perpetrated by patients and providers.
- The prediction of future clinical outcomes.
- The prediction of future resource utilization.

- The prediction of complex cases that can benefit the most from case management.

Nursing Management Applications

Many applications are available for nursing management. In addition to those associated with the use of general-purpose applications software, other applications might include a calendar of events, a nursing management minimum data set (NMMDS), and the HR information system.

A calendar can be useful in supplying nursing personnel with dates and times of staff meetings, committee meetings, and educational events (see Exhibit 21-20).

Educational events would include continuing education, annual review, and patient education. The calendar could be an Internet browser–based application that is available on the organization's intranet. This would provide for simple point-and-click access to events and their details from any personal computer, at work or home. Information for the calendar could be linked to and provided from the organization's information systems such as the HR system. Through the use of these calendar links, employees could actively schedule themselves for meetings or classes. When they choose an event such as an educational class, their names could be added to the class role and automatic notifications could be sent to their nurse managers.

EXHIBIT 21-20
Example of a Nursing Calendar

Nursing Calendar				OCTOBER 200x
Monday	**Tuesday**	**Wednesday**	**Thursday**	**Friday**
2 Nursing Orientation 0800 Nursing Council 1300	**3**	**4** Diabetes Management 1430	**5** Understanding Nutrition 1430	**6**
9 Body Mechanics 0730 Body Mechanics 1930	**10** Annual Education 0800 CPR 1300	**11**	**12** 6th Floor Staff Meeting 1515	**13** Antibiotic Therapy 0730 Antibiotic Therapy 1930
16 ACLS Class 0800 Patient Monitoring 0800 Infusion Pumps 1300	**17**	**18** Understanding ECGs 0730 Understanding ECGs 1930	**19** Quality Improvement 1200	**20** Hospital Picnic 1100
23 Body Mechanics 0730 Body Mechanics 1930	**24** CPR 1300	**25** CCU Staff Meeting 1515	**26**	**27** Antibiotic Therapy 0730 Antibiotic Therapy 1930
30 IV Certification 0900	**31** Halloween Party 1530			

The NMMDS is a research-based management data set available from the American Organization of Nurse Executives. The NMMDS has 17 elements clustered around three broad categories of environment, nurse resources, and financial resources. "It is a means by which data about the context and support of direct healthcare delivery are organized, classified, managed, accessed, and researched. The principle behind the NMMDS is that nurse executives need hard data to make the difficult quality decisions that need to be made in today's operating environment."[27] Implementing the NMMDS empowers nursing management with specific costs and quality data to answer questions related to areas such as outcomes of critical paths, turnover rates of personnel, nurse satisfaction, personnel ratings, budgets, and productivity. The NMMDS provides data to compare time periods.[28]

The management of HR can be a formidable task for today's health care organizations. The collection and manipulation of information associated with this management can require significant time and manpower in itself. The development and implementation of the HR information system can be a blessing to the organization and professionals who manage these resources.

Front-end components can be established to analyze information related to all of the job applicants who apply to the organization and the advertising and recruitment of these applicants. Some information needs to be retained on everyone who applies for any job position. This information can be useful for understanding the professional market. There are also concerns about equal opportunity based on race or disability. Applications analysis can show how many people apply for a position by these indicators. See Exhibit 21-21 for an example report. Advertising analysis can provide recruitment information related to the method and placement of advertisements. See Exhibit 21-22 for an example report.

Information on persons who are hired can be pulled from the applications analysis component and added to the permanent employee database. This database is the central foundation of the HR system, and it maintains all of the relevant information related to employees and their positions, from the moment they are hired until they are terminated. See Exhibit 21-23 for an example of a termination report. This database can be used to maintain information about personnel with special skills or credentials, and it can identify employees facing license renewal deadlines and those who need additional training. Additional components can be integrated into the HR system to collect and report information on employee education, time, and attendance.

The educational component would maintain all of the information associated with the education of employees. See Exhibit 21-24 for an example of an employee education report. This information can also meet the reporting needs of the institution as to the requirements of the state board of nursing and the Joint Commission on Accreditation of Healthcare Organizations. Education elements may include the following[29]:

- New employee orientation
- Clinical specialty courses
- Continuing education offerings
- Competency validation of skills
- Nursing station in-service education
- Annual required reviews

The time and attendance component would maintain the information associated with employees' work, vacation, holiday, and sick time. The information here produces timesheets. From the HR system, information can be exported and imported to the hospital and nursing information systems. It may also be exported to general-purpose microcomputer application software for various purposes.

EXHIBIT 21-21
Example of an Application Analysis Report

APPLICATIONS ANALYSIS REPORT FOR THE MONTH OF SEPTEMBER 200x

POSITION		F	M	AM	AS	BA	CA	HI	PI	DIS	VET	DVET
01412	Registered nurse	3	0	0	0	2	1	0	0	0	0	0
02456	Registered nurse	2	0	0	0	1	1	0	0	0	0	0
02457	Registered nurse	6	2	0	1	2	4	1	0	0	0	0
11923	Licensed practical nurse	7	0	0	0	5	2	0	0	0	0	0
15934	Assistant administrator	3	12	0	0	1	14	0	0	0	0	0
22921	Unit secretary	11	1	0	1	8	3	0	0	1	0	0
23110	Education specialist	5	2	0	0	2	5	0	0	0	1	0

EXHIBIT 21-22

Example of an Advertisement Analysis Report

ADVERTISEMENT ANALYSIS REPORT FOR THE MONTH OF SEPTEMBER 200X

ADD NO.	PLACEMENT	DATE	RN	LPN	PHR	PT	RT	CLK	MG	OTH
1622	Channel 5	09/01/xx	3	2	0	0	1	0	0	5
1633	Channel 10	09/01/xx	1	1	1	0	0	1	0	2
1734	Newspaper	09/03/xx	1	1	1	1	0	0	1	1
1775	Internet	09/03/xx	2	0	2	0	1	0	1	1
1622	Channel 5	09/08/xx	0	0	0	0	1	3	0	1
1633	Channel 10	09/08/xx	2	0	0	1	0	1	0	2
1734	Newspaper	09/10/xx	5	1	1	1	1	0	1	3
1775	Internet	09/10/xx	0	0	0	1	1	0	0	2
1622	Channel 5	09/15/xx	1	1	0	0	2	0	0	7
1633	Channel 10	09/15/xx	0	3	2	0	1	1	0	6
1734	Newspaper	09/17/xx	1	3	3	0	1	4	0	5
1775	Internet	09/17/xx	3	2	1	0	1	0	0	1
1734	Newspaper	09/24/xx	2	0	0	0	1	0	1	0
1755	Internet	09/24/xx	1	0	0	0	1	0	2	0

EXHIBIT 21-23

Example of an Employee Termination Report

EMPLOYEE TERMINATION REPORT FOR THE MONTH OF SEPTEMBER 200X

POSITION	NAME	TITLE	DATE	REASON
00356	Johnson, Mary J.	Registered nurse	09/26/xx	Q
10234	Armstrong, Helen M.	Licensed practical nurse	09/08/xx	Q
16212	Mims, Janet K.	Registered nurse	09/13/xx	F
17335	Baker, Donald M.	Registered nurse	09/05/xx	Q
17366	Smitherman, Carolyn S.	Registered nurse	09/22/xx	R
18549	Jackson, Melanie J.	Unit secretary	09/01/xx	Q
18675	Hanson, Marcus K.	Respiratory therapist	09/29/xx	Q

Ethical, Legal, and Security Issues

Certain ethical issues are involved in the use of technology in nursing. *Ethical* means conforming to professional standards of conduct. "Privacy means control over exposure of self or information about oneself and freedom from intrusion. Privacy denotes the right of an individual to decide how much personal information to share. It includes a right to secrecy of information and protection against the misuse or release of this information."[30] *Confidentiality* means being entrusted with the privacy of others that was shared with you in confidence. The relationship of the three terms can be expressed as a patient entrusting privacy to a professional who has an ethical responsibility to maintain the confidentiality of that privacy.

Legal issues associated with automation may involve the confidentiality of patient information and the risks associated with clinical decision-making based on computerized information. One method of addressing these issues is by maintaining professional standards. Information systems should be designed, developed, and implemented to validate patient outcomes and support professional nursing standards. Thus, computer technology for nursing use needs to be based on nursing input from start to finish. Basing computer technology on nursing input requires the use of expert nurses who have sufficient clinical, theoretical, education, research, and management expertise to adequately represent professional standards. It also requires a unified nursing profession that can specify clear design criteria and professional standards guidelines.[31]

EXHIBIT 21-24
Example of an Employee Education Report

EMPLOYEE EDUCATION REPORT

EMPLOYEE NAME:	JONES, MARY L.
POSITION NUMBER:	353367
NURSING UNIT:	MICU

COURSE TYPE	DESCRIPTION	DATE COMPLETE	EVAL CODE	CLASS HOURS	CLINICAL HOURS	CONTACT HOURS
C	Antibiotic therapy	10/27/xx	S			1.0
	Understanding ECGS	10/18/xx	S			2.0
	Subtotal Continuing Education					3.0
I	Patient monitoring	10/16/xx	S	4.0		
	Infusion pumps	10/16/xx	S	1.0		
	Subtotal In-Service Education			5.0		
O	Personnel	10/02/xx	S	2.0		
	Fire and safety	10/02/xx	S	3.0		
	Infection control	10/02/xx	S	3.0		
	Legal issues	10/03/xx	S	4.0		
	Cardiopulmonary resuscitation	10/04/xx	S	4.0		
	Information systems	10/06/xx	S	8.0		
	Unit orientation	10/27/xx	S		120.0	
	Subtotal Orientation			24.0	120.0	
S	IV Certification	10/30/xx	S	3.0		
	Subtotal Skills Competency			3.0		
	Totals			32.0	120.0	3.0

Nurses should also be capable of assessing and managing the legal risks associated with automated information management. Computer data should be examined, analyzed, interpreted, and appraised. Forced selections and unclear logic should be questioned. Nurses should not hold as fact the belief that clinical decision-making based on the use of technology results in better patient care.

The American Nurses Association, the American Medical Records Association, and the Canadian Nurses' Association offer guidelines and strategies for minimizing legal risks associated with automated charting[32]:

- Never give your computer password to anyone.
- Do not leave a computer terminal unattended after you have logged on.
- Follow procedure for modifying mistakes. Computer entries are part of the permanent medical record and cannot be deleted.
- Do not leave patient information displayed on a screen for others to see.
- Keep track of printed information about patients, and dispose of it appropriately when it is no longer needed.
- Follow your institution's confidentiality policies and procedures.

Automation in nursing also involves security issues. Security means the level to which hardware, software, and information is safe from abuse and unauthorized use or access, whether accidental or intentional. From a management standpoint, professionals need to be aware that security must be overseen from physical, operational, and ethical viewpoints.

Physical security deals with the control of access to hardware, assessment and determination of environmental threats, and prevention of loss. Operational security deals with the threats to information. It includes the assessment and prevention of unauthorized access or use of information, the policies and procedures governing the management of information, and the procedures required for recovery from loss of information. Ethical security deals with the individual's ability to conform to professional standards of conduct, which means that nurses must respect the privacy of information. They must accept and enforce all guidelines that are imposed for the maintenance of physical and operational security of computer systems.

Nurses should be aware of various security measures that may be built into information systems. One of the first things that should be present is the ability to perform auditing, which means leaving a trail of who did what, where, and when. Logs can record when and where the system is accessed and by whom. This same information can be captured when vital information is created, modified, or deleted. Once this information is captured, standard procedures should be in place for the routine auditing of this information.

A significant amount of security may be associated with an individual's computer ID. Every individual should be assigned his or her own personal ID. This ID should have the person's name, title, department, security level, and menu linked to it. There should be a password that protects the ID and is known only by the user. Procedures should be in place to force users to change their passwords every 30 to 90 days and allow them to change passwords more often on their own as desired. Also, a number of each user's old passwords should be stored for comparison purposes, and the user should not be allowed to reuse these passwords.

The security level should be implemented in a hierarchical manner from administrator to nursing assistant. The security level can be a range of numbers from largest to smallest that can be tested to determine who can perform particular functions. Menus that determine the capability to interact with the system should be developed and assigned based on departmental and job requirements.

Summary

The intent of this chapter is to provide an overview of nursing and information technology. The Internet has brought us to a point where we feel that the computer has come of age. We have a vision of tomorrow where everything and everyone is connected. Today, the computer has become an everyday tool for handling information. We feel the impact of their usage throughout our daily lives. Those in health care have come to realize the benefit computers provide in the support of clinical communication and documentation and in the management of today's complicated financial environment.

Computers are used to support and run highly complex information systems that have tremendous capabilities for the manipulation and storage of information. Virtually any nursing process can be augmented or implemented through the use of information technology. There are systems that assist nursing in documenting patient care, order processing, clinical decision-making, and patient and professional education. Other general-purpose application software is also available for personal productivity enhancement. Nurses have needs for document preparation, number crunching, and record keeping. They are also finding that graphics, multimedia, and communications are invaluable tools for presentations and educational support.

We must also not forget the human side of nursing, the compassion we have for our clients. We have ethical and moral responsibilities to protect the privacy that they have entrusted to us. Maintaining the security of information is an active and ongoing duty. As overseers of this information, we must not think of it as our right to know, but as our privilege to know.

APPLICATION EXERCISES

EXERCISE 21-1   Discuss the technologic changes that you have experienced and how you believe they have influenced your life.

EXERCISE 21-2   Discuss the current information technology environment you are working in or are being exposed to in health care. Identify changes that you expect to see in the next 5 years.

EXERCISE 21-3   Which type of computer network(s) do you use within your organization? Identify the various discrete computers (servers with information systems) attached to the network of your organization. Try to develop a graphical representation of the hardware and software environments.

EXERCISE 21-4   What role does the Internet have in the information technology environment of your organization? Identify and discuss the resources available to nursing through the Internet.

EXERCISE 21-5   Identify and discuss information technology used by various nursing personnel (unit secretary, registered nurses, nursing management, and clinical specialists) in your organization. Include personal computer applications, information systems, and diagnostic equipment.

EXERCISE 21-6   Identify and discuss the development of various applications using personal computer applications software. Pick a project and implement it.

EXERCISE 21-7   Identify an area of information management (in your current nursing environment) that is not automated, and develop a proposal for obtaining an information system for it.

EXERCISE 21-8   Discuss your views on ethics, privacy, confidentiality, and security. Which security measures do you interact with in your environment? Is there room for improvement?

NOTES

1. R. L. Rutsky, "Techno-Cultural Interaction and the Fear of Information," *Style* (summer 1999), 267.
2. E. Feretic, "Never Too Old," *Beyond Computing* (April 2000), 8.
3. M. Hagland, "Buyers and Sellers," *Health Management Technology* (April 1997), 20–23.
4. *The American Heritage Dictionary of the English Language, Third Edition* (Houghton Mifflin Company, 1996).
5. "Welcome to 2010," *Business Week* (6 March 2000), 102.
6. J. Blackford, "The Future of Computing: For 500,000 Years, Technology has Advanced While People Remained the Same. In the Next Millennium, the Human Race Plays Catch-up," *Computer Shopper* (December 1999), 319.
7. F. J. Derfler, Jr., "Virtual Private Networks," *PC Magazine* (4 January 2000), 146.
8. R. C. Coile, Jr., "The Digital Transformation of Health Care," *Physician Executive* (January–February 2000), 8–15.
9. J. Ferry, "Virtual Doctors on the Horizon in Seattle," *The Lancet* (11 September 1999), 926.
10. C. Schreiber, "For Your Eyes Only: HHS Aims to protect Patient Confidentiality," *HealthWeek* (3 April 2000), 1, 15.
11. Microsoft Word 2000 (Redmond, WA: Microsoft Corporation, 1999).
12. *Newsweek* (20 September 1999), 58.
13. H. W. Gottinger, "Computers in Hospital Care: A Qualitative Assessment," *Human Systems Management* (fall 1984), 324–345.
14. L. Curtin, "Nursing: High Touch in a High-Tech World," *Nursing Management* (July 1984), 7–8.
15. Ibid.
16. P. McKenzie-Sanders, "The Central Focus of the Information Age," *Business Quarterly* (winter 1983), 87–91.
17. D. F. Carr, "Meeting of the Minds," *Internet World* (15 May 2000), 45.
18. R. X. Fischer and S. P. Singh, "Checklist for a Good Contract for IT Purchases," *Health Management Technology* (March 2000), 14.
19. D. Raths, "Managing Your Three-Ring Circus: The Role of Project Manager is Complex and Risky, but Getting a Grip on Your Staff and Project Processes Can Help Ensure Success," *InfoWorld* (13 March 2000), 93.
20. S. Steinacher, "Organized Data Boosts Corporate IQ: Make Effective Business Decisions in Less Time by Creating a Data Warehouse," *InfoWorld* (8 November 1999), 65.
21. S. L. Roberts-Witt, "Knowledge Management: Know What You Know," *PC Magazine* (1 July 2000), 165.
22. S. Biafore, "Predictive Solutions Bring More Power to Decision Makers," *Health Management Technology* (November 1999), 12.
23. B. H. Waldo, "Decision Support and Data Warehousing Tools Boost Competitive Advantage," *Nursing Economics* (March–April 1998), 91–93.
24. A. H. Rosenstein, "Inpatient Clinical Decision-Support Systems Determining the ROI," *Healthcare Financial Management* (February 1999), 51(5).
25. V. L. Sauter, "Intuitive Decision-Making," *Communications of the ACM* (June 1999), 109.
26. S. Biafore, op. cit.
27. R. L. Simpson, "What Good are Advanced Practitioners if Nobody at the Top Knows Their Value?" *Nursing Administration Quarterly* (summer 1997), 91(2).
28. D. Huber, L. Schumacher, and C. Delaney, "Nursing Management Minimum Data Set (NMMDS)," *Journal of Nursing Administration* (April 1997), 42–48.

29. J. E. Robinette and P. S. Weitzel, "Design and Development of a Computerized Education Records System," *Journal of Continuing Education in Nursing* (July–August 1989), 174–182.

30. C. A. Romano, "Privacy, Confidentiality, and Security of Computerized Systems," *Computers in Nursing* (May–June 1987), 99–104.

31. L. K. Woolery, "Professional Standards and Ethical Dilemmas in Nursing Information Systems," *Journal of Nursing Administration* (October 1990), 50–53.

32. P. Iyer, "Computer Charting: Minimizing Legal Risks," *Nursing* (May 1993), 86.

REFERENCES

Amadio, J. "Share and Share Alike." *Entrepreneur* (February 2000), 59.

Andrieu, M. "A Better Future for Work?" *OECD Observer* (summer 1999), 53.

Baxter, B. "Exploring Newsgroups." *Nursing* (February 1997), 26(1).

Braue, D. "Network Your Business." *Australian PC World* (April 1998), 72(5)

Brekka, T. "Select Mobile Computers Tailored to Healthcare Environment." *Health Management Technology* (December 1995), 48(2).

Chernicoff, D. P. "Networking History in a Nutshell." *PC Week* (12 September 1994), 12(4).

Cini, A. "The Networking Bowl." *Digital Age* (March 1996), 22(6).

Craft, N. "No Touch Technique." *British Medical Journal* (3 February 1996), 318(2).

Dash, J. "Users Take Cautious Approach to 'E-Health'." *Computerworld* (17 April 2000), 10(1).

Domrose, C. "Virtual Nurse: The Internet is Expanding Health Care Possibilities." *HealthWeek* (24 January 2000), 16.

Hayes, F. "100 Years of IT." *Computerworld* (5 April 1999), 74(1).

Howe, D. *The Free On-line Dictionary of Computing* (2000).

Kilgore, C. "Movement Toward Internet-Based Patient Records." *Family Practice News* (15 January 2000), 65.

Moschella, D. "Ten Turning Points in the IT Industry's History." *Computerworld* (13 December 1999), 33(1).

Muehleman, F. "Computer Firsts Paved Way Long Before PC Became PC." *Triangle Business Journal* (22 October 1999), 41.

Rowh, M. "Casting Your Net." *Office Systems* 99 (August 1999), 11(1).

Sanborn, S. "Internet Milestones." *InfoWorld* (4 October 1999), 34.

Satava, R. "Emerging Technologies for Surgery in the 21st Century." *Archives of Surgery* (November 1999), 1197–202.

Stevens, L. "Health Care Turns to the Web." *InternetWeek* (1 May 2000), 33–37.

Telingator, S. "Merging Healthcare and the Internet in the New Century." *Health Management Technology* (April 2000), 42.

Vetter, R., and Kroeker, K. L. "The Internet in the Year Ahead." *Computer* (January 1998), 143(2).

APPENDIX 21-1
Example of an Employee Education Report

ABEND: Abnormal end of task.

Algorithm: A prescribed set of rules for the solution of a problem in a finite number of steps.

Artificial intelligence: The capability of a machine that can proceed or perform functions that are normally concerned with human intelligence, such as learning, adapting, reasoning, self-correction, and automatic improvement.

Batch processing: A system that takes a set of jobs from disk, executes them, and returns the results to disk, all without human intervention. Can be scheduled and executed at a later date and time.

Binary: The number system based on the 2 choices of 0 and 1.

Bit: The smallest unit of data, a binary digit of 0 or 1.

Buffer: Intermediate storage, used in input/output operations to temporarily hold data/information.

Bug: A mistake or error in a computer program.

Byte: A set of eight adjoining bits thought of as a unit.

Cache: A storage buffer that contains frequently accessed instructions and data.

Central processing unit (CPU): The part of the computer that controls all of the other parts. It consists of a control unit, an arithmetic and logic unit, and memory (registers and cache).

Character: A letter, digit, or other symbol that is used as part of the representation of data. A byte.

Compact disc (CD): A type of disk storage that uses magneto-optical recording and lasers.

CRT (cathode ray tube): Cathode ray terminal. A display terminal used as an input/output station.

Data: A representation of numbers or characters in the form suitable for processing by a computer.

Database: A collection of files or tables.

Database management system: A specialized type of software used for the organization, storage, and retrieval of data in a database.

Disk: Disc. Round, flat magnetic media used for the storage of data.

(continued)

Downtime: The elapsed time when a computer is not available for use. It may be scheduled for maintenance or unscheduled because of machine or program problems.

Expert system: An application that contains a knowledge base and a set of algorithms or rules that have been derived from human expertise to provide assistance in decision-making.

Extranet: An extension of an organization's intranet, over the Internet, enabling communication between the institution and people it deals with.

Field: A unit of data within a record.

File: A collection of related data with a given structure.

Forecasting: Predicting the future by an analysis of data.

GUI (graphical user interface): A user interface to a computer based on graphics.

Hardcopy: Printed computer output in the form of reports and documents.

Hardware: The physical computer equipment.

Information systems: Computer systems designed to store and manipulate information for communication and decision support.

Input/Output (I/O): The transfer of data between an external source and internal storage.

Interface: The point at which independent systems or computers interact.

Internet: A worldwide network of computer networks that use the TCP/IP network protocols to facilitate data transmission and exchange.

Intranet: A privately maintained computer network that can be accessed only by authorized persons, especially members or employees of the organization that owns it.

Key: A field or fields within a record that make that record unique with respect to other records in a file.

Kilobyte (KB): 1,024 bytes.

Local area network (LAN): Two or more computers connected for local resource sharing.

Mainframe computer: A large computer capable of being used and interacted with by hundreds of users, seemingly simultaneously.

Megabyte (MB): 1,024 kilobytes.

Microcomputer: A small computer built around a microprocessor.

Minicomputer: A mid-size computer that is smaller and less powerful than a mainframe but larger and more powerful than a microcomputer.

Modeling: A representation of a complex system used as a basis for simulation to allow for the prediction and understanding of its behavior.

Modem: A device that converts digital data from a computer to an analog signal that can be transmitted on a telecommunications line and that converts received analog transmissions to digital data.

Multimedia: The combination of different elements of media, such as text, graphics, audio, video, animation, and sound.

Multitasking: A mode of operation that provides for the concurrent execution of two or more tasks.

Online processing: A system that provides for the immediate, interactive input and processing of data at that time.

Operating system: Software designed to control the hardware of a specific computer system to allow users and application programs to utilize it.

Printer: A terminal or peripheral that produces hard copy or printed output.

Program: A set of computer instruction directing the computer to perform some operation.

Random access: A storage technique whereby a file can be addressed and accessed directly at its location on the media, or a record can be addressed and accessed directly within a file.

Record: A group of related fields of data treated as a unit.

Robotics: The science or study of mechanical devices designed to perform tasks that might be otherwise done by humans.

(continued)

Sequential access: A storage technique whereby a file can be addressed and accessed only after all those before it on the media have been, or a record can be addressed and accessed only after all those before it in the file have been.

Simulation: Attempting to predict aspects of the behavior of some system by creating an approximate model of it.

Software: A program or set of programs written to tell the computer hardware how to do something.

Spread sheet: A specialized type of software for manipulation of numbers.

Table: A collection of related records in a database management system.

Trend: A systematic pattern of change over time.

User-friendly: Software considered easier to use for novices.

Voice communication: Interaction with a computer by voice recognition.

Word processor: A specialized type of software for the manipulation of words to produce printed material.

CHAPTER 22

The Nurse Manager of Staff Development

Nancy C. McDonald, EdD, RN
DISTINGUISHED TEACHING PROFESSOR
SCHOOL OF NURSING
AUBURN UNIVERSITY AT MONTGOMERY
MONTGOMERY, AL

Nursing students and nurses are adults whose learning is based on principles of adult learning embodying critical thinking.

LEARNING OBJECTIVES AND ACTIVITIES

- Distinguish among the characteristics of the adult learner.
- Explain the staff development process.
- Describe an andragogical approach to program design.
- Differentiate among the characteristics of learning.
- Describe the role of the teacher in adult education.
- Describe the role of the learner in adult education.
- Use evaluation procedures in adult education.
- Apply the Critical Thinking-Learning Model in staff development.

CONCEPTS: Staff development, andragogy, Critical Thinking-Learning Model of staff development, facilitator, evaluation.

MANAGER BEHAVIOR: Maintains a staff development staff to meet the legal and accreditation requirements for personnel competency.

LEADER BEHAVIOR: Assesses learning needs of nursing staff and implements the Critical Thinking-Learning Model of staff development.

Introduction

Staff development educators are challenged to provide creative and consistent high-quality education to adult learners who practice nursing in an environment of rapid advances in technology, budget constraints, and sophisticated performance improvement techniques.[1] Nurse managers frequently perform the staff development role, sometimes as director of nursing in a small health care organization, perhaps as a nurse manager, or from other management positions.

Staff development is based on a philosophy of adult education that uses teaching-learning principles and concepts that apply to people who have a combination of responsibilities, including family and financial obligations, employment commitment, and identified areas of interest or specialization. Nurses are adult learners who combine many of these traditional adult responsibilities with the demands of increasingly complex societal and health care provider roles.

Philosophy of Adult Education

Staff development programs are designed to motivate adult learners to consider the learning process as a natural part of living. People are born into society devoid of knowledge. From the day they are born until the day they die, they are part of a society whose institutions are constantly changing. People are capable of learning during this entire life span. Cross believes that "Lifelong learning means self-directed growth. It means acquiring new skills and powers—the only true wealth which you can never lose. It means investment in yourself. Lifelong learning means the joy of discovering how something really works, the delight of becoming aware of some new beauty in the world, the fun of creating something, alone or with other people."[2]

Lifelong learning is essential in nursing because of the rapid changes in the health care delivery system and the changing roles of nursing within that system. Knowledge acquired in basic nursing education programs quickly becomes obsolete. Nursing is influenced by public policy, technology, and societal and economic changes.

Technology, which continually increases in complexity and scope, is a major force motivating nurses to pursue lifelong learning. Nurses must adjust quickly to the demands associated with high-tech skills in many areas. Effective staff development programs respond to the needs of nurses practicing under increased demands.

Educators and nurse managers planning staff development programs consider that nurses also have lifelong learning needs related to the processes of physical, cultural, political, and spiritual maturation. One of the weaknesses of staff development programs has been their narrow emphasis on the major field of study. Continuing education that focuses on education of the whole person will promote the development of free, creative, and responsible nursing personnel.

Staff development programs to educate the whole person are aimed at building competencies for performing various roles in life, which were identified by Malcolm Knowles (1978) in his classic work as friend, citizen, individual (self), family member, worker, and leisure-time user.[3] For example, nurses are adult citizens of the communities in which they live. It is appropriate that educational systems provide them with skills to enhance their participation in social institutions and assist in the assumption of responsibilities, rights, and privileges within their communities and larger social-political structures.

Motivation may be seen as the energy that causes adults to strive toward competence in matters that they hold to be important. A common culture is created when the staff development educator values and engages the needs of adults. "Adult learners have never been more diverse and we as teachers must be attuned to the influence of diversity and culture on motivation and hence on learning."[4]

The Staff Development Process

Staff development offerings focus on developing nursing skills and knowledge within a comprehensive program that includes orientation, in-service education, continuing education programs, and job-related counseling. Orientation introduces employees to new situations and includes content related to philosophies, goals, policies, procedures, personnel benefits, role expectations, and physical facilities. Employees need orientation each time their roles change.

Staff development also includes job-related counseling, which involves promoting the professional growth of employees by assisting them to deliver their best job performance. Counseling also includes promotion possibilities and assistance in obtaining formal training.

In-service education provides learning experiences in the work setting for the purpose of refining and developing new skills and knowledge related to job performance. These learning experiences usually are narrow in scope and brief because they are aimed at only one competency or knowledge area.

A learning experience might be developed to introduce nursing staff in cardiac care to a new, more sophisticated monitoring device.

Continuing education programs are planned and organized around learning experiences in a variety of settings that are intended to build on the educational and experiential bases of the nurse. Continuing education offerings often give nurses new approaches to health care delivery and enhance practice, education, administration, research, and theory development.[5] Examples include workshops, conferences, self-learning modules, and seminars.

Philosophy

The organization needs a statement of beliefs about how it will accomplish its staff development program. The staff development philosophy should relate to the mission and philosophy of the organization of which it is a part. The statement of philosophy should be written by a representative group, not by an individual, and be accepted by staff and administrators.

In writing a philosophy for staff development for health care professionals, the group needs to address its beliefs with regard to the following areas:

1. How learning takes place
2. Teaching methods
3. Employees' responsibility for their own learning
4. Organizational responsibility for providing staff development
5. Clients' right to health care

Exhibit 22-1 is an example of a staff development statement of philosophy.

Organization

A staff development program can function under many organizational models, depending on the philosophy of the agency. A centralized model would have an agencywide staff development department, and the educational staff might consist of nurses or educators who are not nurses. In this model, all departments collaborate in determining and planning the job needs of their staff. The centralized model facilitates scheduling and use of equipment and may prevent duplication of effort. The

> **EXHIBIT 22-1**
> **Department of Nursing Service Staff Development**
>
> **PHILOSOPHY**
>
> The philosophy of Staff Development is in agreement with the philosophy of the Department of Nursing Service.
>
> We recognize that quality health care depends to a large degree on the knowledge, skills, attitudes, and activities of practicing health care personnel. An effective Staff Development program is necessary to assist nursing personnel to maintain and improve competency as new knowledge, technology, and environmental changes continue to emerge.
>
> We believe that the responsibility for identifying learning needs, providing opportunities for meeting these needs, and evaluating the effectiveness of learning activities lies not only with the learner but also with Nursing Service Administration. The Department of Staff Development should provide support services in assisting the staff in becoming more knowledgeable and competent in fulfilling role expectations.
>
> Staff Development supports decentralization of education programs. We acknowledge that the development of personnel is best accomplished through the provision of informal as well as formal learning opportunities. Individual competencies and expertise should be utilized in educational programs. The development and implementation of programs may be carried out by, or in collaboration with, nursing staff clinicians whenever possible.
>
> We believe that education is a continuous process that begins with graduation and entry into practice. We recognize that much adult learning involves changes in attitudes and self-image and assisting the learner to accept change and be a change agent. We believe that Staff Development should strive to inculcate nursing personnel with an awareness of the commitment to and value of continuous learning, professional accountability, and professional involvement.
>
> November 200x
> Revised November 200x
> Revised November 200x

Source: Courtesy of the University of South Alabama Medical Center, Mobile, AL.

main criticism of this model is separation of educational staff from nursing staff and perpetuation of the us-against-them attitude.

In a decentralized model, the nursing department has its own organized in-service or staff development department. The nursing staff development department may then adopt a centralized or decentralized model. The strength of a decentralized model is that the specific needs identified by an area can be addressed. The major areas of concern in decentralization are the use and scheduling of classrooms, potential duplication of effort, and the cost of providing multiple small programs.

There is a trend toward decentralization of as many functions as possible in health care organizations.

Personnel

Nursing service administrators are responsible for staff development to promote quality client care. The following are among their responsibilities:

- Providing financial and human resources.
- Establishing policies for staff development.
- Providing release time, finances, or both for staff to attend continuing education offerings.
- Motivating employees to assume responsibility for their own professional development.
- Providing mechanisms to identify staff growth needs.
- Evaluating the effects of staff participation in continuing education offerings on quality of client care.

The staff development coordinator is an administrator and a teacher who is able to communicate and establish trust, has knowledge and skills in adult education, has knowledge of training resources and subject matter, and understands the program planning process. As an administrator, the coordinator understands organizational theory and has skills in budgeting, personnel management, and group process. As a teacher, the coordinator has educational skills in diagnosing learning needs, developing learning objectives and lesson plans, and selecting and using appropriate teaching techniques.

The professional development staff is selected by the coordinator to work on planning, implementing, and evaluating staff development programs. The size of the staff depends on the size of the agency. In small agencies the coordinator may be the only staff member. These personnel may be totally decentralized to the unit level. Having support staff who are qualified and in adequate numbers is essential for effective staff development.

Advisory Committees

An advisory committee can be useful for identifying needs and resources and for planning programs. Members of the committee should represent all fields of practice in the agency. Other members may include people with needed expertise. Committee members may increase participation because they can communicate the purpose of staff development programs directly to the people they represent.

Budgets

The staff development coordinator is responsible for developing and implementing the budget with input from staff. The amount of monies allocated for staff development depends on staff size, the number of new employees that may be anticipated, and the resources that are already in existence. The agency administration will demonstrate a commitment to staff development by allocating adequate funds for salaries, staff time for training, periodicals, books, software, audiovisuals, and outside educational resources.

Andragogical Approach to Program Design

The characteristics of adult learners require an andragogical approach to curricular development and teaching in staff development programs. *Andragogy* is the art and science of helping adults learn, in contrast to *pedagogy*, the teaching of children. The andragogical approach assumes that the learners themselves are the facilitators who create a climate that motivates their own achievement.[6]

When staff development programs are designed for nurses, the shift from the traditional teacher-centered approach, in which the focus is on information-giving and the teacher, to a student-centered approach, in which the focus is on active learning and the student, requires a fundamental change in the role of the teacher. The *didactic* (information-giving) teacher is replaced by a facilitator of learning, and the creation of an environment for student learning becomes the new prerequisite. These changes have major implications in terms of staff development, recognizing that this environment is unlikely to be effective if teachers are not able to take on new roles.[7]

The flexibility or level of structure is also important in program design. Cavanagh suggested that tightly structured training programs are incongruent with an andragogical approach. Basic learning principles of cardiopulmonary resuscitation programs are examined in this study, with findings that showed a rapid loss of practical skills and knowledge after these highly structured training programs.[8]

It is evident that traditional pedagogical approaches to staff development are less effective than is an individual approach based on professional career development.[9] However, programs that teach highly specialized, concrete skills tend to use a more pedagogical approach than do programs that emphasize intellectual exploration. This tendency may need to be addressed in the early planning phase of program design and by putting compensatory measures in place.

Mutual Diagnosis of Needs

Effective staff development programs begin with a needs assessment of the learners.

> **A common mistake of staff development planners is to assume they know what adults need to learn. This assumption may lead to an unsuccessful educational program.**

Adults are interested and motivated when they enter educational programs because of perceived needs they have identified. Adult learners have a perception of the level of competency they want to achieve and the knowledge they need for better performance in their personal lives or work settings. If adult learners' needs differ from those perceived by staff development planners, participation in the educational offerings will be decreased or nonexistent. A training program is a waste of time and money if it does not increase the efficiency and effectiveness of workers.[10] As a result, educational needs assessment is the first step in adult education programming.

Needs Assessment Methods

Staff development planners decide on a method of assessment that will meet their purposes. The following factors should be considered before designing a needs assessment survey:

1. Target population
2. Development time
3. Cost
4. Financial and human resources
5. Analysis time
6. Anonymity
7. Objectivity

The needs survey should address content, design of learning activities, and learners' background. Content relates to the specific topics of interest to the learners. Design of learning activities covers areas such as planning when individuals can attend courses and the types of learning options (such as workshops or modules) that would best facilitate their learning.[11]

When considering a method of assessment, it is important to address the needs of the organization and learner. Organizational needs are influenced by factors such as the standards of the Joint Commission for Accreditation of Healthcare Organizations (JCAHO), the American Nurses Association (ANA) Standards for Continuing Education, consumer needs, standards of practice, and the philosophy and objectives of the institution. If staff developers ignore these needs, they may lose the support of the sponsoring organization.

Questionnaire or Survey

A questionnaire is perhaps the most frequently used method for assessing needs. Questions on the survey tool may be either forced choice, which allows selection of one of several categories of context needs, or open-ended, which allows more freedom of response. An example of an open-ended question is: "If I could learn more about stress management, I would like to learn. . . ." The survey tool should be designed with a combination of the two types of questions.

A pilot test of the survey is done to ensure that questions are clear and that the data gathered are complete and relevant. Individuals completing the pilot survey are asked to comment on whether they understood the questions, how long it took them to complete the questionnaire, and whether other areas should be added. Their responses are then analyzed by a group and necessary changes made to the questionnaire.

The advantages of the questionnaire include ease and convenience of administration and ease of computing the results. Disadvantages include the cost of data collection and analysis. Also, if a mailed questionnaire yields a low return, the data may not result in a representative sample. Exhibit 22-2 is one example of a broad-scale questionnaire.

Observation

When used with other methods, observation is an effective way to assess needs. A nurse manager or clinical specialist can observe personnel and perhaps identify learning needs. The effectiveness of this technique is increased when a standardized observation guide is used.

EXHIBIT 22-2
Broad-Scale Questionnaire

How can Staff Development help meet your needs over the next year? Please answer the following questions. This is an anonymous survey.

Check most appropriate.

1. I am:
   - _____ a. RN
   - _____ b. LPN
   - _____ c. NA
   - _____ d. WC
2. I work in the following type of nursing area:
   - _____ a. Medical
   - _____ b. Surgical
   - _____ c. Orthopedic/Neuro
   - _____ d. Obstetrical
   - _____ e. Pediatric
   - _____ f. Neonatal
   - _____ g. Emergency room
   - _____ h. Operating room
   - _____ i. Other (specify)_____
3. I have worked in my nursing area for:
   - _____ a. less than 3 months
   - _____ b. 4 to 11 months
   - _____ c. 1 to 3 years
   - _____ d. 4 to 6 years
   - _____ e. over 6 years
4. What is the best time of day for you to attend in-service programs?
   - _____ a. mornings
   - _____ b. afternoons
   - _____ c. evenings
5. What is the best day for you to attend in-service programs?
   - _____ a. Monday
   - _____ b. Tuesday
   - _____ c. Wednesday
   - _____ d. Thursday
   - _____ e. Friday
   - _____ f. Saturday

Circle the most appropriate response, according to your interest, for the following in-service education programs:

4 = I am highly interested.
3 = I am interested.
2 = I am somewhat interested.
1 = I have no opinion or don't know.
0 = I have no interest.

6. 4 3 2 1 0   Respiratory care

7. 4 3 2 1 0   Wound management

8. 4 3 2 1 0   Stress management

9. 4 3 2 1 0   Nursing and the law

10. 4 3 2 1 0   Communication skills

11. 4 3 2 1 0   Nursing process

12. 4 3 2 1 0   Use of computers in nursing

13. 4 3 2 1 0   Death and dying

14. 4 3 2 1 0   Body image

15. 4 3 2 1 0   Cost care

16. What other topics would you like included in in-service education programs? _____
_____

A disadvantage of this method is that observations are subjective and can produce incomplete data. For instance, a nurse observed to be charting incorrectly may be doing so because of lack of time, not faulty knowledge of the procedure.

Interview

Interviewing of a sample representing the target population is a method that can be used to gather valuable information about needs. Interviews can clarify ambiguous data gathered through surveys. Respondents often feel more comfortable expressing feelings verbally than in writing. A disadvantage is that data collected are difficult to sort, measure, and report.

Open Group Meetings

Learning needs can be assessed in group discussions when a resource person is available with questions to focus the group on the topic. The resource person should be skilled in the group process technique so that all group members can be aided in expressing their learning needs clearly. This method can be time-consuming and of limited value if group members are hesitant about speaking out.

Analysis of Professional Literature

A systematic review of the previous 6 to 12 months of pertinent journals is an excellent means to identify trends and compare national information with the leader's own setting. This method is inexpensive and can be present- or future-oriented. On the negative side, a review of literature is time-consuming because it involves analyzing and synthesizing many articles to find trends. Also, a time lag is involved in publication.

Competency Model

A competency model is a valuable means for discovering the needs of an individual. In building a competency model, a series of statements are developed that identify expected performance or behavior. After the competencies are refined to small units that reflect only single behaviors, individuals can then compare their performance with each behavior. Staff developers can help individuals identify gaps between their level of competency and the desired level. Individuals can then participate in learning activities to close the gaps.

Employee Performance Appraisals

The performance appraisal can be an effective method for identifying needs if done in a positive way. Appraisals should avoid confrontation, be meaningful instead of demeaning, and be a worthwhile activity that develops staff. People should be encouraged to state their own hopes and aspirations and identify their learning needs. The rater and the ratee have a clear picture of duties and demands of the job and current abilities and level of performance. The rater and ratee then identify gaps between the desired and the actual levels of performance. Staff development programs are then designed to improve performance or prepare the employee for a new position.

Mutual Planning

Once needs are identified and priorities set, appropriate learning experiences are designed. Adult learners are able to help plan the educational offerings. Professional nurses are more committed to an activity when they have been involved in the decision-making process. Nurses see themselves as self-directed and may resist a staff development program that is imposed on them by the establishment. A committee that represents all subgroups is one mechanism for mutual planning. The nursing service administrator or the education coordinator is responsible for appointing the planning committee.

Translating Learning Needs into Goals

The planning committee should be involved in setting goals for the learning experience. Because developing goals is often a difficult part of the planning process, the staff development director will assist the committee.

Goals provide intent and direction for movement.[12] Goals are important in providing a basis for planning learning activities, selecting methods and materials, and defining and organizing content. For goals to serve as workable tools, certain guidelines should be followed:

- Goals should be centered on the learner, not the teacher. For example, "The student will understand selected concepts of shock," should replace "The instructor will present selected concepts of shock."
- Goals do not dictate specificity but may simply indicate a general aim. Goals may be inexact and imprecise as long as intent is provided.
- One overall goal may be sufficient for a training program if it is stated broadly. For example, an appropriate goal for a program on care of patients with gastrostomy tubes could be: "The learner will employ care and critical thinking in addressing specific human needs of the patient and family dealing with a gastrostomy tube."

Critical Thinking-Learning Model

A model for teaching adult learners that emphasizes collaboration between teacher and learner was developed by McDonald. The conceptual basis for this model, called the Critical Thinking-Learning Model, is an open system of simultaneous interaction between teacher, learner, and the teaching-learning environment. (See Exhibit 22-3.) The model shows the continual influence of each component on all other components, even when no overt interaction is taking place. This model represents a departure from the linear interaction of traditional teaching in which response from the student occurs as a result of stimulus from the teacher. The Critical Thinking-Learning Model shows a balance of influence from all components, with no single component dominating the exchange. Core elements are considered central to each component and are necessary for the outcome of critical thinking to occur. Each component contains five basic characteristics, as seen in Exhibit 22-4.

Teaching-Learning Environment

The core element in the teaching-learning environment is dialogical. This concept places the process of dialogue as the central focus in the classroom as opposed to the traditional lecture method. (See Exhibit 22-5.) To arrive at the desired outcome of critical thinking, students must be able to relate their new ideas and experiences to previous knowledge. Students must be able to share, justify, and validate their new understanding. Dialogue implies a struggle for insight into possible alternatives and a consideration of new perspectives. The development of critical thinking involves the acting on and sharing of knowledge through discourse. This rational process takes place in the creative and unpredictable environment that occurs with dialogic classes.[13]

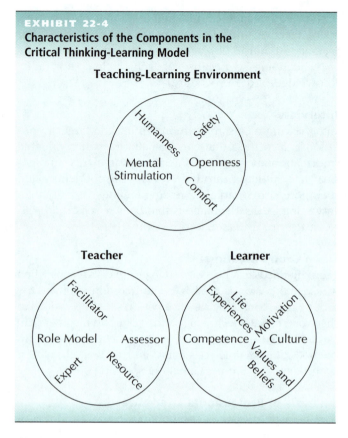

EXHIBIT 22-4

Characteristics of the Components in the Critical Thinking-Learning Model

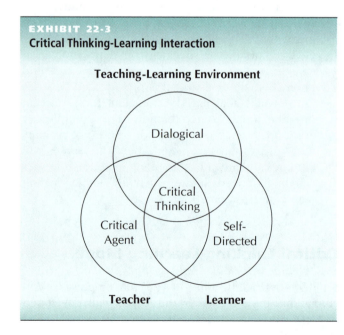

EXHIBIT 22-3

Critical Thinking-Learning Interaction

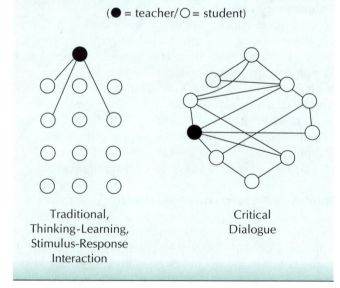

EXHIBIT 22-5

Comparison of Traditional, Stimulus-Response Interaction, and Critical Dialogue

Source: Created by Nancy McDonald for research study, "The Measurement of Selected Aspects of Critical Thinking."

Five characteristics are necessary for the provision of a teaching-learning environment that supports the process of critical thinking and learning: comfort, openness, mental stimulation, safety, and humanness.

Comfort

When a working adult student arrives at class to participate in learning activities, demanding work schedules and responsibilities are already surrounding the learning experience. The teacher must take into consideration factors such as fatigue and distraction, or simply the role change that accompanies adult learners to the classroom. An environment that provides for comfort is a first step in promoting collaboration between teacher and student.

Comfortable seating, good lighting, access to beverages, and thermostat control can make a difference between actively attending to learning activities and simply enduring a class session. This attention to environmental factors is particularly applicable in the longer class sessions that are typical of programs structured for adult learners.

Openness

Establishment of a community in the classroom creates free and open interaction between teacher and student. A circular seating arrangement for students and teacher promotes a nonlinear sharing of power. The dialogue that is central to critical thinking occurs more easily when all members of the class are visible to each other.

Activities that encourage sharing among students are appropriate at the initial class session. If students are asked to repeat other students' names and name their favorite foods and fun activities, attention is more likely to be focused away from self. The teacher should be included in this ice-breaking exercise, which offers valuable information related to the culture, background, and values of the students. The experience that each adult learner brings to the classroom can be identified during these get-acquainted exercises and used later as a resource among students.

Unique experiences and life skills can contribute to the teaching-learning process, as well as enhance the confidence of the participants.

Mental Stimulation

Classes that begin with a mental warm-up assist with the transition of adults from working professionals to students. The following activities stimulate thinking:

1. Round robin sessions in which students name things involving threes (*examples:* triangles, butcher-baker-candlestick maker, French hens).

2. Round-robin sessions in which students name things involving time (*examples:* ETA, time-out, Greenwich mean time).

3. Nine-dots experiment in which students try to draw four continuous straight lines through dots (• • •)
(• • •)
(• • •)

4. A Mensa genius quiz (*example:* Five men raced their cars on a racing strip. Will did not come in first. John was neither first or last. Joe came in one place after Will. James was not second. Walt was two places below James. In what order did the men finish?)

Involving students in problem-solving can be facilitated through the use of small groups to encourage participation from each member and provide an opportunity for students to get to know one another. Having participants form groups by counting off by twos or threes around the room separates dependent partners (all the number ones become a group, all the number twos become a group, and so on), which minimizes visiting and promotes individual involvement. Students who have not had the opportunity to talk can then engage in dialogue and learn from one another.

The infusion of humor and pleasure into the learning experience can minimize stress and stimulate learning. Humor in the classroom promotes a community atmosphere and a sense of ease and relaxation. Care should be taken to establish an environment safe from ridicule. Humor is funny only when self-esteem is not threatened.

Safety

As do all students, adult learners need to build personal confidence in classroom performance and feel comfortable as part of the group. Students are often fearful that expressing thoughts or questions might reveal inadequacies or inappropriate thinking. A technique helpful in reducing this fear or discomfort is to have each student respond to a specific concept by writing the answer and then sharing the answer with a classmate. Working in pairs initially enables students to test ideas and questions, modify responses, and develop confidence before interacting with the larger group. Pairing each student with a different classmate for several of these exercises establishes a known support base and provides a network with other students.

An environment that is safe and nonthreatening is essential to the development of critical thinking. The response of the teacher to each student and to the group must convey respect, caring, and support. A student who fears reprisal, humiliation, or embarrassment will be unlikely to voice opinions or engage in dialogue. Adult learners are often fearful of the unknown and are usually eager to establish credibility and make a good impression.

The learning environment must be supportive of the efforts of adults while providing an atmosphere that supports humor and enjoyment of the learning experience.

Humanness

A person-centered approach to the teaching-learning process means emphasizing the competence of the learners. Teachers who are not afraid to show that they are human value each student's personal choice, responsibility, and contribution to the process of learning. Humanness pervades all interactions within the teaching-learning environment. Human qualities that are essential for the teacher to possess include valuing the student as a fellow human being, regardless of the quality or quantity of classwork; trusting the student to engage in self-discovery; being genuine in responses and interactions; and offering empathic understanding.

The Learner

Self-direction is the core element for the learner in the Critical Thinking-Learning Model. The element of self-direction is intimately related to critical thinking and must be present for the student to be a critical thinker. Responsibility for the internal process of cognition rests with the learner and is a precondition for the development of understanding and knowledge. Each learner who participates in the critical thinking-learning process brings life experiences, competence, motivation, culture, and values and beliefs to the educational experience.[14]

Life Experiences

Adult learners are individuals who have accumulated experience, skills, and wisdom through the process of living. These students are not as malleable as are 20-year-olds and may be more resistant to change. In the Critical Thinking-Learning Model, reciprocal interaction occurs in a continuous process in which the teacher learns from the student and vice versa. Life experiences of adult students are a valuable resource for the teaching-learning process. Teachers who recognize and use this resource enrich the process and help build the self-esteem of the learners.

Competence

The educator of adults who subscribes to the concept of critical thinking and learning must assume that each student is competent to engage in active learning, unless individual performance over time proves otherwise.

Creative thinking is an inherent characteristic of human beings, but it may have been suppressed by rigid and punitive methods encountered in previous educational experiences. Development of competence to assume individual responsibility for learning may be necessary before students can become responsible for personal learning. The teacher should challenge the tendencies toward convergent thinking, give positive feedback for risk taking or creative thinking, and encourage consideration of alternative solutions.

Brainstorming is a process that develops competence in self-discovery and critical thinking. No response generated during the exercise of brainstorming can be seen as incorrect, no viewpoint or statement must be justified, and all members of the group are given the opportunity to participate. This process frees students from censoring others' or their own responses. Divergent rather than convergent thinking is encouraged by rewarding uninhibited and outrageous thinking.

Strategies such as brainstorming encourage and release the competence for active learning that is present in the nature of human beings.

Motivation

Adult learners return to the classroom for various reasons. Identifying these motivators can help the learner develop and maintain the initiative needed to engage in critical thinking activities. Insight into intrinsic and extrinsic aspects of motivation to learn can promote integration of new ideas and highlight the approaches best suited for the exploration of these ideas. Understanding individual motivators can enable teacher and student to anticipate and adjust to the stress and anxiety that may accompany new learning experiences.

Styles of learning can be diagnosed through tools and measurement scales such as those previously described. Students who can understand personal methods of learning are more able to choose approaches that facilitate critical thinking-learning. Preferences, habits, and aptitudes of each student ideally should be identified to enable teacher and students to select effective strategies for learning.

Culture

The cultural background is the basis for many of the assumptions, values, and beliefs held by an individual. Political stances, life choices, and much of behavior in general are grounded in the time and place of birth and maturation. During the process of becoming aware of personal choices, students must examine the scripts inherited from acculturation.

Students may experience for the first time the basis of personal choices when engaging in critical thinking-learning. In this process, students question and challenge rules that have governed past actions. The disruption and discomfort that result from this process are part of the examination of previously held assumptions.

The open interchange of the Critical Thinking-Learning Model indicates that self-directed learning includes the learner's right to challenge both the teacher's assumptions and the learner's personal assumptions. This interchange should never be conducted in an autocratic or intimidating manner by teacher or by student.

When familiar assumptions, such as those resulting from cultural influence, are the launching point for the critical thinking-learning process, students are able to respond specifically and with familiarity. Easily identifiable areas of questioning will be more readily broached than are sophisticated or complicated conceptual areas.

Values and Beliefs

Many individuals believe that absolute truths exist, and some individuals are certain of what these truths are. The emotional responses that result from challenging personal values and beliefs may be difficult for individual students, the group, and the facilitator or teacher. An environment of safety, trust, and caring must exist for adult learners to engage in critical thinking-learning related to personal commitments.

As with all groups of people, the classroom will have individuals who are more developed or mature and who more readily exhibit skepticism, analysis, and divergent thinking. Those students who have not yet reached this level of self-discovery cannot be forced into using imaginative thought. The teacher of adults can only support, challenge, and offer alternatives to those learners who are resistant to the process. Acceptance of the values and beliefs of others must be role-modeled by the teacher, who continues to offer ways to achieve self-insight into students' values and beliefs.

The Teacher

The teacher is the catalyst for the process of critical thinking-learning and must function as a critical agent to provide diversity of thinking, disagreement, and the challenging ideas in the classroom. In leading students toward critical thinking, the teacher must engage in activities that identify and challenge students' assumptions and assist them in imagining and exploring alternatives. Unnecessary criticism and unrealistic utopianism must be avoided.[15]

Facilitator

Effective listening skills are crucial to the collaborative process between student and teacher in the Critical Thinking-Learning Model. Attention to body language and nonverbal communication is as important as is attending to the spoken interchanges among fellow students and between student and teacher. Effective listening assists students in clarifying concepts and problem-solving. Responding specifically and thoughtfully to a student's viewpoint indicates that the teacher values that individual, which enhances the individual's self-esteem.

Learning can be facilitated through specific classroom activities, such as the use of case studies, team learning, or role playing. Case studies can be developed by students whose life experiences apply to the concepts being studied. Dialogue then involves the entire class in examining and analyzing the application of the case study to class content.

Team learning is a process using groups of students who are assigned specific areas of content and then share the concepts with the class. Assignments can be made sufficiently in advance to allow the teams to plan and organize the presentation. All students are given the opportunity to contribute knowledge and expertise. This exercise also develops cooperative work and leadership abilities.

Role playing involves assigning a subject or content to be studied and acted out. Several students can participate as a group in the center of a circle of classmates. Observers may chart the interaction of role players, then participate in an assessment and discussion at the conclusion of the activity to provide learning and feedback.

Role Model

One of the most common means of learning throughout life is by role modeling. Educators of students of all ages are aware of the influence exerted by behavior and of the importance of demonstrating positive qualities in the teaching-learning environment.

In the application of critical thinking to role modeling, positive behaviors demonstrated by the teacher include encouraging criticism of their actions, refusing to evade difficult questions, and being flexible in changing requirements or behaviors as a result of student input.

Resource

The role of teacher as resource begins with the collaboration process in which learning projects and contracts are identified in the learning environment. Once goals are established, the teacher serves as a resource and then guides the student toward other resources appropriate for achievement of these goals. Student learning styles can be used as a basis for selecting human and other resources, as well as methods to promote goal achievement. Emphasis should be placed on adjusting resource selection to meet individual strengths and weaknesses.

Resources for personal communication include friends, faculty, other students, and experts in the area to be examined. Professional journals, textbooks, videotapes, and cassettes are also available as resources. Teachers should guide students toward appropriate methods for achievement of goals while individualizing resources for the learning environment. Methods for meeting goals range from random approaches to trial-and-error methods and from sequential to structured approaches. Management plans are often useful in assisting students to map goals, presentations, and resources or for simply organizing time.

Expert

Lecture is rarely used in the Critical Thinking-Learning Model, but if deemed necessary by the teacher, it can be appropriate if limited to time frames of 10 to 20 minutes. Lecturing frees students from active learning and, if lengthy, is not assimilated. Activities that promote student involvement in the learning process are crucial to critical thinking. The teacher as expert in the teaching-learning process uses methods to minimize passivity and promote activity in the learning process.

Assessor

A needs assessment conducted at the first class session provides information related to the classroom. Students are also given the opportunity at this time to recognize and appreciate the knowledge they and their fellow students bring to the learning experience. The teacher in the role of assessor may then explore ways to use student expertise for teaching-learning.

The motivation or willingness to learn is an area that the teacher must address in the role of assessor. When the adult learner has already identified the need to learn, goal achievement is more likely to occur. Motivation may be intrinsic or extrinsic. When the student engages in learning for the sake of learning, motivation is intrinsic or occurs for personal motives. Extrinsic motivation is based on external, or social, motives and occurs when the student engages in learning for other personal reasons.

During evaluation procedures, the teacher functions as assessor, although the role may be simplified if grade contracts are used. Students and teacher may collaborate to set standards of evaluation or may also evaluate the abilities of students against set criteria. Self-analysis is another method of evaluation that students may use to assess goal achievement. Targeting areas and expertise that need developing or improving should follow assessment by teacher and students.

Teaching Methods

To maximize learning, staff should be aware of three important aspects involved in teaching adult learners.

1. Collaboration between teacher and student is essential for active learning to occur. Learning should be a shared activity in which teacher and students have responsibilities. Learning is more apt to take place when students are active participants. Teaching as a collaborative effort may be viewed as negotiating meaning rather than imparting ready-made knowledge.

2. Critical thinking may be seen as a basic principle of adult education. This process is one of logical reasoning that involves the recognition of assumptions underlying beliefs and behaviors and justification for ideas and actions. Information should be analyzed to make sense of external experiences. Critical thinking demands comprehension. Students are conditioned to be passive when a teacher begins to lecture. Lecture should not be used as a way to challenge students' thinking. The wealth of experience brought to the classroom by adult learners can be incorporated into critical thinking activities that result in greater involvement with the learning experience.

3. Self-directed learning has an important place in the educational activities of adults. Adults have a deep need to be self-directing, which involves being able to make decisions and manage personal experiences. The teacher should determine what the student already knows and must be open about the intent to share responsibility for learning.

Evaluation Procedures

Evaluation is essential to provide staff with information to improve programs or determine whether training programs should be continued. Each course, seminar, class, or workshop is evaluated when it is completed to determine whether the program met the needs for which it was designed. Evaluation includes the learner as well as the program.

Learner Evaluation

Adult learners should have a sense of progress toward their goals and should be involved in evaluating their learning. Teachers should involve learners in developing mutually acceptable criteria and methods for measuring progress toward the learning objectives. When objectives are written in behavioral terms, the standard for evaluation is included in each objective. It can then be observed whether the knowledge, skill, attitude, or practice is accomplished.

When measuring learning, a before-and-after approach should be used so that learning can be related to the training program. When possible, learning should be measured objectively, such as by a written test. Also, when practical, a control group should be compared with the experimental group that receives the training.

Three types of techniques can be used to evaluate learning:

1. Observation of skills or behavior is often useful. Observation guides need to be developed, and observers need to be told specifically what they should be scrutinizing. Validity may be a problem if learners perform in a particular way because they are being observed or if the perception of the observer is incorrect.

2. Paper-and-pencil methods, such as true-false, multiple-choice, or fill-in-the-blank tests are frequently used. Pretesting and posttesting should be done so that comparisons can be made. For some students, tests produce anxiety, which may contribute to poor test results.

3. Unobtrusive measures, when used with other evaluation data, can be valuable. Examples of unobtrusive measures are chart reviews, audits, wear of textbook pages, or numbers of staff using self-directed learning modules.

Program Evaluation

The content, process, and method of a program offering should be evaluated. A survey or questionnaire is often used to elicit participants' reaction to the program. The following information can be obtained by a survey:

- What the participants liked or disliked about the program.
- Whether the faculty and speakers were prepared.
- Whether objectives were met.
- How well the program was organized.
- Whether the facilities were adequate.

- Suggestions for improvements.
- Suggestions for future programs.

Problems can arise when questionnaires are too long or unwieldy for the participants to complete or for the person who must tabulate them. The following guides are useful for preparing questionnaires:

- Determine what you want to find out and avoid unnecessary questions.
- Design the form so that most reactions can be tabulated by a computer.
- Make the form anonymous.
- Give participants the opportunity to make additional comments.
- Perform a pilot-test of the questionnaire on a sample target audience.

Exhibit 22-6 is an example of an evaluation questionnaire.

Summary

The purposes of staff development include the improvement of care given to clients and of participants' quality of life. Nurse managers who present successful staff development programs understand and apply principles of adult education. Staff members, as adult learners, are self-directed and want to be involved in diagnosing their learning needs, developing objectives, and evaluating their own learning. Adult learners have a wide variety of experiences on which to build new learning and are looking for experiential types of teaching techniques that allow them to share their knowledge. They want educational programs that are problem-centered and can be applied in their work or life roles.

Nurse managers as teachers in staff development programs are facilitators of learning. This role is enhanced when the educator possesses attributes such as openness, flexibility, and spontaneity.

EXHIBIT 22-6
Evaluation Questionnaire

PURPOSE
To provide feedback to program planners so presentations can be improved.
Complete the following anonymously.
Evaluation of the Burn Therapy course, August 12. Circle the number representing your feelings about each statement.

	STRONGLY DISAGREE	DISAGREE	AGREE	STRONGLY AGREE	NO OPINION
1. The content presented is applicable to my work.	1	2	3	4	5
2. The goals of the program were clear to me.	1	2	3	4	5
3. The content presented reflected the goals.	1	2	3	4	5
4. The content presented was what I expected.	1	2	3	4	5
5. The content was valuable to me.	1	2	3	4	5

EXHIBIT 22-6

	STRONGLY DISAGREE	DISAGREE	AGREE	STRONGLY AGREE	NO OPINION
6. The instructor's presentation was clear and informative.	1	2	3	4	5
7. The instructor made good use of audiovisuals.	1	2	3	4	5
8. The level of presentation was too theoretical.	1	2	3	4	5
9. The level of presentation was not practical.	1	2	3	4	5

Please respond to the following questions:

10. What were the most positive aspects of this presentation?

_____

_____

11. What did you like best about the presentation?

_____

_____

12. Please make any other comment or suggestion.

_____

_____

13. Suggestions for future presentations.

_____

_____

APPLICATION EXERCISES

EXERCISE 22-1

Staff development programs should be aimed at preparing individuals for various life roles and for maintaining competence in those roles. Identify three roles filled by nurses and give examples of staff development programs that will assist them in coping with these social roles and related tasks.

EXERCISE 22-2

Write a philosophy of staff development for your unit or organization.

EXERCISE 22-3

Staff development planners do careful needs assessments before designing programs. Locate a needs survey done in your organization.

- Is it adequate?
- How has it been used?
- What would you do to improve it?

EXERCISE 22-4 Locate the goals of two staff development programs for your unit or organization. If they are not learner-centered, change them to make them so.

EXERCISE 22-5 Design a questionnaire to evaluate an in-service or continuing education program presented in your workplace. Use it, and analyze the results.

EXERCISE 22-6 Refer to the Critical Thinking-Learning Model in this chapter. Evaluate a staff development program using this model as a standard. Analyze the results and make a management plan to correct any deficiencies.

NOTES

1. D. I. O'Very, "Self-Paced: The Right pace for Staff Development," *The Journal of Continuing Education in Nursing* (July–August 1999), 182–187.
2. K. Cross, *Adults as Learners* (San Francisco: Jossey-Bass, 1982), 16.
3. M. Knowles, *The Adult Learner: A Neglected Species*, 2nd ed. (Houston: Gulf Publishing, 1978).
4. R. J. Wlodkowski, *Enhancing Adult Motivation to Learn*, Rev. ed. (San Francisco: Jossey-Bass, 1999).
5. G. Furze and P. Pearcey, "Continuing Education in Nursing: A Review of the Literature," *Journal of Advanced Nursing*, 29(2), (1999), 355–363.
6. M. Knowles, *Andragogy in Action* (San Francisco: Jossey-Bass, 1984).
7. J. A. Spencer and K. R. Jordan, "Learner Centered Approaches in Medical Education," *British Medical Journal* (May 1999), 1280–1283.
8. S. J. Cavanagh, "Educational Aspects of Cardiopulmonary Resuscitation (CPR) Training," *Intensive Care Nursing*, 6 (1990), 38–44.
9. J. R. Beeler, P. A. Young, and S. M. Dull, "Professional Development Framework," *Journal of Nursing Staff Development* (November–December 1990), 296–301.
10. M. Moore and P. Dutton, "Training Needs Analysis," *Academy of Management Review* (July 1978), 532–545.
11. R. C. Swansburg, *Nursing Staff Development: A Component of Human Resource Development* (Boston: Jones and Bartlett, 1995).
12. J. E. Gould and E. O. Bevis, "Here There Be Dragons," *Nursing and Health Care* (March 1992), 126–133.
13. S. D. Brookfield, "Passion, Purity, and Pillage: Critical Thinking About Critical Thinking," *Adult Education Research Conference Proceedings* (Athens, GA: The University of Georgia, 1990), 25–30.
14. P. C. Candy, *Self-Direction for Lifelong Learning* (San Francisco: Jossey-Bass, 1991).
15. D. R. Garrison, "Critical Thinking and Adult Education: A Conceptual Model for Developing Critical Thinking in Adult Learners," *International Journal of Lifelong Education* (October–December 1991), 287–303.

REFERENCES

Bowen, M., K. J. Lyons, and B. E. Young. "Nursing and Health Care Reform: Implications for Curriculum Development." *Journal of Nursing Education*, 39(1), (2000), 27–33.

Facione, N. D., and P. A. Facione. "Externalizing the Critical Thinking in Knowledge Development and Clinical Judgment." *Nursing Outlook*, 44 (1996), 129–136.

Fowler, L. P. "Improving Critical Thinking in Nursing Practice." *Journal for Nurses in Staff Development*, 14(4), (1998), 183–187.

French, P., and D. Cross. "An Interpersonal-Epistemological Curriculum Model for Nurse Education." *Journal of Advanced Nursing*, 17 (1992), 83–89.

Greenwood, J. "Critical Thinking and Nursing Scripts: The Case for the Development of Both." *Journal of Advanced Nursing*, 31(2), (2000), 428–436.

Hadley, C. S. "Capitalizing on Nursing Creativity." *AWHONN Lifelines* (August–September 1999), 47–49.

Haislett, J., R. B. Hughes, G. Atkinson, and C. L. Williams. "Success in Baccalaureate Nursing Programs: A Matter of Accommodation?" *Journal of Nursing Education* (February 1993), 64–70.

Kintgen-Andrews, J. "Critical Thinking and Nursing Education: Perplexities and Insights." *Journal of Nursing Education* (April 1991), 152–157.

Lindeman, C. "A Vision for Nursing Education." *Creative Nursing*, 2(1), (1996), 5–12.

Nielsen, B. B. "Applying Andragogy in Nursing Continuing Education." *Journal of Continuing Education in Nursing* (July–August 1992), 148–151.

Maynard, C. A. "Relationship of Critical Thinking Ability to Professional Nursing Competence." *Journal of Nursing Education*, 35, 1 (1996), 12–18.

Padberg, R. M., and L. F. Padberg. "Strengthening the Effectiveness of Patient Education: Applying Principles of Adult Education." *Oncology Nursing Forum*, 17(1) (1990), 65–69.

Rew, L. "Acknowledging Intuition in Clinical Decision Making." *Journal of Holistic Nursing*, 18(2) (2000), 94–113.

CHAPTER 23

Conflict Management

Enrica Kinchen Singleton, DrPH, MBA, RN
PROFESSOR OF NURSING
SCHOOL OF NURSING
SOUTHERN UNIVERSITY AND A & M UNIVERSITY
BATON ROUGE, LA

LEARNING OBJECTIVES AND ACTIVITIES

- Analyze causes of conflict.
- Make plans to manage conflict.
- Use techniques or skills for managing conflict.

CONCEPTS: Conflict, organizational conflict, interterritorial conflict, interdisciplinary conflict, defiant behavior, conflict management, assertiveness, mediation.

MANAGER BEHAVIOR: Uses organizational policy to meet the legal requirements for mediating conflicts.

LEADER BEHAVIOR: Develops organizational policies and procedures to prevent conflict and to involve peer review in cases of protracted conflict.

Introduction

There is potential for conflict in any organization in which people interact. Health care institutions include many interacting groups: staff (professional, administrative, and ancillary) with staff, staff with physicians, staff with patients, staff with families and visitors, and so on. These interactions may lead to conflicts.

Conflict relates to human feelings, including feelings of neglect, of being viewed as taken for granted, of being treated like a servant, of not being appreciated, of being ignored, of being overloaded, and other instances of perceived unfairness. Conflict relates to ignoring an individual's self-esteem and worth. The individual's feelings may build from anger to rage. During this time, overt behaviors such as brooding, withdrawing, arguing, instigating unrest among staff, or

fighting can be observed. The individual can let feelings and behavior interfere with job performance, resulting in carelessness, mistakes in areas of responsibility, and reduced productivity for the unit of service.

An atmosphere of uncertainty in the health care environment has resulted from the rapid changes in health care, including the dismantling of the traditional structures in health care organizations, uncertainties advanced by changes in roles and role relationships among traditional health care personnel, and uncharted and evolving relationships with new categories of health care workers. Under these conditions, conflict is a certainty. *Conflict* is defined as[1]:

> An expressed struggle between at least two interdependent parties, who perceive incompatible goals, scarce rewards, interference from the other party in achieving their goals. They are in a position of opposition in conjunction with cooperation.

Causes of Conflict

Organizational Conflict

According to Barker, "organizational conflict arises because of rapid and unpredictable change, new technological advances, competition for scarce resources, differences in cultures and belief systems, and the variety of human personalities."[2] Managers need to understand the concept of conflict, its antecedents, and impact on personnel relationships, management, and resolution.

Bennis indicates that conflict in organizations is inevitable. Conflict can be destructive or useful, depending on how it is handled by the leader. Conflict derives from misinformation and misperception: one party has information that the other does not have, or the parties have different information. Bennis states that "leaders do not avoid, repress, or deny conflict, but rather see it as an opportunity. . . . They don't feel threatened, they feel challenged."[3]

Stevens indicates that the three most often cited potential sources of conflict are human shortcomings, interpersonal failure, and the nature of an organization (not the people in it)."[4] Also, individuals as well as departments often oppose one another to gain prestige, power, or resources, or to show dominance.[5]

Marriner states that conflict arises because individuals have divergent views of their own power and authority and ambiguous jurisdictions. Conflict increases with the need for consensus, the number of organizational levels, the number of specialties, an increase in the degree of associations, and increased degree of dependence of some parties on others. When separation in time and space exists, factionalism is fostered and communication barriers impede understanding. Even though policies, procedures, and rules regulate behavior, make relationships more predictable, and decrease arbitrary decisions; they impose controls over individuals that are likely to be resisted by those who value autonomy.[6]

Antecedent Sources of Conflict

Conflict may develop from a number of antecedent sources, including the following[7]:

- Incompatible goals.
- Distribution of scarce resources when individuals have high expectations of rewards.
- Regulations, when an individual's need for autonomy conflicts with another's need for regulating mechanisms.
- Personality traits, attitudes, and behaviors.
- Interest in outcomes.
- Values.
- Roles, when two individuals have equal responsibilities but actual boundaries are unclear, or when they are required to simultaneously fill two or more roles that present inconsistent or contradictory expectations.
- Tasks, when outputs of one individual or group become inputs for another individual or group, or outputs are shared by several individuals or groups.

Intraterritorial and Interterritorial Conflicts

Conflicts that originate within one person, group, or territory are called, respectively, intrapersonal, intragroup, or intraterritorial conflict.[8] In some instances, these categories overlap and some types of conflict cross levels.

These levels of conflict tend to increase in complexity and interdependence. "We tend to homogenize differences within boundaries of our groups, and exaggerate the differences across boundaries." There is less chance for conflict between people who have their own resources and perform entirely different tasks directed toward completely separate goals.[9] Nurse managers have limited resources, and those of health care organizations are diminishing, thus adding to existing stressors.

Intraterritorial Conflict

Evidence of conflict within hospitals is increasing. Nurses and nonprofessional personnel have gone on strike, conflicts between administrators and medical staff are portrayed in the media, and hospital-client conflicts are increasing as consumers level charges of inefficiency and inattention to their expectations. Managers at all levels face increased interpersonal and departmental conflicts. Also the decrease in inpatient census has forced managers to seek cost savings as they work with diminished resources. Hospital administrators are demanding more accountability and pressuring managers to think in terms of cost-benefit ratios, cost accounting, and marketing strategies. Reviews and audits by external agencies are more frequent and exacting.[10]

Conflict occurs in the health care workplace because of changing attitudes of employees. The contemporary professional expects collegiality, cooperation, and participatory management. Authoritarian management results in worker defiance, undermines employment relationships, and reduces work force capability.[11]

Interterritorial Conflict

Physicians view the physician-patient relationship as primary and all other care as secondary. With advanced practice registered nurses and physician assistants providing primary care in some areas, conflict is not unusual. However, in settings where roles have been defined, conflict has been reduced.

Physician-government conflict was stimulated with the enactment of the Medicare-Medicaid legislation of 1965. The government and other payers insist that care can be provided under certain conditions for a certain price, an approach that challenges the physician's decision-making power in approaching patient care.[12] Strong leadership is needed to clearly establish the boundaries of the payers for care and the providers of care and to define the factors related to the compensation of providers. Changes in the marketplace have increased competition among health care providers, requiring increased productivity, improved service, and conflict resolution to maintain a market advantage. Increased competition has increased the need for research and new methods of patient treatment and management and has increased professionalization.[13]

According to Wenzel, "the best described conflict within the health care institution is that between physician and hospital management." The clash results from the physician's need to work with freedom and the organization's need for integration.[14] However, with the current emphasis on reducing the costs of health care delivery, health care administrators are fostering a communication style with physicians that is more consultative and collaborative. These efforts should help physicians become more aware of the business side of the enterprise.

Patient-physician conflict increases as patients move from submissive acceptance of care to questioning and challenging recommendations. Patients are asking questions about ordered tests and the need for a second opinion. Business and industry—as payers concerned with the economics of providing care—contribute to this conflict by encouraging employees to examine their bills to see that they accurately reflect tests and treatments ordered by physicians and received by patients.

Physicians face litigation when there are untoward results from treatment or surgery. Malpractice allegations cause physicians to have conflict with lawyers. Wenzel asserts that as the disciplines reason and solve problems, "medicine seeks objective truths, while the law employing the adversary system seeks relative truths."[15]

Nurses and Conflict

Nurses experience some of the same categories of intragroup conflict as do physicians. Nursing is now "experiencing increased competition for status from a proliferation of allied health professionals, many of whom enjoy higher standards of education, pay and autonomy."[16] There can be conflict between the following:

- Nurses and the hospital as employer, as attested to by nurses going on strike.
- Nurses and physicians, because of overlapping roles, nurses' desire for collegiality, and changing role relationships as nurses achieve increased levels of education.
- Nurses and lawyers, as nurses act as expert witnesses and are increasingly named defendants in malpractice litigation.
- Nurses and patients, as patients seek more participation in care decisions.
- Nurses and families, as families buy into the concept of family-centered care.
- Nurses and those in other disciplines during efforts to establish collaborative role relationships.
- Nurses and government because of governmental resistance to paying nurse-providers directly.

- Nurses and assistive personnel, as roles are being defined and identities of care providers become less clear.
- Nurses and nurses because of differences in educational levels and philosophies about care delivery models.

Nurses and Intradisciplinary Conflict

Intradisciplinary conflict has the potential to be a serious problem for nurse administrators. The overriding cause of conflict among nurses stems from their major knowledge-assessing modes:

1. The empirical mode, which uses the senses and inductive reasoning.
2. The noetic mode, which uses intuitive feelings and abductive reasoning.
3. The rational mode, which uses defined standards or rules and deductive reasoning.

Each individual has a predisposition to use a particular style or a combination of the three. One research study shows a resulting dissimilar interpretation of reality that may lead to conflict between nurse managers and clinical nurses.

> Failure to resolve intradisciplinary conflict in nursing will "inevitably debilitate both the profession and patients."[17]

Intrapersonal Conflict and Redesign of Delivery Systems

Nurses are expected to experience intrapersonal conflict as delivery systems are restructured. Their education or employment experiences may cause them to have a preference for a particular nursing delivery modality. For example, nurses may have learned primary nursing in school and used that modality in the work setting. Acceding to the use of another modality challenges their values and comfort level. Research studies evaluating outcomes using functional, team, primary, and modular models are inconclusive and often contradictory.[18]

Currently, nurses are involved in project management, also referred to as product-line management, service-line management, or program management. This decentralized organizational approach uses teams of specialists to achieve specific objectives in a specific time, especially when rapid change is needed. Team membership may cross vertical and horizontal lines. With its multiple disciplines, specialists, treatments, and types of cancer, oncology is appropriate as a product line.[19] As rapid changes in health care delivery continue, the incidences of project management should increase. Other models, such as case management in which nurses use critical paths to direct the care of hospitalized patients, will continue to evolve.

Nurses and Other Disciplines: Interdisciplinary Conflict

Studies suggest that interdisciplinary team members see themselves[20]

> . . . primarily as representatives of their respective disciplines rather than as members of a whole that transcends individual disciplines. Perspectives are splintered rather than united. . . . In the conflictual situations . . ., the perspective of a more technical and high-status discipline (psychology) prevailed.

Interdisciplinary Conflict and Organizational Complexity

Guy studied the interdisciplinary concept as it relates to organizational complexity. She compared the amount of conflict among professionals at a less complex psychiatric hospital and at a more complex psychiatric hospital. She concluded that complexity increases conflict even within homogenous disciplines. She indicates the following[21]:

> The more complex hospital may have the luxury of tolerating more diverse groups of employees, since they are divided into organizational components and do not have to interact very much. In comparison, the small hospital has fewer resources. . . . Everyone is in closer view of top management, and less diversity is tolerated. The smaller hospital socializes employees to tow the line, while more complex hospitals don't stress such adherence to constraining norms and preferences. . . . The more complex facility doesn't rely on as much interaction nor group decision making.

Guy says that "appointing professional staff to interdisciplinary hospital committees should be recognized for what it is: representation of groups rather than one representative view of each discipline." She further states, "the interaction of different disciplines won't necessarily lead to conflict . . ., there will be more conflict among staff at complex hospitals simply as a result of the complexity."[22]

Conflict Between the Patient's Family and Hospital Staff

Abramson, Donnelly, King, and Mallick have discussed the conflict that may arise within families during the course of discharge planning. They indicated that the impact of illness on the lives of patients and families is a major factor in the development of disagreements. Responses depend on life stage, the patient's age and factors related to the family such as degree of change required in the social situation, capacity for role flexibility, and problem-solving skills. Citing the research of Donnelly and King, they noted the disagreements among family members but that "7.9 percent of the disagreements were among hospital staff only rather than between staff and patients and/or family members."[23]

Early attention to staff input for discharge planning is especially important in a climate in which the minimum length of stay for hospitalized patients is encouraged. According to Lowenstein and Hoff, "Nurse administrators face major challenges in establishing care delivery systems that emphasize and encourage creative nursing approaches to discharge planning,"[24] In their study of registered nurses' involvement in discharge planning in eight hospitals, nurses were divided in their perception of whether nurses or social workers had primary responsibility for discharge planning. Only 88 nurses (39%) had attended an interdisciplinary team meeting. In this situation, nurses are probably experiencing role ambiguity and confusion. Inherent in this situation is the potential for conflict within nursing and between nursing and other disciplines.

Nursing Dislocation and Redesign

According to Porter-O'Grady, many hospitals and nursing leaders are indifferent about the centrality of nursing and strongly advocate a decreased nursing leadership role in favor of a multidisciplinary integrated approach. He says[25]:

> At times, there seems to be a tacit embarrassment regarding any concerted effort to enumerate the critical role of nursing and nurses in leading change in institutional settings. There has even been discussion suggesting that the creation of a universal, nonaligned caregiver might be in the best interest of the health care system. This thinking . . . is flawed. There must be someone who is concerned with the integration and continuum of patient services."

This would include attention to continuous quality improvement, cost containment, and patient-focused care.

Clearly, the role of the nurse will continue to change, as will the various modalities for restructuring patient care. However, the lack of role clarity will continue to be a major source of conflict as health care personnel establish different roles and relationships. Because resistance is a definitive part of the change process, it may become a major tactic for nurses if they perceive their influence diminishing within the developing interdisciplinary framework.

Defiant Behavior

Defiant behavior can create conflict. It produces guilt feelings in the person to whom it is directed. The nurse manager should take the position that the person expressing defiance is responsible for the conflict. Defiance is a threat to rational dialogue; it violates the acceptable protocols for adult interaction.

The defiant person challenges the authority of the nurse manager through obstinate and intransigent behavior. This behavior may be both verbal and nonverbal.

Murphy describes three versions of the defier. The first is the competitive bomber, who simply refuses to work. Such people mutter statements that translate into "Go to the devil." They scowl and will walk away from the nurse manager or even off the job.[26] Competitive defiers can aggressively undermine the workplace environment and plan deliberate assaults. They comment about unfair and terrible working conditions, manipulation, and lousy schedules. These behaviors are done to provoke managerial response. When a response to these behaviors is not elicited from the nurse manager, defiers sulk and pout to win the pity of peers or even higher management.

The second defier is the martyred accommodator, who uses malicious obedience. Such persons work and cooperate but do so mockingly and contemptuously. They complain and criticize to enlist the support of others.

A third category of defier is the avoider. These defiers avoid commitment and participation. They do not respond to the nurse manager. When conditions change, they avoid participation.[27]

Stress

Conflict leads to stress, fear, anxiety, and disruption in professional relationships. These conditions can, in turn, increase the potential for conflict. Stressors include "having too little responsibility, lack of participation in decision making, lack of managerial support, having to keep up with increasing standards of performance, and coping with rapid technological change." The costs of stress in 1973 were estimated at 1% to 3% of the U.S. Gross National Product.[28] Most likely, given the current climate in organizations, these costs have risen.

Confrontations, disagreements, and anger are evidence of stress and conflict. Stress and conflict are caused by poorly expressed relationships among people, including unfilled expectations.

Stress in patients leads to iatrogenic ailments, complications, and delayed recovery. It may be created by depression and anxiety. Stressed staff members cannot cope with stressed patients. Stressed staff display inefficiency, job dissatisfaction, and insensitive care. Staff, like patients, can develop iatrogenic ailments. Families, like patients, can add to stress when they are not managed appropriately. Increased stress for patients and staff members decreases effective use of staff time. These problems increase patient care costs because they increase the length of the illness and decrease nursing efficiency and effectiveness. In the future, these patients may go somewhere else for care, whether on their own initiative or the recommendations of physicians, relatives, friends, or acquaintances.[29]

Space

When nurses work in crowded spaces they must constantly interact with other staff members, visitors, and physicians. This is particularly true in crowded critical care units. Such conditions cause stress that leads to burnout and high turnover rates.

Physician Authority

Physicians are trained to be the major decision makers in patient care. Today's nurses want to be more independent, to have professional responsibility and accountability for patient care. Nurses spend more time with patients than physicians do and often have valid proposals for altering therapeutic measures. Physicians sometimes ignore nurses' suggestions or indicate they do not want feedback. Nurses become angry as their self-worth diminishes. Communication fails, particularly two-way communication.[30]

Gender

Gender is another source of interpersonal conflict in that men and women negotiate differently. According to Tannen, men are concerned with higher or lower hierarchical order as determined by indicators of status, such as privilege, income, or reputation. Women place more emphasis on how well they can relate to others.[31] Marcus says that when the importance of status is changed in a profession with a history of hierarchical ordering and when expectations, such as men presuming that all women are their subordinates and women believing that all men are superficial, the environment is ripe for conflict. According to Marcus, when a man seeks to "interact relationally, men find him suspicious and women find him clumsy. And when a woman plays the hierarchical game, women see her as disloyal and men find her disingenuous."[32] Astute managers must be aware of the potential influence of gender when they are seeking to resolve conflict.

Beliefs, Values, and Goals

Incompatible perceptions or activities create conflict. This is particularly evident when nurses hold beliefs, values, and personal goals different from those of nurse managers, physicians, patients, visitors, families, administrators, and so on. Nurses' values may boil over into conflicts related to ethical issues involving do not resuscitate orders, callous statements that belittle human worth, abortion, abuse, acquired immunodeficiency syndrome, and other problems. Personal goals may conflict with organizational goals, particularly with regard to staffing, scheduling, and the climate within which nurses work.

Nurses who must violate their personal standards will lash out at the system. Violating personal standards is demeaning to nurses and causes loss of self-esteem and emotional stress. They must know that they are valued and that their beliefs, values, and personal goals are respected. Like other people, nurses act to protect their personal or public image when confronted. They respond in terms of others' expectations of them because they want approval. They will defend their rights and their professional judgments. The ego is easily bruised and becomes a big problem in conflict. Defense becomes more heated when one or both parties to a conflict are uninformed or manipulated. When nurses are not recognized or respected, they feel helpless. They feel hopeless when they are unable to control the situation.[33]

Other Causes[34]

Change creates conflict that, in turn, impedes change. People who are not prepared for change feel threatened. They respond by fighting or failing to support the change.

Organizational climate and leadership style can create conflict when different managers set conflicting rules. Disciplinary problems can result from inadequate orientation and training and poor communication.

Off-the-job problems affect work performance, which leads to disciplinary problems and conflict. These problems include marital discord, drug use, alcoholism, mental stress, and financial concerns.

Age can create stress and conflict. As employees age they increasingly resent scrutiny of their work. Clinical nurses cannot always keep up with the physical demands of work as they grow older. They become fearful of not being able to compete with younger nurses and build up resentment that can lead to conflict.

Nurse managers are professional managers and directors of clinical nursing practice. They must cope with forces internal and external to the nursing organization. Pressures include cost containment, effectiveness of patient care, collective bargaining, consumer awareness and involvement, regulating agencies, entry-level qualifications, scope of practice, and mandated continuing education.

Computers are programmed to perform many of the management activities in business and industry. Hospitals are implementing nursing management information systems. Centrally controlled departments are being replaced with ad hoc task forces, project teams and small autonomous business units. Downsizing of the organization is the result, with decentralization and fewer levels of management, thus increasing the pressures to increase the output without increasing the number of managers. Managers face increased accountability and more demanding performance evaluations. The remaining managers become anxious, insecure, and doubtful about the future, resulting in malaise and conflict. As hospitals implement nursing management information systems, nurse managers are affected.

People who have been discriminated against, such as members of racial minorities, may be especially sensitive to real or imagined slights. They may respond with confrontation, defensiveness, anger, and other conflict-producing behaviors.

Persistent racial prejudice and discrimination are also important sources of workplace conflict.

Characteristics of Conflict

The characteristics of a conflict situation are[35]:

- At less two parties (individuals or groups) are involved in some kind of interaction.
- Mutually exclusive goals or mutually exclusive values exist, either in fact or as perceived by the parties involved.
- Interaction is characterized by behavior destined to defeat, reduce, or oppress the opponent or to gain a mutually designated victory.
- The parties face each other with mutually opposing actions and counteractions.
- Each party attempts to create an imbalance or relatively favored position of power vis-à-vis the other.

Conflict in health care organizations can be viewed from a structural or political perspective. From the structural perspective, conflict interferes with the accomplishment of organizational purposes. Bolman and Deal state that "hierarchical conflict raises the possibility that the lower levels will ignore or subvert management directives. Conflict among major partisan groups can undermine an organization's effectiveness and the ability of its leadership to function."[36]

Within a hierarchy, authorities have the responsibility to resolve conflict between individuals or departments that they cannot resolve and to adjudicate the conflict so that the final decision is consistent with the organization's goals.

Conflict Management

Discipline

In using discipline to manage or prevent conflict or to correct undesirable employee behavior, the nurse manager must know and understand the organization's rules and regulations on discipline. Rules and regulations must be clear, reasonable, and work related. Rules that are unreasonable or reflect personal bias invite infractions.

The following rules will help in managing discipline[37]:

1. Discipline should be progressive.
2. The punishment should fit the offense, be reasonable, and increase in severity for violation of the *same* rule.
3. Assistance should be offered to resolve on-the-job problems.
4. Tact should be used in administering discipline.
5. The best approach for each employee should be determined. Managers should be consistent and should not show favoritism.
6. The individual should be confronted and not the group. Disciplining a group for a member's violation of rules and regulations makes the other members angry and defensive, increasing conflict.
7. Discipline should be clear and specific.
8. Discipline should be objective; stick to facts.
9. Discipline should be firm; stick to the decision.
10. Discipline produces varied reactions. When emotions run high, conclude the session and schedule a second meeting.
11. The nurse manager performing the discipline should consult with the employee's immediate supervisor. Sometimes a manager's decision will be overruled. When managers work within the boundaries of official authority, however, the instances of being overruled should be minimal.
12. Nurse managers should build respect, trust, and confidence in their ability to handle discipline.

Consider Life Stages

Most organizations will have nurses at all life stages in their employ. Conflict can be managed by supporting individual nurses in attaining goals that pertain to their life stages. Three developmental stages are[38]:

1. In general, in the young adult stage, nurses are establishing careers. Nurses at this stage may be pursuing knowledge, skills, and upward mobility. Conflict may be prevented or managed by facilitating career advancement.
2. In general, during middle age, nurses become reconciled with achievement of their life goals. These nurses often help develop the careers of nurses younger than they.
3. In general, after age 55 years, nurses are thinking in terms of completing their work and retiring. Egos and ideals are integrated with accomplishments.

Communication

Communication is an art that is essential to maintaining a therapeutic environment. It is necessary in accomplishing work and resolving emotional and social issues. Supervisors prevent conflict with effective communication and should make it a way of life. To promote communication that prevents conflict, do the following[39]:

1. Teach nursing staff members their role in effective communication.
2. Provide factual information to everyone: be inclusive, not exclusive.
3. Consider all the aspects of situations: emotions, environmental considerations, and verbal and nonverbal messages.
4. Develop these basic skills:
   a. Reality orientation, by direct involvement and acceptance of responsibility in resolving conflict.
   b. Physical and emotional composure.
   c. Positive expectations that generate positive responses.
   d. Active listening.
   e. Giving and receiving information.

Active Listening

Active or assertive listening is essential to managing conflict. In order to be sure that their perceptions are correct, nurse managers can paraphrase what the angry or defiant employee is saying. Paraphrasing clarifies the message for both. Paraphrasing can help cool off the situation because it gives the employee time and the opportunity to hear the supervisor's perceptions of the emotions expressed.

Active assertive listening is sometimes called *stress listening*. Powell suggests these techniques for stress listening[40]:

1. Do not share anger; it adds to the problem. Remain calm and matter-of-fact.
2. Respond constructively in both verbal and nonverbal language. Be cheerful but sober. Maintain eye contact. Prevent interruptions. Bring problems into the open. Make the employee comfortable. Act serious. Always be courteous and respectful.
3. Ask questions and listen to the answers. Determine the reasons for the anger.
4. Separate fact from opinion, including your own.
5. Do not respond hastily. Plan a response.
6. Consider the employee's perspective first.

7. Help the employee find the solution. Ask questions and listen to responses. Do not be paternalistic.

Solving problems of angry confrontation requires stress listening. The nurse manager guides the process to a joint solution.

Quality Circles

Quality circles are considered an important approach to improving employees' behavior, increasing motivation, and reducing stress. They have been used with participatory management programs, standing committees, leadership development programs, exercise classes, career ladders, job enrichment, and nursing grand rounds.[41]

In one hospital, quality circles reduced turnover from 37.6% to 20% in two years.

Assertiveness Training

Assertive nurses, including managers, will stand up for their rights while recognizing the rights of others. They are straightforward and know that they are responsible for their thoughts, feelings, and actions. Assertive nurses also know their strengths and limitations. Rather than attack or defend, assertive nurses assess, collaborate, support, and remain neutral and nonthreatening. They can accept challenges and prevent conflict by helping others deal with their own anger.

Assertiveness can be taught through staff development programs. In these programs nurses are taught to make learned thoughtful responses, to know when to say no, even to the boss. They learn to hold people to a standard and to know when to accept responsibility rather than to blame others. When they are dissatisfied, they do something to increase their satisfaction. Most assertive behaviors can be learned with the use of case studies, role playing, and group discussion.

When they finish their training, assertive nurses will use positive comments to reinforce expectations that others do their jobs. They will use praise and consideration to promote wellness and positive individual behavior. Nurse managers learn that direct communication of support to staff members increases staff job satisfaction.

Assertive nurses focus on data and issues when offering constructive criticism to the boss or constructive feedback to the staff, which encourages dialogue and produces solutions to problems rather than conflict. They ask for assistance or delay when it is needed.

People generally respond positively to assertion and negatively to aggression; however, some people respond negatively to assertion.[42]

Assessing the Dimensions of the Conflict

Greenhalgh has developed a system for assessing the dimensions of conflict. He views conflict as having been managed when it does not interfere with ongoing functional relationships. Participants in a conflict must be persuaded to rethink their views. A third party must understand the situation empathetically from the participants' viewpoints. The conflict may be the result of a deeply rooted antagonistic relationship.

Greenhalgh's Conflict Diagnostic Model has seven dimensions, each with a continuum from "difficult to resolve" to "easy to resolve." Once the dimensions of the conflict have been assessed, those viewpoints that fall in the "difficult to resolve" domain should be shifted to the "easy to resolve" domain (see Exhibit 23-1).[43] Although this model is presented from the perspective of managing conflict in organizations, it can be used in diagnosing conflict inherent in other situations, such as family violence.

Issue in Question

It has been stated previously that values, beliefs, and goals are difficult issues to bring to a reasonable compromise. Principles fall into the same category because they involve integrity and ethical imperatives. The third party must persuade the conflicting parties to acknowledge each other's legitimate point of view. The question is: "How can principles be maintained while saving the organization and its employees?"

Size of the Stakes

The size of the stakes can make conflict hard to manage. When change threatens somebody's job or income, the stakes are high. The third party must try to keep egos from being hurt and gain some idea of what will be a satisfactory settlement to the parties. The parties ask: "If I give in now, what will I have to give up in the future?" Action may be postponed, if necessary, if solutions will create precedents that have the potential for causing future conflicts.

Interdependence of the Parties

People must view resources in terms of interdependence. However, if one group sees no benefits from the way resources are distributed, the members will be antagonistic. A positive-sum interdependence of mutual gain is needed.

Continuity of Interaction

Conflict is reduced in long-term relationships. Managers should opt for continuous, not episodic, interaction.

Structure of the Parties

Strong leaders who unify constituents to accept and implement agreements reduce conflict. When informal

EXHIBIT 23-1
Conflict Diagnostic Model

	VIEWPOINT CONTINUUM	
DIMENSION	DIFFICULT TO RESOLVE	EASY TO RESOLVE
Issue in question	Matter of principle	Divisible issue
Size of stakes	Large	Small
Interdependence of the parties	Zero sum	Positive sum
Continuity of interaction	Single transaction	Long-term relationship
Structure of the parties	Amorphous or fractionalized, with weak leadership	Cohesive, with strong leadership
Involvement of third parties	No neutral third party available	Trusted, powerful, prestigious, and neutral
Perceived progress of the conflict	Unbalanced: One party feeling the more harmed	Parties having done equal harm to each other

Source: L. Greenhalgh. "Managing Conflict." *Sloan Management Review* (summer 1986), 47. Reprinted by permission. Copyright © 1986, Sloan Management Review Association. All rights reserved.

coalitions occur, their representatives should be involved in finding and implementing agreements.

Involvement of Third Parties

Conflicts are difficult to resolve when participants are highly emotional and resort to distorted irrational arguments, unreasonable stances, impaired communication, or personal attacks. Such conflicts can be resolved with a prestigious, powerful, trusted, and neutral third party. The third party can be an outside consultant, mediator, or arbitrator. The inside manager who acts as a judge or arbitrator causes polarization; inviting a third party makes the resolution public. Third parties must be involved, when the nurse manager, as party to a conflict, cannot resolve it.

Perceived Progress of the Conflict

Both parties should be convinced that that the score is equal and enough suffering has occurred.

Techniques or Skills for Managing Conflict

Aims

When involved in managing and resolving conflict, the nurse manager should aim to broaden the staff's understanding of the problem. Staff members should be helped to see the big picture rather than the limited perspective of each party and to voice their opinions about any number of acceptable alternative solutions to the conflict. The manager should then work on a compromise to stimulate the interaction and involvement of the

parties, another aim of conflict management. Other aims include better decisions and commitment to decisions that have been made.

Strategies[44]

Avoidance

Avoidance is a strategy that allows conflicting parties to calm down. The nurse manager involved in a conflict can sidestep the issue by saying, "Let's both take time to think about this and set up a time for a future talk." This approach allows both parties to cool down and gather information. Avoidance can be used when the issue is not critical. Avoidance also can be used when the potential damage of immediate confrontation outweighs the benefits, in which case a third party may be involved. Certainly, the nurse manager as a third party can tell the parties to a conflict: "I want you both to go on with your work while I take time to determine the facts and analyze them." A future meeting should then be set, with a not-too-distant date.

Accommodation

The nurse manager who is party to a conflict can accommodate the other person by yielding and placing the other's needs first. This strategy is particularly effective when the issue is more important to the other person. Accommodation maintains cooperation and harmony and develops subordinates by allowing them to make decisions.

Competition

Nurse managers as supervisors can exert the power of their position at a subordinate's expense. Doing so enforces the rule of discipline. It is an assertive position that does not foster commitment to conflict resolution on the part of the subordinate.

Compromise

Taking a middle ground may resolve a conflict. This temporary strategy should be used when time is needed to work out a permanent satisfactory position. A compromise that leaves both parties dissatisfied is not a good one.

Collaboration

When both parties collaborate to solve conflict, they will both be satisfied. This is especially true of important issues in which integration of insights is needed. Collaboration takes time and energy. A consensual solution wins full commitment.

One of the areas in which collaboration could resolve conflict is that of physician-nurse relationships. The findings of one study undertaken to "examine the personal, organizational and managerial factors that contribute to nurse-physician collaboration on patient care units," are[45]:

1. There was a weak inverse relationship between collaboration and length of employment (personal factor).
2. There was no significant relationship between collaboration and education (personal factor).
3. Although turnover was low due to the system's rewards, productivity was low also (organizational factor).
4. There was low physician involvement in hospital affairs (organizational factor).
5. There was a significant positive relationship between primary nursing and collaboration (organizational factor).
6. There was greater collaboration on critical care units (organizational factor).
7. Collaboration and trust were increased by open communication, managed conflict, and meetings (managerial factor).
8. Collaboration increased with control of organizational stress (managerial factor).
9. Orientation, in-service education, and discussion with all groups produced position collaboration (managerial factor).
10. Positive collaboration was related to standardization of work and skills, supervision, mutual adjustment, and group methods, including rounds (managerial factor).

One could conclude that collaboration contributes to satisfaction among nurses.

Managerial and organizational factors are more important to achieving collaboration than are personal factors.

Resolving Conflict Through Negotiation

Negotiation is probably the most rapidly growing technique for handling conflict. According to Hampton, Summer, and Webber, negotiation includes bargaining power, distributive bargaining, integrative bargaining, and mediation. They are defined as follows[46]:

- *Bargaining power.* Refers to another person's inducement to agree to your terms.
- *Distributive bargaining.* What either side gains at the expense of the other. Most labor management bargaining falls into this category.
- *Integrative bargaining.* Negotiators reach a solution that enhances both parties and produces high joint benefits. Each party looks out for its own interests, with the focus shifting to problem-solving, that is, from reducing demands to expanding the pool of resources.
- *Mediation.* Mediators attempt to eliminate surrender as a demand. They encourage each party to acknowledge that they have injured the other but are also dependent on each other.

Mediation

Mediation is a part of negotiation, but also is a more intense strategy in its own right. The mediator is often brought into the process when the parties are locked in a positional posture. According to Marcus, the mediator must determine whether it is possible to get the parties to talk and, if so, to construct an adaptive process that will move them from confrontation, to cooperation, to resolution.[47] Marcus says mediation includes "premeditation appropriateness, premeeting investigation and party buy-in, party meeting, issue clarification, option building, option assessment, movement toward mutually acceptable solutions, and resolution and implementation."[48] In each phase, the mediator simultaneously engages in investigation, empathy, neutrality, managing the interaction, inventiveness, and persuasion. Because mediation is voluntary, either party can suspend or postpone the mediation. The mediator is without authority to impose a resolution. When a decision has been imposed on one or both parties as a function of legal, moral, organizational, or clinical considerations and there is no room for negotiation, then mediation is improper and it is fraudulent to suggest that there is room for discussion.[49]

Specific Skills

The following is a list of skills that are useful in managing or preventing conflict. Some ideas were mentioned earlier. The manager should[50]:

1. Establish clear rules or guidelines and make them known to all.
2. Create a supportive climate with a variety of options. This makes people feel comfortable about making suggestions. It energizes them, promoting creative thinking and leading to better solutions. It strengthens relationships.
3. Tell people they are appreciated. Praise and confirmation of worth are important to everyone for job satisfaction.
4. Stress peaceful resolution rather than confrontation. Build a bridge of understanding.
5. Confront when necessary to preserve peace. Do so by educating people about their behavior. Tell them the behavior you perceive, what is wrong with it, and how it needs to be corrected.
6. Play a role that does not create stress or conflict. Do not play an ambiguous and fluctuating role that creates confusion among employees.
7. Judge timing that is best for all. Do not postpone an action indefinitely.
8. Keep the focus on issues and off personalities.
9. Keep communication two way. Tune in to the message, to correct interpretation, and to the feeling level of the employee. Reassure people by listening to them vent. Listen for the real or underlying problem.
10. Emphasize shared interests.
11. Separate issues and confront those that are important to both parties.
12. Examine all solutions and accept the one that is most acceptable to both parties.
13. Avoid overriding your better judgment, becoming defensive, reprimanding the individual, cutting off further expressions of feelings, and monopolizing the conversation. These responses increase frustration and are ineffective management techniques.
14. When conflict is evident at decision-making or implementation stages, work to reach an agreement. Commit to a course of action that serves some interests of all parties. Seek agreement rather than power.
15. Understand barriers to cooperation or resolution and focus on the dynamics of conflict to resolve it.
16. Distinguish between defiant behavior and normal on-the-job mistakes. Defiance is usually an individual behavior. Determine who the defier is, and prepare for the confrontation emotionally and intellectually. Deal with one defiant person at a time. Establish authority and competence. Interview privately; teach, evaluate, resolve, guide, and deal with the defier. Do this immediately, and follow up in two days. Discuss behavior and consequences,

including possible termination, keeping calm and steady. Assume adults have a sense of courtesy and cooperation. When challenged, respond on the spot and stand your ground. Then move to a private area or remove yourself from the scene.
17. Be a sponge to a verbal charge by an angry person.
18. Determine who owns the problem. Take responsibility for it as if you own it, and say thanks.
19. Determine needs that are being ignored or frustrations that require recognition and nurturing.
20. Help distinguish demands from dreams.
21. Build trust by listening, clarifying, and allowing the challenges to unwind completely. Give feedback to make sure you understand. Let people know you care and that you trust them. Indicate recognition of other viewpoints and willingness to work to improve the relationship. Be factual. Ask for feedback. Work out a common bridge of "must" items. When an employee has a valid point, recognize it, apologize if need be, and be genuine.
22. Renegotiate problem-solving procedures to forestall further anger, distrust, and defensiveness.

Results of Conflict Management

If attention is given to the role of the nurse manager in creating a climate for productive work by nurses, many of the causes of conflict will be eliminated. Knowledge and skills related to managing conflict when it occurs are essential to the role of nurse manager.

Conflict can be a constructive and positive source of energy and creativity when properly managed. Otherwise, conflict can cause an environment to become dysfunctional and destructive, draining energy and reducing both personal and organizational effectiveness. It can destroy initiative or creativity. Conflict can cause hostile and disruptive behavior, loss of team spirit, and loss of desire to work toward common goals. It can result in deadlock and stalemate. Managed conflicts do not escalate.[51]

Summary

The interrelationships among nurses and other personnel, patients, and families offer the potential for conflict. Therefore, nurse managers should know how to manage conflict.

Causes of conflict include defiant behavior, stress, crowded space, physician authority, and incompatibility of values and goals.

Conflict can be prevented or managed by discipline; consideration of people's life stages; purposive communication, including active listening; use of quality circles; provision of assertiveness training for nurse managers; and assessment of the dimensions of conflict.

Aims of conflict management include broadening understanding about problems, increasing alternative solutions, achieving a working consensus on decisions, and genuine commitment to the decisions that are made. Specific strategies include avoidance, accommodation, competition, compromise, collaboration, negotiation, and mediation. In addition, nurse managers can learn and use specific skills to prevent and manage conflict.

Conflict management keeps conflict from escalating, makes for a productive work environment, and can make conflict a positive or constructive force.

APPLICATION EXERCISES

The following exercises can be done in groups of students or employees. Form groups of five to eight persons. Select a leader to keep the group moving and a recorder to write the plan or report. Refer to the chapter text for techniques and skills for assessing and managing conflict.

EXERCISE 23-1

Case Study. You are called to a unit to resolve a conflict between an RN and LPN. They are shouting at each other in the hallway. The RN is the supervisor of the LPN. As you approach them you hear the following dialogue:

RN: I asked you to get Mr. W. ready to go to x-ray, and you ignored me. The transport person was here and left because you would not help him.

LPN: I was busy with Mrs. L., and could not leave her. Why didn't you get Mr. W. ready? You apparently knew about it.

RN: It was your job. I assigned Mr. W. to you.

LPN: I do my own work and part of yours. You are the RN. You are supposed to be the leader on this floor.

RN: Don't get sarcastic with me. I don't have to put up with it. I'm going to call the supervisor and report you for your insolence.

LPN: My insolence! Go ahead and report me! I'll tell the supervisor what a lazy bitch you are!

Outline a plan to deal with this conflict. You may use the following format:

1. What is (are) the cause(s) of the conflict?
2. Assess the dimensions of the conflict using Greenhalgh's Conflict Diagnostic Model.
3. Decide on aims, strategies, and specific skills for resolving the conflict. List them.

EXERCISE 23-2

Case Study. During the P.M. change-of-shift report an RN calls in ill and the staffing office says she cannot be replaced. This leaves only one RN, Mrs. K., for 26 patients. Mrs. K. says, "If you do not get another RN for this unit, I am going to quit this job. I will not do it this shift, but I will not put up with this constant shortage of help. I don't care if it is an RN, but I should have people with some skills to get the patients cared for. The reason everyone quits around here is because they are overworked, underpaid, and the hospital management does not give a damn. The place needs to be investigated."

Outline a plan to deal with this conflict. You may use the following format:

1. What is (are) the cause(s) of the conflict?
2. Assess the dimensions of the conflict using Greenhalgh's Conflict Diagnostic Model.
3. Decide on aims, strategies, and specific skills for resolving the conflict. List them.

EXERCISE 23-3

Case Study. A surgeon and a scrub nurse get in an argument during an operation. The surgeon tells the scrub nurse she is stupid and he does not want her to ever scrub for him again. The scrub nurse says that she is totally competent but that he expects her to read his mind. She says, "If you don't quit badgering me, I'm going to sue you and this hospital!" This comment leads to escalation of the dialogue into a shouting match.

Outline a plan to deal with this conflict. You may use the following format:

1. What is (are) the cause(s) of the conflict?
2. Assess the dimensions of the conflict using Greenhalgh's Conflict Diagnostic Model.
3. Decide on aims, strategies, and specific skills for resolving the conflict. List them.

EXERCISE 23-4

Describe a recent instance of a conflict in which you were involved. Was it resolved satisfactorily? Can the group help in finding a better solution? Discuss.

EXERCISE 23-5

Do a library computer search on conflict management. Look at indices of nursing, business, and management periodicals. Prepare an abstract on two recent publications. The abstract should describe the value of the publication to the performance of the nurse manager.

NOTES

1. J. H. Frost and W. W. Wilmot, "Making Conflict Work for You," In E. C. Hein and M. J. Nicholson, eds., *Contemporary Leadership Behaviors: Selected Readings* (Philadelphia: J. B. Lippincott, 1944), 338.
2. A. M. Barker, *Transformational Nursing Leadership: A Vision for the Future* (Baltimore: Williams & Wilkins, 1990), 47.
3. W. Bennis, *Why Leaders Can't Lead* (San Francisco: Jossy-Bass, 1990), 158.
4. B. J. Stevens, *The Nurse Executive* (Rockville, MD: Aspen, 1985), 214.
5. J. M. Richardson, "Management of Conflict in Organizations," *Physician Executive* (January–February 1991), 41.
6. A. Marriner, *A Guide to Nursing Management* (St. Louis: C. V. Mosby, 1984), 177–178.
7. P. J. Decker and E. J. Sullivan, *Nursing Administration: A Micro/Micro Approach for Effective Nurse Executives* (Norwalk, CT: Appleton & Lange, 1992), 551
8. Ibid.
9. D. R. Hampton, C. E. Summer, and R. A. Webber, *Organizational Behavior and the Practice of Management* (Glenview, IL: Scott, Foresman, 1987), 620–622.
10. L. G. Bertinasco, "Strategies for Resolving Conflict," *The Health Care Supervisor* (July 1990), 35–37.
11. G. W. Mauer and K. M. Cramer, "Unresolved Conflicts Entail Opportunity Costs," *Physician Executive* (March–April 1987), 7–10.
12. F. J. Wenzel, "Conflict: An Imperative for Success," *The Journal of Medical Practice Management* (April 1986), 252–259.
13. G. W. Mauer and K. M. Cramer, op. cit.
14. F. J. Wenzel, op. cit.
15. Ibid.
16. L. G. Bertinasco, op. cit.
17. K. A. Noble and R. Rancourt, "Administration and Intradisciplinary Conflict within Nursing," *Nursing Administration Quarterly* (summer 1991), 36–42.
18. C. L. Anderson and E. Hughes, "Implementing Modular Nursing in a Long-Term Care Facility," *The Journal of Nursing Administration* (June 1993), 29–35.
19. M. K. Hermann, J. Alexander, and J. T. Kiely, "Leadership and Project Management," In P. J. Decker and E. L. Sullivan, *Nursing Administration: A Micro/Micro Approach for Effective Executives* (Norwalk, CT: Appleton & Lange), 571.
20. R. G. Sands, J. Stafford and M. McClelland, "'I Beg to Differ': Conflict in the Interdisciplinary Team," *Social Work in Health Care* 14(3), (1990), 55–72.
21. M. E. Guy, "Interdisciplinary Conflict and Organizational Complexity," *Hospital & Health Services Administration* (January–February 1986), 111–121.
22. Ibid.
23. J. S. Abramson, J. Donnelly, M. A. King, and M. D. Mallick, "Disagreements in Discharge Planning: A Normative Phenomenon," *Health and Social Work* (February 1993), 58–59; J. Donnelly and M. King, "Extent and Type of Disagreement about Discharge Planning," op. cit., 61.
24. A. Lowenstein and P. S. Hoff, "Discharge Planning: A Study of Nursing Staff Involvement," *The Journal of Nursing Administration* (April 1994), 45–50.
25. T. Porter-O'Grady, "The Real Value of Partnership: Preventing Professional Amorphism," *The Journal of Nursing Administration* 24 (2), (1994), 11–15.
26. E. C. Murphy. "Managing Defiance," *Nursing Management* (May 1984), 67–69.
27. Ibid.
28. D. R. Faulconer and V. B. Goldman, "Managerial Stress," *Nursing Administration Quarterly* (winter 1983), 32.

29. E. C. Murphy, "Communication and Wellness: Managing Patient/Staff Relationships," *Nursing Management* (October 1984), 64–68.

30. G. S. Wlody, "Communicating in the ICU: Do you Read Me Loud and Clear?" *Nursing Management* (September 1984), 54, 56–58.

31. D. Tannen, *You Just Don't Understand: Women and Men in Conversation* (New York: Ballantine, 1990), 155–156.

32. L. J. Marcus with B. C. Dorn, P. B. Kritek, V. C. Miller, and J. B. Wyatt, *Renegotiating Health Care: Resolving Conflict to Build Cooperation* (San Francisco: Jossey-Bass, 1995), 247.

33. M. B. Silber, "Managing Confrontations: Once More into the Breach," *Nursing Management* (April 1984), 54, 56–58.

34. E. C. Murphy, "Practical Management Course," *Nursing Management* (March 1987), 76–77; American Hospital Association, *Role, Functions, and Qualifications of the Nursing Service Administrator in a Health Care Institution* (Chicago: AHA, 1978); R. Zemke, "The Case of the Missing Managerial Malaise," *Training* (November 1985), 30–33; M. A. Palich. "What Supervisors Should Know About Discipline," *Supervisory Management* (October 1983), 21–24; L. Greenhalgh, "SMR Forum: Managing Conflict," *Sloan Management Review* (summer 1986) 45–51.

35. A. C. Filley, "Types and Sources of Conflict." In M. S. Berger, D. Elhart, S. C. Firsich, S. B. Jordan, and S. Stone, eds., *Management for Nurses: A Multidisciplinary Approach* (St. Louis: C. V. Mosby, 1980), 154–165.

36. L. G. Bolman and T. E. Deal, *Reframing Organizations: Artistry, Choice, and Leadership* (San Francisco: Jossey-Bass, 1991), 199.

37. M. A. Palich, op. cit.

38. E. C. Murphy, "Practical Management Course."

39. E. C. Murphy, " Communication and Wellness."

40. J. T. Powell, "Stress Listening: Coping with Angry Confrontations," *Personnel Journal* (May 1986), 27–29.

41. D. R. Faulconer and V. B. Goldman, op. cit.

42. C. C. Clark, "Assertiveness Issues for Nursing Administrators and Managers," *Journal of Nursing Administration* (July 1979), 20–24.

43. L. Greenhalgh, op. cit.

44. H. K. Baker and P. I. Morgan, "Building a Professional Image: Handling Conflict," *Supervisory Management* (February 1986), 24–29.

45. A. C. Alt-White, M. Charns, and R. Strayer, "Personal, Organizational, and Managerial Factors Related to Nurse-Physician Collaboration," *Nursing Administration Quarterly* (fall 1983), 8–18.

46. D. R. Hampton, C.E. Summer, and R. A. Webber, *Organizational Behavior and the Practice of Management* (Glenview, IL: Scott, Foresman, 1987), 635–639.

47. L. J. Marcus, with B. C. Dorn, P. B. Kritek, V.G. Miller, and J. B. Wyatt, op. cit.

48. Ibid., 341–342.

49. Ibid., 361.

50. H. K. Baker and P. I. Morgan, op. cit.; E. C. Murphy, "Practical Management Course." In R. Lamkin, "Communicating Effectively," *B & E Review* (July 1984), 16; H. K. Baker and P. Morgan, "Building a Professional Image: Using 'Feeling Level' Communication," *Supervisory Management* (January 1986), 20–25; E. C. Murphy, "Managing Defiance"; L. Greenhalgh, op. cit; M. B. Silber, op. cit.

51. H. K. Baker and P. I. Morgan, "Building a Professional Image: Handling Conflict."

REFERENCES

Filmer, D. "Improving Communications in Large Organizations." *Work and People* (February 1985), 12–14.

Levenstein, A. "Negotiation vs. Confrontation." *Nursing Management* (January 1984), 52–53.

Swansburg, R. C., and P. W. Swansburg. *Strategic Career Planning and Development for Nurses.* (Rockville, MD: Aspen, 1984).

Templeton, J. "For Corporate Vigor, Plan a Fight Today." *Sales Management, The Marketing Magazine* (15 June 1969), 32–36.

APPENDIX 23-1
Conflict Resolution Questionnaire: How Do You Deal with Conflict?

Used with permission: Jean and Jock McCellan August 30, 2000.

Answer the questions below as a way of examining how you deal with conflict. Members of Jock McCellan's class on conflict resolution (Quinebaug Valley Community–Technical College, Danielson, CT) designed the survey. The questions are based primarily on the methods recommended by Dudley Weeks in *The Eight Essential Steps to Conflict Resolution* (Los Angeles: Jeremy Tarcher, 1992), and on principles in the book by Roger Fisher and William Ury, *Getting to Yes* (Penguin Books, 1991).

INSTRUCTIONS

Rate each of the following statements using the ratings from 1 to 5 below to indicate how often you do as the statement says. Please write your responses in the far left-hand column. Answer the questions to portray your most usual way of dealing with conflicts such as those at home or work. Do not take long on any question. Give your initial reaction. The more honest your answers, the more usable the results will be. When you are through, go to Scoring the Conflict Resolution Questionnaire.

(continued)

1. Almost never   3. Half the time
2. Occasionally   4. Usually   5. Almost always

(Answer/Score)

1. ___/___   I feel that conflict is a negative experience.
2. ___/___   When I resolve a conflict, it improves my relationship.
3. ___/___   I am afraid to enter into confrontations.
4. ___/___   I feel that in conflicts someone will get hurt.
    V ___
5. ___/___   When I prepare to meet to discuss a conflict, I try to arrange for a mutually acceptable time and setting.
6. ___/___   I feel the location where a conflict takes place is important.
7. ___/___   I try to make people feel comfortable when meeting with them about a conflict.
8. ___/___   When I start to discuss a conflict with the other party, I choose my opening carefully to establish positive realistic expectations.
    A ___
9. ___/___   I state my true feelings when dealing with conflict.
10. ___/___   During a conflict, I ask questions to clarify a statement that I'm not sure of.
11. ___/___   I try to be aware of how my negative and positive self-perceptions influence the way I deal with conflict.
12. ___/___   In a conflict, my actions are based on how I think the other person perceives me.
    C ___
13. ___/___   I feel that only my needs are important.
14. ___/___   I feel that for a relationship to last, the needs of both parties must be considered.
15. ___/___   In a conflict, I try to distinguish between real needs and desires.
16. ___/___   In order not to harm the relationship, I may temporarily put aside some of my own less important personal wants.
    N ___
17. ___/___   I share my positive attitude, hoping the other person will do the same.
18. ___/___   I find it necessary to overpower others to get my own way.
19. ___/___   I am aware that the other person may need to feel in control of the conflict.
20. ___/___   In a conflict, I believe there should be no upper hand.
    P ___
21. ___/___   I find it easy to forgive.
22. ___/___   I bring up old issues from the past during a new conflict.
23. ___/___   When dealing with a conflict, I consider the future of the long-term relationship.
24. ___/___   In a conflict, I try to dominate the other party.
    F ___
25. ___/___   I listen with an open mind to alternative options.
26. ___/___   I feel there is just one way to solve a problem.
27. ___/___   When dealing with conflict, I have preconceived notions about the other party that I am unwilling to let go of.
28. ___/___   I can accept criticism from others.
    O ___
29. ___/___   I feel that winning the war is more important than winning the battle.
30, ___/___   I strive for a complete and genuine resolution of a conflict rather than settling for a temporary agreement.
31. ___/___   When dealing with a conflict, I have a predetermined solution to the outcome.
32. ___/___   I feel the need to control an argument.
    D ___

(continued)

33. ___/___   If I had my way, I win, you lose.
34. ___/___   When in a conflict with someone, I ask them to explain their position.
35. ___/___   I bargain to resolve conflict.
36. ___/___   At the end of a conflict, it matters to me that the other person's needs have been met as well as my own.

    M ___

37. ___/___   I express anger constructively.
38. ___/___   In difficult conflicts, I would consider requesting a third-party facilitator.
39. ___/___   I overlook my partner's anger so I can focus on the real issues of the conflict.
40. ___/___   I feel it is okay to agree to disagree on specific issues in a conflict.

    X ___

    Total _____

Using the same 1 to 5 scale above, how often do you feel you are effective at resolving conflicts in a way that builds your long-term relationships with other parties?

___   1.   Almost never

___   2.   Occasionally

___   3.   Half the time

___   4.   Usually

___   5.   Almost always

SCORING THE CONFLICT RESOLUTION QUESTIONNAIRE

1. **Reverse the scores for the 12 questions that give high scores for unrecommended responses.**
   Dudley Weeks says some responses to conflict lead to resolutions that build a relationship, and some do not. All 40 questions need to be on the same scale, giving a high number for desirable or effective responses and a low score for ineffective ones. However, 12 of the questions are worded so that ineffective answers get a "5" instead of a "1." For example, question #1 reads, "I feel that conflict is a negative experience." Weeks would say that someone who answers "Almost always", a "5," will probably have difficulty approaching a conflict, and that this will reduce the person's effectiveness. Therefore, that response deserves a low score, and the "5" needs to be reversed to a "1." Doing this for the 12 questions will ensure that all scores will be consistent, with higher scores going to better responses.

   Please reverse the scores for the following questions: 1, 3, 13, 18, 22, 24, 26, 27, 31, 32, 33, and 35. Reverse the scores by looking at the responses given in the left-hand column and writing in reverse scores in the right-hand column as follows:

Answer:		Score:
5	becomes	1
4	becomes	2
3	remains	3
2	becomes	4
1	becomes	5

2. **For questions that do not need to be reversed.**
   For questions that do not need to be reversed, write the same number given in the left-hand answer column in the right-hand score column.

3. **Compute subtotals and the total.**
   The 40 questions are in groups of four, based on topics in Weeks's book. Add the scores for each group of four, and put the result in the blank. (The letter is an abbreviation for the topic of that group.) Then add the subtotals, and enter the result in the "Total" blank.

4. **Interpret the results, and learn from them.**
   The higher your scores, the more effective you are likely to be at finding resolutions that meet everyone's real needs and that build your long-term relationships. Of the 10 subtotals, which were the highest? These are probably areas where you are effective. Which subtotals were the lowest? These are probably areas where you might try a different approach.

   Choose two or three of the questions with the lowest scores, and try out behaviors that might make you more effective at resolving conflicts productively.

CHAPTER 24

Controlling or Evaluating

Russell C. Swansburg, PhD, RN

LEARNING OBJECTIVES AND ACTIVITIES

- Define the term *controlling*, or *evaluating*.
- Describe the relationship of controlling (evaluating) to the other major functions of management: planning, organizing, and directing (leading).
- Illustrate the use of controls as management tools.
- Illustrate the use of standards for controlling or evaluating.
- Demonstrate controlling (evaluating) techniques.
- Use a set of standards to evaluate the controlling (evaluating) function of a nursing agency or unit.

CONCEPTS: Controlling, evaluating, standards, Gantt chart, performance evaluation and review technique (PERT), benchmarking.

MANAGER BEHAVIOR: Uses legal and accreditation standards to control and evaluate all activities of the organization.

LEADER BEHAVIOR: Obtains input from representative nursing personnel to develop and implement a master control plan incorporating legal and accreditation standards.

Introduction

The final element of management defined by Fayol is control, which he defined as[1]

> . . . verifying whether everything occurs in conformity with the plan adopted, the instructions issued, and principles established. It has for its object to point out weaknesses and error in order to rectify them and prevent recurrence.

Urwick has defined controlling or evaluating as "seeing that everything is being carried out in accordance with the plan which has been adopted, the orders which have been given, and the principles which have been laid down."[2] Urwick referred to three principles[3]:

1. The principle of uniformity ensures that controls are related to the organizational structure.
2. The principle of comparison ensures that controls are stated in terms of the standards of performance required, including past performance. In this sense, controlling means setting a mark and examining and explaining the results in terms of the mark. Today this is called benchmarking.
3. The principle of exception provides summaries that identify exceptions to the standards.

It is important that controlling be done on a factual basis. When issues arise people should be made to meet with each other and settle them through direct contact. To stimulate cooperation, employees need to participate from the beginning. Nurse managers can teach employees to cooperate across departmental lines and to let reason and common sense prevail.[4] Management authors, including nurses, have described the controlling process as follows[5]:

1. Establish standards for all elements of management in terms of expected and measurable outcomes. These are the yardsticks by which achievement of objectives are measured.
2. Apply the standards by collecting data and measuring the activities of nursing management, comparing standards with actual care.
3. Make any improvements deemed necessary from the feedback.

4. Keep the process continuous for all areas, including:
   a. Management of the nursing division and each subunit.
   b. The performance of personnel.
   c. The nursing process and product.

The controlling process may be expressed as a formula:

$$Ss + Sa + F + C \longrightarrow I$$

Where Standards set + Standards applied + Feedback + Correction yield Improvement.

According to Peters, vision, symbolic action, and recognition make up a control system in the truest sense of the word. Peters also stated "what gets measured gets done."[6]

Controlling as a Function of Nursing Management

Control is "the management function in which performance is measured and corrective action is taken to ensure the accomplishment of organizational goals."[7] Control includes coordination of numerous activities: decision-making related to planning and organizing activities and information from directing and evaluating each worker's performance. Control is also viewed as being concerned with records, reports, organizational progress toward aims, and effective use of resources. Control uses evaluation and regulation; controlling is identical to evaluation.[8] Koontz and Weihrich defined controlling as "the measurement and correction of the performance in order to make sure that enterprise objectives and the plans devised to attain them are accomplished."[9]

Systems Theory

Feedback and adjustment comprise the control element of nursing management. Output is described or defined in terms of the patient in the patient care model and is measured by quality indicators and outcomes. In case management, these indicators are predicted and met on a timed basis. Discharge planning will take note of them. When the outcomes or indicators fall short, the information is fed back to the clinical nurses who make adjustments in the case management plan and the process controlled by the critical path. Both the patient and nurse are system inputs, whereas throughput consists of nursing actions related to patient outcomes and managerial actions related to setting goals for nurses' behavior. *Quality management* is the process by which the nursing product or process is measured and action prescribed to correct deficiencies.

Similarly, systems theory can be applied to performance evaluation of the registered nurse as output. Input is still the patient and the nurse, with throughput the managerial actions related to goals for nurse behavior. A performance results contract between clinical nurse and nurse manager spells out agreed-on performance goals or results. When they are not being met, the nurse manager discusses the deficiency with the clinical nurse and they agree on corrective actions. In an open system the process is continuous.

An effective control system has standards, measuring tools, and a surveillance process culminating in corrective action. A quality control program for measuring patient care will have these same components.[10]

Controlling is the second physical act of administration, the first physical act being directing. It is the fourth and final element of the administrative composite process (ACP), planning and organizing being the conceptual acts. All functions of management—planning, organizing, directing, and controlling—occur simultaneously. Inputs would include resources other than the clinical nurse, such as supplies, equipment, and plant, plus all of the direct and indirect cost elements used in achieving the outputs.[11]

> **Nurse managers will use staffing reports, budget status reports, and other information to control the functioning system. These reports are both monitoring devices and feedback to the clinical nurses and care managers.**

Controls as Management Tools

In the process of measuring the degree to which predetermined goals are achieved and of applying necessary corrective actions to improve performance, policies and procedures are used as standards. Also, observations, questions, patient charts, patients, and health care team members serve as sources of data. Corrective actions can be corroborative, disciplinary, or educational.[12] In the process of feedback, a positive experience will stimulate motivation and contribute to the growth of employees.[13]

Controls are management tools for improving performance. Among the controls are rules that are needed to let people know what is expected of them and how functions are to be coordinated. Communication as information is essential to control. Self-control is essential to managerial control because it is the highest form of control. Self-control includes being up-to-date in knowledge, giving clear orders, being flexible, understanding reasons for behavior, helping others improve, increasing problem-solving skills, standing calm under pressure, and planning ahead. Employees should be told the facts in language that they understand and words that have the intended meaning. Effective nursing managers set limits and make them known to their employees. Then, when the line is crossed, the appropriate disciplinary action can be taken. The latter is achieved by corrective action that is consistently applied after checking the facts.[14]

Controls can be separated into two elements: mechanical and sociological. There are three stages of control, the first two being the mechanical elements and the third the sociological element[15]:

1. A predetermined definition of standards for a level of performance.
2. Measurement of current performance against the standards.
3. Corrective action when indicated.

Nurse managers will avoid the unintended consequence of control, that is, noncompliance. Because control can be perceived as a threat from unwanted power and authority, it can trigger defense mechanisms such as aggression and repression. Lemin advocated the following approaches to control by McGregor: time, a high degree of mutual trust, a high degree of mutual support, open and authentic communications, clear understanding of objectives, respect for differences, utilization of member resources, and a supportive environment. These approaches will lead to conflict resolution, changed beliefs and attitudes, genuine innovation, genuine commitment, strengthened management, and prevention of unintended consequences of control.[16]

The following are ten characteristics of a good control system; controls[17]

1. Must reflect the nature of the activity.
2. Should report errors promptly.
3. Should be forward looking.
4. Should point out exceptions at critical points.
5. Should be objective.
6. Should be flexible.
7. Should reflect the organizational pattern.
8. Should be economical.
9. Should be understanding.
10. Should indicate corrective action.

Nurse managers will remain aware that the best way to ensure the quality of nursing services provided in the patient units is to establish philosophy, standards of care, and objectives. At least two of these, philosophy and objectives, involve planning, further evidence that the major functions of management take place simultaneously.[18] Controlling mechanisms also include accreditation procedures, consultants, evaluation devices, rounds, reports, inspections, and nursing audits.[19]

Nurses activate the processes of control. This function involves the use of power and should be used by nurse managers to promote openness, honesty, trust, competence, and even confrontation. This function also involves value systems, ethical decision-making, self-control, professional self-regulation, and control by an aggregate of professionals. The processes of control function is emerging as a system of quality control programs. The dimensions of quality management programs are quality of care, including accessibility, beliefs, and attitudes of patients about health care; structure of health care; processes of care; professional competence; outcomes of care; and self-regulation. Audits and budgets are the major techniques of control.[20]

Control functions can be differentiated among levels of managers. For example, the nurse manager of a unit is concerned with short-range operational activities, including daily and weekly schedules, assignments, and effective use of resources. This nurse manager also keeps records of absences and incidents and prepares personnel appraisals, which are control activities subject to quick changes.

Two measurement methods are used to assess achievement of nursing goals: task analysis and quality control. In task analysis, the nurse manager inspects the motions, actions, and procedures laid out in written guidelines, schedules, rules, records, and budgets. Task analysis is a study of the process of giving nursing care. It measures physical support only; a few tools have been developed to do task analysis in nursing. In quality control the nurse manager is concerned with measurement of the quality and effects of nursing care. The American Nurses Association (ANA), the Joint Commission on Accreditation of Healthcare Organizations (JCAHO), and other organizations have developed mechanisms or models for measuring nursing care. Many quality management techniques are referred to as audits.[21]

Standards

A prime element of the management of nursing services is a system for evaluation of the total effort, including evaluation of the management process, the practice of nursing, and all nursing care services. Evaluation requires standards that can be used as the yardsticks for gauging the quality and quantity of services. The key source for these standards, which are available for both management and practice, is the ANA, whose publications include Scope and Standards for Nurse Administrators and Standards of Clinical Nursing Practice. Several functional yardsticks can be developed using these source documents. These documents can be of assistance in developing the objectives of the division of nursing and of each unit and clinic. Objectives are developed into operational or management plans, and systematic and periodic review of accomplishment of these objectives will be part of the evaluation system. In addition, a management evaluation system can be developed with a similar format. The nurse executive and other nurse managers can effect further evaluation through development of criteria for nursing rounds.

Performance standards can be used for individual performance, and criteria can be developed for collective evaluation of patient care. The latter may include the standards for use during nursing rounds as well as the criteria for the quality management program.

Standards are established criteria of performance, planning goals, strategic plans, physical or quantitative measurements of products, units of service, labor hours, speed, cost, capital, revenue, program, and intangible standards.[22] They have also been defined as "an acknowledged measure of comparison for quantitative or qualitative value, criterion, or norm, . . . a standard rule or test on which a judgment or decision can be based." Nursing managers develop, in collaboration with clinical nurses, the "clinical nursing criteria against which to measure patient outcomes and the nursing process."[23] These standards are stated as patient outcomes, nursing care processes, incident reviews, and evidence-based practice.[24]

The eight categories of standards are[25]:

1. Physical standards. An example would be using patient acuity ratings to establish nursing hours per patient day.
2. Cost standards. Cost per patient day for supplies would be an example.
3. Capital standards. A new program of monetary investment, such as a patient teaching staff, would be included here.
4. Revenue standards. Include the revenue per hour of nursing care received by patients.

5. Program standards. For example one designed to develop a new nursing service for changing clients' behavior regarding exercise, eating, or other health activities.
6. Intangible standards. Staff development costs in nursing are one example. Another example, in the absence of detailed patient classification studies, the staffing standard for nursing homes is expert opinion.
7. Goals are frequently used as standards in nursing management. Intangible standards are being replaced by goals, including those for qualitative measurements.
8. Strategic plans, as control points for strategic control, also are used as standards. As nurse managers increase their involvement in strategic planning, they will need to perform strategic control.

Schoessler described a process for preparing documentation for a JCAHO visit, including a system for maintaining ongoing documentation that is being adapted to changes in JCAHO standards. Such a system ensures that standards are kept up-to-date and prevents last-minute crisis preparation for JCAHO visits. Exhibit 24-1 is an example of a program grid for addressing staff education standards.[26]

Self-study is also a method of meeting JCAHO safety requirements. Employees are held accountable for meeting the standard and are tested to verify competency.[27] Programs are written and distributed by education personnel. Records are maintained on education cards or by computer. Self-study methods can be used to meet other standards.

Measuring productivity is a function of the controlling process. To perform this measure, management establishes a measurement of productivity as the standard for each department and unit. Inputs are computerized and reported to appropriate cost-center managers each month. Productivity measurement tools should be

EXHIBIT 24-1
Program Grid

PROGRAM	MAINTAIN COMPETENCE	DEVELOP NEW COMPETENCE	RESPOND TO QA FINDINGS	NEEDS ASSESSED THROUGH*	EVALUATION OCCURRED THROUGH†	STAFF CONTRIBUTE THROUGH‡
Oncology Workshop	X			I/N	S/E	I/P/D
Advanced Life Support	X			I/P	S/E/P	I
Critical Care Residency		X		I/N	S/E/P	I/P/D
Discharge Planning		X	X	C	S/Q	I

*P = Pretest	†P = Posttest	‡I = Identifying needs of staff
I = Interview	S = Skill demonstration	P = Planning and presentation
N = Needs survey	Q = QA audit	D = Directing unit-based programs
C = Changed or new procedure	E = Evaluation form	S = Sharing information from out-of-house workshops

Source: M. Schoessler. "Preparing Documentation for a JCAHO Visit." *Journal of Nursing Staff Development* (September–October 1991), 217. Reprinted with permission of J. B. Lippincott.

developed, with input from the people being measured. This development may be done locally or through consultation. Nursing departments with computerized patient classification systems often have accurate productivity indices and reporting. Tools to evaluate productivity of independent nurse practitioners are available.[28]

Exhibit 24-2, Operational Plan, is an example of an evaluation or controlling plan for nursing services.

Controlling Techniques

Although evaluation operational plans are controlling techniques, other specific controlling techniques can be developed. These techniques include planned nursing rounds by nurse managers from all levels, checklists from the ANA Scope and Standards of Nurse Administrators, ANA Standards of Clinical Nursing Practice, JCAHO "Accreditation

---

EXHIBIT 24-2
Operational Plan

MISSION STATEMENT TO WHICH OBJECTIVE APPLIES
The division of nursing has a stated philosophy and has objectives. Personnel of each department or unit within the division will have their own philosophy and will set up their own objectives. The objectives will be continuously evaluated and a written statement as to progress will be sent to the chair's office each August and February.

PHILOSOPHY STATEMENT TO WHICH OBJECTIVE APPLIES
We believe that a continuous evaluation of the activities of the division of nursing is necessary to assess how effectively the needs of the patients are being met and to take action to improve nursing service when indicated. Research must be performed, and the results must be analyzed, adapted, and implemented to modify nursing procedures and practices for the attainment of more effective patient care.

OBJECTIVE 6
The patient benefits from close nursing supervision of all nonprofessional personnel who give patient care, and the patient benefits from continuous evaluation of the nursing care given and of performances of all nursing service personnel based on professional standards.

PLANS FOR ACHIEVING OBJECTIVE	ACTION AND ACCOUNTABILITY	TARGET DATES	ACCOMPLISHMENTS
1. Plan and execute a system of continuous evaluation and appraisal of nursing services	1. Make complete rounds throughout the hospital at least once a day from nursing office. Establish a system of formal nursing rounds by chair, assistants, and clinical nursing coordinators monthly.	Apr. 23, 200x	Being done.
	2. Do a monthly nursing audit. Have committee chair brief the chair of the division of nursing afterward.	Dec. 1, 200x	Criteria for major nursing diagnosis outcomes completed. Committee combined with other disciplines. Criteria applied to four nursing diagnosis outcomes with retrieval by medical records personnel and corrective actions taken.
	3. Develop standards for patient care. Use ANA Standards of Clinical Nursing Practice for evaluating patient care. Obtain copies for all head nurses.	Jan. 1, 200x	Obtained. Being incorporated into system by committee of staff nurses. Will cross-check with job performance standards.
	4. Develop standards for personnel performance.	Dec. 31, 200x	Completed for clinical nurses I, II, and III, charge nurse, in-service education coordinator, clinical coordinator, chair and assistants, operating room supervisor and staff nurses, public health nurse, and rehabilitation nurse.

(continued)

EXHIBIT 24-2 *(continued)*

PLANS FOR ACHIEVING OBJECTIVE	ACTION AND ACCOUNTABILITY	TARGET DATES	ACCOMPLISHMENTS

	5. Set up a system whereby managers attend
	   a. Change-of-shift reports.
	   b. Unit conferences
	   c. Unit in-service programs.
		July 1, 200x	Receiving reports and need to plan for their use. Will discuss with managers.

	6. Review and use ANA Scope and Standards for Nurse Administrators to develop an evaluation and inspection checklist.	Dec. 1, 200x	
2. Study organization	1. Reorganize as needed. Have organization chart printed.	July 1, 200x	Done as hospital policy.
	2. Write policy on unit policies and procedures.	July 1, 200x	Done as nursing operating instruction 160-2-4.
3. Establish a counseling program for all nursing personnel	1. Program counseling sessions for all head nurses. Have them do the same for those they supervise. 2. Use the job performance standards.	Jan. 1, 200x	All done once by Jan. 1, 200x.

Manual for Hospitals," and other published standards of third-party payers such as Medicare and Medicaid.

Nursing Rounds

An effective controlling technique for nursing managers is planned nursing rounds, which can be placed on a schedule and can include all nursing personnel. Rounds cover issues such as patient care, nursing practice, and unit management. To be effective, the results should be discussed with appropriate nursing personnel in a follow-up conference. Part of the evaluation process takes place as a result of the communication occurring during the rounds. Exhibit 24-3 shows a protocol for planned monthly nursing rounds.

EXHIBIT 24-3
Protocol for Planned Monthly Nursing Rounds

1. The chair, assistant chair, and other appropriate nursing personnel will make nursing rounds monthly.
2. Time is 10:00 to 11:00 a.m. unless otherwise indicated.
3. Schedule:

UNIT	DAY
1F	1st Tuesday
2A	1st Wednesday
2B	1st Thursday
2F	2nd Tuesday
ICU	2nd Wednesday
4A	2nd Thursday
3A	2nd Friday
3-OB	3rd Tuesday, 10:30 to 11:30 a.m.
3F	3rd Wednesday
4B	3rd Thursday, 11:00 a.m. to 12:00 noon
5A, CCU	4th Tuesday
5B	4th Wednesday

4. All unit nursing personnel are welcome to attend these rounds with their head nurse. Patient care needs come first. The following areas will be covered as rounds are made to each patient's bedside:
   a. Nursing histories
   b. Nursing care plans
   c. Nursing notes
   d. Nurses' signatures on necessary documents
5. Other management areas of note will be discussed after bedside rounds:
   a. Equipment and supplies
   b. Staffing and assignments
   c. Narcotic registers

Nursing Operating Instructions

Nursing operating instructions or policies become standards for evaluation and controlling techniques (see Exhibit 24-4).

The ANA Scope and Standards for Nurse Administrators can be developed into a checklist for evaluating the management processes of nursing services. Exhibit 24-5 shows a format for converting these standards into a usable control tool.

The ANA Standards of Clinical Nursing Practice can be implemented in several ways. One way is to convert these into a checklist as in Exhibit 24-5. The entire set of standards can be developed into a checklist along these lines. Written protocols should be developed to implement a program for the evaluation process. Another way these protocols may be implemented is by using them to develop the evaluation standards, as in Exhibit 24-6.

Gantt Charts

Early in the twentieth century, Henry L. Gantt developed the Gantt chart as a means of controlling production. The chart, which is usually used for production activities, depicts a series of events essential to the completion of a project or program.

Exhibit 24-7 shows a modified Gantt chart that could be applied to a major nursing administration program or project. The five major activities identified are segments of a total program or project. The chart could be applied to a project such as implementing a modality of primary nursing or implementing case management. The following are possible nursing activities for a project:

EXHIBIT 24-5

Format for Converting the ANA Scope and Standards for Nurse Administrators into a Usable Control Tool

STANDARD NO. _____ :

Measurement Criteria	Yes	No
(List)		

- Gather data.
- Analyze data.
- Develop a plan.
- Implement the plan.
- Evaluate, give feedback, and modify the plan as needed.

Exhibit 24-7 is only an example. Application of this controlling process by nurse managers would be specific to the project or program, and the time elements for the various activities would vary. Also, using subcategories of activities with estimated completion times could modify these five major activities. The nurse manager's goal is to complete each activity or phase on or before the projected date.

Critical Control Points and Milestones

Master evaluation plans should have *critical control points*, specific points in production of goods or services at which the nurse administrator judges whether the objectives are being met qualitatively and quantitatively. Critical control points tell whether the plan is progressing satisfactorily. They pinpoint successes and

---

EXHIBIT 24-4

Operating Instructions

1. Special care units will maintain policies and procedures relative to their mission. (These procedures will be reviewed, updated, and signed at least annually.)
   a. Intensive care unit
   b. Critical care unit
   c. Newborn/intensive care unit nursery
   d. Renal dialysis
2. Special care units will maintain a list of equipment needed to achieve their mission.
3. Supplies and equipment
   a. Blount resuscitator will have percent adaptor to increase oxygen concentration.
   b. Ambu resuscitator will have tail on to increase oxygen concentration.
   c. Humidification will not be used with oxygen with Ambu resuscitator.
   d. Trays from Central Sterile Supply will be returned as soon as used so that instruments will not be lost or misplaced.

EXHIBIT 24-6

Standards for Evaluating the Controlling (Evaluating) Function of Nursing Administration of a Division, Service, or Unit

1. An evaluation plan exists and is used for each nursing department, service, or unit.
2. Each evaluation plan is specific to the needs and activities of the individual department, service, or unit.
3. Evaluation findings are given in immediate feedback to subordinate nursing personnel.
4. Standards are accurate, suitable, and objective.
5. Standards are flexible and work when changes are made in plans and when unforeseen events and failures occur.
6. Standards mirror the organizational pattern of the nursing division, service, or unit.
7. Standards are economical to apply and do not produce unexpected results or effects.
8. Nursing personnel know and understand the standards.
9. Application of the standards results in correction of deficiencies.

EXHIBIT 24-7
Modified Gantt Chart

Nursing action

	Jan	Feb	Mar	Apr	May	Jun	Jul	Aug	Sep	Oct	Nov	Dec

Note: Five nursing actions are needed to complete a program planned to start in January and end in December. In Exhibit 24–8, these five actions are translated into milestones and critical control points.

failures and their causes. Critical control points tell managers whether they are on target with regard to time, budget, and other resources. *Milestones* are segments or phases of specific activities of a project or program that are projected to occur within a time frame.

Exhibit 24-8 represents a modified Gantt chart with networks of milestones and critical control points.

The critical path is

$$1 \rightarrow 2 \rightarrow 3 \rightarrow 4 \rightarrow 5 \rightarrow 6 \rightarrow 7 \rightarrow 8 \rightarrow 9 \rightarrow 17 \rightarrow 18.$$

Line 5 represents evaluation of all other nursing actions. This illustration is a simplified version of a control technique. Case management also uses critical paths with milestones and control points. Any major nursing program could have dozens or even hundreds of milestones and critical control points. This system

also is known as the program evaluation and review technique (PERT).

Application of the milestone technique involves establishing a network of controllable pieces when planning a project or program. Each piece of the project or program is also allocated a prorated portion of the total budget. A nurse manager could use this technique to evaluate the actual expenditure amount versus the estimated budget at the end of each step of activity (or monthly) of the project or program. These will be the critical control points, as each would culminate in the achievement of a milestone. Each event may represent a budgeting allocation, a period of time or time span, or a continuum of several or all of these. Bar graphs are frequently used to depict milestone budgeting. Budgeting is a major controlling technique in any of its forms.[29]

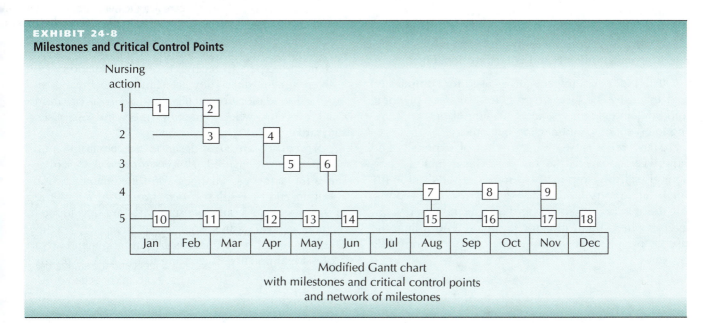

EXHIBIT 24-8
Milestones and Critical Control Points

Nursing action

Modified Gantt chart
with milestones and critical control points
and network of milestones

Program Evaluation and Review Technique, or PERT

The program evaluation and review technique was developed by the Special Projects Office of the U. S. Navy and applied to the planning and control of the Polaris weapon system in 1958. The PERT system worked then, it works today, and it has been widely applied as a controlling process in business and industry.

PERT uses a network of activities, each of which is represented as a step on a chart. A time measurement and an estimated budget should be worked out that include the following[30]:

1. Finished product or service desired.
2. Total time and budget needed to complete the project or program.
3. Start and completion dates.
4. Sequence of steps or activities required to accomplish the project or program.
5. Estimated time and cost of each step or activity.
6. Three paths for steps 4 and 5:
   a. Optimistic time.
   b. Most likely time.
   c. Pessimistic time.
7. Calculation of the critical path, the sequence of the events that would take the longest time to complete the project or program by the planned completion date. This is the critical path because it will leave the least slack time.

Why should nurse managers use the PERT system for controlling?

- It forces planning and shows how the pieces fit for all nursing line managers involved.
- It establishes a system for periodic evaluation and control at critical points in the program.
- It reveals problems and is forward looking.

The PERT system generally is used for complicated and extensive projects or programs such as planning and implementing a system of nursing diagnoses, nursing interventions, and nursing outcomes.

Many records are used to control expenses and otherwise conserve the budget. These include personnel staffing reports, overtime reports, monthly financial reports, and expense and revenue reports. All these reports should be available to nurse managers to help them monitor, evaluate, and adjust the use of people and money as part of the controlling process.[31]

> **Multiple sites exist on the Internet as resources for information on controlling techniques, including Gantt and PERT charts. Many software programs are available for using these tools (www.guysoftware.com/index.htm).**

Benchmarking

Benchmarking is an offshoot of quality management and a technique whereby an organization seeks out the best practices in its industry to improve its performance. Benchmarking is a standard, or point of reference, in measuring or judging factors such as quality, values, and costs. The following are examples of benchmarks that could apply to nursing[32]:

- Establishing a skill mix of nursing employees to obtain the highest quality of patient care at the lowest cost, which is called *vertical leveraging. Horizontal leveraging* uses cross-training to boost productivity. If the average for the industry were a ratio of 60% registered nurses to 40% other nursing personnel, the institution would make a decision to meet or exceed this ratio.
- An operating room utilization rate of 80% or higher if the industry rate is 75%.
- An average turnover time between cases of 15 minutes if the industry rate is 20 minutes.
- A reduction of 10% from the average-for-industry cost of supplies per patient day.
- A reduction of 50% from the average-for-industry rate of hospital-acquired infections.

> **Standards of practice and standards of care are the benchmarks for nursing practice in all domains.**

Standards of care define the levels of care that a patient can expect to receive in a given situation or on a given nursing unit. They are clinical benchmarks and are the foundation for quality improvement programs. Quality occurs when personnel meet the established standards.

Structure standards describe the environment in which care is delivered. *Process standards* describe a series of activities, changes, or functions that bring about an end or result. *Clinical standards*, a subgroup of the process and outcome standards, are developed to include clinical issues specific to areas of practice. These include both standards of care and standards of professional practice. According to the ANA, *standards of care* are authoritative statements describing a competent level of practice. *Standards of professional practice* are authoritative statements describing a competent level of behavior in the professional role.[33] *Outcome standards* are the results to be achieved.

Standards of practice to be achieved are used to structure the quality management program. They are linked to policy and procedure development and to job descriptions and performance appraisals. Implementation of standards is done through use of generic nursing care plans and the computer. Computers provide generic nursing care plans and nursing diagnoses, interventions, and outcomes. Exhibit 24-9 is an example of a generic nursing care plan.[34]

> **Benchmarking is enhanced when quality teams perform at the highest level of service by sharing their best practices and processes with similar committee teams in other institutions and organizations.**

EXHIBIT 24-9
Generic Nursing Care Plan

ST. JOHN MEDICAL CENTER
Medical Excellence • Compassionate Care

GENERAL SURGERY

DATE	NURSING DIAGNOSIS/PROBLEMS	INIT	INTERVENTIONS/ DISCHARGE PLANS	GOALS	DATE RESOLVED
	☐ Anxiety related to fear of surgical procedure as evidenced by: ☐ call light on frequently ☐ multiple questions ☐ inability to sleep ☐ _____		☐ Preoperative teaching method _____ ☐ Provide reassurance and comfort _____	☐ Patient will express feelings of comfort and decreased anxiety	
	☐ Alteration in comfort related to surgical procedure as evidenced by: ☐ protecting the surgical site ☐ inability to stand upright ☐ shallow respiration ☐ _____		☐ Position for comfort _____ ☐ Instruct patient on splinting of incision ☐ Anticipate patient's needs for analgesics	☐ Pain is minimized/controlled with good muscle relaxation and ventilation	

Source: M. McAllister. "A Nursing Integration Framework Based on Standards of Practice." *Nursing Management* (April 1990), 31. Reprinted with permission.

Quality management is a necessary element of benchmarking. The following are some benefits of benchmarking:

- Goals and objectives are set, and full team support to meet them is obtained.
- Performance regarding practices, processes, and outcomes is continually improved.
- Commitment and accountability for excellence exist.
- New approaches are sought out, learned, and adapted to.
- Organizational communication is improved.
- Clinical governance is improved.
- Patient satisfaction is improved.

The benchmarking program includes planning during team meetings, collection of specific data, data analysis to determine gaps, integration through keeping all team members informed, action, and follow-up and monitoring.[35]

Master Control Plan

To fulfill this important management function, nurse managers can use a master control or evaluation plan. It can be a general plan for all, with each manager adding specific items for his or her own management area. A sample basic master control plan in depicted in Exhibit 24-10.

EXHIBIT 24-10
Master Control Plan

OBJECTIVE 1
Inspect for and identify the presence of written, current, and practical statements of mission, philosophy, vision, and objectives for the division of nursing and each of its component units. The statements should reflect the purposes of the health care organization and give direction to the nursing care program.

Actions

1. The written statements of mission, philosophy, and objectives were current (reviewed or revised within past year).
2. They existed for the division of nursing and for each department, ward, unit, and clinic.
3. They were written by appropriate nursing personnel, representative of people who will accomplish them.
4. The philosophy reflected the meaning of clinical practice.
5. The philosophy was developed in collaboration with consumers, employees, and other health care workers.
6. The objectives were specified, written in behavioral terms, and achievable.
7. They guided the process of implementing the philosophy.
8. They were used for orientation of newly assigned personnel and were otherwise widely distributed and interpreted.
9. They supported the mission, philosophy, and objectives of the institution.
10. Nursing personnel knew the rights of individuals and served as advocates for these rights.

OBJECTIVE 2
Inspect for and identify the presence of written operational or management plans for accomplishment of the objectives of the division of nursing and each of its component units.

Actions

1. The written operational or management plans were current (entries within past 30 days).
2. They existed for the division of nursing and for each department, ward, unit, and clinic.

3. They included specific actions to be taken to achieve objective, target dates, and names of personnel assigned responsibility for each action.
4. They were used to evaluate progress; accomplishments were listed.

OBJECTIVE 3
Inspect for and identify the presence of an organizational plan for the division of nursing and each of its component units.

Actions

1. The organizational plan was current; it agreed with actual organization when checked.
2. It existed for the division of nursing and for each department, ward, unit, and clinic.
3. It showed the relationships among component parts, spelling out the major functions of each, and it showed relationships with other services.
4. The organizational plan supported the mission assigned to personnel.
5. All nursing functions were managed by the nurse administrator.

OBJECTIVE 4
Inspect for and identify the presence of adequate policies and procedures for guidance of personnel of the division of nursing and each of its component units.

Actions

1. Policies and procedures of the division of nursing and of each department, ward, unit, and clinic were current (reviewed within past year).
2. Policies and procedures did not duplicate those of higher echelons.
3. Policies and procedures were not obsolete, restrictive, or inappropriate in context.
4. Content of location of policies and procedures was known by people who needed this information.
5. Policies and procedures for special care units included.

(continued)

EXHIBIT 24-10 (continued)

a. Function and authority of unit director.
b. Admission and discharge criteria.
c. Criteria for performance of special procedures, including cardiopulmonary resuscitation, tracheostomy, ordering of medications, administration of parenteral fluids and other medication, and the obtaining of blood and other laboratory specimens.
d. The use, location, and maintenance of equipment and supplies.
e. Respiratory care.
f. Infection control.
g. Priorities for orders for laboratory tests.
h. Standing orders, if any.
i. Regulations for visitors and traffic control.
6. The nursing annex to the disaster plan was current and included
a. Recall procedures.
b. Assignment procedures.
c. Training plan.

OBJECTIVE 5
Inspect for and identify the presence of job descriptions and job standards for all personnel throughout the division of nursing.

Actions

1. Job descriptions and job standards existed and were current throughout the division of nursing (reviewed within past year).
2. Nursing personnel participated in formulating them.
3. Nursing personnel were classified according to competence, and salaries were commensurate with qualifications and positions of comparable responsibility within the agency and the community.
4. Job descriptions were used for purposes of counseling and helping employees to be productive.
5. They were used for orientation of newly assigned personnel.
6. They described the functions, qualifications, and authority of each position identified in the organizational plan.
7. They were readily available and known to each employee.
8. There was a designated nurse leader for the division of nursing who was a registered nurse with educational and experiential qualifications in nursing practice and the administration of nursing services.

OBJECTIVE 6
Inspect for and identify the presence of a master staffing plan for the division of nursing and each of its component units.

Actions

1. A master staffing plan existed and was current for the division of nursing and each department, ward, unit, or clinic. It showed authorized versus assigned personnel and was reviewed at least monthly.
2. Adequate personnel policies existed to give guidance to nursing personnel in the planning of time schedules and to allow for mobility so that personnel could be matched to jobs.
3. Avenues of communication existed to give input from nursing personnel to the nurse administrator regarding staffing problems.
4. An active plan existed for sponsoring newly assigned personnel and for identifying their special training and experience and their desired assignments.

OBJECTIVE 7
Inspect for and identify the presence of a planned counseling program for all personnel of the division of nursing.

Actions

1. The nurse executive had a planned program for counseling with managers, including charge nurses.
2. Counseling occurred at least every six months on a scheduled basis.
3. Charge nurses counseled with individual staff members on a scheduled basis at least once every six months.
4. The counseling process included discussion of progress toward personal objectives, and revisions resulted from the sessions. Job standards were reviewed, and special educational and experience goals were discussed and acted on.
5. Records of counseling sessions were available and were reviewed.
6. A career progression plan was operational.

OBJECTIVE 8
Inspect for and identify the presence of a system of evaluation of nursing activities in the division of nursing and each of its component units.

Actions

1. A system for evaluation of the division of nursing and each of its departments, wards, units, and clinics was in operation.
2. Change-of-shift reports and ward conferences were being periodically evaluated (at least once every six months).
3. Management plans indicated current evaluation of accomplishment of objectives (within past 30 days).
4. Management personnel, including the nurse executive, made planned ward rounds at least monthly and checked all aspects of department, ward, unit, or clinic management, including

(continued)

EXHIBIT 24-10 *(continued)*

a. Narcotic registers
b. Nursing histories
c. Nursing care plans
d. Nursing notes
e. Drug levels and security
f. Supplies and equipment
g. Assignment procedures
h. Patient records

5. The quality assurance program was in effect, and at least one problem per month had been evaluated since June 1.
6. There was provision for inclusion of other health care disciplines and consumers in evaluating the nursing care programs.
7. Results of evaluation were used to assess planning for change.

OBJECTIVE 9

Inspect for and identify the representation of division of nursing personnel on institution-wide and departmental boards, committees, and councils.

Actions

1. The division of nursing was represented on institution-wide boards, committees, and councils whose activities affected nursing personnel directly.
   a. Social actions
   b. Personnel boards such as awards and benefits
2. Nursing service committees had specific objectives.
3. Membership was current and representative of all appropriate segments of the nursing staff.
4. Minutes of meetings reflected progress toward objectives and follow-up of problems.

OBJECTIVE 10

Inspect for and identify the existence of a working public relations program that serves as a means of communication between personnel of the division of nursing and the community they serve.

Actions

1. Evaluation programs existed to tell consumers of the nursing services available to them and to receive feedback from consumers on the types of services they needed.
2. There was a planned program to publicize nursing activities and recognize contributions and accomplishments of nursing personnel.

OBJECTIVE 11

Inspect for and identify the existence of a planned program for training and continuing education for all division of nursing personnel.

Actions

1. Written statements of mission, philosophy, and objectives existed and were current (reviewed within past year).

2. An operational or management plan for the accomplishment of objectives was current (entries made within past 30 days).
3. The plan listed activities, set priorities and target dates, assigned responsibility, and provided for continuous evaluation.
4. The plan provided for identification of training and continuing education needs, including input from participants, translation of needs into objectives, and the accomplishment of objectives.
5. An orientation program existed and included philosophy and objectives of organization and nursing service, personnel policies, job descriptions, work environment, clinical practice policies and procedures, and operational policies and procedures.
6. Supplemental classes were taught to meet on-the-job training needs.
7. Training programs were documented.
8. The program supported career advancement.

OBJECTIVE 12

Inspect for and identify the existence of procedures and policies for providing needed primary nursing care to patients.

Actions

1. Collection of data on each patient was sufficient to permit identification and assessment of the patient's needs and to institute an individual plan of care. Included were admission data and patient's nursing history.
2. The nursing care plan included the nursing diagnosis, prescription for care, and patient's teaching needs.
3. The plan was used to provide care to the patient, and there was an ongoing reassessment of the patient's needs with appropriate changes made in the plan of care.
4. There was evidence that nursing actions required by physicians' orders, nursing care plans, and hospital policies were accomplished appropriately. Observations of patient's progress and response to actions were made and recorded.
5. There was evidence of interpretation and implementation of the ANA *Standards of Clinical Nursing Practice*.
6. Nursing administration had a plan for reviewing the requirements for giving credentials to individuals and health care organizations and for participating in their implementation.
7. Guidelines existed for assignment of personnel based on level of competence.
8. There were policies to use unit managers and ward clerks to perform clerical, managerial, and indirect service roles.
9. Nursing administration provided resources to accomplish primary nursing care to patient: facilities, equipment, supplies, and personnel.

Summary

Controlling or evaluating is an ongoing function of nursing management occurring during planning, organizing, and directing activities. Through this process, standards are established and then applied, followed by feedback that leads to improvements. The process is kept continuous.

Each nurse manager should have a master plan of control that incorporates all standards related to these actions. This plan can be applied to obtain immediate feedback and meet the objectives of control established for the unit, department, or division. The plan will verify results, provide instructions, and apply principles of uniformity, comparison, and exception.

Controls include policies, rules, procedures, self-control or self-regulation, discipline, rounds, reports, audits, evaluation devices, task analysis, quality control, and benchmarking. They should reflect the nature of the activity and be forward looking, objective, flexible, economical, and understandable. Controls should lead to continuous action.

Standards are the yardsticks for evaluation and include ANA Scope and Standards for Nurse Administrators and Standards of Clinical Nursing Practice. Other standards include management plans, goals, programs, costs, revenues, and capital. Physical standards use Gantt charts, critical control points, milestones, and PERT. Each nurse manager should have a master evaluation plan.

APPLICATION EXERCISE

EXERCISE 24-1   With a group of your peers or colleagues, use Exhibits 24-6 and 24-10 to discuss developing a new evaluation plan for a nursing cost center. Incorporate the standards from both exhibits. How can they be measured? Modify them if need be. Use your final product to evaluate the cost center.

NOTES

1. H. Fayol, *General and Industrial Management*, translated by C. Storrs (London: Sir Isaac Pitman & Sons, 1949), 107.
2. L. Urwick, *The Elements of Administration* (New York: Harper & Row, 1944), 105.
3. Ibid., 107–110.
4. Ibid., 113–117.
5. Koontz and H. Weihrich, *Management*, 5th ed. (New York: McGraw-Hill, 1990), 394–395; R. M. Hodgetts, *Management: Theory, Process, and Practice*, 5th ed. (Orlando, FL: Harcourt Brace 1990), 226–229; R. M. Fulmer and S. G. Franklin, *Supervision: Principles of Professional Management*, 2nd ed. (New York: Macmillan, 1982), 214–216; H. S. Rowland and B. L. Rowland, *Nursing Administration Handbook*, 4th ed. (Gaithersburg, MD: Aspen, 1997), 15–16, 35–44; P. F. Drucker, *Management: Tasks, Responsibilities, Practices* (New York: Harper & Row, 1973), 495–505; A. Marriner-Tomey, *Guide to Nursing Management and Leadership*, 5th ed. (St. Louis: Mosby 1996), 379; D. C. Mosley, P. H. Pietri, and L. C. Megginson, *Management: Leadership in Action*, 5th ed. (New York: HarperCollins, 1996), 492–512.
6. T. Peters, *Thriving on Chaos* (New York: Harper & Row, 1987), 587, 593.
7. S. Rowland and B. L. Rowland, op. cit., 40.
8. T. Kron and A. Gray, *The Management of Patient Care: Putting Leadership Skills to Work*, 6th ed. (Philadelphia: W. B. Saunders, 1987), 100
9. H. Koontz and H. Weihrich, op. cit.; 393.
10. B. S. Barnum and M. Kerfoot, *The Nurse as Executive*, 4th ed. (Gaithersburg, MD: Aspen, 1995), 229.
11. C. Arndt and L. M. D. Huckebay, *Nursing Administration: Theory for Practice with a Systems Approach*, 2nd ed. (St. Louis: C.V. Mosby, 1980), 22–46.
12. P. Franck and M. Price, *Nursing Management*, 2nd ed. (New York: Springer Publishing, 1980), 135.
13. M. L. Holle and M. E. Blatchly, *Introduction to Leadership and Management in Nursing* (Monterey, CA: Wadsworth Health Services Division, 1982), 178–185.
14. A. Levenstein, *The Nurse as Manager*, M. J. F. Smith, ed. (Chicago: S-N Publications, 1981), 17–33.
15. B. Lemin, *First Line Nursing Management* (New York: Springer, 1977), 47–51.
16. Ibid.
17. R. M. Fulmer and S. G. Franklin, op. cit., 216–217.
18. G. Ramey, "Setting Standards and Evaluating Care," S. Stone et al., eds., *Management for Nurses* (St. Louis: C. V. Mosby, 1976), 79.
19. H. M. Donovon, *Nursing Service Administration: Managing the Enterprise* (St. Louis, MO: 1975), 160–169.
20. M. Beyers and C. Phillips, *Nursing Management for Patient Care*, 2nd ed. (Boston: Little, Brown, 1979), 109–141.
21. L. M. Douglass, *The Effective Nurse: Leader and Manager*, 5th ed. (St. Louis: C. V. Mosby, 1986), 245–278.
22. H. Koontz and H. Weihrich, op. cit., 394–395.
23. J. M. Ganong and W. L. Ganong, *Nursing Management*, 2nd ed. (Gaithersburg, MD: Aspen, 1980), 191.
24. M. A. Rosswurm and J. H. Larrabee, "A Model for Change to Evidence-Based Practice," *Image: The Journal of Nursing Scholarship*, 31(4), 1999, 317–322; P. Matthews, "Planning for Successful Outcomes in the New Millennium," *Topics in*

Health Information Management, (February 2000), 55–64; M. S. Silver, "Incident Review Management: A Systemic Approach to Performance Improvements," *Journal of Healthcare Quality* (November–December 1999), 21–27.

25. H. Koontz and H. Weihrich, op. cit., 396–398; C. Harrington, C. Kovner, M. Mezey, J. Kayser-Jones, S. Burger, M. Mohler, R. Burke and D. Zimmerman, "Experts Recommend Minimum Nurse Staffing Standards for Nursing Facilities in the United States," *Gerontologist* (February 2000), 5–16.

26. M. M. Schoessler, "Preparing Documentation for a JCAHO Visit," *Journal of Nursing Staff Development* (September–October 1991), 215–219.

27. A. Haggard, "Using Self-Studies to Meet JCAHO Requirements," *Journal of Nursing Staff Development* (July–August 1992), 170–174.

28. D. R. Kearnes, "A Productivity Tool to Evaluate NP Practice: Monitoring Clinical Time Spent in Reimbursable Patient-Related Activities," *Nurse Practitioner* (April 1992), 50, 52, 55.

29. H. Koontz and H. Weihrich, op. cit., 424; R. M. Hodgetts, op. cit., 243; M. Beyers and C. Phillips, op. cit., 134–135; H. S. Rowland and B. L. Rowland, op. cit., 36; R. M. Fulmer and S. G. Franklin, op. cit., 221–227; http://www-mmd.eng.ac.uk/people 9/17/2000; http://gracie.santarosa.edu, 9/17/2000.

30. H. Koontz and H. Weihrich, op. cit., 424–428, R. M. Hodgetts, op. cit., 240–242; http://www.criticaltools.com 9/17/2000; http://www.infosystems.eku.edu, 9/17/2000

31. J. M. Ganong and W. L. Ganong, op. cit., 257.

32. P. Patterson, "Benchmarking Study Identifies Hospitals Best Practices," *OR Manager* (April 1993), 11, 14–15.

33. American Nurses Association, *Standards of Clinical Nursing Practice* (Washington, DC: 1991).

34. M. McAllister, "A Nursing Integration Framework Based on Standards of Practice," *Nursing Management* (April 1990), 28–31.

35. J. A. Murray and M. H. Murray, "Benchmarking: A Tool for Excellence in Palliative Care," *Journal of Palliative Care* 8(4), (1992), 41–45; N. Woomer, C. O. Long, C. Anderson, and E. A. Greenberg, "Benchmarking in Home Health Care: A Collaborative Approach," *Caring* (November 1999), 22–28; S. McGowan, D. Wynaden, N. Harding, A. Yassine, and J. Parker, "Staff Confidence in Dealing with Aggressive Patients: A Benchmarking Exercise," *Australia New Zealand Journal of Mental Health Nursing* (September 1999), 104–108; C. R. Voyles and K. B. Boyd, "Criteria and Benchmarks for Laparoscopic Cholecystectomy in a Free-Standing Ambulatory Center," *JSLS*

(October–December 1999), 315–318; D. Gardner and C. Winder, "Using Benchmarking to Improve Organizational Communication," *Quality Assurance* (October–December 1998), 201–211; "Nurse Staffing Law May Herald Benchmarks," *Healthcare Benchmarks* (December 1999), 137–138; B. C. Johnson and M. J. Chambers, "Foodservice Benchmarking: Practices, Attitudes, and Beliefs of Foodservice Directors," *Journal of the American Dietetic Association* (February 2000), 175–182; C. E. Bucknall, I. Ryland, A. Cooper, I. I. Coutts, C. K. Connolly and M. G. Pearson, "National Benchmarking as a Support System for Clinical Governance," *Journal of Royal College of Physicians London* (January–February 2000), 52–56.

REFERENCES

American Nurses Association. *Scope and Standards for Nurse Administrators* (Washington, DC, 1995).

Balle, M. "Making Bureaucracy Work." *Journal of Management in Medicine* 13(2–3), (1999) 190–200

Coombs, C. R., N. F. Doherty, and J. Loan-Clarke. "Factors Affecting the Level of Success of Community Information Systems." *Journal of Management in Medicine* 13(2–30), (1999) 142–153.

Dreachslin, J. L. "Diversity Leadership and Organizational Transformation: Performance Indicators for Health Services Organizations." *Journal of Healthcare Management* (November–December 1999), 427–439.

Jones, L. "Integrating Research Activities, Practice Changes, and Monitoring and Evaluation: A Model for Academic Health." *Quality Review Bulletin* (July 1991), 229–239.

Kurec, A. S. "Recruiting, Interviewing, and Hiring the Right Person." *Clinical Laboratory Management Review* (September–October 1999), 251–261.

"Patient Satisfaction Measures More Meaningful with New Standardized Surveying System." *Data Strategic Benchmarks* (October 1999), 149–153

Swansburg, R.C. *Management of Patient Care Services* (St. Louis: Mosby 1976).

Walker, J., A. Brooksby, J. McInerny, and A. Taylor. "Patient Perceptions of Hospital Care: Building Confidence, Faith and Trust." *Journal of Nursing Management* (July 1998), 193–200.

Ziegler, J. C., and N. K. Van Ellen. "Implementation of a National Nursing Standards Program." *Journal of Nursing Administration* (November 1992), 40–46.

Total Quality Management

Russell C. Swansburg, PhD, RN

> Improve quality (and) you automatically improve productivity. You capture the market with lower price and better quality. You stay in business and you provide jobs. It's so simple.
>
> W. Edwards Deming[1]

LEARNING OBJECTIVES AND ACTIVITIES

- Describe the elements of total quality management.
- Discuss Deming's 14 points of a theory of management.
- Discuss Deming's seven deadly diseases related to his theory of management.
- Distinguish among examples of common and special causes of variation.
- Apply the Deming (Shewhart) cycle.
- Make a Pareto diagram using categories and measures of your choice.
- Do a fishbone diagram to isolate the causes of a problem.
- Identify nursing's internal and external customers.
- Prepare a total quality matrix related to current cultural examples within your workplace.
- Form and use a quality circle to identify, analyze, and solve a problem within your workplace.

CONCEPTS: Total quality management (TQM), Deming (Shewhart) cycle, Pareto diagram, internal customer, external customer, Theory Z, quality circle.

MANAGER BEHAVIOR: Uses select elements of a total quality management (TQM) theory in controlling or evaluating organizational performance.

LEADER BEHAVIOR: Applies the principles of a total quality management (TQM) theory as the foundation for controlling or evaluating organizational performance.

Introduction

In total quality management (TQM), quality is a state of mind, a work ethic involving everyone in the company.[2]

TQM has been described "as a way of life that they (business leaders) believe can ensure the survival of American business."[3] Among the elements of TQM are decentralization and *participative management*, that is, the process of making decisions at lower levels in the organizational hierarchy. This process involves every employee in making management contributions: It allows them to fix things instead of being treated like robots. TQM reduces or eliminates adversarial relationships.[4] Other elements of TQM are matrix management and management by objectives (MBO), statistical analyses, team building, quality circles, and Theory Z.

Many U.S. managers blame workers, taxes, government regulations, and the decay of society, among other things, for productivity problems. W. Edwards Deming, an early advocate of the principle of management for quality, found that 80% to 85% of problems are with the system; only 15% to 20% are with workers. Workers should be told this and given the freedom to speak and contribute as thinking, creative human beings. Deming's theory of management includes 14 points (see Exhibit 25-1). Deming also warned against the seven deadly diseases that decrease productivity and profitability because they destroy employee morale (see Exhibit 25-2).

> Total quality management and benchmarking should be integral parts of strategic and operational planning.[5] TQM does not compromise organizational effectiveness; TQM improves effectiveness and contributes to an enterprise increasing market share of business.[6]

> **EXHIBIT 25-1**
> **Deming's 14 Points**
>
> 1. Create constancy of purpose toward improvement of product and service. Everyone should have a clear goal every day, month after month. Satisfy the customer and reduce variation so all employees do not have to constantly shift their priorities.
> 2. Adopt a new philosophy by learning how to improve systems in the presence of variation, thus reducing variation in materials, people, processes, and products. End tampering and overreacting to variation.
> 3. Cease dependence on inspection to achieve quality by thoroughly understanding the sources of variation in processes and working to reduce variation.
> 4. End the practice of awarding business on the basis of price tag alone. Instead, minimize total cost by working with a single supplier.
> 5. Improve constantly and forever every process for planning, production, and service. Everyone uses PDCA (plan-do-check-act) cycle.
> 6. Institute training on the job. Know methods of performing tasks and standardize training. Accommodate variation in ways people learn.
> 7. Adopt and institute leadership. Work to help employees do their jobs better and with less effort. Learn which employees are within the system and which are not. Support company goals, focus on internal and external customers, coach, and nurture pride in workmanship.
> 8. Drive out fear, including fear of reprisal, fear of failure, fear of providing information, fear of not knowing, fear of giving up control, and fear of change. Fear makes accurate data nonexistent.
> 9. Break down barriers among staff areas, between departments. Promote cooperation. What is the constant, common goal?
> 10. Eliminate slogans, exhortations, and targets for the work force. Improvement requires changed methods and processes. Leaders change the system.
> 11. Eliminate numerical quotas for the work force and numerical goals for management. All people do not work at the same level of speed. There will be variation. Use realistic production standards. Eliminate management by objectives and use a system that rewards people's efforts toward improvement.
> 12. Remove barriers that rob people of pride of workmanship. Eliminate the annual rating or merit system.
> 13. Institute a vigorous program of education and self-improvement for everyone. This can be any education that improves self-esteem and potential to contribute to improvements in existing processes and advances in technology.
> 14. Put everyone in the company to work to accomplish the transformation.

Source: Reprinted from *Out of the Crisis* by W. Edwards Deming by permission of MIT and The W. Edwards Deming Institute. Published by MIT, Center for Advanced Engineering Study, Cambridge, MA 02139. Copyright 1986 by The W. Edwards Deming Institute. Dr. Deming rejected the concept of TQM, saying it was undefined.

> **EXHIBIT 25-2**
> **Deming's Seven Deadly Diseases**
>
> 1. Lack of constancy of purpose.
> 2. Emphasis on short-term profits.
> 3. Evaluation of performance, merit rating, or annual review.
> 4. Management by use of only visible figures.
> 5. Mobility of management.
> 6. Excessive medical costs.
> 7. Excessive costs of liability.

Source: Reprinted from *Out of the Crisis* by W. Edwards Deming by permission of MIT and The W. Edwards Deming Institute. Published by MIT, Center for Advanced Engineering Study, Cambridge, MA 02139. Copyright 1986 by The W. Edwards Deming Institute.

Application of Deming's Theory

According to Piczak, General Douglas McArthur summoned W. Edwards Deming to set up quality circles for the Japanese in 1950.[7] When Deming presented the quality methods to 45 Japanese industrialists, they applied the methods. "Within six weeks, some of the industrialists were reporting gains of as much as 30 percent without purchasing any new equipment."[8]

Using Deming's methods, managers and workers have a natural division of labor: The workers do the work of the system, while the managers improve the system. Thus, the potential for improving the system is never ending. Because workers know where the potential for improving the system lies, consultants are not needed. Managers know the system is subject to great variability and that problem events occur randomly. The common language for managers and workers is elementary statistics, which all workers learn.[9]

The Language Is Statistics

Variation

Deming used and advocated the use of the language of statistics to identify which problems are caused by workers and which by the system. The most-used statistical tool is that of variation, which measures whether an activity is under control or, if not, to what degree it is out of control. Statistics enable workers to control variation by teaching them to work more intelligently. The common language of statistics stimulates discussion between workers and bosses at quality circle meetings.[10] Variation is the concept that distinguishes normal routine changes in a process from unusual, abnormal changes that can be attributed to specific causes. Variations in performance are attributable mostly to the system. Deming, in examples, found 400% variation in performance attributable to the system.[11]

According to Deming, Shewhart, and others, there are chance (common) causes and special (assigned) causes of variation. *Chance causes* are common causes that are the fault of the system. They are system variations such as process input or conditions that are ever present and cause small, random shifts in daily output. These variations occur in 90% of cases and require fundamental system change by management. Chance causes are controlled causes. A system totally influenced by controlled variation or common causes is said to be in statistical control.

Special, or assigned, causes are specific to a particular group of workers, an area, or a machine. *Special causes* are uncontrolled variations resulting from assignable causes or sources. Special causes occur in less than 10% of cases. A special cause requires the local work force to find the source and take preventive action. Special causes require obtaining timely data to effect changes that will prevent bad causes and keep good causes happening (see Exhibit 25-3).

Management by action uses the Deming (Shewhart) cycle (see Exhibit 25-3). The cycle should be kept in constant motion and used at all levels of the organization. Reports should conform to the new system.[12]

Training in statistical process control takes the guesswork out of what is really happening in the operation. Statistical process control aims to prevent errors by identifying where they occur. The process is then tightened to improve the outcome. In looking at safety systems, Smith indicated that 85% to 90% of problems have common causes (the system), whereas only 10% to 15% of problems have special causes (employees). Using control charts to determine whether the causes of accidents are common or special leads to development of methods to prevent accidents. Employees can then set goals to reduce the special causes.[13]

Variation is a part of everything—of supplies used by nurses, employee performance, and many other activities. Other causes exist in addition to common and special causes. One cause is tampering or making unnecessary adjustments to compensate for common-cause variations. Another cause is structural variation, resulting from seasonal patterns and long-term trends.[14]

Data Analysis

Quality is not just another fad. Just as business and industry must have high-quality standards to compete in international markets, institution of TQM at every level of the process in the U.S. health care industry will support its expansion to provide at least an affordable safety net for all citizens. Deming states that quality must be defined and employees trained to deliver quality products and services. According to Deming, we should "measure the variations in a process in order to pinpoint the causes of poor quality and then how to gradually reduce those variations."[15]

Quality control should be on-line rather than end-of-line control. On-line quality control is achieved by sampling products during the process to determine how to correct those variations that result in the product deviating from the acceptable range. Quality improves as variability decreases.[16] Statistical charts are used to plot variations from the ideal in the production process and determine the right course to correct those variations.

Pareto charts are one example of control charts (see Exhibit 25-4). The Pareto principle states that most effects come from relatively few causes. Of rework, 80% of costs come from 20% of the possible causes. The Pareto principle is one of the most powerful decision tools available. Among the data that can be plotted on Pareto charts for nursing services are wasted time; number of jobs that have to be redone; customer inquiries; and number of errors, accidents, incidents, infections, and complications.[17]

When constructing Pareto diagrams, one should place the most frequent cause at the left and arrange the remaining in descending order of occurrence. The impact on the system becomes obvious, as does the priority for fixing it. A double Pareto diagram can be used to contrast two areas, for example, the use of flexible work shifts before and after improvement. One must recognize what data are useful. Group consensus should be used to identify important causes and problems. Nominal group technique may be used[18]:

1. Give each person ten 3-by-5 cards.
2. Have each person write causes and problems on the cards, one pair for each card.
3. Have each person rate the causes by importance, with 10 being the most and 1 being the least important.
4. Compile numbers for each cause.
5. Construct a Pareto chart.

Pareto charts may be used to plot reasons that nurses leave an agency. Reasons may be constructed using the National Commission on Nursing report or a career book and exit interviews.

Calculating system variations on process data allows control limits to be set, with variations being expected in the process as a result of aggregate common causes. Data may be plotted on a graph to show

EXHIBIT 25-3

Application of the Deming (Shewhart) PDCA Cycle to Total Quality Management

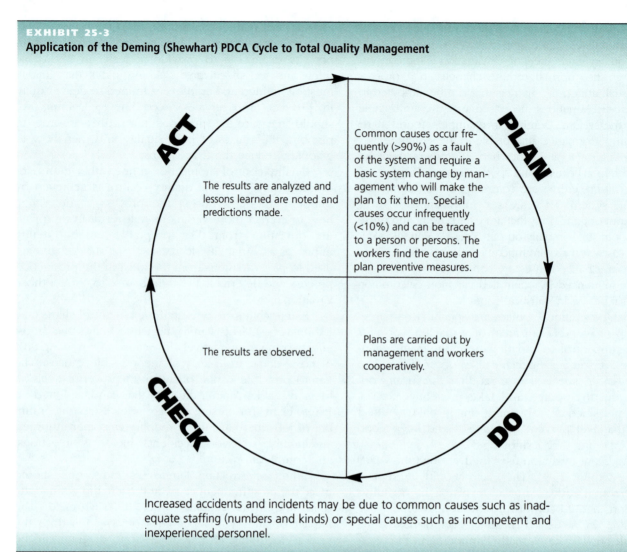

PLAN: Common causes occur frequently (>90%) as a fault of the system and require a basic system change by management who will make the plan to fix them. Special causes occur infrequently (<10%) and can be traced to a person or persons. The workers find the cause and plan preventive measures.

DO: Plans are carried out by management and workers cooperatively.

CHECK: The results are observed.

ACT: The results are analyzed and lessons learned are noted and predictions made.

Increased accidents and incidents may be due to common causes such as inadequate staffing (numbers and kinds) or special causes such as incompetent and inexperienced personnel.

EXHIBIT 25-4

Generalized Pareto Diagram

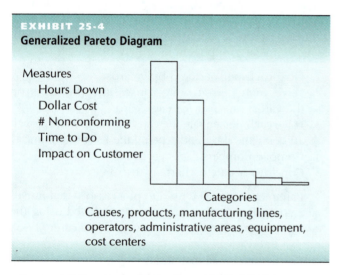

Measures
   Hours Down
   Dollar Cost
   # Nonconforming
   Time to Do
   Impact on Customer

Categories

Causes, products, manufacturing lines, operators, administrative areas, equipment, cost centers

Source: J. T. Burr, Center for Quality and Applied Statistics, Rochester Institute of Technology, One Lomb Memorial Dr., P. O. Box 9887, Rochester, NY 14623-9887. Reprinted with permission.

upper control limits (UCL) and lower control limits (LCL). When all points fall within these lines, variations are due to common causes and one should not tamper with them (see Exhibit 25-5).

It is common but incorrect to treat all causes of variance as special and to tamper with them although the special causes of variation are but 10% of all causes. All data should be plotted on control charts, including performance appraisals, which are often based on a system of common-cause variation. Plotting data reveals who performs at a level outside the system, that is, above (UCL) or below (LCL) the control limits. One should learn what causes an employee to perform outside the system (below the control limits) and correct the cause by fixing the system. Dispense with praise-and-blame sessions, study the performance appraisal system, find the special causes, and prevent them from recurring. When all causes are common causes, ways to improve the variation in the system should be studied. Thus,

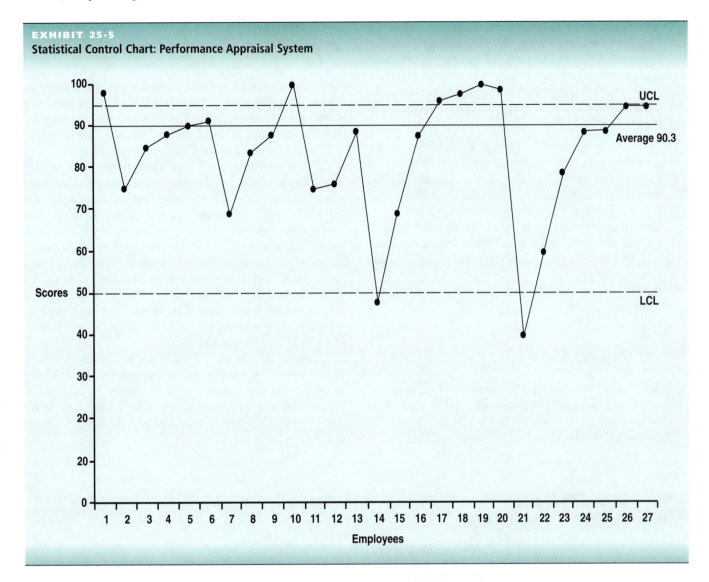

EXHIBIT 25-5

Statistical Control Chart: Performance Appraisal System

employees will work in an environment that facilitates their being able to improve by correcting special causes of variation. Also remember to remove barriers to pride of workmanship such as annual or merit ratings.[19]

Cohen describes seven basic teamwork tools used in quality function development at Digital Equipment Corporation (DEC) as a structural method for planning[20]:

1. Scatter diagrams
2. Histograms
3. Check sheets
4. Pareto diagrams
5. Run charts
6. Control charts
7. Cause-and-effect diagrams

These are problem-solving tools as contrasted to physical tools. Teams solve problems by analyzing data of past events through data analysis, cause-and-effect analysis, and process management. In nursing, quality function develop-

ment could prepare a structured list of a patient's needs (a nursing diagnosis) and evaluate each proposed service and function (nursing intervention) according to the impact or outcome it has in meeting this patient's needs. Physical tools are technology-based. They include spread sheet programs, electronic calculators, telephones, word-processing software, and all the materials needed to give nursing care to patients. Physical tools do not solve problems.[21]

Seven new tools about the future are used at DEC to make decisions (that analyze relationships between ideas and activity):

1. Affinity diagrams
2. Relational diagrams
3. True diagrams
4. Matrix diagrams
5. Program decision process charts
6. Arrow diagrams
7. Matrix data analyses

As illustrated by Cohen, these tools can could be used by nurse leaders during the planning process.[22]

Fishbone analysis can be used in conjunction with Pareto analysis, and each may be used separately. Fishbone analysis has been successfully used at the Rotor Clip Company, Somerset, New Jersey, as a problem-solving technique as follows[23]:

1. Involve all employees having knowledge of the problem, product, or service.
2. Express the problem in the simplest terms possible.
3. Divide the problem into potential problem areas. Draw a fishbone structure (see Exhibit 25-6).
4. Use brainstorming techniques to identify reasons for the problem (refer to Chapter 15, Committees and Other Groups). Assign reasons to appropriate problem areas.
5. Review all the causes, and decide on and test the solution.

Other Quality Gurus

In addition to Deming, who is considered by many to be the pioneer in quality management, other early wise persons in the field include Joseph Juran, Philip B. Crosby, and Genichi Taguchi.

Joseph Juran

To Juran, quality means fitness to serve, doing it right the first time to meet customers' needs, and freedom from deficiencies. Quality means employee involvement, with management leading the effort in planning, control, and improvement so that requirements are met. It means identification of customers and their needs in a product-by-product and step-by-step process.[24]

Juran describes leadership that charts a new course that breaks with traditional management. This new course applies quality management to all functions at all levels of the enterprise and incorporates the exercise of personal leadership and participation by top managers. All managers would be educated in quality management techniques. There would be an all-pervasive unity in which everyone knows the direction of the new course and is stimulated to go there. The resisting forces are multiple functions, levels in hierarchy, and product lines.[25] All of these resisting forces are prominent in health care agencies.

Juran's philosophy of quality is based on three major premises: quality planning, quality control, and quality improvement. According to Juran, "Quality planning creates a process for meeting established goals under operating conditions." Quality planning includes the following[26]:

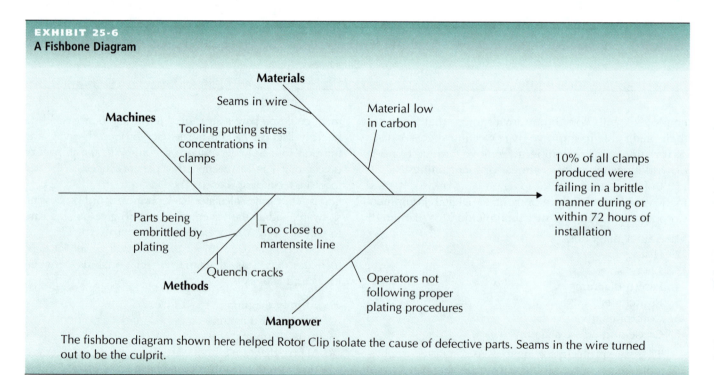

EXHIBIT 25-6
A Fishbone Diagram

The fishbone diagram shown here helped Rotor Clip isolate the cause of defective parts. Seams in the wire turned out to be the culprit.

Source: B. Rudin. "Simple Tools Solve Complex Problems." *Quality* (April 1990), 50. Reprinted with permission from *Quality*, a publication of Hitchcock/Chilton Publishing, a Capital Cities/ABC, Inc., Company.

- Identify customers, both internal and external
- Determine customer needs
- Develop product features that respond to customer needs
- Set goals that meet needs of customers and suppliers
- Develop process to produce the product features
- Prove process meets quality goals during operations

Quality control, the second activity of the quality process, is performed by operations personnel who put the plan into effect by identifying deficiencies, correcting them, and monitoring the process. Quality control includes the following[27]:

- Choose what to control
- Choose units of measurement
- Establish measurement
- Establish standards of performance
- Measure actual performance
- Interpret the difference
- Take action on the difference

The third and final premise of the Juran philosophy is quality improvement, which should be purposeful and in addition to quality control. Quality improvement includes the following[28]:

- Prove the need for improvement
- Identify projects for improvement
- Organize to guide the projects
- Diagnose to find the causes
- Provide remedies
- Prove remedies are effective under operating conditions
- Provide for control to hold the gains

According to Juran, the quality trilogy can be grafted onto the strategic planning process. A corporate task force may be set up to design appropriate training. A quality planning council can be established for policies, goals and plans, resources, and performance reviews, thus incorporating quality into the merit rating system. Goals would be written for the future, for the marketplace, and for competition. The entire infrastructure would be used in this process, which would require putting money into quality improvement. Juran even suggested the creation of a new role of quality controller to[29]:

- Assist management in preparing strategic funding goals
- Set means of reporting performance against quality goals
- Evaluate competitive quality and market trends
- Design and introduce needed revisions in quality planning, quality control, and quality improvement
- Conduct training to assist company personnel in carrying out the assessory change

Philip B. Crosby

Crosby earned his spurs as a quality guru at International Telephone and Telegraph (ITT). He defines quality as "conformance to requirements," the first of his four absolutes. If the process is done right the first time, there is no need to redo it. Management sets the requirements and supplies the wherewithal to employees to do the job by encouraging and helping.[30]

Crosby's second absolute is that the system of quality is prevention rather than appraisal. His third absolute is a performance standard of zero defects. A policy should be to deliver defect-free products on time. Other quality gurus, notably Deming and Taguchi, do not advocate zero defects, which they view as focusing on numbers rather than on the quality process.

The fourth and final Crosby absolute is that the measurement of quality is the cost of nonconformance, because service companies spend half of their operating expenses on the cost of doing things wrong. Achieving these absolutes should be a constant priority. It requires the determination of management and the commitment of the entire organization. It requires the training and education of all employees as part of a continual, formal preparation of the organization for the future. Everyone should be taught the common quality language. All people are trainable, interested, and ambitious. When they know and understand management's policy, employees will make TQM work. All levels of management are trained early.

Culture and climate are important to achieving Crosby's absolutes. A climate of innovation is created because continuous innovation keeps customers coming back. The organizational culture often must be changed to raise every person's basic expectations. A small group of people may be used to keep ethics and integrity on the up-and-up. People come to believe that quality is as important and has the same importance as does financial management. An attitude that fosters change is created. If managers think and operate in terms of quality, they will change the culture and create a climate of consideration for people, employees, customers, suppliers, and the community.

Crosby's strategy uses a nontechnical approach, beginning with an awareness campaign and a focus on behavior among people. During the campaign the organization is stripped down to examine it for problems, to identify and satisfy the customers, to eliminate waste, and to instill pride and teamwork. By policy, every department and unit has a quality strategy and a quality function. All managers participate in TQM; it becomes a part of how they think, feel, and act. Nurse managers may want to use Crosby's Quality Management Maturity Grid to measure the quality assurance aspects of their departments or units and then extend its use to other units (see Exhibit 25-7).

Genichi Taguchi

The Taguchi method focuses on "robust quality" of service to meet customer performance expectations every time, even under severe operating or environmental conditions. Taguchi invented the theory of robust quality, which says that the product should be robust enough to achieve high quality despite fluctuations on the production lines. Taguchi's approach to quality control involves complicated mathematical formulas.[31]

The theory of robust quality is important to nursing insofar as it may be used to produce the supplies and equipment nurses use. Clinical nurses would be interested to know whether Taguchi's methods have been used in developing products they are evaluating. The theory of robust quality also could be applied to the nursing process in a research and development project. Variance in the application of the nursing process using various nursing modalities, nursing diagnoses, and nursing care standards (including interventions and outcomes), could be studied using the theory of robust quality. The object of this theory is to reduce the things that can go wrong in applying the theory of nursing. Thus, the objective is to minimize variations around the customer's (patient's) performance requirements.

In education, the theory of robust quality could be applied to prevent students failing courses and nurses failing state boards. The goal would be to make the educational system work harmoniously. Thus, college faculty would work in harmony with high-school faculty to reduce problems with student placement in subjects such as English and mathematics.

Taguchi opposes the goal of zero defects, saying that robustness begins from meeting exact targets consistently, whereas the goal of zero defects stops only within a certain tolerance. He uses an orthogonal array, a system of product development using signal-to-noise ratios. This system balances the levels of performance demanded by customers against the many variables, or noises, affecting performance. Once the level of performance demanded by patients as customers is determined, it can be balanced against the many variables in the health care system that affect it. The robust service would be one that meets a determined ratio of the mean total divided by the standard deviation. This robust service minimizes the average of the squared deviations from the target averaged ones over the different customer-use conditions. This system verification test would need to be tested through nursing research to establish a model for application to nursing.[32]

To begin with, on entering the system customers would be asked their expectations of providers. Nursing literature is short on customer expectations and long on provider-imposed prescription. If variance in the production of nursing services is to be reduced, the variances must be identified.[33]

Zeroing in rapidly on the variation in nursing care delivery will distinguish the bad part from the good and sustain quality.

One takes the best of the theory of total quality management and applies it assiduously. The best approach is to develop a pervasive philosophy that continuous improvement by all employees and managers is both desirable and possible.

Customers

The customer is the focus of TQM philosophy. One should first find out what the customer wants, then describe it, then meet it exactly. The service that meets the customer's needs provides the income to the supplier, be it an educational institution or a health care agency. Quality is freedom from waste, trouble, and failure. One endeavors to meet and exceed customers' needs and expectations, then continues to improve.[34]

> Although TQM techniques have not always produced significant change in organizational performance, customers demand an enhanced focus on continuous quality improvement.[35] Many failures of TQM result from a lack of managers understanding the complexity of making changes in organizations with multiple subcultures and interests.[36] Covance Laboratories achieved this cultural change through quality assurance practices that improved efficiency, productivity, and customer and employee satisfaction.[37] An unrelenting effort toward continuous improvement in health care will result in unflinching customer loyalty, sustainable growth, and impressive performance.[38]

Internal and External Customers

In TQM, there are both internal and external customers, all of whom should be given service. In nursing management, the external customers are patients, employers, and the community. These customers will be satisfied by quality care that produces a patient improved to the point of being discharged and able to get on with his or her life. A patient facing death wants a quality of care to make his or her remaining time peaceful. The employer

EXHIBIT 25-7
Quality Management Maturity Grid

MEASUREMENT CATEGORIES	STAGE ONE: UNCERTAINTY	STAGE TWO: AWAKENING	STAGE THREE: ENLIGHTENMENT	STAGE FOUR: WISDOM	STAGE FIVE: CERTAINTY
Management understanding and attitude	No comprehension of quality as a management tool. Tend to blame quality department for "quality problems."	Recognize that quality management may be of value but not willing to provide money or time to make it all happen.	While going through quality improvement program, learn more about quality management; becoming supportive and helpful.	Participating. Understand absolutes of quality management. Recognize personal role in continuing emphasis.	Consider quality management an essential part of company system.
Quality organization status	Quality is hidden in manufacturing engineering departments. Inspection probably not part of organization. Emphasis on appraisal and sorting.	A stronger quality leader is appointed but main emphasis is still on appraisal and moving the product. Still part of manufacturing or other.	Quality department reports to top management, all appraisal is incorporated, and manager has role in management of company.	Quality manager is an officer of company; effective status reporting and preventive action. Involved with consumer affairs and special assignments.	Quality manager is on board of directors. Prevention is main concern. Quality is a thought leader.
Problem handling	Problems are fought as they occur; no resolution; inadequate definition; lots of yelling and accusation.	Teams are set up to attack major problems. Long-range solutions are not solicited.	Corrective action communication established. Problems are faced openly and resolved in an orderly way.	Problems are identified early in their development. All functions are open to suggestion and improvement.	Except in unusual cases, problems are prevented.
Cost of quality as percentage of sales	Reported: Unknown Actual: 20%	Reported: 3% Actual: 18%	Reported: 8% Actual: 12%	Reported: 6.5% Actual: 8%	Reported: 2.5% Actual: 2.5%
Quality improvement actions	No organized activities. No understanding of such activities.	Trying obvious "motivational" short-range efforts.	Implementation of the 14-step program with thorough understanding and establishment of each step.	Continuing the 14-step program and starting Make Certain.	Quality improvement is a normal and continued activity.
Summation of company quality posture	"We don't know why we have problems with quality."	"Is it absolutely necessary to always have problems with quality?"	"Through management commitment and quality improvement we are identifying and resolving our problems."	"Defect prevention is a routine part of our operation."	"We know why we do not have problems with quality."

"It isn't a business of hanging up a whole bunch of signs and doing a whole bunch of things; it's a matter of instituting new policy, telling everyone this is the way we're going to do it."

Source: B. J. Deutsch. "A Conversation with Philip Crosby." *Bank Marketing* (April 1991), 25. Reprinted with permission from the Bank Marketing Association.

wants knowledgeable and skilled workers; the community wants a productive citizen.

Internal customers are those who interact with each other within and among departments and disciplines. Internal customers to nursing are those departments that contribute to patient care such as pharmacy, radiology, and medical laboratory. Clinical nurses are customers of nurse managers, admission services, and others. For each organization, the goal of quality care is defined by each self-managed team and possibly by an interdepartmental team. Quality takes time. It is here to stay. The customer should be satisfied quickly and economically if nurse managers are to stay in business. Business, including that of nursing, focuses on core customers and learns from them. This core of customers includes those who generate a profit and inspire nurses to their best ideas and highest motivation.[39]

The focus of TQM is harmony, not competition or adversarial relations. The optimal system of delivering patient care is achieved when all managers and workers function as teams. The next shift in nursing is also an internal customer. Quality control focuses on satisfying such customers, not confronting them. The continual quest for improvement would reduce variation caused by confrontation, adversarial relationships within and among departments, and disharmony. These things can be done by developing information and using statistical tools to analyze it.[40]

Quality improves nursing services because it reduces costs and keeps customers happy. Even in a recession, customers buy quality products and services. Quality is not a program but a philosophy and a way of life. It is a survival issue. Traditional management is "out"; quality management is "in." It is customer-oriented, decentralized, and empowering.[41] Quality nurses aim for world-class quality of care, which entails learning to deal with the most difficult patients and families. Nurse managers would facilitate the capability of clinical nurses to deal with difficult customers.

Nurse managers and practitioners decide who their customers are, internal and external, by projecting a path through the health care system at the following potential input points of nursing services: definition, production, delivery, and follow-up. Nursing personnel identify customers of their services at each of these points.[42]

Teamwork is absolutely essential. Teamwork will include cross-functional teams and an open, trusting, cooperative relationship. It will involve self-managed teams that perform multiple functions and that schedule their own work, develop budgets, and deal directly with customers. The teams will be trained to develop needed relationships, do networking, deal with vendors, and manage projects.[43]

> To make TQM effective requires appropriate development of a responsive and supportive organizational environment, change in management culture, teamwork, focus on customers, and continuous feedback to staff.[44] Among the processes that have affected enterprises positively are fundamental changes that stress teamwork and customer over turf and hierarchy.[45]

Successful customer relations requires constant training and educational programs. The need for staff development will continue to increase as nursing deals with improved technology, greater product reliability, a customer-service orientation, and flexibility in adapting to change. Nurse managers will continue to move decisions down the chain of command to all associates or team members. An educated and well-trained work force is a nursing imperative. Every team member will need the skills of reading, understanding mathematics, and conveying ideas.[46]

Each nursing associate will know the status of the work entering the nursing station, how to handle the customer in the workstation, and what the next internal customer requires. Such a quality system requires massive and continuous training to prevent errors. Authority and responsibility for quality of nursing care reside in the workstation, where associates will take pride in craftsmanship, group output and ownership of the process.[47]

According to Peters, 3% of gross revenues should be spent on training to produce quality products and services. CEOs who put customers first put employees first. Employees will continue to learn new skills and knowledge to be marketable.[48]

Leadership

Leadership is discussed in great detail in Chapter 18; however, its importance to TQM requires mention here. Leadership is an essential element of the theory and philosophy of TQM. It transcends the process, requiring a people-oriented leadership style, cooperation in all ventures, and win-win relationships.[49] Such leadership will include all persons who work in nursing.

Total quality management requires total commitment by top management because it is a long-range process. TQM focuses on the achievement of top quality in every relationship with every customer. Leadership will make each worker a "business person" with commitment to total responsibility for patient care. Each worker will be cross-trained and have access to all information. Each worker will have customers and be a manager.[50]

Long-term leadership is needed to achieve continuous improvement of productivity and services for the consumer. Continuous improvement requires innovation and investment in research and education, long-range planning, and focus on the future. Long-term leadership is needed to maintain constancy of purpose and common purpose, part of which is to stay in business and provide jobs. Leadership oversees the mental revolution required when TQM becomes the process, with its constant focus on training and instruction. Leadership focuses on goals and conserves productive energy by efficient direction; it builds quality with every stage of production, beginning with the purchase of high-quality raw materials.[51]

If managers do not attend to quality in today's health care environment, they will lose their leadership to someone else. Deming indicates that leadership aims to improve the performance of person and machine, to improve quality, to increase output, and to provide pride of workmanship. According to Bryce, Juran states that leadership will be of the hands-on type and will provide the breakthroughs.[52]

Leaders have a clear set of values and the integrity to institutionalize them. This occurred at LTV Steel, in Cleveland, Ohio, where integrated process management was the model of the quality process improvement implemented. As a result, LTV Steel went from a bottom-quality steel producer to a top-quality company. It did this by establishing a culture in which workers were obsessed with customer satisfaction, innovation became the norm, people were turned on throughout the organization, and common-sense systems were used.[53] Successful nursing leadership will change climate and culture to foster TQM.

Techniques that leaders can use to improve relationships with suppliers, customers, and other partners include: (1) installing a companywide negotiation infrastructure to apply the knowledge gained from forging past agreements to improve future ones (managed care contracts especially), (2) creating broadened measures to evaluate negotiators' performance beyond matters of cost and price, (3) drawing a clear distinction between elements of an individual deal and the nature of the ongoing relationship between the parties, and (4) making negotiators feel comfortable walking away from a deal when it's not in the company's best interests.[54]

Culture and Climate

Total quality management requires a favorable environment for total quality behavior in which values are shared as worthwhile or desirable, and beliefs as truth. All employees in such an environment, including top management, believe in focusing on customers, both internal and external. Management believes in an employee focus, teamwork, safety, and candor. Total involvement exists because individual employees are empowered to identify and solve problems. A process focus exists that prevents rather than fixes errors and problems.[55]

The total quality culture exists in a warm, friendly climate in which employees feel good about themselves, others, and their work. Employees in such a culture trust managers, who facilitate their work and treat them as equals who have intellectual and creative abilities. Fear has been driven out through leadership that has promoted teamwork, respect, and trust. All employees feel empowered to speak freely and to suggest changes. The heroes of the culture include employees who accept blame even though they are not at fault, who frequently defend employees of other departments or units, and who model total quality behavior to all customers. Myths and artifacts that may be eliminated include all titles from name tags, business cards, and nameplates. Rites and rituals that may be changed in a total quality culture include abolishing reserved parking and increasing the visibility of managers throughout the workplace. Management has expended great effort to create a strong total quality culture that has thickness, breadth, and clarity of ordering.[56]

Linkow suggests changing the culture through a total quality culture matrix tool (see Exhibit 25-8) that follows these steps[57]:

1. Describe the current culture through group brainstorming and interviewing.
2. Establish seven core total quality values and beliefs.
3. Correlate core values and beliefs with the current culture.
4. Determine the strength of the current culture.
5. Identify targets for culture change. These will be core values and beliefs with negative or nonexistent correlation or that are low in strength.
6. Use groups to change the culture.
7. Use external threats to mobilize internal forces of change.

O'Boyle indicates that U.S. managers of Japanese plants are frustrated with the Japanese concepts of consensus building and shared decision-making. Over 350,000 Americans work for Japanese companies in the United States. In the corporate culture of these plants, the workers are called "associates" or "team members." Teamwork, harmony, and consensus are stressed. Presidents have the same kinds of metal desks as do secretaries and in the same offices. There are no executive dining rooms, reserved parking, special bonuses, or stock options.

EXHIBIT 25-8
Total Quality Culture Matrix

Cultural Media	Current Culture Examples	Customer Focus	Employee Focus	Teamwork	Safety	Candor	Total Involvement	Process Focus	Symbols
Heroes	Employee who got out of a hospital bed for important meeting with a client	●	△	△	△				
	Person who left his family on vacation to work with client	●	△	△					
	Understudy steps in at last minute for sick "star" and makes resoundingly successful presentation to tough clients	●		○					● = highly correlated
Myths and Artifacts	No titles on business cards		○	○			○		○ = correlated
	Stories of failures with clients are told with relish		○			●			
	Employees do whatever it takes to satisfy the client	●	△						△ = negatively correlated
Rites and Rituals	Anyone may be interrupted at any time		△	○			○		
	When a problem is identified a list of solutions is brainstormed by a group			●			○		
	CEO walks through headquarters many afternoons asking, "What are you working on?"		○	●			○		

Strength of Culture		Customer Focus	Employee Focus	Teamwork	Safety	Candor	Total Involvement	Process Focus	
Thickness		●	△	○	△	○	○	△	● = high
Extent of Sharing		●	○	●	△	●	○	△	○ = medium
Clarity of Ordering		●	○	●	△	○	○	△	△ = low

Core Values/Beliefs

Source: Reprinted with permission of P. Linkow, Interaction Associates, Cambridge, Massachusetts.

When business is poor, the employer educates workers in analytical and statistical procedures. Productivity is up 50%, and costs are down 55%. Almost 100% quality has been achieved. Factories are immaculate, well lit, ergonomically designed, and air-conditioned. Warm-up exercises are used to help eliminate back and wrist injuries. Workers rotate jobs every two hours and maintain output. There are 24-hour childcare facilities. Bosses provide direction, guide group decision-making, and facilitate continuous improvement.[58]

We view reality from the perspective of our own culture. U.S. business and industry is imbued with the values of the upper-middle-class White male. There have been few changes in these beliefs and values in the past 60 years. Superior nursing leadership performance will assimilate the following principles used by Japanese managers:

1. Take competition seriously. Short-staffed, overworked American nurses have surrendered many

primary nursing activities to other professions and occupations while retaining the clerical tasks. Drucker blames the nurse shortage on nurses performing nonnursing duties.[59]

2. Put society's needs first even before one's own. Power is not black and white, win or lose. Nurses should build coalitions, faith, and trust to provide society with nursing that is kind, caring, compassionate, and trustworthy.

3. Provide long-term support for employees. Encourage preceptorship or mentorship for a decade: provide advice, emotional support, career counseling, and help with organizational problems. Develop managerial talent. Prepare replacements. Pursue lifelong learning for self-improvement. Become familiar with tasks and responsibilities of other professional groups within the organization.

4. Use consensus decision-making. Take time to involve employees in making decisions that affect them. Consensus building is time-consuming but eliminates the need to "sell" decisions. Start at the bottom, and go up.[60]

Florida Power & Light went from the worst to the best electric utility in United States by using TQM. Its middle managers became "facilitators" who coaxed team members to look for and solve problems. In a major training effort, 230 employees were trained in a five-week course in advanced statistical process control. Eight hundred employees studied basic statistics, and all 15,000 employees learned how to interpret data. The company launched a policy deployment management system of strategic planning, budgeting, and management with short- and long-range goals set at every level by consensus and involvement of every employee. It held expos to share solutions and awards banquets. A company goal was to win the Deming Prize, and it did! Although Deming advocated abandoning slogans, they were effective when developed by the company's own employees. One slogan was "In God we trust; the rest, bring data."[61]

Geyer states that the real dangers to economic wellness in the United States today are the following:

- Businesses and industry have not worked and planned for quality products and services.
- Solutions of public officials are not the right ones.
- Corporate executives get huge salaries even when businesses fail.
- Employees become unemployed.
- Japanese and German economies soar because of a community of spirit and personal interest.[62]

Nursing organizations within institutions should have ideals, vision, and values.

Like other sectors of the economy, health care organizations must have sound business plans that attack the status quo and entrenched players, and find new technologies that improve or replace earlier ones. "The economic, social, and cultural factors underlying the new economy are rock solid."[63]

Theory Z Organizations

Theory Z organizations focus on consensual decision-making. The leadership style of such organizations is a democratic one that includes decentralization, participatory management, employee involvement, and an emphasis on quality of life. Leaders are managers who concentrate on developing and using their interpersonal skills. This theory has been attributed to William Ouchi.[64]

Using Theory Z management, an "organization can significantly benefit from facilitating the creative ideas and input of the members of that organization."[65]

Theory Z management and TQM are closely interrelated. Both start with planning that includes emphasis on staff development to improve quality of staff members and their work. These theories start with a statement of philosophy that embodies the elements of both theories and proceed to the training of managers. Theory Z and TQM both require a long-term relationship between the organization and the employees. The organization invests in the employee by caring, by focusing on career needs, and by assisting employees to integrate their work and home lives through childcare centers, wellness programs, recreational opportunities, shift options, counseling, and opportunities for career development. Results have included production of generalists who can do more than one job, a turnover rate reduced from 30% to 4%, unity because of the greater independence of nurses, reduced interdepartmental conflicts, reduced costs, improved risk management, and improved quality.[66]

Quality Circles

Quality circles (QCs) are a participatory management technique that uses statistical analyses of activities to maintain quality products. The technique was initiated in Japan after World War II through the teaching of Deming, an American. The concept is to use statistical analysis to make quality improvements. Workers are taught the statistical concepts and use them through trained, organized, structured groups of four to 15 employees, called QCs. Group members share common interests and problems and meet on a regular basis, usually an hour a week. They represent other employees from whom they gather information to bring to the meetings.[67]

The QC process is widespread in Japan, and this has raised Japanese manufacturing to worldwide eminence. It involves workers in decision-making. QCs have spread to major U.S. manufacturers and some U.S. health care institutions. QCs are similar to other elements of participatory management. Employees are trained to identify, analyze, and solve problems. Involved in the process, employees make solutions work because they identify with ownership. As a result of being recognized, they develop good will toward their employers.

Quality circles are effective when facilitators, leaders, and members are trained in group dynamics and QC techniques. Leaders act as peers to generate ideas to improve operations and eliminate problems. In the process, all QC members reach consensus before decisions are recommended or implemented. Training occurs during subsequent meetings.[68]

The objects of QCs are participation, involvement, recognition, and self-actualization among clinical nurses caring for patients. Output from the objects of QCs contributes to the knowledge base of human behavior and motivation, which is important to the development of nursing management theory. This theory will be learned and used by nurse managers concerned with developing job satisfaction of professional nurses in delivering quality nursing care.

Quality circles should meet successful group design guidelines, including the following[69]:

1. Participation groups process or have access to the necessary skills and knowledge to address problems systematically. All actors in the process receive training. Support people participate only as needed.
2. Formalized procedures enhance the effectiveness of the group, including adherence to formal meeting schedules and systematic record-keeping.
3. To promote communication, participation groups are integrated horizontally and vertically with the rest of the organization. Accomplishments are publicized through award dinners and in-house newsletters. Organized higher-level support groups hear the ideas of lower-level groups. All are limited by usual formal and informal communication mechanisms and routes.
4. Groups are a regular part of the organization and not a special or extra activity. They are composed of members of natural work groups. Results are measured in terms of ongoing organizational objectives and goals.
5. Normal accountability processes operate using the same skills, habits, and expectations as those in general organizations.
6. Groups manage themselves and are assisted by leaders and facilitators who are peer-group members.

7. Participation occurs in areas such as decisions about job enrichment; hiring; training in problem-solving skills, management skills, and business conditions; pay based on skill mastery; gain sharing; and union management relationships based on mutual interests.

Research indicates that productivity and morale improve greatly when employees participate in decision-making and planning for change. It is important that participation include goal setting, because participation will lead to higher levels of acceptance and performance. This research has been supported by meta-analysis. Research also shows that highly nonparticipatory jobs cause psychological and physical harm.

It is an ethical imperative to prevent harm by enabling employees to participate in work decisions.

Mental health is positively influenced by feelings of interest, a sense of accomplishment, personal growth, and self-respect.[70] Nurse managers will use this knowledge in managing clinical professional nurses.

Nursing staff who participate in selecting managers increase nursing support, management knowledge and skills, and nurses' ability to write resumes and prepare for interviews. Management's knowledge of the nursing staff increases also. Conflict and favoritism decrease; the chances of the new manager's effectiveness increase. Such participation by nursing staff can be stressful to manager candidates, however, because it is time-consuming.[71]

According to Piczak, Deming set up QCs for the Japanese in 1950. QCs are focus groups and often survive in hostile environments. They are not an end in themselves. In 1985, over 90% of Fortune 500 companies were using QCs. In Japan, QCs use statistical methods, meet on their own time, and are given financial rewards. In the United States QCs are voluntary; share an area of responsibility; and meet, discuss, analyze, and propose solutions to quality goals or problems and other programs.

Quality circles use the techniques of Pareto analysis, histograms, graphing, control charts, stratification, scatter diagrams, brainstorming, cause-and-effect diagrams, run analysis, and conflict resolution. A budget of $20,000 to $25,000 is needed as a start-up fund. Success factors of QCs include management commitment and involvement, labor union involvement, training, and patience. Tangible benefits include improved quality, increased productivity, and increased efficiency. Intangible benefits include improved work life quality, job security, morale, and job satisfaction.[72]

Quality circles should have themes, should know how to select or recognize the themes they will work on, then assist with implementation of the solution.[73]

Performance Appraisal

Performance Appraisal (PA) has long been touted as a key management tool for evaluating worker productivity. Not so, said Deming, who advocated their abolition. PA is the most serious of Deming's deadly diseases that stand in the way of TQM. PA embodies a win-lose philosophy that destroys people psychologically and poisons healthy relationships. A win-win philosophy emphasizes cooperation, participation, and leadership directed at continuous improvement of quality.[74]

The traditional purposes of PA include compensation, counseling, training and development, promotion, staff planning, retention, discharge, validation of selection techniques, motivation through feedback, and documentation for legal protection.[75] These purposes tend to be overshadowed by the negative consequences of PA, which include the following[76]:

- PA is usually ineffective in counseling an employee on developmental issues when that employee knows a salary increase hangs on a favorable evaluation. Shortcomings are blamed on other factors.
- Too often, PA is used to control employees.
- There are no good production records available for many jobs. This is very true of nursing.
- PAs lack validity.
- PAs eventually become regimented.
- PAs typically define results and not the process.
- PAs encourage the status quo and discourage autonomy, innovation, and creativity. (The typical employee response is ". . . but I met the standards."
- Employees who feel they did the job, although their appraisals do not agree, feel they have been treated unfairly.
- PAs can be inhumane, hostile, aggressive acts that hurt or destroy people.

Deming's system provides for three ratings for PAs using process data. Using the statistic of variation, ratings will fall within the system, outside the system on the high side, and outside the system on the low side. If the rating is[77]:

- Within the system, pay by seniority.
- Outside the system on the high side, give merit pay.
- Outside the system on the low side, coach or replace.

The assumption of TQM is that employees want to do better and will do better with the motivation of participation, adequate work tools, and training. Employees share the vision of the quality process and products. They develop broad-based skills through shared efforts and responsibilities. The team concept fosters trust, effective communication, and cooperation. Let the team develop the PA system and keep it separate from pay and promotion through gain-sharing or equal profit sharing.[78]

Abolishing or simplifying the PA system will free up many resources. The PA system can be replaced with a system of education and leadership that does a better job of selecting employees initially, provides quality training and education, fosters a colleague or team relationship, and uses the company's formula for pay raises for all employees that form a system. A long conference of three to four hours can be held at least once a year with each employee to foster help and better understanding of the employee's performance.[79]

Salaries, wages, and bonuses can be based on market rates needed to replace employees, accumulation of skills and responsibilities, seniority, and sharing in the welfare and prosperity of the entire organization. Promotion to new positions can be based on special assignments that contain elements of the new job, assessment centers to screen applicants, and involvement of customers of the new job. Employees should help develop plans for change in compensation. Compensation should not be reduced for any group in the organization. Improvement should be part of the job, not the reward. Continuous learning of employees should be rewarded. Profit sharing or bonuses should be awarded on a companywide basis rather than to a single person or department.[80]

General Motors has dropped forced ratings altogether to focus on employee development. American Cyanamid substituted forced ratings with a progress review system, with categories of exceptional, good, and unacceptable. "Compensation would be raised based on position in the salary range for good, a lump sum bonus equal to fixed percentages of their salaries for exceptional, and no raise for unacceptable." The company learned that pride rather than money was the biggest motivator of performance. The U.S. Air Force did away with PA at McClellan Air Force Base in Sacramento, California. A gain-sharing plan resulted in savings of $500,000 and $1 million, respectively, for the first two quarters of 1987.[81]

Application of Total Quality Management to Nursing

Before deciding to apply the principles of TQM to nursing, top managers should learn the theory of TQM. TQM can be implemented in nursing with or without implementation in the total organization. If there is a source of knowledge of TQM theory within the organization, it may be tapped first. Doing so will give recognition to employees as experts within their own organization.

Schonberger suggests that using outside persons to interpret quality is not effective.[82]

All members of the lead team should read *Out of the Crisis*, in which Deming describes his theory of TQM and the deadly diseases of management and recommends a management philosophy. Then the team can write its management plan for implementing TQM. The process will be never ending, because quality is a complicated construct and producing high-quality nursing services is a complicated process.

The first goal of a nursing management plan is to write the stated purpose of nursing service so that it is constant and provides a clear goal for everyone for every day, month after month. This is the first of Deming's 14 points (refer to Exhibit 25-1). All 14 points should be discussed by the lead team. The management plan should list activities to achieve each of these points. Teams can be assigned to develop plans for the following:

- Assessing the culture and climate and making plans to change them.
- Planning for training in statistical methods, with particular emphasis on variance.
- Improving supplier relationships.
- Breaking down interdepartmental barriers.
- Developing realistic production standards.
- Transforming the entire nursing organization.

Quality management should be decentralized so that practicing nurses own quality and apply the processes needed to deliver quality nursing service. Nurses would develop quality methods to check the application of the nursing process to patients, check process and outcomes, and fix deficits (variation) in the process. When necessary, these nurses subject the nursing process to Pareto and fishbone analyses. They may repeat the process at more specific levels to identify the solution to a problem. Nurses will "commit to 'do right' principles: maintain control of every process, post quality evidence on the walls, brook no compromises, find a way to check every unit (where checks are necessary), fix their own mistakes, and assess continual involvement in quality-improvement projects."[83]

Traditional American management theory "motivates employees by fear (principally of losing their jobs), by requiring them to meet quotas, and by attempting to maximize their merit increases. Deming's principles require a fundamental change in American habits."[84]

Habits are based on immediate consequences of behavior, on short-term success. Their long-term consequences and subsequent problems have been very destructive. Management habits often cause problems. Well-established destructive habits of management can be changed. The following are six principles for making changes:

1. The individual manager or leader must perceive a need to change, must genuinely admit and accept that he or she must change, and must commit to the change. Unfortunately, managers or leaders often do not perceive a need for change unless their business is in serious trouble.
2. The change must be voluntary, not coercive.
3. The change process requires a philosophical base, a statement of beliefs about how people will be managed. If TQM is to be implemented, the philosophical base may be a statement of beliefs that include all or some of Deming's 14 points. The leader who implements this change process acts as teacher and planner and is the object of a process called "transference."
4. The change process requires the support of others participating in the same process. Thus, a group interacts, shares insights and feelings, and provides social support while implementing a philosophy of TQM.
5. The process should be broken down into steps that can be accomplished in sequence. The nurse leader should aim for at least one quick success, make a road map or plan, and provide education and communication.[85]
6. The daily routine needs to be changed until the desired behavior is accomplished habitually and with little external decision.[86]

Today's manager is "a high-tech management-trained individual with a focus on profitability through quality and a sensitive, but widely encompassing, utilization of work force talent."[87] Committed to TQM, this manager leader knows that if quality is improved, productivity will be improved.

The following are some goals for this new breed of nurse leader:

1. Change the management style and operating climate.
2. Do the job right the first time to meet and exceed customers' expectations.
3. Stop producing waste, stop sorting good from bad to avoid poor products or services to customers, stop paying people to produce waste. Innovate and excite the customer with high-quality services.
4. Look at the waste standards and spoilage problems of nursing.
5. Identify and eliminate performance inhibitors and continuously improve productivity.
6. Use process data to change methods, techniques, and technology to create improvements.
7. Replace boss-imposed solutions with group interaction.
8. Eliminate as many layers of management and support personnel as possible. Replace with integrated, self-governing work teams.
9. Train managers to be coaches, trainers, and information resources.

10. Reach out and involve customers and suppliers.[88]
11. Recognize that all improvements take place project by project.
12. Publish quality goals with names of projects and names of team members to fix responsibility and give rights to teams. Review progress on projects.[89]
13. Constantly work to improve the work system for employees by providing better tools and raw materials and building a culture of trust.
14. Scrap quality control departments, numerical goals, and quotas. Give workers the right to shut down the production line if the quality of the product is in jeopardy. Spot and fix defects in the process. Give authority to practicing nurses.
15. Drive out fears by throwing out or simplifying worker performance evaluations.
16. Learn to live without enemies. Get workers to cooperate, not compete.[90]
17. Use plan-do-check-act (PDCA). Hospital Corporation of America hospitals use a quality improvement strategy called FOCUS-PDCA[91] (Also see Exhibit 25-3):
    a. Find opportunity for improvement.
    b. Organize a team that knows the process.
    c. Clarify current knowledge of the process.
    d. Uncover root causes of process variations.
    e. Start an improvement cycle based on theory.
    f. Plan the process improvement.
    g. Do the improvement.
    h. Check the results against the theory.
    i. Act on the process and theory.

Exhibit 25-9 summarizes several successful applications of TQM in U. S. firms.

One estimate is that 40% of operating costs of service industries is spent on errors.[92] Hospital and nursing administrations make the commitment and create the environment for making quality improvement happen.

Total quality management has its detractors, including managers involved in downsizing and restructuring U. S. business and industry. Executives who are committed to TQM are making it work, for example, at Xerox, Motorola, Federal Express, Harley-Davidson, and others. Many executives claim that TQM costs more than it is worth. The theory of TQM is solidly integrated into the theory of human resources development as the management theory that will produce the most motivated and productive workers. It takes true leadership to make it work.

The literature abounds with examples of application of TQM in health care systems. Rush-Presbyterian-St. Luke's Medical Center in Chicago started implementing TQM in 1987. Its program centered on the establishment of professional standards for clinical services. Rush examined various industrial models of quality management to identify the elements of the model that would strengthen

its own quality initiatives. The employees were trained in TQM concepts and empowered to make improvements in their work. The corporation required a cultural change that focused on a vision and unrelenting pursuit of realization of that vision.

To accomplish a change in the culture of this organization, a combined emphasis was placed on training, measurement, and communications. Among the improvements noted were a reduction in the preparation time to pick up a neonatal infant from a referring hospital, a reduction in the number of incomplete medical records following hospital discharge, a reduction in the x-ray repeat rate, and a reduction in patient delays in radiology. Rush management acknowledges that TQM has worked because the employees were willing to try something new.[93]

McEachern, Schiff, and Cogan outline the application of continuous quality improvement (CQI) to direct patient care. The goal of the CQI process is to improve direct patient care. The principles used are the customer's knowledge level, process focus, and statistical mindedness. Three methods of developing direct patient care teams are[94]:

1. Following the interest of an individual who usually becomes the team leader.
2. Organizing the top 25 diagnosis-related groups by functional body systems or major functional processes.
3. Forming of teams by clinicians.

Winter Park Memorial Hospital is one of the hospitals that early on experimented in applying the TQM guidelines of industrial business to the health care industry. Encouraged by the Joint Commission on Accreditation of Healthcare Organizations and supported by the Hospital Corporation of America, Winter Park examined practices over five years dealing with patient and employee issues. The hospital decided that, because of competition in their area, TQM would be able to help it compete in the marketplace.

With Philip Crosby serving as consultant, health care quality management issues were introduced to the Winter Park administration. Crosby's philosophy that all work is a process that produces an outcome helped Winter Park begin to understand the 14 necessary actions to achieve TQM.

A medical staff quality council was formed but was not initially involved in any of the TQM efforts. Medical staff members did not accept the results or the proposed changes readily until they began to learn about TQM. As a result, the medical council actively participated in the TQM movement at Winter Park.[95]

Health care institutions are finding that between 40% and 60% of all therapeutic effects can be attributed to placebo and Hawthorne effects. These are code words for caring and concern. Kindness prevents

EXHIBIT 25-9
Total Quality Management (TQM) Examples

DEPARTMENT OF VETERANS AFFAIRS, PHILADELPHIA

Initiated TQM with concept of veterans as customers. Established cross-functional teams and involved middle management so they were not threatened by new ideas and won their trust. Start-up training costs were $75,000: 2-hour orientation class for every employee run by division managers; 40-hour quality improvement course in group dynamics, analytical tools, hypothetical problem solving for 50 percent of employees; 24-hour course for team members to act as team facilitators; and series of 2-hour modules teaching clerks and staffers to welcome change, and suggest new ideas. Teams with IDs listing team and members' names. Success: $168,000 saved on loan default processor improvements; people believe their ideas are being heard, and people relate to other's jobs.

Source: E. Penzer. "A Philadelphia Story." *Incentive* (July 1991), 33–34, 36.

BRAZOSPORT MEMORIAL HOSPITAL

Brazosport Memorial Hospital established a quality improvement process of quality orientation, continuous process improvement, and total employee involvement. A quality improvement council of top administrators developed a policy with employee input: "It is our commitment at BMH to promote genuine pride in excellence among our employees and other professionals in order to continuously improve the quality and value of the services provided to achieve customer satisfaction." A definition of quality states: "Providing health care services which are continuously improved to meet the needs and expectations of our patients, physicians, employees, payers and the community we serve." Employees are encouraged to speak freely about hospital operations and generate ideas for improvement. They are encouraged to collect and analyze data in process improvement. Questionnaires are sent every six months to 300 former patients to assess quality. Process includes quality improvement teams, training, changes including management style, commitment, stress on ideas, and networking among others.

Source: M. L. Lynn. "Deming's Quality Principles: A Health Care Application." *Hospital & Health Services Administration* (spring 1991), 111–120.

PUBLISHERS PRESS

Assessed the organization's working environment through employee surveys. Provided three-week training course in SPC for all middle managers. All employees trained in Deming's philosophy. Process improvement team (PIT) members were trained to change the work culture to eliminate fear and lack of communication. Because employee input and experience was considered important, the culture was changed to make the employees want to get involved. Teams

of owners and experts met 1–2 hours a week to determine internal customers and suppliers of the process chosen for study. Teams decided where process began and ended, applied process components, measured process input, and made change as needed. They validated prioritized objectives and diagrammed process control charts. Brainstorming led to action plan for improvement. New PITs form, old PITs disband when processes improve. Statistical improvements take months. Had 17 percent error reduction in order entry and 20 percent in film spoilage. Process requires coach, not judge, and interaction between managers and employees.

Source: G. A. Ferguson. "Printer Incorporates Deming—Reduces Errors, Increases Productivity." *Industrial Engineering* (August 1990), 32–34.

GENERAL MOTORS

Adopted Deming's philosophy to transform GM's culture. Results included decreased parts transport from 5 days to 31 hours and with 35 percent fewer shipping racks and fewer rail cars. Applied successfully to re-engineering an engine to decrease variance.

Source: J. P. White. "No More Excuses." *The Wall Street Journal* (21 November 1991), 1, A6.

INGERSOLL MACHINE TOOL

"But in the machine tool segment of manufacturing, Ingersoll has faced hard times and has shown that top management's involvement in a quality program can keep a company competitive in world markets."

Ingersoll made an unstinting investment in new technology. They expanded during recession by integrating computers into manufacturing systems. They expanded production capacity and made a commitment to employees, thus preparing for a business upturn. They kept a skilled and knowledgeable work force intact, as well as a shop full of new, modern, updated, and accurate machines. Everyone learned to work a little more effectively. Through planning and commitment to quality on a long-term basis, they sold machines to Hitachi, Fuji, and Honda and competed worldwide.

Ingersoll has a philosophy of original design. Their mission is defined in the quality policy statement "we achieve quality . . . when we successfully design and build to specifications that accurately . . . define our customers' needs." Ingersoll spent money to develop inspection equipment. They developed supplier evaluation programs, annual quality improvement programs, continuous training of workers to upgrade quality skills, and process evaluations for SPC.

Source: J. Wolak. "From the Top." *Quality* (August 1988), 14–15.

LEVI STRAUSS

Levi Strauss will attempt to keep its plants in the U.S. by restructuring. Assembly lines will be replaced by self-

(continued)

EXHIBIT 25-9 *(continued)*

managed teams of 30 to 50 workers who will make an entire product. Team members will learn a variety of skills. The restructuring process requires much time and training. Workers will help make decisions, and they will make the teamwork system successful because they believe in it. They will run the factories, hire colleagues, set their own hours, and purchase their own thread and equipment: empowerment and flattened organizational structure with the workers in control. There will be programs to help workers pay for child care. Dress will be informal, and managers will be called by their first names in a casual culture. They will provide quality products for satisfied customers. There will be decreased injuries and increased profits.

Mission Statement. The mission of Levi Strauss & Co. is to sustain responsible commercial success as a global marketing company of branded casual apparel. We must balance goals of superior profitability and return on investment, leadership market positions, and superior products and service. We will conduct our business ethically and demonstrate leadership in satisfying our responsibilities to our communities and to society. Our work environment will be safe and productive and characterized by fair treatment, teamwork, open communications, personal accountability, and opportunities for growth and development.

Aspiration Statement. We all want a Company that our people are proud of and committed to, where all employees have an opportunity to contribute, learn, grow, and advance based on merit, not politics or background. We want our people to feel respected, treated fairly, listened to, and involved. Above all, we want satisfaction from accomplishments and friendships, balanced personal and professional lives, and to have fun in our endeavors.

When we describe the kind of LS&CO we want in the future, what we are talking about is building on the foundation we have inherited: affirming the best of our Company's traditions, closing gaps that may exist between principles and practices, and updating some of our values to reflect contemporary circumstances.

What type of leadership is necessary to make our aspirations a reality?

Teamwork and Trust. Leadership that exemplifies directness, openness to influence, commitment to the success of others, willingness to acknowledge our own contributions to problems, personal accountability, teamwork and trust. Not only must we model these behaviors, but we must also coach others to adopt them.

Diversity. Leadership that values a diverse workforce (age, sex, ethnic group, etc.) at all levels of the organization, diversity in experience, and a diversity in perspectives. We have committed to taking full advantage of the rich backgrounds and abilities of all our people and to promote a greater diversity in positions of influence. Differing points of view will be sought; diversity will be valued and honesty rewarded, not suppressed.

Recognition. Leadership that provides greater recognition—both financial and psychic—for individuals and teams that contribute to our success. Recognition must be given to all who contribute: those who create and innovate and also those who continually support the day-to-day business requirements.

Ethical Management Practices. Leadership that epitomizes the stated standards of ethical behavior. We must provide clarity about our expectations and must enforce these standards throughout the corporation.

Communication. Internally, leadership that builds an environment in which information is actively shared, sought, and used in ways that lead to empowerment that works, improved performance, and meaningful feedback. Externally, leadership that strengthens our corporate reputation with key stakeholders. All communications should be clear, timely, and honest.

Empowerment. Leadership that promotes ways of working in which responsibility, authority, and accountability for decision making are held by those closest to products and customers, and every employee has the necessary perspective, skills, and knowledge to be successful in his or her job. We all share responsibility for creating the environment that will nurture empowerment at all levels of the organization.

In an interview with Robert Howard for the *Harvard Business Review*, Robert Haas, the CEO of Levi, stated, "A company's values—what it stands for, what its people believe in—are crucial to its competitive success." He went on to say, "Because we value open and direct communication, we give people permission to disagree."

Note: Mission Statement and Aspiration Statement used courtesy Levi Strauss Associates, Inc., San Francisco, California.

Source: J. Kever. "People Power." *San Antonio Light* (12 July 1992), A1, A10–12; Editorial, "Levi's Plan to Tailor Production Fits U.S. Manufacturing Needs." *San Antonio Light* (6 February 1992), C8; P. Konstam. "Levi's New System Can Save U.S. Jobs." *San Antonio Light* (5 February 1992), D1; R. Howard. "Values Make the Company: An Interview with Robert Haas." *Harvard Business Review* (September–October 1990), 133–144.

MARS

Mars, Inc., is a multibillion-dollar, world-class company that is a leader in candy, pet food, rice, and other products. At the Mars company there are no assigned parking spaces for anyone. There are no offices or partitions between desks. Offices have a concentric structure, with the president and staff at the center and others fanning outward. Senior officers are totally visible and accessible. Time clocks are at doors,

EXHIBIT 25-9 *(continued)*

and everyone, including owners, punches in. An employee who punches in on time gets a 10 percent punctuality bonus.

Communications at Mars are personal and immediate. Memos are not written and electronic mail goes unused. Factories are spotless and shining, with efficient, high-speed lines. Employees, including managers, wear white uniforms and white hats in production areas. Otherwise dress is casual for all. Employees are highly paid, nonunion, loyal, and proud. Quality is an obsession and is everyone's responsibility. All Mars employees get the same annual step increase. There are only six pay levels, with vice presidents all receiving approximately the same salary. People can be easily transferred from business unit to business unit and from function to function.

Mars is a true quality culture. It maintains state-of-the-art technology. Equipment is valued at replacement cost. The company uses a unique equation called ROTA (return on total assets) that accounts for inventory turns and asset utilization.

The business acumen of the Mars family has created great personal wealth for them. They are listed in *Fortune*, June 28, 1993, as among the world's 101 richest people.

Source: C. J. Cantoni. "Quality Control from Mars." *The Wall Street Journal* (27 January 1992), A10.

USAA

USAA, which is based in Texas, is a Fortune 500 insurance and financial services company. Over 20,000 employees work in all branches of the United Services Automobile Association.

USAA was started in 1922 by military officers. McDermott came as CEO in 1968, lured away from his post as dean of the United States Air Force Academy. At that time 40 percent of employees quit each year. Many jobs were mundane and low-paying, and management was untrained. McDermott believed that technology had to be developed to make dull jobs easier. Also, employees "had to be made to feel they were part of something special if they were to make the company's customers feel the same way."

The corporate culture of USAA includes the following:

- A community recreation complex where employees leave work to play softball on two manicured diamonds; soccer on a lush, green field; basketball on two outdoor courts outfitted with scoreboards and bleachers; tennis courts; and volleyball courts.
- A sense of community, enthusiasm, not-too-serious competition, a sense of sportsmanship, and a given sense of purpose.
- An employee health clinic.

- Encouragement of employees to participate in the external community as mentors to students.
- A 286-acre "campus" in San Antonio and another large one in Phoenix, AZ.
- A headquarters structure that rivals the Pentagon in square footage and consumes more than $4 million in gas and electricity per year.
- A work experience that gives pleasure, satisfaction, and psychic income.
- Stress on teamwork and common goals, even though the organization is highly structured and insists on adherence to protocol.
- A take-care-of-its-own attitude reflected in its pay, benefits, perks, and working conditions, including a four-day work week.
- A state-of-the-art plant and equipment. The computer operation handles over 8 million transactions a day and is linked via cable and satellite with field offices in other cities.
- Training and conference rooms that include the company's own television production facility, the latest in video technology, production of video press releases, training videos, a USAA news program that runs on its own closed-circuit network, documentaries for use by the insurance industry, and 50 to 60 hours a month of teleconferencing.
- Comfortable workstations and high-tech equipment.
- Facilities to increase fitness and improve wellness.
- First-rate cafeterias. Employees are offered a "dinner express" from 3 to 6 p.m. They take home 3,000–4,000 dinners each week.
- A credit union and the USAA Federal Savings Bank.
- College courses; job-related courses have tuition paid by USAA.
- A company-owned store for employees.
- A local post office branch, which processes more than 350,000 pieces of mail daily.
- A day-care facility serving 300 employees' children up to age 5. "Having a well-adjusted child in a quality day-care arrangement reduces stress on employees who have children."

The whole idea is to make employees happy and productive. They are! Turnover is down to 8.5 percent a year. USAA's customers are happy and the company is highly profitable and expanding. It is poised for the future.*

Source: *M. Tolson. "USAA, TX 78228." *San Antonio Light* (23 September 1990), A1, A12; **L. Hicks. "USAA to Erect Day Care Facility." *San Antonio Express-News* (12 May 1994), 1E.

(continued)

EXHIBIT 25-9 *(continued)*

DIALYSIS CENTER, LINCOLN, NEBRASKA

At the Dialysis Center of Lincoln, NE, after implementation of TQM the following changes occurred:

	1987–1988	1990–1991
Employee satisfaction survey	40%	92%
Staff turnover	70%	5%
Absenteeism	8 days/yr/ employee	2.5 days/yr/ employee
Medicare statement of deficiencies	7 pages	3 pages

Source: M. Churchill. "Employees Are Also Our Customers." *ANNA Journal* (April 1992), 152.

MOTOROLA

Motorola is one of the best-managed companies in the world. Part of this is due to their commitment to TQM, termed "six sigma quality." With only 3.4 mistakes per one million parts produced, Motorola attempts to measure every task performed by its 120,000 employees. It calculates $1.5 billion saved by reducing defects and simplifying procedures during 1993.

Source: R. Henkoff. "Keeping Motorola on a Roll." *Fortune* (18 April 1994), 67–68, 70, 72, 74, 77–78.

malpractice suits. Quality of life is improved by esteem-enhancing interventions. Attention, information in the form of follow-up summaries of visits, and surroundings all contribute to improved quality of care and life.[96]

The U. S. health care industry will solve its problems by producing a higher-quality product more efficiently.[97] TQM techniques combined with motivational management techniques and critical thinking strategies provide a conceptualization of clinical teaching and learning.[98]

Summary

Total quality management is fast replacing old concepts of management. It is a system that empowers the worker. TQM has evolved from the work of W. Edwards Deming who found that 85% to 90% of problems are due to the system (common causes) and only 10% to 15% are due to employees (special causes). Through the use of statistical methods such as variation, the common causes can be separated from the special causes, and workers can themselves fix the special causes during the process of production. Application of the philosophy and theory of TQM leads to increased productivity and profitability.

Among the data analysis tools that are used to fix causes are the Pareto chart or diagram, the fishbone diagram, the master diagram, and the cause-and-effect diagram. In addition to Deming, other TQM gurus include Joseph Juran who describes quality as "fitness to use"; Philip B. Crosby, who defines quality as "conformance to requirements"; and Genichi Taguchi, who developed the theory of robust quality. All of these theories are having a profound effect on U. S. management.

TQM focuses on customer satisfaction and includes the notion of internal and external customers. If the customer is going to radiology for a special procedure, the nurse's next internal customer is radiology. Clients, families, and communities are external customers.

Leadership is the paramount qualification for success in TQM. It is leadership that will change the culture and climate of the business to give workers the training they need to participate in planning, make decisions, be creative, and improve productivity through improvement of quality of products and services. It is a leadership that fosters self-esteem and eliminates formal barriers to cooperation such as job titles, unfair pay practices and performance appraisals, and divisive perquisites of office.

Total quality management is the new wave of nursing management. It is a proven theory waiting for broad application.

APPLICATION EXERCISES

EXERCISE 25-1 Using a team representing nurse managers and clinical nurses, examine the purpose of a nursing division. How long has the purpose existed? Has the purpose been constant over time? Does it need changing? Examine a definition of total quality management and decide whether a change in purpose is needed. Will the change affect nursing services? Is this desirable? Make a management plan for accomplishing the agreed-on purpose and for communicating it to all employees.

EXERCISE 25-2 Using a team that represents both nursing leaders within the organization and customers, construct a questionnaire for measuring external customer satisfaction. If one is currently available, review it and make changes only if changes are needed. Use the questionnaire to measure external customer satisfaction with nursing. Analyze the results using statistical applications, and plan for changes to improve external customer satisfaction.

EXERCISE 25-3 Using a team that represents nursing leaders within the organization and internal customers of nursing, identify problems and make plans to fix them. Aim for cooperation and win–win fixes.

EXERCISE 25-4 Using a team representing nursing leaders within the organization, discuss abolishing the current performance appraisal system. Decide how to identify the three categories of performance of Deming: within the system, outside the system (high), and outside the system (low).

EXERCISE 25-5 Using a team representing nursing leaders within the organization, identify a major problem. Decide on the data to be collected and the statistical methods to be applied. Proceed to gather and analyze data and solve the problem.

EXERCISE 25-6 Using a team representing nursing leaders within the organization, discuss abolishing job descriptions. Outline on one 5-by-8-inch card the qualifications for appointment to a nursing job. On another card, outline the qualifications for promotion.

EXERCISE 25-7 Using a team representing nursing leaders within the organization, describe the culture of the organization. Decide which beliefs and values need to be changed. Make a plan for changing them.

EXERCISE 25-8 Use Juran's three major premises of quality planning, quality control, and quality improvement to do a quality plan for a nursing division or unit. Use the activities itemized in this chapter under these premises.

EXERCISE 25-9 Make a plan for a quality circle using the guidelines described in this chapter.

NOTES

1. J. Oberle, "Quality Gurus: The Men and Their Message," *Training* (January 1990), 47–52.
2. J. J. Kaufman, "Total Quality Management," *Ekistics* 336 (May–June) 1989 and 337 (July–August 1987), 182–187.
3. P. Konstam, "Quality Should Begin at Home," *San Antonio Light* (1 March 1992), D1.
4. Ibid.; R. Boissoneau, "New Approach to Managing People at Work," *The Health Care Supervisor* (July 1989), 67–76.
5. M. M. Yasin, K. A. Meacham, and J. Alavi, "The Status of TQM in Healthcare," *Health Marketing Quarterly*, 15(3) 1998, 61–84.
6. M. M. Yasin and J. Alavl, "An Analytical Approach to Determining the Competitive Advantage of TQM in Health Care," *International Journal of Health Care Quality Assurance Inc. Leadership Health Service,* 12(1), (1999), 18–24.
7. M. W. Piczak, "Quality Circles Come Home," *Quality Progress* (December 1988), 37–39.
8. M. Tritus, "Deming's Way," *Mechanical Engineering* (January 1988), 28.
9. Ibid., 26–30.
10. Ibid.
11. W. J. Duncan and J. G. Van Matre, "The Gospel According to Deming: Is It Really New?" *Business Horizons* (July–August 1990), 3–9.
12. A. E. Francis and J. M. Germels, "Building a Better Budget," *Quality Progress* (October 1989), 70–75.
13. T. A. Smith, "Why You Should Put Your Safety System Under Statistical Control," *Professional Safety* (April 1989), 31–36.
14. B. L. Joiner and M. A. Gaudard, "Variation, Management, and W. Edwards Deming," *Quality Progress* (December 1990), 29–39.
15. L. A. Heinzlmeir, "Under the Spell of the Quality Gurus," *Canadian Manager* (spring 1991), 22–23.
16. Ibid.
17. J. T. Burr, "The Tools of Quality Part VI: Pareto Charts," *Quality Progress* (November 1990), 59–61.
18. Ibid.
19. B. L. Joiner and M. A. Gaudard, op. cit.
20. L. Cohen, "Quality Function Deployment: An Application Perspective from Digital Equipment Corporation," *National Productivity Review* (summer 1988), 197–208.
21. Ibid.
22. Ibid.
23. B. Rudin, "Simple Tools Solve Complex Problems," *Quality* (April 1990), 50–51.
24. L. A. Heinzlmeir, op. cit.; SV, "Quality Can't Be Delegated," *Supervision* (May 1988), 6–7.
25. J. M. Juran, "Universal Approach to Managing for Quality," *Executive Excellence* (May 1989), 15–17.
26. Ibid.
27. Ibid.
28. Ibid.
29. Ibid.
30. G. S. Vasilash, "Crosby Says Get Fit for Quality," *Production* (January 1981), 51–52, 54; L. A. Heinzlmeir, op. cit; J. Oberle, op. cit; B. J. Deutsch, "A Conversation with Philip Crosby," *Bank Marketing* (April 1991), 22–27; P. B. Crosby, *Quality without Tears: The Art of Hassle-Free Management* (New York: McGraw-Hill, 1984).
31. C. R. O'Neal, "Its What's Up Front That Counts," *Marketing News* (4 March 1991), 9, 28; O. Port, "How to Make It Right the First Time," *Business Week* (8 June 1987), 142–143.
32. G. Taguchi and D. Clausing, "Robust Quality," *Harvard Business Review* (January–February 1990), 65–75.
33. D. Schaaf, "Beating the Drum for Quality," *Quality* (March 1991), 5–6, 8, 11–12.
34. M. Schrage, "Fire Your Customers," *The Wall Street Journal* (16 March 1992), A12.
35. L. H. Friedman and D. B. White, "What is Quality, Who Wants It, and Why?" *Management Care Quarterly* (autumn 1999), 40–46.
36. N. G. Bloor, "Organizational Culture, Organizational Learning and Total Quality Management: A Literature Review and Synthesis," *Australian Health Review*, 22(3), (1999), 162–179.
37. N. Centanni, M. Monroe, L. White, and R. Larson, "Quality Beyond Compliance," *Quality Assurance*, 7(1), (1999), 17–35.
38. E. E. Scheuing, "Achieving Excellence: Creating Customer Passion," *Hospital Materials Management Quarterly* (August 1999), 76–87.
39. D. Schaff, op. cit.
40. G. Rex Bryce, "Quality Management Theories and Their Application," *Quality* (January 1991), 15–18.
41. "What's Next On the Quality Agenda?" *Quality* (March 1991), 42.
42. C. R. O'Neal, op. cit.
43. T. Peters, "Family Gives 'Teams' Plenty of Experience," *San Antonio Light* (12 November 1991), E3.
44. G. Isouard, "The Key Elements in the Development of a Quality Management Environment for Pathology Services," *Journal of Quality Clinical Practice* (December 1999), 202–207.
45. M. Hammer and S. Stanton, "How Process Enterprises Really Work," *Harvard Business Review* (November–December 1999), 108–118, 216.
46. P. Konstam, "Making Productivity Grow Takes Work," *San Antonio Light* (1 January 1992), 1E.
47. J. J. Kaufman, op.cit.
48. T. Peters, "Plenty Left to Do for U.S. Economy," *San Antonio Light* (14 January 1992), B9.
49. Ibid.
50. T. Peters, "Turn Your Workers Into Business People," *San Antonio Light* (26 November 1991), E3.
51. W. J. Duncan and J. G. Van Matre, op. cit.
52. G. R. Bryce, op. cit.
53. R. H. Slater, "Integrated Process Management: A Quality Model," (January 1991), 27–31.
54. D. Ertel, "Turning Negotiation into a Corporate Capability," *Harvard Business Review* (May–June 1999), 55–60, 62–70, 213.
55. P. Linkow, "Is Your Culture Ready for Total Quality?" *Quality Progress* (November 1989), 69–71.
56. Ibid.
57. Ibid.
58. T. F. O'Boyle, "Two Worlds," *The Wall Street Journal* (27 November 1991), 1.
59. L. H. Clark, Jr., "Service Center Faces Task of Cutting Costs Without Trimming Quality of Its Product," *The Wall Street Journal* (2 April 1992), B9A.
60. D. E. Hendricks, "Avoiding Cultural Myopia: What The Japanese Can Teach Nurses About Management," *Nursing Leadership* (June 1982), 11–15.
61. L. Dusky, "Anatomy of a Revolution," *Executive Excellence* (May 1991), 19–20.
62. G. A. Geyer, "Blame Game Avoids U.S. Sickness," *San Antonio Light* (26 December 1991), B7.
63. W. A. Sahlman, "The New Economy is Stronger Than You Think," *Harvard Business Review* (November–December 1999), 99–106, 216.
64. W. G.Ouchi, *Theory Z* (Reading, MA: Addison-Wesley, 1981).
65. M. N. Adair and N. K. Nygard, "Theory Z Management: Can It Work for Nursing?" *Nursing & Health Care* (November 1982), 489–491.
66. Ibid.

67. The theory of quality circles was actually developed by Frederick Herzberg and F. Edwards Deming of the United States approximately 50 years ago, S. Johnson, "Quality Control Circles: Negotiating an Efficient Work Environment," *Nursing Management* (July 1985), 34A–34B, 34D–34G; A. M. Goldberg and C. C. Pegels, *Quality Circles in Health-Care Facilities* (Gaithersburg, MD: Aspen, 1984).

68. Ibid.

69. S. A. Morhman and G. E. Ledford, Jr., "The Design and Use of Effective Employee Participation Groups: Implication for Human Resource Management," *Human Resource Management* (winter 1985), 413–428.

70. M. Sashkin, "Participative Management Remains an Ethical Imperative," *Organizational Dynamics* (spring 1986), 62–75.

71. N. Ertl, "Choosing Successful Managers: Participative Selection Can Help," *Journal of Nursing Administration* (April 1984), 27–33.

72. M. W. Piczak, op. cit.

73. D. Schaaf, op. cit.

74. R. D. Moen, "The Performance Appraisal System: Deming's Deadly Disease," *Quality Progress* (November 1989), 62–66.

75. Ibid.

76. S. M. Moss, "Appraise Your Performance Appraisal Process," *Quality Progress* (November 1989), 58–60.

77. L. E. Mainstone and A. S. Levi, "Fundamentals of Statistical Process Control," *Journal of Organizational Behavior, Management*, 9(1), (1987), 5–21.

78. S. M. Moss, op. cit.

79. R. D. Moen, op. cit.

80. Ibid.

81. Ibid.

82. R. J. Schonberger, "The Quality Concept: Still Evolving," *National Productivity Review* (winter 1986–87), 81–86.

83. Ibid., 82.

84. B. Carder, "Kicking the Habit," *Quality Progress* (March 1991), 87–89.

85. Ibid.

86. F. Alemi, D. Neuhauser, S. Ardito, L. Headrick, S. Moore, F. Hekelman, and L. Norman, "Continuous Self-Improvement: Systems Thinking in a Personal Context," *Joint Commission Journal of Quality Improvement* (February 2000), 74–86.

87. W. C. Lamporter, "The New Breed," *American Printer* (July 1991), 28–31.

88. Ibid.

89. SV, op. cit.

90. B. Richmond, "Auto Advice is Good School of Thought," *San Antonio Light* (11 January 1992), 1B.

91. D. Burda, "Provider Looks to Industry for Quality Models," *Modern Healthcare* (15 July 1988), 24–26, 28, 30, 32.

92. F. F. Jespersen, "Once More With Feeling: Quality Starts at the Top," *Business Month* (August 1989), 65–66.

93. M. E. Sinioris, "TQM: The New Frontier for Quality and Productivity Improvement in Health Care," *Journal of Quality Assurance* (September–October 1990), 14–17.

94. J. E. McEachern, L. Schiff, and O. Cogan, "How to Start a Direct Patient Care Team," *Quality Review Bulletin* (June 1992), 191–200.

95. J. M. Hughes, "Total Quality Management in a 300-Bed Community Hospital: The Quality Improvement Process Translated to Health Care," *Quality Review Bulletin* (September 1992), 311–318.

96. T. Peters, "Good Service Vital to Health Care, Too," *San Antonio Light* (10 November 1992), B2.

97. J. L. Haughom, "Transforming U. S. Health Care: The Arduous Road to Value," *Topics in Health Information Management* (February 2000), 1–10.

98. L. J. Massarweh, "Promoting a Positive Clinical Experience," *Nurse Educator* (May–June 1999), 44–47.

REFERENCES

Arikian, V. L. "Total Quality Management: Applications to Nursing Service." *Journal of Nursing Administration* (June 1991), 46–50.

Cole, R. "What Was Deming's Real Influence?" *Mechanical Engineering* (January 1988), 49–51.

Dobyns, L., and C. Crawford-Mason. *Quality or Else: The Revolution in World Business* (New York: Houghton Mifflin Company, 1991).

Duncan, R. P., E. C. Fleming, and T. G. Gallati. "Implementing a Continuous Quality Improvement Program in a Community Hospital." *Quality Review Bulletin* (April 1991), 106–112.

Eddy, D. M., and J. Billings. "The Quality of Medical Evidence: Implications for Quality of Care." *Health Affairs* (spring1988), 19–32.

Eubanks, P. "The CEO Experience: TQM/CQI." *Hospitals* (5 June 1992), 24–36.

Ferketish, B. J., and J. W. Hayden. "HRD & Quality: The Chicken or the Egg?" *Training & Development Journal* (January 1992), 39–42.

Gitlow, H.S., S. J. Gitlow, A. Oppenheim, and R. Oppenheim. "Telling the Quality Story." *Quality Progress* (September 1990), 41–46.

Kaluzny, A. D., C. P. McLaughlin, and K. Simpson. "Applying Total Quality Management Concepts to Public Health Organizations." *Public Health Reports* (May–June 1992), 257–263.

Konstam, P. "'Quality' Should Begin at Home." *San Antonio Light* (1 March 1992), D1.

Ludeman, K. "Using Employee Surveys to Revitalize TQM." *Training* (December 1992), 51–57.

Mathews, J., and P. Katel. "The Cost of Quality." *Newsweek* (7 September 1992), 48–49.

McCabe, W. J. 1992. "Total Quality Management in a Hospital." *Quality Review Bulletin* (April 1992), 134–140.

McCormick, V. E. "Software Helps with Hard Decisions." *Training* (August 1991), 23–24.

McLaughlin, C. P., and A. D. Kaluzny. "Total Quality Management in Health: Making It Work." *Health Care Management Review,* 15(3), (1990), 7–14.

Meisenheimer, C. "The Customer: Silent or Intimate Player in the Quality Revolution." *Holistic Nurse Practitioner* (April 1991), 39–50.

Walton, M. "Deming's Parable of the Red Beads." *Across the Board* (February 1987), 43–48.

Williams, R. "Putting Deming's Principles to Work." *The Wall Street Journal* (4 November 1991), A18.

Woods, M. D. "New Manufacturing Practices: New Accounting Practices." *Production and Inventory Management Journal* (Fourth Quarter 1989), 8–12.

CHAPTER 26

Quality Management

Beverly Blain Wright, RNC, CNA, CPHQ

QUALITY MANAGEMENT PROJECT COORDINATOR
UNIVERSITY OF SOUTH ALABAMA MEDICAL CENTER
MOBILE, ALABAMA

LEARNING OBJECTIVES AND ACTIVITIES

- Define *quality management*.
- Differentiate among components of a quality management program.
- Describe the structure of a quality management program.
- Differentiate among tools for collecting and analyzing quality management data.

CONCEPTS: Quality management, structure audit, process audit, outcome audit.

MANAGER BEHAVIOR: Provides resources to meet the requirements of accreditation for quality management.

LEADER BEHAVIOR: Uses results of research to support accountability of nurses through education and assurance that they deliver quality patient care.

Introduction

As discussed in Chapter 24 on controlling, a master evaluation or control plan is needed to evaluate the total program of any nursing department, service, or unit. One of the most critical components of such a plan will be a quality management program. A key element of quality management is continuous improvement. As the costs of hospital and all aspects of health care continue to grow, it becomes essential that quality management programs truly establish standards to maintain and, indeed, deliver quality care. A primary assumption is that nursing must be accountable to the client for the care rendered by its practitioners.

Quality assurance (QA) programs began in hospitals in the 1960s, with voluntary implementation of nursing audits. Initially, nursing QA programs were designed to set standards for nursing care delivery and establish criteria by which to evaluate these standards. The term has emerged in the health care field as a synonym for evaluation, or as a significant evaluative activity. Kirk describes the relationship between QA, quality control (QC), and quality improvement (QI). *Quality assurance* defines performance measurements and compares actual processes and outcomes to clinical and satisfaction indicators. *Quality control* involves performance management and maintenance and includes systematic methods of ensuring conformance to a desired standard or norm. *Quality improvement* is concerned with performance development and is ongoing, involved with fixing problems now, costly mistakes in the future, and fostering breakthroughs.[1]

Programs for QA, QC, and QI are integrated and now include additional focal points of service quality and customer satisfaction. These elements must be incorporated into any QA program if it is to be a success. Matching the expectation of the service with that which is actually experienced by the customer defines the link between service quality and customer satisfaction. In other words, if the customer's perception is that the expectation of the service has been met or exceeded, the service is generally considered a quality one, and thus one has a satisfied customer.[2] Being ever watchful of client satisfaction of services provided is essential in all QA programs.

The Joint Commission on Accreditation of Healthcare Organizations (JCAHO) purports that from its initial form of retrospective, time-limited audits, the process has evolved to its current form of ongoing monitoring using well-chosen process and outcome indicators. In the same vein, the QI process must be a never-ending cycle.[3] According to Deming, this cycle must employ statistical QC, and the development of a "bedrock philosophy of management" is critical to ensure an enduring process of QI.[4] It is the blending and balancing of caring and providing such care around which a well thought-out quality management program is built. This program is a major part of the evaluation phase of the nursing management process.

Part of evaluation involves the understanding of the vision and purpose the organization serves for its clients, employees, customers, and the community. The leadership role in providing this vision is ultimately critical to how well management's vision is translated into well-written and understood objectives and outcomes. In addition, one would be remiss if efficiency (the cost of achieving objectives) were not considered in the model. QA not only incorporates evaluation but also involves its use to secure improvement.

Components of a Quality Management Program

A quality management program is composed of the following components:

1. Clear and concise written statements of purpose, philosophy, values, and objectives.
2. Standards or indicators for measuring the quality of care.
3. Policies and procedures for using such standards for gathering data. These polices define the organizational structure for the program.

4. Analysis and reporting of the data gathered, with isolation of problems and variances.
5. Use of the results to prioritize and correct problems and variances.
6. Monitoring of clinical and managerial performance and ongoing feedback to ensure problems stay solved.
7. Evaluation of the quality management system.

These components may be conceptualized in many different ways. Continuous quality improvement (CQI), the essence of quality management, can be conceptualized to illustrate how one component builds on another. Batalden and Stoltz describe a framework for the continual improvement of health care (see Exhibit 26-1), which incorporates underlying knowledge, policy for leadership, tools and methods, and daily work applications.[5] Underlying knowledge incorporates professional and improvement knowledge. Such knowledge includes theory of knowledge and knowledge of a system, variation, and psychology. The mission, vision, guiding principles, and integration of values are critical to the policy for leadership. "For the continual improvement of health care, tools and methods are available that can accelerate building and using knowledge and communicating that understanding to others."[6] Tools and methods can be grouped into four major categories: process and system, group process and collaborative work, statistical thinking, and planning and analysis. Daily work applications include developing models for testing change and making adjustments as well as review of the improvements. Conceptualizing QA and CQI provides the nurse with tools for assisting the nursing department with the overall process.

EXHIBIT 26-1
The Framework for the Continual Improvement of Health Care

UNDERLYING KNOWLEDGE	POLICY FOR LEADERSHIP	TOOLS AND METHODS	DAILY WORK APPLICATIONS
Professional knowledge: • subject • discipline • values	Mission, vision, and quality definition Guiding principles	Process, system Group process and collaborative work	Models for testing change and making improvement Review of improvement
Improvement knowledge: • system • variation • psychology • theory of knowledge	Integration with values	Statistical thinking Planning and analysis	

Source: P. B. Batalden and P. K. Stoltz. "A Framework for the Continual Improvement of Health Care: Building and Applying Professional and Improvement Knowledge to Test Changes in Daily Work." *Joint Commission Journal on Quality Improvement* (October 1993), 426. Oakbrook Terrace, IL: Joint Commission on Accreditation of Healthcare Organizations, 1993, p. 426. Reprinted with permission.

Statement of Purpose, Philosophy, and Objectives

The initial planning of a quality management program includes the development of clear and concise statements of purpose, philosophy, and objectives. The program's purpose and philosophy go hand in hand with the organizational purpose and philosophy and should be interwoven with the value the organization places on quality and continual improvement of the services provided. The JCAHO gives specific guidelines designed to assess and improve quality of client care. In addition, quality improvement theories are recommended to health care organizations to better conceptualize the entire quality management program. Such quality improvement theories include those of Deming, Crosby, Juran, and Senge.[7] An organization need not limit itself to one theory and may incorporate concepts from a wide variety to develop a framework that best fits the organizational purpose, philosophy, and objectives. Every quality management program needs well-articulated objectives, and every study needs a purpose (Exhibit 26-2 gives an example of mission and purpose statements).

Standards for Measuring Quality of Care

Standards define nursing care outcomes, nursing activities, and the structural resources needed. Standards are used to plan and evaluate nursing care. Outcomes include positive and negative indexes. Standards are directed at structure, process, and outcome issues and guide the review of systems function, staff performance, and client care. A number of health care organizations issue indexes. The Health Care Financing Administration (HCFA) annually discloses projected and actual hospital mortality rates by diagnostic-related groups (DRGs). The HCFA outlines physical quality indexes. The JCAHO has issued clinical and organizational performance measures and outcomes under the auspices of QA and QI. The JCAHO requires that the organization have a written plan for assessing and improving quality that describes the objectives, organization, scope, and mechanisms for overseeing the effectiveness of monitoring, evaluating, and improving activities. Such activities include quality of patient care, clinical performance with clinical privileges, pharmacy and therapeutics functions, infection control, utilization review, and risk management. Scoring guidelines are identified, and the organization is judged against its own criteria from individual guidelines.

Other organizations collecting data for quality measurement are the American Hospital Association, Voluntary Hospitals of America, National Committee for Quality Healthcare, and the National Association of Health Data Organizations. These organizations will gather, analyze,

---

EXHIBIT 26-2
Mission and Purpose Statements

MISSION
The mission of the Quality Assurance Plan of the University of South Alabama Medical Center is directly reflective of the mission of the University of South Alabama Medical Center. As stated in the policy, "Functional Plan of Organization of the University of South Alabama Medical Center" (from Mission Statements), the Department of Quality Assurance "ensures that the quality of patient care at the University of South Alabama Medical Center is optimal through a unified program for patient care evaluation activities."

PURPOSE
The purpose of the Quality Assurance Plan of the University of South Alabama Medical Center is to ensure that all patients receive the optimal quality of care.

Source: Courtesy of the University of South Alabama Medical Center, Mobile, AL.

---

and publish data on quality of health care for consumers, employers, and the federal government. The standards will include performance standards for providers (see Exhibit 26-3). The objectives are to achieve improvement in the health status of clients, reduce unnecessary utilization of health care services, and meet specifications of clients and purchasers. These standards will address improvement of health care quality, functions, and processes that must be carried out effectively to achieve good patient care outcomes, patient care, governance, and management. Theory of quality management has been applied in the form of identifying common causes and special causes of performance variation.[8] Outcomes or indexes serve as measures of the value, rank, or degree of excellence (see Exhibit 26-4 and Appendix 26-1).

Policies and Procedures

The third element of a quality management program is the development of policies and procedures for using standards or indicators for gathering data to measure the quality of care. Batalden and Stoltz describe guiding principles that reflect the organization's assumptions about the responsibilities and desired actions of leaders leading to the creation of a positive work environment. It is essential to integrate the leadership policy with the values common to health professionals and underlying health care work; this contributes to shared ownership of the policy by everyone in the organization.[9] The policies and procedures define the organizational structure for the quality management program and will prescribe the tools for gathering data.

EXHIBIT 26-3
Standards for Nursing

DEFINITION OF NURSING CARE
Based on the University of South Alabama Hospitals' mission, USAMC philosophy of Nursing, rules of Alabama State Board of Health Division of Licensure and Certification, and Nurse Practice Act, nursing care at the University of South Alabama Medical Center is defined as those acts received by the patient/significant other from nursing to assist the patient/family to reach the optimal level of wellness. Nursing care is further defined as being under direction of or provided by a Registered Nurse on a 24-hour basis and supports the nursing process as evidenced by documented actual or potential patient/family problems, planned interventions, nursing care provided, and results of interventions for the stated actual/potential problem. Nursing practice is defined by departmental policies, procedures, and standards which direct nursing care within the hospital.

I. POLICY STATEMENT
   Using the nursing process, patients receive nursing care within the guidelines of the following Standards of Care and Standards of Practice. These standards apply to all settings in which nursing care is provided: Medical Surgical Units: 8th, 7th, 6th, 5N, 5S; Labor and Delivery; Post-Anesthesia Care Unit; Operating Room; Special Care Units (SICU, NTICU, SINU, CCU, MICU, CCU II, MINU, ICN/Premature, Burn Center); Obstetrics: High-Risk/Antepartum, Mother-Baby; Newborn Nursery; and Ambulatory Surgery.

II. PURPOSE
   1. To guide the provision of nursing care.
   2. To provide the means by which nursing personnel are evaluated in the provision of nursing care.
   3. To provide the means by which to measure the end results of nursing care through patient outcomes.

III. GENERAL INFORMATION
   1. Nursing standards are used to monitor, evaluate, and initiate actions to improve the delivery of care through quality assessment and improvement.
   2. Standards for Nursing serve as the foundation for the development of policies and procedures.
   3. Standards for Nursing identify important aspects of care; standards of practice; concurrent process; retrospective process; standards of care; concurrent outcome; and retrospective outcome.

Source: Courtesy of the University of South Alabama Medical Center, Mobile, AL.

EXHIBIT 26-4

Measurable Outcomes to Achieve with Verification from Automated Documentation

1. Admission assessment within 24–48 hours
2. All diagnosis and treatment orders fulfilled
3. Discharged in safe physical, emotional, and mental health
4. Discharged with stable vital signs
5. No abnormal diagnostic findings left unattended
6. Normal fluid hydration
7. Continent (urinating and defecating appropriately)
8. Mobile steady gait, without threat of falls
9. Without drug interactions
10. Comfort achieved to the extent possible
11. Without decubitus ulcers and oral mucosal membrane ulcers
12. Capable of bathing, toileting, feeding and dressing self
13. No nosocomial infection
14. No purulent or blood drainage from wounds
15. Patient understands home treatment plan and was satisfied with care given by nursing staff

Source: K. A. McCormick. "Future Data Needs for Quality of Care Monitoring, DRG Considerations, Reimbursement, and Outcome Measurements." *IMAGE: Journal of Nursing Scholarship* (spring 1991), 32. Reprinted with permission.

Organizational Structure

The organizational structure of a QA program is defined by organizational policy encompassing every department and the medical staff. If the organization is large enough, it will have a quality management department. Otherwise, a full- or part-time person is assigned to oversee the program. Quality management programs are designed to meet the needs of the organization and to accomplish the organization's program objectives. The program should have an organizational and functional scheme, which is generally outlined in the policy (as in Appendix 26-1). QA committees often function at the levels of both the organization and the nursing department. Each level should have representation from practitioners because the major focus concerns the quality of patient care and patient care delivery systems.

Committees will usually be defined by policy that includes the purpose, membership, and functions designed to support the quality management program. Clinical nurses generally have hours assigned to accomplish their QA committee functions.

Tools for Collecting Quality Data

Data collection tools may be in the form of questionnaires, rating scales, and interviews. Reliability and validity are important concepts in determining the worth of instruments used to measure variables in a study. *Reliability* is the extent to which an experiment, test, or measurement procedure yields the same results on repeated trials. For example, a scale that measures a person's weight as 100 pounds one minute and as 160 pounds the next would be considered unreliable. *Interrater reliability* refers to the degree to which two raters, operating independently, assign the same ratings for an attribute being measured. *Validity* is the degree to which an instrument measures what it is intended to measure. *Content* (face) *validity* is the degree to which an instrument adequately represents the universe of content.[10]

Tools for collecting quality data should incorporate standards to be measured into the QC and appropriateness measures. Standards alone are not evaluation instruments. Quality assessment and improvement (QAI) are both staff and line functions. QAI entails both QC and appropriateness measures. Cotter defines *quality control measurement* as evaluation of the effectiveness of a nursing strategy that incorporates efficiency, timeliness, and congruence with established criteria describing performance.[11] Cotter defines *appropriateness measurement* as the determination of the necessity of a specific nursing intervention through the evaluation of the client's clinical condition in comparison with objective, predetermined indicators for nursing interventions.[12] With regard to operative and other procedures, JCAHO standards for determining the appropriateness of a procedure for each patient is based on a review of the patient's history, physical status, and diagnostic data; the risks and benefits of the procedures; and the need to administer blood or blood components.[13] Nursing judgments must weigh standard procedures and immediate appropriateness in providing individualized care that restores, stabilizes, or improves the client's health status.[14] QC, appropriateness, and standards are essential to a comprehensive quality assessment program. Various standardized instruments are available. If the QA committee decides to develop new tools, reliability and content validity will need to be determined before implementation.

Nursing Audits

A basic form of quality data collection is the nursing audit. An *audit* is an examination, a verification or accounting of predetermined indicators. There are three basic forms of nursing audits: structure, process, and outcome audits.

Structure Audits

Structure audits focus on the setting in which care takes place. They include physical facilities, equipment, caregivers, organization, policies, procedures, and medical records. A checklist that focuses on these categories measures standards or indicators. Structure can include content such as staff knowledge and expertise in addition to policies and procedures for nursing practice. Content related to specific nursing care to meet established standards are included in nursing process audits.

Process Audits

Process audits implement indicators for measuring nursing care to determine whether nursing standards are met. They are generally task-oriented. Process audits were first used by Maria Phaneuf in 1964 and were based on the seven functions of nursing established by Lesnick and Anderson. The Phaneuf audit is retrospective, being applied to measure the quality of nursing care received by the client after a cycle of care has been completed and the client discharged. The Phaneuf audit has seven subsections[15]:

1. Application and execution of physicians' legal orders.
2. Observations of symptoms and reactions.
3. Supervision of the client.
4. Supervision of those participating in care (except the physician).
5. Reporting and recording.
6. Application and execution of nursing procedures and techniques.
7. Promotion of physical and emotional health by direction and teaching.

The Phaneuf model uses a Likert scoring system. It does not evaluate care recorded.

The Quality Patient Care Scale (Qual PacS) is a process audit that measures the quality of nursing care concurrently with the cycle of care being given. Its six subsections are:

1. Psychosocial—individual
2. Psychosocial—group
3. Physical
4. General
5. Communication
6. Professional implications

In this audit the nurse is evaluated by direct observation in a nurse–client interaction. A 15% sample of nurses on a unit is considered adequate.

Both the Phaneuf and the Qual PacS process audits use the performance of the first-level staff nurse as a standard for safe, adequate, therapeutic, and supportive care.[16]

The Qual PacS audit was developed from the Slater Nursing Competencies Rating Scale. The Slater model references five staff nurses from best to poorest, contains 84 questions, and takes 2.5 to 3 hours to administer per nurse–client interaction. Qual PacS reduced the questionnaire to 68 items.[17] Higgins and associates, using a modified version of the Qual PacS, found that such outcome measures did prove to be a useful and cost-effective method of evaluating patient care inasmuch as they identify problems at the unit level where they can most easily be resolved.[18]

Other open system audits include the Commission on Administrative Service in Hospital (CASH) Scale and the Medicus Corporation Nurses' Audit. These audits also measure or monitor intervention, assessment, and clinical skills.

Outcome Audits

Outcome audits can be concurrent or retrospective. They evaluate nursing performance in terms of establishing client outcome criteria. The National Center for Health Services developed an outcome audit based on Orem's description of nine categories of self-care requirements:

1. Air
2. Water and fluid intake
3. Food
4. Elimination
5. Rest, activity, and sleep
6. Social interaction and productive work
7. Protection from hazards
8. Normalcy
9. Health deviation

These categories are evaluated in terms of the following evidence[19]:

- The requirement is met.
- The client has the necessary knowledge to meet the requirement.
- The client has the necessary skill and performance abilities to meet the requirement.
- The client has the necessary motivation to meet the requirement.

Outcome criteria are set for selected topics. They can evaluate specific aspects of nursing care for particular groups, such as clients with AIDS, residents with brain injury, and long-term care residents. Evans and Ruff describe three measurable consumer-driven variables when evaluating rehabilitation outcomes achieved in acquired brain injury. These variables are identified as residential setting status, living assistance, and productive activity. Residential setting status is rank-ordered of independent functioning from least to most restrictive. Living assistance refers to the amount of time per 24-hour period the client requires supervision or assistance from others, such as a professional paid attendant or family member. Productive activity as a measurable outcome is the primary productive activity in which the client is engaged and includes competitive employment or degree-directed academic or vocational training. It may also include homemaking, volunteer services, avocational activities, or no productive activity.

The outcome variables as described by Evans and Ruff have face validity as outcomes of functional utility, and their value can be reliably assessed using descriptive statistics. These variables are considered important rehabilitation outcomes by clients, family members, and financial providers and have an impact on long-term functioning.[20]

Morbidity, disability, and mortality during and after provision of health care services are nationally recognized outcomes of health care. Nursing assessment and intervention may make a significant difference in the outcome variables such as nosocomial infection rates in high-risk clients.[21] McCormick illustrates the direction of outcomes that patients can have related to the assessment and treatments carried out. The outcome of improvement, stabilization, or deterioration can be facilitated through an automated system if patient data can be quantified in relation to days (see Exhibit 26-4).

Using an automated system may improve production time, but the benefits to nursing are still a challenge with regard to describing health care costs, accessibility, and outcomes of care. McCormick illustrates a model for computerization of QA, which incorporates nursing inputs to affect quality outputs (see Exhibit 26-5). Such inputs include essential elements in a hospitalized patient's nursing record, including demographic information, patient history, physical information, nursing problem list, recovery progress, medications administered, interactions, and drug errors.[22]

Another method of developing outcome criteria includes grouping of items for efficiency: DRGs, specific protocols for treatment, life stages, and like standards. A determination is made as to whether the outcomes are met. When outcomes are not satisfactorily met, deficiencies are identified, corrected, and followed up.

More on Tools

Two major categories of tools and methods that can accelerate building and using knowledge of continual quality improvement of health care are statistical techniques and data analysis tools.[23]

Statistical Techniques

Statistical techniques include measures of central tendency, measures of variability, and tests of significance. Central tendency refers to the middle value and general trend of the numbers. The three most common meas-

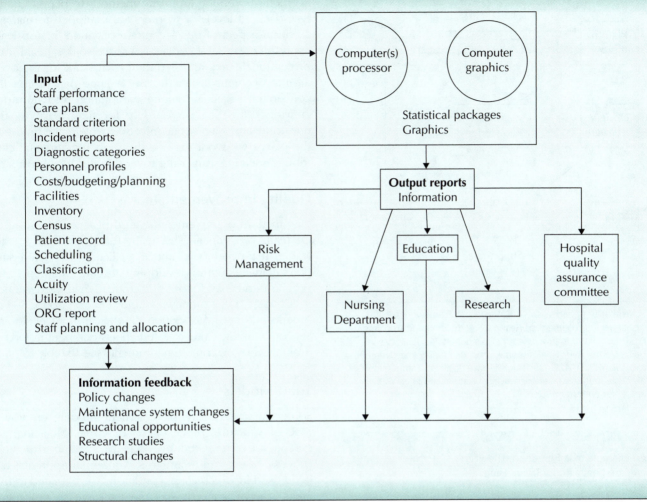

EXHIBIT 26-5
Model for Computerization of Quality Assurance

Input
Staff performance
Care plans
Standard criterion
Incident reports
Diagnostic categories
Personnel profiles
Costs/budgeting/planning
Facilities
Inventory
Census
Patient record
Scheduling
Classification
Acuity
Utilization review
ORG report
Staff planning and allocation

Computer(s) processor
Computer graphics
Statistical packages
Graphics

Output reports
Information

Risk Management
Education
Hospital quality assurance committee
Nursing Department
Research

Information feedback
Policy changes
Maintenance system changes
Educational opportunities
Research studies
Structural changes

Source: K. A. McCormick. "Future Data Needs for Quality of Care Monitoring, DRG Considerations, Reimbursement, and Outcome Measurements." *IMAGE: Journal of Nursing Scholarship* (spring 1991), 32. Reprinted with permission.

ures of central tendency are the mean, the median, and the mode. Measures of variability look at the dispersion of the measures. Three common measures of variability are the range, the standard deviation, and interpercentile measures. The most common measure of interpercentile measure of variability is the interquartile range. Ranking the order of the measures and then dividing the array into quarters determines this. The range of scores comprising the middle 50% is the interquartile range. The t-test, regression analysis, and chi-square tests are tests of statistical significance.[24]

Data Analysis

Data analysis tools may be divided into two types, decision-making tools and relational charts. Brainstorming and multivoting are types of decision-making tools that involve groups or teams. These methods are useful

in generating ideas and then determining the most important item. Several relational charts were discussed in Chapter 25, Total Quality Management. A Pareto diagram, control chart, run chart, fishbone diagram, and process flow chart are popular examples of relational charts used in decision-making.[25]

Exhibit 26-6 illustrates a system map as a graphic tool that may display the various components of a system such as a whole organization, a department or unit within the organization, or even a system of clinical care. With a degree of skill in the use of these tools and methods, workers can obtain and analyze data to validate their ideas about potential improvements and later test the results of implemented changes.[26] Exhibit 26-7 gives an example of a run chart illustrating the effect of a process change on emergency room triage time.

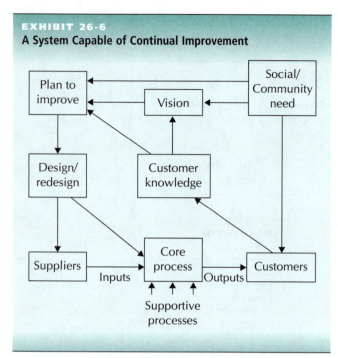

EXHIBIT 26-6
A System Capable of Continual Improvement

Source: P. B. Batalden and P. K. Stoltz. "A Framework for the Continual Improvement of Health Care: Building and Applying Professional and Improvement Knowledge to Test Changes in Daily Work." *Joint Commission Journal on Quality Improvement* (October 1993), 428. Oakbrook Terrace, IL: Joint Commission on Accreditation of Healthcare Organizations, 1993, p. 428. Reprinted with permission.

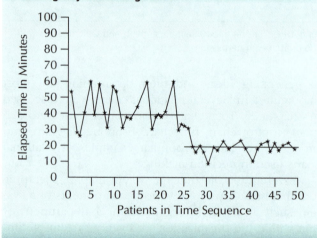

EXHIBIT 26-7
An Example of a Run Chart: The Effect of a Process Change on Emergency Room Triage Time

Source: P. B. Batalden and P. K. Stoltz. "A Framework for the Continual Improvement of Health Care: Building and Applying Professional and Improvement Knowledge to Test Changes in Daily Work." *Joint Commission Journal on Quality Improvement* (October 1993), 436. Oakbrook Terrace, IL: Joint Commission on Accreditation of Healthcare Organizations, 1993, p. 436. Reprinted with permission.

Planning and analysis are conceptual methods that were generally thought to be limited to top-level management. Given the tools and methods to plan and analyze data, all levels of workers are equipped to manage a critical aspect of QI. A central obligation for top leaders is the creation of conceptual space so that health care professionals may redesign their own work for the overall improvement of health care. A large part of creating conceptual space is inviting exploration and nurturing curiosity. "Creating opportunity for new learning and nurturing curiosity about improvement in the midst of the places we work may be the most fundamental contribution leaders can make toward better health care."[27]

Quality Improvement Teams

One method of implementing a QI program is through a QI team or council. This team functions with a team leader, team members, and a facilitator. The team supports management in developing and implementing a QI program and may follow the group dynamics described in Chapter 15, Committees and Other Groups.[28] The American Nurses Association Guidelines for Developing Sets of Outcome Criteria Statements is pertinent in today's evaluation of outcome environment (see Exhibit 26-8).

Triad Models

Some nursing quality management models employ a triad of structure, process, and outcome. Measurement criteria are referenced by code to specific structural, process, or outcome standards. A modular approach has been used in which client conditions were related to five areas: client rights, developmental stage of the client, social groups, therapy-associated needs, and medical diagnoses. Standards for each client group were developed and used to construct the evaluation tool.

The modular design for QA provides discrete components that can be used independently or in different combinations. This design has three modules[29]:

1. Client care standards.
2. Outcome, process, and structure trail.
3. The standard, with derived measurement criteria.

Outcome indicators also include mortality rates, infection rates, and incident reports.

Problem Identification

Analysis and reporting of the data gathered from the evaluation process lead to problem identification and isolation. Evidence comes from primary sources such as the client and nursing personnel, and from secondary

EXHIBIT 26-8
Guidelines for Developing Sets of Outcome Criteria Statements

1. Screening criteria are a crucial factor that, if not met, may indicate a significant deficiency in nursing care.
2. The purpose of screening criteria is to survey a large number of cases and quickly determine acceptable levels of patient outcomes.
3. The outcome stated in the criteria must be possible to achieve.
4. Criteria should be statements of specific outcomes representing optimal achievement.
5. Criteria should be written as specifically as possible, including the time when they are to be measured and the measurement to be used to determine if the criteria have been met.
6. In establishing criteria, one should select the most critical time for the measurement of the identified outcome for a particular patient population.
7. Criteria must be appraisable. However, the ease of measurement should not be used as the sole basis for accepting or rejecting potential criteria. If criteria are important, some assessment can usually be obtained.
8. Criteria should be stated to yield a dichotomous distinction (yes-no).
9. Criteria should be phrased in positive terms (presence of) rather than negative terms (absence of), when applicable.
10. Criteria should be pertinent to the particular patient population under consideration. For example, for the ambulatory patient receiving photocoagulation of the eye, skin care is not a priority. Hence, criteria would not be written for skin care.
11. Criteria should be free from bias. Each patient to whom criteria are applied should be equally likely to be able to meet the criteria. For example, the skin condition of an aged patient and a youth might require different criteria.
12. A set of criteria applicable to a specific patient population may include criteria for outcomes of care for members of the family or significant others.

Establishing criteria is a "pencil and eraser" operation. Criteria will change as values and scientific knowledge change and as health care practices change. Thus criteria should be revised at regular intervals.

Source: *ANA Guidelines for Review of Nursing Care at the Local Level.* © 1977, American Nurses' Association, Washington, DC: 21–22. Reprinted with permission.

sources, including the client's chart and family. Active client and family participation should be part of the process. Quality management addresses current problems. Nurses look for patterns or trends of deviation from normal. They also identify deficiencies relating to other departments that affect nursing care. When a systems approach is taken, problem identification is a team approach and the client and family are major team players.

Problem Resolution

Once problems have been defined and isolated, plans are made to solve them on a priority basis. Critical problems are addressed first, and plans are immediately made and implemented to resolve them. Problems involving the safety and welfare of the client take first priority. Other factors used in determining priority will include severity, frequency, benefit, cost-effectiveness, elimination, reduction, association with professional liability, and impact on accreditation. The first consideration is always based on the impact on client care.[30]

Solutions and corrective action for problems will be assigned to appropriate nursing departments, services, and units. The need is to resolve problems, not just evaluate them.

Monitoring and Feedback

The quality management process is cyclic and requires monitoring of clinical and managerial performance and feedback to ensure that problems stay solved. Follow-up can be expensive and difficult. Its breadth should determine what should be covered. Problems of a multidisciplinary nature, such as those involving occupational therapy, physical therapy, speech pathology, and nursing, can be one consideration.

The cyclic process will continue to set standards of care, take measurements according to those standards, evaluate care from multiple sources, recommend improvements, and, above all, ensure that improvements are carried out.

System Evaluation

Although nurses defend their right to define and regulate the quality of care, they often do not pursue QA activities. A study of nurse managers, staff development nurses, and clinical nurses in ten metropolitan hospitals found that most nurses believed QA involved all levels of nursing personnel but not part of their daily work. Twenty-five percent viewed QA as an accreditation requirement. Peer review and patient care audits ranked low compared with direct patient care activities. Less than 50% of respondents wanted to participate in these activities.

Nurses with formal QA experience were more likely to want to write standards for their specialty, participate in peer review, and be on QA committees. They were more interested in QA associated with direct patient care.[31]

Several models for quality program evaluation have been developed, including the FOCUS-PDCA model (see Chapter 25).

Processes Involved in Quality Management

Nurses who want to control their practice arena believe that quality management is important in accountability. Many groups are seeking evidence that outcomes of nursing care are of good quality and represent a cost-effective use of resources. An excellent example of this is the dialogue currently being maintained with legislators regarding advanced practice nurses' role in health care reform. Nursing's Agenda for Healthcare Reform has been accepted by the President's Committee on Healthcare Reform, and goals such as universal coverage and access to affordable and portable health care will be paramount in any health care plan adopted. Statistics have been frequently cited along with anecdotal reports of nursing's outcomes of quality care (e.g., shorter hospital stays, healthier babies, decreased infection) and improved client satisfaction.

Accountability for nursing practice is still diffused by the employment environment, and this fact must be addressed and corrected by nurses.

Involvement of Practicing Nurses

Practicing nurses can be stimulated to increase their positive attitudes about quality management by direct behavioral experience. Nurse managers should learn why practicing nurses view QA unfavorably. Negative connotations may exist due to lack of executive administrative support, belief that the process is futile without changes in practice, and lack of physician involvement. Correcting and changing these views may be managed by a variety of strategies that include the following:

1. Having practicing nurses identify areas needing improvement.
2. Providing release time for practicing nurses to participate in QA activities, including attendance at committee meetings and time for QA audits.
3. Providing rewards, such as performance results achievement records, that can lead to pay raises, promotions, educational opportunities, or special assignments.
4. Targeting QA to patient care outcomes, the very essence of nursing practice.
5. Involving clinical nurses in management through techniques such as quality circles, employee involve-

ment programs, participatory management, decentralization, "adhocracy," and quality of work life.
6. Establishing a peer review program involving nursing staff at all levels of patient care. Such a program's expectation is to identify outcome criteria based on established standards for nursing practice. Peers determine whether outcomes have been met based on ongoing and retrospective audits. Corrective action is determined by peers based on outcomes being adequately met.

Resources

Quality management programs are labor intensive, requiring efficient and effective use of resources that include personnel, physical plant, supplies, equipment, policies, and procedures. Nurses should be selective in determining areas to be evaluated, considering time and difficulty as well as safety and urgency. They should sample the standards rather than dogmatically evaluate every one. Doing so will require prioritizing standards and even making a decision about whether to eliminate some that are not critical.

Efficiency

Efficiency is concerned with the cost–benefit ratio. Can the appropriate standard be met with a cost acceptable to both consumer and provider?[32] The computer is a labor-saving device for developing and conducting a QA program. Nurse managers will use the computer and teach other practicing nurses to use it. The computer can be used to track the QA process.

Standards will be kept up-to-date and accessible to all units. A loose-leaf notebook or the computer memory is efficient for easy access. Standards should be cross-referenced.

Charts can be labeled so they can be easily retrieved for nursing QA evaluation. Charts can be coded by nursing diagnosis or nursing care standards.[33] In addition, using the long-term care minimum data set (MDS) can be an efficient QA tool for nursing homes. The MDS is a collection of baseline data (physical, social, psychological factors) that can be used to assess, analyze, and plan care for residents in nursing homes. The 1987 Omnibus Budget Reconciliation Act mandated its specific elements.[34]

The following are some elements of efficiency and effectiveness:

1. Identification of the impact of nursing care on the health of the patient, that is, results or outcomes measured in terms of the patient's health status. Do the notes meet such a standard?

2. A program practical enough to be used in all clinical nursing settings.
3. Random, unannounced samples.
4. Nursing personnel who serve on committees long enough to be proficient.
5. Grading by each person administering criteria.
6. Higher patient acuity combined with shorter hospital stays.
7. Interdisciplinary programs so that nurses will not do the work of other disciplines. Nursing is ethically and operationally interdependent with other groups and organizations.
8. Planning for an uncertain future by creating blueprints of scenarios for managing the future, changing the culture of nursing organizations, developing interpersonal skills, and making a creative response to risk taking.[35]
9. Each nurse being held responsible for self-improvement and for delivering a high standard of patient care.

Customer Satisfaction

Customers will be involved in all aspects of a quality management program, including discharge planning. They know what they want and are demanding quality with economy. A study of consumers' perspectives of quality nursing care found that patients' and families' descriptions of quality nursing care fell into two major attributes: (1) practice attributes, and (2) nurse attributes. A smaller number of patients and families identified a third type, practice-setting (structural) attributes. Practice attributes included holistic care, nurse–patient interaction, and effective communication. Nurse attributes identified were personal qualities (kind, nice, friendly, helpful), proficiency, professional character, and commitment to excellence. Practice-setting attributes, although less significant, were effective organization, management, and patient environment.

Overall, clients express a close relationship and frequent contact with the nurse as synonymous with quality nursing care.

Consumer satisfaction as an outcome of QA can be assessed through methods such as patient, family, and nurse interviews or surveys and observation checklists of nurse–patient interactions.[36]

Training and Communication

Training and communication are important elements of a total quality management program. Training includes interpersonal skills, stress management, and conflict management. Learning is a cyclic or continuous process.

Nurse managers who play educator roles develop self-awareness by applying learning principles to their own behaviors. Patient education requires an interdisciplinary team approach.

Communication of QA findings, including problems, resolution of problems, and results, must be clear. Physicians and nursing employees need to be kept up-to-date. Quality must be provided and communicated to be successful, which means that providers and consumers will know the status of the quality of care being rendered.

Quality in the health care marketplace is defined by employers, employee benefit consultants, physicians, and consumers—not by providers (even though physicians are providers, as are hospitals, nurses, and other caregivers). Physicians determine quality because they have control over all orders for diagnosis and treatment procedures. Only half of consumers, employers, and employee consultants differentiate between high- and low-quality hospitals. Two-thirds of physicians do.[37]

Good employee relations and consumer relations programs are necessary for success in the health care marketplace, and their good quality must be communicated. Consumers want quality factors in this order[38]:

1. Warmth, caring, concern
2. Expert medical staff who are concerned, thorough, and successful
3. Up-to-date technology and equipment
4. Specialization or scope of services available
5. Outcome

Research and Quality Management

Nursing QA programs can be combined with research programs. Nursing research is being done in clinical settings to improve patient care outcomes. Research can be sold to nurse managers because it provides prestige, advanced knowledge for nursing professionals, and a database for clinical nursing practice.[39]

Nursing research can be used to evaluate management issues such as staffing, cost management, and staff retention. It produces new knowledge of the relationship between process and outcome. Combining quality management with research makes efficient use of personnel and other resources to link research with a mandatory process; increase the probability that research will relate to patient care; and increase sharing of successful quality management programs with others outside the institution.[40]

Research and quality management complement each other.

Discharge Planning

Schuman, Ostfeld, and Willard studied discharge planning in an acute care hospital. The need for this function was recognized in 1944, and studies indicated that it was still being poorly done 32 years later. The research team indicated that the nurse manager supervises the function of discharge planning by nurses and supports their communication with physicians.[41] The competency required of the nurse manager is to supervise staff nurses, who need to provide discharge planning that makes patients aware of necessary precautions related to diagnosis and therapy; of their medical regimens, including times to take medications and dietary restrictions related to their medication and treatment; and of where to get help as needed. Patients suffer decreased functional capacity after discharge, and discharge planning decreases hospital readmission rates by fostering compliance with therapy. Instructions increase the importance of therapy in the eyes of the patient. Schuman and associates suggested, "Nurses tend to be the most qualified personnel to delineate a patient's nursing needs following discharge and tend also to be aware of the patient's need for ancillary services."[42]

Summary

Quality management programs make certain that the patient care delivered meets established standards. QA programs have as their objective the determination of whether the actual service provided matches predetermined criteria of excellence. Quality management also involves continuous action to eliminate deficiencies in meeting standards. QA is a management process that provides a sound basis for decision-making and problem-solving. Management of care by competent clinical nurses and nurse managers ensures the quality of that care.

APPLICATION EXERCISES

EXERCISE 26-1   Examine the quality management program of a health care agency. How does it address the components outlined previously?

EXERCISE 26-2   Examine the statements of purpose, philosophy, and objectives of a health care agency. Which elements of quality management are evident?

EXERCISE 26-3   Examine the standards for quality management of a nursing entity. How do they meet the outcomes listed in Exhibit 26-4?

EXERCISE 26-4   Identify the tools used for audits in a nursing organization. Use one of them and analyze your results.

NOTES

1. R. Kirk, "The Big Picture Total Quality Management and Continuous Quality Improvement," *Journal of Nursing Administration*, (April 1992), 24–31.
2. J. B. Patterson, "The Client as Customer: Achieving Service Quality and Customer Satisfaction in Rehabilitation," *Journal of Rehabilitation* (October–November–December) 1992, 16–21.
3. P. B. Batalden and P. K. Stoltz, "A Framework for the Continual Improvement of Health Care: Building and Applying Professional and Improvement Knowledge to Test Changes in Daily Work," *Joint Commission Journal on Quality Improvement* (October 1993), 424–450.
4. W. E. Deming, *The New Economics for Industry, Education, Government* (Cambridge, MA: Massachusetts Institute of Technology, Center for Advanced Engineering Study, 1993).

5. P. B. Batalden and P. K. Stoltz, op. cit.

6. Ibid., 434.

7. W. E. Deming, *Out of the Crisis* (Cambridge, MA: MIT Press, 1986); P. B. Crosby, *Quality Without Tears* (New York: McGraw-Hill, 1984); J. M. Juran, *Juran on Planning for Quality* (New York: The Free Press, 1988); P. M. Senge, *The Fifth Discipline: The Art and Practice of the Learning Organization* (New York: Doubleday, 1990).

8. "Standards for Quality Assessment and Improvement," *1995 Comprehensive Accreditation Manual for Hospitals* (Oakbrook Terrace, IL: Joint Commission on Accreditation of Healthcare Organizations, 1994), 219–266.

9. P. B. Batalden and P. K. Stoltz, op. cit.; 434.

10. "Measurement Tools for Analysis," *NAHQ Guide to Quality Management*, 7th ed. (Glenview, IL: NAHQ, 1997), 81–105.

11. K. Cotter, *Quality Review Strategies for Clinical Nursing Practice* (North Hampton, NH: InterQual, 1989), 10.

12. Ibid.

13. *1995 Comprehensive Accreditation Manual for Healthcare Organizations*, op. cit.

14. M. R. Ventura, J. Rizzo, and S. Lenz, "Quality Indicators: Control Maintains: Propriety Improves," *Nursing Management* (January 1993), 46–50.

15. B. J. Curtis and L. J. Simpson, "Auditing: A Method for Evaluating Quality of Care," *Journal of Nursing Administration* (October 1985), 14–21.

16. Ibid.

17. Ibid.

18. M. Higgins, D. McCaughand, and M. Carr-Hill, "Assessing the Outcomes of Nursing Care," *Journal of Advanced Nursing* (May 1992), 561–568.

19. B. J. Curtis and L. J. Simpson, op. cit.

20. R. W. Evans and R. M. Ruff, "Outcome and Value: A Perspective on Rehabilitation Outcomes Achieved in Acquired Brain Injury," *Journal of Head Trauma* (December 1992), 24–36.

21. E. Larson, I. Oram, and E. Hedrick, "Nosocomial Infection Rates as an Indicator of Quality," *Medical Care* (July 1988), 676–684.

22. K. A. McCormick, "Future Data Needs for Quality Care Monitoring, DRG Considerations, Reimbursement and Outcome Measurements," *Image: Journal of Nursing Scholarship* (spring 1991), 29–32.

23. "Measurement Tools for Analysis," op. cit.

24. Ibid.

25. Ibid.

26. P. B. Batalden and P. K. Stoltz, op. cit, 434–438.

27. Ibid., 438.

28. H. S. Rowland and B. L. Rowland, eds., *Nursing Administration Handbook*, 4th ed. (Gaithersburg, MD: Aspen, 1997), 405–428.

29. L. Edmunds, "A Computer Assisted Quality Assurance Model," *Journal of Nursing Administration* (March 1983), 36–43; A. DeLotto, "Examining Quality of Care Becomes Top Industry Priority," *Amherst Quarterly* (winter 1988), 1–3.

30. H. S. Rowland and B. L. Rowland, eds. "Quality Assurance," *Hospital Legal Forms, Checklists, and Guidelines* (Gaithersburg, MD: Aspen, 1988), 26(14), 1–26.

31. S. R. Edwardson and D. I. Anderson, "Hospital Nurses' Evaluation of Quality Assurance," *Journal of Nursing Administration* (July–August) 1983, 33–39.

32. H. S. Rowland and B. L. Rowland, *Nursing Administration Handbook*, op. cit. 424.

33. L. Edmunds, op. cit.

34. J. Spuck, "Using the Long-Term Care Minimum Data Set as a Tool for CQI in Nursing Homes," In J. Dienemann, ed., op. cit., 95–105.

35. R. Allio, "Forecasting: The Myth of Control," Interview with Donald Michal, *Planning Review* (May 1986), 6–11.

36. A. G. Taylor, K. Hudson, and A. Keeling, "Quality Nursing Care: The Consumers' Perspective Revisited," *Journal of Nursing Quality Assurance* (January 1991), 23–31.

37. D. C. Coddington and K. D. Moore, "Quality of Care as a Business Strategy," *Healthcare Forum Journal* (March–April 1987), 29–34.

38. Ibid.

39. E. Larson, "Combining Nursing Quality Assurance and Research Programs," *Journal of Nursing Administration* (November 1983), 32–34.

40. Ibid.

41. J. E. Schuman, A. M. Ostfeld, and H. N. Willard, "Discharge Planning in an Acute Hospital," *Archives of Physical Medicine and Rehabilitation* (July 1976), 343–347.

42. Ibid.

REFERENCES

Bauerhaus, P. I. "Creating a New Place in the Competitive Market." *Nursing Policy Forum* (March–April 1996), 13–20.

Cohen, S. S. "National Committee for Quality Assurance." *Rehab Management* (October–November 1995), 13, 109.

Hutchins, B. "Managing Cost and Quality." *Rehab Management* (April–May 1996), 25–26.

Maciorowski, L. J., E. Lar, and A. Keane. "Quality Assurance: Evaluate Thyself." *Journal of Nursing Administration* (June 1985), 38–42.

Mackelprang, R., and P. B. Johnson. "Managed Care: Balancing Costs, Quality, and Access." *SCI Psychosocial Access* (November 1995), 175–178.

Moore, K. F. "Cost or Quality When Selecting a Health Plan?" *National Policy Forum* (March–April 1996), 24.

Nelson, M. F., and R. H. Christenson. "The Focused Review Process: A Utilization Management Firm's Experience with Length of Stay Guidelines." *Journal of Quality Improvement* (September 1995), 477–487.

Spicer, J. G., M. J. Craft, and K. C. Ross. "A Systems Approach to Customer Satisfaction." *Nursing Administration Quarterly* (spring 1988), 79–83.

Towers, J. "What Do You Know About NCQA?" *Nursing Policy Forum* (May–June 1996), 30.

Wolff, G. M. "Systems Management: Evaluating Nursing Departments as a Whole." *Nursing Management* (February 1986), 40–43.

Ubell, E. "You Can Get Quality Care in an HMO World." *Parade Magazine* (14 September 1997), 10–11.

UNIVERSITY OF SOUTH ALABAMA MEDICAL CENTER
DEPARTMENT OF NURSING

QUALITY ASSESSMENT AND IMPROVEMENT (QAI) PROGRAM

I. POLICY STATEMENT

The University of South Alabama Medical Center Department of Nursing will monitor the provision of nursing care and the results of nursing care in an ongoing and systematic manner following the Quality Assessment and Improvement Program for the Department of Nursing. This program is designed to improve care based on the monitoring and evaluation of structure, practice (process), and care (outcome) standards, and is consistent with the Quality Assessment and Improvement Plan for the University of South Alabama Medical Center.

Nursing quality assessment and improvement activities are reports to the QAI Executive Committee of the University of South Alabama Medical Center.

II. PURPOSE

1. To ensure that the quality of patient care is optimal through a unified program.
2. To provide the process by which the provision of nursing care and end results (patient outcomes) are measured and evaluated against Standards for Nursing.
3. To integrate efforts of physicians and nurses in Special Care Units to continuously improve patient care.
4. To maintain quality care in current use.

III. GENERAL INFORMATION

Structure Standards describe the environment in which safe, effective, and appropriate care takes place, i.e., organization, management, resources, care delivery, productivity, and turnover rate. Structure standards are a form of productivity reporting and are used for management information. Nurse Managers receive daily productivity/variance reports from Nursing Information Systems to assist in monitoring and evaluating structure standards.

Standards of Practice describe the nature and sequence of health care activities and are based on identified important aspects of care. Policies and procedures describe how important aspects of care are carried out.

Standards of Care describe nursing care results for the major patient populations and those patients who receive high-risk, high-volume nursing care.

Care Plans define and describe individual patients' nursing care and expected results.

Quality Care Framework (Exhibit A26-1) clarifies Integration of Standards for Nursing into Quality Assessment and Improvement.

Nursing staff members participate, by way of the Nursing Practice Committee and unit meetings, in the identification of the important aspects of care, identifying the indicators, planning action to improve care, and evaluating the results. All nursing departments participate on CQI teams as assigned.

Each nursing department develops and follows an annual plan for QAI that is maintained on each unit, and copies of which are located in the office of Nursing Administration. The JCAHO 10-step process is the method used to accomplish improvements. Each unit plan is assisted by a matrix—used to simplify and clarify information pertinent to each indicator. (See Exhibit A26-2.)

IV. PROCEDURE

Responsibility. The Nurse Manager is responsible for ensuring the completion of QAI activities.

Scope of Care. This is a 406-bed, level I trauma center that provides nursing care by RNs, LPNs, and NAs 24 hours a day to patients requiring emergency services, interfacility transportation, aeromedical transportation, surgical services, postanesthesia care, labor and delivery, obstetrics, intensive care nursery, neonatal transportation, premature nursery, newborn nursery, medical–surgical nursing, burn center, neurotrauma intensive care, surgical intensive care, renal dialysis, medical intensive care, coronary intensive care, and intermediate nursing care. Medical–surgical pediatric patients are located on 6th and 5th South nursing units. Pediatric patients also receive nursing care in the Burn Center, CCU, and, less frequently, in SICU/NTICU. The scope of care is based on the needs and expectations of the high-risk and high-volume patient who is admitted (Special Care Units) or discharged from each nursing unit. High volume is determined by annual review of diagnoses (DRGs) and by categorizing the diagnoses according to similar patient needs. The largest categories or patient populations having similar needs based on diagnoses are designated as high volume. Patients identified as at-risk are determined by the history of complications within certain groups of patients or for individual patients. In addition to the needs and expectations of the major patient populations, subcategories are identified to reflect those patients who receive problem-prone nursing care and those at risk for developing complications due to their biophysical status.

Important Aspects of Care are identified in addressing the high-volume and/or problem-prone (present a risk

(continued)

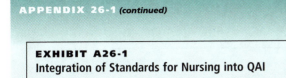

EXHIBIT A26-1
Integration of Standards for Nursing into QAI

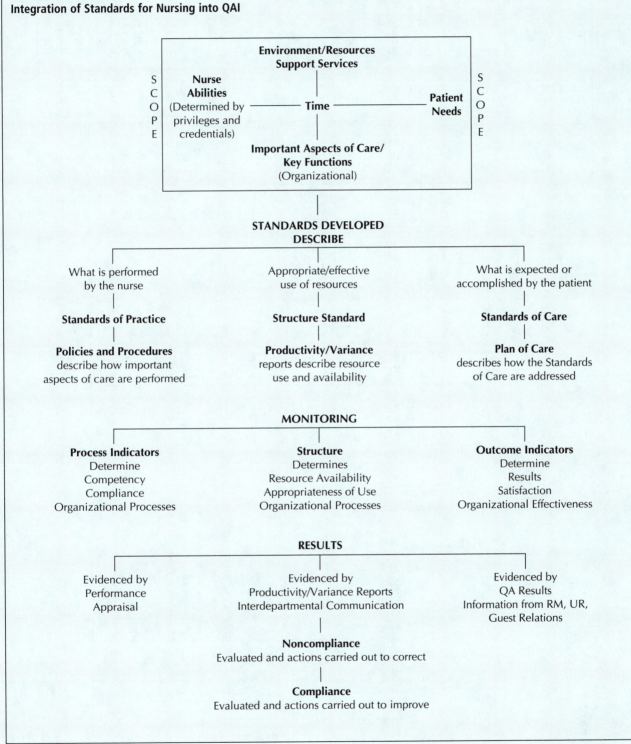

EXHIBIT A26-2
Quality Assurance Monitoring Plan

UNIVERSITY OF SOUTH ALABAMA MEDICAL CENTER

DEPARTMENT: 5th Floor Medical Surgical

QA MONITORING PLAN

KEY FUNCTION	SUBJECT	INDICATOR	DIMENSION PERFORM	DEPARTMENTAL INTERDEPT. SCOPE	PROCESS OUTCOME STRUCTURE TYPE INDIC	RATE COUNT TYPE INDIC	<100%; >0 BENCH # TREND EVAL. TRIGGER	5% 30 ALL SAMPLE SIZE	OBSERVATION CHART REVIEW LOGS; REPORTS COLLECTION METHOD
TX/IM	Restraint	Appropriate restraint documentation (12 criteria)	Res	Departmental	Process	Rate	Trend	All	Chart review
PI/TX	Blood Use	Correct transfusion procedure	Safe	Interdepart.	Process	Rate	Trend	5%	Obs/chrt review
TX	Med Use	Medication errors	Safe/Cont	Interdepart.	P/O	Rate	>0	All	Rep/Chrt review
IC	Stand Prec	Handwashing	Appro	Interdepart.	Process	Rate	Trend	5%	Observation
IC	Stand Prec	Correct handwashing procedure	Effec	Interdepart.	Process	Rate	Trend	5%	Observation
IC	Stand Prec	Appropriate glove use	Appro	Interdepart.	Process	Rate	Trend	5%	Observation
EC	Fall	Patient falls	Safe	Departmental	Process	Rate	Trend	All	Obs/Rep
RI	Satisfac	Patient satisfaction/nursing care	Res	Interdepart.	Outcome	Rate	Trend	10/mo	Questionnaire
TX	Plan	Multidisciplinary Goals/Problem form present	Avail	Interdepart.	Process	Rate	<100%	5%	Chart review
TX	Plan	Goals measurable	Appro	Departmental	Process	Rate	<100%	5%	Chart review
TX	Plan	Patient problems individualized	Appro	Departmental	Process	Rate	<100%	5%	Chart review
TX	Plan	Priorities for care identified each shift	Appro	Departmental	Process	Rate	<100%	5%	Chart review
TX	Plan	Priorities based on goals/problems	Appro/Cont	Departmental	Process	Rate	<100%	5%	Chart review
TX	Provide	Focus note relates to priorities each shift	Appro/Cont	Departmental	Process	Rate	<100%	5%	Chart review
TX	Provide	Problem/goal summary each shift	Appro/Cont	Departmental	Process	Rate	<100%	5%	Chart review
TX	Provide	Evaluation of goal attainment each shift	Appro/Cont	Departmental	Process	Rate	<100%	5%	Chart review
PF	Plan	Knowledge deficit on Goal/Problem form	Appro	Departmental	Process	Rate	<100%	5%	Chart review
PF	Provide	Teaching related to goal documented on MPEP	Appro	Departmental	Process	Rate	<100%	5%	Chart review
RI	Edu	Patient instructed on plans for care & expectations	Res	Departmental	Process	Rate	Trend	5%	Chart review
PE	Fall	Patient assessed for fall risk upon admission	Safe	Departmental	Process	Rate	Trend	5%	Chart review
PE	Pain	Patient assessed for pain upon admission	Res	Departmental	Process	Rate	Trend	5%	Chart review

(continued)

EXHIBIT A26-2 *(continued)*

KEY FUNCTION	SUBJECT	INDICATOR	DIMENSION PERFORM	DAILY WEEKLY MONTHLY / COLLECTION INTERVAL	MONTHLY QUARTERLY / REPORT INTERVAL	DEPT. GROUP / COLLECT BY	DEPT. GROUP / AGGREGATE BY	DEPT. GROUP TITLE / REPORT BY	AA; COMMITTEE EXTERNAL GROUP OTHER DEPT. / REPORT TO
TX/IM	Restraint	Appropriate restraint documentation (12 criteria)	Res	Daily	Quarterly	Staff	QM	QM	AA
PI/TX	Blood Use	Correct transfusion procedure	Safe	Daily	Quarterly	Staff	QM	QM	Bld Use Com
TX	Med Use	Medication errors	Safe/Cont	Daily	Quarterly	Staff	QM	QM	Med Use Com
IC	Stand Prec	Handwashing	Appro	1 Mo/Qtr	Quarterly	Staff	IC	IC NM	IC Committee
IC	Stand Prec	Correct handwashing procedure	Effec	1 Mo/Qtr	Quarterly	Staff	IC	IC NM	IC Committee
IC	Stand Prec	Appropriate glove use	Appro	1 Mo/Qtr	Quarterly	Staff	IC	IC NM	IC Committee
EC	Fall	Patient falls	Safe	Daily	Quarterly	Staff	QM	QM	AA; EC Com
RI	Satisfac	Patient satisfaction/nursing care	Res	Daily	Quarterly	Staff	Satisf Com	Satisf Com	AA
TX	Plan	Multidisciplinary Goals/Problem form present	Avail	Monthly	Quarterly	Nur	DH/QM	DH/QM	AA
TX	Plan	Goals measurable	Appro	Monthly	Quarterly	Nur	DH/QM	DH/QM	AA
TX	Plan	Patient problems individualized	Appro	Monthly	Quarterly	Nur	DH/QM	DH/QM	AA
TX	Plan	Priorities for care identified each shift	Appro	Monthly	Quarterly	Nur	DH/QM	DH/QM	AA
TX	Plan	Priorities based on goals/problems	Appro/Cont	Monthly	Quarterly	Nur	DH/QM	DH/QM	AA
TX	Provide	Focus note relates to priorities each shift	Appro/Cont	Monthly	Quarterly	Nur	DH/QM	DH/QM	AA
TX	Provide	Problem/goal summary each shift	Appro/Cont	Monthly	Quarterly	Nur	DH/QM	DH/QM	AA
TX	Provide	Evaluation of goal attainment each shift	Appro/Cont	Monthly	Quarterly	Nur	DH/QM	DH/QM	AA
PF	Plan	Knowledge deficit on Goal/Problem form	Appro	Monthly	Quarterly	Nur	DH/QM	DH/QM	AA
PF	Provide	Teaching related to goal documented on MPEP	Appro	Monthly	Quarterly	Nur	DH/QM	DH/QM	AA
RI	Edu	Patient instructed on plans for care & expectations	Res	Monthly	Quarterly	Nur	DH/QM	DH/QM	AA
PE	Fall	Patient assessed for fall risk upon admission	Safe	Monthly	Quarterly	Nur	DH/QM	DH/QM	AA
PE	Pain	Patient assessed for pain upon admission	Res	Monthly	Quarterly	Nur	DH/QM	DH/QM	AA

KEY FUNCTION:
PI = Improving Organizational Performance
EC = Environment of Care
IM = Information Management
IC = Infection Control

RI = Patient Rights/Organizational Ethics
PE = Assessment of Patients
TX = Care (Planning/Providing; Anesthesia; Med Use; Nutrition; Op/Invasive; Rehab; Special Tx)
PF = Patient/Family Education

DIMENSION OF PERFORMANCE:
Right thing: Efficacy; Appropriateness
Right thing well: Availability; Timeliness; Effectiveness; Continuity; Safety; Efficiency; Respect and Caring

(continued)

to the patient or nurse) nursing care activities. From the important aspects of care, standards are developed: Standards of Practice, Concurrent Process, Retrospective Process, Standards of Care, Concurrent Outcome, and Retrospective Outcome. Policies and procedures are based on standards determined by the requirements of the major patient populations.

The following generic key functions are important to patient care at the University of South Alabama Medical Center:

Assessment/Reassessment

Care Plan

Implementation/Evaluation

Continuity of Care

Safety/Universal Precautions/Infection Control

Appropriateness

Teaching/Emotional and Spiritual Support

Medication Administration/Treatments

Discharge Preparation

Confidentiality

IV Therapy

Each Nursing Unit has identified aspects of care related to generic standards for quality assessment and improvement.

Indicators. Elements of the high-volume, problem-prone nursing activities that provide evidence as to whether the care provided is of quality are developed into statements called Indicators for each nursing unit. The Indicator Development Form (Exhibit A26-3) is used to operationalize indicators as needed.

Process Indicators measure how well departments and individuals meet stated standards for practice, use the nursing process, and document care.

Outcome Indicators measure specific patient outcomes and direct departments in needed action and changes toward meeting standards of care.

Evaluation Trigger. A value is placed on the results of each indicator to assist in determining if opportunity for improvement exists. When counting events (0, 1, 2, 3, . . .), the evaluation trigger may be >0 signifying that each event is evaluated and action is taken to eliminate the type of occurrence. When using rate-based indicators (numerator–denominator), the evaluation trigger could be stated as <100%, signifying that no less than 100% is expected and actions are taken to correct deficiencies. Another type oif evaluation trigger is the benchmark. The *benchmark* is a measure of best practice for

like populations from other organizations. *Trends* in results may also be used as evaluation triggers. Trending involves at least three consecutive points of data. The goal is to always show improvement. Therefore, actions should be taken for the evaluation of "no trend," "decreasing performance," or "results staying the same."

Collection and Organization of Data. The Nurse Manager or designee sets up an annual Quality Assessment and Improvement Matrix that specifies the sequence and the data to be collected for monitoring. (See Exhibit A26-2.) Data sources include patient charts and questionnaires. Process monitoring may involve staff observation/interview, and outcome monitoring may involve patient/family interview/observation.

Special Care Nursing Units (SICU/NTICU, CCU/MICU, Burn Center, ICN) and medical staff of Special Care Units monitor joint aspects of care and patients, integrating efforts to improve patient care. Nursing concurrently monitors patients applicable to the chosen joint aspect and supplies the medical record number to the medical staff Quality Assurance Coordinator for physician review. Department heads and medical directors discuss findings and opportunities to improve via the Critical Care Committee.

Documentation review classes will be held on Committee Day, the first Tuesday of each month. RNs will be assigned to participate in retrospective review of documentation. Generically, Nursing will monitor 5% of patient admissions for appropriate documentation.

Concurrent monitoring is performed on each nursing unit each month as part of assignments to the nursing staff. Results of monitoring and any adverse effects to the patient as a result of individual performance are addressed and followed up through Nurse Credentialing as part of the Performance Appraisal.

The staff nurse follows Staff Nurse Guidelines for Quality Monitoring (Exhibit A26-4) in using a quality review worksheet or concurrent data sheet for monitoring.

Evaluate. The data is initially evaluated by the Nurse Manager who further involves the staff in evaluation through staff meetings and Nurse Practice Committee Meetings. Evaluation may consist of more intensive review of specific cases or continued monitoring. Concurrent monitoring is advantageous in that the staff nurse who takes corrective action at the time of review is involved in the initial evaluation.

Actions to Improve Care. Methods to resolve problems and improve care identified through monitoring include staff meetings, individual counseling, education,

(continued)

EXHIBIT A26-3
Indicator Development Form

I. Indicator Statement: _____

_____

II. Definition of Terms: _____

_____

III. Type of Indicator: Rate based _____ Process _____

Sentinel event _____ Outcome _____

IV. Rationale

A. Why useful? _____

B. Supportive references: _____

C. Components of quality assessed: _____

V. Description of Indicator Population

A. $\dfrac{\text{(Numerator)}}{\text{(Denominator)}}$: _____

B. Subcategories: _____

VI. Indicator Data Collection Logic

Data Elements   Data Source

VII. Underlying Factors

A. Patient factors: _____

B. Practitioner factors: _____

C. Organization factors: _____

problem-solving with other departments, developing standards, modifying documentation tools, changing departmental/organizational process and related policies, and revision of Quality Assessment. Actions taken will specify who will do what and when.

Specific problems may be referred to standing committees within the department. Problems identified by any staff member that involve any department or activity are documented on a Quality Assurance Problem Reporting Sheet (Exhibit A26-5) and attached with follow-up to the monthly narrative analysis report.

Assess Actions and Document Improvement. A time frame for assessing effectiveness for action is determined. Subsequent findings are reviewed at that time, and further recommendations for action are made if necessary. The QAI Report Grid is completed quarterly for all indicators monitored during the report interval. The Nurse Manager or designee uses the Performance Improvement Report Form (Exhibit A26-6) to complete the report.

Communicate Relevant Information. Information obtained from staff nurse data collection is communicated

EXHIBIT A26-4
Staff Nurse Guidelines for Quality Monitoring

Quality Assurance (QA) monitoring is documented on unit-specific data retrieval sheets by the assigned staff nurse each month. The data retrieval sheets are located on each nursing unit in a QA notebook or in the employee file for QA.

The data retrieval sheets monitor two different aspects of nursing: (1) Standards of practice are monitored by process indicators. Practice/process measures what the nurse does (nursing practice, nursing process) and is stated in terms of "The nurse will. . . ." (2) Standards of care are monitored by outcome indicators. Care/outcome measures the final picture of the patient as a result of nursing/interdepartmental care and is stated in terms of "The patient will . . ." or "The patient can expect. . . ."

The staff nurse retrieves the QA data sheets from the book or file and monitors a patient/chart according to the indicators during a month specified by the Nurse Manager or designee.

The staff nurse uses the column beside the indicator to designate the results of the patient/nurse/chart that is monitored. Each time the indicator is monitored, the adjacent column is used. The month in which the monitoring takes place is written at the top of the page.

The result of monitoring is documented using the following key:

+   Results are compliant

–   Results are not compliant

J   Results are not compliant but are justified

N/A   Results do not apply

When justification (J) is used, the justifier must be written below the standard to which it applies.

Example: The patient was not wearing an identification band because of injuries to the extremities—BUT, *the I.D. band was taped to the head of the bed.*

Example: The nurse did not document confirmation of the enteral feeding tube insertion because M.D.

inserted it and started feedings—BUT *the M.D. documented in the progress notes the confirmation of the feeding tube.*

Not applicable (N/A) is used when a specific indicator does not apply for that patient. Examples would be a patient who has no IV tubing to be changed because the patient has an INT, or the patient is discharged without medications needed at home. In these instances, indicators for IV tubing changed or verbalizing understanding of discharge medications would be N/A.

The staff nurse should seek out the patient populations for which the Standard of Care applies versus monitoring one patient for all outcome indicators.

Examples: An abdominal surgery patient is found to monitor the outcome for abdominal surgery patients; a seizure patient is monitored for outcome of seizure patients; a cardiac patient is found to monitor outcome of cardiac patients; a patient with an IV is found to monitor outcomes for IV therapy; a patient who has been discharged, or is in the process of being discharged, is monitored for discharge criteria and discharge teaching.

This process ensures that the standards are applicable in the majority of situations.

At the end of each month the Nurse Manager or designated staff nurse compiles the information from each data sheet and then returns this sheet to the file or QA book. Indicators are monitored every month until they reach quarterly compliance. At that time another standard and/or indicators may be added by the Nurse Manager or designated staff nurse, depending on problems identified.

The staff nurse participates in identifying standards and indicators by way of staff meetings, the Nursing Practice Committee, or one-to-one conferences with the Nurse Manager or designated staff nurse.

appropriately as per the established communication system. (See Exhibit A26-7.)

Monitoring results of Special Care Units are communicated through the Critical Care Committee and signed by the Medical Director. All nursing units forward monthly QA reports to the Clinical Administrator for Nursing Practice.

Each quarter the Clinical Administrator for Nursing Practice summarizes each unit's specific report into a

Division Report that is signed by the Director of Nursing and the Assistant Administrator for Nursing. Signed original quarterly reports are maintained in the office of Nursing Administration and copies are maintained by the hospital QAI Department.

V. ANNUAL EVALUATION
Quality Assurance for the Department of Nursing and Standards for Nursing are reviewed at least annually

(text continues on p. 580)

APPENDIX 26-1 *(continued)*

EXHIBIT A26-5
Quality Assurance Problem Reporting Sheet

Department: ______________________ Date: ______________________

Initiated by: ______________________ To: ______________________

Problem or concern studied:

____

____

____

How identified and why important (data sources) impact on patient care:

____

____

____

____

Contributing factors:

____

____

Quality goal (after study is completed):

____

____

____

____

Departments involved:

____

____

Referred to department: ______________________ Action taken: ______________________

____

____

____

____

Follow-up plan or recommendations:

____

____

____

Please respond by: ______________________ To: ______________________

Thank you very much. ______________________________ (signature)

(continued)

EXHIBIT A26-6
Example Performance Improvement Report

University of South Alabama Medical Center
Example Performance Improvement Report

DEPARTMENT: _____ US _____

MONTHS: APRIL, MAY, JUNE

| DATE LAST REPORTED AND RESULTS | INDICATORS | ET | FINDINGS: IDENTIFY/CLARIFY | | | | CONCLUSIONS: ANALYZE OR EVALUATE | ACTIONS: REVISE/EDUCATE | MO/YR OF NEXT REPORT |
			SAMPLE	MET	NOT MET	RESULT # OR %			
4/99									
79%	Staff sign off MD orders per P&P	Trend	32	26	6	81%	Results improved 2% and continue to indicate need for further improvement. The initial 20% improvement sustained since 3/97. The six "not met": 4—no time; 2—no date. One nurse identified in three of the "not met" was counseled; no other trend in individual performance. Need to separate signature, time, and date, for more accurate measurement.	Revise indicator to reflect measurement in each area expected (signature, date, time). Communicate improvement and expectations to staff in light of improvement. Continue monitoring to measure effectiveness of actions.	10/99
New	Consent form completed correctly	Trend	18	13	5	72%	Initial measure of GI/CV/OR pre-op consent form completed correctly. Reasons for "not met" continue to vary, and one consent may have more than one problem. Need to separate out reasons for trending.	State actions . . .	
New	Timely completion of (name of) reports: dictated, transcribed, placed on chart. WITHIN 48 HOURS	Trend bench?	42	11	31	26%	26% of venous Doppler studies were placed on the patients record within 48 hours. 15 of the 31 "not met" were dictated for more than 2 days. The other 16 were dictated within 1 day, transcribed the next, but did not get placed on the MR. . . . Findings to IM Committee. . . . Separate out reasons for trending.	State actions . . .	
5	Patient complaints	>0				2	Trend 8–5-2: Improvement noted over last two quarters. Only two complaints this quarter about waiting time. Actions effective (what actions?) Continue . . . in light of improvement.	State actions . . .	
98%	Completion of admission H&P within 24 hours	Trend	38	37	1	97%	Results have been stable for three quarters. (See graphs attached.) The one "not met" was not dated and timed. The physician was notified. Recommend continued monitoring for sustained compliance.	State actions . . .	

_____ _____
Department Head Signature   Date

_____ _____
Assistant Administrator Signature   Date

This document is PRIVILEGED AND CONFIDENTIAL for the University of South Alabama Medical Center Quality Assessment & Improvement Program as prepared and maintained pursuant to the 1975 Code of Alabama: § 6-5-333; § 22-21-8; § 34-24-58.

EXHIBIT A26-7
Communication System

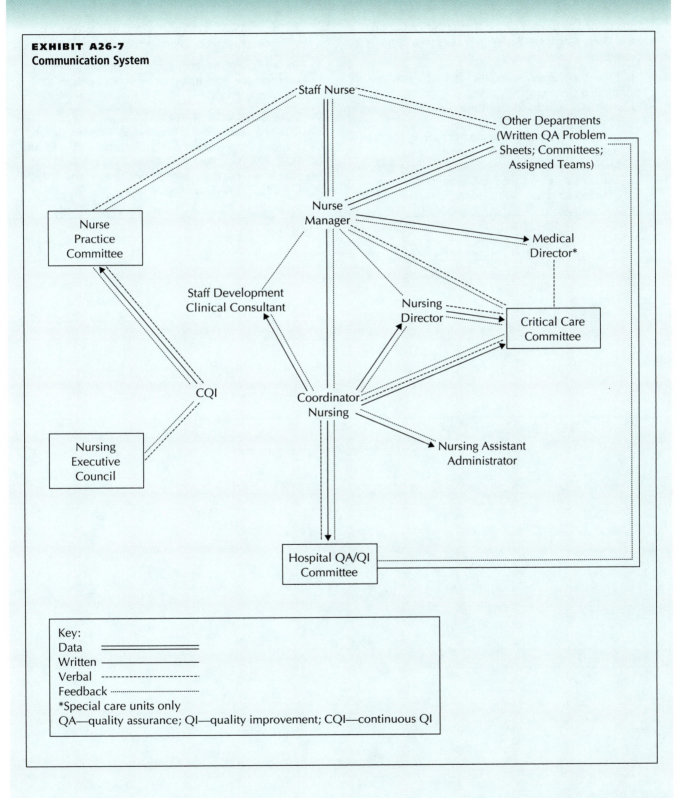

Key:
Data ═══════
Written ─────────
Verbal ------------
Feedback ·············
*Special care units only
QA—quality assurance; QI—quality improvement; CQI—continuous QI

and revised as needed by the Nurse Practice Committee and Nurse Managers. Review and revision of Standards considers:

1. Patient requirements and the effectiveness of the staffing plan.
2. Ability to attract and retain the numbers and types of nursing personnel required.
3. Variance reports that indicate the staffing plan's adequacy or inadequacy to meet patient needs.
4. Monitoring information that relates to the staffing plan.
5. The consistency for the provision of nursing care between units based on Standards.

6. The staff's ability to pursue activities to promote innovation and/or improvement of nursing care.

The annual report will identify any opportunities to improve care, care that improved, and revisions to the plan.

VI. CONFIDENTIALITY STATEMENT
Quality assessment and improvement documents and activities are privileged and confidential for the USAMC Quality Management Program and are prepared and maintained pursuant to the Code of Alabama 1975: 6-5-333, 22-21-8, and 34-24-58.

Source: Reprinted courtesy of the University of South Alabama Medical Center, Mobile, AL.

CHAPTER 27

Legal Principles of Nursing

Russell C. Swansburg, PhD, RN

> Every activity of the nurse in the performance of her nursing services is the subject of potential analysis by the law.
>
> M. J. Lesnik and B. E. Anderson[1]

LEARNING OBJECTIVES AND ACTIVITIES

- Differentiate among the elements of a risk management program.
- Identify the risks professional nurses face regarding malpractice and other torts.
- Outline a plan for professional nurses to use to reduce the risks of legal actions.

CONCEPTS: Nurse practice acts, contracts, torts, negligence, malpractice, assault and battery, false imprisonment, slander and libel, liability, wills.

MANAGER BEHAVIOR: Applies legal principles that manage risks to and reflect the values of the organization and providers of care.

LEADER BEHAVIOR: Applies legal principles that maintain quality nursing care and satisfactory service to customers. This satisfactory service is not only legal but also ethical and moral, reflecting the values of the leader.

Introduction

As nursing has evolved professionally so has the nurse's liability increased. Assuming authority, responsibility, and accountability for their professional practice, professional nurses increasingly are being subjected to scrutiny by state boards of nursing representing the policing power of the state to protect the public welfare. Nurses also increasingly are being subjected to malpractice lawsuits. When nurses become defendants in legal actions, other nurses serve as expert witnesses both for the defense representing the practitioner and the prosecution representing the plaintiff. Expert witnesses testify to the standard of care required of the health care provider and whether it was met. For these reasons, professional nurses need basic knowledge of the legal aspects of nursing.

Nurse Practice Acts

In 1899, nurse leaders in the United States decided[2]

> "that nursing had reached the stage of acknowledged indispensability as an occupation in the care of the ill and convalescent; and further, that this occupation was so intimately bound up with the safety and health of the public that it required regulation and control in the education of those who desired to engage in it. The leaders who inspired the struggle were keenly aware that, since all progress must have a beginning, some effective legislation was better than none at all. Once reform was begun, the pressing need would become more obvious. Time would serve to improve the extent of control, to fill in the gaps, to remedy the errors. The important thing was to get some law on the books."

The first states to enact laws were North Carolina in 1902, and New Jersey, New York, Virginia, Maryland, Indiana, California, Connecticut, and Colorado in 1903.

Nurse practice acts are the policing power of the state. Most states regulate nursing similarly through nurse practice acts. As an example, the acts are laws that define nursing, mandate and set standards for licensure, mandate licensure examinations, regulate schools of nursing, set standards for curricula of schools of nursing, review and require continuing education for licensure renewal, investigate reports of violation of nursing practice, discipline violators of nurse practice laws, and regulate advanced practice nurses.

Nurse practice acts protect the public against negligence and malpractice and other torts. Through their boards of nursing, nurse practice acts discipline violators by probation, revocation of license, and referral to criminal courts. Patients injured by professional nurses also may pursue redress through civil courts.

The first legal principle of nursing is that the professional nurse must qualify for and become licensed in a state to meet the legal requirement for the right to practice professional nursing. Every state in the United States has a mandatory nurse-licensing requirement.

Legal Aspects of Contracts

A *contract*[3] consists of (1) an offer and (2) an acceptance, which constitute (3) the agreement between (4) two or more parties (5) having legal capacity (6) to do or forbear the doing of (7) a legal act for (8) a price, which in legal parlance, is termed "consideration."

Professional nurses make oral and written contracts. They accept or reject offers of employment and make counteroffers. Once an offer is accepted, revocation by either party is a breach of contract. When agents of parties make contracts, the parties to the contract are called principals and those who made the contracts are called agents. An example of this is nurse staffing agencies acting as agents for nurses and hospitals. Professional nurses negotiate those contract terms that will satisfy them: salary, fringe benefits and shift differential; hours of work and shift rotation; moving, housing, travel, and education expenses; and payment of malpractice insurance premiums. It is best to have all contract terms written and signed before accepting a job. Legally, both parties to a contract must live up to the terms of the contract or be subjected to the possibility of civil litigation.

Principle: A principal of a contract cannot require the other principal to commit an illegal act, which is prohibited by law or violates the spirit of the law.

Professional nurses are bound by contracts between unions and employers when such contracts exist. When seeking employment, the professional nurse should ask whether there is a union and the terms of the contract, which would bind him or her.

In this era of managed care, advanced practice nurses may enter into contracts with managed care organizations. When doing so, advanced practice nurses should make sure the following contract categories are covered[4]:

1. The parties are clearly identified.
2. The preface includes statements found in the body of the contract.
3. Terms are defined.
4. Provider duties are specified.
5. Payer-contractor duties are specified.
6. Utilization review is specified.
7. Claims management is specified.
8. Medical records are specified.
9. Provider compensation is specified.
10. Patient duties are specified.
11. Liability issues are specified.
12. Quality issues are specified.
13. Marketing is specified.
14. Insolvency protection is specified.
15. Terms of the contract are specified.
16. Termination conditions are specified.
17. Exclusivity is specified.
18. Other general provisions are specified.

When contracting with managed care organizations and other providers, professional nurses need a sound business plan that keeps them solvent and limits their liability. It is wise to consult an attorney.

Legal Aspects of Torts

Three legal terms that are intertwined are tort, negligence, and malpractice. A *tort* is a civil wrong that can be redressed in a civil proceeding. It includes *negligence*, the doing or nondoing of an act which a reasonable person under similar circumstances would or would not do, and which act or failure to act is the proximate cause of injury. A *proximate cause* is one, which in a natural and continuous sequence produces an event that results in an injury. The last person who could have reasonably prevented the injury from occurring is associated with the proximate cause of injury. *Malpractice* is the unskillful or negligent practice of a professional person whereby the health of a person (patient) is injured (malpraxis).

For a malpractice lawsuit to be successful, the following must exist:

1. There must be a duty between the injured party and the person who allegedly caused the injury.
2. There must be a breach of this duty.
3. The breach of duty must be the proximate cause of the injury.
4. The injured party must have experienced damages or injuries recognized as compensable by law.

One of the earliest and most famous cases of negligence by a nurse was the celebrated Somera case, reported in *The International Review*, July 1, 1930, pp. 325–334. Lorenza Somera, as the head nurse, was directed by the operating surgeon to prepare 10% cocaine with adrenaline for administration to a patient for a tonsillectomy. Miss Somera repeated and verified the order. A few moments after the injection was given, the patient showed symptoms of convulsions and died. The operating surgeon *meant* to say 10% procaine (Novocain). Only Miss Somera was found guilty of manslaughter due to negligence. The negligence consisted of fulfilling an order, which the nurse should have known by reason of her training and experience was an incorrect one. Although the physician was negligent, the cause of death was the nurse's negligence.[5]

When in doubt, obtain confirmation and use caution.

Malpractice suits are endemic in the United States, mostly owing to a multitude of alleged errors. Results of the Harvard Medical Practice Study of 1984 found that at least 4% of hospitalized patients suffer an adverse event, two-thirds of which are preventable. Thus, estimates are that **one million preventable injuries** and **120,000 preventable deaths** from errors occur annually. In 1998, the cost of these adverse events was estimated at $100 billion, which is a conservative estimate.

Evidence indicates that most errors are caused by the system and not the provider of care. However, the provider, that is, the individual practitioner, is usually punished by the system for failure of the system. Punishment results in the provider not reporting errors. Regulatory agencies, employers, and professional organizations need to change this punitive culture to one that redesigns systems and prevents errors.[6] This approach is compatible with the theory of quality management of W. Edwards Deming, covered in Chapter 25.

Because government functions are performed for the public welfare, it is difficult to sue the government. In 1946, the Congress of the United States passed P.L. 601, Title 4, the Federal Torts Claims Act. This law allows persons to sue the federal government for negligence of its employees. The monetary claims are restricted. Most states do not allow lawsuits and are protected by sovereign immunity, that is, the supreme power residing in the people.

Criminal responsibility may ensue from negligence in which the course of conduct is palpably imprudent and unreasonable.[7]

Assault and Battery

Assault and battery are torts that can involve nurses. *Assault* includes[8]

(1) a threat or attempt, (2) coupled with an apparent ability to execute the threat or attempt, (3) to put another in

fear of an immediate offensive or harmful contact (4) which is intended and which is neither consented to nor privileged.

Battery is[9]

(1) the execution of the threat or attempt to commit an assault, or the unlawful touching or striking of another (2) by any means, which results in bodily contact (3) that is intended and is neither consented to nor privileged.

Here is an example of assault and battery. The nurse approaches a patient and tells her he is going to give her a bath. The patient, who is mentally sound, tells the nurse she does not want him to bathe her. After conferring with his supervisor, the nurse proceeds to undress and bathe the patient. When the husband arrives, the patient is in emotional turmoil. The husband gathers the facts and writes a letter of complaint to the administrator, who replies that the patient cannot refuse to be bathed by any competent nurse. The husband consults with a professional nurse acquaintance who determines that the husband will settle for a letter of apology that states that his wife will not be forced to accept being bathed by a nursing employee again. The letter averts a lawsuit.

A nurse who carries out any nursing intervention without the patient's consent, even if the intervention is beneficial, is potentially guilty of professional misconduct. The nurse may be disciplined by the state board of nursing and could be sued by the patient or face an allegation of battery or civil assault.

Other Torts Applicable to Nurses

Other torts that have the potential for occurring in health care and that nurses should be aware of are false imprisonment; slander and libel; and destruction, injury, or loss of another's property.

False imprisonment occurs when a person is[10]

(1) confined or imprisoned by any means, (2) unlawfully by another, (3) for no matter how short a time, (4) with intention to cause such confinement or imprisonment, (5) of which the one confined or imprisoned has knowledge, and which is neither privileged nor consented to.

A person cannot be confined to a psychiatric facility because of exhibiting behavior that is annoying to another person. For example, a husband brings his pregnant wife to the emergency room because she is verbally noisy. The husband wants the physician to admit his wife to the mental health unit because she is keeping him awake at night with her talking. The physician determines that the wife is not dangerous to herself or anyone. The physician follows hospital policy and refers the husband to the courts.

There are many reports of instances of improper restraint of institutionalized residents that constitute false imprisonment and assault and battery.

Slander is[11]

> the (1) malicious (2) utterance by speaking of base or defamatory words concerning another's reputation or profession which tend to expose him to contempt, ridicule or public hatred, (3) are published to another, (4) are intended and are neither true nor privileged.

Libel is[12]

> the (1) malicious (2) utterance either in writing or printing, or by signs, pictures or caricatures, of base or defamatory words concerning another's reputation or profession which tend to expose him to contempt, ridicule or public hatred, (3) are published to another, (4) are intended and (5) are neither true nor privileged.

A person who defames the character of another and causes a loss of professional reputation must be able to prove the truth of the accusation. Truth is the absolute defense to an action in slander and libel. It is difficult for prominent public figures to sue successfully for slander and libel.

Privileged Communication

Certain communications are privileged and cannot be used against the accused in a court of law. These include communication between attorney and client, physician and patient, clergyman and member of congregation, members of a household, and prospective and former employers.

Liability

A person who takes or appropriates another person's property under admittedly wrongful circumstances can be charged with a crime and be subject to civil court action as well. Because nurses are frequently required to handle the property of others, liability for negligence may result if a patient's property is lost or damaged. To avoid a charge of negligence in handling patients' property, the nurse exercises reasonable care and follows the policies and procedures of the employing institution.

Nurses may be asked to witness patient's signatures on legal documents such as wills. The nurse must know the various laws governing witnessing of patients' signatures. Many states have laws defining who can or cannot witness signatures on certain documents. When in doubt, the nurse should not sign and should seek counsel from the institution's legal counsel.

Ignorance of the law is no excuse. When a law exists and the nurse violates it, the nurse is subject to criminal charges.

Expert Witness

In nursing practice, an expert witness is a professional nurse who can speak with authority on a subject, field, and specialty of nursing. As an expert witness, the nurse is a legal participant in litigation involving malpractice. A civil lawsuit alleging that malpractice has taken place is filed against a hospital, nursing home, or individual nurse. The plaintiff's lawyers will often file against the institution, physician, and nurse on the "deep pockets" theory that they will collect damages from the party or parties with the most liability insurance and income or wealth. The alleged victim is the plaintiff, the party making the complaint in civil court. The party alleged to have committed the negligent act is the defendant. The negligent act involves the nurse as expert witness when it is an alleged violation of nursing practice. Each side will have an expert witness.

The expert witness does the following:

- Reviews records, charts, and depositions of other witnesses. Gives opinions based on expert knowledge of standards of nursing care related to all aspects of the care of the patient at the center of the suit.
- Gives depositions under oath. Is well prepared by the attorney with whom she is working. Must remember questions asked and answers given when the case goes to trial because the opposing lawyer will try to confuse the expert witness and cause the jury to doubt the expertise and credibility of the opposing side's expert witness.
- Does a literature search for similar cases plus up-to-date articles related to all medical and nursing aspects of the case.

A nurse becomes an expert when someone related to the case suggests or refers the attorney to the nurse. The attorney and the nurse establish a rapport and make a contract. Together the attorney and the nurse establish a theory of the case. Preparation for the deposition and trial must be thorough, with records thoroughly analyzed by both. The expert nurse not only notes records that support his or her case but those entries, or lack of them, that support the opposition's case.[13] An expert's opinion must have evidentiary—scientific—reliability to be admissible.[14]

Qualifications needed by the expert nurse include clinical experience, formal education (an advanced degree), publication in peer-reviewed journals, ability to speak in terms a jury can understand, good eye contact, a record of accepting cases for plaintiffs and defendants, and participation in professional organizations.

EXHIBIT 27-1

An elderly, blind, woman resident in a nursing home in Alabama fell and broke her hip. The family sued the nursing home for negligence. The resident's chart indicated that the nursing personnel had planned her care with the resident and arranged the furniture in her room and the position of her bed so she could safely go to her chair and to the bathroom. The nursing personnel had carefully documented repeatedly communicating the plan to the resident, and she followed it without incident for more than 2 years.

The plaintiff's lawyer charged that the resident should have been restrained in bed with instructions to call nursing personnel before getting up for any reason. the defendant's lawyer and expert witness prepared and presented a theory of the case that showed documented nursing care planning that had given this resident safe freedom of movement for more than 2 years. The jury believed the expert witness and acquitted the nursing home. Afterward jury members congratulated the expert witness.

Risk Management

Risk management can be defined as a "process that centers on identification, analysis, treatment and evaluation of real and potential hazards."[15] Risk management has its beginnings in transportation and industry, with the present concepts being formed from investigation into aviation and traffic accidents. The primary reasons for these investigations were to determine patterns or causative factors in the accidents and then to eliminate, or at least control, as many factors as possible.[16]

Hayden describes risk management as the risk of financial loss. Specifically, she addresses control of financial loss resulting from legal liability. Financial loss and legal liability can be best understood by the following steps[17]:

1. Identifying patterns and trends of risk through internal audits and claims.
2. Reporting individual risk-related incidents and taking steps to reduce the liability related to them.
3. Developing and engaging in product evaluation systems with appropriate informed consent protocols.
4. Vigilant evaluation of patient care settings to determine risks.
5. Preventing those occurrences likely to be a liability to the organization.

Hayden goes further and describes three aspects of risk identification that should be monitored on a continuous basis[18]:

1. Clinical settings, clinical problems, personnel, and specific incidents involving patients, employees, and visitors.

2. Safety management.
3. Procedures for evaluation and follow-up on identified risks.

In addition, review of pertinent documents such as medical records, incident reports, pharmacy logs, infection control reports, and utilization review reports is paramount to a successful risk management program. Excellent communication skills are essential when interacting with medical and administrative staff and with clients. Substandard communication skills are often the root of a complaint or claim.[19]

The Joint Commission on Accreditation of Healthcare Organizations (JCAHO) recommends the establishment of an integrated risk management–quality assurance program that would provide a more efficient and cost-effective method of evaluation than having two separate functions. The following parameters are incorporated into the JCAHO model for risk management[20]:

1. Continuing education and in-service training.
2. Use of data from a variety of sources, such as patient surveys and feedback from other providers (referring or referral facilities).
3. Improvement of credentialing protocols for practitioners.
4. Development and enforcement of rules, regulations, policies, and procedures.
5. Establishment of written criteria to evaluate risk factors, including follow-up on conclusions reached.

Bennett further describes the importance of both quality improvement and risk management, identifying issues associated with quality patient care, collecting and analyzing data, making recommendations, and evaluating outcomes to prevent reoccurrences and upgrade quality. Avoidance of costly malpractice litigation is as important as is providing safe and quality patient care.[21] Five common reasons for malpractice litigation are injuries to patients resulting from the following[22]:

1. Errors or failures in safety of care that result in patient falls.
2. Failure to identify and document pertinent information (omissions of significant data).
3. Failure to correctly perform treatments or nursing care.
4. Failure to communicate significant data to patients or other therapists.
5. Errors in medications.

Adhering to standards of care (general and specialty nursing) can provide a model for risk management. It is significant to note that quality nursing care is concerned, compassionate, and nurturing. It is often within the context of a therapeutic nurse–patient relationship that problems are solved and errors avoided.

Effective communication is a cornerstone to a therapeutic relationship and is enhanced by active listening, empathy, understanding, and positive reinforcement. When the patient and family truly feel cared about, errors that do occur are considered in the context of this relationship. In addition, the following primary responsibilities of every nurse are essential in preventing malpractice litigation[23]:

1. Practice safely, that is, deliver quality nursing care to all patients.
2. Incorporate effective patient rapport in nursing practice.
3. Keep accurate and complete records.
4. Act reasonably—as all other professional nurses would in the community, the state, and the nation—to give standard nursing care.

The risk manager uses carefully planned public relations; makes private explanations; apologizes when necessary; and collects, prepares, and presents evidence.[24] The risk manager's job duties are further outlined in Exhibit 27-2.

Process

The following process describes an effective risk management program[25]:

1. Identify areas within the organization that expose it to loss.
2. Evaluate the potential loss those exposures represent.
3. Treat the exposure through two broad categories: risk financing and risk control.
4. Reduce the severity of the loss through risk control strategies such as hospital bill write-offs or early investigations of the event.

Employing these strategies is a joint effort of the risk management department along with health care providers, because it is everyone's responsibility to provide a safe environment for the patient. Such strategies include early warning systems, documentation, informed consent, and patient relations.[26]

Early Warning Systems

Early warning systems include strategies that involve acquiring early information and knowledge of the occurrence of an untoward event. Early warning provides an opportunity to evaluate the incident while the circumstances are still very clear. "Early reporting also allows the organization to secure medical records related to the event and equipment that may have malfunctioned and contributed to the event."[27] With computerization, a formal information system may be put in place, with labels for generic screens or occurrence screens that serve as a set of criteria and list the kinds of "red flag" occurrences that indicate a loss.

EXHIBIT 27-2
Risk Manager Competencies

1. Keep an up-to-date manual, including policies, lines of authority, safety roles, disaster plans, safety training, procedures, incident and claims reporting, procedures, and schedule, and description of retention/insurance program.
2. Update programs with changes in properties, operations, or activities.
3. Review plans for new construction, alterations, and equipment installation.
4. Review contracts to avoid unnecessary assumptions of liability and transfer to others where possible.
5. Keep up-to-date property appraisal.
6. Maintain records of insurance policy renewal dates.
7. Review and monitor all premium and other billings and approve payments.
8. Negotiate insurance coverage, premiums, and services.
9. Prepare specifications for competitive bids on property and liability insurance.
10. Review and make recommendations for coverage, services, and costs.
11. Maintain records and verify compliance for independent physicians, vendors, contractors, and subcontractors.
12. Maintain records of losses, claims, and all risk management expenses.
13. Supervise claim-reporting procedures.
14. Assist in adjusting losses.
15. Cooperate with director of safety and risk management committee to minimize all future losses involving employees, patients, visitors, other third parties, property, and earnings.
16. Keep risk management skills updated.
17. Assess the system for causes of errors and adverse events. Fix the system.
18. Use focus groups to identify unreported errors and adverse events. Eliminate punitive organizational culture.
19. Prepare annual report covering status, changes, new problems and solutions, summary of existing insurance and retention aspects of the program, summary of losses, costs, major claims, and future goals and objectives.
20. Prepare an annual budget.

The nurse manager and the clinical staff are often the key players in reporting early warnings. Claims management can be included in the early warning systems. It includes analysis of risk for possible loss frequency and severity, that is, the assessment of potential claims based on data analysis. This information (written and verbal reports) is used to investigate potentially compensable events and losses and their causes, thereby determining liability and settlement value.

Documentation

Documentation strategies are essential to an effective risk management program. The medical record generally serves as a means of determining whether a deviation existed in the standard of care. Contradictions, inconsistencies, and unexplained time gaps in the medical records signal potential problems during litigation. It is recommended that documentation take place as soon after the occurrence as possible and that a minute-by-minute recording is done during the emergency. When time is of the essence, brief notes with times, interventions, and other relevant information should be written on a piece of paper and transferred to the medical records as soon as the crisis is over. Any corrections to the medical record should be done with a thin line drawn through the original entry, dated and initialed. Information should be documented as a factual recording and objectivity should be practiced. Documentation of any instructions given to the patient should also be recorded.

Informed Consent

Informed consent does not involve just the signing of a consent form. This procedure has little relation to the patient's understanding of the procedure to be performed. Informed consent is the provision of enough information to patients to enable them to make a rational decision whether or not to undergo the treatment. The form that is signed, however, is indicative that adequate information has been given to the patient and that understanding and consent have been duly explained. Exceptions to the rule are emergency treatments and situations where such disclosure could potentially adversely affect the patient's medical condition. Informed consent may be sought for diagnosis, nature and purpose of the proposed treatment, risks and consequences of the proposed treatment, and feasible treatment alternatives.

Patient Relations

Patient relations are important; often the deterioration of the professional-to-patient relationship is what leads to malpractice claims. Many large health care organizations employ patient representatives who provide services such as orientating patients and their families to organizational policies, procedures, and services; resolving complaints; making phone calls and mailing letters; and daily follow-up. Volunteers often assist the patient representative.[28]

Incident Reporting

Incident reporting is an effective technique of a good risk management program. The tool itself should be constructed to collect complete and accurate information, including the name, address, age, and condition of the individual involved; exact location, time, and date of the incident; description of the occurrence; physician's examination data; bedrail status; reason for hospitalization; names of witnesses; and extent of out-of-bed privileges.

Use

Incident reports are used to collect and analyze future data for the purpose of determining risk-control strategies. These reports are prepared for any unusual occurrence involving people or property, whether or not injury or damage occurs. Blake describes the use of a multiple causation model in incident report investigation. This theory purports that causes, subcauses, and contributing factors weave together in particular sequences to cause incidents. An incident may have many concomitant causes; therefore, seeking out as many causes as possible and rating them to their proximate or primary influence on the incident may be useful in reducing the chance of the incident recurring. Proximate causes are often referred to as unsafe acts and conditions and are generally the most apparent and closest cause of the incident. Primary causes are procedural in nature, and such causes are discovered though backtracking from the proximate cause.

Blake identifies six principles of risk management related to incident investigation[29]:

Principle I: Each cause of an incident reflects a management problem.

Principle II: One can predict that sets of circumstances will produce incidents. These circumstances can be identified and controlled.

Principle III: In any given group or array, a relatively small number of items will tend to give rise to the largest proportion of results.

Principle IV: The purpose of incident investigation is to locate and define the operational errors that allow incidents to occur.

Principle V: Accountability is the key to effective incident investigation and analysis.

Principle VI: The past performance of an organization or unit tends to forecast its future performance.

Preparation

The incident report is discoverable by the plaintiff's attorney. For this reason, it should be prepared by the involved employee(s) in a timely manner to ensure accuracy and objectivity of reporting. It must be complete and factual. The incident report is corrected in the same manner as any other medical record and should not be altered or rewritten. It should contain no comments criticizing or blaming others. To keep the incident report from being discoverable, it must be sent directly from preparer to attorney to ensure confidentiality. Nurse managers frequently insist on reviewing the report, although they can obtain accurate information from the patient's chart and from conversations with the preparer. The incident report should be prepared in a single copy and should never be placed on the patient's medical record. Exhibit 27-3 lists the dos and don'ts of incident reporting.

Attorneys can prepare abstracts of data from collective incident reports. Thus, attorneys can identify the number of occurrences of particular incidents. The information will be used by the risk manager to do his or her job, for example, in doing trend analysis to establish patterns and in determining needed education and training of personnel to reduce risks.[30]

It may be institutional policy to send the incident report to the risk manager, but an alternative method of notification is better. The preparer can call the risk manager and nurse manager and give them verbal information on the need to investigate and evaluate deviations from the standard of care and for making corrections. To accomplish this, managers will have to establish a climate of trust that supports incident reporting by nurses. The JCAHO requires that incidents be reported.

Accident Reporting

Incidents involving employees are frequently referred to as accidents. The person preparing the accident report should follow the same principles as those for incident reporting. These principles will usually be covered by institutional policy and procedure. Perceptions vary too much to require personnel to discriminate between an incident and accident. Accidents are incidents, and many incidents are accidents.

Infection Control

A major area for quality control and risk management is infection control. Infections acquired in hospitals are termed *nosocomial infections*. Many hospitals will have full-time infection control nurses who investigate all reported nosocomial infections. A source of data is the medical laboratory. It is good policy to have all laboratory reports indicating a positive result for infectious diseases routed to the infection control nurse. The diseases will be investigated and procedures implemented to prevent their spread and future development. Staff development is a major function of infection control. Standards followed are those of the Centers for Disease Control and Prevention.

Other basic principles of law important to nursing include the following[31]:

1. Ignorance of the law is not an excuse for wrongdoing. If a law exists but a person does not know it, that person will not be excused for breaking it.

EXHIBIT 27-3
DOs and DON'Ts of Incident Reporting

DOs

- Report any event involving patient mishap or serious expression of dissatisfaction with care.
- Report any event involving visitor mishap or property.
- Be complete.
- Follow established policy and procedure.
- Be prompt.
- Act to reduce fear by the nursing staff.
- Correct in the same manner as any medical record.
- Include names and identities of witnesses; record their statements on separate pages.
- Report equipment malfunctions, including control numbers. Remove equipment from service for testing.
- Keep the report confidential.
- Report to nurse manager.
- Confer with risk manager.
- Work to provide nursing care to meet established standards.
- Attend all staff development programs.
- Confirm all telephone orders in writing.

DON'Ts

- Place blame on anyone.
- Place report on the patient's chart.
- Make entry about an incident report on the patient's chart.
- Alter or rewrite.
- Report hearsay or opinion.
- Be afraid to consult, ask questions, or complete incident reports. They can be part of your best defense and protection.
- Prescribe in the physician's domain.
- Be cold and impersonal to patients, families, or visitors.

2. Every person is responsible for his or her own actions. The nurse must know cause and effect of all actions or will be subject to suit for malpractice when harm occurs to a patient.

3. A nurse will not carry out an illegal order of a physician or any other health care provider. The nurse must know that the order is a legal one before carrying it out.

4. New nurse graduates must not be assigned to duties beyond their competence.

5. An employer hiring a nurse is required to exercise ordinary, prudent policies and procedures.

6. In the rule of "respondent superior" or the "master–servant" rule, injury by an employee because of negligence makes both employee and employer equally responsible to an injured party. The injured party may sue both employer and employee. Both may not necessarily be found guilty.

7. Professional nurses should carry malpractice insurance. Even when an employer insures an employee, the licensed employee is usually not covered outside the place of employment.

8. Malpractice lititgation can be reduced by documenting telephone advice to patients, improving communication and listening skills, and effectively obtaining patients' informed consent.

9. Malpractice risks are increased when professional nurses supervise unlicensed employees.

10. Knowledge of state laws, such as mandatory reporting of abuse, is important for nurses.

11. Courts have interpreted ERISA (Employee Retirement Income Security Act) to limit physician autonomy and subordinate clinical decision-making to cost-containment decisions made by managed care organizations.

12. Good provider–patient relationships contribute to preventing malpractice suits.

13. Iatrogenic injuries are a significant public health problem that must be addressed by professional nurses.

14. The costs of malpractice litigation can be reduced by managing risks rather than vindicating providers accused of malpractice. Successful risk management techniques include credentialing of professional staff, monitoring and tracking of complaints and incidents, and documenting in the patient's medical record.

15. Medical malpractice appeared in the United States around 1840 and has been sustained by innovative pressures on medicine, adoption of uniform standards, the advent of medical malpractice liability insurance, contingency fees, citizen juries, and the nature of tort pleading.

16. Human errors in clinical nursing practice are common and underreported.

17. With increased credentialing of advanced practice nurses in HMOs, there will be increased liability for their employers and increased need for personal malpractice insurance.

18. The nursing profession appears to hold its licensees to safer standards than does the medical profession; therefore, nurses are disciplined more often and more harshly than are physicians.

19. Personal involvement with patients places the professional nurse in jeopardy for legal action by the state board of nursing.

20. Many charting practices can help decrease the liability risks for nurses.

Ten rules for avoiding going to court are[32]:

1. Know the law.
2. Document everything.
3. Make no negative comments about the patient.
4. Question authority.
5. Stay educated.
6. Manage risks.
7. Don't hurry through discharge.
8. Be discreet.
9. Use restraints wisely.
10. Be kind.

> Tort reform has as its objective reducing the costs of liability insurance premiums for providers and subsequently to the patient. Inherent in this process is the fact that mistakes by providers are withheld from patients even when they result in morbidity and mortality.[33]

Summary

Nurse practice acts orginiated in the United States in 1902, when the first law was enacted by North Carolina. These acts represent the policing power of the state and protect both patients and nurses. With the advance of knowledge and technology, professional nurses are required to have advanced education and training. Lawsuits against torts, such as negligence, are common and require professional nurses to purchase malpractice insurance. Other torts include assault and battery; false imprisonment; slander and libel; and destruction, injury, or loss of property. In the course of their practice, professional nurses may face civil or criminal charges.

In addition to being a defendant, the professional nurse may be called on to act as an expert witness for either the plaintiff or defendant. Employing institutions protect themselves by maintaining risk management departments.

APPLICATION EXERCISES

EXERCISE 27-1   Interview a risk manager. How do the risk manager's job duties compare with those outlined in Exhibit 27-2? What risk prevention strategies does the manager use? What has been the cost of losses caused by negligence during the past year?

EXERCISE 27-2   Examine the incident reporting program in a health care agency. What are its strengths? Its weaknesses? How can it be improved?

NOTES

1. M. J. Lesnik and B. E. Anderson, *Legal Aspects of Nursing* (Philadelphia: Lippincott, 1947), 9.
2. Ibid., 25–26.
3. Ibid., 50
4. J. Nugent, "Managed Care Contract Checklist Redux," *PT: Magazine of Physical Therapy* (March 1995), 34–36.
5. M. J. Lesnik and B. E. Anderson, op. cit., 258; Dr. Ian R. Kerr (http://instruct.uwo.ca/mit/247f/lectures/tort5/index.html#1); www.thegrid.net/agpd/report1.html; www.norcalmutual.com/rm/pages/m2pls1.html.
6. Ibid., 172.
7. Ibid., 181.
8. Ibid.
9. Ibid., 194.
10. Ibid., 202.
11. Ibid.
12. Ibid.
13. R. Cady, "So You Want to be and Expert Witness? Things You Need to Know." *MCN* (January–February 2000), 49
14. Daubert v. Merrell Dow Pharmaceuticals, Inc., 509 U.S. 579, 113 S. Ct. 2786, 125 L. Ed. 2d 469 (1993).
15. Intravenous Nurses Society, "Revised Intravenous Nursing Standards of Practice," *Journal of Intravenous Nursing*, 13(suppl), (1990) s91.
16. J. T. Rogers, *Risk Management in Emergency Medicine* (Dallas: Emergency Medicine Foundation, American College of Emergency Physicians, 1985), 2.
17. L. S. Hayden, "Risk Management Strategies," *Journal of Intravenous Nursing* (September–October 1992), 288–290.
18. Ibid.
19. Ibid.
20. R. Wilkinson and B. J. Moore, eds., *Quality Assurance in Ambulatory Care*, 2nd ed. (Chicago: Joint Commission on Accreditation of Healthcare Organizations, 1990), 25.
21. B. Bennett, "Quality Care Through Risk Management," *Orthopaedic Nursing* (May–June)1993, 54–55.
22. G. Troyer and S. Salman, *Handbook of Health Care Risk Management* (Germantown, MD: Aspen, 1986).
23. B. Bennett, op. cit.
24. D. Joseph and S. K. Jones, "Incident Reporting: The Cornerstone of Risk Management," *Nursing Management* (December 1984), 22–23.
25. T. A. Goldman, "Risk Management Concepts and Strategies," *Journal of Intravenous Nursing* (May–June 1991), 199–204.
26. Ibid.
27. Ibid.
28. Ibid.; "QAs Pave the Way: The Quest for Quality," *Hospital Profiles* (Alabama Hospital Association), (December 1987–January 1988), 1, 4–5.
29. P. Blake, "Incident Investigation: A Complete Guide," *Nursing Management* (November 1984), 37–41.
30. G. W. Poteet, "Risk Management and Nursing," *Nursing Clinics of North America* (September 1983), 457–465. K. H. Henry, ed., *Nursing Administration and Law Manual* (Gaithersburg, MD: Aspen, 1985), 9(39), 1–9.
31. A. V. Irving, "Twenty Strategies to Reduce Risk of a Malpractice Claim," *Journal of Medical Practice Management* (November–December 1998), 130–133; A. Helm, "Liability, UAPs and You." *Director* (winter 1999), 15–16, 29; P. E. Freed and V. K. Drake "Mandatory Reporting of Abuse: Practical, Moral, and Legal Issues for Psychiatric Home Healthcare Nurses," *Issues in Mental Health Nursing* (July–August 1999), 423–436; P. D. Jacobson and S. D. Pomfret. "ERISA Litigation and Physician Autonomy," *JAMA* (February 2000), 921–926; G. F. Klimo, W. J. Daum, M. R. Brinker, E. McGuire, and M. N. Elliot, "Orthopedic Medical Malpractice: An Attorney's Perspective," *American Journal of Orthopedics* (February 2000), 93–97; E. J. Thomas, D. M. Studdert, H. R. Burstin, E. J. Orav, T. Zeena, E. J. Williams, K. M. Howars, P. C. Weiler, and T. A. Brennan, "Incidence and Types of Adverse Events and Negligent Care in Utah and Colorado," *Medical Care* (March 2000), 261–271; L. L. Wilson, and M. Fulton, "Risk Management: How Doctors, Hospitals and MDOs Can Limit the Costs of Malpractice Litigation," *Medical Journal of Australia* (January 2000), 77–80; J. C. Mohr, "American Medical Malpractice Litigation in Historical Perspective," *JAMA* (April 2000), 1731–1737; C. E. Meurier et al., "Understanding the Nature of Errors in Nursing: Using a Model to Analyze Critical Incident Reports of Errors Which Had Resulted in an Adverse or Potentially Adverse Event," *Journal of Advanced Nursing* (July 2000), 202–207; K. Benesch, "Emerging Theories of Liability for Negligent Credentialing in HMOs, Integrated Delivery and Management Care Systems," *Trends in Health Care, Law & Ethics* (fall 1994), 41–42, 28, 45; M. Flaherty, "Crossing the Line: When Nurses Push the Limits," *HealthWeek* (12 October 1998), 14–15; M. Habel, "Documenting Patient Care, Part 1: Requirements, Charting Systems, and Reimbursement," *HealthWeek* (24 January 2000), 10–11; M Habel, Documenting Patient Care, Part 2: Limit Liability, Trends and Computer Chartering," *HealthWeek* (21 February 2000), 10–11.

32. T. Stein, "On the Defensive: More Patients are Naming Nurses in Malpractice Suits," *HealthWeek* (15 May 2000), 1, 18.

33. C. Terhune, "Rules on Reporting Errors in Hospitals Cause Alarm," *The Wall Street Journal* (4 March 1998).

REFERENCES

Brent, N. J. *Nurses and the Law: A Guide to Principles and Application* (Philadelphia: Saunders, 1997).

Cady, R. "So You Want to be an Expert Witness? Things You Need to Know." *MCN American Journal of Maternal Child Nursing* (January–February 2000), 49.

Castledine, G. "Case 34: Patient Consent: Nurse Who Carried Out Manual Evacuation Without Consent." *British Journal of Nursing*, 9(17), (2000), 1123.

Davis, G. S. "Learning the Ropes of Contracting." *Provider* (July 1996), 32–34.

Ginty, M. J., P. S. Golding, and M. B. Jellison. "The Basics of Managed Care Contracting: What Every Nurse Executive Needs to Know." *Aspen's Advisor for Nurse Executives* (May 1995), 1, 4–6.

Goldsmith, C. "Blowing the Whistle: Laws Protect Nurses Who Report Healthcare Fraud." *NurseWeek* (May 2000), 16.

Goodroe, J. H., and D. A. Murphy. "The Algebra of Managed Care." *Hospital Topics* (fall 1994), 14–18.

Gunn, I. P. "Regulation of Health Care Professionals, Part 2: Validation of Continued Competence." *CRNA* (August 1999), 135–141.

Hogue, E. E. "Contracting with Managed Care Providers." *Journal of Home Health Care Practice* (February 1994), 17–23.

Jacobs, L. A. "An Analysis of the Concept of Risk." *Cancer Nursing* (February 2000), 12–19.

Jenkins, M., and D. L. Torrisi. "Nurse Practitioners, Community Nursing Centers,and Contracting for Managed Care." *Journal of the American Academy of Nurse Practitioners* (March 1995), 119–123.

Kinsman, J. "Malpractice Liability in Health Professional Education." *Radiology Technology* (January–February 2000), 239–246

Kroll, M. "Bringing Together Nursing and Law: A Fitting Combination in Today's Health Care Environment." *Health Care Management* (September 1999), 48–52.

Lindberg, G. E. "The Any-Willing Provider Controversy." *Rehab Economics* 8 (6), (1995) 79–81.

Malugaani, M. "Nurse Interrupted: A Disciplinary Action Can Put a Wrinkle in Your Career and Tie You Up in Knots." *HealthWeek* (21 August 2000), 1, 18–19.

Osley, M. "Liability Risks of the Hold Harmless Clause in Managed Care." *Journal of Legal Nurse Consulting* (October 1995), 12–13.

Satinsky, M. A. "Advanced Practice Nurse in a Managed Care Environment." In Hickey, J. V. *Advanced Practice Nursing* (Philadelphia: Lippincott-Raven 1996.), 26–45.

Sheehan, J. G. "Public? Private Information Sharing in Healthcare Fraud Investigations." *Journal of Health Law* (fall 1999), 593–620.

Silver, M. S. "Incident Review Management: A Systemic Approach to Performance Improvements." *Journal of Healthcare Quality* (November–December 1999), 21–27.

Varga, K. "How to Protect Yourself Against Malpractice." *Revolution* (summer 1998), 55–57.

Waidley, E. "Nursing Information Systems, Name Badges." *HealthWeek* (September 1999), 17.

CHAPTER 28

Performance Appraisal

Russell C. Swansburg, PhD, RN

LEARNING OBJECTIVES AND ACTIVITIES

- Define *performance appraisal*.
- Illustrate the purposes of performance appraisal.
- Differentiate among the standards for performance appraisal.
- Illustrate training approaches for performance.
- Distinguish among performance appraisal methodologies.
- Illustrate performance appraisal problem areas.

CONCEPTS: Performance appraisal, performance standards, job analysis, job description, job evaluation, feedback, work redesign, peer ratings, self-ratings.

MANAGER BEHAVIOR: Maintains a system of probationary and annual performance appraisals based on job descriptions as standards.

LEADER BEHAVIOR: Develops a system of performance appraisal that uses a combination of supervisor, peer, and self-ratings. Feedback is provided based on input from the nursing staff. Human resource personnel use job analysis, job evaluation, and work redesign techniques to improve employee productivity.

Introduction

Performance appraisal (PA) is a control process in which employees' performances are evaluated against standards. The literature on PA is voluminous, indicating its value to management. Considerable research has been done on various aspects of the PA process.

Neither employees nor managers like PA. Some employees view PA as being more valued by top management than by themselves and their supervisors. Some managers do not like to do PA because it makes them feel guilty: Did I do justice by the employee? As writers of PAs, managers are concerned that they may "cast something in stone" that is inaccurate, be criticized on written grammar and spelling, say something illegal about the ratee, or may not be able to substantiate their comments.[1] Other managers are afraid of employees' reactions to ratings. Also, PA requires careful planning, information gathering, and an extensive formal interview, which is a time-consuming process. Managers perform activities of short duration, attend ad hoc meetings, perform nonroutine behavior, and focus on current information, which are short-term activities compared with the ongoing PA process.[2] The process is usually not interactive, moves slowly, is passive, is isolated, and is not people-oriented.[3]

Measurement of performance is imprecise. Often the focus is on the format, not the people. In some organizations, the human resource (HR) department sends the rating forms to the departments shortly before the end of the fiscal year. The forms must be completed immediately and are done with little or no training or preparation of the rater or ratee. The result is distrust by employees and dread by managers.

A survey of Fortune 1300 companies (1000 industrial and 300 nonindustrial) indicated that 29% of hourly workers are not evaluated by a formal appraisal system; 39% of respondents indicated that where used, PA systems are "extremely effective" or "very effective." PA systems are underappreciated.[4]

Performance appraisal systems require top management commitment. They can be tied to the planning cycle by relating them to personnel budgets or including them as a management plan. PA systems are most helpful when managers commit to using them for purposes beneficial to both employees and the organization.

Research in PA domains has little effect on the process or the outcome. A suggestion is that research and practice focus on fair and accurate PA as a process before attempting to use it to improve performance.[5]

Performance appraisal literature indicates the following ten results[6]:

1. U. S. industry uses PA systems for an average of 11 years. PA systems had little input from line managers, employees, and customers.
2. Most formats use management by objectives for executives, managers, and professional employees. Trait-based rating scales are the norm for nonexempt employees. Behavioral-anchored rating scales (BARS), forced-choice scales, or mixed standard scales are little used. Executives and hourly employees are least likely to be evaluated.
3. Supervisor ratings are most common. Self, peer, and subordinate ratings are seldom used.
4. Very few organizations allow decisions about PA policies or practice to be made at the level at which they are executed.
5. Some raters receive rater training; however, employees are seldom involved.
6. Only 25% of raters are held accountable for managing the appraisal process.
7. Few employees' opinions about the appraisal process are solicited.
8. Managers are concerned with fairness, justice, and future performance.
9. Of an organizational work force, 60% to 70% is rated in the top two performance levels.
10. A more comprehensive theory of the PA process is needed.

Research indicates that high levels of organizational politics relate to the conscientious job performance of workers.[7]

Purposes of Performance Appraisal

Performance appraisal may be a nurse manger's most valuable tool in controlling human resources and productivity. The PA process can be used effectively to govern employee behavior to produce goods and services in high volume and of high quality. Nurse managers can also use the PA process to govern corporate direction in selecting, training, doing career planning with, and rewarding personnel. The Fortune 1300 survey indicated that 80% used appraisal systems to justify merit increases, provide feedback, and identify candidates for promotion, all of which are considered short-

range goals. These goals were linked to long-range goals of performance potential for succession planning and career planning but could be much more useful in strategic planning. Of these companies 58% used PA to identify strengths and weaknesses, whereas 39% used PA for career planning; 89% used PA for general guidelines for salary increases, whereas only 1% used PA for forced distribution of bonuses. Forced distribution sets a limit on the number of high-level ratings.[8]

In addition to being used for promotions, counseling, training and development, staff planning, retention, termination, selections, and compensations, performance monitoring has been found to make employees effective. It is a managerial tool that can facilitate performance levels that achieve the company's mission and objectives.[9]

Appraisal systems are needed to meet legal requirements, including those for standardized forms and procedures, clear and relevant job analysis, and trained raters. When they do not meet such requirements, disciplinary actions, including termination, do not stand up in court.[10]

Motivation

A goal of PA is to stimulate motivation of the employee to perform the tasks and accomplish the mission of the organization. Promotions, assignments, selections for education, and increased pay are some goals that stimulate this motivation. If PA is to improve performance, the science of behavioral technology as described in Chapter 2, Introduction to Managed Care, should be employed.

Salary Problems

Performance evaluation is used to determine and provide equitable salary treatment. Jobs within groups of professionals, such as engineers, physicians, chemists, physicists, and nurses, have the same basic characteristics. Differences exist in the complexity of jobs. One could say that the job of a nurse assigned to a special care unit is more complex than is that of a nurse assigned to an intermediate care unit. This could be true to the extent that the depth of complexity exists. Contrast this with the complexity of managing the care of an active, intermediate care unit of 20 to 45 patients. The *breadth* of complexity of providing nursing care to many patients who have differing problems and are being treated by many physicians in addition to directing many medical care plans and many nonprofessional workers appears to be equivalent to the *depth* of complexity of intensive nursing care. In fact, some nurses want to be assigned to special care units not because of the dynamics of the situation but because their sphere of operations is encapsulated. Is a nurse in one of these units entitled to a higher salary than a nurse in the other? The job analysts say yes, when special training is required, complicated specialized equipment is being used, and the nurse is required to make more independent and critical judgments.

Certainly, the jobs of all professionals can be evaluated using the yardsticks of conventional PA techniques. However, arguments abound regarding the relationship between PAs and salaries and promotion. Some writers say keep PAs well away from times of salary increases and promotions.[11] In a survey of 875 companies, 32% experimented with some form of performance-based pay, a concept discussed in Chapter 29, Pay for Performance.[12]

Kirkpatrick recommends separating appraisals for merit salary increases from appraisals for performance improvement. Appraisals used for merit salary increases look backward at past performance, look at total performance, compare one individual with others doing same job, are subjective, and are done in an emotional climate. Appraisals used to improve performance look ahead; are concerned with detailed performance; are compared with what is expected regarding standards, goals, and objectives; and are conducted in a calm climate.[13]

For performance reviews related to salary administration, nurse managers would explain to subordinates the basis of decisions. The reviews would be fair and would be totally understood by the managers, who would allow employees to react even to the point of discussing the reviews with higher management. When a high salary increase results, the nurse manager communicates the good news to the employee. Three months should elapse between appraisals for salary administration and those for improved performance.[14]

Expectancy theory states that "the greater a person's expectancy (i.e., subjective probability) that effort expenditure will lead to various rewards, the greater the person's motivation to work hard."[15] Rewards of high value should be obtainable and related to job performance. Employees will repeat rewarded behavior and will be retained, thus maintaining productivity.

Research indicates that productivity increased from 29% to 63% with output-based pay plans versus time-based pay plans. Also, individual incentive plans are better than group incentive plans.[16]

Adequate pay is the most powerful motivator of performance, and people will not work without it. Other financial incentives such as shift differentials, education pay, and certification pay are positive motivators. Research has shown that productivity actually drops with time-based rewards and hourly wages. Good employees will leave rather than work with poorly performing ones. Rewards should be related to job performance. The results can be seen by correlating rewards across individual performances. There should be substantial differences in the rewards.

Kopelman suggests a mixed-consequence system: rewards for good performance, deductions for poor performance. The latter requires coaching, training, counseling, reassigning, or terminating. Important job responsibilities and behaviors deserving of high rewards can be determined from job analysis and should be related to difficult performance standards or goals.[17]

The Xerox Experience

Before 1983, Xerox had a traditional appraisal system, tying merit pay increases to performance rating. Employees were dissatisfied with the lack of an equitable rating distribution. Of employees, 95% were at the level three or four in a four-level rating system. Forced distribution was used to control the numbers of employees above or below a specific level. There were no preplanned objectives, the focus being on the summary rating. A task force was used to develop a performance feedback and development process with the following characteristics[18]:

1. Objectives were set between manager and employee.
2. The evaluation was documented and approved by a second-level manager.
3. An appraisal review was held at the end of 6 months, with review and discussion of objectives and progress. Both manager and employee signed the written report.
4. A final review was held at 1 year.
5. The process emphasized performance feedback and improvements.
6. A merit increase discussion was held 1 to 2 months later.
7. There was agreement on personal goals related to communications, planning, time management, human relations, and professional goals (specialty and job).
8. There were financial and human resource management objectives.
9. Managers were trained in the process.

Regular surveys of the Xerox system indicated that 81% of employees understood their work group objectives better, 84% considered the appraisals to be fair, 72% understood how merit pay was determined, 70% met personal and professional objectives, and 77% favored the system.

Other Purposes

An effective appraisal generates understanding and commitment, leading to productivity. Career development and PA support each other if they share objectives, recognition, concern, and communication. Usually, nurse managers take charge of PA and nurses take charge of career development. They can be brought together for mutual benefits.

Talent development can be a mutual goal and benefit of the two programs. Performance input supports future options and paths for future growth and development of employees.[19]

Accreditation and professional standards may require or suggest the use of performance evaluation.

Performance appraisals can also be used to confirm hiring decisions, particularly when new employees have a probationary period before becoming permanent. This period is crucial because employees can be terminated without the extended termination process. Effective nurse managers will use this period to counsel and coach the employee to perform effectively. The PA will document the process.

Performance appraisal has multiple purposes. Management should determine purposes that fit organizational needs.[20] Perhaps the ultimate purpose of PA is to measure accountability and improve practice standards. In nursing, the delivery of care is a major domain to be evaluated. Evaluation addresses strengths and weaknesses, new or altered policies, and the need for more knowledge. Feedback increases self-awareness and professionalism.[21]

Developing and Using Standards

Performance Standards

Performance standards are derived from job analysis, job descriptions, job evaluation, and other documents detailing the qualitative and quantitative aspects of jobs. Performance standards are established by authority, which may be the agency in which they are used or a professional association, such as the American Nurses Association (ANA). They are measuring sticks for qualitative and quantitative evaluation of the individual's performance. These standards should be based on appropriate knowledge and practical enough to be attained. Like other documents, they must be kept up-to-date.

Job or performance standards for the nurse manager may be developed using the ANA Scope and Standards for Nurse Administrators. Performance standards for a job are written and used to measure the performance of the individual filling the job. Employees should know that these standards are being used and know what they are. They may be asked to bring copies of the standards to their supervisor for scheduled counseling. Employees also may be asked to list their accomplishments in relation to the standards. Doing so makes performance counseling less of a threat and

allows employees to recognize and discuss their accomplishments. Employees may be guided to recognize areas in which their performance falls short and may be encouraged to voice goals for improvement in these areas. This method of using performance standards has been found to be effective.

The ANA Congress for Nursing Practice has developed and published standards of practice in several specialty areas. The ANA Standards of Clinical Nursing Practice can be used in the development of performance standards. Exhibit 28-1 is an example of performance standards for a clinical nurse.

The nurse manager controls nursing productivity with standards that measure nursing performance. Standards are based on history or past experience "and gut-level appraisal by the person in charge."[22] They include establishment of criteria, planning goals, and physical or quantitative measurements of products, units of service, labor hours, speed, and the like.[23]

A *standard* is "a unit of measurement that can serve as a reference point for evaluating results."[24] In collaboration with clinical nurses, nurse managers develop the units of measurement as both process (intervention) and outcome criteria.

Accuracy and fairness of PA come from having an objective, standards-oriented PA plan. The plan should have objectively defined task standards that can be measured in terms of output and observable behavioral change. These performance standards will relate to both the quantity and quality of work, that is, the who, how, when, where, and what is produced. They will include production standards.[25]

Performance evaluation includes standards for experience, complexities of the job, the level of trust, and understanding the work and mission. Friedman recommends developing job standards based on four to eight core responsibilities. For nurse managers, these core responsibilities could be in the major management functions of planning, organizing, directing (leading), and controlling (evaluating). They could also be related to the roles of clinician, teacher, administrator, consultant, and researcher. Finally, these core responsibilities could be related to self-development. Desired behaviors, outputs, or results under each core responsibility are then developed as performance objectives. Objectives are related to or combined with behaviors as standards for performance evaluation.[26]

Standards will include the dimensions of evidence-based nursing practice, measurable outcomes, and accountability.[27]

Job analysis, job descriptions, and job evaluations are important sources of standards for performance evaluation.

EXHIBIT 28-1
Performance Standards—Clinical Nurse

PERFORMANCE STANDARDS

1. *Type of work:* Nursing care of patients
   Major duty: Performs the primary functions of a professional nurse (50% of working hours).
   a. Obtains nursing histories on all newly admitted patients.
   b. Reviews nursing histories of all transfer patients.
   c. Uses nursing histories to make nursing diagnoses determining patients' needs and problems. Using this information:
   d. Initiates a nursing care plan for each patient.
   e. Lists goal(s) for each nursing need or problem.
   f. Writes nursing prescription or orders for each patient to meet each need or problem and goal.
   g. Applies the plan of care, giving evidence of knowledge of scientific and legal principles.
   h. Executes physicians' orders.
2. *Type of work:* Management of nursing personnel
   Major duty: Plans nursing care of patients on a daily basis (14% of working hours).
   a. Rates each patient according to number and complexity of needs and goals.
   b. Knows abilities of each team member.
   c. Makes a daily assignment for each team member.
   d. Discusses assignment with each team member at the beginning of each shift.
      (i) Listens to taped report with team members.
      (ii) Sees that team members review physicians' orders and nursing care plans.
      (iii) Answers questions arising from these activities.
   e. Confers with charge nurse and ward clerk periodically to ascertain whether there are any new orders.
   f. Plans for a team conference at a specific time and place and tells team members.
   g. Incorporates division and unit philosophy and objectives into team activities.
   h. Assists with assignment of LPN and RN students, including them as active team members according to their backgrounds and learning needs.
3. *Type of work:* Management of nursing personnel
   Major duty: Supervises team activities (10% of working hours).
   a. Makes frequent rounds to assist team members with care of patients. At the same time, talks to and observes patients to determine:
      (i) New needs or problems.
      (ii) Progress. Confirms these observations with patient if possible.
   b. Conducts 15- to 20-minute team conference using a specific agenda that has been made known to team members at previous day's conference.
      (i) Involves all team members.

   (ii) Solicits comments on new problems or special problems of patients and updates selected nursing care plans as needed.
   (iii) Assigns roles for next day's team conference.
   c. Writes nursing progress notes and updates remaining nursing care plans.
      (i) Assists technicians with writing notes as needed for training. Otherwise reads and countersigns their notes. Writes own notes.
      (ii) Updates those nursing care plans not done at team conference. Recognizes this is a professional nurse's responsibility.
      (iii) Reads notes of LPNs and RNs.
   d. Communicates nursing service and hospital policies to team members on a daily basis through referral to information such as daily bulletins, minutes of meetings, and changes in regulations.
4. *Type of work:* Management of equipment and supplies
   Major duty: Identifies needs; plans and submits requests for new and replacement equipment and supplies to charge nurse (1% of working hours).
   a. While working with team members identifies malfunctioning equipment and supply shortages and reports same to charge nurse and ward clerk on a daily basis.
   b. Submits requests for new equipment and supplies to charge nurse on a quarterly basis.
5. *Type of work:* Training
   Major duty: Identifies training needs of team members and plans activities to meet needs (5% of working hours).
   a. Identifies specific training needs of individual team members through daily observation of their performance and interviews.
   b. Evaluates performance through use of performance standards. Makes these standards known to each team member, and holds each responsible for meeting standards.
   c. Plans counseling and guidance of each team member on an individual basis and at least quarterly.
   d. Plans and conducts unit in-service education programs at least monthly. Involves team members.
   e. Recommends team members for seminars, short courses, college programs, and correspondence courses.
   f. Thoroughly orients all new team members. Conducts skill inventory during initial interview and plans on-the-job training for those needed skills in which team member is not proficient.
   g. Annually submits budget requests for training materials and programs to charge nurse.
   h. Makes reading assignments and allows time for team members to use library resources.

(continued)

EXHIBIT 28-1 *(continued)*

6. *Type of work:* Planning patient care
   Major duty: Coordinates nursing resources essential to meeting each patient's total needs and goals (5% of working hours).
   a. Consults with patients' physicians daily.
   b. Requests consultations of clinical nurse specialists. This may include clinical nurse specialists in pediatrics, mental health, medical–surgical, radiology, public health, and rehabilitation.
   c. Consults with other personnel as needed, including chaplain, social worker, recreation worker, occupational therapist, physical therapist, pharmacist, and inhalation therapist. Coordinates with physicians and charge nurse as needed.
   d. Supports philosophy of having ward clerks assume nonnursing activities by assisting with their training as needed on a daily basis to help them become proficient in their duties.
   e. Aggressively pursues having ward clerks do administrative tasks and nursing team members perform the primary functions of nursing. The latter most commonly occurs at patients' bedsides.
7. *Type of work:* Teaching patients
   Major duty: Teaches patients to care for themselves after discharge from the hospital (5% of working hours).
   a. Plans teaching as a major rehabilitation goal for each newly admitted patient. Includes it as part of nursing assessment and enters it on the nursing care plan.
   b. Reviews and updates teaching plans daily.
   c. Involves resource people in teaching program.
   d. Refers cases to visiting nurse for follow-up.
   e. Makes follow-up appointments for assessment of progress toward nursing goals with a clinical nurse.
   f. Involves families in teaching as indicated.

8. *Type of work:* Evaluation of care process
   Major duty: Conducts audits of nursing care (3% of working hours).
   a. Audits nursing records on a daily basis.
   b. Performs bedside audit on a weekly basis.
   c. Audits closed charts of discharged patients monthly.
   d. Reviews patient questionnaires.
   e. Discusses results of all audits with team members as a group and on an individual basis.
9. *Type of work:* Personnel administration
   Major duty: Rates performances of team members (2% of working hours).
   a. Writes performance reports.
   b. Discusses reports with individuals to learn their personal goals.
10. *Type of work:* Self-development
    Major duty: Pursues a program of continuing education activities (5% of working hours).
    a. Sets own goals for self-development, including a reading program and a set of educational goals for short courses, conventions, workshops, college courses, and management courses.
    b. Participates in division and departmental in-service education programs.
    c. Participates in nursing service committee activities.
    d. Participates in research projects.
    e. Participates as a citizen in the community through involvement in professional organizations and service projects.
    f. Assumes responsibility for knowledge of, progress in, and utilization of community resources such as:
       (i) Health groups
       (ii) Civic groups
       (iii) General education groups
       (iv) Nursing recruitment
       (v) Others

Job Analysis

Edwards and Sproull list objective performance dimensions developed by management and employees as a necessity for effective performance appraisal. These performance dimensions are developed from job analysis. "Performance criteria should be: (1) measurable through observation of behaviors of the job, (2) clearly defined, and (3) job-related." Nurse managers and nursing employees would agree on the meaning and priority of each measurement. These standards need not be quantifiable but must be keyed to observable behavior[28]:

Observable behavior ⟶ Job analysis ⟶ Job standards

Basing performance appraisal on job analysis makes it more relevant and establishes content validity.[29] Job analysis systematically gathers information about a particular job. It "identifies, specifies, organizes, and displays the duties, tasks, and responsibilities actually performed by the incumbent in a given job."[30] Job analysis begins with identification of the domain or universe of content to be measured. The domain or universe of content may be stated in terms of the tasks to be performed, the knowledge base required, the skills or abilities needed for the work, or personal characteristics deemed necessary.[31] Exhibit 28-2 is a format for gathering data for doing a job analysis.

Job analysis will reveal overlaps among jobs so that they can be modified. It can be used to improve efficiency and proficiency by identifying skills certification, altering staffing levels, reassigning staff, selecting new employees, altering management, establishing training

EXHIBIT 28-2
Job Analysis Questionnaire

TITLE: HEAD NURSE

Check here if you ever do the task in your present job:	Relative time spent <Lo><Avg><Hi>	Training emphasis <Lo><Avg><Hi>
_____ 1. (List DTRs)	123456789	123456789
_____ 2.		

objectives and standards, developing career ladders, and improving job satisfaction.[32]

A procedure for doing job analysis is as follows[33]:

1. Name the job specifically, for example, nurse manager—oncology.
2. Go to the workplace, identify the target nurses working in the job family, and talk to them. Ask these questions:
   a. What are the characteristics of a good nurse manager?
   b. What are the characteristics of a poor nurse manager?
   c. How does a good nurse manager differ from a poor nurse manager?
   d. How does a good nurse manager perform tasks better than others?
   e. Give examples of effective performance by a nurse manager.
   f. Why is this nurse manager effective?
   g. Give examples of ineffective performance by a nurse manager.
   h. Why is this nurse manager ineffective?
   i. Describe a nurse manager who performs the job better than anyone else. Why?
   j. Which job skills would you look for if you had to hire someone to be a nurse manager? Why?
   k. Describe the prior training or experience needed to effectively perform as a nurse manager. Why is this so?
3. Have the job incumbents list all duties, tasks, and responsibilities (DTRs) that they perform. Cover a specific time period.
4. List on index cards all DTRs that the job incumbents perform. Do this by observation for a specific time period that coincides with the period covered in item 3 above. DTRs can be listed one to each index card.
5. Compare the two lists, and aim for a consensus between job incumbents' lists and yours.
6. State the duties, tasks, and responsibilities in specific, clear, behavioral terms.
7. Determine the four to eight categories of job tasks to be used such as managerial, direct care, maintenance, and interpersonal.
8. Classify each DTR into the four to eight core job categories.
9. List the DTRs by priority, and use consensus to improve efficiency.
10. Evaluate DTRs for specificity, indicating how and when they will be performed.
11. Review DTRs with the team, eliminating those with low priority. Rewrite items as needed, making each a unique job skill stated in understandable language.
12. Set standards of performance, including the percentage of time each is to be done.
13. List constraints: education, experience, physical, and emotional.
14. Write a summary of the unique facets of the job.
15. Prepare a job analysis questionnaire and administer it to all personnel with the same job title. (See Exhibit 28-2.)

Research on job analysis information has shown no significant differences between effective and ineffective retail store managers. Research also has shown no significant differences among police officers between high-job-performers' perceptions of the demands of their jobs compared with low-job-performers' perceptions. Because these research studies are few, and inconclusive in relation to the literature on the subject, nursing researchers should do research in these areas. The described method of developing a master inventory of knowledge, skills, and abilities could be used to develop job analysis for other jobs.[34]

Recent downsizing and demassing of organizations have caused managers to plan and restructure the work of those employees remaining. This includes eliminating, simplifying, and combining steps, tasks, or jobs to make work easier and enjoyable. One goal is to reduce stress by eliminating unneeded rules, procedures, reviews, reports, and approvals.

Oryx, a Dallas-based oil and gas company, used teams to eliminate 25% of internal reports and reduced signatures for capital expenditures from 20 to four. It reduced the annual budget time from 7 months to 6 weeks and saved $70 million in operating costs in 1 year.

Another goal is to redesign physical work by analyzing jobs using the overall process described by Denton: observe and understand the current decision-making process; use a flow chart to document decisions; evaluate each decision-making step, both current and proposed; implement the change; and valuate the results after a reasonable time has passed. Money is saved by eliminating ineffective bureaucracy. Sometimes money is saved by adding employees and slowing the production process to improve quality.[35]

Motorola uses these six steps to achieve statistical process control[36]:

1. What do I do?
2. For whom do I work?
3. What do I need to do to do my work better?
4. How can I specifically design my work?
5. How can I do my work better?
6. Do benchmarking: Measure, analyze, and control the improvement process.

Job analysis is used to establish board certification in nursing specialties, ergonomic criteria for shift workers, licensure examination for registered nurses (NCLEX-RN), job descriptions for nurse editors, compensation systems, redesign for effective and efficient systems of care, and develop interviewing techniques for hiring the right applicants.[37]

Job analysis leads to a job description of the work expected by the institution, which can be used for PA.

Job Description

Job Description as a Contract

A job description is a contract that should include the job's functions and obligations and specify the person to whom the employee is responsible. It is a written report outlining duties, responsibilities, and conditions of the work assignment. It is a description of a job and not of a person who happens to hold that job. In 1966, Berenson and Ruhnke wrote[38]:

> That many executives recognize the importance of obtaining good position descriptions is reflected in a survey made several years ago by the American Management Association. In this study, seventy firms reported a median fee of $20,000 paid to management consultants for preparation of their job descriptions. Most significantly, 95 percent of the respondents reported that the expenditure was "definitely worthwhile." In two instances the fee paid for this service approached $100,000.

Most formats for job descriptions include a job title, statements of basic functions (one sentence), scope, duties, responsibilities (areas in which achievements are measured), organizational relationships (for communication),

limits of authority, and criteria for performance evaluation. Job descriptions should be one to two pages long.[39]

Use of Job Descriptions

Job descriptions are used for many purposes, including the following:

- Establishing a rational basis for the salary structure.
- Clarifying relationships among jobs.
- Helping analyze employees' duties.
- Defining the organizational structure and support.
- Reassigning and fixing functions and responsibilities in the entire agency.
- Evaluating job performance.
- Orienting new employees.
- Assisting with hiring and placement.
- Establishing lines of promotion.
- Identifying potential training needs.
- Critically reviewing the existing work practices within the agency.
- Maintaining continuity of all operations.
- Improving the work flow.
- Providing data as to proper channels of communication.
- Developing job specifications.
- Serving as a basis for planning staffing levels.

Many changes in the dynamic environment of a health care agency, such as changes in personnel, departmental or agency objectives, budget, and technology, create the need for periodic review and revision of job descriptions. Time should not be wasted preparing job descriptions that will not be put to use. Job descriptions should be available to all personnel so that they will know the dimensions of their jobs, who in the agency can help them in their work, how their performances will be evaluated, and the opportunities for advancement. To make the data more useful, numerical values may be assigned to the important elements of the specific duties, as in Exhibit 28-1.

To avoid bias, data for job descriptions should be gathered from several sources. Data may be collected by interviewing the job incumbent, having an incumbent keep a log of duties performed during a specific time period, observing the person, and having the person fill out a questionnaire (job analysis).

Role development of nurse specialists is defined in evolving job descriptions of practice from novice to expert. This role development is being shaped by health care policy, particularly that related to managed care; available resources; increased job complexity; and relationships between job satisfaction and organizational climate. The new career models are founded on self-responsibility, entrepreneurial aptitude, vision, and personal empowerment. The case manager nurse of the twenty-first century is forward-thinking, flexible, and solution-oriented.[40]

The person preparing the job descriptions should determine the uses that will be made of them so the needed information may be included. It is probably best to introduce job descriptions during a time of favorable economic outlook when this action will be less threatening to employees. Job descriptions should be introduced to the staff registered nurses first. Managers may fear increased work loads and grievances. It is important to consult with all employees and allow them to discuss, comment on, and recommend changes in the job descriptions for positions. Doing so makes development of job descriptions a cooperative venture, leading to consensus, effective management, and effective performance appraisal. Language used in the job descriptions should be simple and understandable.

Because job descriptions are guides, rigid application can result in negative behavior.

Job descriptions should define minimum standards for effective job performance and employment and should not be too detailed. The catch-all phrase, "Performs other duties as directed" is evasive and should not be put into a job description.

A format is needed for quality and thoroughness of job descriptions. Kennedy recommends the following 11 elements[41]:

1. Header: job title, name and location of incumbent, immediate superiors.
2. Principle purpose or summary; overall contribution of incumbent.
3. Principal responsibilities, including percentage of time spent on each.

4. Job skills: knowledge, skills, and education.
5. Dimension or scope: quantifies areas such as the budget, size of reporting organizations, and impact on the bottom line.
6. Organizational chart.
7. Problem-solving examples.
8. Environment.
9. Key contacts.
10. References guiding the incumbent's actions.
11. Supervision given and received.

Job descriptions can be written to comply with some legal, regulatory, and accrediting requirements, and used to do the following[42]:

1. Meet the licensing laws of the state, rules of accrediting agencies, and Medicare and Medicaid regulations.
2. Determine job ratings and classifications.
3. Determine whether jobs are exempt or nonexempt.
4. Recruit, select, evaluate, and retain employees.

Exhibit 28-3 presents a job description for a bedside nurse in a U.S. hospital around 1887. Exhibit 28-4 is a current job description for a generalized clinical nurse.

Performance Appraisal and Job Descriptions

Tom Peters has a low opinion of job descriptions.[43]

Performance appraisal should be ongoing, based on a simple, written "contract" between the person being appraised and his or her boss. Limit objectives to no more than three per period (quarter, year). Eliminate job descriptions.

Performance appraisal, the setting of objectives, and job descriptions are control devices. As such, they

---

EXHIBIT 28-3

1887 Job Description

In its publication, *Bright Corridor*, Cleveland's Lutheran Hospital published this job description for a bedside nurse in a U.S. hospital in 1887.

In addition to caring for your fifty patients, each bedside nurse will follow these regulations:

1. Daily sweep and mop the floors of your ward; dust the patient's furniture and window sills.
2. Maintain an even temperature in your ward by bringing in a scuttle of coal for the day's business.
3. Light is important to observe the patient's condition. Therefore, each day fill kerosene lamps, clean chimneys, and trim wicks. Wash the windows once a week.
4. The nurse's notes are important in aiding the physician's work. Make your pens carefully; you may whittle nibs to your individual tastes.
5. Each nurse on day duty will report every day at 7:00 A.M. and leave at 8:00 P.M., except on the Sabbath, on which day you will be off from 12:00 noon to 2:00 P.M.

6. Graduate nurses in good standing with the director of nursing will be given an evening off each week for courting purposes, or two a week if you go regularly to church.
7. Each nurse should lay aside from each payday a goodly sum of [her] earnings for her benefits during her declining years, so that she will not become a burden. For example, if you earn $30 a month you should set aside $15.
8. Any nurse who smokes, uses liquor in any form, gets her hair done at a beauty shop, or frequents dance halls will give the director of nurses good reason to suspect her worth, intentions, and integrity.
9. The nurse who performs her labors, serves her patients and doctors faithfully and without fault for a period of 5 years will be given an increase by the hospital administration of $.05 a day, providing there are no hospital debts that are outstanding.

EXHIBIT 28-4
Position Description
TITLE: GENERALIZED CLINICAL NURSE (GCN)

General Description. The GCN is a professional nurse with academic preparation at the BSN level or above, who provides expert nursing care based on scientific principles; delivers direct patient care and serves as a consultant or technical advisor in the area of health professions; and serves as a role model in the leadership, management, and delivery of quality nursing care by integrating the role components of clinician, administrator, teacher, consultant, and researcher.

Qualifications

1. Educational
   a. Graduation from an accredited school of nursing.
   b. Bachelor of Science in Nursing degree required.
2. Personal and professional
   a. Current state professional nursing license.
   b. Knowledge of and experience in preventive care (screening and teaching).
   c. Demonstrated knowledge and competence in nursing, communication, and leadership skills.
   d. Ability to analyze situations, recognize problems, search for pertinent facts, and make appropriate decisions.
   e. Ability to coordinate orientation and continuing education of clinic staff utilizing appropriate teaching strategies.
   f. Ability to apply principles of change, organizational theory, and decision-making.
   g. Membership and participation in professional organizations desirable.
   h. Recognition of civic responsibilities of nursing.
   i. Ability to communicate effectively both in writing and verbally.
   j. Evidence of professional manner and conduct.
   k. Optimum physical and emotional health.

Organizational Relationships. The GCN is administratively responsible and accountable to the nurse administrator. He or she is responsible for assessing, teaching, coordinating, providing appropriate care, and making referrals when necessary.

Activities

1. Clinician
   a. Give direct patient care in selected patient situations and serve as a behavioral model for excellence in practice.
   b. Assist the nursing personnel in assessing individual patient needs and formulation of a plan of nursing care; write nursing orders, when appropriate, for implementation of nursing plan; assist the nursing personnel in documenting the effectiveness of the individualized care.
   c. Set, evaluate, and re-evaluate standards of nursing practice; communicate these standards to the nursing personnel; change standards as necessary.
   d. Evaluate nursing care given to patients within the clinical area (assessing and teaching); when appropriate, make recommendations for improvement of that care.
   e. Function as a change agent; identify the barriers to more comprehensive health care delivery, modify behavior, and introduce new approaches to patient care.
   f. Collaborate with other health care providers and make appropriate referrals when necessary.

2. Teacher
   a. Provide an atmosphere conducive to learning.
   b. Teach appropriate preventive measures to clients.
   c. Direct the orientation of new staff and student nurses to ease their role transition and improve their skills, attitudes, and practices.
   d. Consider the needs of the adult learners (nursing personnel) as well as the clinicians' knowledge and expertise when planning continuing education to the clinical practice.
   e. Initiate or assist with the planning, presenting, and evaluating continuing education programs for clinic staff.
   f. Guide and assist staff and nursing students as they assume the responsibility of patient teaching.

3. Administrator
   a. Function as a change agent and appraise leadership, communication, and change processes in the organization and assist with direct strategies for change as necessary.
   b. Work collaboratively with hospital personnel and other health care providers in planning care and making referrals.
   c. Make recommendations relative to improving patient care and staff and student requirements to the appropriate administrative personnel.
   d. Support and interpret the clinical policies and procedures.

4. Self-Development
   a. Assume responsibility for identifying own educational needs and upgrade deficit areas through independent study, seminar attendance, or requesting staff development programs.
   b. Evaluate own nursing practice and instruction of others and the effect these have on the quality of patient care.

5. Consultant
   a. Conduct informal conferences with nursing personnel concerning patient care of specific health problems,

(continued)

EXHIBIT 28-4 *(continued)*

the problem patient, or other pertinent problems related to nursing as suggested by the staff.

b. Assist personnel to develop awareness of community agencies/resources available in planning patient care.

c. Serve as a resource person to patients and their families.

6. Researcher

a. Determine research problems related to preventive care, nursing clinics, and so on.

b. Conduct research studies to upgrade independent nursing practice.

c. Demonstrate knowledge of the current research applicable to the clinical area, and apply this knowledge in nursing care when appropriate.

d. Research clinical nursing problems through the development and testing of relevant theories, evaluation, and implementation of research findings for nursing practice.

e. Promote interest in reading and reviewing of current publications dealing with the delivery of preventive care to ambulatory patients.

---

are increasingly bureaucratic, run by "experts," and out of touch with the world of human relations, because they promote stability at the expense of flexibility. Most job descriptions are not read or adhered to by successful workers. The alternative is coaching and teaching values.[44]

Job Evaluation

Job evaluation is a process used to measure exact amounts of base elements found in a job. Laws require men and women to be paid equally for equal work requiring equal skill, knowledge, effort, and responsibility under similar working conditions. This factor is important in the fight to achieve pay equity for women and hence for nurses.[45]

Job evaluation rates jobs within a given agency. Although several job evaluation systems exist, The Hay Job Evaluation System is the best known. It was developed in 1951 by the Hay Group, a Philadelphia-based consulting firm, to approve managerial, technical, and professional positions.[46]

The Hay System attempts to measure exact amounts of base elements found in all jobs, including know-how, problem-solving, and accountability. Know-how includes practical procedures, specialized techniques, scientific disciplines, managerial know-how, and human relations skills. Problem-solving includes the thinking challenge created by the environment. Accountability includes freedom to act, input of the job on the corporation, and the magnitude of the job. Observations of use of the Hay System indicate that the percentage of specialized know-how decreases with high-level positions, leaving problem-solving and accountability to be the real pay-off factors.[47]

Work Classification

Helton reports a system for work classification to improve white-collar work. The system includes four categories: specialist, professional, support, and clerical. Professional and specialist jobs involve a significant amount of cognitive effort, are not routine, and are challenging. Criteria used to classify white-collar work are work range, work structure, control, and cognitive effort. Applied to nursing, the nurse with a master's degree would be a specialist; the nurse with a baccalaureate degree a professional, the nurse with a diploma, an associate degree, or a licensed practical nurse a support person; and aides and clerks equivalent to clerical workers. It would be economical to develop or integrate aides and clerks into one job classification.[48]

Job redesign uses job enlargement and job enrichment. Job enlargement uses horizontal loading to add tasks of equal difficulty and responsibility to jobs. Job enrichment uses vertical loading to add tasks that increase the difficulty and responsibility of jobs. Job enlargement and job enrichment have beneficial results, including increased productivity. In 32 experiments involving job redesign, 30 indicated impact; the median increase in productivity was 6.4%. Employee satisfaction increased in 20 cases and was tied to more pay for increased work, plus less supervision and more worker autonomy.

To make job redesign effective, nurse managers need to make accurate diagnosis and real job changes. They need to address technological and personnel system constraints; support autonomy; have a bureaucratic climate; have union cooperation and top management and supervising management support; have individuals ready to fill the jobs; and have contextual satisfaction with pay, supervision, promotion opportunities, and coworkers.[49]

> **Some persons indicate that autonomy and bureaucracy are incompatible; however, bureaucratic activities that support professional nurses' autonomy are desirable.**

Work Redesign

Work redesign needs to encompass the entire nursing care system. Work redesign should incorporate cultural issues, management structure, practice patterns, task and operating system alignment, and commitment to continuous quality improvement. Work redesign is serious work.[50]

A hostile internal culture fostering competition depresses performance because players tend to attempt to beat rivals rather than perform tasks well. The weaker party may give up while the stronger one feels dangerously invincible. Friendly competition is replaced by mistrust, suspicion, and scorn. Change the environment to one of cooperation and higher performance. Outside competition can stimulate employees.[51]

Other suggestions for work redesign include[52]:

- Define the existing culture; identify the desired culture. Identify gaps, and plan to close them consistent with the vision and strategies of the health care system.
- Change structures to those that facilitate autonomy, multidisciplinary teams, new work designs, and participation in reward and risk.
- Change unwanted patient outcomes by identifying and changing practices and processes that create them.
- Because treatment design drives work redesign, gather and analyze data about treatment types and number.
- Redesign operating policies, systems, and jobs. Assess all of them using teams of practitioners who decide which to eliminate, modify, or add. Assess everything.
- Create a customer-supplier model of quality improvement to provide quality and quantity of products and services that customers want. Consider all of these as management work.

Training

Nurse managers should be educated to do effective PAs that will maintain employee productivity. Training will entail coverage of subjects such as motivational environment, appropriate job assignment, proper supervision, establishing job expectancies, appropriate job training, interpersonal relationships, providing feedback, interviewing, coaching, counseling, and PA methods.

Training raters makes PA work. The goal of such training is improved productivity. A training program can give nurse managers a conceptual understanding of PA as a management system for transmitting, reinforcing, and rewarding the behaviors desired by the organ-

ization. Raters need to know how PAs will be used. Research indicates that raters have been found to vary ratings depending on their use. Refresher training is recommended after 1 year. PA training can be conducted with other management development programs.[53]

An effective appraisal system will have an objective, reliable method to evaluate whether raters are qualified. Training of raters should focus on specific evaluating errors. Research indicates that rater training decreases accuracy because the raters become more sensitive to typical rating error and change their responses, thus creating new errors. Training programs should be designed to increase awareness of this fact and correct for it. Raters will be trained to capture all components of an individual's contribution to the organization, including qualitative behavior. All behavior does not reduce to quantitatively measurable performance.[54]

Training based on feedback is specific. Train the raters in behavior observation, documentation of critical performance incidents that support the consensus of a team evaluation, sensitivity to employees in legally protected categories, and performance criteria.[55]

Feedback

Feedback was discussed in Chapter 20, Communication. An analysis of 69 articles reporting 126 experiments in which feedback was applied indicated that feedback with goal setting, behavioral consequences, or both was much more consistently effective than was feedback alone. Daily and weekly feedback produced more consistent effects than did monthly feedback. Also, feedback accompanied by money or fringe benefits of food and gasoline produced improvements in behavior more often than did praise. Graphs were the feedback mechanism producing the highest proportion of consistent effects. The conclusion is that feedback graphically presented at least weekly along with tangible rewards yields effective work performance.[56]

Training will include providing specific feedback to raters on timeliness, completeness, rating errors, and quality and consistency of ratings. Training methods include case studies, role plays, behavioral modeling, discussion, and writing exercises that evaluate actual appraisals, relating them to job descriptions.[57]

Feedback closes the loops by tying together the appraisal process. Feedback informs the ratee of achievements compared with expectations. It must be timely, constructive, and objective, and ensure that the ratee knows and can respond. The goal is to have good results continue by eliminating frustrations, which lead to lowering of goals and performance.[58]

Rater feedback from team evaluation consensus addresses systematic inconsistencies, including unlawful bias. Correction by feedback creates improved accuracy of the system, improved morale, increased worth, and increased productivity. Team evaluation consensus identifies inaccurate raters for directed training or elimination as raters.[59]

Feedback can be provided through coaching, counseling, and interviewing.

Coaching

The appraisal rater is a leader and a coach. Coaching for job performance is similar to coaching for athletic performance. As a coach, the rater does continuous reinforcement of tasks done well and helps with other tasks. In addition, the rater uses knowledge of adult education to train the employees to accomplish assigned work, does two-way communication, and has the necessary resources to do the job.

Coaching can include observing and listening for examples of work, good or bad. The rater coach praises the good and helps improve the bad with a joint action plan. Coaching makes performance evaluation useful.[60]

Coaching is yearlong evaluation and discussion of performance, which eliminates surprises. Progress discussions can be brief, regular, frank, open, and factual and can include the employee's viewpoint. The rater does not try to achieve truth but tries to discuss perceptions. The coach also removes obstacles to satisfactory performance. If the consequences are not working to improve unsatisfactory performance, the coach changes them. The ultimate resort is to transfer or terminate the employee.[61]

Progressive discipline protects the employer from unwarranted liability resulting from discrimination charges and lawsuits but fails to bring about behavioral change in employees to make them fully functioning, committed team members. Employees already perceive PA to be evaluative and judgmental, not developmental. Progressive discipline combined with performance evaluation results in compliant employees. Effective leaders are coaches who gain commitment from employees. Today's employees will put forth effort if stimulated, challenged, and recognized for their efforts. They do not want to be managed; therefore, managers must manage, lead, and coach.

Coaching prevents discipline. The nurse manager as coach is available to observe behavior, provide feedback, and encourage employees to do their best. Coaching is done on a regular basis and is nonjudgmental. Employees believe the coach manager is supporting them to do better, to be successful, to excel.

The following are some characteristics of an effective manager–coach[62]:

- Listens.
- Views the employee as a person.
- Cares about the employee and helps with personal problems.
- Sets a good example.
- Stretches the employee.
- Encourages the employee.
- Helps get the work done.
- Keeps the employee informed.
- Praises the employee for a job well done, and provides criticism in a forthright manner.

An employee, who can do the job as if his or her life depended on it, but does not, needs coaching. Coaching is personal. It is a process that involves time, interviews, observation, feedback, and help to make employees successful. The process may be repeated as necessary.

A written coaching plan is helpful. It should be positive and upbeat. The manager writes the suggestions to be used for employee improvement. These suggestions should not be overstated but should describe behaviors, not characteristics. Appropriate alternative behaviors should be included in all coaching plans and sessions. The rater observes and gives feedback to correct wrong behavior or reinforce improvements by praise, factoring him or herself into the problem as a possible contributor to it. Coaching should be done frequently and feedback given immediately with incremental changes so that employees are not stretched to the breaking point. The goal is to build a relationship that helps an employee do a good job or move on.[63]

Counseling

Counseling can be the most productive function of supervision. Counseling interviews are for the purpose of advising and assisting an individual to grow and develop self-direction, self-discipline, and individual responsibility. The counseling interview is a helping relationship involving direct interaction between the counselor (rater) and the counselee (ratee). In a counseling interview, a personal face-to-face relationship takes place. One person helps another recognize, accept, examine, and solve a certain problem.

Nurse managers can use the counseling interview to offer support and to:

- Help workers develop realistic pictures of themselves, their abilities, their potential, and their deficiencies.
- Explore courses of action.
- Explore sources of assistance.
- Accept incontestable limitations and learn to live with them, whether physical, emotional, or intellectual.
- Make choices and improve capabilities.

Unless they have had special training, most nurse managers are not qualified for in-depth, extensive counseling in areas involving personality structure or analysis of psychological or emotional conditions. Nurse managers must beware of tampering with the psyche of the worker. In such cases, nurse managers should know and be able to recommend sources of help.

Although counseling interviews are conducted to promote desirable behavior, the term *counseling* should not be used synonymously with the term *reprimand*. Reprimands belong more properly in the progress and informational type of interview.

One often hears supervisors say, "I have counseled him on what will happen if he does not improve." This is not counseling; this is informing a worker of the consequences of certain types of behavior or performance.

Three approaches can be used for the counseling interview: directive, nondirective, and elective. When using the directive approach, the interviewer knows in advance what will be discussed. In this approach, the interviewer gives advice, makes suggestions, helps the individual make meaningful decisions, and may even take action on some of the decisions made. This approach can be quite successful in career counseling.

The nondirective approach starts with the individual being counseled on strengths and weaknesses, potential, and problems. The individual takes responsibility for solving the problems; the counselor aids by listening. This approach is ideal for personal counseling but requires skill. The person being counseled says what he or she wants and freely expresses feelings; the interviewer must hide personal feelings and not express personal ideas. The counselor is a mirror only, reflecting the thoughts, ideas, and emotions of the counselee. This technique gives the individual an opportunity to think through problems out loud. Usually the employee will come up with some kind of answer or course of action. In using the nondirective approach, it is most important that there be no interruptions or advice on a course of action.

With the exception of the preemployment interview, it is advisable to keep notes during the interview and write a summary afterward. The summary should indicate any decisions made during the interview and any follow-up action required. A comment should be made in terms of how well the interview accomplished its purpose. No notes should be taken during the preemployment interview, although a summary of the interview and the decision reached should be written up immediately afterward. Taking notes during the interview discourages the applicant and makes it difficult to obtain the information needed.

Career progression depends on present and past duty performance, personal initiative, motivation, professional development, and growth potential. Performance counseling of subordinates is vitally important so they will know where they stand, how well they are doing, and where they can improve. The goal of this counseling is to improve present and future performance, not make a critical examination of the past. The informal day-to-day performance counseling dealing with current activities and immediate performance is important and must be continuous; however, it is not enough. Planned, careful performance counseling, scheduled at regular intervals, is needed to encourage self-improvement and further development. During the counseling interview, the supervisor and subordinate work together to set targets in response to the job description requirements and targets for future job progression. The targets are put into writing, and progress is reviewed at the next session.

Performance counseling results from observation and evaluation of performance based on job standards. Anecdotal records may be kept and will yield facts to support written ratings or reports.

When counseling employees on performance problems the rater uses a problem-solving approach. Such an approach includes reaching agreement that a problem exists, discussing alternative solutions, agreeing on a solution, and following up on progress.[64]

Interviewing

Interviewing is covered in Chapter 8, Human Resource Management Activities. For appraisal interviews, the problem-solving approach is also more effective than are tell-and-see and tell-and-listen methods. High ratee participation produces greater rater satisfaction. The problem-solving rater has a helpful and constructive attitude, does mutual goal setting with the ratee, and focuses on solutions to problems. The rater also acts with the knowledge that being very critical does not improve behaviors.[65]

Good performance appraisal interviews follow these basic guidelines[66]:

- They are based on detailed, specific notes that address accomplishments and shortcomings.
- They produce no surprises from the coach.
- The drafted appraisal is discussed with the ratee and then finalized.
- Work is started and ended with positive accomplishments.
- Needed changes are specified.
- Criticism is respectful.
- Written responses are allowed.
- Staff members are invited to assess the manager's performance.

Topics for performance appraisal review include the following[67]:

- Regular job duties (based on job description).
- Special assignments and miscellaneous projects.
- Service and professional development.
- Working relations.
- Communication skills.

Peer Ratings

Research has shown that an individual's peers, that is, those people the individual works with from day to day, are a more reliable source for identifying the capacity for leadership than are the person's superiors. The armed services have found that peer nominations for leadership are significant predictors of future performance, a finding that could be tested in the nursing population. Democratic procedures, that is, having peers select the person to be promoted, would probably be threatening to many nurse managers. It has been found that peer selection differs little from selections by superiors. Occasionally, peers see a member of their group as a leader when superiors do not. Peer rating is valid when the group members have sufficient interaction and when group membership is reasonably stable over time. Peer rating is also valid if the position is important within the organization. Peer rating does help to identify potential leaders who go unnoticed by superiors. When several individuals are equally qualified for a position, peer ratings may single out the one with the highest informal leadership status.[68]

Peer evaluation may begin in high school with the Peer and Self-Evaluation System (PSES).[69] Peer rating is the professional model of appraisal used by physicians and is gaining interest and use among professional nurses. Peer rating is advocated as part of a system to make PAs more objective, the theory being that multiple ratings will give a more objective appraisal. Ratings can be obtained from multiple managers, project leaders, peers, and even patients.[70]

Peer review is a PA process among persons with similar competencies who are in active practice. These persons critically review the practice of others using established standards of performance.[71] It is self-regulation and supports the principle of autonomy.[72] It consists of colleagues examining the goal-directed care of colleagues with standards that are specific, critical indicators of care written by colleagues.[73]

The purposes of peer review are to measure accountability, evaluate and improve delivery of care, identify strengths and weaknesses, develop new or altered policies, identify a worker's need for more knowledge (competence), increase workers' self-awareness from feedback (critical reflection), and increase professionalism.[74]

Implementation of a peer review rating or evaluation system includes the following[75]:

- Planning by management and clinical nurses. It may be a steering committee representing these categories of nurses plus those from the domains of research and education.
- Having a shared governance type of environment.
- Defining the peer review process and who is a peer.
- Setting goals.
- Outlining the process through consultation with management, HR personnel, and a labor attorney. A decision is made as to who gathers the data. It can be the employee, with a clinical nurse specialist as coordinator. Decisions are also made as to when and how often the interview will be done and how the outcome will be handled.
- Developing a tool using the job description.
- Obtaining multiple inputs: peer reports, self-reports, and coach reports. The manager acts as coach and counselor.

The peer review process may be developed using three distinct phases of establishing a peer review program: familiarization, utilization, and internalization.[76] The phases are outlined in Exhibit 28-5.

A new performance evaluation system is needed for flattened organizations with only one manager for 30 to 100 employees. Peer evaluation meets this need and

---

EXHIBIT 28-5
Three Phases of Peer Review

PHASE I: FAMILIARIZATION
Characterized by the development of trust, the talking through of the process and its related problems, and the realization that performance, not human worth, is being evaluated.

PHASE II: UTILIZATION
Marked by trial-and-error responses. Objectives are refined. Colleagues become more open with each other. The peer review process takes a sharper focus.

PHASE III: INTERNALIZATION
Occurs with complete actualization of the entire peer review process. Staff no longer feel threatened. Objectives are well-defined. On-site, hands-on evaluations are conducted, charts audited, and results discussed in peer review conferences. If indicated, findings are acted on.

Source: M. E. Jacobs and J. D. Vail. "Quality Assurance: A Unit-Based Plan." *Journal of the Association of Nurse Anesthetists* (June 1986), 265–271. Reprinted with permission.

when done within a team should be anonymous. Peers are more knowledgeable of each other's performance. Peer review can improve teamwork. Rigg recommends using one rating category of overall capability, with a bell-shaped curve ranking criteria. Written comments are made for only those results falling outside the range.[77]

Peer review can be taught using videotapes developed locally. Studies of peer review indicate that professional nurses view it favorably, although some consider it a threat to friendship, time-consuming, and artificially inflated. It does not always change the level of staff satisfaction with PAs. Because nurses are more often directly accountable to their employers than to their customers, peer review requires strong management support.[78]

A survey of advanced practice nurses indicated peers evaluated only 17.5% with the most frequent evaluation parameters being appropriateness of care, patient satisfaction, patient outcomes, and patient volumes. Patient outcomes fell into four categories: clinical end points, complications, compliance, and functional status.[79]

Appendix 28-1 is a peer review evaluation tool.

Self-Rating

Self-rating is another method of performance appraisal that is little used. In the Fortune 1300 study, immediate supervisors did 96% of appraisals.[80] Problems with self-raters are the same as with supervisor raters, indicating the need for training of both.[81]

Employee-developed PAs have been found to be tougher than those of supervisors. Employees are the subject-matter experts and do wider coverage of their jobs. Proactive, they establish expectations beforehand. Appraisal interviews are done after self-evaluation, with a common agenda and without surprises; therefore, conversations are more productive. Objectives are under the employee's control. Because they come from employees and supervisors, the job elements and performance indicators are legally defensible and broad in perspective, and elicit employee commitment.[82]

Self-evaluation can be developed by using small groups. Having a good job description facilitates development of good behavioral expectation appraisal forms that become customized for each position. The HR department can provide a facilitator and other support. Questions that will facilitate performance indicators are[83]:

- Think of who has been most effective at this element or task. What behaviors and results can you cite to support your choice?

- Think of the behaviors or results that made you say to yourself, "It would be good if everyone did that."
- What are the tricks of the trade related to this task or element?
- Think about times when you perform this task well and other times when you are not as successful. What causes the difference?
- How is the average performer different from the excellent one?
- If you were training someone, what would you emphasize?

Self-rating has been found to be threatening because the employee must place him or herself in view of others. Self-rating is a participatory management approach supported by research. Employees who view the organization as being open are more favorable to participating in PAs.[84]

Employees can be trained to research their own performance and the work environment. They can do self-assessments of and then analyze goals and expectations. Employees can also be trained to influence management communication skills to obtain information and advice, express their needs, and learn the style of influence to use on the manager. Thus, employees become protégés of proactive performers.[85]

Although self-appraisals increase employee understanding of performance feedback and provide unique information, they are little used. To be effective, self-evaluation should measure similar attitudes, as do evaluations by supervisors. Self-appraisals should measure actual performance, relate to same time period as the criterion, be done by individuals who are experienced in self-evaluation, and be tied to a criterion group (coworkers).

Somers and Birnbaum studied a sample of 198 staff nurses in a large urban hospital. They found "no evidence of leniency error or restriction of range in self-appraisal job performance." Convergence between self- and supervisory ratings was also evident and was interpreted as an effect of *halo error*, that is, a tendency to rate all employees as outstanding. Self-rating requires employees be trained in its use and a focus on core job skills to make it work.[86]

A two-part format for self- and peer evaluation is depicted in Appendix 28-1. The objective of the emergency medical services unit using this format was to determine competence. Qualification for peer evaluation included the amount of time peers worked together. Results indicated the following[87]:

- Peers rated partners higher than partners rated themselves in intubation, ECG recognition, advanced cardiac life support, skills as an emergency medical technician (EMT)–paramedic, and skills as an EMT–ambulance.

- Self-ratings were higher than were peer ratings in communication, scene management, trauma, patient assessment, and report-rating skills, which are more subjective areas.
- Both peer and self-ratings indicated that patients who were system abusers received the lowest quality of care and that the higher the socioeconomic group the better was the care received.

Research indicates that employee ratings do not differ by age; however, supervisors may view the capabilities of younger employees more positively than those of older employees.[88]

Peer and supervisor ratings have been found to be relatively highly correlated; self-supervisor and self-peer ratings are only moderately correlated. In an assessment center study, peer evaluations were better predictors of subsequent job advancement than were other ratings, including self-ratings. Peer and self-ratings predicted management potential. Behavioral information was important to peer and self-evaluation.[89]

Other Rating Methodologies

Other rating methodologies are less common than are supervisor, peer, and self-ratings. Other rating methods include team evaluation consensus (TEC), behavior-anchored rating scales (BARS), and task-oriented performance evaluation system (TOPES). These methodologies measure job-related behaviors.

Team Evaluation Consensus, or TEC

Team evaluation consensus uses multiple raters, a method claimed to minimize rater bias and inaccuracies. TEC uses peers, managers, and immediate supervisors for a total of two to eight raters. Direct comparisons are made with other employees or with performance benchmarks of "outstanding" or "consistently exceeds."[90]

Behavior-Anchored Rating Scales, or BARS

Behavior-anchored rating scales list specific descriptors of good, average, and poor performance for each of several to many job aspects. Extensive analysis is required to develop these descriptions, making them time-consuming and difficult to develop. Returns are small.[91]

Descriptions of particular jobs are used to identify key job elements. Key job elements are used to develop descriptive statements of good and bad behavior. An individual's behavior is rated by closeness to behavior descriptions for key job elements (performance dimensions). Job elements, in turn, lead to behavior descriptions for each category of excellent, good, average, poor, and unacceptable, and finally lead to rating of an individual's behavior.

Raters and ratees develop the description list. Personnel time makes BARS expensive to develop. There is no composite performance score. The system is defensible in court. There have been favorable employee response and performance improvement. The results of BARS are more realistic because this system is less threatening than are most PA systems. See Exhibit 28-6 for an example of BARS performance dimensions.[92]

EXHIBIT 28-6
Behavior-Anchored Rating Scales (BARS) Performance Dimension: Patient Relations

Excellent	1. Employee always treats patients with dignity and cheerfulness, respecting their individual needs while performing professional duties. Employee receives frequent favorable comments from patients under his or her care.
Good	2. Employee treats patients with dignity and respect without becoming involved in their individual problems. Employee receives occasional favorable comments from patients.
Average	3. Employee is impersonal with patients, tending their medical needs but avoiding personal interaction. Employee is the subject of few comments by patients.
Poor	4. Employee becomes impatient with patients and is concerned more about performing his or her tasks than being of assistance to patient's nonmedical needs. Employee generates some complaints from patients.
Unacceptable	5. Employee is antagonistic toward patients, treating them as obstacles or annoyances rather than individuals. Employee generates frequent complaints from patients and causes them considerable upset.

Source: S. C. Bushardt and A. R. Fowler, Jr. "Performance Evaluation Alternatives." *Journal of Nursing Administration* (October 1988), 42. Reprinted with permission of J. B. Lippincott.

Task-Oriented Performance Evaluation System, or TOPES

The task-oriented performance evaluation system concentrates on job tasks rather than behavior, although it is behaviorally based because it measures task accomplishments. TOPES is also legally defensible because it relates directly to the job. Job tasks are weighted for a composite performance score. Employees can be compared across jobs. TOPES is more objective than are other methodologies because it can be used to measure quantifiable performance. Task elements are evaluated by statements that support an excellent, good, average, weak, or unacceptable rating. The score on each task is multiplied by its weight, and scores are added for a composite score.[93] See Exhibit 28-7 for a TOPES task scale.

Problem Areas in Performance Evaluation

It is largely assumed that merit-rating systems of performance evaluation help to develop subordinates and attest to their readiness for pay increases, promotions, selected assignments, or penalties. When such systems have been scrutinized, three main problem areas have been found[94]:

1. Subordinates have not been motivated to want to change.
2. Even when people recognize a need for change, they are unable to do so.
3. Subordinates become resentful and anxious when the merit system is conscientiously implemented.

Effectiveness

Contrast two situations in which the same job standards are applied. In the first situation, the subordinate is handed a completed rating form and is told to read and sign it. She does so but immediately appeals to the next highest level of supervision. The subordinate says that this rating is the lowest she has received in her 15-year career and that she has never been told the quality of her performance was slipping. Although the situation is resolved in favor of the subordinate, she is no longer satisfied to work for the supervisor and must be transferred.

In the other situation, the job standards are discussed with the subordinate before they are used. The subordinate is asked to identify those performance factors and responsibilities that are really important to the success of the unit. She is asked also to write out the goals of her job as she sees them. The goals are fully discussed between the supervisor and subordinate. Progress is discussed at the request of the subordinate and at stated intervals. As a result, the subordinate is assisted in planning educational activities that she will accomplish in preparation for the career she desires.

Which of the two situations meets the criterion of an effective PA?

Weaknesses

Many pitfalls and deficiencies exist in the PA process. Many managers defend PA as a system for improving performance. As used, it probably has negative influences because most people know their shortcomings better than does a supervisor. Criticisms by people who have not been adequately trained to manage an appraisal system cause employees to be anxious and frustrated, to feel themselves failures, and, in some cases, to withdraw.

The rater is influenced by the most recent period of performance, an influence that may be positive or negative. Without objective measurements and records, raters tend to focus on the few outstanding activities

EXHIBIT 28-7
Task Scale: Generic

Excellent	5. Performance of this task is superior in nature leaving little or no room for improvement. An individual performing at this level is eligible for the maximum individual rewards available.
Good	4. Performance is better than that of the average employee but does allow for improvement. An employee performing at this level is eligible for moderate individual rewards.
Average	3. Performance is acceptable, meeting the basic requirement of the task involved but leaving substantial room for improvement. An average employee is eligible for system but not individual rewards.
Weak	2. Performance is barely adequate to meet task requirements. It needs substantial improvement in quality and/or efficiency. An employee performing at this level is not eligible for any rewards.
Unacceptable	1. Performance fails to meet minimum standards and must be immediately improved. Failure to improve will subject the employee to disciplinary action and eventual dismissal.

Source: S. C. Bushardt and A. R. Fowler, Jr. "Performance Evaluation Alternatives." *Journal of Nursing Administration* (October 1988), 43. Reprinted with permission of J. B. Lippincott.

that are vivid in their minds. Personal feelings can influence raters, causing positive "halo" or negative "horns" effects. In many instances, the performance is appraised without clear job definitions, job descriptions, and job standards. The employee seldom knows the yardsticks by which performance is being measured. Raters are either lenient or tough, causing a great variance in value judgments. Attitudes about whether the employee deserves a pay increase influence the rater. Some managers believe that all employees are average, and they project their beliefs by rating everyone the same.[95]

Other rating errors include the following:

- Leniency–stringency error. The rater tends to assign extreme ratings of either poor or excellent.
- Similar-to-me error. The rater rates according to how he or she views him or herself.
- Central tendency error. All ratings are at the middle of the scale.
- First impression error. The rater views early behavior that may be good or bad and rates all subsequent behaviors similarly.

Other problems of PA include racial bias, focus on longevity, and complacency of managers. In their usual form, PAs are intrinsically confrontational, emotional, judgmental, and complex. A survey of 360 managers in 190 corporations on the PA process indicated the following[96]:

- 69% viewed objectives as unclear.
- 40% saw some payoff.
- 29% saw minimal benefits.
- 45% were only partially involved in setting objectives for their own performance.
- 81% said regular progress reviews were not conducted.
- 52% said guidelines for collecting performance data were haphazard or nonexistent.
- Only 19% viewed PA as properly planned.
- Only 37% viewed meetings as highly productive.
- 30% saw no worthwhile results.

Performance appraisals are extrinsically affected when format is improper due to lack of manager preparation, confusion about objectives, once-a-year activity; and overreliance on forms. There also is the extrinsic area of inappropriate values and attitudes: avoidance of conflict to avoid unpleasantness; lack of respect by failing to take the appraisal seriously; and misuse of power, causing the ratee to be beaten down, resentful, and uncommitted.[97]

The Future

Deming advocated the abolition of PAs. PA is the deadliest of Deming's deadly diseases that stand in the way of quality management. PAs embody a win-lose philosophy that destroys people psychologically and poisons healthy relationships. A win-win philosophy emphasizes cooperation, participation, and leadership, directed at continuous improvement of quality.[98]

Deming's system provides for three ratings for PA using process data. Using the statistic of variation, ratings will fall within the system, outside the system on the high side, or outside the system on the low side. If the rating is within the system, pay should be according to seniority; if outside the system on the high side, pay should be based on merit; and if outside the system on the low side, the employee should be coached or replaced.[99]

Effective Management of Performance Appraisals

How do we overcome these pitfalls or deficiencies? First, we must be aware of them. Second, we can learn the management by objectives approach and treat people as people. As a result, employees will know by which yardsticks they will be measured. The PA will be a joint project. It will be a helpful situation for rater and ratee. If the situation is working correctly, ratees usually will push themselves.

A complex and lengthy evaluation form has not proved effective in rating personnel. Many managers have reduced their rating system to a limited checklist and a write-up that asks for strengths and weaknesses, with specific examples to justify each. Many managers will agree to the following 23 principles for a rating system:

1. The system should be simple and effective, efficient and administratively feasible.
2. The procedures and uses of the system should be understood and agreed on by line management and the employees being rated.
3. Factors to be rated should be measurable and agreed on by managers and subordinates.
4. Raters should understand the purpose and nature of the performance review. They should be taught to use the system, observe, and write notes, including a critical incident file; organize notes and write evaluations that include examples of evidence; edit their reports; and conduct effective review interviews.
5. Raters should understand the meanings of the dimensions rated, including the dimensions' relative weights. Managers are reported to be able to distinguish among only three levels of performance: poor, satisfactory, and outstanding.
6. Criticism should promote warmth and the building of self-esteem for both ratee and rater.
7. The process should be organized and used to manage employees on a daily basis according to their needs to be coached.

8. Praise or suggestions for improvement should be done at the time of the event.

9. Standards of performance should be set and modified at the time of the event.

10. Performance standards should be valid, reliable, and fair.

11. Managers should be rewarded for good performance evaluation skills.

12. Professionally accepted procedures should be used for job analysis, development of job-related observable performance criteria, and job classifications. Fairness is ensured when processes are applied systematically and uniformly throughout the organization.

13. A fair employment posture committed to equal opportunity should be used. A conscientious and equitable appraisal system reduces lawsuits and ensures fairness and confidence. Such a system should be congruent with administrative and legal guidelines.

14. Work output, not habits and traits such as loyalty, should be measured *unless* the habits or traits are described by specific examples of observed behavior.

15. Quality, constant innovation, and functional barrier distraction should be emphasized.

16. Appraisal should be less time-consuming through time management: daily feedback, preparation time for annual or semiannual evaluation, execution time that is spread out, and group time for consultation and coordination of appraisal criteria with peers. The last provides for fairness and equity throughout the organization.

17. The number of performance categories should be small, and no forced ranking should be used. Raters should keep it simple: 10% to 20% of the total, superior (bonus x 2); 70% to 85%, satisfactory (bonus); and 5% to 10%, questionable or unsatisfactory (no bonus).

18. The form and process should be kept simple: a one- to two-page written contract drafted with the subordinate and containing one to two specific annual or semiannual objectives, one to two personal, group, or team growth or career-enhancement objectives, one to two objectives to improve skills, and one objective related to the team's strategic theme (such as quality improvement). The manager should use open-ended prose as the format, do formal reviews bimonthly or more often, and be able to recall the content of each contract.

19. Performance goals should be straightforward, emphasizing the manager's desired results and considering what is important to the continuing success of the business.

20. Pay decisions should be made public. No one will be embarrassed if there is equity.

21. Formal appraisal should be made a small part of overall recognition that includes listening, celebrating, pay, and involvement.

22. Multiple ratings, including those of ratees' subordinates, should be used.[100]

23. To get employees to buy into performance improvement, managers should create a relationship to both individual and organizational performance improvement and, in turn—to add value to the success of each individual—the department and the organization; identify a measurement for each critical point in the process; and present reports and celebrate monthly at staff meetings.[101]

Summary

Performance appraisal is a major component of the evaluating or controlling function of nursing management. Both raters and ratees dislike it. If used appropriately and conscientiously, the PA process will govern employee behavior to produce goods and services in high volume and of high quality.

The purposes or uses of PA are multiple. In nursing, PA is used to motivate employees to produce high-quality patient care. The results of performance appraisal are often used for promotion, selection, and termination, and to improve performance.

Performance appraisal is a part of the science of behavioral technology and should be viewed as part of that body of knowledge that relates to the management of human behavior. Nurse managers need this knowledge to manage the clinical nurse effectively and efficiently as a human resource.

When used for merit pay increases, which is a retrospective use, PA should be separated from that which looks to the future. Output-based pay plans are more effective than are time-based pay plans.

Performance appraisal should be done as a system with:

1. Clearly defined performance standards developed by rater and ratee.
2. Objective application of the performance standards, with both rater and ratee measuring the ratee's performance against the standards.
3. Planned interval feedback with agreed-on improvements when indicated.
4. A continuous cycle. (Raters and ratees should trust each other.)

Job analysis and job description are essential instruments of behavior technology used in PA that provide objectivity and discriminate among jobs.

Coaching, counseling, and interviewing are skills of an effective PA system. In addition to supervisor ratings, PA can include peer ratings, self-ratings, TEC, BARS, and TOPES.

Problems with PA systems include poor preparation of raters and ratees, problems of recency, halo and horns effects, lack of use of standards, leniency–stringency errors, similar-to-me errors, central tendency errors, and first impression errors.

A simple, well-planned PA system can be devised. It will be successful when understood by employees and will require considerable supervisory effort using nursing management theory.

APPLICATION EXERCISES

EXERCISE 28-1   Determine the extent to which a nurse manager exhibits coaching behavior. Apply it to yourself or have a group of peers apply it to themselves, and use the results for discussion.

EXERCISE 28-2   Within a group of peers discuss whether the performance appraisal system is too complicated. If it is, how can it be simplified and still meet accreditation and legal requirements. Are these requirements keeping the system too complicated? If so, how?

EXERCISE 28-3   Within a group of peers, discuss how the job descriptions can be modified consistent with the vision of the organization. The goal is to make them objective and usable.

NOTES

1. S. Krantz, "Five Steps to Making Performance Appraisal Writing . . .," *Supervisory Management* (December 1983), 7–10.
2. R. Zemke, "Is Performance Appraisal a Paper Tiger?" *Training* (December 1985), 24–32.
3. S. Krantz, op. cit.
4. C. J. Fombrun and R. L. Land, "Strategic Issues in Performance Appraisal: Theory and Practice," *Personnel* (November–December 1983), 23–31.
5. B. P. Moroney and M. R. Buckley, "Does Research in Performance Appraisal Influence the Practice of Performance Appraisal? Regretfully Not!" *Public Personnel Management* (summer 1992), 185–195.
6. R. D. Bretz, G. T. Milkovich, and W. Read, "The Current State of Performance Appraisal Research and Practice: Concerns, Directions and Implications," *Journal of Management* (June 1992), 321–352.
7. W. A. Hochwarter, L. A. Witt, and K. M. Kacmar, "Perceptions of Organizational Politics as a Moderator of the Relationship Between Conscientiousness and Job Performance," *Journal of Applied Psychology* (June 2000), 472–478.
8. C. J. Fombrun and R. L. Land, op. cit.
9. C. E. Schneier, A. Geis, and J. A. Wert, "Performance Appraisals: No Appointment Needed," *Personnel Journal* (November 1987), 80–87.
10. R. Zemke. op. cit.
11. A. Levenstein, "Feedback Improves Performance," *Nursing Management* (February 1984), 65–66.

12. R. Zemke. op. cit.
13. D. L. Kirkpatrick, "Performance Appraisal: When Two Jobs Are Too Many," *Training* (March 1986), 65, 67–69.
14. Ibid.
15. R. E. Kopelman, "Linking Pay to Performance Is a Proven Management Tool," *Personnel Administrator* (October 1983), 60–68.
16. Ibid.
17. Ibid.
18. N. R. Deets and D. T. Tyler, "How Xerox Improved Its Performance Appraisals," *Personnel Journal* (April 1986), 50–52.
19. B. Jacobson and B. L. Kaye, "Career Development and Performance Appraisal: It Takes Two to Tango," *Personnel* (January 1986), 26–32.
20. K. J. Kelly, "Administrator's Forum," *Journal of Nursing Staff Development* (September–October 1990), 255–257.
21. J. Jambunathan, "Planning a Peer Review Program," *Journal of Nursing Staff Development* (September–October 1992), 235–239.
22. R. M. Fulmer and S. G. Franklin, *Supervision: Principles of Professional Management*, 2nd ed. (New York: Macmillan 1982), 214–215.
23. H. Koontz and H. Weihrich, *Management*, 9th ed. (New York: McGraw Hill, 1988), 490–494.
24. J. M. Ganong and W. L. Ganong, *Nursing Management*, 2nd ed. (Gaithersburg, MD: 1980), 191.
25. B. Blai, "An Appraisal System That Yields Results," *Supervisory Management*, November 1983, 39-42.

26. M. G. Friedman, "10 Steps to Objective Appraisals," *Personnel Journal* (June 1986), 66–71.

27. B. Rambur, "Fostering Evidence-Based Practice in Nursing Education," *Journal of Professional Nursing* (September–October 1999), 270–274; S. L. Aliotta, "Focus On Case Management: Linking Outcomes and Accountability," *Topics in Health Information Management* (February 2000), 11–16; A. J. Frankel and H. Heft-LaPorte, "Tracking Case Management Accountability: A Systems Approach," *Journal of Case Management* (fall 1998), 105–111.

28. M. R. Edwards and J. R. Sproull, "Safeguarding Your Employee Rating System," *Business* (April–June 1985), 17–27.

29. S. Price and J. Graber, "Employee-Made Appraisals," *Management World* (February 1986), 34–36.

30. D. Ignatavicius and J. Griffith, "Job Analysis: The Basis for Effective Appraisal," *The Journal of Nursing Administration* (July–August 1982), 37–41.

31. J. Dienemann and C. Shaffer, "Faculty Performance Appraisal Systems: Procedures and Criteria," *Journal of Professional Nursing* (May–June 1992), 148–154.

32. J. Markowitz, "Managing the Job Analysis Process," *Training and Development Journal* (August 1987), 64–66.

33. D. Ignatavicius and J. Griffith, op. cit.; J. Markowitz, op. cit.; E. P. Prien, I. L. Goldstein, W. H. Macey, "Multidomain Job Analysis: Procedures and Applications," *Training and Development Journal* (August 1987), 68–72.

34. P. R. Coaly and P. R. Sackett, "Effects of Using High—Versus Low—Performing Job Incumbents as Sources of Job Analysis Information," *Journal of Applied Psychology* (August 1987), 434–437.

35. D. K. Denton, "Redesigning a Job by Simplifying Every Task and Responsibility," *Industrial Engineering* (August 1992), 46–48.

36. Ibid.

37. J. G. Turner, K. M. Kolenc, and L. Docken, "Job Analysis 1996: Infection Control Professional," *American Journal of Infection Control* (April 1999), 145–157; B. J. Burgel, E. M. Wallace, S. D. Kemerer, and M. Garbin, "Certified Occupational Health Nursing. Job Analysis in the United States," *AAOHN Journal* (November 1997), 581–591; G. Costa, "Guidelines for the Medical Surveillance of Shift Workers," *Scandinavian Journal of Work Environment Health*, 24 (suppl 3), (1998), 151–155; N. L. Chornick and C. J. Yocom, "NCLEX Job Analysis Study: Questionnaire Development," *Journal of Nursing Education* (March 1995), 101–105; N. L. Chornick and A. L. Wendt, "NCLEX–RN: From Job Analysis Study to Examination," *Journal of Nursing Education* (October 1997), 378–382; S. S. Blancett, "Nursing Journalism Leadership," *Nursing Administration Quarterly* (fall 1997), 16–22; M. N. Wolfe and S. Coggins, "The Value of Job Analysis, Job Description and Performance," *Medical Group Management Journal* (May–June 1997), 42–44, 46–48, 50–52; V. S. Conn, N. K. Davis, and L. G. Occena, "Analyzing Jobs for Redesign Decisions," *Nursing Economics* (May–June 1996), 145–150;

38. C. Berenson and H. O. Ruhnke, "Job Descriptions: Guidelines for Personnel Management," *Personnel Journal* (January 1966), 14–19.

39. P. R. Webb and R. J. Cantone, "Performance Evaluation: Triumph or Torture?" *Journal of Home Health Care Practice* (February 1993), 14–19.

40. R. M. Kleinpell, "Evolving Role Descriptions of the Acute Care Nurse Practitioner," *Critical Care Nursing Quarterly* (February 1999), 9–15; S. J. Quaal, "Clinical Nurse Specialist: Role Restructuring to Advanced Practice Registered Nurse,"

Critical Care Nursing Quarterly (February 1999), 37–49; L. Nemeth, "Leadership for Coordinated Care: Role of a Project Manager," *Critical Care Nursing Quarterly* (February 1999), 50–58.

41. W. R. Kennedy, "Train Managers to Write Winning Job Descriptions," *Training and Development Journal* (April 1987), 62–64.

42. H. S. Rowland and B. L. Rowland, eds. *Hospital Legal Forms, Checklists, and Guidelines* (Gaithersburg, MD: Aspen, 1987), 23: 28.

43. T. Peters, *Thriving on Chaos* (New York: Harper & Row, 1987), 596–597.

44. Ibid.

45. A. Waintroob, "Comparable Worth Issue: The Employers Side," *The Hospital Manager* (July–August 1985), 6–7.

46. TNA's Professional Services Committee, "Nurses and the Comparable Worth Concept," *Texas Nursing* (April 1985), 12–16.

47. "How to Establish the Comparable Worth of a Job: Or One Way to Compare Apples and Oranges," *California Nurse* (March–April 1982), 10–11; TNA's Professional Services Committee, op. cit.

48. B. R. Helton, "Will the Real Knowledge Worker Please Stand Up?" *Industrial Management* (January–February 1987), 26–29.

49. R. G. Kopelman, "Job Redesign and Productivity: A Review of the Evidence," *National Productivity Review* (summer 1985), 237–255.

50. C. J. Bolster, "Work Redesign: More Than Rearranging Furniture on the Titanic," *Aspen's Advisor for Nurse Executives* (August 1991), 4–7.

51. R. M. Kanter, *When Giants Learn to Dance* (New York: Simon & Schuster, 1990), 75–82.

52. C. J. Bolster, op. cit.

53. D. C. Martin and K. M. Bardol, "Training the Raters: A Key to Effective Performance Appraisal," *Public Personnel Management* (summer 1986), 101–109.

54. R. Edwards and J. R. Sproull, op. cit.

55. Ibid.

56. F. Balcazar, B. L. Hopkin, and Y. Suarez, "A Critical, Objective Review of Performance Feedback," *Journal of Organizational Behavior Management* (fall 1985–winter 1985–86), 65–89.

57. D. C. Martin and K. M. Bardal, op. cit.; M. G. Friedman, op. cit.

58. T. A. Ratcliffe and D. J. Logsdon, "The Business Planning Process: A Behavioral Perspective," *Managerial Planning* (March–April 1980), 32–38.

59. M. R. Edward and J. R. Sproull, op. cit.

60. C. E. Schneier, A. Geis, and J. A. Wert, op. cit.

61. V. D. Lachman, "Increasing Productivity Through Performance Evaluation," *The Journal of Nursing Administration* (December 1984), 7–14.

62. L. P. Frankel and K. L. Ofuzo, "Employee Coaching: The way to Gain Compliance," *Employment Relations Today* (autumn 1992), 311–320.

63. Ibid.

64. V. D. Lachman, op. cit.

65. D. C. Martin and C. M. Bardol, op. cit.

66. S. Wilbers, "Performance Reviews Can be Easier," *San Antonio Express-News* (23 May 1993), 3G.

67. Ibid.

68. G. S. Booker and R. W. Miller, "A Closer Look at Peer Ratings," *Personnel* (January–February 1966), 42–47.

69. P. S. Strom, R. D. Strom and E. G. Moore, "Peer and Self-Evaluation of Teamwork Skills," *Journal of Adolescence* (August 1999), 539–553.

70. M. G. Friedman, op. cit.

71. J. Jambunathan, op. cit.

72. J. B. Jurf, L. Ecoff, W. Haley, P. L. Keegan, and P. A. Williams, "First Steps Toward Peer Review," *Journal of Nursing Staff Development* (July–August 1992), 184–186.

73. M. E. Jacobs and J. D. Vail, "Quality Assurance: A Unit-Based Plan," *Journal of the Association of Nurse Anesthetists* (June 1986), 265–271.

74. Ibid.; J. Jambunathan, op. cit.

75. M. E. Jacobs and J. D. Vail, op. cit.; J. B. Jurf, L. Ecoff, W. Haley, P. L. Keegan, and P. A. Williams; J. Jambunathan, op. cit.

76. Ibid.

77. M. Rigg, "Reasons for Removing Employee Evaluations from Management Control," *Industrial Engineering* (August 1992), 17.

78. J. Jambunathan, op. cit., J. Jurf, L. Ecoff, W. Haley, P. L. Keegan, and P. A. Williams, op. cit.

79. A. C. Gregg and K. C. Bloom, "Performance Evaluation and Patient Outcomes Monitored by Nurse Practitioners and Certified Nurse-Midwives in Florida," *Clinical Excellence in Nursing Practice* (September 1999), 279–285.

80. C. J. Fombrun and R. L. Land, op. cit.

81. R. Zemke, op. cit.

82. S. Price and J. Graber, "Employee-Made Appraisals," *Management World* (February 1986), 34–36; M. A. Andrusyszyn, "Faculty Evaluation: A Closer Look at Peer Review," *Nurse Education Today* (December 1990), 410–414.

83. Ibid.

84. M. P. Lovrich, "The Dangers of Participative Management: A Test of Unexamined Assumptions Concerning Employee Involvement," *Review of Public Personnel Administration* (summer 1985), 9–25.

85. B. Jacobson and B. L. Kaye, op. cit.

86. M. J. Somers and D. Birnbaum, "Assessing Self-Appraisal of Job Performance as an Evaluation Device: Are the Poor Results a Function of Method or Methodology?" *Human Relations* (October 1991), 1081–1091.

87. J. Ballinger and J. Ferko III, "Peer Evaluations," *Emergency* (April 1989), 28–31.

88. B. I. Van der Heijden, "Professional Expertise of Higher Level Employees; Age Stereotyping in Self-Assessments and Supervisor Ratings," *Tijdschr Gerontol Geriatr* (April 2000), 62–69.

89. I. H. Shore, L. H. Shole, and G. C. Thornton III, "Construct Validity of Self- and Peer Evaluation of Performance Dimensions in an Assessment Center," *Journal of Applied Psychology* (February 1992), 42–54.

90. M. R. Edwards and J. R. Sproull, op. cit.

91. R. Zemke, op. cit.; M. R. Edwards and J. R. Sproull, op. cit.

92. S. C. Bushardt and A. R. Fowler, Jr, "Performance Evaluation Alternatives," *Journal of Nursing Administration* (October 1988), 40–44.

93. Ibid.

94. W. M. Fox, "Evaluating and Developing Subordinates," *Notes and Quotes* (April 1969), 4.

95. J. C. Coyant, "The Performance Appraisal: A Critique and an Alternative," *Business Horizons* (June 1973), 73–78.

96. R. E. Lofton, "Performance Appraisal: Why They Go Wrong and How to Do Them Right," *National Productivity Review* (winter 1985), 54–63.

97. Ibid.

98. R. D. Moen, op. cit.

99. L. E. Mainstone and A. S. Levi, "Fundamentals of Statistical Process Control," *Journal of Organizational Behavior Management* 9, (1), (1987), 5–21.

100. S. Krantz, op. cit.; D. C. Martin, and K. M. Bardol, op. cit.; C. Logan, "Praise: The Powerhouse of Self-Esteem," *Nursing Management* (June 1985), 36, 38; M. G. Friedman, op. cit.; C. E. Schneier, J. A. Geis, and J. A. Wert, op. cit.; M. R. Edwards and J. R. Sproull, op. cit.; E. Y. Breeze, "The Performance Review," *Manage* (May 1968), 6–11; J. Dienemann and C. Shaffer, op. cit.; T. Peters, op. cit.

101. P. A. MacFalda, "Performance Improvement: How to Get Employee Buy-In," *Radiology Management* (January–February 1998), 35–44.

REFERENCES

Anthony, C. E., and D. del Bueno. "A Performance-Based Development System." *Nursing Management* (June 1993), 32–34.

Ballengee, N. B. "Developing a Performance Appraisal System." *Management Accounting* (September 1990), 52–54.

Barker, P., S. Jackson, and C. Stevenson. "The Need for Psychiatric Nursing: Towards a Multidimensional Theory of Caring." *Nursing Inquiry* (June 1999), 103–111.

Barnett, J., and G. Anderson. "Performance Appraisal Revived." *Senior Nurse* (December 1987), 20–22.

Bernarden, H. J., D. K. Cooke, and P. Villanova. *Journal of Applied Psychology* (April 2000), 232–236.

Brooks, B. A., and M. Madda. "How to Organize a Professional Portfolio for Staff and Career Development." *Journal of Nurses Staff Development* (January–February 1999), 5–10.

Carson, K. P., R. L. Cardy, and G. H. Dobbins. "Upgrade the Employee Evaluation Process." *HR Magazine* (November 1992), 88–92.

Chu, N. L., and J. A. Schmele. "Using the ANA Standards as a Basis for Performance Evaluation in the Home Health Care Setting." *Journal of Nursing Quality Assurance* (May 1990), 25–33.

Davis, D. S., A. E. Greig, J. Burkholder, and T. Keating. "Evaluating Advance Practice Nurses." *Nursing Management* (March 1984), 44–47.

Ernst, E., and K. L. Resch. "Reviewer Bias Against the Unconventional? A Randomized Double-Blind Study of Peer Review." *Complement Therapy Medicine* (March 1999), 19–23.

Ethridge, J. R. "Criteria for Evaluating Performance: An Empirical Study for Nonprofit Hospitals." *Health Care Supervisor* (September 1990), 49–56.

Findley, H. M., W. F. Giles, and K. W. Mossholder. "Performance Appraisal Process and System Facets: Relationship with Contextual Performance." *Journal of Applied Psychology* (August 2000), 634–640.

Fouracre, S., and A. Wright. "New Factors in Job Evaluation." *Personnel Management* (May 1986), 40–43.

Goodale, J. G. "Improving Performance Appraisal." *The Business Quarterly* (autumn 1992), 65–70

Goodson, J. R., and G. W. McGee. "Enhancing Individual Perceptions of Objectivity in Performance Appraisal." *Journal of Business Research* (June 1991), 293–303.

Hagenstad, R. "Integrating Values into the Interviewing and Selection Process." *Seminars in Nurse Management* (March 1995), 16–26.

Herbert, G. R., and D. Doverspike. "Performance Appraisals in the Training Needs Analysis Process: A Review and Critique." *Public Personnel Management* (fall 1990), 253–270.

Hough, L. M., and F. L. Oswald. "Personnel Selection: Looking Toward the Future—Remembering the Past." *Annual Review of Psychology* 51(2000), 631–664.

Idaszak, J. R., and F. Drasgow. "A Revision of the Job Diagnostic Survey: Elimination of a Measurement Artifact." *Journal of Applied Psychology* (February 1987), 69–74.

Keuter, K., E. Byrne, J. Voell, and E. Larson. "Nurses' Job Satisfaction and Organizational Climate in a Dynamic Work Environment." *Applied Nursing Research* (February 2000), 46–49.

King, G. B. "Performance Appraisal on the Automated Environment." *Journal of Library Administration* (Mid-winter 1990), 195–204.

Kirby, P. "An Aberration: Supervisors Who Like Performance Appraisal?" *Supervision* (October 1992), 14–17.

Klimaski, R., and L. Inks. "Accountability Forces in Performance Appraisal." *Organizational Behavior and Human Decision Processes* (April 1990), 194–208.

Lawler, F. E. III. "What's Wrong with Point Factor Job Evaluation?" *Management Review* (November 1986), 44–48.

Lee, M. A. "How to Use Job Analysis Technique." *Restaurant Management* (April 1987), 84–85.

Longnecker, C. O., and S. J. Goff. "Performance Appraisal Effectiveness: A Matter of Perspective." *SAM Advanced Management Journal* (spring 1992), 17–23.

Mann, L. M., C. F. Burton, M. T. Presti, and J. E. Hirsch. "Peer Review in Performance Appraisal." *Nursing Administration Quarterly* (summer 1990), 9–14.

Manshor, A. T., and T. J. Kamalanabhan. "An Examination of Raters' and Ratees' Preferences in Process and Feedback in Performance Appraisal." *Psychology Reports* (February 2000), 203–214.

Martin, D. C., and K. M. Bectal. "The Legal Ramifications of Performance Appraisal: An Update." *Employee Relations Law Journal* (autumn 1991), 257–286.

Martin, R. K. "The Role of the Transplant Advanced Practice Nurse: A Professional and Personal Evolution." *Critical Care Nursing Quarterly* (February 1999), 69–76, 86.

Mathes, K. "Will Your Performance Appraisal System Stand Up in Court?" *HR Forum* (August 1992), 5.

McCarthy, J. P. "A New Focus on Achievement." *Personnel Journal* (February 1991), 74–76.

McCloskey, J. C., and B. McCain. "Nurse Performance: Strengths and Weaknesses." *Nursing Research* (September–October 1998), 308–313.

McGee, K. G. "Making Performance Appraisal a Positive Experience." *Nursing Management* (August 1992), 36–37.

Meyer, A. L. "A Framework for Assessing Performance Problems." *The Journal of Nursing Administration* (May 1984), 40–43.

Mossholder, K. W., W. F. Giles, and M. A. Weslowski. "Information Privacy and Performance Appraisal: An Examination of Employee Perceptions and Reactions." *Journal of Business Ethics* (February 1991), 15–156.

Murphy, K. R. "Criterion Issues in Performance Appraisal Research Behavioral Accuracy versus Classification Accuracy." *Organizational Behavior and Human Decision Processes* (50: 1991), 45–50.

Murphy, K. R., B. A. Gannett, B. M. Herr, and J. A. Chen. "Effects of Subsequent Performance on Evaluation of Previous Performance." *Journal of Applied Psychology* (August 1986), 427–431.

Nathan, B. R., A. M. Mohrman, Jr., and J. Milliman. "Interpersonal Relations as a Context for the Effects of Appraisal Interviews on Performance and Satisfaction: A Longitudinal Study." *Academy of Management Journal* (June 1991), 352–369.

Neuman, G. A., and J. Wright. "Team Effectiveness: Beyond Skills and Cognitive Ability." *Journal of Applied Psychology* (June 1999), 376–389.

Odiorne, G. S. *Strategic Management of Human Resources* (San Francisco: Jossey-Bass, 1984).

Parlish, C. "A Model for Clinical Performance Evaluation." *Journal of Nursing Education* (October 1987), 338–339.

Pelle, D., and L. Greenhalgh. "Developing the Performance Appraisal System." *Nursing Management* (December 1987), 37–40, 42, 44.

Philp, T. "Getting Down to Some Serious Work on Staff Appraisal." *CA Magazine* (June 1992), 26, 28.

Reed, P. A., and M. J. Kroll. "A Two-Perspective Approach to Performance Appraisal." *Personnel* (October 1985), 51–57.

Ramsey, P. G., J. D. Carline, L. L. Blank, and M. D. Wenrich. "Feasibility of Hospital-Based Use of Peer Ratings to Evaluate the Performances of Practicing Physicians." *Academic Medicine* (April 1996), 364–370.

Richmond, B. "Teachers Must Stand Up to School Board Group." *San Antonio Light* (12 December 1992), F5.

Rotarius, T., and A. Liberman. "Objective Employee Assessments: Establishing a Balance Among Supervisory Evaluations." *Health Care Management* (June 2000), 1–6.

Schnake, M. G., and M. P. Dumler. "Affective Response Bias in the Measurement of Perceived Task Characteristics." *Journal of Occupational Psychology* (June 1985), 159–166.

Schwarz, J. K. 1999. "Assisted Dying and Nursing Practice." *Image Journal of Nursing Scholarship* 31(4); (1999), 367–373.

Strickland, D., and O. C. O'Connell. "Saving Your Career in the 21st Century." *Journal of Case Management* (summer 1998), 47–51.

Thomas, P. A., K. A. Gebo, and D. B. Hellmann. "A Pilot Study of Peer Review in Residency Training." *Journal of General Internal Medicine* (September 1999), 551–554.

Waldman, D. A., and R. S. Kenett. "Improve Performance by Appraisal." *HR Magazine* (July 1990), 66–69.

Weingard, M. "Establishing Comparable Worth Through Job Evaluation." *Nursing Outlook* (March–April 1984), 110–113.

Williams, S. L., and M. L. Hummert. "Evaluating Performance Appraisal Instruments Dimensions Using Construct Analysis." *Journal of Business Communication* (spring 1990), 117–133.

Wren, K. R., and T. L. Wren. "Legal Implications of Evaluation Procedures for Students in Healthcare Professions." *AANA Journal* (February 1999), 73–78.

Zawackie, R. A., and C. A. Norman. "Breaking Appraisal Tradition." *Computerworld* (1 April 1991), 78.

APPENDIX 28-1
Peer Review Evaluation Format

CONFIDENTIAL (NONDEPARTMENTAL) SELF-EVALUATION

Name _____ Age _____ Sex _____
Time of EMT-P Certification: _____ years _____ months

A B C D F	Knowledge		A B C D F
☐ ☐ ☐ ☐ ☐	EMT-A Knowledge	ACLS Knowledge	☐ ☐ ☐ ☐ ☐
☐ ☐ ☐ ☐ ☐	EMT-P Knowledge	Trauma Knowledge	☐ ☐ ☐ ☐ ☐

A B C D F	Skill Competency		A B C D F
☐ ☐ ☐ ☐ ☐	EMT-A Skill Competency	EKG Recognition	☐ ☐ ☐ ☐ ☐
☐ ☐ ☐ ☐ ☐	EMT-P Skill Competency	Intubation Competency	☐ ☐ ☐ ☐ ☐
☐ ☐ ☐ ☐ ☐	ACLS Skill Competency	Trauma Skill Competency	☐ ☐ ☐ ☐ ☐
☐ ☐ ☐ ☐ ☐	Report Writing	Scene Management Skills	☐ ☐ ☐ ☐ ☐
☐ ☐ ☐ ☐ ☐	Patient Assessment Skills	Communication Skills	☐ ☐ ☐ ☐ ☐

A B C D F	Quality of Care When Encountering . . .		A B C D F
☐ ☐ ☐ ☐ ☐	Lower Socioeconomic Groups	Intoxicated Patients	☐ ☐ ☐ ☐ ☐
☐ ☐ ☐ ☐ ☐	Higher Socioeconomic Groups	System Abusers	☐ ☐ ☐ ☐ ☐
☐ ☐ ☐ ☐ ☐	Patients of Different Race	Homosexual Patients	☐ ☐ ☐ ☐ ☐
☐ ☐ ☐ ☐ ☐	Drug Abusers		

A B C D F	Other		A B C D F
☐ ☐ ☐ ☐ ☐	Fair Treatment of Partner	Motivation Level	☐ ☐ ☐ ☐ ☐
☐ ☐ ☐ ☐ ☐	Ability to Relate to Patients	Compassion for Patients	☐ ☐ ☐ ☐ ☐
☐ ☐ ☐ ☐ ☐	Decision-Making Under Overwhelming Conditions		
☐ ☐ ☐ ☐ ☐	Stress Management Skills/Emotional Stability		
☐ ☐ ☐ ☐ ☐	Overall Quality of Patient Care		

CONFIDENTIAL (NONDEPARTMENTAL) EVALUATION OF COLLEAGUE

Colleague Evaluated: _____ His/Her Sex _____ Age _____
Approximate Time of Colleague's EMT-P Certification: _____ years _____ months
Number of Shifts Worked With Colleague (last six months): _____
Time of Your EMT-P Certification: _____ years _____ months   Your Sex _____ Age _____

A B C D F	Knowledge		A B C D F
☐ ☐ ☐ ☐ ☐	EMT-A Knowledge	ACLS Knowledge	☐ ☐ ☐ ☐ ☐
☐ ☐ ☐ ☐ ☐	EMT-P Knowledge	Trauma Knowledge	☐ ☐ ☐ ☐ ☐

A B C D F	Skill Competency		A B C D F
☐ ☐ ☐ ☐ ☐	EMT-A Skill Competency	EKG Recognition	☐ ☐ ☐ ☐ ☐
☐ ☐ ☐ ☐ ☐	EMT-P Skill Competency	Intubation Competency	☐ ☐ ☐ ☐ ☐
☐ ☐ ☐ ☐ ☐	ACLS Skill Competency	Trauma Skill Competency	☐ ☐ ☐ ☐ ☐
☐ ☐ ☐ ☐ ☐	Report Writing	Scene Management Skills	☐ ☐ ☐ ☐ ☐
☐ ☐ ☐ ☐ ☐	Patient Assessment Skills	Communication Skills	☐ ☐ ☐ ☐ ☐

A B C D F	Quality of Care When Encountering . . .		A B C D F
☐ ☐ ☐ ☐ ☐	Lower Socioeconomic Groups	Intoxicated Patients	☐ ☐ ☐ ☐ ☐
☐ ☐ ☐ ☐ ☐	Higher Socioeconomic Groups	System Abusers	☐ ☐ ☐ ☐ ☐
☐ ☐ ☐ ☐ ☐	Patients of Different Race	Homosexual Patients	☐ ☐ ☐ ☐ ☐
☐ ☐ ☐ ☐ ☐	Drug Abusers		

A B C D F	Other		A B C D F
☐ ☐ ☐ ☐ ☐	Fair Treatment of Partner	Motivation Level	☐ ☐ ☐ ☐ ☐
☐ ☐ ☐ ☐ ☐	Ability to Relate to Patients	Compassion for Patients	☐ ☐ ☐ ☐ ☐
☐ ☐ ☐ ☐ ☐	Decision-Making Under Overwhelming Conditions		
☐ ☐ ☐ ☐ ☐	Stress Management Skills/Emotional Stability		
☐ ☐ ☐ ☐ ☐	Overall Quality of Patient Care		

EMT–A—emergency medical technician–ambulance
EMT–P—emergency medical technician–paramedic
ACLS—advanced cardiac life support

Source: J. Ballinger and J. Ferko, III. "Peer Evaluation." *Emergency* (April 1989), 31. Reprinted with permission of *Emergency* magazine.

CHAPTER 29

Pay for Performance

Russell C. Swansburg, PhD, RN

> If you want more, then work more.
>
> John A. Parnell[1]

LEARNING OBJECTIVES AND ACTIVITIES

- Distinguish among the major types of pay for performance.
- Identify the criteria being used in a pay-for-performance plan.
- Discuss the design of a pay-for-performance plan.

CONCEPTS: Pay for performance, merit pay, gain-sharing.

MANAGER BEHAVIOR: Bases all pay increases on a merit pay system.

LEADER BEHAVIOR: Employs a variety of pay-for-performance compensation plans as a part of the annual budget.

Introduction

Pay for performance is based on equity theory, expectancy theory, the law of effect, and psychological fulfillment. Equity theory indicates that people want to be treated equally and fairly by employers. Expectancy theory says that people believe they can achieve certain levels of performance and, if they do, they expect to be rewarded. The Law of Effect states that behavior will be rewarded when repeated. Equity theory, expectancy theory, and the law of effect, individually or combined, apply when the employee says, "I believe that when I increase my efforts or inputs to produce sustained greater outputs my employer will increase my rewards." Increased pay that is linked as a reward to increased employee inputs and outputs is termed *pay for performance*. When used effectively, the compensation system rewards superior, excellent, and satisfactory performance. People per-

ceive an imbalance in this theory when they put forth greater effort than others but receive the same rewards. They perceive compensation to be inequitable, and pay becomes a dissatisfier.[2] Pay for performance is an incentive program that links pay to employee or corporate performance.[3]

Performance, not longevity, is fast becoming the basis for pay increases in institutions of all sizes. This may apply only to the managerial staff, or it can apply down to the lowest-paid employees in an organization.[4]

Since the recession of 1982, pay for performance has become the mode for pay increases in business and industry. Of 1,080 Canadian companies surveyed in 1990, 64% indicated they would use a merit-only pay increase in 1991; 32% would use a general-plus-merit system for pay increases.[5] A 1990 survey of 250 manufacturers indicated that 76% had incentive-based programs.[6] A 1993 survey of 2,000 U.S. companies indicated that 6% of this sample did pay for performance.[7]

> Results of longitudinal research conducted by the Italian National Health Service indicate that performance-related pay for health service professionals requires a careful implementation process to be a powerful tool at management's disposal to increase employees' performance and commitment.[8]

Expected Outcomes

Expectancy theory postulates that individuals will choose among alternatives in a rational manner to maximize expected rewards. A study designed to test subjects' choice of a pay plan from among piece rate, fixed rate, and bonus concluded the following[9]:

- Pay choice has a strong impact on subjects' behavior.
- High-ability individuals choose a piece-rate plan or a bonus plan over a fixed-rate plan.
- Individuals tend to choose a pay plan that maximizes their expected rewards.
- Pay choice results in higher pay satisfaction.

Studies of managers and administrators show a positive relationship between pay-for-performance perception and pay satisfaction. A pay rate higher than that of the outside market also results in greater employee satisfaction. Pay system fairness is a function of factors that pertain to organizational justice such as participation in pay system development, perceived fairness of allocation procedures, and greater understanding of the pay system.[10]

A company's ability to compete and company-employee relations are improved by creatively managed compensation systems. Performance-based pay affects profitability, with profits increasing when high or good performance is rewarded with pay incentives. Variable pay affects profitability more than does base pay.[11]

There may be a limit to the ratio of pay for performance. A study of 75 college students that related performance to 0%, 10%, 30%, 60%, or 100% of base pay as incentive indicated that whereas 0% produced no significant incentive, "the productivity of subjects in the 10%, 30%, 60% and 100% incentive groups did not differ. They all produced significant incentive."[12]

Compensation is a part of business strategy. A direct link exists between compensation and achievement of established goals. Increased compensation is an incentive for employees to do well. An employee will work to achieve predetermined goals if there are predetermined rewards.[13]

The following are some reasons for basing pay on performance[14]:

1. Increases job satisfaction. Subordinates who are involved in developing a work plan feel ownership of the process; as a result, they will work harder to make their plan successful.
2. Reduces absenteeism.
3. Increases productivity. Workers will perform clearly identified behaviors that are rewarded. (Mediocrity should not be rewarded.)
4. Decreases voluntary turnover, which says, "I believe I am worth more. Other employers will pay me more."
5. Improves the quality of the employee mix. This system attracts and keeps higher-level performers.

Zenger reported on a study of 984 engineering employees of two large U. S. high-technology companies. The study found that offering pay incentive awards confirmed that "extremely high and moderately low performers are likely to remain in firms offering these contracts while moderately high and extremely low performers are likely to depart." The contracts with these companies aggressively rewarded extreme performance and largely ignored moderate performance limits. To correct this, the employer can design a system to retain above-average performers and reduce turnover for only the extremely low performers.[15]

Pay for performance rewards what is valued by the employer, which may be time-in-grade and longevity. In a competitive business environment, however, employers are more apt to value new job skills and new knowledge by paying more for performance that demonstrates their use than for longevity.[16]

Types of Compensation Programs

Exhibit 29-1 lists the major types of compensation programs.[17]

Pay-for-Performance Process

The following are elements of a pay-for-performance process[18]:

1. Compensation should be part of the strategic planning process. When done with employees or their representatives as part of a task force, the compensation plan is more apt to be perceived as fair and to elicit employees' trust.

   Company mission, philosophy, objectives, vision, values, and business plans can be guides to developing a compensation plan. Decisions are made on how to link compensation to employee or company performance and hence to individuals versus groups. It is best to use more than one kind of incentive. The plan should be customized to the organizational culture and core values of a pay system. An obvious link exists between effort and performance and the need for rewards. The organization should consider the need for change and the level(s) of organizational participation. The current compensation system should be assessed for gaps, holes, and overfunding. Potential plan types should then be assigned to close the gaps.
2. Goals should be carefully set. They should be achievable to avoid system errors. When goals are set with employees, they assume ownership of the goals. Organizational performance goals may relate to improving employee motivation, engendering a culture of employees who genuinely care about organizational effectiveness, and tying labor costs

EXHIBIT 29-1

Major Types of Pay-for-Performance (Compensation) Programs

TYPE	CHARACTERISTICS
Merit pay	Probably most common. Usually a percentage of base pay. Sometimes part of a pay raise—a percentage for merit and a percentage for longevity. Pay raises are established for each job or group of jobs. Progression at fixed intervals based on observation of performance. Standards of employees' success are not established a priori. When given as a merit bonus, it is not added to base pay. An individual incentive plan.
Gain-sharing	A profit-sharing plan, usually a group incentive plan. A specific share of the organization's profits is distributed to a group of employees based on production measures, financial performance, and quality of service. (See also Chapter 16, "Decentralization and Participatory Management.")
Cash or lump-sum bonuses	Usually a share of the profits. Also a group incentive. May be a uniform bonus paid to all or most employees organizationwide.
Pay for knowledge	Pay is linked to learning new skills and being able to work at a higher level or at more than one specialty.
Employee stock ownership plans (ESOPs)	Profit-sharing plan. Some pay cash from interest and dividends. Most are deferred plans. See Chapter 16, "Decentralization and Participatory Management." Risky link between pay and performance for these plans. The direct pay contingency is typically quite small and linked to company performance.
Individual incentive	Compensation is paid for individual performance.
Small group incentive	Each member of a group is compensated for achieving predetermined objectives.
Instant incentive	Individual compensation for noteworthy achievements.
Recognition programs	Performance awards to individuals or groups. May be money, educational programs, vacation/travel, certificates, or other symbolic award.

to the organization's ability to pay specific amounts. Goals should be made job specific. Exhibits 29-2 and 29-3 give examples of criteria for establishing a pay-for-performance plan and policy.

3. Standards for measurement should be precise because they are the benchmarks against which performance is met. Participants should be able to influence standards. Standards may include the following:

- Quality standards related to total quality management or continuous quality improvement for eliminating defects or errors.
- Safety standards related to all customers, internal and external.
- Attendance standards such as pay for unused sick time or paid days off.
- Productivity standards related to volume of inputs versus outputs.
- A pay-for-performance matrix (see Exhibit 29-4).
- Job descriptions that include specific objectives of each position and measure the accomplishments of those objectives. Job descriptions can be developed with input from incumbents. When job descriptions are related to pay for knowledge, new technology may require help from experts and outside vendors. End results of these job descriptions include items such as

EXHIBIT 29-2

Criteria Established for the Pay-for-Performance Plan

- The plan must create or better establish a link between pay and plant and division performance (performance should be a factor in considering appropriate wage adjustments).
- The plan must provide a fair and equitable method of compensation or rewards to attract, retain, and motivate good employees.
- The plan should be based on criteria that allow employees to contribute to and have an impact on the organization's objectives.
- Costs of the plan must be consistent with the financial state of the business.
- The plan should be consistent with plant and division objectives.
- The plan must fit the culture of the organization.
- The plan should provide a stable level of compensation to foster commitment among participants.
- The plan should involve a high level of communication and employee participation.

Source: Reprinted by permission of publisher, from J. P. Guthrie and E. P. Cunningham. "Pay for Performance for Hourly Workers: The Quaker Oats Alternative." *Compensation & Benefits Review* (March–April © 1992), 20. American Management Association, New York. All rights reserved.

The Pay-for-Performance Policy

- If wages are more than 5% greater than the market average, then the annual hourly wage adjustment will be a lump sum determined by the performance matrix (0–6.5% cash bonus of last 12 months' wages).
- If wages are less than 5% greater than the market average, then an across-the-board annual adjustment, determined by the performance matrix, will be given. It is, however, our policy to keep wages at 5% above the market average.

Source: Reprinted by permission of publisher, from J. P. Guthrie and E. P. Cunningham. "Pay for Performance for Hourly Workers: The Quaker Oats Alternative." *Compensation & Benefits Review* (March–April © 1992), 20. American Management Association, New York. All rights reserved.

Summary of Pay-for-Performance Matrix

1. Financial (0–2% possible payout)
   a. Raw materials
      Meet (lower) target rate = 0.5% payout
      Meet (higher) target rate = 1% payout
   b. Conversion
      Meet (lower) target rate = 0.5% payout
      Meet (higher) target rate = 1% payout
2. Safety (0–1% possible payout)
   Safety goals:
   a. OSHA incidence rate (target rate)
   b. Days away severity rate (target rate)
   c. Lost workdays case incidence rate (target rate)
      Achieve two of three safety rates = 0.5% payout
      Achieve all three safety rates = 1% payout
3. Quality (0–1% possible payout)
   a. Comply with target specifications = 0.5% payout
   b. Meet reduction target in plant controllable complaints = 0.5% payout
4. Sanitation (0–1% possible payout)
   a. Make an excellent rating on corporate audits = 0.5% payout
   b. Quality assurance audits meet absolute/variance standards = 0.5% payout
5. Focus (0–1% possible payout)
   a. This will change from year to year to reflect an area of special emphasis during the upcoming pay-for-performance cycle
6. Division performance (0–0.5% possible payout)
   a. Division meets operating income goal = 0.5% payout

Source: Reprinted, by permission of publisher, from J. P. Guthrie and E. P. Cunningham. "Pay for Performance for Hourly Workers: The Quaker Oats Alternative." *Compensation & Benefits Review* (March–April © 1992), 22. American Management Association, New York. All rights reserved.

"trained and motivated crew" and "safety." Each end result has one to three or four measures of accomplishment, such as "responsiveness to customer's needs" and "number of machine break-

downs." Preparation to meet pay for knowledge includes massive training efforts that may be done in cooperation with vendors, consultants, and educational institutions. An extensive set of training modules can be developed so that training is directly related to the job description.

- Organizational performance: profitability and financial performance.
- Management by objectives.
- Critical incidents: innovation, new products and services, market penetration, and targets.
- Economic value added (EVA). Some companies are awarding bonuses and stock options to managers on the basis of EVA, which is a way of increasing a company's real profitability. EVA equals the operating profits minus taxes minus the total annual cost of capital. The cost of capital includes interest paid on borrowed capital (less the deductible tax) plus equity capital, the money provided by the shareholders. Equity includes investment in human capital. A positive EVA means wealth is being created, whereas a negative EVA means that capital is being destroyed. EVA can be used for service businesses. EVA can be raised by using less capital and giving shareholders higher dividends. Stock prices go up.
- Cooperation among individuals or groups.
- Specific competencies, such as the ability to communicate, customer focus, dealing with change, interpersonal skills, team relationships, and leadership.
- Cultural diversity.

4. An objective performance appraisal system needs to be established that measures the achievement of the standards as employee outputs. The following are some examples:
   - Completion of specific education and training programs.
   - Absence or reduction (including prevention) of accidents, injuries, and illnesses, and measurable reduced pollution.
   - Specific problems solved.
   - Reduced supply inventories and supply use.
   - Reduced patient stays.
   - Increased responsibility.
   - Reduced costs.
   - Demonstrated mastery of knowledge, skills, and abilities.

Supervisors should be trained to use the performance appraisal (PA) system effectively. The PA system must be objective. Some companies separate PAs from salary reviews. During PAs career development—improvement, job skills, and career growth—

is the focus. During the salary review the focus is on worth—objectives and potential to learn new skills—is the focus.

Performance standards should not be confused with results or accomplishments. If cultural diversity is a standard that is measured and rewarded, it will be accomplished.

5. A plan needs to be chosen (see Exhibit 29-1). The structure should be tailored to the performance dimensions of the job.

6. Needed policies and procedures for implementing the plan must be written and communicated to the participants. All employees need to understand the system, that is, what it is and how it works. Exhibit 29-5 suggests guidelines for performance-based salary increases.

7. The plan is then implemented and monitored.

8. The effectiveness of the plan is evaluated.

Exhibit 29-6 summarizes the process for designing a pay-for-performance plan.

> Successful gain-sharing programs address the primary issues of employee involvement and a formula for bonus payout. After careful planning, Boulder Community Hospital instituted a gain-sharing program called "Encore! Quality Share." The plan involved employees from all levels of the organization, educational seminars for new employees, and orientation to the plan for new employees. Evaluation indicates success and the need for safeguards against complacency.[19]

Group Versus Individual Plans

Group Plans

Group incentive plans include small groups or work units where rewards are allocated for group performance exceeding predefined standards, productivity improvement plans, and profit-sharing plans. These plans are designed to encourage teamwork and coop-

eration with shared profits, information, responsibility, accountability, and participation in decision-making.

Group variable pay is used for meeting goals based on collaborative performance and teamwork and thus encourages communication. Quality can become a team sport and a win–win situation. Group variable pay is flexible and can respond to multiple goals and measures and to change. Group variable pay should be funded independently of other pay plans.[20]

Most compensation plans tend to be indecisive. People expect to be rewarded when they increase their output because of work redesign. Managers act as their coaches and facilitators in the process.[21]

Teams, not individuals, increasingly are being rewarded for good work that results in innovation, increased cost control, and higher morale. Team leaders or managers set up worthwhile goals that are easy to measure. Everyone from plant manager on down receives the same annual raise for achieving or exceeding goals. The percentage of pay is set by goals that may be divided between those of the unit and organization. Employees are involved in designing team-based incentive programs. A trusting work relationship is needed. Some companies have teams of 25 to 50 employees who supervise themselves; they have no time clock and no foreperson. After a 3-month probation period, teams take over evaluation. When employee performance is substandard, the team recommends improvement programs, probation, or termination. The team helps hire new employees. Team members identify free riders and layabouts.[22]

Individual Plans

Individual merit pay can create internal competition for pay raises and the withholding of information from each other by competing employees. It encourages individuals to try to improve the system on their own, a difficult job to accomplish. Individual merit pay also uses individual quality outcome measures, which are difficult to develop meaningfully. It encourages a microfocus, decreases flexibility, and produces anxiety.[23]

> Stars are best rewarded individually with career development, promotional tracking, and distinguished service awards. Be sure their performance is not distractive if they achieve at the expense of others.[24]

Competency Model

Individual accomplishments are temporary and variable, whereas competencies and salaries are additive over time. Competency reflects individual performance; accomplishments can result from individual or group efforts. A value-added pay system combines base salary to employee competency and rewards individual or

EXHIBIT 29-5 Guidelines for Performance-Based Salary Increases		
APPRAISAL FACTOR	**WEIGHT**	**SALARY INCREASE**
Unsatisfactory	0–20 points	0%
Satisfactory	21–41 points	3%
Excellent	42–62 points	5%
Superior	63+ points	7%

Source: J. T. Browdy. "Performance Appraisal and Pay for Performance Start at the Top." *Health Care Supervisor* (April 1989), 31–41. Reprinted with permission.

EXHIBIT 29-6
Designing a Pay-for-Performance Plan

The following principles, objectives, and design standards provide a framework; each organization can tailor the specific pay-for-performance programs that are compatible with its environment.

OVERALL PRINCIPLES

Pay-for-performance programs should

- Be designed to ensure that each unit's programs meet overall corporate policies, thereby supporting the overall philosophy and intentions of the firm.
- Offer decentralized units within the firm the operational flexibility to strengthen pay for performance in ways that take into account their unique circumstances while simultaneously adhering to corporate personnel policies and strategy.

All pay-for-performance programs must

- Adhere to the philosophy of a meritocracy.
- Ensure fair employee/labor relations.
- Improve the firm's quality of services and operations.
- Support corporate personnel strategies and philosophy.
- Be consistent with and supported by the appropriate corporate compensation system.
- Be cost effective/affordable.
- Maintain/enhance the reputation and legitimacy of the firm.

SPECIFIC PROGRAM OBJECTIVES

Each unit's pay-for-performance program must be designed to

- Help improve the unit's quality of services and performance.
- Sharpen employees' focus on unit purposes and results.
- Contain costs/enhance affordability.
- Support fair labor/employee relations.
- Take advantage of the unit's unique features.
- Adhere to and be consistent with corporate personnel policies.

PROGRAM DESIGN STANDARDS

To ensure a technically sound design, companies should follow these design standards:

Objective(s)	Make objectives specific yet flexible.
Measures	Specify appraisals, measures, and results to measure objectives.
Eligibility	Specify which employees are eligible, which are not, rationales, etc.
Funding	Examine how the plan will be funded and its effects on labor costs.
Data sources	Detail information systems that exist or need to be developed to support measurements.
Labor/Employee relations	Specify how employees and/or their units will participate in the plan.
Payouts	Specify the nature of payouts, timing, etc.
Simulation of scenarios	Give a detailed analysis of payouts/nonpayouts and anticipated effects under various conditions.
Modifications/Termination	Consider how the program will or can be adapted and/or terminated as conditions change.
Dispute-resolution procedures	Specify how issues will be handled.
Communications/Expectations management	Consider how employees and managers will understand and react to the plan; anticipate effects on employee satisfaction. Communicate how participants can influence achievement.
Administration	Consider ease of administration and administrative roles and responsibilities.
Fit with total compensation	Keep in mind that pay-for-performance programs are part of a total compensation approach. Ensure that these programs are not conceived in isolation from rest of the firm's pay system.
Evaluation of effects	Detail how the effects of plan on the unit's mission will be evaluated.
Measurements	Ensure that these are known and understood by participants. Make them as simple as possible. Ensure that documentation enables examination or audit.

team accomplishment with one-time lump-sum awards. Employees are paid and rewarded for actual accomplishments, and fixed payroll costs are reduced. As employees move through competency levels, the salaries are planned to reflect this. Thus, employees are paid what they are worth to the organization. Employees who exceed goals add value to their positions. The value-added compensation approach is motivational and controls costs.[25]

Benner's research, using the Dreyfuss Model of Skills Acquisition, could be used as the competency model for a pay-for-performance system. Base pay would mirror the five levels of proficiency: novice, advanced beginner, competent, proficient, and expert. A nurse who bettered the time line for achieving a higher level of proficiency could be paid a lump-sum bonus for the accomplishment.[26] Exhibit 29-7 is a simplified pay-for-competency plan.

Peer Review

The subjectivity of pay for performance can be partially eliminated by peer review. At one Motorola plant, employees are working on peer review for pay. In the early stages, peer review represented 20% of annual pay, with a goal of 50%. Employees vote on one another's performance, putting enormous pressure on fellow workers to perform better. Under the Motorola pay system, all factory workers reach a maximum base pay after 39 weeks on the job. The rest of their pay is based on their individual performance.[27]

Pay Designs

Many employees are willing to risk fat bonuses for superb results. The risk is that bonuses go down with recession. Bonuses hold down fixed costs; merit raises increase costs, driving up retirement benefits.[28]

A study by Schwab and Olson produced the following findings[29]:

A conventional merit system achieves a considerably better link between pay and performance than does a bonus system with periodic adjustments in base wages. A bonus system without periodic adjustments in base wages also performs less well than a conventional merit system, because merit systems benefit from the consistency of true performance over time. One surprising finding is that even a very substantial error in the measurement of performance has only a modest effect on the pay performance correlation.

Rewards should be consistent, fair, and timely and should relate to work. They should also be ample.[30] In a pay-for-performance system, the outcomes include increased productivity from "overpaid" performers and rewards for underpaid performers.[31]

> Money to fund some programs has come from senior managers who gave up their bonuses. Other companies use money from attrition.[32]

The Quaker Oats pet food plant at Lawrence, Kansas, paid employees 5% to 10% above market to attract and retain above-average employees and remain nonunion.[33] Exhibit 29-8 illustrates the Quaker Oats pay-for-performance policy. To achieve maximal effect on employees, base pay must be kept at a level at or above the industry average. Also, labor costs must be reduced by using incentives not added into base pay (see Exhibit 29-9).

EXHIBIT 29-7

SIMPLIFIED PAY-FOR-COMPETENCY PLAN

	PERFORMANCE CRITERIA*					
	COMMON SKILLS	PRIMARY CRAFT SKILLS	BLENDED CRAFT SKILLS	PROCESS EQUIPMENT SKILLS	LEADERSHIP & TEAM SKILLS	WAGES
Skill block III	[1]	[1]	40%	100%	100%	$ _____
Skill block II	[1]	100%	20%	66%	66%	$ _____
Skill block I	100%	50%	0	33%	33%	$ _____
Entry level	Specific skills, experiences, and/or aptitudes and abilities required to enter					

Notes
*Participant must demonstrate the required skills (performance criteria) in each category of the skill block prior to moving into the next skill block.
[1] Continued proficiency in previously demonstrated skills.
% Percent of total skills listed in the category.

SOURCE: R. M. Williamson. "Reward What You Value and Reach New Maintenance Levels." Reprinted from *Plant Engineering* (12 August 1992), 118, with permission of Reed Publishing USA, © 1992.

EXHIBIT 29-8
The Pay-for-Performance Policy: An Illustration

Employee: Ed Norton
Hourly wage: $12.00
Annual salary: Ed worked 1,900 hours at regular pay and 100 hours of overtime.
(1,900 × $12.00) + (100 × $18.00) = $24,600

SCENARIO 1 (A):
- Performance matrix determines payout of 5.5%.
- Lawrence plant is 6.25% above the "market."
- Since plant wages are greater than 5% above market, payout takes form of lump sum, based on Ed's total earnings for the previous year.
- Ed's lump sum payment = $1,353 ($24,600 × .055).

SCENARIO 1 (B):
- Performance matrix determines payout of 5.5%.
- Lawrence plant is 4.5% above the "market."
- Since plant wages are less than 5% above market, payout takes the form of a base wage increase.
- Ed's adjusted hourly wage = $12.66 ($12.00 × 1.055).

Source: Reprinted, by permission of publisher, from J. P. Guthrie and E. P. Cunningham. "Pay for Performance for Hourly Workers: The Quaker Oats Alternative." *Compensation & Benefits Review* (March–April © 1992), 21. American Management Association, New York. All rights reserved.

EXHIBIT 29-9
Does Performance-Based Pay Matter?

LEVEL OF PERFORMANCE MEASUREMENT

	INDIVIDUAL	GROUP
Added into base	Merit	
Not added in	Awards	Gain-sharing
	Piece rates	Profit sharing
	Commissions	Stock options
	Bonuses	

Source: Reprinted, by permission of publisher, from G. Milkovich and C. Milkovich. "Strengthening the Pay-for-Performance Relationship: The Research." *Compensation & Benefits Review* (November–December © 1992), 56. American Management Association, New York. All rights reserved.

How to Do a Merit Pay Increase

Merit is a term that is becoming increasingly associated with performance and pay increases for nurses. Merit means that employees receive what they deserve. Pay and rewards are based on the degree of competence employees demonstrate in performing their jobs. Merit systems can include both rewards and punishments. The general goal of a merit performance and pay system is to reward people on an incremental scale so that the top

achievers or performers are paid the highest salaries. A merit pay system must have four components:

1. Individual performance standards
2. Measurement scales
3. A budget
4. An award procedure

Merit pay increases are an employee incentive program. Employees who have their competencies developed, encouraged, and recognized have better attitudes about their work and their employers. These employees will work to achieve organizational objectives that are supportive of their personal objectives. Merit rewards or punishments are extrinsic. The reward or punishment can be in the form of promotion, praise, recognition, criticism, social acceptance or rejection, or fringe benefits.[34]

Many of these rewards or punishments are activated with a total merit pay system. Extrinsic rewards need to be associated with the intrinsic rewards that come from employees' participation in making decisions about their work and the conditions under which they will perform their work. Professional nurses want control of their nursing practice. They want to participate in management decisions about how they will accomplish this. As a result, they will receive intrinsic rewards from having made the organization successful, because they have contributed to that success.

Performance Standards

Individual performance standards are written criteria developed by the supervisor in conference with the individual to be evaluated. They evolve from an established, more generalized set of job performance criteria, the job description. These performance standards are tailored to the individual's abilities and goals and to the common expectations of the individual and that person's supervisor. These standards should be measurable, and they should be objectively applied. The supervisor and employee can both observe or know that the standards have been met. These standards can be written in the format of a performance results contract related to the job description. Exhibit 29-10 represents a division of nursing policy. The procedure for implementing this policy involves use of a job description and a performance results contract (See Exhibit 29-11.)

Measurement Scales

The weights assigned to each key results area can be in terms of units or percentages. It is more practical to assign up to 1.0 unit to each key results area and determine the percentage of achievement at the annual or final conference. Doing so allows objectives to be added, modified, or deleted without readjusting the percentage

---

EXHIBIT 29-10

Policy and Evaluation of Personnel Performance

All nursing service employees will have a criteria-based performance evaluation as follows:

1. Initiated on employee orientation.
2. At the end of the probationary period (6 months).
3. Annually (to be initiated during the following evaluation period for all employees). The annual performance evaluation will be cosigned by the head nurse or supervisor and employee, and filed in the employee's personnel file.

4. When an employee terminates employment or transfers there shall be an evaluation conference. A completed performance results contract will be cosigned by the employee and head nurse/supervisor, then placed in the personnel file.

Conferences and renegotiations concerning the criteria-based performance evaluation may occur as often as the employee/supervisor deem necessary.

Source: Courtesy of the University of South Alabama Medical Center, Mobile, AL.

EXHIBIT 29-11

Sample Performance Results Contract

1. SCOPE OF RESPONSIBILITY

As clinical nurse consultant, assumes responsibility to improve the quality of health care received by the patient in the defined clinical area of expertise through role modeling, teaching, consultation, and research. The consultant assists nursing personnel to achieve their full potential and satisfaction in providing effective, efficient, and individualized care to patients and their families. The clinical nurse consultant is self-directive, determining the priorities of the role through inter- and intradisciplinary collaboration. Evaluates own practice based on the attainment of individual objectives. Responsible to the director of nursing for staff development.

2. KEY RESULTS AREAS

PERFORMANCE RESULTS	INDIVIDUAL'S PERFORMANCE
1. Schedule monthly meetings with head nurse of each unit to discuss needs and to plan for utilization of clinical consultant in meeting those needs.	I would like to see more assertive behavior in this area. Meetings were often put off and not enough consistent follow-up—head nurses to set a time. 8%
2. Present in-service for each area as contracted with head nurses.	Observations and needs should be made by both parties in setting up classes. This area has improved since January in some units. 7%
3. Work with department members to evaluate and revise nursing orientation program.	Done. New schedule completed. Meeting held—head nurses of 5th, 6th, 7th, and 8th floors. 10%
4. Orient new staff to orientation program.	Worked with [Name]. 10%
5. Coordinate nursing orientation program with Staff Development, Personnel Relations, and Nursing Service.	Continuous need for smooth coordination and double-checking on dates. 9%
6. Review and revise medication exam as necessary.	Recommendation made to [Name]. 10%
7. Assist in teaching CPR as directed.	Class taught as scheduled. 10%
8. Continue to coordinate and present Drug Update.	Aminoglycoside (antihypertensive agents, penicillin—March) Series started in September—was delayed in starting. Need for assertion in meeting this objective. 9%
9. Present classes based on needs survey.	Equipment Fair done. Coordinated with [Name]. 10%
10. Participate in critical care course—present emergency reinsertion of tracheostomy tube.	Content approved by Alabama Board of Nursing. Very poor evaluations from second class, with many negative comments written and verbalized. 7%

(continued)

EXHIBIT 29-11 *(continued)*

COMPLETE FOR TERMINAL EVALUATION ONLY

	EXCELLENT	GOOD	FAIR	POOR
Attendance				
Initiative				
Quantity of work				
Cooperation				
Eligible for rehire ____ Yes ____ No				

3. AUTHORITY CODES
A. Does without reporting
B. Does and reports
C. Gets approval before doing
D. Participates in
E. Recommends to supervisor
F. Assists supervisor under direction

SUMMARY

[Name] has been flexible in coming in for classes on 3-11 and 11-7 shifts. Has completed most of the areas on the performance contract satisfactoirily. Is generally well received by new employees and helpful in their orientation to USAMC.

I would like for [Name] to take more initiative and to be more assertive in identifying needs with the head nurses of the clinical units and in addressing those needs promptly and cionsistently. [Name] has been active in emergency admission unit and I would like to see more activity on 6th and 9th floors and the Burn Unit.

I would also ask [Name] to address concerns and questions to me directly.

Director Staff Development   May 8, 200x

Source: Courtesy of the University of South Alabama Medical Center, Mobile, AL.

weight. In Exhibit 29-12, the weights are the numbers assigned to each key results area. The total of these is 100. If the employee achieves 90, then the percentage of achievement for merit pay purposes is 90%. This percentage is used to allocate budgeted wage and salary increases.

Budget

Personnel pay increases are usually projected in the operational budget represented by the excerpt in Exhibit 29-12. They can be related to increases in the consumer price index, to the marketplace, or to the financial status of the institution. The financial status must be a major consideration. The human resources department usually prepares a cost analysis by position (Exhibit 29-13). This cost analysis is the bridge for merit pay increases for the total nursing division.

Award Procedure

Nurse administrators take all performance results contracts for each category of nursing personnel and add

EXHIBIT 29-12
Calculating Merit Increase for RTN II Positions

PERCENT	AMOUNT	PERCENT	AMOUNT
100	$1,008	71	$716
99	998	70	706
98	988	69	696
97	978	68	685
96	968	67	675
95	958	66	665
94	948	65	655
93	937	64	645
92	927	63	635
91	917	62	625
90	907	61	615
89	897	60	605
88	887	50	504
87	877	40	403
86	867	30	302
85	857	20	202

Source: Courtesy of the University of South Alabama Medical Center, Mobile, AL.

EXHIBIT 29-13
Budget for 4% Merit Pay Increase

POSITION CLASSIFICATION	HOSPITAL NURSING POSITIONS					
	FTE FILLED	TOTAL CURRENT SALARIES	COST	FTE VACANT	TOTAL CURRENT SALARIES	COST
Licensed practical nurse	84.50	$1,108,339	$ 44,334	9.00	$110,021	$ 4,401
RTN I—clinical level I	249.00	4,607,379	184,295	18.00	312,794	$12,512
RTN I—clinical level II	14.00	292,921	11,717	1.00	20,255	810
RTN I—clinical level IIII	1.00	22,755	910	0.00	0	0
RTN I (working supervisor)	45.00	893,820	35,753	0.00	0	0
Registered teaching nurse II	20.00	443,126	17,725	2.00	38,438	1,538
Nursing service supervisor I	11.50	266,910	10,676	2.00	40,228	1,609
	425.00	$7,635,250	$305,410	32.00	$521,736	$20,869
Total cost: Annual			$305,410			$20,869
Monthly			$ 25,451			$ 1,739

Source: Courtesy of the University of South Alabama Medical Center, Mobile, AL.

up the percent totals for all persons (for the nurse in Exhibit 29-12, this was 90%.) The total for registered teaching nurse II (RTN II) was 1.911%. This number is divided into the total budgeted dollars for RTN II, which was $19,263 (the sum of the amounts for filled and vacant positions labeled "Cost" in Exhibit 29-13). For each percent, each person in this category will be allocated $10.08. A person who receives a 90% merit pay increase will receive 90 × $10.08 = $907.20 (see Exhibit 29-14). This amount is transferred to a personnel action memorandum and processed through payroll. Each employee is told by the supervisor how much merit pay he or she will receive.

The Process

Step 1. Employee and supervisor have a conference at an appointed time to establish the key results (objectives) that the employee will accomplish over an agreed-on period of time. These results will include organizational objectives from the supervisor and personal objectives of the employee. Each will come to the conference table prepared to present the objectives in an atmosphere of mutual trust and cooperation. At this conference the wording of the key results areas will be negotiated, weights will be assigned to each, time frames will be established, controls or reporting authority will be established, and the approximate date will be set for the next evaluation conference.

Step 2. A definitive date is established, and the next conference is held. At this conference the supervisor and employee discuss progress in accomplishment of key results areas. The supervisor and employee modify objectives by negotiation, discard those they agree are no longer relevant, add new ones as needed, and discuss and record progress in

EXHIBIT 29-14
Standards for Evaluation of Pay-for-Performance Programs

1. There are pay-for-performance programs.
2. They were developed with input from employees.
3. They are based on company philosophy, goals, objectives, and vision.
4. They have policies and procedures.
5. The goals are job-specific.
6. There are standards for measurement.
7. They are linked to an objective performance appraisal system.
8. Rewards are linked to effort and performance.
9. Employees are informed about the programs.
10. Employees trust the programs.
11. Managers are well-trained and skilled in administering the programs.
12. The programs are funded or budgeted.
13. An evaluation program is in place to monitor the programs.
14. Productivity and performance outcomes are being measured.
15. The plans are accomplishing the stated objectives.

the accomplishment of each objective. This conference and all succeeding ones can be scheduled at earlier dates on supervisor or employee request.

Step 3: Conferences are scheduled at 1- to 3-month intervals until the probationary period is completed, the annual rating is required, or the employee transfers or terminates. At these times the contract is summarized, signed by employee and supervisor, and filed in the employee's personnel folder. The weights assigned by negotiated discussion are totaled, and a number is assigned. This number is used in allocating the merit pay increase.

As has been discussed earlier, merit pay is a difficult procedure to accomplish because employees may not agree with the outcome. Also, supervisors are hesitant to make decisions that give employees variable pay increases. Some experts suggest that merit PA for pay be separated from PA done for other purposes. The authors have found that the two can work together when planned, communicated, and fairly applied.

Summary

Incentive programs are very common in organizations. The trend is to link pay to employee or corporate performance. Doing so motivates employees to increase productivity, especially when tied to operational measures such as attendance, quality, and safety. The most common individual performance-based pay plans are merit, awards, piece rates, and commissions. Gain-sharing,

profit sharing, and stock options are the most common performance-based group awards. Bonuses are common as both individual and group awards. In many instances, merit pay is added to base pay; whereas other awards are given on a one-time basis and are less expensive over time.

A pay-for-performance plan should be communicated well, have measures that can be influenced by participants, be consistent and fair, provide ample and timely rewards linking them to work, and be trusted.

Participants in a pay-for-performance plan often risk the choice of earning less for the chance to earn more later through higher retirement benefits. Pay for performance starts with reduced wages and salaries, although the base should equal or slightly exceed the industry standard.

Equity theory, expectancy theory, and the Law of Effect are the basis for pay for performance. People expect equal pay for equal work, and increased rewards for increased output.

Teams are effective in implementing pay-for-performance plans.

Merit pay increases are designed to reward employees for past performance based on the degree to which they meet their job standards. Merit pay increases include use of individual performance standards developed by individual employees and their supervisors. A measurement scale is used to quantify the degree by which the employee meets the agreed-on standards. A budget is established to pay for the merit pay increase based on award procedures known to both employees and supervisors.

APPLICATION EXERCISES

EXERCISE 29-1   Use Exhibit 29-14 to evaluate the pay-for-performance programs in a health care organization. These may be individual awards, such as merit awards, piece rate, or individual commissions, or they may be group awards, such as gain-sharing, profit sharing, stock options, or bonuses.

How can the programs be improved? Make a management plan for improving them and present it to your supervisor and the director of human resources.

EXERCISE 29-2   If a pay-for-performance program does not exist in your organization, prepare a proposal for one. Present it to your supervisor and the director of human resources. You may want to do this as a group exercise.

NOTES

1. J. A. Parnell, "Five Reasons Why Pay Must Be Based on Performance," *Supervision* (February 1991), 6–8.

2. S. H. Appelbaum and B. T. Shapiro, "Pay for Performance: Implementation of Individual and Group Plans," *Management Decision: Quarterly Review of Management Technology* (November 1992), 86–91.

3. J. Grossmann, "Pay, Performance and Productivity," *Small Business Reports* (October 1992), 50–59.

4. J. D. Browdy, "Performance Appraisal and Pay for Performance Start at the Top," *Health Care Supervisor* (April 1989), 31–41.

5. S. H. Appelbaum and B. T. Shapiro, op. cit.

6. J. Grossmann, op. cit.

7. S. Tully, "Your Paycheck Gets Exciting," *Fortune* (1 November 1993), 83–84, 88, 95, 98.

8. P. Adinolfi, "Performance-Related Pay for Health Service Professionals: The Italian Experience," *Health Service Management Research* (November 1998), 211–220.

9. Jiing-Lih Farh, R. W. Griffith, and D. B. Balkin, "Effects of Choice of Pay Plans on Satisfaction, Goal Setting, and Performance," *Journal of Organizational Behavior*, 12, (1991), 55–62.

10. M. P. Miceli, I. Jung, J. P. Near, and D. B. Greenberger, "Predictions and Outcomes of Reactions to Pay-for-Performance Plans," *Journal of Applied Psychology* (April 1991), 508–521.

11. G. Milkovich and C. Milkovich, "Strengthening the Pay-Performance Relationship: The Research," *Compensation & Benefits Review* (November–December 1992), 53–62.

12. C. J. Frisch and M. A. Dickinson, "Work Productivity as a Function of the Percentage of Monetary Incentives to Base Pay," *Journal of Organizational Behavior Management*, 11(1); (1990), 13–33.

13. S. Berger and J. Moyer, "Launching a Performance-Based Pay Plan," *Modern Healthcare* (19 August 1991), 64.

14. J. A. Parnell, op. cit.

15. T. R. Zenger, "Why Do Employers Only Reward Extreme Performance? Examining the Relationships Among Performance, Pay, and Turnover," *Administrative Science Quarterly* (June 1992), 198–219.

16. R. M. Williamson, "Reward What You Value and Reach New Maintenance Performance Levels," *Plant Engineering* (13 August 1992), 113–114.

17. S. H. Appelbaum and B. T. Shapiro, op. cit.; J. Grossman, op. cit.; M. A. Conte and D. Kruse, "ESOPs and Profit-Sharing Plans: Do They Link Employee Pay to Company Performance?" *Financial Management* (winter 1991), 91–100; D. P. Schwab and C. A. Olson, "Merit-Pay Practice Implications for Pay-Performance Relationships," *Industrial and Labor Relations Review* (February 1990), 237S–2555S; D. W. Jones and M. C. Hanser, "Putting Teeth into Pay-for-Performance Programs," *Healthcare Financial Management* (September 1991), 32, 34–35, 40, 42.

18. J. Grossmann, op. cit., S. H. Appelbaum and S. H. Shapiro, op. cit., J. P. Guthrie and E. P. Cunningham, "Pay for Performance for Hourly Workers: The Quaker Oats Alternative," *Compensation and Benefits Review* (March–April 1992), 18–23; G. J. Meng, "Using Job Descriptions, Performance and Pay Innovations to Support Quality: A Paper Company's Experience," *National Productivity Review* (spring 1992), 247–255; "Performance Reviews Key in Pay for Performance and Pay," *The Wall Street Journal* (10 May 1993), B1; G. Milkovich and C. Milkovich, op. cit.; S. Berger and J. Moyer, op. cit., S. Tully, "The Real Key to Creating Wealth," *Fortune* (20 September 1993), 38–39, 44–45, 48, 50; B. P. MacLean, "Value-Added Pay Beats Traditional Merit Programs," *Personnel Journal* (September 1990), 46, 48–50, 52; J. Greenwald, "Workers: Risks and Rewards," *Time* (15 April 1991), 42–43; L. Thornburg, "Pay for Performance: What You Should Know," *HR Magazine* (June 1992), 58–61; L. Thornburg, "How Do You Cut the Cake?" *HR Magazine* (October 1992), 66–68, 70, 72; K. A. McNally, "Compensation as a Strategic Tool," *HR Magazine* (December 1992), 38–40; J. D. Browdy, op. cit.

19. M. E. Hopkins, "Gainsharing: Providing Incentives for Process Improvement," *Radiology Management* (fall 1995), 46–51.

20. P. K. Zingheim and J. R. Schuster, "Linking Quality and Pay," *HR Magazine* (December 1992), 55–59.

21. C. Harris, "Work Redesign Calls for New Pay and Performance," *Hospitals* (5 October 1992), 56, 58, 60.

22. L. M. Sixel, "Team Incentives Gain Popularity as Reward Method," *San Antonio Express-News* (24 July 1994), 8H.

23. P. K. Zingheim and J. R. Schuster, op. cit.

24. L. Thornburg, June 1992, op. cit.

25. B. P. MacLean, "Value-Added Pay Beats Traditional Merit Programs," *Personnel Journal* (September 1990), 46–52.

26. P. Benner, *From Novice to Expert* (Menlo Park, CA: Addison Wesley, 1984).

27. F. Swoboda, "Motorola Tests Peer Review of Performance for Pay," *San Antonio Express-News* (24 July 1994), 8H.

28. S. Tully, "Your Paycheck Gets Exciting," op. cit.

29. D. P. Schwab and C. A. Olson, op. cit.

30. L. Thornburg, "How Do You Cut the Cake?" op. cit.

31. S. H. Appelbaum and B. T. Shapiro, op. cit.

32. L. Goff, "Working Harder to Get the Same Raise," *Computerworld* (2 March 1992), 76.

33. J. P. Guthrie and E. P. Cunningham, op. cit.

34. D. McGregor, *Leadership and Motivation* (Cambridge, MA: The MIT Press, 1966), 203–204.

REFERENCES

Editorial. "Executive Pay: It Doesn't Add Up." *Business Week* (26 April 1993), 122.

McBride, A. B., S. Nieman, and J. Johnson. "Responsibility-Centered Management: A 10-Year Nursing Assessment." *Journal of Professional Nursing* (July–August 2000), 201–209.

Index